FUNDAMENTAL PHARMACOLOGY

for Pharmacy Technicians

Jahangir Moini, MD, MPH, CPhT
Professor and Former Director, Allied Health Sciences, including the Pharmacy

Technician Program,
Everest University
Melbourne, Florida

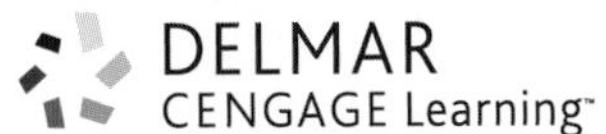

Fundamental Pharmacology for Pharmacy Technicians by Jahangir Moini

Vice President, Career and Professional Editorial:
William Brottmiller

Director of Learning Solutions:
Matthew Kane

Acquisitions Editor:
Tari Broderick

Managing Editor:
Marah Bellegarde

Senior Product Manager:
Darcy M. Scelsi

Editorial Assistant:
Anthony Souza

Vice President, Career and Professional Marketing:
Jennifer McAvey

Marketing Manager:
Kristin McNary

Marketing Coordinator:
Erica Ropitsky

Production Director:
Carolyn Miller

Production Manager:
Andrew Crouth

Content Project Manager:
Katie Wachtl

Senior Art Director:
Jack Pendleton

Technology Project Manager:
Ben Knapp

For more information, contact **Cengage Delmar Learning, 5 Maxwell Drive, Clifton Park, NY 12065**
Or find us on the World Wide Web at http://www.delmarlearning.com
For permission to use material from this text or product, contact us by
Tel (800) 730-2214
Fax (800) 730-2215
www. Cengagerights.com
permissionrequest@cengage.com

Library of Congress Cataloging-in-Publication Data: 2008937977

ISBN 10: 1-4180-5357-0

ISBN 13: 978-1-4180-5357-4

Delmar Cengage Learning
5 Maxwell Drive
Clifton Park, NY 12065-2919
USA

Cengage Learning products are represented in Canada by Nelson Education, Ltd.

For your lifelong learning solutions, visit **delmar.cengage.com**

Visit our corporate website at **www.cengage.com**

Notice to the Reader

Publisher does not warrant or guarantee any of the products described herein or perform any independent analysis in connection with any of the product information contained herein. Publisher does not assume, and expressly disclaims, any obligation to obtain and include information other than that provided to it by the manufacturer. The reader is expressly warned to consider and adopt all safety precautions that might be indicated by the activities described herein and to avoid all potential hazards. By following the instructions contained herein, the reader willingly assumes all risks in connection with such instructions. The publisher makes no representations or warranties of any kind, including but not limited to, the warranties of fitness for particular purpose or merchantability, nor are any such representations implied with respect to the material set forth herein, and the publisher takes no responsibility with respect to such material. The publisher shall not be liable for any special, consequential, or exemplary damages resulting, in whole or part, from the reader's use of, or reliance upon, this material.

Printed in Canada
1 2 3 4 5 6 7 13 12 11 10 9 8

Dedication

This book is dedicated to

my wonderful wife of thirty years,

Hengameh.

Contents

Section II Pharmacology Related to Specific Body Systems and Disorders

Section IV Pharmacology for Specific Populations

Preface

Introduction

Pharmacology is one of the most challenging aspects of study for pharmacy technicians. The study of pharmacology requires thorough knowledge of anatomy and physiology, chemistry, pathology, psychology, and sociology. This book clearly connects pharmacology with pathophysiology in order to foster a complete understanding of these sciences. Though pharmacology is a difficult topic, the approach of this book illuminates its key principles as well as the more complex points that must also be mastered.

In today's health care, drug therapy is of the utmost importance, but is also a complicated area of understanding. The field of pharmacology is always changing. Pharmacy technicians who deal with pharmacology must continually improve in their knowledge with regular review and updating of the latest advancements.

Organization of Content

This book is organized into four units that focus on the general aspects of pharmacology, followed by organizations of chapters by body system and related disorders. The final unit concerns pharmacology for specific populations. There are a total of 26 chapters, followed by appendices, a glossary, and index. In each chapter, drugs are discussed related to their mechanisms of action, indications, adverse effects, contraindications, precautions, and drug interactions. At the end of the book, there are also 30 additional case studies with multiple questions.

The classification of drugs according to their related body systems allows the text to easily reference tables, figures, and other items so that the intended effects of each drug may be related to the pertinent parts of the body. Terminology that is new to each chapter is highlighted in *Medical Terminology Reviews* that help the student to better understand and break down new terms into their component parts.

Features

Each chapter contains an outline of the key topics, a glossary of important terms (which are **bolded** in the chapter text), and objectives that the student must be able to meet upon completion of the reading. Overviews and anatomy reviews serve to introduce the student to the key concepts of the chapter as well as related anatomical structures and functions. Figures serve to accurately illustrate chapter principles, organs, drug functions, and related information. Accurate tables focus on key drugs and related topics that must be fully understood in order to master each chapter's content. The chapters conclude with a summary of information, followed by "Exploring the Web," which lists pertinent Internet websites for additional study. Finally, unique varieties of review questions with accompanying answer keys are provided. Included in the review questions are short scenarios with Critical Thinking questions.

Current Drug Information

All of the included drug information was current and up-to-date at the time of the writing of this book. It is important to remember that drug information changes frequently, and to always verify this information before any preparation, compounding, or administration occurs. You should always consult a current *Physician's Desk Reference, Facts and Comparisons,* or the package inserts accompanying a drug. Pharmacists and physicians may also be able to provide current drug information.

Resources

This book is accompanied by a StudyWare CD-ROM that provides additional questions and activities for students such as multiple choice, fill-in-the-blank, concentration, word building, and a *Jeopardy*-style quiz game. An additional audio library is provided for definitions and proper pronunciations of drug names.

Instructor Resources

This book is accompanied by an Electronic Classroom Manager, which contains PowerPoint slides for all chapters, and a test bank of additional questions. It is also accompanied by an instructor's manual and a student workbook.

Acknowledgments

The author would like to acknowledge the following individuals for their time and efforts in aiding him in the reviewing and editing of the book.

Maggie Daley, PharmD
Pharmacist Consultant
Melbourne, Florida

Mahkameh Moini, DMD
Dental Practitioner
West Palm Beach, Florida

Stephanie K. Mullin, RN, MSN, CPNP
Pediatric Nurse Practitioner
Medical College of Wisconsin
Children's Hospital of Wisconsin
Milwaukee, Wisconsin

Norman Tomaka, CRPh, LHRM
Consultant Pharmacy Services
Melbourne, FL
and
President, Florida Pharmacy Association

Greg Vadimsky, Pharmacy Technician
Melbourne, Florida

Reviewers

Lisa Barnes, MBA, B. Pharm
Assistant Professor, Pharmacy Practice
Skaggs School of Pharmacy at The University of Montana
Missoula, Montana

Barbara Lacher, BS, RPhTech, CPhT
Assistant Program Director, Associate Professor
Pharmacy Technician Program
North Dakota State College of Science
Wahpeton, North Dakota

Paula Lambert, BS, CPhT
Pharmacy Technology Instructor
North Idaho College
Coeur d'Alene, Idaho

Michelle McCranie, CPhT
Pharmacy Technology Instructor
Ogeechee Technical College
Statesboro, Georgia

James Mizner, RPh, MBA
Pharmacy Technician Program Director
Applied Career Training
Arlington, Virginia

Phillip Penrod, BS, AA.AA, CPhT
Medical Department Chair
Florida Metropolitan University
Tampa, Florida

Diana Rangaves, PharmD, RPh
Pharmacy Technician Program, Lead Instructor
Santa Rosa Junior College
Santa Rosa, California

Dr. John J. Smith, EdD
Associate Dean, Health Sciences
Corinthian Colleges, Inc.
Santa Ana, California

About the Author

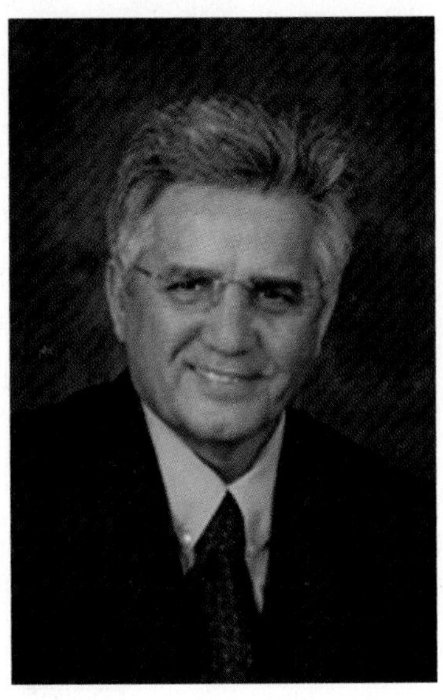

Dr. Moini was assistant professor at Tehran University School of Medicine for nine years teaching medical and allied health students. The author is a professor and former director (for 15 years) of allied health programs at Everest University. Dr. Moini established, for the first time, the associate degree program for pharmacy technicians in 2000 at EU's Melbourne campus. For 5 years, he was the director of the pharmacy technician program. He also established several other new allied health programs for EU. As a physician and instructor for the past 35 years, he believes that pharmacy technicians must be knowledgeable about pharmacology, and have confidence in their duties and responsibilities in order to prevent medication errors.

Dr. Moini is actively involved in teaching and helping students to prepare for service in various health professions, including the roles of pharmacy technicians, medical assistants, and nurses. He worked with the Brevard County Health Department as an epidemiologist and health educator consultant for 18 years, offering continuing education courses and keeping nurses up to date on the latest developments related to pharmacology, medications errors, immunizations, and other important topics. He has been an internationally published author of various allied health books since 1999.

SECTION I

GENERAL ASPECTS OF PHARMACOLOGY

CHAPTER 1

Introduction to Pharmacology, Drug Legislation, and Regulation

OBJECTIVES

After completing this chapter, the reader should be able to:

1. Define the key terms.
2. Explain the four stages of drug product development.
3. Explain the differences between the DEA and the FDA.
4. Name the first drug act passed in the United States for consumer safety, and give the year it was passed.
5. Distinguish between legend drugs, over-the-counter drugs, and controlled substances.
6. Summarize the provisions of the Controlled Substances Act of 1970, and define the C-I to C-V schedules.

GLOSSARY

Clinical pharmacology – an area of medicine devoted to the evaluation of drugs used for human benefit

Controlled substances – drugs recognized by the Drug Enforcement Agency (DEA) as having abuse potential

Drug Enforcement Agency (DEA) – the government agency concerned with controlled substances that enforces laws against drug activities, including illegal drug use, dealing, and manufacturing

Food and Drug Administration (FDA) – the branch of the U.S. Department of Health and Human Services that is responsible for the regulation of foods, drugs, cosmetics, and medical devices

Genetic engineering – techniques wherein genes from one organism are spliced into the chromosomes of another organism; also known as recombinant DNA technology

Investigational new drug (IND) application – an application for human drug testing that is submitted to the FDA once enough data has been collected on a new drug

Legend drug – a prescription drug

Narcotics – drugs that produce a sedative or pain relieving affect

Over-the-counter (OTC) – nonprescription drugs

Pharmacology – the science concerned with drugs and their sources, appearance, chemistry, actions, and uses

Recombinant DNA technology – techniques wherein genes from one organism are spliced into the chromosomes of another organism; also known as genetic engineering

OUTLINE

Overview

Pharmacology is defined as the study of the sources, appearance, chemistry, actions, uses, and manufacturing of drugs and medications. This chapter presents a basic overview of the history of pharmacology, drug development, and drug legislation affecting the dispensing and use of medications.

The History of Pharmacology

Historical records show that drug use has long been a part of human culture worldwide. A historical timeline showing major pharmacological developments provides a continuum that may be divided into three distinct periods: the age of natural substances, the age of synthetic substances, and the age of biotechnology.

Medical Terminology Review

pharmacology
pharmac/o = drugs, medicine
-logy = the study of
the study of drugs or medicine

The Age of Natural Substances

The age of natural substances is characterized by the use of plant derivatives (e.g., morphine, which is derived from opium). The use of natural substances evolved in China and Egypt. In 1875, George Ebers found one of the earliest written records of medicinal uses of plants in Egypt, the Ebers Papyrus. This document was written around 1500 B.C. It contained formulas for more than 800 remedies. About 2000 B.C., the Chinese began developing an interest in herbs as having value in the cure of diseases. Theophrastus, an early Greek philosopher and scientist (about 300 B.C.), wrote about observations on the classification of plants by their various parts.

The Age of Synthetic Substances

The age of synthetic substances is characterized by the mass production of synthetic medicines and drug screening techniques (e.g., antibiotics and insulin). The period from 1350 to 1650 A.D. (the later stages of the Middle Ages) is known as the Renaissance. During this period, Swiss-born physician Theoprastus Philippus Aureolus Bombastus von Hohenheim, also known as Paracelsus, began to emphasize a chemical rather than a botanical orientation to medicine. He believed that disease was a chemical manifestation and should be treated chemically.

The production of synthetic substances for medicinal uses continued into the twentieth century. It was at this time that synthetic drugs began to be mass-produced relatively cheaply in pharmaceutical laboratories. Once the molecular structure of a natural drug is identified, it may be more convenient to synthesize it wholly in the laboratory instead of extracting it in its natural form, or else modify it chemically for better absorption, greater effectiveness, or fewer side effects.

The Age of Biotechnology

Biotechnology is defined as the use of proteins from cells and tissues from humans, animals, and plants to produce medicines and therapeutic treatments. These proteins are highly complex compounds where the functional characteristics are determined by subtle chemical bonds and structural arrangements. Biotechnological techniques involve the manipulation of these bonds and structural arrangements from microbial and human genetic material. A human gene can be inserted into one bacterium or fungal cell, which in turn, divides to produce a colony in which each microbe contains the gene. This process is referred to as **recombinant DNA technology** or **genetic engineering** and was put into practice in the early 1970s. The best clinical example of this includes substances used in hormone replacement therapy (e.g., insulin and growth hormone).

DRUG PRODUCT DEVELOPMENT

In the United States, the development of new drugs and drug therapies can take anywhere from seven to fifteen years. The **Food and Drug Administration (FDA)**, a branch of the U.S. Department of Health and Human Services, is responsible for the regulation of foods, drugs, cosmetics, and medical devices. The FDA oversees the approval of new drugs, over-the-counter and prescription drug labeling, and standards related to the manufacture of drugs. The FDA considers a new chemical entity as an active pharmaceutical ingredient that has not been approved for marketing in the United States. Before a drug is approved for sale, it must go through several phases of drug product development.

- Pre-clinical Investigation (Stage 1)
  Animal pharmacology and toxicology data are obtained to determine the safety and effectiveness of the drug. It takes about one to three years, with the average being approximately eighteen months. An **investigational new drug (IND) application** for human testing is submitted to the FDA once enough data has been collected on the new drug.
- Clinical Investigation (Stage 2)
  Clinical testing on humans takes place in three different phases called clinical phase trials. This is the longest part of the drug approval process and involves **clinical pharmacology**, an area of medicine devoted to the evaluation of drugs used for human benefit. Clinical phase trials are essential because responses among patients vary. If a drug appears to be effective without causing serious side effects, approval for marketing may be accelerated, or the drug may be used for treatment immediately in special cases, with careful monitoring. In any case, an IND must be submitted before a drug is allowed to proceed to the next stage of the approval process. During the clinical phase trials, healthy volunteers are

used in large groups of selected patients to determine drug toxicity and tolerance. The trial phase takes about two to ten years with the average being five years.

- Investigational New Drug (IND) Review (Stage 3)
  A review of the IND is the third stage of drug approval. During this stage, the final phase of clinical trials and testing may continue, depending on the results obtained from preclinical testing. If the IND is approved, the process continues to the final stage. If the IND is rejected, the process stops until concerns are addressed. This stage takes about two months to seven years. The average is twenty-four months.
- Postmarketing Studies (Stage 4)
  Postmarketing surveillance is the fourth stage of the drug approval process. It takes place after clinical trials and the IND review process have been completed. Testing in humans is continued to check for any new side effects in larger and more diverse populations. Some adverse effects take longer to appear and are not identified until a drug is used by large numbers of patients.

Removal of a Drug from the Market

The FDA holds annual public meetings to hear comments from patients and professional and pharmaceutical organizations about the effectiveness and safety of new drug therapies. If the FDA discovers a serious problem, it will require that a drug be withdrawn from the market and its use discontinued.

Prescription Drugs

A prescription drug is a medication that can only be legally dispensed to a patient with a written order (prescription) from a physician or another individual licensed to prescribe medications. Most prescription drugs are so designated by the FDA; however, states can also designate specific drugs or devices as prescription items. Prescription drugs may only be dispensed by a pharmacist, pharmacy technician under direction of a pharmacist, or by the prescriber. Prescription drugs are also called **legend drugs**.

Nonprescription Drugs

When drugs are used over long periods of time and demonstrate "wide" margins of safety, prescription drugs may become nonprescription or **over-the-counter (OTC)** drugs. Unlike prescription drugs, OTC drugs do not require a physician's order. Patients may treat themselves safely if they carefully follow the instructions included with these OTC drugs. If patients do not follow these guidelines, OTC drugs can have serious side effects.

Controlled Substances

A **controlled substance** is a medicinal product that has a high potential for abuse and is regulated by the **Drug Enforcement Agency (DEA)**, a part of the U.S. Department of Justice. The DEA is tasked with the enforcement of laws regulating drug activities, illegal drug use, illegal drug dealing and sale, and illegal manufacture of drugs. A controlled substance can only legally be obtained with a physician's prescription. Many **narcotics**, drugs producing sedative or pain relieving affects, are classified as controlled substances.

Federal Drug Legislation

Many laws and regulations have been enacted during the past century regulating pharmacy practice. These laws include: the Pure Food and Drug Act; the Harrison Narcotic Act; the Pure Food, Drug, and Cosmetic Act; and the Comprehensive Drug Abuse Prevention and Control Act. These laws have been passed to control the use of prescription drugs, nonprescription drugs, and controlled substances.

The Pure Food and Drug Act of 1906

The Pure Food and Drug Act was the government's first attempt to control and regulate the manufacture, distribution, and sale of drugs. Before this law, the purity and potency of many drugs were questionable, and some of these agents were even dangerous for human consumption.

The Harrison Narcotic Act of 1914

The Harrison Narcotic Act regulated the importation, manufacture, sale, and use of opium, codeine, and their derivations and compounds. Before this law, any narcotic could be purchased without a prescription. In 1970, the Harrison Narcotic Act was replaced by the Comprehensive Drug Abuse Prevention and Control Act.

The Pure Food, Drug, and Cosmetic Act of 1938

In 1938, further amendments were made to the Pure Food and Drug Act of 1906, resulting in the Pure Food, Drug, and Cosmetic Act, which created the FDA. The FDA provided additional control over the manufacture and sale of cosmetics. Under this act, manufacturers must be concerned with the purity, strength, effectiveness, safety, and packaging of drugs. Foods and cosmetics are also regulated. By this act, the FDA has the power to approve or deny new drug applications and even to conduct inspections to ensure compliance. The FDA approves the investigational use of drugs on humans and ensures that all approved drugs are safe and effective.

Key Concept

The FDA is concerned with general safety standards in the production of drugs, foods, and cosmetics. It is responsible for the approval and removal from the market of many products.

Key Concept

The DEA is concerned with controlled substances only, and enforces laws against drug activities, including illegal drug use, dealing, and manufacturing.

Drugs are frequently added, deleted, or moved to one schedule or another. The DEA determines if a drug should be moved from one schedule to another.

The Comprehensive Drug Abuse Prevention and Control Act of 1970

The Comprehensive Drug Abuse Prevention and Control Act, also called the Controlled Substances Act (CSA), regulates the manufacture, distribution, and dispensation of drugs with a potential for abuse. This law deals with control and enforcement of pharmaceuticals and places this control and enforcement under the jurisdiction of the DEA.

The CSA classifies drugs with the potential for abuse into five schedules designated with a C and a Roman numeral (I–V) to indicate their level of control (Table 1-1). Drugs in Schedule I have the highest potential for abuse and addiction. Those in Schedule V have the least potential for abuse. Records must be kept on the transactions of all pharmaceuticals that are classified as controlled substances. This is also regulated by the DEA.

TABLE 1-1 Schedules of Controlled Substances

Schedule	Manufacturer's Label	Abuse Potential	Prescription Requirement	Examples
I	C-I	high; no accepted medical use	no prescription permitted	heroin, LSD (lysergic acid diethylamide), marijuana, mescaline, and peyote
II	C-II	high; accepted medical use	prescription required; no refills permitted without a new written prescription	codeine, fentanyl, methadone hydrochloride, methamphetamine, methylphenidate, morphine, and opium (deodorized)
III	C-III	moderate; accepted medical use	prescription required; 5 refills permitted in 6 months	certain drugs compounded with small quantities of narcotics; also other drugs with strong potential for abuse (Tylenol® with codeine), and certain barbiturates
IV	C-IV	low; accepted medical use	prescription required; 5 refills permitted in 6 months	barbital, chloral hydrate, chlordiazepoxide, diazepam, and pentazocine hydrochloride
V	C-V	low; accepted medical use	no prescription required for individuals 18 or older unless quantities are greater than 4 fluid ounces.	cough syrups with codeine, diphenoxylate hydrochloride with atropine sulfate, and kaolin/pectin/opium

SUMMARY

Pharmacology deals with the discovery, chemistry, effects, uses, and manufacturing of drugs. History shows that drug use has long been a part of human culture worldwide. Three distinct periods in the development of pharmacology have included: the age of natural substances, the age of synthetic substances, and the age of biotechnology.

The development of a new drug is controlled by the FDA, and consists of several phases. Drug product development is a long and difficult process, taking anywhere from seven to fifteen years.

In the past century, Congress has passed many laws to control and regulate the importation, manufacture, sale, and use of drugs. Any new drug that is developed must be safe and effective for the human body.

EXPLORING THE WEB

Visit ***www.drugs.com***

- Look for information on drugs going through drug trials for FDA approval. Choose one drug and review the study and approval process from start to finish.

Visit ***www.fda.gov***

- Search using the term drug development. Review documents and articles that provide details about the process of developing new drugs.
- Search using the term pulled drugs/Review articles on why drugs may be pulled off the market and how this is determined.

Visit ***www.napra.org***

- Click on "Federal Drug Legislation." Review the information on the Controlled Drugs and Substances Acts as well as the Food and Drugs Acts.

REVIEW QUESTIONS

Short Answer

1. What types of drugs are listed in the C-II and C-V schedules?

____

____

2. Define the role of the DEA.

____

____

3. List three responsibilities of the FDA.

____

____

____

4. In what year was the first major U.S. drug act passed and what was it called?

____

____

5. Define the following:

   a. The Controlled Substances Act (CSA)

   ____

   b. The Pure Food and Drug Act of 1906

   ____

   c. The Harrison Narcotic Act of 1904

   ____

   d. Legend drugs

   ____

Multiple Choice

1. The drugs with the highest potential for abuse and addiction, which are not accepted for medical use, are classified as which of the following schedules?

   A. I
   B. II
   C. IV
   D. V

2. Which of the following agencies oversees controlled substances and prosecutes individuals who illegally distribute them?

   A. FDA
   B. CDC
   C. DHHS
   D. DEA

3. Which of the following was the first period of historical drug development?

   A. synthetic substances
   B. natural substances
   C. biotechnical substances
   D. genetic engineering

4. The FDA is a branch of which department that controls all drugs for legal use?
   - A. U.S. Department of Health
   - B. U.S. Department of Health and Human Services
   - C. U.S. Department of Agriculture
   - D. U.S. Department of Labor

5. The best clinical example of a "genetic engineering" substance is which of the following?
   - A. insulin
   - B. penicillin
   - C. aspirin
   - D. vitamin A

6. Which type of schedule drugs has a high potential for abuse but is currently accepted for medical treatment in the United States?
   - A. Schedule I
   - B. Schedule II
   - C. Schedule III
   - D. Schedule IV

7. Which of the following drug schedules do heroine, LSD, and marijuana fall into?
   - A. Schedule IV
   - B. Schedule III
   - C. Schedule II
   - D. Schedule I

8. Stage 1 of drug product development may take:
   - A. 2-7 months
   - B. 18-24 months
   - C. 1-3 years
   - D. 2-10 years

9. Which of the following phases of drug product development may be improved as a result of equipment, regulatory, supply, or market demands?
   - A. Stage 1
   - B. Stage 2
   - C. Stage 3
   - D. Stage 4

10. Which of the following laws was the first to regulate the importation, manufacture, sale, and use of narcotic drugs?
    - A. Harrison Narcotic Act
    - B. Pure Food, Drug, and Cosmetic Act
    - C. Controlled Substances Act
    - D. Pure Food and Drug Act

11. An investigational new drug application for human testing is submitted to which of the following?

- **A.** DEA
- **B.** DHHS
- **C.** FDA
- **D.** JCAHO

12. Which of the following federal laws may control the use of prescription drugs, nonprescription drugs, and controlled substances?

- **A.** The Harrison Narcotic Act
- **B.** The Comprehensive Drug Abuse Prevention and Control Act
- **C.** The Pure Food and Drug Act
- **D.** All of the above

Matching

_____ **1.** Schedule C-I	**A.** low abuse potential; accepted medical use
_____ **2.** Schedule C-II	**B.** moderate abuse potential; accepted medical use
_____ **3.** Schedule C-III	**C.** high abuse potential; accepted medical use
_____ **4.** Schedule C-V	**D.** high abuse potential; no accepted medical use

Critical Thinking

Tom is a student in the pharmacy technician program who is taking the final exam for law and ethics. Many of his questions are related to federal drug acts.

1. What would be the correct name of the act that regulates the importation, manufacturing, sale, and use of opium, codeine, and their derivations and compounds?

2. Which agency has the power to approve or deny new drug applications?

3. What was the first federal drug act Congress passed in 1906?

CHAPTER 2 Drug Sources and Dosage Forms

OBJECTIVES

After completing this chapter, the reader should be able to:

1. Differentiate between the chemical name, generic name, and trade name of drugs.
2. Explain the classification of drug sources.
3. Name three animal sources of drugs.
4. Distinguish between engineered and synthetic drug sources.
5. Describe the various dosage forms of drugs.
6. Distinguish between syrups and elixirs.

OUTLINE

Drug Names

Drug Sources

- Plant Sources
- Animal Sources
- Mineral Sources
- Synthetic Sources
- Engineered Sources

Dosage Forms of Drugs

- Solid Drugs
- Semisolid Drugs
- Liquid Drugs
- Gaseous Drugs

GLOSSARY

Aromatic water – a mixture of distilled water with an aromatic volatile oil

Buffered tablet – a type of tablet manufactured to prevent irritation of the stomach

Caplet – a tablet shaped like a capsule

Capsule – a solid dosage form in which the drug is enclosed in either a hard or soft shell of soluble material

Chemical name – a drug's full name, that refers to its complete chemical makeup

Cream – a semisolid emulsion of either the oil-in-water or the water-in-oil type, ordinarily intended for topical use

Elixir – a clear, sweetened, flavored, hydroalcoholic liquid medication intended for oral use

Emulsion – a system containing two liquids that cannot be mixed together in which one is dispersed in the form of very small globules throughout the other

Enteric-coated tablet – a tablet covered in a special coating to protect it from stomach acid, allowing the drug to dissolve in the intestines

Fluidextract – a pharmacopoeial liquid preparation of vegetable drugs, made by filtration, containing alcohol as a solvent or as a preservative, or both

Gel – a jelly or the solid or semisolid phase of a colloidal solution

Gelcap – an oil-based medication that is enclosed in a soft gelatin capsule

Generic name – a drug not protected by a trademark, but regulated by the FDA. Also called the *official name*

Granule – a very small pill, usually gelatin- or sugar-coated, containing a drug to be given in a small dose

Liniment – a liquid preparation for external use, usually applied by friction to the skin

Lozenge – a small, disk-shaped tablet composed of solidifying paste containing an astringent, an antiseptic, or an oil-based drug used for local treatment of the mouth or throat and is held in the mouth until dissolved; also known as a troche

Mixture – a mutual incorporation of two or more substances, without chemical union, in which the physical characteristics of each of the components are retained

Ointment – a semisolid preparation usually containing medicinal substances and is intended for external application

Pill – a small, globular mass of soluble material containing a medicinal substance to be swallowed

Plaster – a solid preparation that can be spread when heated and then becomes adhesive at the temperature of the body

Powder – a dry mass of minute separate particles of any substance

Solution – a liquid dosage form in which active ingredients are dissolved in a liquid vehicle

Spirits – alcoholic or hydroalcoholic solutions of volatile substances

Suppository – a small, solid body shaped for ready introduction into one of the orifices of the body other than the oral cavity (e.g., rectum, urethra, or vagina), made of a substance, usually medicated, that is solid at ordinary temperature but melts at body temperature

Suspension – a liquid dosage form that contains solid drug particles floating in a liquid medium

Sustained release (SR) capsule – a capsule with a controlled release of the dosage over a special period of time

Syrup – a liquid preparation in a concentrated aqueous solution of a sugar used for medicinal purposes or to add flavor to a substance

Tablet – a solid dosage form containing medicinal substances with or without suitable diluents

Tincture – an alcoholic solution prepared from vegetable materials or from chemical substances, used as a skin disinfectant

Trade name – brand name given to a drug by its manufacturer (such drugs are marked with the symbol®). Trade names are also called *proprietary* or *brand* names

Troche – a small, disk-shaped tablet composed of solidifying paste containing an astringent, antiseptic, or oil-based drug used for local treatment of the mouth or throat and is held in the mouth until dissolved; also known as a lozenge

Overview

The pharmacy technician must be familiar with many different forms of medication. There are varieties of sources from which drugs are derived and forms in which drugs are prepared. A working knowledge of these sources and forms will aid the pharmacy technician in understanding how drugs are used and administered.

Drug Names

It is not unusual for each drug entity to be known by several designations. Usually, a single drug may have up to three names: chemical, generic, and trade. The first type of name, usually applied to compounds of known composition, is the **chemical name**. For substances of plant or animal origin that cannot be classified as pure chemical compounds, scientific identification is given in terms of precise biochemical or zoological names. Chemical names are generally not useful to the physician, pharmacist, or other users of the drug.

When a new drug is proven to be useful through successive research stages to the point at which it appears that it may become a marketable product, a **trade name** is developed by the manufacturer. Properly registered trade names become the legal property of their owners, are protected by copyright laws, and cannot be used freely in the public domain. These two types of names do not fulfill the need for a single, simple, informative designation available for unrestricted public use. The nonproprietary name is the only name intended to function in this capacity.

Medical Terminology Review

biochemical
bio = life; living systems
chemical = drug; agent
drug created from a living system

The nonproprietary name often is referred to as the **generic name.** A generic name is the official name of the drug. This name is much simpler than the chemical name, and it is not protected by copyright. The use of generic names is encouraged over trade names to avoid confusion. Generic drugs are cheaper than brand name drugs. They are usually easier to remember and less complicated. However, because generic drug formularies may be different, the inert ingredients may be somewhat different and consequently may affect the ability of the drug to reach the target cells and produce an effect.

Key Concept

Chemical names and generic names are unique to each drug – there is only one chemical name and one generic name for any specific drug. However, any drug may have dozens of trade (or brand) names, with similar ingredients.

Drug Sources

There are basically five sources of drugs: plants, animals (including humans), minerals or mineral products, synthetic (chemical substances), and engineered drugs (investigational drugs). Today, chemicals and even human tissues such as those used in stem-cell therapy can be manipulated to create new drug sources.

Plant Sources

Plant sources are grouped by their physical and chemical properties. Alkaloids are organic compounds combined with acids to make a salt. Nicotine, morphine sulfate, and atropine sulfate are examples of these chemical compounds. An important cardiac glycoside is digoxin. Digoxin is made from digitalis, a derivative of the foxglove plant.

Medical Terminology Review

alkaloid
alkal = alkaline
oid = compound
an alkaline based compound

Animal Sources

Animal sources, such as the body fluids and glands of animals, can act as drugs. The drugs obtained from animal sources include enzymes such as pancreatin and pepsin. Hormones such as thyroid and insulin are also from animal sources.

Mineral Sources

Minerals from the earth and soil are used to provide inorganic materials unavailable from plants and animals. They are used as they occur in nature. Examples include iron, potassium, silver, and gold, which are used to prepare medications. Sodium chloride (table salt) is one of the best-known examples in this category. Gold is used to prevent severe rheumatoid arthritis, and coal tar is used to treat seborrheic dermatitis and psoriasis.

Synthetic Sources

New drugs may come from living organisms (organic substances) or nonliving materials (inorganic substances). These drugs are called synthetic or manufactured drugs. They are created through the application of chemistry and biology. Because they are not found in nature, these medications come from artificial substances. Common examples of synthetic drugs include meperidine (Demerol®), sulfonamides, and oral contraceptives. Certain organic drugs such as penicillin are semisynthetic and are made by altering their natural compounds or elements. Some drugs are both organic and inorganic, such as propylthiouracil, which is an antithyroid hormone.

> ***Medical Terminology Review***
>
> **inorganic**
> *in* = not
> *organic* = relating to living organisms
> not related to live organisms

Engineered Sources

The newest area of drug origin is gene splicing or genetic engineering. The newer forms of insulin for use in humans have been produced with this technique. Other engineered drugs include: tissue plasminogen activator, growth hormones, cancer drugs, and drugs that combat HIV. The replacement of missing or nonfunctional genes is an emerging area of genetic engineering.

Dosage Forms of Drugs

Pharmaceutical principles are the underlying physiochemical principles that allow a drug to be incorporated in a pharmaceutical dosage form such as tablets and solutions. These principles apply whether the drug is extemporaneously compounded by the pharmacist or manufactured for commercial distribution as a drug product. Drug dosage forms are classified according to their physical state and chemical composition. They may include gases, liquids, solids, and semisolids. Some substances can undergo a change of state or phase, from solid to liquid states (melting) or from liquid to gaseous states (vaporization). Certain drugs are soluble in water, some are soluble in alcohol, and others are soluble in a mixture of liquids.

> ***Medical Terminology Review***
>
> **physiological**
> *physio* = relating to nature or physiology
> *chemical* = drug; agent
> drug related to nature

Solid Drugs

Intermolecular forces of attraction are stronger in solids than in liquids or gases. Solid drugs include tablets, pills, plaster, capsules, caplets, gelcaps, powder, granules, troches, or lozenges (Figure 2-1).

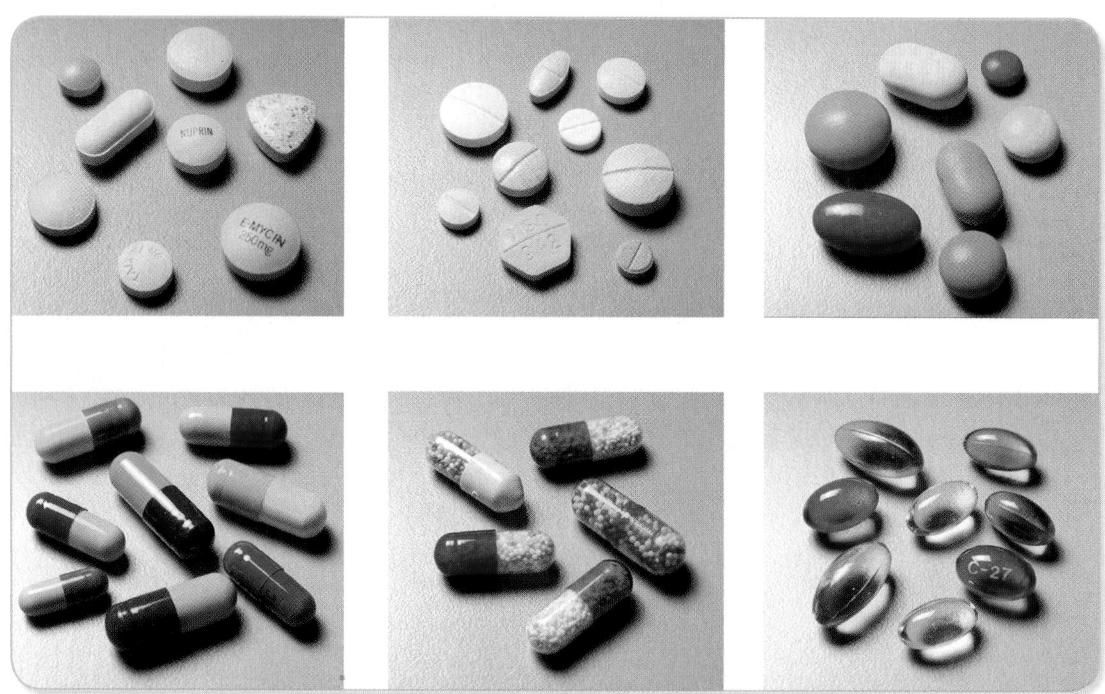

Figure 2-1 Solid dosage forms.

Tablet

A **tablet** is a pharmaceutical preparation made by compressing the powdered form of a drug and bulk filling material under high pressure (Figure 2-1). Most tablets are intended to be swallowed whole for dissolution and absorption from the gastrointestinal tract. Some are intended to be dissolved in the mouth or dissolved in water. Many times tablets are mistakenly called pills. Tablets come in various sizes, shapes, colors, and composition. The various forms of tablets include chewable, sublingual, buccal, enteric-coated, and buffered tablets.

Key Concept

Enteric-coated tablets are often given to patients who cannot take certain medications, such as aspirin, which are irritating to the stomach. For example, many elderly people who have stomach ulcers cannot tolerate aspirin unless it has an enteric-coating.

Medical Terminology Review

nitroglycerin
nitro = nitrate; nitrogen
glycerin = preparation obtained from fats and oils
drug preparation containing nitrogen

Chewable tablets *must* be chewed. They contain a flavored or sugar base. Chewable tablets are commonly used for antacids and antiflatulents, and for children who cannot swallow medication. Sublingual tablets must be dissolved under the tongue for rapid absorption. An example is nitroglycerin for angina pectoris. Buccal tablets are placed between the cheek and the gum until they are dissolved and absorbed. An **enteric-coated tablet** has a special coating to protect against stomach acid, allowing the drug to dissolve in the alkaline environment of the intestines. A **buffered tablet** can prevent ulceration or severe irritation of the stomach wall. Antacids have been added to reduce irritation to the stomach by the active ingredients. Some tablets are coated with a volatile liquid that is meant to dissolve in the mouth, such as antacid tablets.

Pill

A single-dose unit of medicine made by mixing the powdered drug with a liquid, such as syrup and rolling it into a round or oval shape is called a **pill**.

Plaster

Any composition of a liquid and a powder that hardens when it dries is called a **plaster**. Plasters may be solid or semisolid. An example is the salicylic acid plaster used to remove corns.

Capsule

A **capsule** is a medication dosage form in which the drug is contained in an external shell (Figure 2-1). Capsule shells are usually made of hard cylindrical gelatin and enclose or encapsulate powder, granules, liquids, or some combinations of these. Liquids may be placed in soft gelatin capsules, such as vitamin E capsules and cod liver oil capsules. They are used when medications have an unpleasant odor or taste. Capsules can be pulled apart, and the entire contents can be added as powder to food for individuals who have difficulty swallowing. Some forms of capsules come with a controlled-release dosage and are used over a defined period of time. These are called **sustained-release (SR)** or timed-release capsules. These drugs should never be crushed or dissolved, because this would negate their timed-release action.

Caplet

A **caplet** is shaped like a capsule but has the form of a tablet. The shape and film-coated covering make swallowing easier.

Gelcap

A **gelcap** is an oil-based medication that is enclosed in a soft gelatin capsule (Figure 2-1).

> ***Medical Terminology Review***
>
> **chloride**
> *chlor = chlorine*
> *ide = compound*
> substance containing chlorine

Powder

A drug that is dried and ground into fine particles is called a **powder**. An example is potassium chloride powder (Kato Powder).

Granule

A small pill, usually accompanied by many others most commonly encased within a gelatin capsule is called a **granule**. In most cases, granules within capsules are specially coated to gradually release medication over a period of up to 12 hours (Figure 2-1).

Troche or Lozenge

A hard or semisolid dosage form containing a medication intended for local application in the mouth or throat is called a **troche** or **lozenge**. These are flattened disks. Typically, a troche is placed on the tongue or between the cheek and gum and left in place until it dissolves. The medications most commonly administered by means of troches include cough suppressants and treatments for sore throat.

Semisolid Drugs

Semisolid drugs are often used as topical applications. These drugs are soft and pliable. Semisolid drugs include suppositories, ointments, and gels.

Suppository

A bullet-shaped dosage form intended to be inserted into a body orifice is called a **suppository**. Suppositories contain medication usually intended for a local effect at the site of insertion. Suppositories maintain their shape at room temperature but melt or dissolve when inserted. The most common sites of administration for suppositories are the rectum, vagina, and urethra.

Ointment

An **ointment** is a semisolid, greasy medication intended for external application, usually by rubbing (Figure 2-2). Medications that may be administered in ointment form include anti-inflammatory drugs, topical anesthetics, and antibiotics. Examples are zinc oxide ointment and Ben-Gay® ointment.

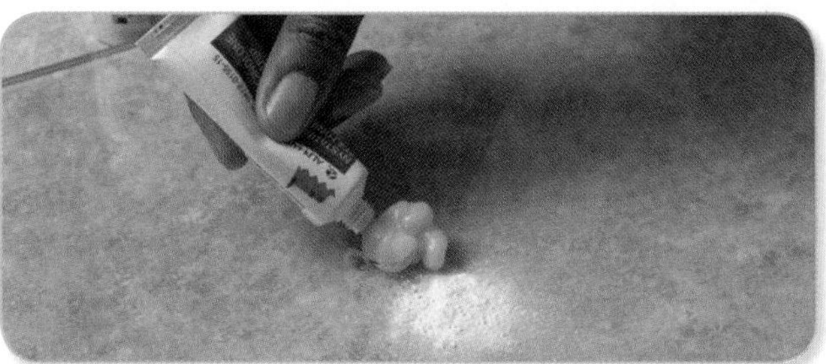

Figure 2-2 Semisolid dosage forms.

Cream

A **cream** is a semisolid preparation that is usually white and nongreasy; it has a water base. It is applied externally to the skin or administered via an applicator intravaginally.

Gel

A **gel** is a jelly-like substance that may be used for topical medication. Some gels have a high alcohol content and can cause stinging if applied to broken skin.

Liquid Drugs

Liquid preparations include drugs that have been dissolved or suspended. Examples of liquid drugs are syrups, spirits, elixirs, tinctures, fluid extract, liniments, emulsions, solutions, mixtures, suspension, aromatic waters, sprays, and aerosols (Figure 2-3). They are also classified by site or route of

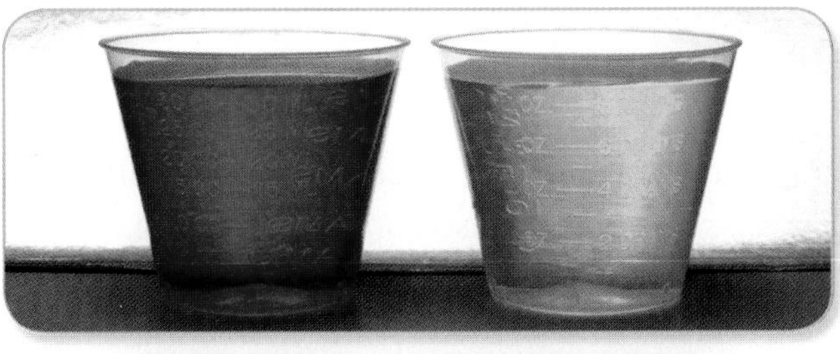

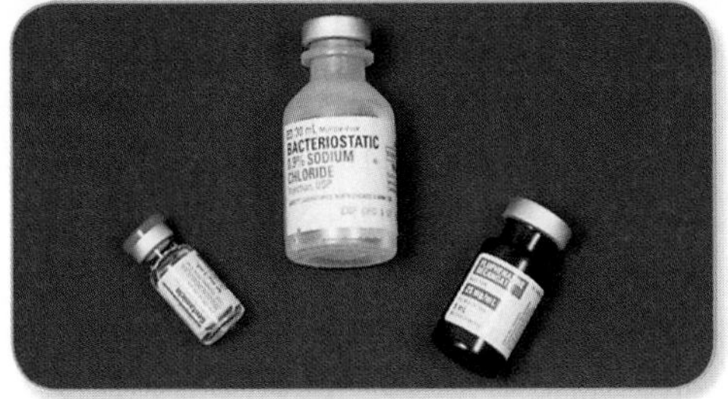

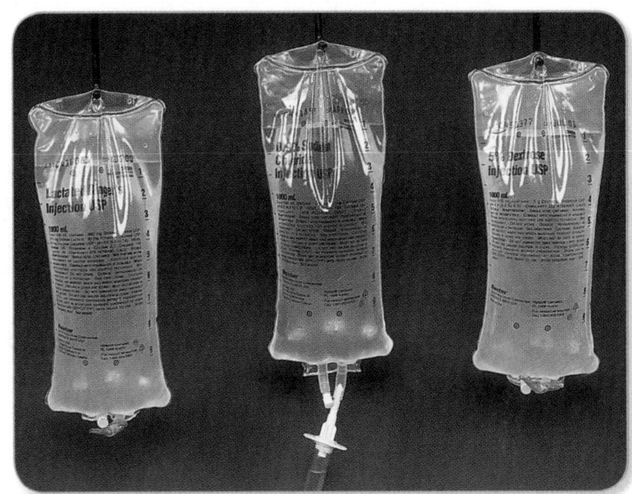

Figure 2-3 Liquid dosage forms.

> ***Key Concept***
>
> *Liquid drugs are very popular for use in children because other oral forms, such as tablets and capsules, are harder to swallow. Children have far less difficulty in taking liquid drugs.*

administration such as local (topical) on or through the skin, through the mouth, through the eye (ophthalmic), through the ear (otic), or through the rectum, urethra, or vagina. Liquid drugs may also be administered systemically by mouth or by injection throughout the body.

Syrup

A drug dosage form that consists of a high concentration of a sugar in water is called a **syrup**. It may or may not have medicinal substances added (e.g., simple syrup, ipecac syrup).

Solution

A **solution** is a drug or drugs dissolved in an appropriate solvent. An example of a solution is normal saline, which is salt dissolved in water.

Spirit

An alcohol-containing liquid that may be used pharmaceutically as a solvent is called a **spirit**. It is also known as essence (e.g., essence of peppermint, camphor spirit).

Elixir

A drug vehicle that consists of water, alcohol, and sugar is known as an **elixir**. It may or may not be aromatic and may or may not have active medicinal properties. The alcohol content makes elixirs convenient liquid dosage forms for many drugs that are only slightly soluble in water. In these cases, the drug is first dissolved in alcohol and the other elixir components are added. All elixirs contain alcohol (e.g., terpin hydrate elixir, phenobarbital elixir). Elixirs differ from tinctures in that they are sweetened. They should be used with caution in patients with diabetes or a history of alcohol abuse.

Tincture

A **tincture** is an alcoholic preparation of a soluble drug, usually from plant sources. In some cases, the solution may also contain water (e.g., iodine tincture, digitalis tincture).

Fluidextract

A concentrated solution of a drug removed from a plant source by mixing ground parts of the plant with a suitable solvent, usually alcohol, and then separating the plant residue from the solvent is called a **fluidextract**. Typically, 1 mL (1 cc) contains 1 g of the drug. Fluidextracts are not intended to be administered directly to a patient. Instead, they are used to provide a source of drug in the manufacture of final dosage forms. Only vegetable drugs are used (e.g., glycyrrhiza fluidextract).

Liniment

A **liniment** is a mixture of drugs with oil, soap, water, or alcohol, intended for external application with rubbing. Most liniments are counterirritants intended to treat muscle or joint pain (e.g., camphor liniment, chloroform liniment).

Emulsion

A pharmaceutical preparation in which two agents that cannot ordinarily be combined are mixed is called an **emulsion**. In the typical emulsion, oil is dispersed inside water, however they can also be water dispersed inside oil. Most creams and lotions are emulsions (e.g., Petrogalar Plain).

Mixtures and Suspensions

In a **mixture** or a **suspension**, an agent is mixed with a liquid but not dissolved. These preparations must be shaken before the patient takes them. An example is Milk of Magnesia®.

Aromatic Water

In pharmacy, a mixture of distilled water with an aromatic volatile oil is called an **aromatic water**. Aromatic waters may be used for medicinal purposes (e.g., peppermint water, camphor water).

Gaseous Drugs

Pharmaceutical gases include the anesthetic gases such as nitrous oxide and halothane. Compressed gases include oxygen for therapy (Figure 2-4) or carbon dioxide.

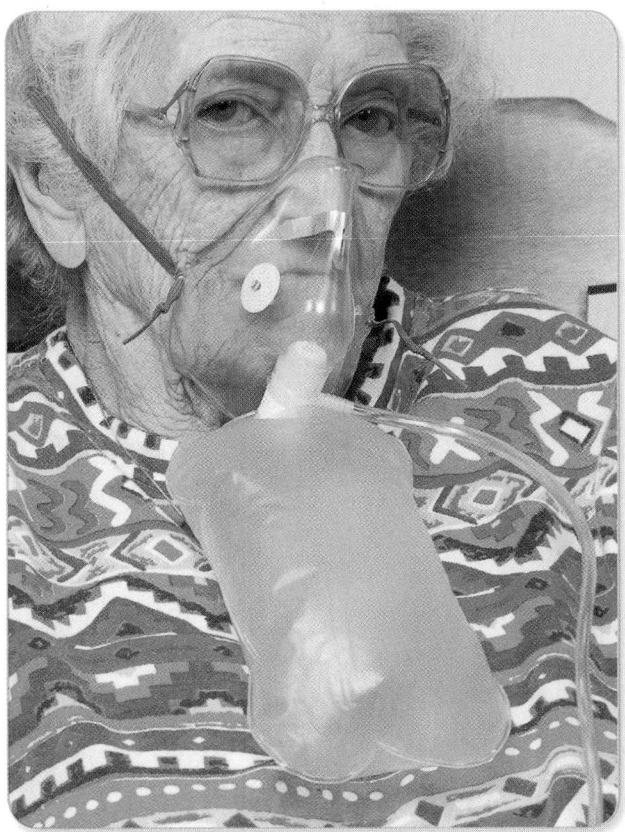

Figure 2-4 Gaseous dosage forms.

Summary

A single drug may have up to three names: chemical, generic, and trade. There is only one chemical name and one generic name for each drug, whereas a drug may have several trade names, with similar ingredients in each marketed drug product.

Drug sources may include: plants, animals (including humans), minerals, synthetics (chemical substances), and engineered drugs (investigational drugs). Drug dosage forms are classified according to their physical state and chemical composition. They may include solids, semisolids, liquids, and gases. Some substances may change from solid to liquid states (melting) or from liquid to gaseous states (vaporization). Certain drugs are water soluble, some are soluble in alcohol, and others are soluble in a mixture of liquids.

Exploring the Web

Visit ***www.fda.gov***

- Search using the term dosage forms defined. Review information that outlines the characteristics of the dosage forms.
- Search for the various drug sources and review information related to the drugs derived from those sources.

Visit ***www.ismp.org***

- Review information listed under the link "Medication Safety Tools and Resources." Discover the common types of errors that can occur with drugs and what strategies can be used to avoid them.

Visit ***www.mapharm.com***

- Click on "medical drug sources." What additional information can you find here on the various forms of medications available?

Review Questions

Multiple Choice

1. Which of the following is an important cardiac glycoside?

A. nicotine
B. digoxin
C. morphine sulfate
D. atropine sulfate

2. Tablets are mistakenly called:
   A. pills
   B. powders
   C. buffered
   D. gelcaps
3. Which of the following is an example of semisolid drugs?
   A. caplets
   B. gelcaps
   C. gels
   D. granules
4. Which of the following is an example of plant drug sources?
   A. insulin
   B. pepsin
   C. meperidine
   D. morphine
5. Any composition of a liquid and a powder that hardens when it dries is called a:
   A. capsule
   B. plaster
   C. gelcap
   D. granule
6. Which of the following is an example of spirits?
   A. phenobarbital liquids
   B. peppermint and camphor liquids
   C. iodine and digitalis liquids
   D. Milk of Magnesia®
7. A preparation that can be used rectally is called a:
   A. powder
   B. gel
   C. pill
   D. suppository
8. A solution containing alcohol is called a(n);
   A. emulsion
   B. solution
   C. syrup
   D. elixir
9. A small, disk-shaped medication, which is composed of a solidifying paste and used for local treatment is called a(n):
   A. lozenge
   B. liniment
   C. ointment
   D. gelcap

10. Nicotine, morphine sulfate, and atropine sulfate are examples of which of the following compounds?

A. engineered (investigational drugs)
B. animals or humans
C. plants
D. synthetics

11. Which of the following is an advantage of generic drugs over equivalent trade-name drugs?

A. less toxic
B. absorbed slower
C. taste better
D. cheaper

12. A dry mass of minute separate particles of any substance is called a:

A. powder
B. plaster
C. pill
D. granule

Matching

_____	**1.** Not intended to be administered directly to a patient	**A.** emulsion
_____	**2.** A bullet-shaped dosage form intended to be inserted into a body orifice	**B.** aromatic water
_____	**3.** A drug or drugs dissolved in an appropriate solvent	**C.** ointment
_____	**4.** Can prevent ulceration or severe irritation of the stomach wall	**D.** buccal tablet
_____	**5.** An alcoholic preparation of a soluble drug, usually from plant sources	**E.** buffered tablet
_____	**6.** A semisolid, greasy medication intended for external application, usually by rubbing	**F.** tincture
_____	**7.** Placed between the cheek and the gum until dissolved	**G.** capsule
_____	**8.** A mixture of distilled water with a volatile oil	**H.** solution
_____	**9.** Shells usually made of hard cylindrical gelatin	**I.** suppository
_____	**10.** Most creams and lotions	**J.** fluidextract

Critical Thinking

A pharmacist decides to switch from a trade-name drug that was ordered by a physician to a generic-equivalent drug instead.

1. What advantages does this substitution have for the patient?
2. What disadvantages might the switch cause?
3. What must the pharmacist do before switching from a trade-name drug to a generic-equivalent drug?

CHAPTER 3

Biopharmaceutics

OUTLINE

OBJECTIVES

After completing this chapter, the reader should be able to:

1. Describe the mechanisms of drug action and define pharmacokinetic and pharmacodynamic.
2. Explain the importance of the first-pass effect.
3. Explain the significance of the blood-brain barrier to drug therapy.
4. Identify the major processes by which drugs are eliminated from the body.
5. Describe the process of filtration, secretion, and reabsorption for renal excretion of drugs.
6. Describe factors affecting drug action.
7. Explain how rate of elimination and plasma half-life (t ½) are related to the duration of drug action.
8. Define idiosyncratic and anaphylactic reactions.

GLOSSARY

Absorption – the movement of a drug from its site of administration into the bloodstream

Active transport – a process that moves particles in fluid through membranes from a region of lower concentration to a region of high concentration

Agonist – the drug that produces a functional change in a cell

Anaphylactic reaction – a severe, life-threatening allergic reaction to a drug

Antagonist – the drug blocks a functional change in the cell

Antimetabolite – a substance that is produced to alter the actions of liver enzymes

Bioavailability – measurement of the rate of absorption and total amount of drug that reaches the systemic circulation

Biotransformation – the conversion of a drug within the body; also known as metabolism

Diffusion – the process of particles in a fluid moving from an area of higher concentration to an area of lower concentration, resulting in an even distribution of the particles in the fluid

Dose-effect relationship – the relationship between drug dose and blood, or other biological fluid concentrations

Drug clearance – elimination rate over time divided by the drug's concentration

Excretion – the process whereby the undigested residue of food and waste products of metabolism are eliminated, material is removed to regulate composition of body fluids and tissues, or substances are expelled to perform functions on an exterior surface

Filtration – the movement of water and dissolved substances from the glomerulus to the Bowman's capsule

First-pass effect – drugs reaching the liver where they are partially metabolized before being sent to the body

Glomerular filtration rate (GFR) – the rate of filtration in the kidneys

Half-life – the time it takes for the plasma concentration (e.g., of a drug) to be reduced by 50 percent

Hepatic portal circulation – the circulation of blood through the liver

Idiosyncratic reaction – experience of a unique, strange, or unpredicted reaction to a drug

Lipid solubility – the ability to dissolve in a fatty medium

Metabolism – the conversion of a drug within the body; also known as biotransformation

Passive transport – the most common and important mode of traversal of drugs through membranes; diffusion

Pharmacodynamics – the study of the biochemical and physiological effects of drugs

Pharmacokinetics – the study of the absorption, distribution, metabolism, and excretion of drugs

Placebo – sugar pill

Reabsorption – the movement of water and selected substances from the tubules to the peritubular capillaries

Target sites – the areas where a drug's greatest action takes place at the cellular level

Tolerance – reduced responsiveness of a drug because of adaptation to it

Tubular secretion – the active secretion of substances such as potassium from the peritubular capillaries into the tubules

Overview

Drugs differ widely in their biochemical and physiological properties, as well as their mechanisms of action. In clinical applications, a drug must be absorbed, transported to the target tissue or organ, and then it must penetrate into the cell membranes, their organelles, and alter the ongoing processes. The drug may be distributed to a number of tissues, bound or stored, then metabolized to inactive or active products. Then it must be excreted. The usual route of drug administration, distribution, and elimination are factors in the effectiveness of a drug's ability to produce a desired outcome. The principles explaining the manner in which drugs act within the body are explained in this chapter.

PHARMACOKINETICS

Pharmacokinetics is the study of the action and movement of drugs within the body, including the mechanisms of absorption, distribution, metabolism, and excretion of drugs. It defines the processes by which the body ingests a drug, breaks down the drug, distributes it throughout the body, uses it, and then excretes the waste products of the drug.

> ***Medical Terminology Review***
>
> **pharmacokinetics**
> *pharmac/o = drugs, medicine*
> *-kinet- = movement*
> *-ic = pertaining to*
> the movement of drugs through the body

Drug Absorption

The movement of a drug from its site of administration into the bloodstream is **absorption**. In most cases, this is the first step the body takes to begin processing a drug. For absorption to occur, a drug must be transported across one or more biological membranes to reach the blood circulation. This process can take place via passive (diffusion) or active transport.

Passive Transport

The most common and important mode of traversal of drugs through membranes is **passive transport** or **diffusion**. Diffusion is the process in which particles in a fluid move from an area of higher concentration to an area of lower concentration, resulting in an even distribution of the particles in the fluid (Figure 3-1). This mechanism requires little or no energy. In the body, diffusion depends upon **lipid solubility** (ability to be dissolved in a fatty substance) of the drug. Cell membranes consist of a fatty bi-layer through which drugs must pass for diffusion to occur. Agents that are relatively lipid-soluble diffuse more rapidly than less lipid-soluble drugs.

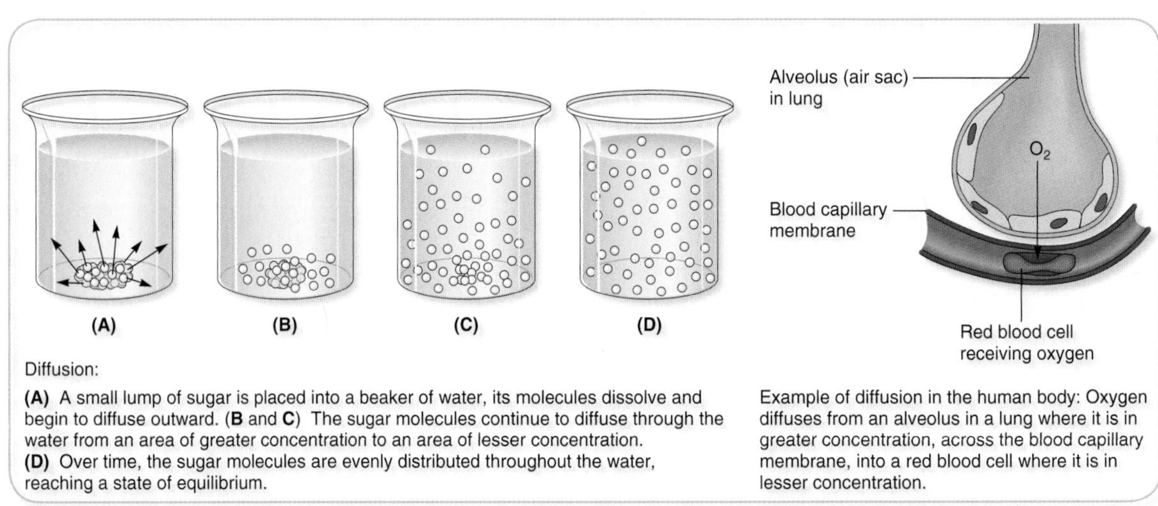

Figure 3-1 The process of diffusion.

Active Transport

Active transport is a process that moves particles in fluid through membranes from a region of lower concentration to a region of high concentration. It uses specific carrier molecules (proteins) in the cell membranes and requires energy (Figure 3-2).

Absorption of Medications Through the Digestive System

Oral administration of drugs is the most convenient, economical, and common route of administration. Absorption of most drugs administered orally takes place through the digestive system. Drugs given orally are usually absorbed across the stomach or upper intestinal wall and enter blood vessels

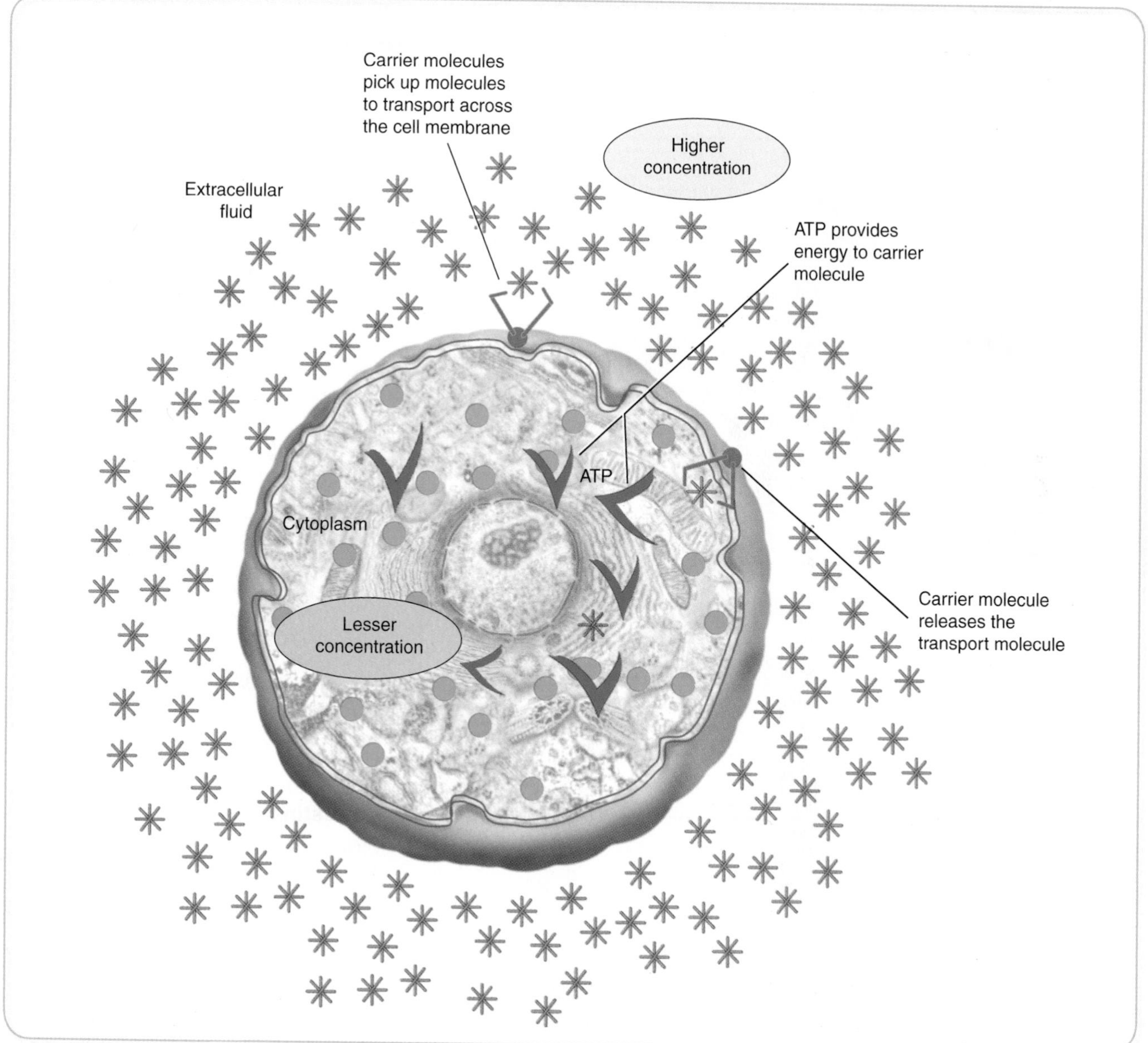

Figure 3-2 Active transport.

> **Medical Terminology Review**
>
> **hepatic**
> *hepat/o = liver*
> *-ic = pertaining to*
> related to the liver

of **hepatic portal circulation** (Figure 3-3). Hepatic portal circulation carries blood directly to the liver where it is immediately exposed to metabolism by the liver enzymes before reaching the systemic circulation. This exposure is called the **first-pass effect**; the drug reaches the liver, where it is partly metabolized before being sent to the body for systemic effects. Drugs that are administered parenterally or sublingually do not undergo a first-pass effect. Therefore, parenteral medications are often given in lower doses than those given orally.

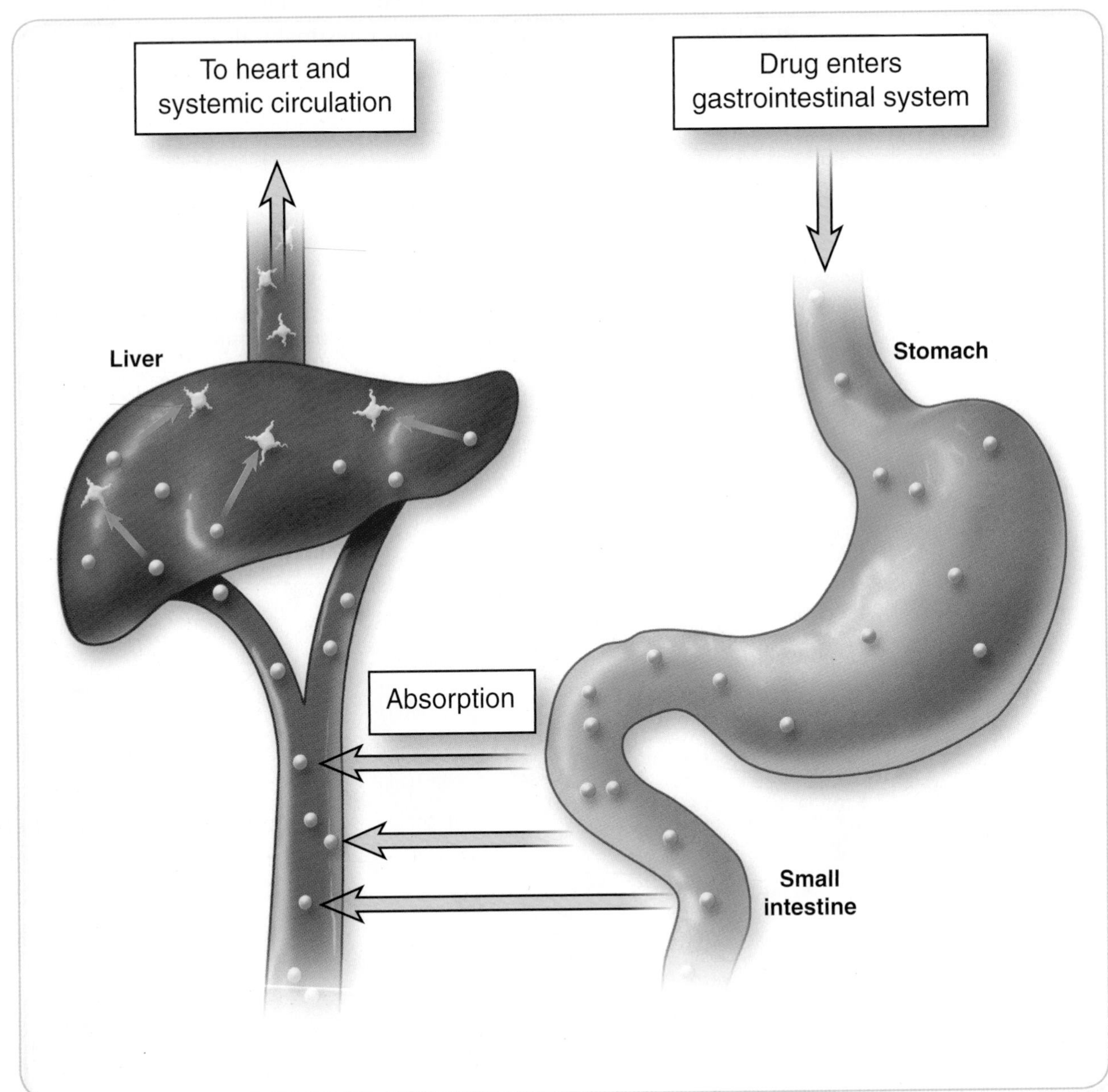

Figure 3-3 First-pass effect. Drugs are absorbed from the small intestine into the portal vein. From the portal vein, the drugs travel to the liver where they are metabolized into inactive forms. The drugs then leave the liver to be distributed through general circulation.

Factors Influencing Absorption

There are many factors that may alter the rate of absorption of drugs into the body. Such factors to consider are the acidity of the stomach, presence of food in the stomach, dosage of drugs, bioavailability, and the routes of administration.

- Acidity of the Stomach
  Drugs with an acidic pH, such as aspirin, are easily absorbed in the acid environment of the stomach, whereas alkaline medications are more readily absorbed in the alkaline environment of the small intestine. Milk products and antacids tend to change the pH of the stomach. Therefore, some drugs are not absorbed properly. The infant who is taking formula or milk may need to take medications on an empty stomach because the regular feedings will change the stomach acid level.

- Presence of Food in the Stomach
  The presence of food in the stomach or intestine can have a profound influence on the rate and extent of drug absorption. Food in the stomach decreases the absorption rate of medications, while an empty stomach increases the rate. Sometimes the drug must be put into effect quickly, requiring the stomach to be empty. If the medication causes irritation of the stomach, food should be eaten to serve as a buffer and decrease irritation.

- Dosage of Drugs
  Drugs administered in high concentrations tend to be more rapidly absorbed than those administered in low concentrations. The relationship between drug dose and blood, or other biological fluid concentrations, is called the **dose-effect relationship**.

- Drug Bioavailability
  Bioavailability is a term that indicates measurement of both the rate of drug absorption and total amount of drug that reaches the systemic blood circulation from an administered dosage form. The route of drug administration in this matter is essential. If a drug is administered by intravenous injection, all of the dose enters the blood circulation. This is not true for drugs administered by other routes, especially for drugs given orally. Solid drugs such as tablets and capsules must dissolve. This is a major source of difference in drug bioavailability. Poor solubility of a drug or incomplete absorption of a drug in the gastrointestinal tract, and rapid metabolism of a drug during its first pass through the liver are other factors that influence bioavailability.

Medical Terminology Review

sublingual
sub- = under
lingu/o = tongue
-al = pertaining to
under the tongue

buccal
bucc/o = cheek
-al = pertaining to
related to the cheek

subcutaneous
sub- = under
cutaneous = of the skin
under the skin

- Routes of Administration

  Absorption will vary based upon the route of administration. Some oral drugs are administered sublingually (under the tongue) or buccally (inner lining of cheek); these drugs are absorbed through the mucous membranes directly into the bloodstream to protect the drug from decomposition and deterioration in the stomach or liver. Topical drugs may be absorbed through several layers of skin for local absorption. For example, nitroglycerin commonly is applied to the skin in the form of an ointment or transdermal patches; it is absorbed rapidly, and provides sustained blood levels. When the drug is injected directly into the bloodstream (vein or artery) and distributes throughout the body, it acts rapidly; the process of absorption is bypassed. The drug may be injected deeply into a skeletal muscle. The rate of absorption depends on the vascularity of the muscle site, and the lipid solubility of the drug. If it is injected beneath the skin, drug absorption is less rapid, because the subcutaneous region is less vascular than the muscle tissues.

Medical Terminology Review

lymphatic
lymph/o = lymph
-ic = pertaining to
related to the lymph

Key Concept

Sedatives, antianxiety drugs, and anticonvulsants readily cross the blood-brain barrier to produce their actions on the central nervous system.

Alcohol, cocaine, caffeine, nicotine, and certain prescription drugs easily cross the placental barrier and can potentially harm the fetus.

Drug Distribution

The process by which drug molecules leave the bloodstream and enter the tissues of the body is called distribution. When a drug reaches the bloodstream, it is ready to travel through blood, lymphatics, and other fluids to its site of action. Drugs interact with specific receptors. Some drugs are frequently bound to plasma proteins (albumin) in the blood. If these drugs are bound to albumin, they are known as inactive drugs, while those that are unbound are called pharmacologically-active drugs. If binding is extensive and firm, it will have a considerable impact upon the distribution and excretion of the drug in the body. Only when the protein molecules release the drug can it diffuse into the tissues, interact with receptors, and produce a therapeutic effect. The brain and placenta possess special anatomical barriers that prevent many chemicals and drugs from entering. These barriers are referred to as the blood-brain barrier and fetal-placental barrier.

Medical Terminology Review

hepatocyte
hepat/o = liver
-cyt = cell
liver cell

Drug Metabolism

Drug **metabolism** is a chemical reaction wherein a drug is converted into compounds, and then easily removed from the body. It occurs once the drug reaches the liver, before the drug reaches its intended site within the body. Most drugs are acted upon by enzymes in the body, and are converted to metabolic derivatives during metabolism. The process of conversion is called **biotransformation**. The liver is the major site of biotransformation. Many biotransformations in the liver occur in the smooth endoplasmic reticulum of the hepatocytes. Liver enzymes react with the drugs creating metabolites. The majority of these metabolites are inactive and toxic. Drug metabolism

Key Concept

Patients with liver disease may require lower dosages of a drug, or a drug that does not undergo biotransformation in the liver.

influences drug action, such as duration of drug action, drug interactions, drug activation, and toxicity or side effects. In most cases, biotransformation can terminate the pharmacological action of the drug and increase removal of the drug from the body.

Drug Excretion

The final step of pharmacokinetics is **excretion**, which is the removal of drugs from the body. Drugs may be excreted from the body by many routes, including urine, feces (unabsorbed drugs, and those secreted in the bile), saliva, sweat, milk, lungs (alcohols and anesthetics), and tears. Any route may be important for a given drug, but the kidney is the major site of excretion for most drugs. Unchanged drugs or drug metabolites can be eliminated by the kidneys. The main role of the kidney is to remove all non-natural and harmful agents in the bloodstream while keeping a balance of other natural substances. Kidney impairment can significantly prolong drug action and causes drug toxicity. Renal excretion of drugs and their metabolites may undergo three processes: (1) filtration, (2) secretion, and (3) reabsorption.

Drug Filtration

Urine formation begins in the glomerulus and Bowman's capsule in the kidneys. **Filtration** causes water and dissolved substances to move from the glomerulus into Bowman's capsule. Filtration occurs when the pressure on one side of a membrane is greater than the pressure on the opposite side. Small substances such as water, sodium, potassium, chloride, glucose, uric acid, and creatinine move through the wall of the glomerulus very easily. These substances are filtered in proportion to their plasma concentration. In other words, if the concentration of a particular substance or drug in the plasma is high, many of these substances are filtered (Figure 3-4). Approximately one-fifth of the plasma reaching the kidney is filtered. The rate of filtration is referred to as the **glomerular filtration rate (GFR)** and is normally 125–130 milliliters per minute (mL/min).

Medical Terminology Review

peritubular
peri- = *around*
tubular = *related to tubes*
around or near tubes

Drug Secretion

Although most of the water and dissolved substances enter the tubules of the kidneys as a result of filtration across the glomerulus, a second process moves very small amounts of substances from the blood into the tubules. This is called **tubular secretion**. It involves the active secretion of substances such as potassium ions (K^+), hydrogen ions (H^+), uric acid, the ammonium ion, and drugs from the peritubular capillaries into the tubules. Secretion occurs primarily in the proximal convoluted tubule (Figure 3-4). This is an active process mediated by two carrier systems, one specific for organic acids and one specific for organic bases. Therefore, the pH of the urine may affect the rate of drug excretion by changing the chemical form of a drug to one that can be more readily excreted or to one that can be reabsorbed. Penicillins

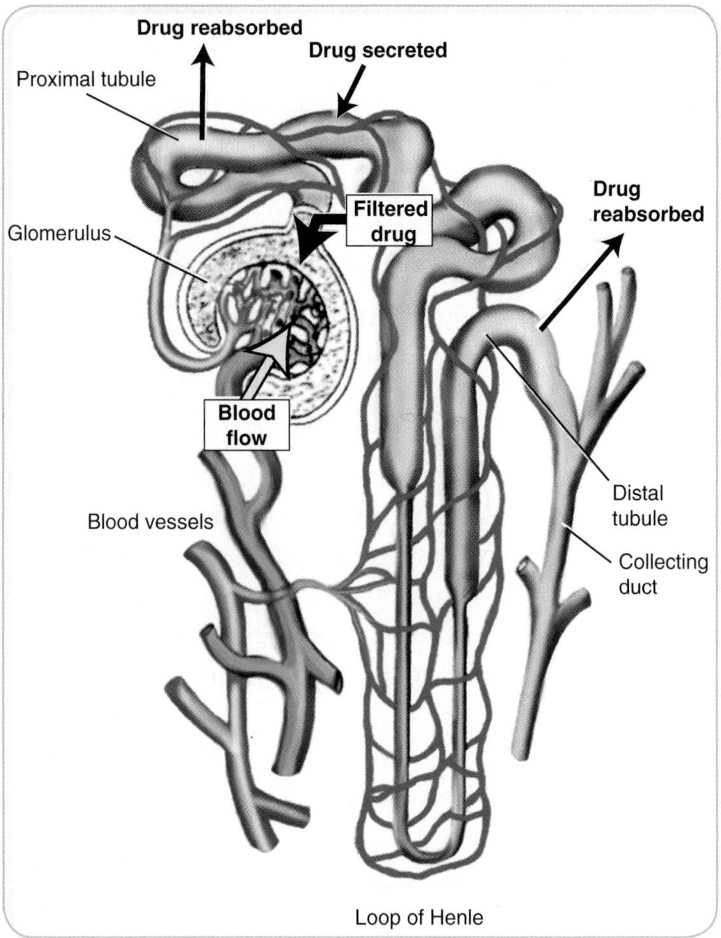

Figure 3-4 Renal excretion of drugs. Note sites where drugs are secreted and reabsorbed.

or barbiturates are weak acids, and available as sodium or potassium salts. These agents can be better excreted if the urine pH is less acid.

On the other hand, any drug which is available as sulfate, hydrochloride, or nitrate salts, such as atropine or morphine, can be excreted better if the urine is more acidic. By altering the pH of urine, increased elimination of certain drugs can be facilitated, thus preventing prolonged action or overdosage of a toxic compound. Another technique to alter the rate of excretion of a drug is to produce a competitively blocking effect. For example, probenecid may be used to block the renal excretion of penicillin. This prolongs the effect of the antibiotic by maintaining a higher therapeutic plasma level. Secretions of drugs are active transport systems. They require energy and may become saturated.

Drug Reabsorption

Reabsorption may occur throughout the tubules of the nephrons (Figure 3-4). It causes water and selected substances to move from the tubules into the peritubular capillaries. The mechanism is passive diffusion, therefore, only the unionized form of a drug is reabsorbed.

It is dependent upon its lipid solubility. For example, the kidneys selectively reabsorb substances such as glucose, proteins, and sodium, which they have already secreted into the renal tubules. These reabsorbed substances return to the blood.

Drug Clearance

Drug clearance describes drug elimination (excretion plus metabolism). It is defined as elimination rate over time divided by the drug's concentration. Drug clearance can also be described as being equal to the volume of fluid completely cleared of a drug per a unit of time. It is usually expressed in mL/minute or L/hour. Plasma clearance divided by blood clearance equals blood concentration divided by plasma concentration. Total clearance equals the sum of clearances of individual body processes. The eliminated drug amount is proportional to the clearance of the respective elimination process.

Pharmacodynamics

Pharmacodynamics is the study of the biochemical and physiological effects of drugs. It is also defined as the study of a drug's mechanism of action. After administration, most drugs enter the blood circulation, and expose almost all body tissues to their possible effects. All drugs produce more than one effect in the body. The primary effect of a drug is the desired or therapeutic effect. Secondary effects are all other effects, whether desirable or undesirable (causing harmful effects), produced by the drug. Most drugs have an affinity for certain organs or tissues, and exert their greatest action at the cellular level in those specific areas, which are called **target sites.**

Most often, there are links between pharmacokinetics and pharmacodynamics that demonstrate the relationship between drug dose and blood, or other biological fluid concentration. The pharmacologic response by itself does not provide information about some very important determinants of that response; for example, dose, drug concentration in plasma or at the site of action. Pharmacokinetic and pharmacodynamics can determine the dose-effect relationship (see Figure 3-5).

Drug Action

Drugs produce their effects by altering the normal function of the cells and tissues of the body. They do not create new cellular functions. Instead, they change existing cellular functions. Drug action is generally described relative to a physiological state that was in existence when a drug was administered. Some drugs accumulate in specific tissues because they have an affinity for a tissue component. The most common way that drugs exert their

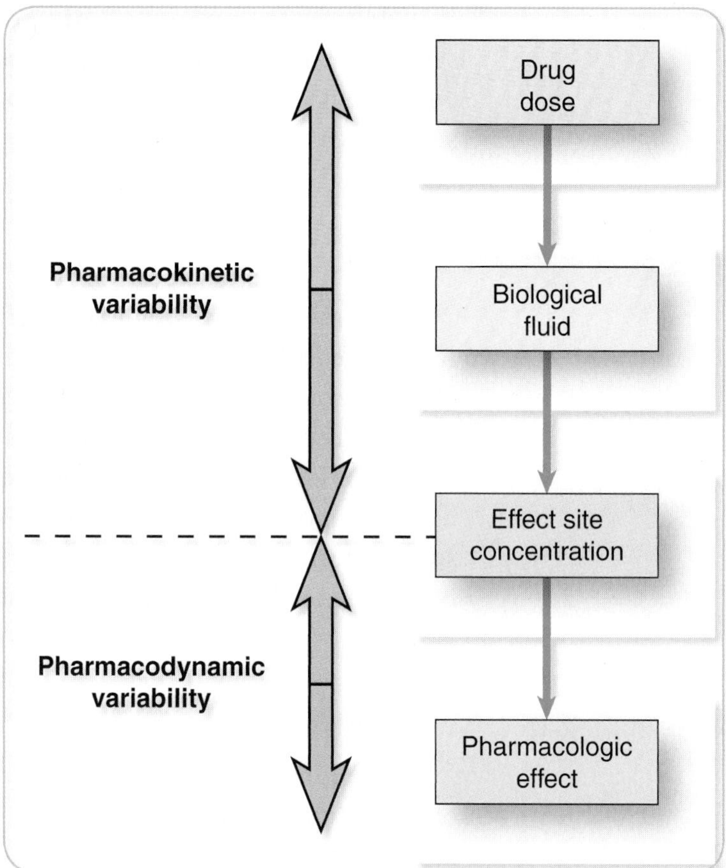

Figure 3-5 The dose-effect relationship.

action is by forming chemical bonds with certain receptors in the body. This usually occurs only if the drug and its receptor have a compatible chemical shape. Drugs with molecules that fit precisely into a given receptor elicit a comparable drug response and are known as **agonists**. Those that do not fit perfectly produce only a weak response or no response at all (Figure 3-6).

Not all drugs that bind to specific cells cause a functional change in the cell. These drugs act as **antagonists** to the natural process and work by blocking a sequence of biochemical events.

Some drugs may act by affecting the enzyme functions of the body. When drugs are metabolized in the liver, they produce **antimetabolites**. These antimetabolites interrupt or inhibit the actions of particular enzymes, thus producing a desired therapeutic effect.

Factors Affecting Drug Action

There are various factors that are important in determining the correct drugs for a patient, such as drug half-life, age, sex, body weight, time of day administered (diurnal), presence of illnesses, psychological factors, tolerance, toxicity of drugs, idiosyncrasy, and drug interactions.

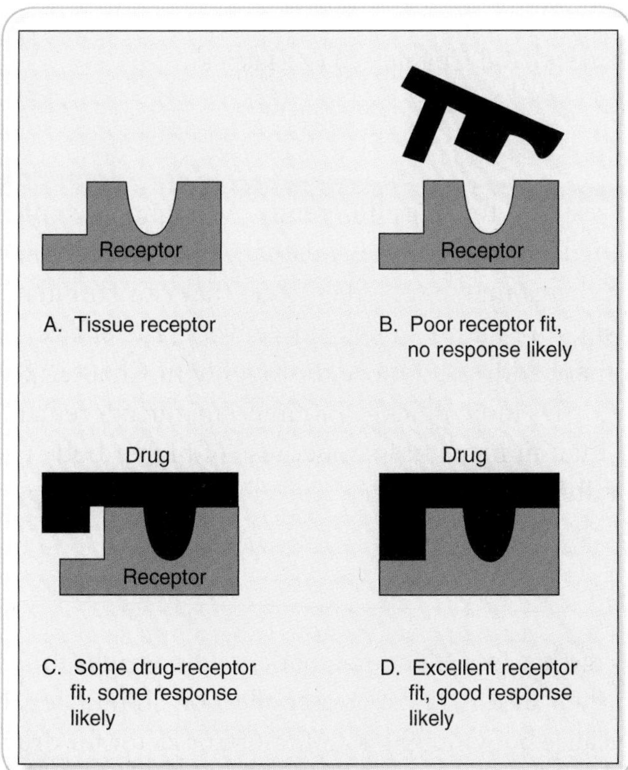

Figure 3-6 Drug-receptor interaction. Binding with specific receptors occurs only when the drug and its receptors have a compatible chemical shape.

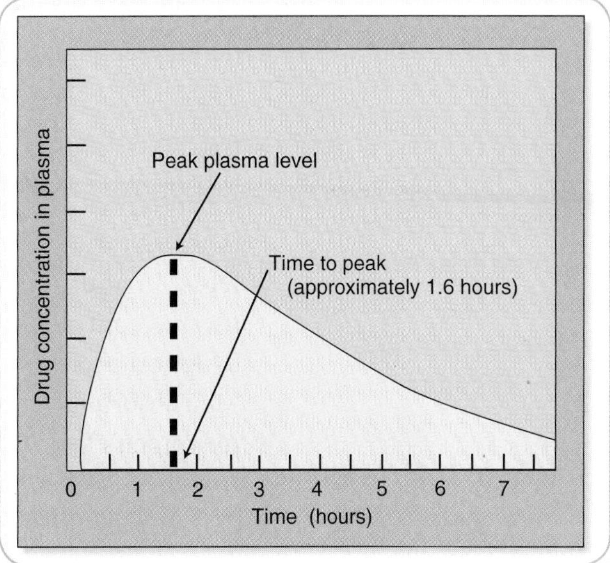

Figure 3-7 Plot of drug concentration in plasma versus time after single oral administration of a drug.

Drug Half-Life

The **half-life** of a drug is a related measurement used to ensure that maximum therapeutic dosages are given. The half-life of a drug is the time it takes for the concentration of the drug in plasma to be reduced by one-half (50 percent). It is an indication of how long a medication will produce its effect in the body. The larger the half-life value, the longer it takes for a drug to be eliminated. This is one of the most common methods used to explain drug actions. The half-life of each drug may be different: for example, a drug with a short half-life, such as two or three hours, will need to be administered more often than one with a long half-life, such as eight hours. Another method of describing drug action is by the use of graphic depiction of the plasma concentration of the drug versus time (see Figure 3-7).

Age

Newborns and elderly individuals show the greatest effects of a drug's actions. Because of their ages and either immature or impaired body systems, they are more sensitive to medications that affect the central nervous system, and are at risk for developing toxic drug levels. Calculations of drug dosages for these two groups must be carefully measured, and treatment usually starts with very small doses. These factors are discussed in greater depth in Chapter 25 (pediatrics) and Chapter 26 (geriatrics).

Sex

Both men and women respond to drugs differently. A pregnant woman is at risk for taking some medications because of damage to the developing fetus. In addition, certain drugs may have side effects that can stimulate uterine contractions, causing premature labor and delivery. The effects of drugs on pregnant women are addressed more thoroughly in Chapter 24. Men absorb intramuscular drugs more quickly. Intramuscular drugs remain in women's tissues longer than in men's tissues, because of higher body fat content. Women and men differ in the way they are affected by other types of drugs as well.

Body Weight

Basically, the same dosage has less effect on a patient who weighs more than the normal range for their height, and a greater effect on an individual who weighs less. This is because body weight is an important factor for drug action, and some medication doses must be adjusted based on body weight. Pediatric medications are designed for the body weight or body surface of children. If adult medications are used for children, the correct dosage must be calculated and adjusted for the child's body weight.

Diurnal Body Rhythms

Diurnal (during the day) body rhythms play an important part in the effects of some drugs, because they can affect the intensity of a person's response to a drug. For example, sedatives given in the morning will not be as effective as when administered before bedtime. On the other hand, corticosteroid administration is preferred in the morning, because this best mimics the body's natural pattern of corticosteroid production and elimination.

Key Concept

Acute or chronic illnesses of the liver in elderly patients may cause severe toxicity. For example, diazepam may cause coma in severely liver-damaged patients when given in average doses.

Presence of Illnesses

Patients with liver or kidney disease may respond to drugs differently, because the body is not able to detoxify and excrete chemicals properly. The liver and kidneys are the major sites of elimination of chemical substances. Other illnesses that affect the physical health of the liver and kidneys must also be considered.

Psychological Factors

Psychological factors involve how patients feel about the drug(s) they are prescribed, and the different ways they respond to them. If an individual believes in the therapy, even a **placebo** (sugar pill, or sterile water thought to be a drug) may help to bring about relief. Some patients cooperate in following the directions for a specific drug, and a patient's mental attitude can reduce or increase an expected response to a drug.

Tolerance

Tolerance is the phenomenon of reduced responsiveness to a drug. The body becomes so adapted to the presence of the drug that it cannot function properly without it. The only way to prevent drug tolerance from occurring is to avoid the repeated use of a drug. The signs of drug tolerance consist of an increased amount required by the body to achieve the desired effects. Certain drugs that stimulate or depress the central nervous system are prone to causing drug tolerance.

Drug Toxicity

Almost all drugs are capable of producing toxic effects. There is a range between the therapeutic dose of a drug and its toxic dose. This range is measurable by the therapeutic index, which is used to explain the safety of a drug. The therapeutic index is expressed in the form of a ratio:

$$\text{Therapeutic Index (TI)} = \frac{\text{median lethal dose:} \quad LD_{50}}{\text{median effective dose:} \quad ED_{50}}$$

The larger the difference between the two doses, the greater the therapeutic index. For example, if the therapeutic index is 3 (such as 30 mg ÷ 10 mg), it means that three times the dose of a drug will be lethal to a patient.

Idiosyncratic Reactions

When a patient has experienced a unique, strange, or unpredicted reaction to a drug, this is termed an **idiosyncratic reaction**. Idiosyncratic reactions may be caused by underlying enzyme deficiencies from genetic or hormonal variation.

Drug Interactions

Drug interactions are defined as effects of medications taken together. When two or more drugs are prescribed together, this generally results in one of the following:

1. The drugs have no effects on each other's action.
2. The drugs increase each other's effect.
3. The drugs decrease each other's effect.

Any of these results may also be affected by the ingestion of food. Most drugs do not interact with other drugs or food, but when such interactions do occur, some may be life-threatening. Plasma protein binding can be a source of drug interaction if several drugs compete for binding sites on protein molecules. Drug interactions may result in elevated concentrations of drugs by displacement of protein-bound drugs or by reduced rates of drug disposition, therefore, resulting in toxic drug concentrations.

Some drug interactions are wanted, and the medications are prescribed together to produce the desired effect. For example, probenecid is given with penicillin to increase the absorption of penicillin. Other interactions are unintended and unwanted, producing possible dangers for the patient. Drug interactions may also cause a more rapid drug disappearance, with plasma concentrations decreasing to below minimum effective values. For example, some antibiotics make birth control pills less effective.

Side Effects and Adverse Effects of Drugs

Side effects are usually referred to as mild but annoying responses to the medication. Adverse reactions or adverse effects usually imply more severe symptoms or problems that develop because of a drug. Adverse effects may require the patient to be hospitalized, or may even threaten the patient's life. Certain side effects such as nausea may disappear if the dosage is reduced. Some side effects such as drowsiness may go away after the patient takes the medication for a while. Occasionally, side effects are very problematic, thus the dispensing of the drug to the patient is stopped or changed to a different drug. An example of this can be hyperactivity or inability to sleep, bleeding, nephrotoxicity, or hepatoxic development.

Hypersensitivity or Allergy

Allergies or hypersensitivity reactions are another unpredictable reaction that some drugs such as aspirin, penicillin, or sulfa products may cause in some patients. Hypersensitivity reactions generally occur when a patient has received a drug and the body has developed antibodies against it. After this process of antibody production, if the patient is re-exposed to the drug, the antigen-antibody reaction produces, itching, hives, rash, or swelling of the skin. This is a common type of allergic reaction.

Anaphylactic Reaction

An **anaphylactic reaction** to a drug is a severe form of allergic reaction that is life threatening. The patient develops severe shortness of breath, and may even have cardiac collapse. An anaphylactic reaction is a medical emergency because the patient may suffer paralysis of the diaphragm, swelling of the oropharynx, and an inability to breathe.

Summary

A biologic response is induced within a living organism when a drug is administered to that organism. This chapter reviews the study of the absorption, distribution, metabolism, and excretion of drugs. It also reviews the study of the biochemical and physiological effects of drugs. The mechanisms of drug action depend on several factors that affect pharmaceutical, pharmcokinetic, and pharmacodynamic phases. Drug interaction is another major consideration. Multiple-drug therapy should never be employed without a convincing indication that each drug is beneficial and less harmful. In addition, drugs may induce side effects or adverse reactions. An adverse drug effect is more serious and its effect is unintended, undesirable, and often unpredictable.

Exploring the Web

Visit ***www.aafp.org***

- Search using the term drug interactions. What common foods may interfere with the actions of some drugs? What drugs when taken together may cause adverse effects?
- Search using the term adverse drug reactions. What information can you find related to identifying and reducing these reactions?

Visit ***www.fda.gov***

- Search using the following terms: drug absorption, drug distribution, drug metabolism, drug excretion. What additional information can you find to help reinforce your understanding of these concepts?

Visit ***www.medscape.com***

- Click on the link "pharmacists." Review the resources available on this page.

Visit ***www.nlm.nih.gov/medlineplus***

- Become familiar with the resources and information available at this site.

Review Questions

Multiple Choice

1. For action to occur, a drug must be ______________, transported to tissues or organs, and penetrate cell membranes.
   - **A.** filtered
   - **B.** secreted
   - **C.** absorbed
   - **D.** therapeutic

2. The study of the action of drugs within the body is known as:
   A. metabolism
   B. pharmacokinetics
   C. pharmacology
   D. pharmacodynamics

3. The most common and important mode of traversal of drugs through membranes is:
   A. filtration
   B. transportation
   C. diffusion
   D. transaction

4. Idiosyncratic reactions may be caused by which of the following factors?
   A. genetics
   B. obesity
   C. gender
   D. age

5. The process by which drug molecules leave the bloodstream and enter the tissues of the body is called:
   A. solubility
   B. distribution
   C. suitability
   D. concentration

6. The process of converting drugs to metabolic derivatives during metabolism is known as:
   A. ionization
   B. binding
   C. excretion
   D. biotransformation

7. The major site of excretion for most drugs is the:
   A. spleen
   B. sweat glands
   C. gall bladder
   D. kidney(s)

8. A second process that moves very small amounts of substances such as potassium and hydrogen from the blood into the renal tubules is known as:
   A. tubular secretion
   B. pH alteration
   C. increased elimination
   D. blocking effect

9. Which of the following is the study of the biochemical and physiological effects of drugs?

   A. pathophysiology
   B. pharmacology
   C. pharmacodynamics
   D. pharmacokinetics

10. A drug that has a specific affinity for a particular cell receptor is known as the:

    A. antagonist
    B. agonist
    C. blocker
    D. biochemical event

11. Which of the following pharmacokinetic phases may cause a major problem in patients with liver impairment?

    A. excretion
    A. distribution
    C. absorption
    D. metabolism

12. All of the following factors may influence the effectiveness of drug therapy, except:

    A. time of administration
    B. route of administration
    C. food-drug interaction
    D. temperature

13. Sedatives given in the morning will not be as effective as when they are administered before bedtime. This is due to the effect of:

    A. diurnal (during the day) body rhythms
    B. nocturnal (during the night) body rhythms
    C. corticosteroids
    D. placebos

14. The phenomenon of reduced responsiveness to a drug is known as:

    A. adaptation
    B. toxicity
    C. tolerance
    D. therapeutic index

15. When a patient has experienced a unique, strange, or unpredicted reaction to a drug, this reaction is called:

    A. hormonal
    B. idiosyncratic
    C. hypersensitive
    D. biologic

Fill in the Blank

1. A mechanism whereby drugs are absorbed across the intestinal wall and enter into blood vessels known as the hepatic portal circulation is called ______________.
2. The effectiveness of a drug in producing a more intense response as its concentration is increased is known as ______________.
3. The study of how the body responds to drugs and natural substances is called ______________.
4. The rate of filtration is referred to as the ______________.
5. Lipid-soluble drugs enter the central nervous system ______________.
6. ______________ and elderly individuals show the greatest effects of a drug.
7. Sugar pills or sterile water are thought to be a drug referred to as a ______________.

Critical Thinking

A 75-year-old man was diagnosed with a urinary tract infection and a high fever. After the results of a urine culture, his physician ordered IV gentamicin 2 mg/kg loading dose, followed by 3–5 mg/kg/day in divided doses. Consider the nephrotoxicity of this agent to elderly patients, and answer the following questions.

1. What formula should be used to calculate drug toxicity?
2. Since the patient is 75 years old, what precautions must the physician take in calculating the correct dosage?
3. Besides nephrotoxicity, name the other potential adverse effects of this drug for elderly patients.

SECTION II

PHARMACOLOGY RELATED TO SPECIFIC BODY SYSTEMS AND DISORDERS

CHAPTER 4

Drug Therapy for the Nervous System: Antipsychotic and Antidepressant Drugs

OBJECTIVES

After completing this chapter, the reader should be able to:

1. List the main parts of the brain.
2. Describe the principal functions of the cerebrum and hypothalamus.
3. List the major chemical transmitters of the CNS.
4. Describe the major role of acetylcholine in the CNS.
5. Explain the role of dopamine in the brain.
6. Define schizophrenia, bipolar disorder, and depression.
7. List major groups of drugs that are used for schizophrenia.
8. Identify the drugs used for bipolar disorder.
9. List three major groups of drugs used to treat depression.
10. Describe the major adverse effects of MAOIs.

GLOSSARY

Acetylcholine – a neurotransmitter that plays a major role in cognitive function and memory formation as well as motor control

Anorexia nervosa – an eating disorder characterized by a psychological fear of being overweight; view of body image is distorted

Antidepressants – drugs used to treat depression

Antipsychotic drugs – the major therapeutic modality for psychotic disorders; also known as neuroleptic drugs

Bipolar disorder – a type of mental illness characterized by periods of extreme excitation, or mania, and deep depression.

Bulimia nervosa – an eating disorder characterized by recurrent (at least

OUTLINE

(*continues*)

OUTLINE (*continued*)

twice a week) episodes of binge eating, during which the patient consumes large amounts of food and feels unable to stop eating

Dementia – a chronic deterioration of intellectual function and other cognitive skills severe enough to interfere with the ability to perform activities of daily living

Depression – a mood disorder

Dopamine – a neurotransmitter that is naturally produced in the brain, affecting motor control, memory, attention span, the ability to problem solve, motivation, pleasure, and creative thought

Extrapyramidal – nerves in the brain that control movement

Gamma-aminobutyric acid (GABA) – a neurotransmitter distributed throughout the brain and spinal cord; now considered to be the major inhibitory neurotransmitter in the CNS, acting to modulate the activity of excitatory pathways

Glutamate – an amino acid that acts as a neurotransmitter and is a key molecule in cellular metabolism, playing an important role in the body's disposal of excess or waste nitrogen

Hallucinations – false or distorted sensory experiences that appear to be real perceptions

Mania – a severe medical condition characterized by extremely elevated mood, energy, and unusual thought patterns; a characteristic of bipolar disorder

Monoamine oxidase inhibitor (MAOI) – a class of drug effective for the treatment of depression

Neuroleptic drugs – the major therapeutic modality for psychotic disorders; also known as antipsychotic drugs

Neurotransmitter – a biochemical that is formed in and released from a neuron in order to stimulate or inhibit the actions of another cell

Nocturnal enuresis – nighttime bedwetting

Norepinephrine – a neurotransmitter that regulates appetite, sleep, arousal, mood, temperature, and hormone release

Schizophrenia – a mental illness characterized by distortion of reality, disorganized thought patterns, social withdrawal, hallucinations, and poor judgment

Selective serotonin reuptake inhibitor (SSRI) – a class of drugs used as antidepressants; they block resorption of serotonin in nerve cells in the brain

Serotonin – a neurotransmitter that regulates appetite, sleep, arousal, mood, temperature, and hormone release

Serotonin syndrome – a rare condition resulting from intentional self-poisoning with serotonin, use of the drug therapeutically, or from inadvertent drug interactions characterized by progressively worsening symptoms such as: mental confusion, shivering or muscle twitching, sweating or fever, hallucinations, hypertension, tachycardia, headache, tremor, nausea, diarrhea, coma, and death; also known as serotonin toxicity

Serotonin toxicity – a rare condition resulting from intentional self-poisoning with serotonin, use of the drug therapeutically, or from inadvertent drug interactions characterized by progressively worsening symptoms such as: mental confusion, shivering or muscle twitching, sweating or fever, hallucinations, hypertension, tachycardia, headache, tremor, nausea, diarrhea, coma, and death; also known as serotonin syndrome

Tricyclic antidepressant (TCA) – a class of antidepressants; they inhibit reabsorption of serotonin, norepinephrine, and dopamine in the brain

Overview

The human brain is an extremely complex organ. It is responsible for all affective (emotional) and cognitive (thinking) processes, and is as capable of coordinating bodily functions (eating, sleeping, walking, talking) as it is of pursuing abstract thought. Sometimes imbalances in mental functioning occur that can result in one of a number of brain disturbances, producing disorders such as schizophrenia, depression, anxiety, or parkinsonism. The onset of such conditions can make normal functioning within society difficult, if not impossible. The use of psychopharmacology in the treatment of these conditions may be a necessary part of the reintegration of affected individuals in the community.

Mental health problems involve significant dysfunction in the areas of behavior or personality that interfere with a person's ability to function. Biochemical and structural abnormalities in the brain appear to contribute to the pathologies. Many disorders have a genetic component. Stressors may play a role in the development of mental illness. Psychotic illnesses include the more serious disorders such as schizophrenia, delusional disorders, and some affective or mood disorders. Many patients with psychotic disorders receive large doses of drugs with significant adverse effects. Other common mental disorders include anxiety, insomnia, and panic disorders, which are less severe but nevertheless disruptive.

Anatomy Review

The nervous system is composed of the brain, spinal cord, and nerves (Figures 4-1 and 4-2).

- The nervous system has two divisions: the central nervous system (CNS) and the peripheral nervous system (PNS).
- The brain and spinal cord make up the CNS. The nerves make up the peripheral nervous system.
- The brain is divided into specific regions; each region is responsible for the performance of specific functions within the body (Figures 4-3A and 4-3B).
- The brain consists of four parts: the cerebrum, diencephalon (thalamus and hypothalamus), cerebellum, and brain stem.
- The main functions of the cerebrum include the controlling of consciousness, memory, emotions, sensations, and voluntary movements.

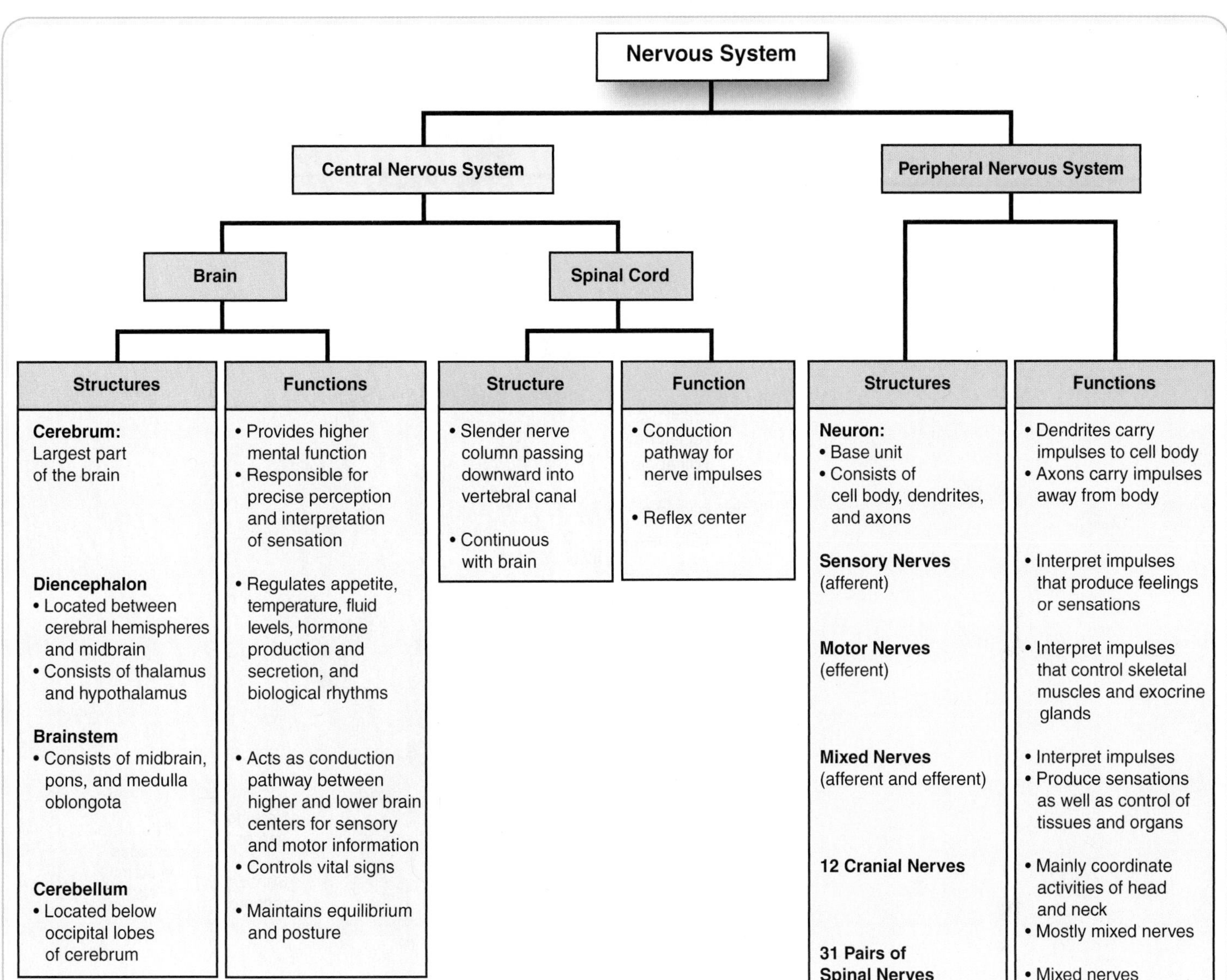

Figure 4-1 Overview of the structure and function of the nervous system.

- The thalamus receives sensory stimuli (except the sense of smell), relaying them to the cerebral cortex.
- The hypothalamus (located just below the thalamus) activates, controls, and integrates the peripheral autonomic nervous system. It also controls endocrine system processes, body temperature, appetite, sleep, and other sensory functions.
- The cerebellum, attached to the brain stem, maintains muscle tone, and coordinates balance and movement.
- The brain stem controls blood pressure, respiration, pulse, and other body functions; it connects the hypothalamus with the spinal cord.

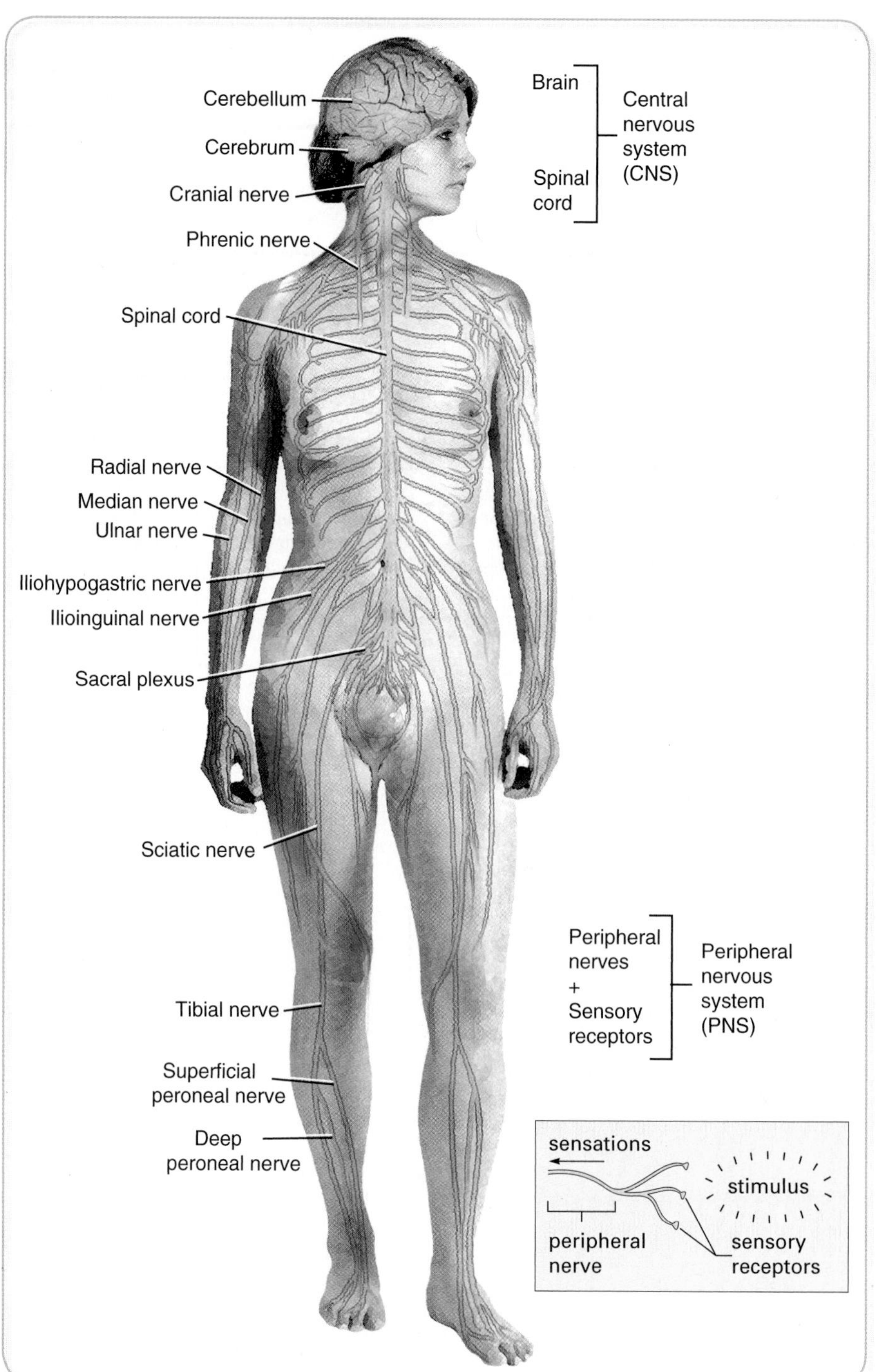

Figure 4-2 The nervous system.

- The basic functional unit of the nervous system is the neuron (Figure 4-4).
- There are three types of nerves: sensory nerves transmit information that produces sensation and feelings, motor nerves transmit

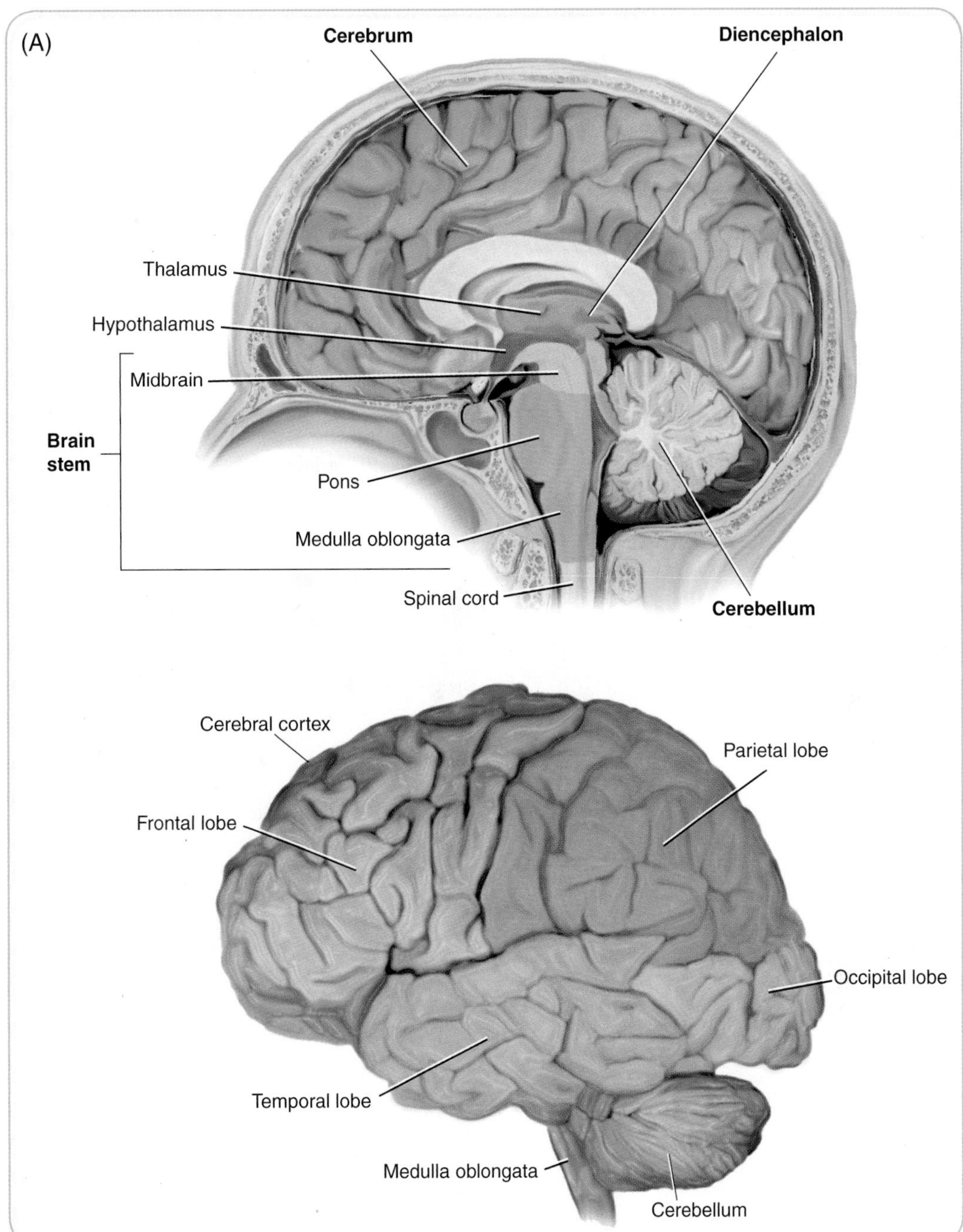

Figure 4-3A Divisions of the brain and related functions.

information that produces movement and function, mixed nerves transmit information that produces both sensation and movement.

- The spinal cord provides a two-way communication system between the brain and body parts outside of the nervous system (Figure 4-5).

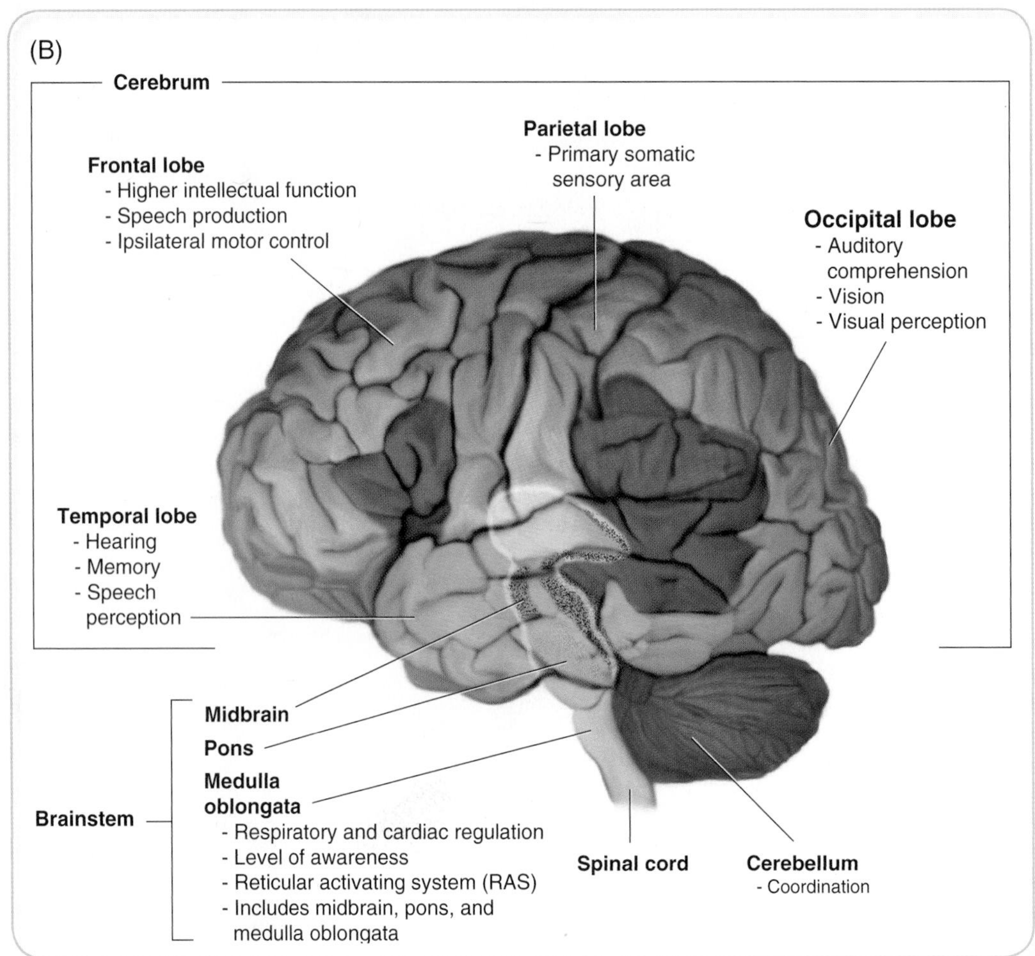

Figure 4-3B Divisions of the brain and related functions.

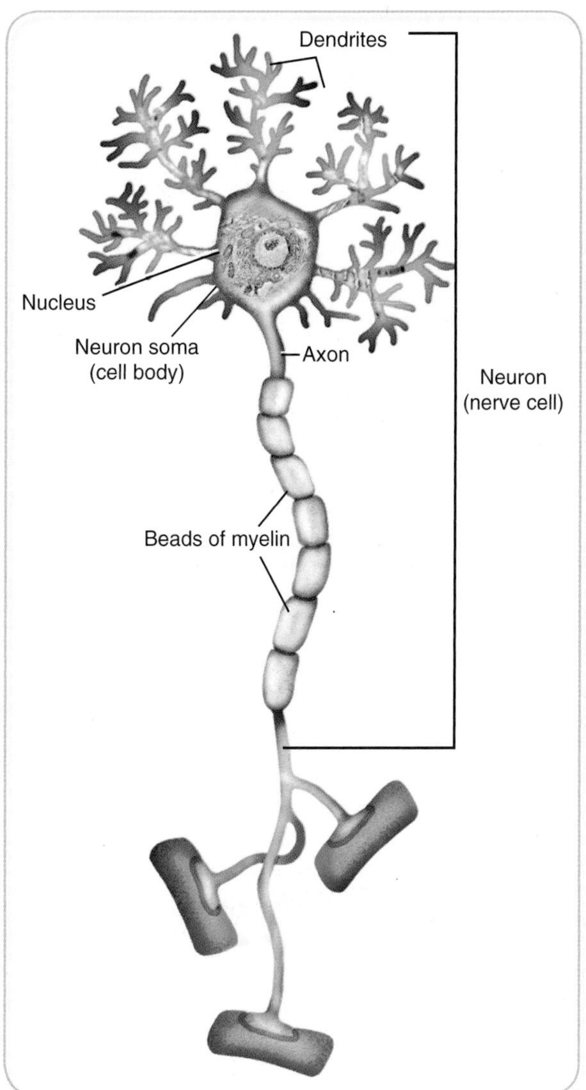

Figure 4-4 The neuron.

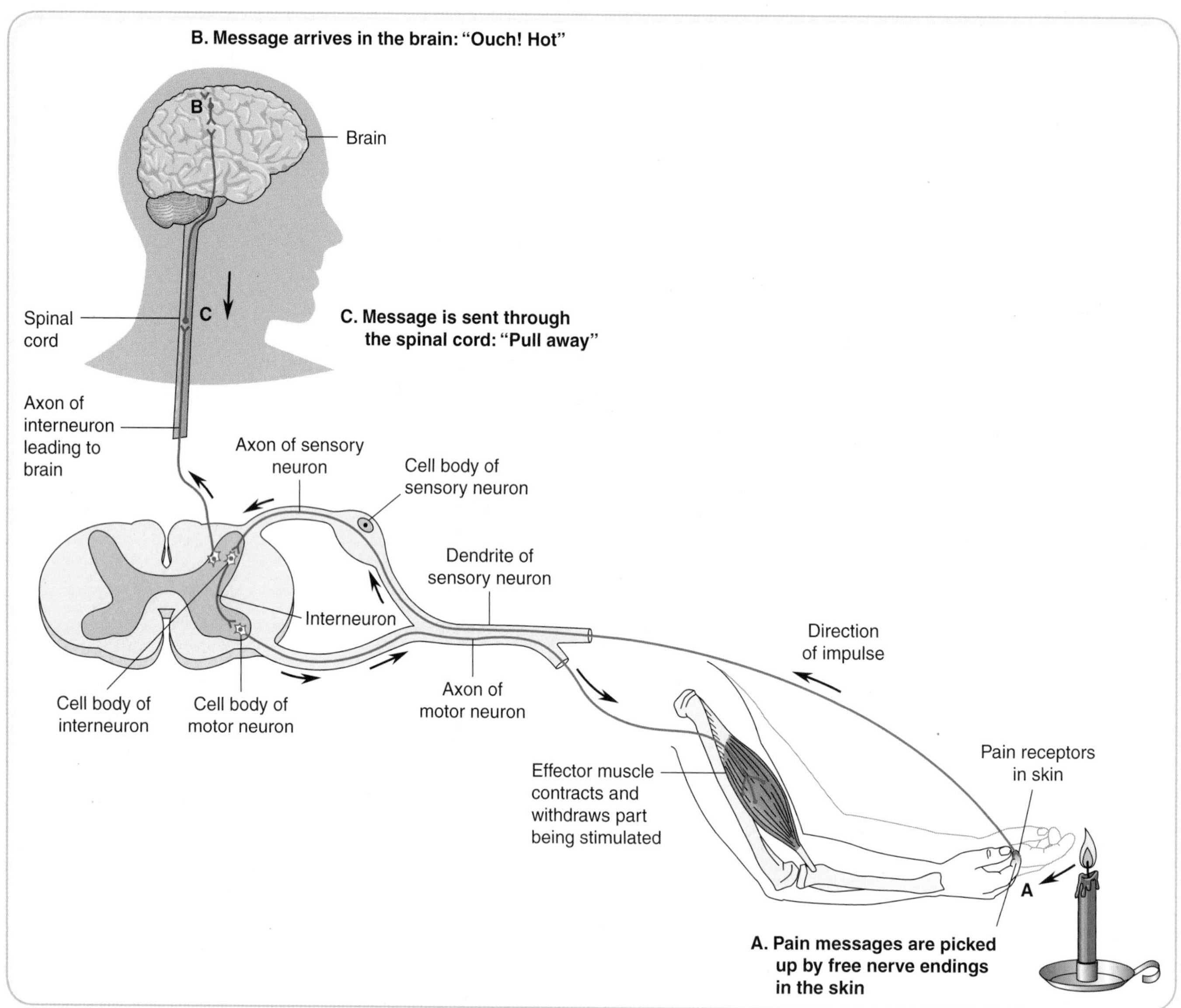

Figure 4-5 The two-way communication system of the brain and nerve function.

Neurotransmitters

The term **neurotransmitter** is defined as a biochemical that is formed in and released from a neuron in order to stimulate or inhibit the actions of another cell. Examples of neurotransmitters include acetylcholine, dopamine, noradrenaline, serotonin, glutamate, and GABA. Disorders in the production and function of neurotransmitters may contribute to psychiatric illnesses.

Acetylcholine

Acetylcholine plays a major role in cognitive function and memory formation as well as motor control. It was the first neurotransmitter to be identified. Acetylcholine allows neurons to communicate with each other. This neurotransmitter is released by the axon terminals in response to a nerve impulse. In relation to motor function, the release of acetylcholine will cause a change in the muscle cell and elicit a contraction of the muscle, producing movement.

Dopamine

Dopamine is a naturally produced agent that, in the brain, functions as a neurotransmitter. Dopamine release and dopamine levels within the brain affect motor control, memory, attention span, the ability to problem solve, motivation, pleasure, and creative thought. Alterations in dopamine production and secretion play a role in disorders such as Parkinson's disease (see Chapter 7), attention deficit disorder, and schizophrenia. It is also believed to play a role in addiction to drugs.

Norepinephrine and Serotonin

Both **norepinephrine** and **serotonin** seem to be involved in similar functions within the brain: regulation of appetite, sleep, arousal, mood, temperature, and hormone release.

Norepinephrine is also known as noradrenaline. As a stress hormone, it affects parts of the human brain where attention and responding actions are controlled. It is released from the medulla of the adrenal glands as a hormone into the blood, but is also a central and sympathetic nervous system neurotransmitter.

Serotonin is a neurotransmitter synthesized in the CNS as well as the gastrointestinal tract. It is believed to play an important role in regulating anger, aggression, body temperature, mood, sleep, vomiting, sexuality, and appetite. It was initially identified as a vasoconstrictor present in blood serum, and it was from here that its name was derived. Serotonin (also known as 5-hydroxytryptamine or 5-HT) may also have a role in pain perception and behavior. It acts as an inhibitory neurotransmitter.

A rare condition known as **serotonin syndrome**, also known as **serotonin toxicity**, can result from intentional self-poisoning with serotonin, use of the drug therapeutically, or from inadvertent drug interactions. This condition includes progressively worsening symptoms such as: mental confusion, shivering or muscle twitching, sweating or fever, hallucinations, hypertension, tachycardia, headache, tremor, nausea, diarrhea, coma, and death.

Glutamate

Glutamate is an amino acid, however, not one of the essential amino acids. It is a key molecule in cellular metabolism. Glutamate plays an important role in the body's disposal of excess or waste nitrogen. It is important for the ability to perceive taste sensations.

> ***Medical Terminology Review***
>
> **glutamate**
> *glutam = glutamic acid*
> *ate = salt or ester*
> a salt containing glutamic acid

Glutamate is distributed throughout the CNS. It is considered the major excitatory CNS neurotransmitter. It can stimulate a number of receptor types in the brain and spinal cord. Glutamate is involved in the facilitation of learning and memory. The brain is very vulnerable to glutamate-mediated over-excitation. This results in excitotoxicity, which causes cell integrity to be disrupted and nerve cells to die. Excitotoxicity has been demonstrated in strokes and some neuro-degenerative diseases. Glutamate has also been implicated in the development of epilepsy (see Chapter 9).

Gamma-Aminobutyric Acid

Gamma-aminobutyric acid (GABA) is distributed throughout the brain and spinal cord. It is now considered to be the major inhibitory neurotransmitter in the CNS and it acts to modulate the activity of excitatory pathways. It is formed from the excitatory neurotransmitter glutamate. Motor control, consciousness, levels of arousal, and memory formation are all inhibited by GABA.

GABA has mostly excitatory effects during early development. It has been purported to increase the amounts of human growth hormone. It is unknown if GABA can cross the blood-brain barrier.

MENTAL DISORDERS

Mental illness is defined as any disturbance of emotional equilibrium, as manifested in maladaptive behavior and impaired functioning of behavior or personality. Biochemical and structural abnormalities in the brain appear to contribute to these disorders. Some of these disorders have a genetic component. Stressors may play a role in the development of these types of illnesses. Psychotic illnesses include the more serious disorders such as schizophrenia, bipolar disorder, and depression. Other common mental disorders including dementia and eating disorders (discussed here) as well as anxiety and sleep disorders (discussed in Chapter 5), are less severe but nevertheless disruptive.

Schizophrenia

Schizophrenia is a mental illness characterized by distortion of reality, disorganized thought patterns, social withdrawal, **hallucinations**, and poor judgment. Schizophrenia is one of the most devastating forms of mental illnesses. It occurs in approximately 1 percent of the population.

Schizophrenia includes a variety of syndromes, presented differently in each individual. Although the cause of this disorder has not been fully determined, some common changes do occur in the brains of patients suffering from schizophrenia, including reduction of the cortex (outer portion) of the temporal lobes, enlargement of the third and lateral ventricles, excessive dopamine secretion, and decrease blood flow to the front of the brain.

The cause of schizophrenia may be genetic, along with brain damage in the fetus caused by perinatal complications or viral infections in the mother during pregnancy. The onset of schizophrenia usually occurs between ages 15 and 25 in men, and between 25 and 35 in women. Stressful events appear to initiate the onset and recurrence of the disorder.

Medical Terminology Review

schizophrenia
schizo = split
phrenia = mind condition
condition in which the mind is divided

perinatal
peri = around
nat = birth
-al = pertaining to
around the time of birth

Bipolar Disorder

Bipolar disorder is a mental illness characterized by periods of extreme excitation or **mania**, and deep depression. It is not commonly understood why it takes months to move from one of these extremes to the other. Some patients have predominantly manic episodes or predominantly depressive episodes. Few patients experience the classic swing from mania to depression and back. Bipolar disorder is also called manic-depressive illness.

Depression

Depression is classified as a mood disorder, of which there are several subgroups. Major depression, or unipolar disorder, is a chemical deficit within the brain, and a precise diagnosis is based on biologic factors or personal characteristics. The causes of depression include genetic and psychosocial stressors. Depression may also occur as a reactive episode, a response to a life event, or secondarily to many systemic disorders (including cancer, diabetes, heart failure, and AIDS). This condition is a common problem, and many patients with milder forms may be misdiagnosed and not receive treatment.

Eating Disorders

Anorexia nervosa is a complex psychological state characterized by the fear of being overweight. Often, patients' perceptions are distorted to the extent that they believe they are overweight despite appearing emaciated to others. Without proper treatment, anorexia nervosa may be fatal.

Bulimia nervosa is another eating disorder that is characterized by recurrent (at least twice a week) episodes of binge eating, during which the patient consumes large amounts of food and feels unable to stop eating. This is followed by inappropriate compensatory effects to avoid weight gain, such as self-induced vomiting, laxative or diuretic abuse, vigorous exercise, or fasting.

Dementia

Dementia is a chronic deterioration of intellectual function and other cognitive skills severe enough to interfere with the ability to perform activities of daily living. Dementia may occur at any age and can affect young people as the result of injury or hypoxia. However, it is mostly a disease of the elderly.

Antipsychotic Drugs

Antipsychotic drugs, also called **neuroleptic drugs**, are a major therapeutic modality for psychotic disorders, often in conjunction with psychotherapy and psychosocial rehabilitation. The antipsychotic drugs (conventional and atypical agents) are listed in Table 4-1.

TABLE 4-1 Antipsychotic Drugs

Generic Name	Trade Name	Route of Administration	Average Adult Dosage
Conventional Agents			
chlorpromazine hydrochloride	Thorazine®	PO, IM, IV, PR (suppository)	50–400 mg/day
fluphenazine	Prolixin®	PO, IM	1–30 mg/day
haloperidol	Haldol®	PO, IM	1–50 mg/day
loxapine succinate	Loxitane®	PO	10–160 mg/day
molindone	Moban®	PO	15–225 mg/day
perphenazine	Trilafon®, Etrafon®	PO	12–24 mg/day
pimozide	Orap®	PO	1–10 mg/day
prochlorperazine	Compazine®	PO, IM, PR	2.5–25 mg/day
thioridazine hydrochloride	Mellaril®	PO	50–800 mg/day
thiothixene hydrochloride	Navane®	PO	6–60 mg/day
trifluoperazine	Stelazine	PO, IM	4–60 mg/day
Atypical Agents			
aripiprazole	Abilify®	PO	10–15 mg/day
clozapine	Clozaril®, Fazaclo®	PO	300–900 mg/day
olanzapine	Zyprexa®	PO, IM	5–20 mg/day
quetiapine fumarate	Seroquel®	PO	50–400 mg/day
risperidone	Risperdal®	PO, IM	2–6 mg/day
ziprasidone hydrochloride	Geodon®	PO, IM	40–120 mg/day

Mechanism of Action

Antipsychotic drugs act by blocking receptors for dopamine, acetylcholine, histamine, and norepinephrine. The current suggestions are that conventional antipsychotic drugs suppress symptoms of psychosis by blocking dopamine receptors in the brain.

Medical Terminology Review

antipsychotic
anti = against
psych/o = mind
tic = pertaining to
against the mind

neuroleptic
neuro = nerve
lep = seizure, attack
tic = pertaining to
attack of the nerves

Key Concept

Antipsychotic drugs do not alter the underlying pathology of schizophrenia. Therefore, treatment is not curative.

Indications

Schizophrenia is the primary indication for antipsychotic drugs. These agents effectively suppress symptoms during acute psychotic episodes and, when taken chronically, can greatly decrease the risk of relapse. Selection among these drugs is based primarily on their adverse effect profiles, rather than on therapeutic effects.

In addition to their antipsychotic properties, some of these drugs, such as prochlorperazine, are also used as antiemetics. Chlorpromazine is used for treating hiccups and lithium for managing bipolar disorders. Small doses of neuroleptics can be effective to control acute agitation in the elderly.

Adverse Effects

Antipsychotic drugs frequently cause a wide variety of adverse effects, which include dry mouth, blurred vision, urinary retention, orthostatic hypotension, tachycardia, sedation, headache, and behavior changes. These drugs may also produce agitation, confusion, lethargy, and paranoid reactions. Antipsychotic agents commonly cause adverse effects related to excessive **extrapyramidal** (nerves in the brain controlling movement) activity (or parkinsonian signs). Involuntary muscle spasms in the face, neck, arms, or legs (dystonia) may be present. Tardive dyskinesia may be present, such as chewing or grimacing, repetitive jerky or writhing movements of the limbs, tremors, or a shuffling gait. Extrapyramidal effects usually diminish with a decreased dosage of the antipsychotic medication.

Contraindications and Precautions

Antipsychotic drugs are contraindicated in patients with a known hypersensitivity, severe depression, blood dyscrasias, liver dysfunction, severe hypotension or hypertension, and Parkinson's disease.

Safe use of antipsychotic drugs during pregnancy and lactation has not been established. These agents in pregnancy are category C (except for clozapine, which is category B).

Antipsychotic agents should be used with caution in patients with glaucoma, asthma, epilepsy, prostatic hypertrophy, peptic ulcer, renal dysfunction, and in those who have been exposed to extreme heat.

Drug Interactions

Antipsychotic medications may have drug interactions with antihistamines, alcohol, tranquilizers, narcotics, and barbiturates. They may result in additive CNS depression.

Mood Altering Drugs

Bipolar disorder was formerly known as manic-depressive illness. According to the National Institutes of Health, more than 5.7 million Americans are suffering from this disease. Bipolar disorder is a chronic condition that requires treatment for life.

Bipolar disorder is treated with three major groups of drugs: mood stabilizers, antipsychotics, and antidepressants. The mainstays of therapy are lithium and valproic acid, drugs with the ability to stabilize mood. In addition, benzodiazepines are commonly used for sedation. Antipsychotic drugs were discussed before, and antidepressants will be discussed later in this chapter. The following is a discussion of mood stabilizers.

The principal mood stabilizers are lithium and two drugs originally developed for epilepsy: valproic acid and carbamazepine (see Chapter 8). Lithium has a low therapeutic index. As a result, toxicity can occur at blood levels only slightly greater than therapeutic levels. Accordingly, monitoring of lithium levels is mandatory.

Mechanism of Action

Key Concept

Lithium is not a true antipsychotic drug, but it is used in regulating the severe fluctuations of the manic phase of bipolar disorder.

The precise mechanism of action of lithium is unknown. The lithium ion behaves in the body much like the sodium ion, but its exact mechanism of action is unclear. Lithium competes with various physiologically important cations: Na^+, K^+, Ca^{++}, and Mg^{++}. At the synapse, it accelerates catecholamine destruction, inhibits the release of neurotransmitters, and decreases sensitivity of postsynaptic receptors.

Indications

Lithium is a drug of choice for controlling acute manic episodes in patients with bipolar disorder, and for long-term prophylaxis against recurrence of mania or depression. In manic patients, lithium reduces euphoria, hyperactivity, and other symptoms, but does not cause sedation. Anti-manic effects begin five to seven days after the onset of treatment, but full benefits may not develop for two to three weeks.

Adverse Effects

Adverse effects of lithium, such as nausea, diarrhea, abdominal bloating, and anorexia are common but transient. The other adverse effects include fatigue, muscle weakness, headache, confusion, memory impairment, polyuria, and thirst. Lithium-induced tremors can be augmented by stress and fatigue.

Contraindications and Precautions

Lithium is contraindicated in patients with known hypersensitivity, in those with significant cardiovascular or kidney disease, brain damage, dehydration, or sodium debilitation. Lithium is also contraindicated in pregnancy, especially during the first trimester (category D), lactation, and in children younger than 12 years of age.

Lithium should be used with caution in older adults and in patients suffering from thyroid disease, epilepsy, cardiac disease, dehydration, diarrhea, renal impairment, and seizure disorders.

Drug Interactions

Diuretics promote sodium loss and can thereby increase the risk of lithium toxicity. Nonsteroidal anti-inflammatory drugs can increase lithium levels and increase renal reabsorption of lithium. Anticholinergics can cause urinary hesitancy coupled with lithium-induced polyuria.

ANTIDEPRESSANTS

Medical Terminology Review

unipolar
uni = one
polar = pole; mood
one mood

Key Concept

Antidepressant effects may not be observed for up to four weeks after treatment begins.

As previously mentioned in this chapter, depression is classified as a mood disorder with several subgroups. Severe depression, or unipolar disorder, is endogenous (originating from within), and a precise diagnosis is based on biologic factors or personal characteristics. Etiologic factors include genetic, developmental, and psychosocial stressors. Bipolar disorder involves alternating periods of depression and mania. Depression may also occur as an exogenous or reactive episode, a response to a life event, or secondarily to many systemic disorders, including cancer, diabetes, heart failure, and systemic lupus erythematosus.

The scene is now set to discuss the action of **antidepressant** drugs in the context of nerve physiology within the brain. Four major drug classifications are used to treat depression, which include: tricyclic antidepressants, selective serotonin reuptake inhibitors (SSRIs), monoamine oxidase inhibitors (MAOIs), and atypical antidepressant drugs (see Table 4-2).

TABLE 4-2 Drugs Used to Treat Depression

Generic Name	Trade Name	Route of Administration	Average Adult Dose
Tricyclic Antidepressants (TCAs)			
amitriptyline hydrochloride	Elavil®, Enovil®	PO	75–100 mg/day (max: 150–300 mg/day)
amoxapine	Asendin®	PO	200–400 mg/day
desipramine hydrochloride	Norpramin®	PO	75–100 mg/day (max: 300 mg/day)
doxepin hydrochloride	Sinequan®	PO	30–150 mg/day h.s. (max: 300 mg/day)
imipramine hydrochloride	Tofranil®	PO	75–100 mg/day (max: 300 mg/day)
maprotiline	Ludiomil®	PO	25–150 mg/day
nortriptyline hydrochloride	Aventyl®	PO	25 mg t.i.d.-q.i.d. (max: 150 mg /day)
protriptyline	Vivactil®	PO	15–40 mg/day in 3-4 div. doses (max: 60 mg/day)
trimipramine	Surmontil®	PO	75–100 mg/day (max: 300 mg/day)
Selective Serotonin Reuptake Inhibitors (SSRIs)			
citalopram hydrobromide	Celexa®	PO	Start at 20 mg/day (max: 40 mg/day)
escitalopram oxalate	Lexapro®	PO	10 mg/day (max: 20 mg/ day after 1 wk)

(continues)

TABLE 4-2 Drugs Used to Treat Depression—*continued*

Generic Name	Trade Name	Route of Administration	Average Adult Dose
fluoxetine hydrochloride	Prozac®	PO	20 mg/day in a.m. (max: 80 mg/day)
fluvoxamine	Luvox®	PO	Start at 50 mg/day (max: 300 mg/day)
paroxetine	Paxil®	PO	10–50 mg/day (max: 60 mg/day)
sertraline hydrochloride	Zoloft®	PO	Start at 50 mg /day (max: 200 mg/day)
Monoamine Oxidase Inhibitors (MAOIs)			
isocarboxazid	Marplan®	PO	10–30 mg/day (max: 30 mg/day)
phenelzine	Nardil®	PO	15 mg t.i.d. (max: 90 mg/day)
tranylcypromine	Parnate®	PO	30 mg/day (20 mg in a.m. and 10 mg in p.m.) (max: 60 mg/day)
Atypical Antidepressants			
bupropion hydrochloride	Wellbutrin®	PO	75–100 mg t.i.d. (max: 450 mg/day)
mirtazapine	Remeron®	PO	15 mg/day h.s. (max: 45 mg/day)
nefazodone hydrochloride	Serzone®	PO	50–100 mg b.i.d. (max: 600 mg/day)
trazodone hydrochloride	Desyrel®, Trialodine®	PO	150 mg/day (max: 600 mg/day)
venlafaxine	Effexor®	PO	25–125 mg t.i.d.

Tricyclic Antidepressants

Historically, **tricyclic antidepressants** (TCAs) were the first choice in the treatment of depression, until SSRI's entered the market. The term tricyclic derives from the common three-ringed structure of the drug molecule itself.

Mechanism of Action

Tricyclic antidepressants inhibit the reuptake of serotonin and noradrenaline into nerve terminals (Figure 4-6).

> ***Medical Terminology Review***
>
> **tricyclic**
> *tri = three*
> *cyclic = related to cycles, circles, rings*
> three cycles

Indications

Tricyclic antidepressants are mainly used for major depression, and imipramine may be used for the treatment of **nocturnal enuresis** (nighttime bedwetting) in children.

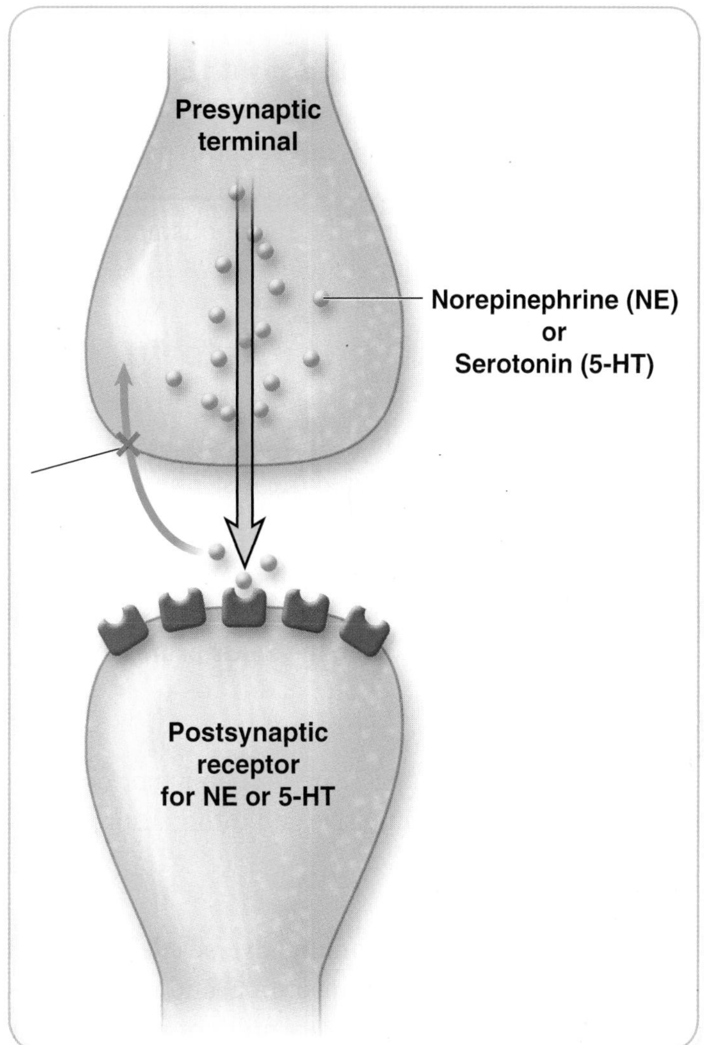

Figure 4-6 Mechanism of action for tricyclic antidepressants.

Adverse Effects

Common adverse effects of tricyclic antidepressants include dry mouth, blurred vision, postural hypotension, constipation, and urinary retention. Other adverse effects may be sedation, drowsiness, cardiovascular symptoms (such as dysrhythmias), and extreme hypertension.

Contraindications and Precautions

The TCAs are contraindicated in patients with known hypersensitivity to these drugs. They are also contraindicated in patients with glaucoma, hypertrophy of prostate gland, and during pregnancy or lactation.

Like other antidepressants, the tricyclics should be used with caution in patients who have heart disease (angina or paroxysmal tachycardia), hepatic or renal dysfunction, or a history of seizures.

Drug Interactions

The TCAs, with concurrent use of other CNS depressants, including alcohol, may cause sedation. If taking clonidine, patients may experience a decrease in the antihypertensive effects of the drug and are at an increased risk for CNS depression. Cimetidine (a histamine blocking agent) may prevent the metabolism of imipramine, leading to increased serum levels and toxicity.

Selective Serotonin-Reuptake Inhibitors

Selective serotonin-reuptake inhibitors (SSRIs) are antidepressants that have had a tremendous impact on prescribing patterns. They are now considered the first-line drugs in the treatment of major depression.

Mechanism of Action

SSRIs block the presynaptic amine reuptake pump, as do the TCAs. However, the SSRIs primarily affect serotonin reuptake (see Figure 4-7).

Indications

SSRIs are used in major depression and may be prescribed for obsessive-compulsive and eating disorders.

Adverse Effects

Common adverse effects of SSRIs include headache, vomiting, diarrhea, nausea, insomnia, and nervousness. Generally, the adverse effects of SSRIs are relatively mild, of shorter duration, and cease as treatment continues. Cardiac toxicity and the risk of death after overdose are less likely than with the TCAs.

Contraindications and Precautions

SSRIs are contraindicated in patients with known hypersensitivity to these agents and during pregnancy. SSRIs should be used with caution in patients with hepatic or renal dysfunction, diabetes mellitus, and during lactation.

Drug Interactions

Concurrent use of SSRIs with benzodiazepines may cause increased adverse CNS effects. Beta blockers may cause decreased elimination of SSRIs, resulting in hypotension or bradycardia. Clozapine, phenytoin, and theophylline may interact with SSRIs and decrease their elimination and their toxicity.

Monoamine Oxidase Inhibitors

Monoamine oxidase inhibitors (MAOIs) were the first drugs approved for the treatment of depression.

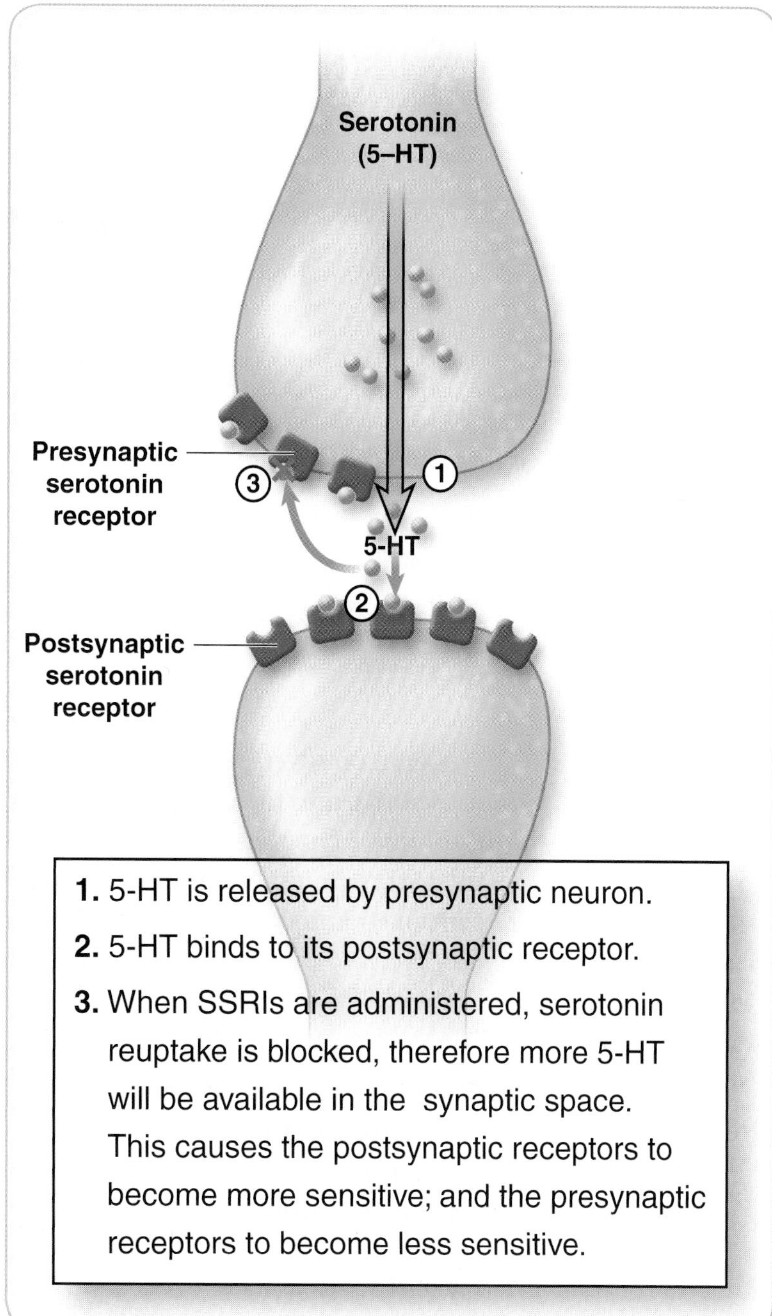

Figure 4-7 Mechanism of action for SSRIs.

Mechanism of Action

MAOIs inhibit monoamine oxidase (an enzyme) that stops the actions of dopamine, norepinephrine, epinephrine, and serotonin. Therefore, these drugs intensify the effects of norepinephrine in adrenergic synapses.

Indications

MAOIs are used to manage symptoms of depression not responsive to other types of pharmacotherapy. The effect of these drugs may continue for two to three weeks after therapy is discontinued.

TABLE 4-3 Foods that Contain Tyramine

Type of Food	Tyramine-Containing Foods
alcohol	beer, wines (especially red wines and Chianti)
dairy products	cheese (except for cottage cheese), sour cream, yogurt
fruits	avocados, bananas, canned figs, papaya products (including meat tenderizers), raisins
meats	beef or chicken liver, bologna/hot dogs, meat extracts, pate, pepperoni, pickled or kippered herring, salami, sausage
other	chocolate
sauces	soy sauce
vegetables	pods of broad beans (fava beans)
yeast	all yeast or yeast extracts

Adverse Effects

Common adverse effects of the MAOIs include dizziness, vertigo, dry mouth, nausea, diarrhea or constipation, loss of appetite, orthostatic hypotension, and insomnia. Hypertensive crisis (severe hypertension) may occur if ingesting foods containing tyramine while taking MAOIs. Table 4-3 lists foods that contain tyramine.

Contraindications and Precautions

MAOI agents are contraindicated in patients with known hypersensitivity to these drugs; in patients with hepatic or renal disease, hypertension, congestive heart failure, cerebrovascular disease, and in the elderly. MAOI drugs should be used with caution in patients with liver dysfunction, diabetes, hyperthyroidism, and history of seizures.

Drug Interactions

MAOIs may interact with other antidepressant drugs such as SSRIs and TCAs, resulting in elevation of body temperature and seizures. Meperidine should be avoided with MAOIs due to increased risk of respiratory failure or hypertensive crisis.

Atypical Antidepressants

Atypical antidepressants are also called miscellaneous agents. They are frequently prescribed to alleviate symptoms of depression for patients with bipolar disorder. Atypical antidepressants are chemically unrelated to other antidepressants. They include trazodone, mirtazapine, and bupropion.

Mechanism of Action

Atypical antidepressants inhibit the reabsorption of serotonin and norepinephrine. They elevate mood by increasing the levels of dopamine, serotonin, and norepinephrine in the central nervous system.

Indications

Atypical antidepressants are indicated for mental depression. Since bupropion has been associated with increased risk of seizures, it is not the agent of first choice. It is also used as an adjunct for smoking cessation. Venlafaxine is also used for generalized anxiety disorder and social anxiety disorder.

Adverse Effects

Common adverse effects of atypical antidepressants include dry mouth, blurred vision, dizziness, headache, nausea, vomiting, orthostatic hypotension, increased appetite, and insomnia.

Contraindications and Precautions

Atypical antidepressants are contraindicated in patients with known hypersensitivity to these agents. These drugs should be avoided in patients with hepatic diseases, pregnancy (category C), lactation, suicidal thoughts, and in children less than 8 years of age.

Atypical antidepressants must be used cautiously in patients with renal failure, hepatic impairment, history of mania, acute closed-angle glaucoma, cardiac disorders, hypertension, hyperthyroidism, and history of seizures or seizure disorders.

Drug Interactions

Atypical antidepressants may increase metabolism of carbamazepine, cimetidine, phenytoin, and phenobarbital. They may increase incidence of adverse effects of levodopa and MAOIs. They may cause additive cognitive and motor impairment with alcohol or benzodiazepines, and increase risk of hypertensive crisis with MAOIs. Antihypertensive agents may potentiate hypotensive effects of atypical antidepressants. Levels of digoxin or phenytoin may be increased if used concurrently. Levels and toxicity of ketoconazole, indinavir, and ritonavir may be increased with concurrent use.

Summary

The nervous system is composed of two divisions: the CNS (brain and spinal cord) and the peripheral nervous system (nerves). The major parts of the human brain are the cerebrum, diencephalon, brainstem, and cerebellum. The cerebrum is involved in motor and sensory function, and is the seat of intellect. The diencephalon comprises the thalamus, which acts as an information sorting area, and hypothalamus, which is an integration area for visceral functioning. The brainstem contains control centers for heart rate, respiratory rate, and blood pressure. The cerebellum controls muscle tone and posture, and facilitates smooth and coordinated muscle movements. Acetylcholine, dopamine, noradrenaline, serotonin, and GABA are key neurotransmitters in the brain.

Antipsychotics are used in the treatment of psychoses such as schizophrenia, dementia, and restlessness. All antipsychotics exert their effect on dopamine receptors and antagonize dopaminergic activity in the CNS. Antipsychotics have a diverse and potentially debilitating adverse effect profile.

Depression is a state of profound sadness. It can be reactive, in response to a life event, or endogenous, without an apparent trigger. Antidepressant drugs act by raising the levels of one or both of these neurotransmitters. This is achieved by blocking a subtype of postsynaptic serotonin receptors (selective serotonin receptor blockers) or MAOIs.

Exploring the Web

Visit ***www.fda.gov***

- Search using the term antipsychotics. Look for drug information sheets for patients. You can also search for information on specific drug names for additional information on specific drugs.

Visit ***www.mentalhealth.com***

- Click on the link "disorders." Choose one of the disorders discussed in the text and research what is known about the disorder and the treatments that are used to address it.

Visit ***www.nimh.nih.gov***

- Choose one of the disorders discussed in the text and research what is known about the disorder and the treatments that are used to address it.

Visit ***www.nlm.nih.gov/medlineplus***

- Choose one of the types of drugs discussed in the chapter and research the uses, mechanisms of action, adverse effects, contraindications and precautions, and drug interactions to further your understanding of the drug. Make index cards with the pertinent information to help you review and study.

Visit *www.rxlist.com*

- Bookmark this site to be used as a reference. It is one of several drug information sites available on the Web. What additional websites are available for drug information? Make sure the sites are reputable.

Review Questions

Multiple Choice

1. Which of the following parts of the brain is responsible for the precise perception and interpretation of sensation?
   A. cerebellum
   B. cerebrum
   C. diencephalon
   D. brainstem
2. Which of the following disorders is the *primary* indication for antipsychotic drugs?
   A. insomnia
   B. anxiety
   C. manic-depressive
   D. schizophrenia
3. Lithium is a *drug of choice* for controlling which of the following mental disorders?
   A. schizophrenia
   B. restlessness
   C. acute manic episodes
   D. brain injury
4. Which of the following antidepressants have relatively mild adverse effects, and are the *newest* of these drugs?
   A. monoamine oxidase inhibitors
   B. tricyclic antidepressants
   C. atypical antidepressants
   D. selective serotonin reuptake inhibitors
5. Which of the following neurotransmitters is distributed *throughout* the central nervous system?
   A. GABA
   B. dopamine
   C. acetylcholine
   D. serotonin

6. Which of the following is the largest part of the brain?
   A. hypothalamus
   B. cerebellum
   C. brainstem
   D. cerebrum

7. Which of the following neurotransmitters is involved in hormone release, motor control, behavior, and emesis?
   A. serotonin
   B. dopamine
   C. acetylcholine
   D. GABA

8. Which of the following neurotransmitters' functions within the brain is *similar* to noradrenaline?
   A. dopamine
   B. GABA
   C. serotonin
   D. acetylcholine

9. Bipolar disorder involves alternating periods of which of the following?
   A. depression and insomnia
   B. depression and mania
   C. depression and anxiety attacks
   D. insomnia and anxiety

10. Which of the following is the *cure* for schizophrenia?
    A. lithium
    B. chlorpromazine
    C. benzodiazepine
    D. no cure

Matching

_____ 1. Involved in the facilitation of learning and memory	A. dopamine
_____ 2. Plays a major role in cognitive function and memory function	B. serotonin
_____ 3. Involved in behavior and emesis	C. GABA
_____ 4. Formed from the excitatory neurotransmitter glutamate	D. acetylcholine
_____ 5. Principally involved in the regulation of sleep	E. glutamate

Fill in the Blank

1. Serotonin is also known as 5-hydroxytryptamine or ________________.
2. Antipsychotic drugs are also called ________________ drugs.

3. Schizophrenia is one of the most devastating forms of ______________.
4. Lithium is used for managing ______________ disorders.
5. Bipolar disorder was formerly known as ______________ illness.
6. The principal mood stabilizer is ______________.
7. SSRIs are now considered the first-line drugs in the treatment of ______________.

Critical Thinking

A 45-year-old female has been diagnosed with major depression based on biologic factors and personal characteristics. Her physician has several options for prescribing the best drugs to treat her. These are TCAs, SSRIs, MAOIs, and atypical antidepressants.

1. Which of these classes of antidepressants is the drug of choice?
2. Which of these classes of drugs are the newest types of antidepressants?
3. If the patient is taking MAOIs, which type of foods would be contraindicated?

CHAPTER 5

Drug Therapy for the Nervous System: Antianxiety and Hypnotic Drugs

OBJECTIVES

After completing this chapter, the reader should be able to:

1. Identify the major classifications of anxiety disorders.
2. Describe the difference between a sedative or anxiolytic and a hypnotic.
3. Identify the various types of anxiolytics and hypnotics.
4. Explain the problems associated with anxiolytics and hypnotics.
5. List four benzodiazepine-like drugs and their mechanisms of action.
6. Discuss the therapeutic effects and adverse effects of the major barbiturates.
7. Explain miscellaneous drugs that are used for insomnia.

OUTLINE

GLOSSARY

Antianxiety agents – drugs that relieve anxiety; also known as anxiolytics

Anxiety – state of apprehension and autonomic nervous system activation resulting from exposure to a nonspecific or unknown cause

Anxiolytics – drugs that relieve anxiety; also known as antianxiety agents

Compulsion – a ritualized behavior or mental act that a patient is driven to perform in response to his or her obsessions

Barbiturates – drugs that depress multiple aspects of central nervous system function and can be used for sleep, seizures, and general anesthesia

Benzodiazepines – drugs of first choice for treating anxiety and insomnia

Buspirone – an anxiolytic drug that differs significantly from the benzodiazepines

Generalized anxiety disorder – difficult-to-control, excessive anxiety that lasts six months or more

Hypnotics – drugs given to promote sleep

Insomnia – the inability to fall asleep or stay asleep

Melatonin – an important hormone secreted from the pineal gland that is believed to induce sleep

Obsession – a recurrent, persistent thought, impulse, or mental image that is unwanted and distressing, and comes involuntarily to mind despite attempts to ignore or suppress it

Obsessive-compulsive disorder – anxiety characterized by recurrent, repetitive behaviors that interfere with normal activities or relationships

Panic attacks – of sudden onset, reaching peak intensity within ten minutes; symptoms may include trembling, shortness of breath, heart palpitations, chest pain (or chest tightness), sweating, nausea, dizziness (or slight vertigo), light-headedness, hyperventilation, paresthesias (tingling sensations), and sensations of choking or smothering

Panic disorder – anxiety characterized by intense feelings of immediate apprehension, fearfulness, and terror

Post-traumatic stress disorder – anxiety characterized by a sense of helplessness and the re-experiencing of a traumatic event

Sedative-hypnotics – drugs that when given in lower doses, produce a calming effect, and when given in higher doses, produce sleep

Social anxiety disorder – characterized by an intense, irrational fear of situations in which one might be scrutinized by others, or might do something that is embarrassing or humiliating; also known as social phobia

Social phobia – characterized by an intense, irrational fear of situations in which one might be scrutinized by others, or might do something that is embarrassing or humiliating; also known as social anxiety disorder

Overview

Anxiety disorders are common occurrences in society today. These disorders can prove stressful and disruptive to those suffering from them. There are a variety of anxiety disorders for which drug therapy may be therapeutic. Antianxiety drugs or hypnotics are the most common classifications of medications that may be used to treat these disorders.

> ***Medical Terminology Review***
>
> **preanesthetic**
> *pre = before*
> *an- = without, not*
> *-esthesi/o = feeling, sensation*
> *-tic = pertaining to*
> a drug administered before an anesthetic

Sleep disturbances are also extremely common. If continuous, they have the potential to seriously disrupt normal day-to-day living. Many people suffering from a sleep disorder want to turn to drugs to solve their problem. The use of drugs in many of these situations is usually undesirable.

Many of the medications discussed in this chapter are also administered as muscle relaxants, preanesthetic medications, anticonvulsants, and therapeutic aids in psychiatry.

Anxiety

According to the Anxiety Disorders Association of America, anxiety disorders are the most common psychiatric illnesses in the United States, affecting 40 million people, with a higher incidence of anxiety seen in women than in men. **Anxiety** is an uncomfortable state that has both psychological and physical components. The psychological component can be characterized with terms such as fear, apprehension, dread, and uneasiness. The physical component may exhibit as tachycardia, palpitations, trembling, dry mouth, sweating, weakness, fatigue, and shortness of breath. Fortunately, anxiety disorders respond well to treatment either with behavior therapy, psychotherapy, or drug therapy.

> ***Medical Terminology Review***
>
> **tachycardia**
> *tachy- = fast, rapid*
> *cardia = the heart*
> rapid heart beat

Anxiety disorders may be classified as generalized anxiety disorder, panic disorder, obsessive-compulsive disorder, social anxiety disorder, or post-traumatic stress disorder. Brief explanations of the different types of anxiety follow.

Generalized Anxiety Disorder

Generalized anxiety disorder is a chronic condition characterized by uncontrollable worrying. Most patients with generalized anxiety disorder also have another psychiatric disorder, usually depression. The hallmark of this disorder is unrealistic or excessive anxiety about several events or activities (e.g., work or school performance). Generalized anxiety disorder may last for six months or longer.

Panic Disorder

Panic disorder is characterized by recurrent, intensely uncomfortable episodes known as **panic attacks**. Panic attacks have a sudden onset, reaching peak intensity within ten minutes. Symptoms may include trembling, shortness of breath, heart palpitations, chest pain (or chest tightness), sweating, nausea, dizziness (or slight vertigo), light-headedness, hyperventilation, paresthesias (tingling sensations), and sensations of choking or smothering. These symptoms typically disappear within 30 minutes. Many patients go to an emergency department because they think they are having a heart attack. Some patients experience panic attacks daily; others have only one or two per month. According to the *American Journal of Psychiatry*, the incidence of panic disorders in women is two to three times that seen in men. Onset of panic disorder usually occurs in the late teens or early twenties.

Obsessive-Compulsive Disorder

Obsessive-compulsive disorder is a potentially disabling condition characterized by persistent obsessions and compulsions that cause marked distress, consume at least one hour per day, and significantly interfere with daily living. An **obsession** is defined as a recurrent, persistent thought, impulse, or mental image that is unwanted and distressing, and comes involuntarily to mind despite attempts to ignore or suppress it. A **compulsion** is a ritualized behavior or mental act that a person is driven to perform in response to his or her obsessions.

Social Anxiety Disorder

Social anxiety disorder, formerly known as **social phobia**, is characterized by an intense, irrational fear of situations in which one might be scrutinized by others, or might do something that is embarrassing or humiliating. Exposure to the feared situation almost always elicits anxiety. As a result, the person avoids the situation, or, if it cannot be avoided, endures it with intense anxiety. Manifestations include blushing, stuttering, sweating, palpitations, dry throat, and muscle tension.

Social anxiety disorder is one of the most common psychiatric disorders and the most common anxiety disorder. This disorder typically begins during the teenage years, and if left untreated, is likely to continue lifelong.

Post-Traumatic Stress Disorder

Post-traumatic stress disorder develops following a traumatic event that elicited an immediate reaction of fear, helplessness, or horror. It is more common in women than in men, and is the fourth most common psychiatric disorder. Traumatic events that involve interpersonal violence (e.g., assault, rape, or torture) are more likely to cause post-traumatic stress disorder than are traumatic events that do not (e.g., car accidents or natural disasters).

Sleep Disorders

Insomnia is the inability to fall asleep or stay asleep. Difficulty in falling asleep or disturbed sleep patterns both result in insufficient sleep. Sleep disorders are common and may be short in duration or may be longstanding. They may have little or no apparent relationship to other immediate disorders. Sleep disorders can be secondary to emotional problems, pain, physical disorders, and the use or withdrawal of drugs. Excess alcohol consumed in the evening can shorten sleep and lead to withdrawal effects in the early morning.

> ***Medical Terminology Review***
>
> **insomnia**
> *in = lack of*
> *somnia = ability to sleep*
> lacking the ability to sleep

Sedatives and Hypnotics

The **sedative-hypnotics** are agents that depress central nervous system (CNS) function. These drugs are widely used primarily to treat anxiety and insomnia. Agents given to relieve anxiety are known as **antianxiety agents** or **anxiolytics**. They were previously known as tranquilizers. Drugs given to promote sleep are known as **hypnotics**. The distinction between antianxiety and hypnotic effects is often a matter of dosage. Sedative-hypnotics relieve anxiety in low doses and induce sleep in higher doses. Therefore, a single drug may be considered both an antianxiety agent and a hypnotic agent, depending upon the reason for its use and the dosage employed.

Sedative-hypnotic drugs include barbiturates, benzodiazepines, and benzodiazepine-like drugs. Anxiety and insomnia are treated primarily with the benzodiazepines. Benzodiazepines are used primarily for one condition (generalized anxiety disorder). In contrast, the selective serotonin reuptake inhibitors (SSRIs) are now used for all anxiety disorders. It should be noted that, although SSRIs were developed as antidepressants, they are highly effective against anxiety (with or without depression). SSRIs are discussed in Chapter 4.

TABLE 5-1 First-Line Drugs for Anxiety Disorders

Type of Anxiety Disorder	Benzodiazepines	SSRIs	Others
Generalized Anxiety Disorder	alprazolam	escitalopram oxalate	buspirone hydrochloride
	chlordiazepoxide	paroxetine hydrochloride	venlafaxine hydrochloride
	clorazepate dipotassium	paroxetine mesylate	
	diazepam		
	lorazepam		
	oxazepam		
Panic Disorder	alprazolam	paroxetine	
	clonazepam	sertraline hydrochloride	
	lorazepam		
Obsessive-Compulsive Disorder		citalopram hydrobromide	
		escitalopram oxalate	
		fluoxetine hydrochloride	
		fluvoxamine maleate	
		paroxetine	
		sertraline hydrochloride	
Post-Traumatic Stress Disorder		paroxetine	
		sertraline hydrochloride	

Key Concept

Elderly patients need smaller doses of hypnotics because, in some instances, a sedative dose may produce sleep.

Table 5-1 shows the first-line drugs that are used for specific anxiety disorders. Table 5-2 shows sedative-hypnotics, including barbiturates, benzodiazepines, and miscellaneous agents used to treat anxiety and insomnia.

Benzodiazepines

Benzodiazepines are the drugs of first choice for treating anxiety and insomnia. The popularity of the benzodiazepines as sedatives and hypnotics stems from their clear superiority over the alternatives, such as barbiturates and other general CNS depressants. The benzodiazepines are safer than the general CNS depressants and have a lower potential for abuse.

Mechanism of Action

The mechanism of action of benzodiazepines on the CNS appears to be closely related to their ability to potentiate GABA (gamma-aminobutyric acid)-mediated neural inhibition. Recent research has identified specific

TABLE 5-2 Drugs for Anxiety and Insomnia

Generic Name	Trade Name	Route of Administration	Average Adult Dosage
Barbiturates (Short-Acting)			
pentobarbital	Nembutal®	PO	Sedative: 20–30 mg b.i.d. -t.i.d. Hypnotic: 120–200 mg/day
secobarbital	Seconal®	PO	Sedative: 100–300 mg/day in 3 div. doses Hypnotic: 100–200 mg/day
(Intermediate-Acting)			
amobarbital	Amytal®	PO	Sedative: 30–50 mg b.i.d. -t.i.d. Hypnotic: 65–200 mg (max: 500 mg/day)
aprobarbital	Alurate®	PO	Sedative: 40 mg t.i.d. Hypnotic: 40–160 mg/day
butabarbital	Butisol®	PO	Sedative: 15–30 mg t.i.d.-q.i.d. Hypnotic: 50–100 mg h.s.
(Long-Acting)			
mephobarbital	Mebaral®	PO	Sedative: 32–100 mg t.i.d.
phenobarbital	Luminal®	PO	Sedative: 30–120 mg/day
Benzodiazepines			
alprazolam	Xanax®	PO	0.25–2 mg t.i.d.
chlordiazepoxide	Librium®	PO	5–25 mg t.i.d.-q.i.d.
clonazepam	Klonopin®	PO	1–2 mg/day in div. doses (max: 4 mg/day)
clorazepate dipotassium	Tranxene®	PO	15 mg/day h.s. (max: 4 mg/day)
diazepam	Valium®	PO	2–10 mg b.i.d.-q.i.d.
estazolam	ProSom®	PO	1 mg h.s. (max: 2 mg prn)
flurazepam	Dalmane®	PO	15–30 mg h.s.
halazepam	Paxipam®	PO	20–40 mg t.i.d.-q.i.d.
lorazepam	Ativan®	PO	1–3 mg b.i.d.-t.i.d.
oxazepam	Serax®	PO	10–30 mg t.i.d.-q.i.d.
quazepam	Doral®	PO	7.5–15 mg h.s.
temazepam	Restoril®	PO	15 mg h.s.
triazolam	Halcion®	PO	0.125–0.25 mg h.s. (max: 0.5 mg/day)

(*continues*)

TABLE 5-2 Drugs for Anxiety and Insomnia—*continued*

Generic Name	Trade Name	Route of Administration	Average Adult Dosage
Benzodiazepine-like Drugs			
eszopiclone	Lunesta®	PO	2–3 mg h.s.
ramelteon	Rozerem®	PO	8 mg within 30 min of h.s.
zaleplon	Sonata®	PO	5–10 mg h.s.
zolpidem tartrate	Ambien®	PO	10 mg h.s.
Miscellaneous Drugs: Antiseizure Medication			
valproic acid, (divalproex sodium, sodium valproate)	Depakote®, Depakene®, Depacon®	PO PO PO	250 mg t.i.d. (max: 60 mg/kg/day)
Special Anxiolytic			
buspirone hydrochloride	BuSpar®	PO	7.5–15 mg in div.doses (max: 60 mg/day)
Beta Blockers (rarely indicated for treatment of anxiety)			
atenolol	Tenormin®	PO	25–100 mg 1x/day
propranolol hydrochloride	Inderal®	PO	40 mg b.i.d. (max: 320 mg/day)

binding sites for benzodiazepines in the CNS, and has established the close relationship between the sites of action of the benzodiazepines and GABA.

Indications

Benzodiazepines are useful for the short-term treatment panic disorder, generalized anxiety, phobias, and insomnia. Chlordiazepoxide (Librium) and diazepam (Valium) are the most widely prescribed in medicine. The benzodiazepines are categorized as Schedule IV drugs. Benzodiazepines are also used in absence seizures and myoclonic seizures. Parenteral diazepam is used to terminate status epilepticus.

Adverse Effects

> ***Medical Terminology Review***
>
> **ataxia**
> *a- = without, not*
> *tax/o = order*
> *-ia = condition*
> without muscular coordination

Adverse effects of benzodiazepines are drowsiness, ataxia, impaired judgment, dry mouth, fatigue, visual disturbances, rebound insomnia, and development of tolerance. Overdosage may result in CNS and respiratory depression as well as hypotension and coma. Gradual withdrawal of these drugs is recommended. Although the use of any of the benzodiazepines during pregnancy is likely to cause fetal abnormalities, flurazepam is entirely contraindicated during pregnancy. Benzodiazepines produce considerably less physical dependence and result in less tolerance than barbiturates.

Key Concept

A child born to a mother taking benzodiazepines can develop withdrawal symptoms after birth.

Contraindications and Precautions

Benzodiazepines are contraindicated in patients with known hypersensitivity to the drugs. Benzodiazepines are also contraindicated in patients with acute narrow-angle glaucoma, psychosis, liver or kidney disease, and neurological disorders.

Benzodiazepines should be used cautiously during pregnancy (category D), and in elderly or debilitated patients.

Drug Interactions

Benzodiazepines increase CNS depression with alcohol and omeprazole. They also increase pharmacological effects if combined with cimetidine, disulfiram, or hormonal contraceptives. The effects of benzodiazepines decrease with theophyllines and ranitidine.

Benzodiazepine-like Drugs

Nonbenzodiazepines have become quite popular as sleep aids. They are not indicated for anxiety (see Table 5-2).

Mechanism of Action

Benzodiazepine-like drugs are structurally different from the benzodiazepines, but nonetheless share the same mechanism of action. They all act as agonists at the benzodiazepine receptor site on the GABA receptor-chloride channel complex. These drugs are highly effective hypnotics, and have a low potential for tolerance, dependence, or abuse. Ramelteon has a unique mechanism of action that activates the receptors of **melatonin**.

Indications

Benzodiazepine-like drugs, especially zolpidem (Ambien) and buspirone (BuSpar) are widely used for sleep disorders and anxiety. Buspirone is discussed in detail later in this chapter. Benzodiazepine-like drugs are approved only for short-term management of insomnia, except eszopiclone, which was approved by the FDA in 2005 with no limitation on how long it can be used. Ramelteon is approved for treating chronic insomnia, and long-term use is permitted.

Key Concept

Ramelteon is the only sedative-hypnotic not regulated as a controlled substance.

Adverse Effects

Zolpidem has adverse effects similar to those of benzodiazepines. Daytime drowsiness and dizziness are the most common, and these occur in only 1 to 2 percent of patients. At therapeutic doses, benzodiazepine-like drugs cause little or no respiratory depression. Safety during pregnancy has not been established.

> ***Medical Terminology Review***
>
> **myalgia**
> *My/o = muscle*
> *-algia = pain*
> muscle pain

Zaleplon and eszopiclone are well tolerated. The most common side effects are headache, nausea, drowsiness, dizziness, myalgia, and abdominal pain.

Ramelteon can increase levels of prolactin and reduce levels of testosterone. As a result, the drug has the potential to cause galactorrhea, amenorrhea, reduced libido, and fertility problems.

Contraindications and Precautions

Benzodiazepine-like drugs are contraindicated in patients with a known hypersensitivity, acute narrow-angle glaucoma, shock, and psychoses. These drugs are also contraindicated in patients with acute alcoholic intoxication, depressed vital signs, and in comatose patients.

> ***Medical Terminology Review***
>
> **metabolite**
> *metabol = metabolism*
> *ite = produced substance*
> substance produced through metabolism

Benzodiazepine-like agents are contraindicated in patients during pregnancy (category B) and the drug metabolite freely crosses the placenta. These drugs are used with caution in patients who have impaired liver or kidney function, and in the elderly.

Drug Interactions

Benzodiazepine-like drugs cause less additive CNS depression than other antianxiety drugs, but should still be avoided with concurrent use of a CNS depressant. Buspirone may increase serum digoxin levels, increasing the risk of digitalis toxicity.

Barbiturates

The **barbiturates** depress multiple aspects of CNS function and can be used for sleep, seizures, and general anesthesia. Barbiturates cause tolerance and dependence, have high abuse potential, and are subject to multiple drug interactions. Moreover, barbiturates are powerful respiratory depressants that can be fatal in overdose. Because of these undesirable properties, barbiturates are used much less than in the past, having been replaced by newer and safer drugs—primarily the benzodiazepines and benzodiazepine-like drugs. However, although their use has declined greatly, barbiturates still have important applications in seizure control and anesthesia.

> ***Medical Terminology Review***
>
> **anesthesia**
> *an- = without*
> *-esthesia = sensation, feeling*
> without sensation

Mechanism of Action

All barbiturates exert a depressant effect on the CNS. These drugs act by changing the action of GABA, the primary inhibitory neurotransmitter in the brain. Barbiturates mimic the effects of GABA by stimulating an influx of chloride ions that interact with the GABA receptor through chloride channel molecules. When the receptors of barbiturate are stimulated, chloride ions move into the cells, therefore suppressing the ability of neurons to fire.

Indications

Barbiturates are used as sedatives and as hypnotics (short term, up to two weeks) for insomnia. Long-term treatment with certain barbiturates is prescribed for generalized tonic-clonic and cortical focal seizures. They are also indicated for emergency control of some acute convulsive episodes such as status epilepticus, eclampsia, meningitis, tetanus, and toxic reactions to local anesthetics. Thiopental and other highly lipid-soluble barbiturates are given to induce general anesthesia. Unconsciousness develops within seconds of IV injections. After prolonged use of barbiturates, withdrawal symptoms may occur.

Medical Terminology Review

neonatal
neo = *new*
natal = *pertaining to birth*
new birth, newborn

Phenobarbital and mephobarbital are used for seizure disorders, congenital hyperbilirubinemia, and neonatal jaundice. Indications for intermediate-acting barbiturates are regional anesthesia, sedation, and hypnosis. Ultra-short-acting barbiturates are used for intravenous general anesthesia.

Adverse Effects

Barbiturates may cause numerous adverse effects on several different body systems. The manifestation of adverse effects includes ataxia, drowsiness, dizziness, and hangover effect. Some patients may have nausea and vomiting, insomnia, constipation, headache, night terrors, and faintness. Long-term use of barbiturates may cause bone pain, anorexia, muscle pain, and weight loss.

Contraindications and Precautions

Barbiturates are contraindicated in patients with known hypersensitivity to these agents, pregnancy (category D), or lactation. Barbiturates are also contraindicated in parturition, fetal immaturity, and uncontrolled pain.

Barbiturates should be used cautiously in patients with liver or kidney impairments and those with neurological disorders. These drugs are used with caution in patients with pulmonary disorders and in hyperactive children.

Drug Interactions

Barbiturates increase serum levels and therapeutic and toxic effects with valproic acid. They also increase CNS depression with alcohol, narcotic analgesics, and antidepressants. Barbiturates decrease effects of the following drugs: theophyllines, oral anticoagulants, β-blockers, doxycycline, griseofulvin, corticosteroids, hormonal contraceptives, and metronidazole.

Miscellaneous Drugs

There are several CNS drugs used for anxiety and insomnia that are categorized as miscellaneous drugs. These agents are chemically unrelated to either benzodiazepines, benzodiazepine-like drugs, or barbiturates.

The antiseizure drug valproate (Chapter 8), the beta blockers atenolol and propranolol (Chapter 11), and the CNS depressant buspirone are also used for anxiety or sleep disorders (see Table 5-2). Buspirone is unique and is commonly prescribed for antianxiety.

Buspirone

Buspirone (BuSpar) is an anxiolytic drug that differs significantly from the benzodiazepines. Buspirone is as effective as the benzodiazepines and has three distinct advantages:

- It does not cause sedation
- It has no abuse potential
- It does not intensify the effects of CNS depressants

Mechanism of Action. The anxiolytic effect of buspirone is mainly on the brain's D_2-dopamine receptors. It has agonist effects on presynaptic dopamine receptors. It also has a high affinity for serotonin receptors.

Indications. Buspirone is prescribed for management of anxiety disorders and for short-term treatment of generalized anxiety.

Adverse Effects. Buspirone is generally well tolerated. The most common reactions are dizziness, nausea, headache, nervousness, lightheadedness, and excitement. The drug is nonsedating and does not interfere with daytime activities.

Contraindications and Precautions. Buspirone is contraindicated in patients with known hypersensitivity to this medication. It is also contraindicated with concomitant use of alcohol and buspirone. Safety during pregnancy (category B), labor, delivery, lactation, and in children younger than 18 years is not established. Buspirone should be used with caution in patients with moderate to severe renal or hepatic impairment.

Drug Interactions. Blood levels of buspirone can be greatly increased by erythromycin and ketoconazole. Levels of buspirone can also be increased by grapefruit juice. Buspirone does not enhance the depressant effects of alcohol, barbiturates, and other general CNS depressants.

Summary

Sedatives affect the CNS, which can relieve anxiety, hence they are often called anxiolytics. Hypnotic is the term used to describe a substance that induces sleep. Both anxiety and insomnia are extremely common in the United States.

There are three major groups of anxiolytics and hypnotics: barbiturates, benzodiazepines, and benzodiazepine-like drugs. Benzodiazepines act on the GABA receptor complex. These drugs are relatively nontoxic, but can have several undesirable adverse effects. With most anxiolytics, the antianxiety effect is related to their sedative effect. The use of barbiturates as hypnotics is no longer advised, and they are gradually being phased out from use. Their availability today is mainly because some are still used in the treatment of epilepsy, and as anesthetics. Hypnotic drugs should be used for short-term therapy only.

Nonbenzodiazepine drugs have become very popular as sleep aids. They are not indicated for anxiety use. Benzodiazepine-like drugs are structurally different from the benzodiazepines, but their mechanism of action is the same. Nonbenzodiazepine drugs, especially zolpidem and buspirone, are widely used for anxiety and sleep disorders.

Miscellaneous drugs that are used for anxiety and insomnia are chemically unrelated to either benzodiazepines or barbiturates. These agents include antiseizure drugs (valproate) and beta blockers (atenolol and propranolol).

Exploring the Web

Visit ***www.medicinenet.com***

- Search using the term post-traumatic stress disorder. Review relevant articles related to the treatment of this disorder.

Visit ***www.nlm.nih.gov***

- Choose one of the disorders discussed in this chapter and research the treatments used to address the disorder.

Visit ***www.usdoj.gov***

- Search using the term benzodiazepines. Look for information published by the DEA on this drug. What are the concerns with use of this drug? What is the potential for abuse?

Review Questions

Multiple Choice

1. Which of the following are the first-line drugs used in the treatment of anxiety and insomnia?
   A. benzodiazepines and barbiturates
   B. benzodiazepines and SSRIs
   C. benzodiazepines and MAOIs
   D. benzodiazepines and chloral hydrate
2. Which of the following is the main concern for a patient that stopped taking barbiturates suddenly?
   A. shock
   B. hypotension
   C. severe withdrawal
   D. respiratory depression
3. Which of the following may increase the effects of sedatives?
   A. chocolate
   B. cheese
   C. nicotine
   D. alcohol
4. Benzodiazepines act by binding to the GABA receptor of which of the following channel molecules?
   A. chloride
   B. sodium
   C. potassium
   D. calcium
5. Generalized anxiety disorder may last for:
   A. 3 weeks
   B. 6 weeks
   C. 3 months
   D. 6 months
6. Symptoms of panic disorder typically disappear within:
   A. 30 seconds
   B. 30 minutes
   C. 30 days
   D. 90 days
7. Benzodiazepine-like drugs are the preferred agents for treating:
   A. insomnia
   B. depression
   C. panic disorder
   D. obsessive-compulsive disorder

8. Which of the following benzodiazepine-like drugs may increase levels of prolactin and reduce levels of testosterone?

A. ramelteon
B. zolpidem
C. zaleplon
D. all of the above

9. The newest drugs used for anxiety and sleep disorders include which of the following?

A. Nembutal and Depakote
B. Seconal and Inderal
C. Tofranil and Librium
D. BuSpar and Ambien

10. Adverse effects of zolpidem (Ambien) are similar to which of the following?

A. antihypertensives
B. barbiturates
C. benzodiazepines
D. beta blockers

11. The indications for barbiturates have declined greatly, but they still have important applications in which of the following disorders or conditions?

A. insomnia
B. major depression
C. anxiety
D. anesthesia

12. Which of the following hormones is believed to induce sleep?

A. prolactin
B. thyroxin
C. melanin
D. melatonin

13. The trade name of diazepam is:

A. Librium
B. Valium
C. Xanax
D. Serax

14. The generic name of Luminal is:

A. butabarbital
B. pentobarbital
C. phenobarbital
D. secobarbital

15. Long-term treatment with certain barbiturates is prescribed for which of the following disorders?

A. insomnia
B. anxiety attacks
C. general anesthesia
D. generalized tonic-clonic seizures

Fill in the Blank

1. Benzodiazepines are the drugs of first choice for treating ______________ and ______________.
2. Barbiturates cause tolerance and ______________.
3. All barbiturates act by changing the action of ______________.
4. Panic disorder is known as ______________.
5. The sedative-hypnotics are used primarily to treat ______________ and ______________.
6. Antianxiety agents were previously known as ______________.
7. Barbiturates are contraindicated in pregnancy because they are in category ______________.

Critical Thinking

Kaleen is a nurse who was injured in a car accident on her way home from the hospital where she works. She was hospitalized for three weeks and developed post-traumatic stress disorder after approximately six months.

1. What would be the first-line drug for this condition?
2. If she also developed a panic disorder, does her physician have to change her medication or add other drugs to her regimen?
3. If her physician is prescribing the correct first-line drug, what would be the most severe adverse effect?

Drug Therapy for the Autonomic Nervous System

CHAPTER 6

OUTLINE

OBJECTIVES

After completing this chapter, the reader should be able to:

1. Describe the subdivisions of the ANS.
2. Explain the various types of receptors.
3. Differentiate sympathomimetics from sympatholytic agents and give two examples for each.
4. Outline five beta$_2$-adrenergic drugs.
5. Explain the action of adrenergic blockers.
6. Describe the use of cholinergic agonist drugs.
7. Differentiate between cholinergics and cholinergic blockers.
8. Explain the major adverse effects of anticholinergic drugs.
9. Explain the contraindications of cholinergic blockers.
10. List three neurotransmitters that employ the ANS.

GLOSSARY

Adrenergic blocker agents – drugs that antagonize the secretion of epinephrine and norepinephrine from sympathetic terminal neurons; also known as sympatholytics

Adrenergic receptor – receptors that mediate responses to epinephrine (adrenaline) and norepinephrine

Alpha-receptors – an adrenergic receptor; there are two types: alpha$_1$ and alpha$_2$

Beta-receptors – an adrenergic receptor; there are two types: beta$_1$ and beta$_2$

Catecholamines – a group of chemically related compounds having a sympathomimetic action

Cholinergic receptor – receptors that mediate responses to acetylcholine

Congenital megacolon – congenital dilation and hypertrophy of the colon due to reduction in motor neurons of the parasympathetic nervous system, resulting in extreme constipation, and if untreated, growth retardation; also known as Hirschsprung's disease

Cycloplegia – paralysis of the ciliary muscles of the eye, resulting in loss of visual accommodation

Dopamine receptors – an adrenergic receptor

Epinephrine – a major transmitter released by the adrenal medulla

Iritis – inflammation of the iris

Miosis – contraction of the pupil of the eye

Mydriasis – dilation of the pupil

Necrosis – death of a group of cells or tissues

Norepinephrine – the chemical transmitter released by all postganglionic neurons of the sympathetic nervous system

Parasympathomimetic – producing effects similar to those produced when a parasympathetic nerve is stimulated

Pheochromocytoma – a usually benign tumor of the adrenal medulla or the sympathetic nervous system in which the affected cells secrete increased amounts of epinephrine or norepinephrine

Somnolence – prolonged drowsiness that may last hours to days

Sympatholytic – inhibiting or opposing adrenergic nerve function; sympatholytic agents are also known as *adrenergic blocker agents*

Sympathomimetic – adrenergic, or producing an effect similar to that obtained by stimulation of the sympathetic nervous system

Uveitis – inflammation of the uvea (the vascular middle layer of the eye, including the iris, ciliary body, and choroid)

Overview

The peripheral nervous system regulates both voluntary and involuntary functions in the human body. This chapter focuses on those drugs that are used to regulate and control disorders in the involuntary functions. The therapeutic agents discussed here are used to treat many disorders and conditions such as hypertension, hypotension, asthma, dysrhythmia, glaucoma, and even runny nose.

Anatomy Review

- The peripheral nervous system has two divisions the somatic nervous system (SNS) and the autonomic nervous system (ANS) (Figure 6-1).
- The SNS regulates voluntary or conscious functions such as motor movement.
- The autonomic nervous system regulates all involuntary functions such as secretion of hormones; contraction of the heart muscle, blood vessels and bronchioles; and the ability to move substances through the digestive tract.
- The ANS can be further divided into the sympathetic and parasympathetic nervous systems (PNS) (Figures 6-2 and 6-3).

Nervous System
Central Nervous System (CNS)
Peripheral Nervous System (PNS)
Brain
Receives and processes sensory information, initiates responses, stores, memories generates thoughts and emotions
Spinal cord
Conducts signals to and from the brain, controls reflex activities
Motor Neurons
CNS to muscles and glands
Sensory Neurons
Sensory organs to CNS
Somatic Nervous System
Controls voluntary movements
Autonomic Nervous System
Controls involuntary responses
Sympathetic Division
"Fight or Flight"
Parasympathetic Division
"Rest or Digest"

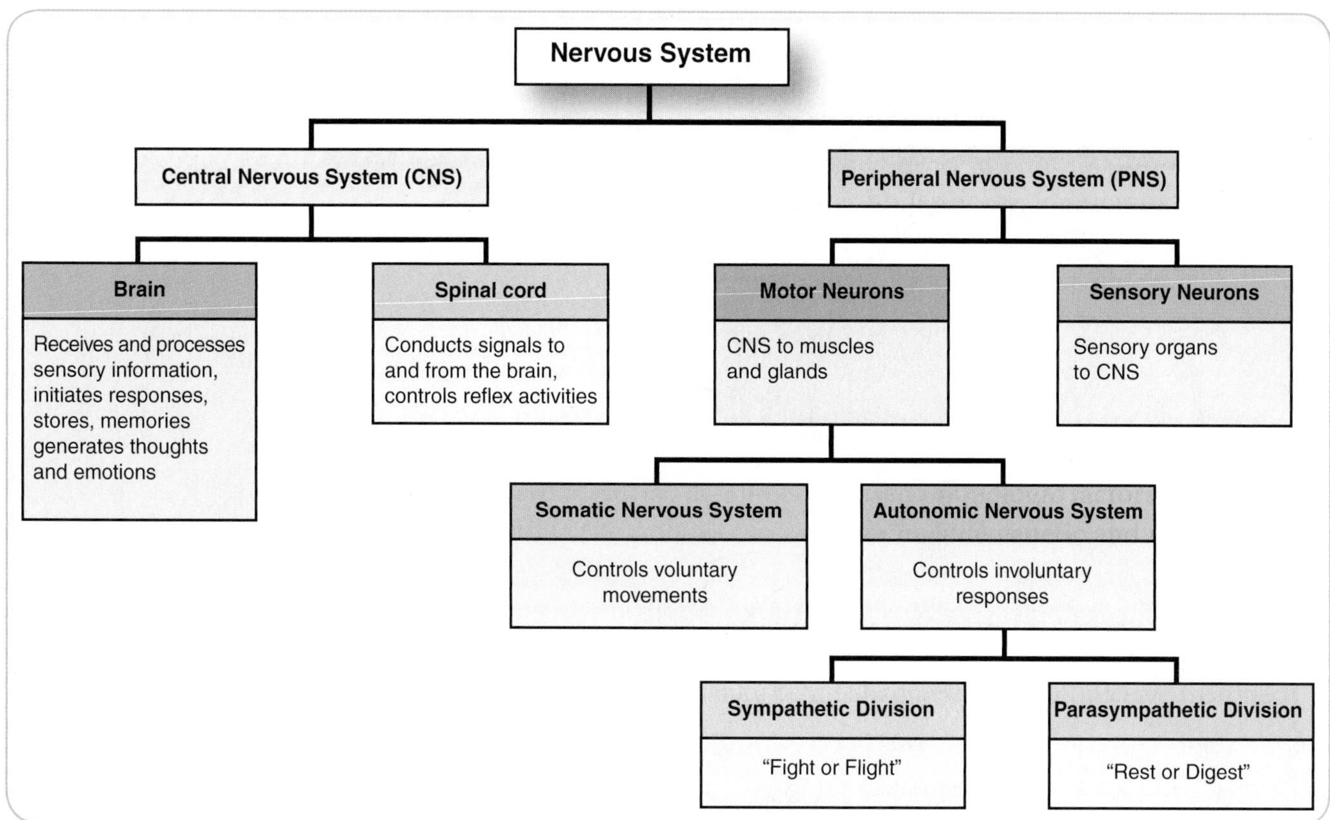

Figure 6-1 Divisions of the nervous system.

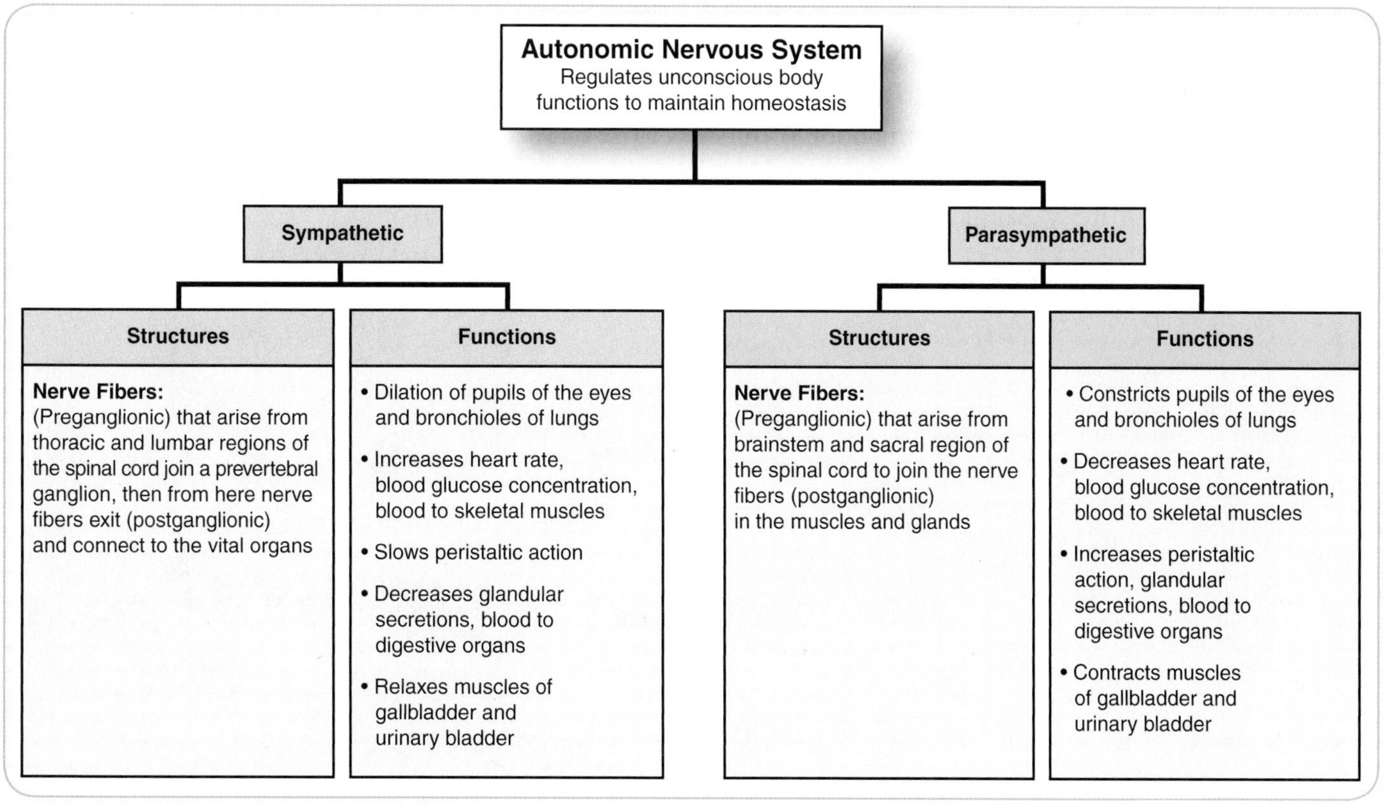

Autonomic Nervous System
Regulates unconscious body functions to maintain homeostasis
Sympathetic
Parasympathetic
Structures
Nerve Fibers:
(Preganglionic) that arise from thoracic and lumbar regions of the spinal cord join a prevertebral ganglion, then from here nerve fibers exit (postganglionic) and connect to the vital organs
Functions
• Dilation of pupils of the eyes and bronchioles of lungs
• Increases heart rate, blood glucose concentration, blood to skeletal muscles
• Slows peristaltic action
• Decreases glandular secretions, blood to digestive organs
• Relaxes muscles of gallbladder and urinary bladder
Structures
Nerve Fibers:
(Preganglionic) that arise from brainstem and sacral region of the spinal cord to join the nerve fibers (postganglionic) in the muscles and glands
Functions
• Constricts pupils of the eyes and bronchioles of lungs
• Decreases heart rate, blood glucose concentration, blood to skeletal muscles
• Increases peristaltic action, glandular secretions, blood to digestive organs
• Contracts muscles of gallbladder and urinary bladder

Figure 6-2 The autonomic nervous system.

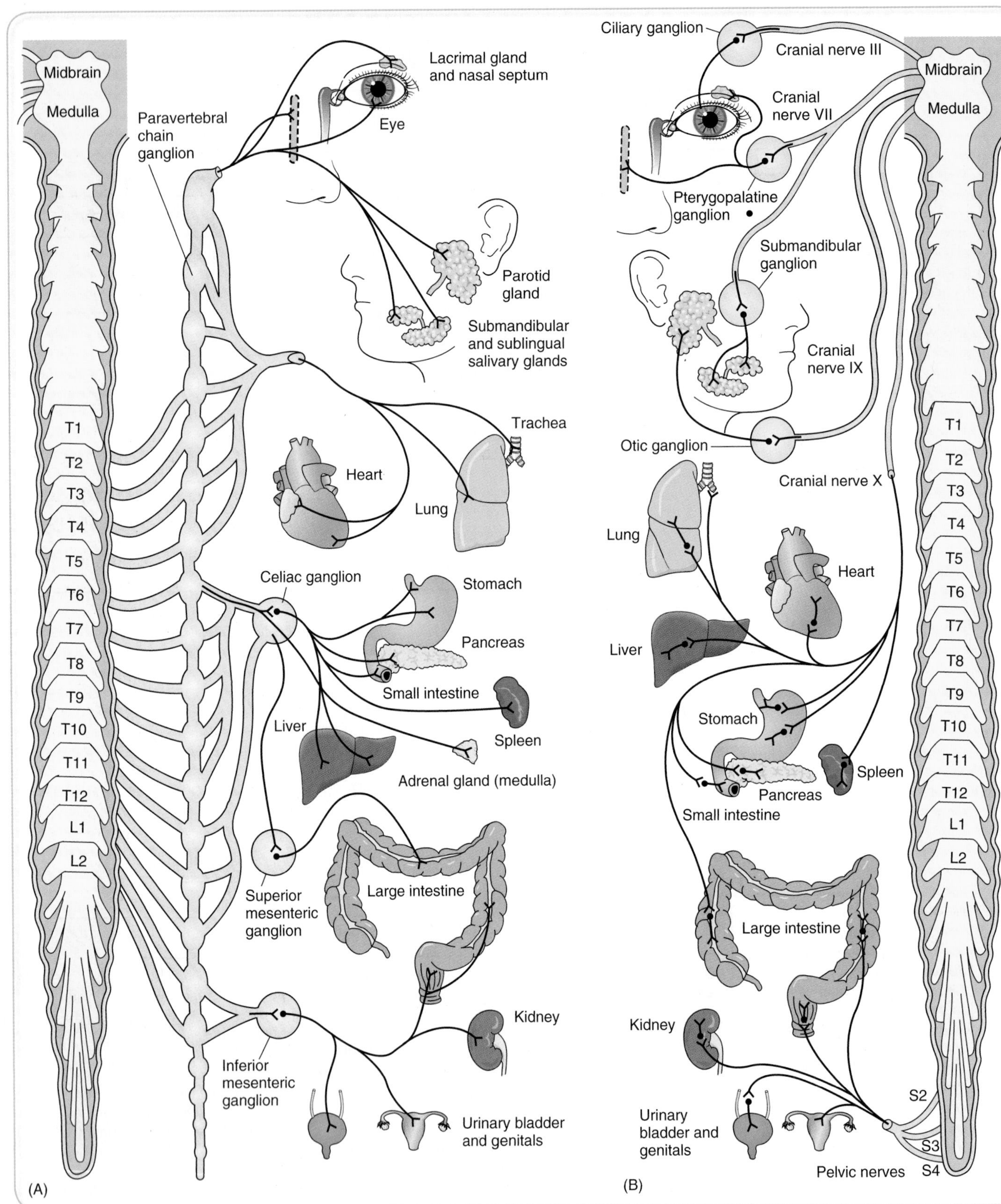

Figure 6-3 (A) The sympathetic division of the autonomic nervous system (B) The parasympathetic division of the autonomic nervous system.

- These divisions work antagonistically, for example, activation of the sympathetic division will increase heart rate while activation of the parasympathetic division will decrease heart rate.
- The sympathetic division responds in emergencies or during stressful situations and is called the fight-or-flight response.
- The parasympathetic division responds as a restorative function and is called the rest-and-digest response.

Neurotransmitters Associated with the Autonomic Nervous System

In previous chapters, neurotransmitters are discussed related to the role alterations that these neurotransmitters play in psychiatric illnesses and the treatments of these illnesses. This chapter focuses on the role of neurotransmitters in the involuntary functions of the body regulated by the autonomic nervous system. The three main neurotransmitters discussed are acetylcholine, norepinephrine, and epinephrine. Any given junction in the autonomic nervous system uses only one of these transmitter substances. A fourth compound, dopamine, may also serve as a transmitter, but this role has not been demonstrated conclusively.

In order to understand the mechanism of action of drugs that act upon these neurotransmitters, it is necessary to know the identity of the transmitter employed at each of the junctions of the autonomic nervous system (Figure 6-4).

Acetylcholine is the chemical transmitter employed at most junctions of the ANS as well as at the skeletal muscles. Acetylcholine is the transmitter released by:

1. All preganglionic neurons of the PNS
2. All preganglionic neurons of the SNS
3. All postganglionic neurons of the PNS
4. Most postganglionic neurons of the SNS that go to sweat glands
5. All motor neurons to skeletal muscles

Norepinephrine is the chemical transmitter released by all postganglionic neurons of the SNS. The only exceptions are the postganglionic sympathetic neurons that go to sweat glands, which employ acetylcholine as their transmitter. **Epinephrine** is a major transmitter released by the adrenal medulla.

Medical Terminology Review

preganglionic
pre = before
ganglionic = nerve tissue masses
nerves that lead to nerve tissue masses

postganglionic
post = after
ganglionic = nerve tissue masses
nerves that lead to the specific organs

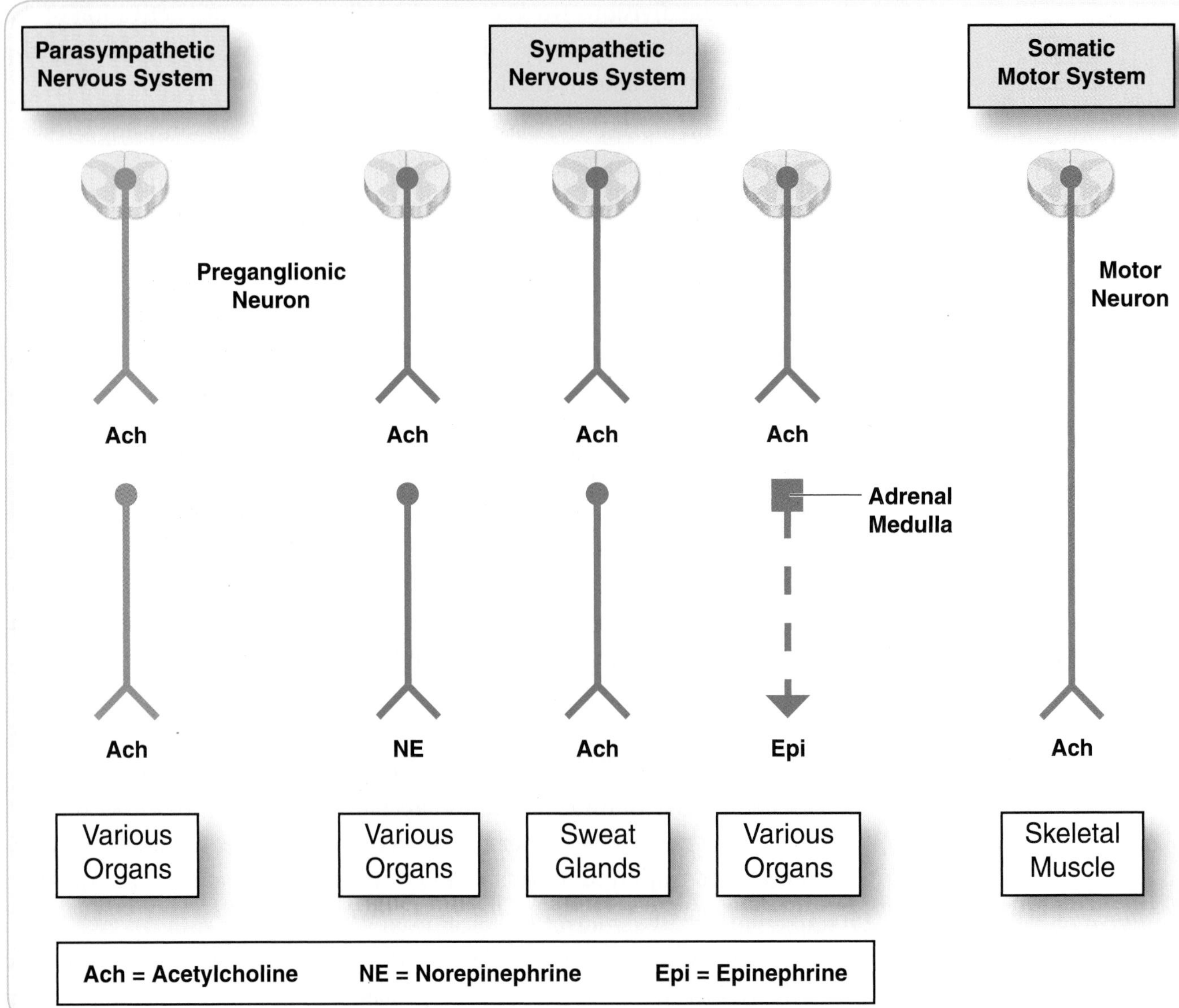

Figure 6-4 Chemical transmitters employed at specific junctions of the peripheral nervous system.

Receptors

The peripheral and autonomic nervous systems work through various types of receptors. Understanding these receptors is essential to understanding nervous system pharmacology.

There are two basic types of receptors associated with the PNS: adrenergic and cholinergic receptors. Each of these receptors is divided into different subtypes. Activation of each subtype of these receptors causes a characteristic set of physiological responses. Some drugs affect all receptor subtypes while others only affect one type of receptor. Different doses of a drug may activate one type of receptor, while increased doses may activate other receptor subtypes. It is important to memorize the various receptor types and their responses.

Cholinergic Receptors

Cholinergic receptors are defined as receptors that mediate responses to acetylcholine. These receptors mediate responses at all junctions where acetylcholine is the transmitter. There are three major subtypes of cholinergic receptors, which are referred to as nicotinic$_N$, nicotinic$_M$, and muscarinic.

Adrenergic Receptors

Adrenergic receptors are defined as receptors that mediate responses to epinephrine (adrenaline) and norepinephrine. These receptors mediate responses at all junctions where norepinephrine or epinephrine is the transmitter. Adrenergic receptors are divided into two types: **alpha-receptors** (α-receptors) and **beta-receptors** (β-receptors). Alpha-receptors are divided into alpha$_1$ and alpha$_2$ receptors, and beta-receptors are divided into beta$_1$ and beta$_2$ receptors.

In addition to the four major subtypes of adrenergic receptors, there is another adrenergic receptor type, referred to as the **dopamine receptor**. Dopamine receptors respond only to dopamine, a neurotransmitter found primarily in the CNS. Tables 6-1 and 6-2 summarize functions of cholinergic and adrenergic receptor subtypes.

TABLE 6-1 Cholinergic Receptor Subtype Functions

Receptor Subtype	Location	Response to Receptor Stimulation
nicotinic$_N$	all autonomic nervous system ganglia and the adrenal medulla	stimulation of both parasympathetic and sympathetic postganglionic nerves and release of epinephrine from the adrenal medulla
nicotinic$_M$	neuromuscular junction	contraction of skeletal muscle
muscarinic	all parasympathetic target organs:	
	eyes	contraction of the ciliary muscle focuses the lens for near vision, and contraction of the iris sphincter muscle causes **miosis** (contraction of the pupil)
	heart	decreased rate
	lungs	constriction of bronchi and increased secretions
	GI tract	salivation, increased gastric secretions, increased intestinal tone and motility, defecation
	sweat glands	generalized sweating
	urinary bladder	increased bladder pressure, relaxation of smooth muscles and sphincter, allowing urine to leave the bladder
	sex organs	erection
	blood vessels	vasodilation

TABLE 6-2 Adrenergic Receptor Subtype Functions

Receptor Subtype	Location	Response to Receptor Stimulation
$alpha_1$	eyes	contraction of the radial muscle of the iris causes **mydriasis** (pupil dilation)
	arteries	constriction
	veins	constriction
	male sex organs	ejaculation
	prostate capsule	contraction
	bladder	contraction of bladder and sphincter
$alpha_2$	presynaptic nerve terminals	inhibition of transmitter release
$beta_1$	heart	increased rate and force of contraction
	kidneys	renin release
$beta_2$	arterioles of the:	
	heart	dilation
	lungs	dilation
	skeletal	dilation
	muscles of:	
	bronchi	dilation
	uterus	relaxation
	skeletal	increased contraction
	muscle liver	glycogenolysis (the breakdown of glycogen into glucose, releasing it back into the circulating blood in response to a very low blood sugar level)
dopamine	kidneys	dilation of kidney vasculature

Drugs Affecting the Autonomic Nervous System

Drugs that affect the ANS may be classified into four categories:

- Sympathomimetics (Adrenergics)
- Sympatholytics (Adrenergic blockers)
- Parasympathomimetics (Cholinergics)
- Parasympatholytics (Anticholinergics)

Key Concept

Although dopamine receptors are classified as adrenergic, these receptors do not respond to epinephrine or norepinephrine.

Sympathomimetics (Adrenergic Drugs)

Sympathomimetic agents are also called adrenergic agonists. These agents produce their effects by activating adrenergic receptors. Since the SNS acts through these same receptors, responses to adrenergic agonists and responses to stimulation of the SNS are very similar.

Adrenergic agonist drugs may affect both alpha- and beta-receptors. The classification seems confusing, therefore, adrenergic drugs on each receptor will be discussed separately. Selected adrenergic agonist drugs are listed in Table 6-3.

Medical Terminology Review

Sympathomimetic

sympatho = *related to the sympathetic nervous system*
mimetic = *an agent that mimics*
a drug agent that mimics the actions of the sympathetic nervous system

TABLE 6-3 Sympathomimetics (Adrenergic Drugs)

Generic Name	Trade Name	Route of Administration	Average Adult Dosage
albuterol	Proventil® Ventolin®	PO, Inhalation	PO: 2.4 mg 3-4 times/day; Inhalation: 1-2 q4-6h
dobutamine	Dobutrex®	IV	2.5-10 mcg/kg/min
dopamine hydrochloride	Intropin® Dopamine®	IV	2-5 mcg/kg/min
epinephrine	EpiEZPen®, Primatene Mist Suspension ®	SC, Inhalation	SC: 0.1-0.5 mL of 1:1000 q10-15 min prn; Inhalation: 1 inhalation q4h prn
isoproterenol hydrochloride	Isuprel® Dispos-a-Med®	IV, MDI	IV: 0.01-0.02 mg prn; MDI: 1-2 inhalations 4-6 times/day
metaproterenol sulfate	Alupent® Metaprel®	PO, MDI, Nebulizer	PO: 20 mg q6-8h; MDI: 2-3 inhalations q3-4h; Nebulizer: 5-10 inhalations
methyldopa	Aldomet®	PO, IV	PO/IV: 250-500 mg bid or tid
norepinephrine bitartrate	Levarterenol® Levophed®	IV	Start with 8-12 mcg/min; maintenance dose 2-4 mcg/min
oxymetazoline	Afrin®	Intranasal	2-3 drops or 2-3 sprays of 0.05% solution bid
phenylephrine hydrochloride	Neo-Synephrine® Alconefrin®	IM, IV, SC	IM/SC: 1-10 mg q10-15 min prn; IV: 0.1-0.18 mg/min
pseudoephedrine hydrochloride	Sudafed® Cenafed®	PO	60 mg q4-6h
ritodrine	Yutopar®	PO, IV	PO: 10 mg q2h; IV: 50-350 mcg/min
salmeterol xinafoate	Serevent®	Inhalation	2 inhalations of aerosol (42 mcg) bid
terbutaline sulfate	Brethine® Brethaire®	PO, Inhalation, SC	PO: 2.5-5 mg tid; Inhalation: 2 inhalations q4-6h; SC: 0.25 mg q15-30 min up to 0.5 mg in 4h

Mechanism of Action

Adrenergic drugs stimulate both $alpha_1$ and $beta_2$ receptor sites. The alpha-adrenergic receptor sites are located in the smooth muscle of blood vessels, the gastrointestinal tract, and the genitourinary tract. They produce vasoconstriction when stimulated by adrenergic drugs. The $beta_1$-adrenergic receptors are located in the heart muscle. When stimulated by adrenergic drugs, they produce increased contractility (resulting in increased heart rate).

$Beta_2$-adrenergic receptors in the respiratory system, located in the bronchial muscle, produce bronchodilation when stimulated by adrenergic agents.

Medical Terminology Review

hemostasis
hemo = related to blood or bleeding
stasis = slowing or stopping
slowing or stopping bleeding

Indications

Adrenergic agonist drugs that affect alpha-adrenergic receptors are used in patients with hypotension, hemostasis, to relieve nasal congestion, as adjuncts to local anesthesia (to reduce bleeding), and for dilation of the pupils (which facilitates eye examinations and ocular surgery). The beta-adrenergic drugs are used in the treatment of asthma and bronchitis.

Adverse Effects

All of the adverse effects caused by $alpha_1$ activation result directly or indirectly from vasoconstriction. The most common adverse effects include hypertension, **necrosis** (death of a group of cells or tissues) if an IV line is employed to administer an $alpha_1$ agonist, and slowness of the heart rate.

Common adverse effects of beta-adrenergic drugs include headache, tremors, mild leg cramps, nervousness, fatigue, hypertension, palpitation, nausea, vomiting, and shortness of breath.

Contraindications and Precautions

Adrenergic drugs are contraindicated in patients with known hypersensitivity to these agents. These drugs are also contraindicated in the elderly, who are more sensitive to the effects of adrenergic drugs. These drugs should not be given to patients with symptoms such as blurred vision, seizures, chest pain, and palpitations.

Alpha-adrenergic drugs are contraindicated in children younger than 2 years of age. Safe use during pregnancy (category C) or lactation is not established.

Beta adrenergic drugs are contraindicated in cardiac arrhythmias associated with tachycardia, hyperthyroidism, pregnancy (category C), and lactation.

Adrenergic drugs should be used with caution in older adults, hypertension, cardiovascular disorders (including coronary artery disease), hyperthyroidism, and diabetes.

Drug Interactions

No clinically significant drug interactions have been established for alpha-adrenergic agents. Beta-adrenergic drugs may interact with general anesthetics (especially cyclopropane and halothane).

Sympatholytics (Adrenergic Blockers)

Sympatholytic agents (or **adrenergic blocker agents**) produce many of the same responses as the parasympathomimetics. These drugs are the most commonly prescribed class of autonomic drugs. Adrenergic blocker agents are also effective on all adrenergic alpha- and beta-receptors. Selected adrenergic antagonists or adrenergic blockers are listed in Table 6-4.

TABLE 6-4 Sympatholytics (Adrenergic Blockers)

Generic Name	Trade Name	Route of Administration	Average Adult Dosage
acebutolol	Sectral®	PO	400-800 mg/day
atenolol	Tenormin®	PO	25-50 mg/day
carteolol	Cartrol®	PO	2.5 mg once/day
carvedilol	Coreg®	PO	3.125 mg b.i.d.
doxazosin mesylate	Cardura®	PO	1-16 mg h.s.
esmolol hydrochloride	Brevibloc®	IV	500 mcg/kg loading dose followed by 50 mcg/kg/min
metoprolol tartrate	Lopressor®	PO	50-100 mg/day
nadolol	Corgard®	PO	40 mg once/day
phentolamine	Regitine®	IM, IV	IM/IV: 5 mg 1-2h before surgery
prazosin hydrochloride	Minipress®	PO	Start with 1 mg h.s., then 1 mg b.i.d. or tid
propranolol hydrochloride	Inderal®	PO, IV	PO: 10-40 mg b.i.d.; IV: 0.5-3 mg q4h prn
sotalol hydrochloride	Betapace®	PO	40-160 mg b.i.d.
tamsulosin hydrochloride	Flomax®	PO	0.4 mg q.d. 30 min. after a meal
terazosin	Hytrin®	PO	1-5 mg/day
timolol maleate	Blocadren®, Timoptic®	PO	10-60 mg b.i.d.

Medical Terminology Review

sympatholytic
sympatho = related to the sympathetic nervous system
lytic = opposing effects
a drug that acts to oppose the actions of the sympathetic nervous system

Mechanism of Action

Adrenergic blockers reduce delivery of **catecholamines** to the adrenergic receptors by disrupting catecholamine synthesis, storage, or release.

Indications

Adrenergic blockers are used in treatment of hypertension, dysrhythmias, angina, heart failure, glaucoma, and migraines.

Adverse Effects

Adverse effects of adrenergic blockers include orthostatic hypotension, edema, headache, dizziness, vertigo, **somnolence** (prolonged drowsiness), fatigue, nervousness, and anxiety. These agents may also cause abdominal pain, nausea, vomiting, diarrhea, and exacerbation of peptic ulcer.

Adverse effects of beta-adrenergic blockers include respiratory disturbances, bradycardia, peripheral vascular insufficiency, palpitations, postural hypotension, behavioral changes, blurred vision, and dry eyes.

Contraindications and Precautions

Alpha adrenergic blockers are contraindicated in patients with known hypersensitivity to these agents, and those patients with hypotension or syncope. Safe use during pregnancy (category D) or in children is not established.

Beta adrenergic blockers are contraindicated in patients with sinus bradycardia, heart failure, peripheral vascular disease, hypotension, or pulmonary edema. Safety during pregnancy (category D) or lactation is not established.

Alpha adrenergic blockers must be used cautiously in patients with hepatic impairment, renal disease, or lactation.

Beta adrenergics are used with caution in hypertensive patients with congestive heart failure controlled by digitalis, and with diuretics, in vasospastic angina, asthma, bronchitis, emphysema, major depression, diabetes mellitus, impaired renal function, myasthenia gravis, hyperthyroidism, pheochromocytoma, and in older adults.

> ***Medical Terminology Review***
>
> **pheochromocytoma**
> *pheo = dusky or gray*
> *chromo = related to chromaffin cells*
> *cytoma = cell tumor*
> a pigmented tumor of the chromaffin cells (adrenal gland)

Drug Interactions

Atropine and other anticholinergics may increase absorption of adrenergic blockers from the gastrointestinal (GI) tract.

Parasympathomimetics (Cholinergic Drugs)

Parasympathomimetic or cholinergic agonist drugs are able to mimic action of the PNS. Table 6-5 shows selected parasympathomimetic drugs.

Mechanism of Action

Some cholinergic drugs increase concentration of acetylcholine at cholinergic transmission sites, which prolongs and exaggerates their action. Others produce reversible cholinesterase inhibition and have direct stimulant action on voluntary muscle fibers.

Indications

Cholinergic agonist drugs are used most commonly in glaucoma by inducing miosis. Specific muscarinic agonist drugs may be used in the treatment of atonic constipation, **congenital megacolon**, and in postoperative or postpartum adynamic intestinal ileus. Bethanechol has been used to increase the tone of the lower esophageal sphincter in the diagnosis or treatment of reflux esophagitis. Muscarinic agonists are useful in the treatment of nonobstructive urinary retention and neurogenic atony of the urinary bladder with retention. Cholinergic agonist drugs are also used for dysrhythmias and for Alzheimer's disease.

TABLE 6-5 Parasympathomimetics (Cholinergic Drugs)

Generic Name	Trade Name	Route of Administration	Average Adult Dosage
bethanechol chloride	Urecholine®	PO	10-50 mg b.i.d. to q.i.d.
cevimeline hydrochloride	Evoxac®	PO	30 mg t.i.d.
neostigmine	Prostigmin®	PO, IM, IV	PO: 15-375 mg/day; IM: 0.022 mg/kg; IV: 0.5-2.5 mg slowly
physostigmine salicylate	Antilirium®	IM, IV	IM/IV: 0.5-3 mg
pilocarpine hydrochloride	Isopto Carpine®, Salagen®	PO, Ophthalmic	PO: 5-10 mg t.i.d.; Ophthalmic: 1 drop of 1-2% solution in affected eye q5-10 min for 3-6 doses
pyridostigmine	Mestinon®	PO	60 mg-1.5 g/day
rivastigmine tartrate	Exelon®	PO	1.5-6 mg b.i.d.
tacrine	Cognex®	PO	10 mg q.i.d.

Adverse Effects

Undesirable effects of cholinergic agonist drugs include flushing, sweating, abdominal cramps, difficulty in visual accommodation, headache, and convulsions (at high doses). Specific GI adverse effects include epigastric distress, diarrhea, involuntary defecation, nausea and vomiting, and colic. Other adverse effects are asthma and excessive salivary, nasopharyngeal, and bronchial secretions.

Contraindications and Precautions

Cholinergic agonist drugs are contraindicated in patients with known hypersensitivity to these agents: hypertension, coronary insufficiency, **pheochromocytoma** (benign tumor of adrenal medulla that increases production of epinephrine and norepinephrine), hyperthyroidism, asthma, and peptic ulcer.

Muscarinic drugs should be used cautiously in patients with hypertension, coronary disease, asthma, and hyperthyroidism.

Drug Interactions

Procainamide, quinidine, atropine, and epinephrine antagonize the effects of bethanechol. Beta-adrenergic agonists may cause conduction disturbances that may have additive effects with cholinergic drugs.

Neostigmine antagonizes effects of tubocurarine, atracurium, procainamide, quinidine, and atropine. Physostigmine may antagonize effects of echothiophate and isoflurophate.

Parasympatholytics (Anticholinergics or Cholinergic Blockers)

All parasympathetic effectors, some sympathetic effectors, all autonomic ganglia, and voluntary muscles bear cholinergic receptors. As a consequence, cholinergic drugs may affect the function of both divisions of the autonomic nervous system. Anticholinergic drugs are shown in Table 6-6.

Mechanism of Action

Cholinergic blockers act by selectively blocking all muscarine responses to acetylcholine, whether excitatory or inhibitory. Cholinergic blockers depress the CNS and relieve rigidity and tremor of Parkinson's syndrome.

TABLE 6-6 Parasympatholytics (Anticholinergics or Cholinergic Blockers)

Generic Name	Trade Name	Route of Administration	Average Adult Dosage
atropine sulfate	Atropisol®, Isopto Atropine®	IV, IM, SC, Ophthalmic	IV/IM/SC: 0.4–0.6 mg 30-60 min before surgery; Ophthalmic: 1-2 drops t.i.d.
benztropine mesylate	Cogentin®	PO	0.5-6 mg/day
cyclopentolate	Cyclogyl®	Topical	1 drop of 1% solution in eye 40-50 min. before procedure, followed by 1 drop in 5 min.
dicyclomine hydrochloride	Bentyl®	PO, IM	PO: 20-40 mg q.i.d.; IM: 20 mg q.i.d.
glycopyrrolate	Robinul®	PO, IM, IV	PO: 1-2 mg t.i.d.; IM/IV: 0.1-0.2 mg as single dose t.i.d. or q.i.d.
ipratropium bromide	Atrovent®	Inhalation	2 inhalations of MDI q.i.d. at no less than 4h intervals
oxybutynin	Ditropan®	PO	5 mg b.i.d. or t.i.d.
propantheline	Pro-Banthine®	PO	15 mg 30 min. a.c. and 30 mg h.s.
scopolamine	Hyoscine®, Transderm-Scop®	PO, IM, IV, SC	PO: 0.5-1 mg; IM/IV/SC: 0.3-0.6 mg
tiotropium bromide	Spiriva®	Inhalation	Inhale the contents of one capsule daily using hand inhaler device provided

Antisecretory action of cholinergic blockers includes suppression of sweating, lacrimation, salivation, and secretions from the nose, mouth, and bronchi.

Indications

Cholinergic blockers are used as adjuncts in the symptomatic treatment of GI disorders (i.e., peptic ulcer, pylorospasm, GI hypermotility, irritable bowel syndrome, and spastic disorders of the biliary tract). Cholinergic blockers are prescribed to produce mydriasis, **cycloplegia** (paralysis of the ciliary muscles of the eye) before refraction, and for the treatment of anterior **uveitis** (inflammation of the middle layer of the eye) and **iritis** (inflammation of the iris). These agents are also used in general anesthesia, bradycardia, or asystole during CPR.

Adverse Effects

The main adverse effects of cholinergic blockers include headache, ataxia, dizziness, excitement, irritability, convulsions, drowsiness, fatigue, weakness, mental depression, confusion, disorientation, hallucinations, hypertension or hypotension, ventricular fibrillation, inability to swallow, difficulty passing urine, skin eruption, and loss of power in the ciliary muscles of the eye.

Contraindications and Precautions

Cholinergic blockers are contraindicated in patients with hypersensitivity to belladonna alkaloids, syenchiae, angle-closure glaucoma, parotitis, obstructive uropathy, intestinal atony, paralytic ileus, obstructive GI tract diseases, severe ulcerative colitis, toxic megacolon, tachycardia, acute hemorrhage, or myasthenia gravis. Safety during pregnancy (category C) or lactation is not established.

Cholinergic blockers are used with caution in patients with myocardial infarction, hypertension or hypotension, coronary artery disease, congestive heart failure (CHF), and irregular heart rhythms. Other conditions wherein cholinergic blockers should be used cautiously include: gastric ulcer, GI infections, hiatal hernia with reflux esophagitis, hyperthyroidism, chronic lung disease, and hepatic or renal disease. These blockers should be used cautiously in the following types of patients: older adults, debilitated patients, children under the age of 6 years, Down syndrome patients, those with autonomic neuropathy or spastic paralysis, children with brain damage, those exposed to high environmental temperatures, and in patients with fever.

Drug Interactions

Cholinergic blockers may interact with amantadine, antihistamines, tricyclic antidepressants, quinidine, and procainamide, which may add to the anticholinergic effects. The effects of levodopa are decreased with cholinergic blockers. Methotrimeprazine may precipitate extrapyramidal effects. The antipsychotic effects of phenothiazines are decreased due to decreased absorption.

Key Concept

Because the thermal regulatory system in elderly patients declines, hyperthermia is possible with anticholinergics. This happens because these drugs decrease sweating.

Summary

The portion of the PNS serving involuntary effectors is called the autonomic nervous system or ANS. The sympathetic and parasympathetic nervous systems are subdivisions of the ANS.

Three neurotransmitters play a role in the functions regulated by the autonomic nervous system: acetylcholine, norepinephrine, and epinephrine. Dopamine may also serve as a nervous system transmitter.

There are two basic types of receptors associated with the ANS: cholinergic receptors and adrenergic receptors. There are three major subtypes of cholinergic receptors, which are referred to as $nicotinic_N$, $nicotinic_M$, and muscarinic. There are four major subtypes of adrenergic receptors, which include $alpha_1$, $alpha_2$, $beta_1$, and $beta_2$.

Drugs that affect the ANS may be classified into four categories: sympathomimetics (adrenergic agonists), sympatholytics (adrenergic blockers), parasympathomimetics (cholinergic agonists), and parasympatholytics (anticholinergics).

Exploring the Web

Visit ***http://cvpharmacology.com***

- Click on the link "vasodilators." Research additional information on this drug class and the variations of drugs within this class. Record your findings to help further your understanding of the topics discussed in this chapter.

Visit ***www.anaesthetist.com***

- Click on the link "autonomic physiology." Read additional information about the autonomic nervous system to enhance your understanding of its functions.

Visit ***www.pharmacology2000.com***

- Click on the link "Chapter 4: Autonomic Introduction." Explore the discussions related to the autonomic nervous system and the drug classes that affect this system.

Review Questions

Multiple Choice

1. Dopamine, epinephrine, and isoproterenol are classified as which of the following types of drug?

A. sympatholytics
B. anticholinergics

C. adrenergics
D. cholinergic-blockers

2. Which of the following agents are used to treat patients with myasthenia gravis?
   A. sympathomimetics (adrenergics)
   B. sympatholytics (adrenergic blockers)
   C. parasympatholytics (anticholinergics)
   D. parasympathomimetics (cholinergics)
3. Propranolol, metoprolol, and atenolol are:
   A. parasympathomimetics
   B. adrenergic drugs
   C. anticholinergic drugs
   D. beta-adrenergic blocking drugs
4. Elderly patients receiving anticholinergic drugs should be monitored closely for which of the following adverse effects?
   A. hyperthermia
   B. diuresis
   C. bradycardia
   D. hypothermia
5. The ANS employs all of the following neurotransmitters, *except*:
   A. epinephrine
   B. serotonin
   C. norepinephrine
   D. acetylcholine
6. Sympathomimetic drugs are also known as:
   A. cholinergics
   B. anticholinergics
   C. adrenergics
   D. adrenergic blockers
7. Which of the following adrenergic receptor subtypes may cause mydriasis?
   A. $alpha_1$
   B. $alpha_2$
   C. $beta_1$
   D. $beta_2$
8. Dobutamine is used to treat cardiac decompensation because of its action as a(n):
   A. beta adrenergic
   B. adrenergic blocking agent
   C. anticholinergic
   D. cholinergic
9. Atenolol may best be described as a(n):
   A. $beta_2$-adrenergic blocker
   B. $alpha_1$-adrenergic blocker

C. $beta_1$-and $beta_2$-adrenergic blocker
D. $beta_1$-adrenergic blocker

10. Which of the following agents is indicated for the treatment of anterior uveitis and iritis?
A. timolol
B. atropine
C. nadolol
D. bethanechol

11. Which of the following drugs are contraindicated in patients with hypertension, asthma, hyperthyroidism, and peptic ulcer?
A. cholinergic agonists
B. anticholinergics
C. adrenergic blockers
D. adrenergic agonists

12. Which of the following describes pilocarpine?
A. direct-acting mydriatic agent
B. direct-acting miotic agent
C. reduces the delivery of catecholamine
D. stimulates alpha receptor sites

13. Which of the following agents is classified as a sympatholytic?
A. neostigmine (Prostigmin)
B. cevimeline (Evoxac)
C. pilocarpine (Isopto Carpine)
D. prazosin (Minipress)

14. Which of the following statements is true of scopolamine?
A. it is an anticholinergic
B. it is an anticoagulant
C. it is a thrombolytic agent
D. it is an adrenergic blocker

15. Which of the following agents is used prior to anesthesia?
A. scopolamine
B. cyclopentolate
C. atropine
D. oxybutynin

True or False

_____ 1. All of the adverse effects caused by $alpha_1$ activation result in vasoconstriction.

_____ 2. Sympathomimetics are also called adrenergic blockers.

_____ 3. Adrenergic blockers are used in the treatment of hypotension.

_____ 4. The sympathetic nervous system's responses are also called rest-and-digest responses.

_____ **5.** Norepinephrine is released by all postganglionic neurons of the sympathetic nervous system.

_____ **6.** Muscarinic cholinergics may cause miosis.

_____ **7.** Adrenergic agonist drugs may affect both alpha- and beta-receptors.

_____ **8.** Prostigmin is the trade name of neostigmine.

_____ **9.** All preganglionic neurons of the parasympathetic nervous system release acetylcholine.

_____ **10.** Acetylcholine is a major transmitter released by the adrenal medulla.

Critical Thinking

A 61-year-old man has been diagnosed with glaucoma. He has recently had abdominal surgery. He has developed postoperative adynamic intestinal ileus.

1. Which class of autonomic nervous system drugs is the best for glaucoma and postoperative adynamic intestinal ileus?
2. If the patient is taking the drug of choice for these two conditions, what would be the most common adverse effects?
3. If the patient has asthma and hyperthyroidism, can the drug of choice still be used?

CHAPTER 7

Drug Therapy for Parkinson's and Alzheimer's Diseases

OBJECTIVES

After completing this chapter, the reader should be able to:

1. Identify the most common degenerative diseases of the CNS.
2. Explain the cause of Parkinson's disease.
3. Classify the drugs that are used for the treatment of Parkinson's disease.
4. Describe the roles of dopamine and acetylcholine in Parkinson's disease.
5. Identify the characteristics of dopamine and levodopa.
6. Discuss the actions and adverse effects of dopaminergic drugs when used in the treatment of Parkinson's disease.
7. Discuss the actions and contraindications of cholinergic blocker drugs when used in the treatment of Parkinson's disease.
8. Identify the characteristics of Alzheimer's disease.
9. Explain the role of acetylcholinesterase inhibitors in the treatment of Alzheimer's disease.

GLOSSARY

Alzheimer's disease – a disorder causing severe cognitive dysfunction in older persons in which the brain experiences atrophy (shrinkage) and exhibits senile plaques

Atrophy – wasting away or "without development"

Basal nuclei – clusters of nerve cells at the base of the brain; responsible for body movement and coordination

Bradykinesia – a decrease in spontaneity and movement, as seen in Parkinson's disease

Corpus striatum – a layer of nervous tissue within the brain

Encephalitis – inflammation of the brain's connective tissue framework

Parkinson's disease – a neurological syndrome usually resulting from deficiency of dopamine because of degenerative, vascular, or inflammatory changes in the basal ganglia

Substantia nigra – pigmented cells in the midbrain responsible for the production of dopamine

Tremor – repetitive, often regular, oscillatory movements caused by alternate, or synchronous, but irregular contraction of opposing muscle groups

OUTLINE

Overview

Degenerative diseases of the central nervous system (CNS) include Alzheimer's disease, multiple sclerosis, Huntington's chorea, and Parkinson's disease. In this chapter, focus will be on Parkinson's and Alzheimer's diseases, which are more common than other related diseases and affect millions of people (mostly elderly patients) in the United States.

Parkinson's Disease

Medical Terminology Review

bradykinesia
brady = slow
kinesia = ability of movement
slowing in the ability to move

Parkinson's disease is a progressive degenerative disorder affecting motor function through the loss of extrapyramidal activity. This disease is characterized by muscle **tremor**, muscle rigidity, and **bradykinesia**, and disturbances of posture and equilibrium are often present (see Figure 7-1).

According to the National Parkinson's Alliance, it is estimated that as many as 1.5 million Americans have Parkinson's disease. This disorder causes dysfunction and changes in the **basal nuclei** (clusters of nerve cells at the base of the brain), principally in the **substantia nigra** (pigmented cells in the midbrain responsible for the production of dopamine). In this condition, a decreased number of neurons in the brain secrete dopamine, an inhibitory neurotransmitter, leading to an imbalance between excitation and inhibition in the basal nuclei. The cause of the disease is not fully understood, but it is believed to be associated with an imbalance of the neurotransmitters acetylcholine and dopamine in the brain (see Figure 7-2).

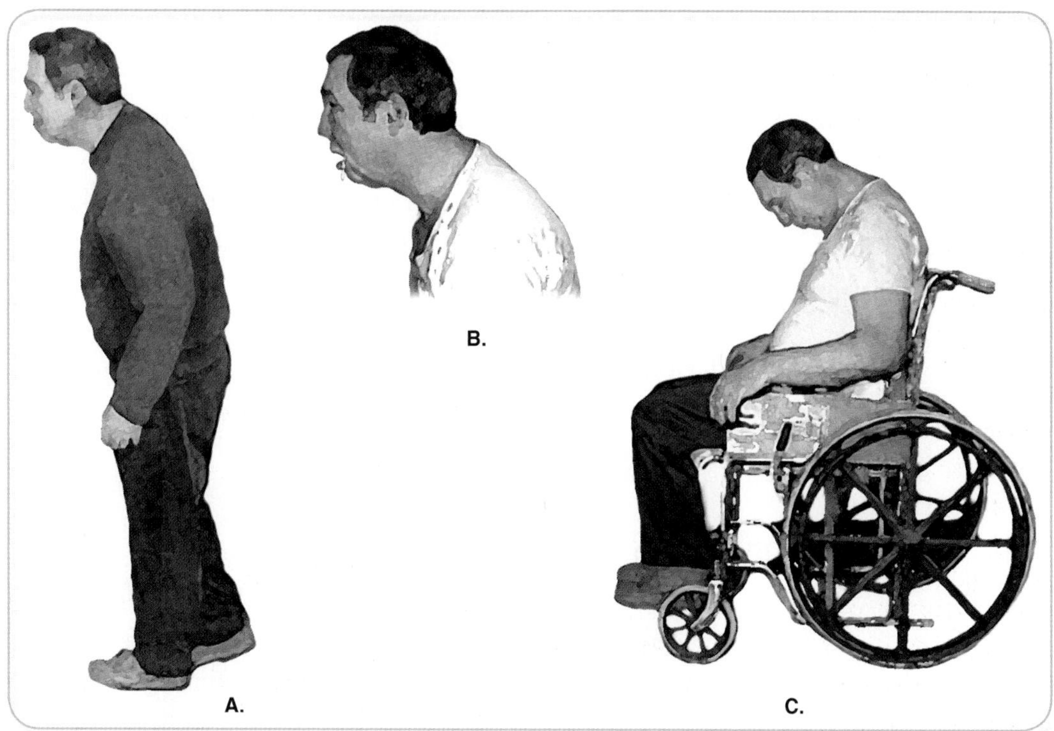

Figure 7-1 Parkinson's disease is characterized by a shuffling gait and early postural changes.

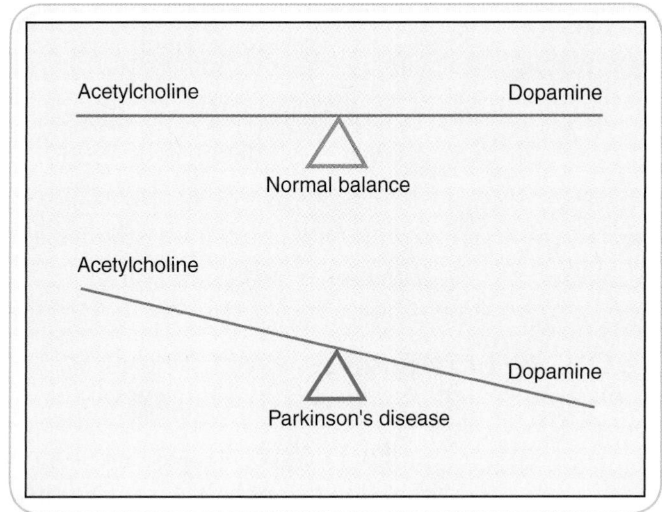

Figure 7-2 Dopamine imbalance exhibited in Parkinson's disease.

The excess stimulation affects movement and posture by increasing muscle tone and activity, leading to resting tremors, muscular rigidity, difficulty in initiating movement, and postural instability. Parkinson's disease usually develops after age 60 and occurs in both men and women. It may occur following **encephalitis**, trauma, or vascular disease. Drug-induced Parkinson's disease is particularly linked to use of phenothiazines (e.g., chlorpromazine). Pharmacotherapy is often successful in reducing some of the distressing symptoms of this disease.

> ***Medical Terminology Review***
>
> **encephalitis**
> *encephal = brain*
> *itis = inflammation*
> inflammation of the brain

Pharmacotherapy for Parkinson's Disease

Several drugs can be used for Parkinson's disease; the goal of drug therapy for this condition is to increase the ability of the patient to perform daily activities. Pharmacotherapy does not cure Parkinson's disease, but it can dramatically reduce symptoms in some patients.

Anti-parkinsonism drugs are administered to restore the balance of dopamine and acetylcholine in the **corpus striatum** (layers of nervous tissue in the brain). Dopaminergic drugs and anticholinergics (cholinergic blockers) are the mainstays of anti-parkinsonism (see Tables 7-1 and 7-2).

> ***Medical Terminology Review***
>
> **dopaminergic**
> *dopamin = dopamine*
> *ergic = related to*
> drugs affecting dopamine

Dopaminergic Drugs

The group of drugs classified as dopaminergic drugs are used to increase dopamine levels in the brain. Levodopa is the drug of choice for Parkinson's disease. Levodopa is a precursor of dopamine formation and stimulates this process.

TABLE 7-1 Dopaminergic Drugs for Parkinsonism

Generic Name	Trade Name	Route of Administration	Average Adult Dosage
amantadine hydrochloride	Symmetrel®	PO	200 mg/day or 100 b.i.d.
bromocriptine mesylate	Parlodel®	PO	1.25–2.5 mg/day (max: 7.5 mg/day in div. doses)
carbidopa-levodopa	Sinemet®	PO	1 tablet of 10 mg carbidopa/ 100 mg levodopa, or 25 mg carbidopa/100 mg levodopa t.i.d. (max: 6 tablets/day)
levodopa	Larodopa®	PO	500 mg–1 g/day, may be increased by 750 mg q3–7 days
pergolide mesylate	Permax®	PO	Start with 0.05 mg/day for 2 days, increase by 0.1–0.15 mg/day q3 days for 12 days, then increase by 0.25 mg every third day (max: 5 mg/day)
pramipexole	Mirapex®	PO	Start with 0.125 mg t.i.d. for 1 week; double dose for the next week, increasing by 0.25 mg/dose t.i.d. q week to a max dose of 1.5 mg t.i.d.
ropinirole hydrochloride	Requip®	PO	Start with 0.25 mg t.i.d., increasing by 0.25 mg/dose t.i.d. q week to a max dose of 1 mg t.i.d.
selegiline hydrochloride	Carbex®, Eldepryl®	PO	5 mg/dose b.i.d. – Note: doses greater than 10 mg/day are potentially toxic
tolcapone	Tasmar®	PO	100 mg t.i.d. (max: 600 mg/day)

TABLE 7-2 Anticholinergic Drugs for Parkinsonism

Generic Name	Trade Name	Route of Administration	Average Adult Dosage
benztropine mesylate	Cogentin®	PO	0.5–1 mg/day, increasing p.r.n. (max: 6 mg/day)
biperiden hydrochloride	Akineton®	PO	2 mg/day to q.i.d.
diphenhydramine hydrochloride	Benadryl®	PO	25–50 mg t.i.d.-q.i.d. (max: 300/day)
procyclidine hydrochloride	Kemadrin®	PO	2.5 mg t.i.d. pc; may increase to 5 mg t.i.d. if tolerated, with an additional 5 mg at bedtime (max: 45–60 mg/day)
trihexyphenidyl	Artane®, Trihexy®	PO	1 mg for day 1; doubled for day 2; increased by 2 mg q3–5 days up to 6–10 mg/day (max: 15 mg/day)

Mechanism of Action

Dopaminergic agents restore the neurotransmitter dopamine in the extrapyramidal region of the brain. Levodopa can cross the blood-brain barrier, but dopamine cannot. Therefore, dopamine by itself is not used for the treatment of Parkinson's disease. The mechanism of action of amantadine and selegiline in the treatment of Parkinsonism is not fully understood.

Indications

Levodopa is considered the drug of choice for Parkinson's disease. Either carbidopa is combined with levodopa, or they are prescribed as two separate drugs. Amantadine is less effective than levodopa as a drug therapy for Parkinson's disease, but more effective than the cholinergic blockers. Amantadine is given alone or in combination with another anti-parkinsonism drug with cholinergic activity. Amantadine is also indicated for drug therapy for viral disorders.

Adverse Effects

Adverse effects of levodopa include increased, uncontrollable rhythmic hand shaking or trembling, grinding of teeth (bruxism), muscle incoordination, numbness, fatigue, and headache. Levodopa may also cause upright position hypotension, tachycardia, hypertension, nausea, vomiting, dry mouth, bitter taste, and hepatotoxicity.

Adverse effects of bromocriptine include headache, dizziness, vertigo, fainting, sedation, nightmares, and insomnia. It may also produce blurred vision, hypertension, palpitation, arrhythmias, nausea, vomiting, and diarrhea. The most serious adverse effects of amantadine are orthostatic hypotension, congestive heart failure, depression, psychosis, convulsions, leukopenia, and urinary retention.

Medical Terminology Review

hepatotoxicity
hepato = liver
toxicity = state of being toxic or poisonous
liver poisoning

leukopenia
leuk/o = white
-penia = decrease in
decrease in white blood cells

Key Concept

Hallucinations occur commonly in older adults when taking dopamine receptor agonists.

Contraindications and Precautions

The dopaminergic drugs are contraindicated in patients with known hypersensitivity to these agents. Levodopa should be avoided in patients with narrow-angle glaucoma, those receiving an MAO inhibitor (MAOI) and during lactation.

Dopaminergic drugs are used with caution in patients with renal or hepatic disease, bronchial asthma, cardiovascular disease, and peptic ulcer. These agents should be used cautiously during pregnancy (category C) and lactation.

Key Concept

Patients taking levodopa should be monitored for orthostatic hypotension and cardiac arrhythmias, and also watched for psychiatric disturbances.

Drug Interactions

Levodopa increases therapeutic effects and possibility of a hypertensive crisis with MAOIs. Withdrawal of MAOIs is necessary at least 14 days before levodopa therapy is started. Levodopa exhibits decreased efficacy with pyridoxine (vitamin B_6) and phenytoin.

Key Concept

Patients taking levodopa should avoid foods and medications containing substantial amounts of pyridoxine (vitamin B_6).

Cholinergic Blockers

Cholinergic blockers, or anticholinergic drugs, are able to change the balance between dopamine and acetylcholine in the brain.

Mechanism of Action

Cholinergic blockers act by inhibiting excess cholinergic stimulation of neurons in the brain. Anticholinergic drugs inhibit acetylcholine in the central nervous system.

Indications

Cholinergic blockers are used as adjunctive therapy to relieve Parkinsonism symptoms and in the control of drug-induced disorders such as postural tremor and chorea.

Medical Terminology Review

dysuria
dys- = *difficult*
-uria = *characteristic of urine*
difficult urination

Adverse Effects

Cholinergic blockers produce dry mouth, blurred vision, sedation, dizziness, tachycardia, and constipation. Other adverse effects include urinary retention, dysuria, muscle weakness, confusion, disorientation, and skin rash.

Key Concept

Elderly people are very sensitive to anticholinergics, and these drugs must be used only when the patient can be carefully observed, because confusion and disorientation are often reported.

Contraindications and Precautions

Anticholinergic drugs are contraindicated in patients with known hypersensitivity to these agents. These drugs are also contraindicated in those with peptic ulcers, duodenal obstruction, glaucoma (angle-closure), prostatic hypertrophy, myasthenia gravis, and an extreme dilation of the large intestine.

Anticholinergic drugs should be used cautiously in patients with cardiac arrhythmias, hypertension, hypotension, and liver or kidney dysfunction.

Drug Interactions

Cholinergic blockers interact with many drugs. These agents should not be taken with alcohol, MAO inhibitors (MAOIs) tricycline, procainamide, phenothiazines, or quinidine because of combined sedative effects.

Alzheimer's Disease

Alzheimer's disease (senile disease complex) has been demonstrated to be one of the most common causes of severe cognitive dysfunction in older persons. Pathologically, the brain experiences **atrophy** (shrinkage) and exhibits senile plaques. The exact cause of Alzheimer's disease is unknown, but current theories include loss of neurotransmitter stimulation by choline acetyltransferase.

Alzheimer's disease is a devastating illness characterized by progressive memory failure, impaired thinking, confusion, disorientation, personality changes, restlessness, speech disturbances, and the inability to perform routine tasks. Unfortunately, the disease is incurable and, according to the American Health Assistance Foundation, affects about 350,000 new individuals per year in the United States. The current pharmacotherapy is focused on improving cognitive functioning or limiting the disease progression and controlling symptoms. In Alzheimer's disease, acetylcholine is decreased (this chemical substance is necessary for neurotransmission and for forming memories). There is no specific test for this disease; therefore, a definitive diagnosis is possible only upon autopsy.

Pharmacotherapy for Alzheimer's Disease

The FDA has approved only a few medications for Alzheimer's disease. Table 7-3 lists drugs used for the treatment of this disease. These agents are classified as acetylcholinesterase inhibitors.

Mechanism of Action

Acetylcholinesterase inhibitors are centrally acting agents, leading to elevated acetylcholine levels in the brain. Therefore, their action slows the neuronal degradation that occurs in Alzheimer's disease, and improves memory in cases of mild to moderate Alzheimer's dementia. Patients should receive pharmacotherapy for at least six months prior to assessing the maximum benefits of drug therapy.

Indications

Acetylcholinesterase inhibitors are used in the treatment of mild to moderate dementia of the Alzheimer's type.

TABLE 7-3 Drugs Used to Treat Alzheimer's Disease

Generic Name	Trade Name	Route of Administration	Average Adult Dosage
donepezil hydrochloride	Aricept®	PO	5–10 mg h.s.
galantamine hydrobromide	Razadyne®	PO	Start with 4 mg b.i.d. (at least 4 weeks); increase by 4 mg b.i.d. q4wk to 12 mg b.i.d. (max: 8–16 mg b.i.d.)
rivastigmine tartrate	Exelon®	PO	Start with 1.5 mg b.i.d. with food; increase by 1.5 mg b.i.d. q2wk if tolerated to 3–6 mg b.i.d. (max: 12 mg b.i.d.)
tacrine	Cognex®	PO	10 mg q.i.d.; increase in 40 mg/day increments q6wk (max: 160 mg/day)

Adverse Effects

There is a significant risk of liver damage from using tacrine, but increases in liver enzymes (which indicate damage) can be monitored with regular blood tests. Adverse effects of acetylcholinesterase inhibitors generally include nausea and vomiting, diarrhea, heartburn, muscle pain, and headache. Donepezil may cause darkened urine. Other adverse effects of acetylcholinesterase inhibitors include an inability to sleep, a sudden drop in blood pressure, depression, irritability, and headache.

Contraindications and Precautions

Key Concept

Ginkgo is a natural remedy, and one of the oldest known herbs in the world. Gingko extract is most commonly used in treating dementia. Adverse effects include gastrointestinal upset, muscle cramps, bleeding, and headache.

Acetylcholinesterase inhibitors are contraindicated in patients with known hypersensitivity to these agents. Acetylcholinesterase inhibitors are also contraindicated in patients with liver or kidney impairment, in pregnancy (category B), and lactation.

Acetylcholinesterase inhibitors should be used cautiously in patients with cardiac disorders, asthma, enlargement of the prostate, a history of seizures or GI bleeding, and renal or hepatic disease.

Drug Interactions

Donepezil and tacrine increase effects and risk of toxicity with theophylline and cholinesterase inhibitors. They decrease effects of anticholinergics and increase risk of GI bleeding with NSAIDs. Phenobarbital, phenytoin, dexamethasone, and rifampin may speed elimination of donepezil. Tacrine may prolong the action of succinylcholine.

Summary

Parkinson's and Alzheimer's diseases are among the most common degenerative diseases of the CNS. Multiple sclerosis and Huntington's chorea are other degenerative diseases. **Parkinson's** disease is a degenerative disorder of the CNS resulting in the death of neurons that produce dopamine. It affects over 1.5 million Americans. Parkinson's disease is primarily seen in patients over the age of 60, and occurs in both men and women.

The goal of drug therapy for Parkinson's disease is to increase the ability of the patient to perform daily activities. Anti-parkinsonism agents are given to restore the balance of dopamine and acetylcholine in the brain. Dopaminergic drugs and anticholinergics are the mainstays of anti-parkinsonism.

Alzheimer's disease is another degenerative disorder of the CNS, and is characterized by progressive memory failure, impaired thinking, confusion, disorientation, and speech disturbances. It is very common, and affects about 350,000 new individuals per year in the United States. In Alzheimer's disease, acetylcholine (which is necessary for forming memories) is decreased. Unfortunately, the disease is incurable. The FDA has approved only a few medications for Alzheimer's disease to reduce its symptoms. These drugs are known as acetylcholinesterase inhibitors.

Exploring the Web

Visit ***http://jaapa.com***

- Find the August 2006 issue, and read the article "Pharmacotherapy for Parkinson's Disease: Current Options, Promising Future Therapies."

Visit ***www.alz.org***

- Learn more about Alzheimer's disease and review information on treatments and research related to pharmacological therapies.

Visit ***www.nlm.nih.gov***

- Click on the link "Medline Plus". Search for additional information on Parkinson's disease and Alzheimer's disease.

Review Questions

Multiple Choice

1. Which of the following drugs may induce Parkinson's disease?

   A. pyridoxine (vitamin B_6)
   B. chlorpromazine
   C. dopamine
   D. levodopa

2. The mechanism of action of amantadine in the treatment of Parkinsonism is
   - A. to inhibit the effect of GABA
   - B. to prevent the production of dopamine
   - C. to inhibit the effect of acetylcholine
   - D. unknown
3. Which of the following agents is the drug of choice for Parkinson's disease?
   - A. levodopa
   - B. aspirin
   - C. amantadine
   - D. pyridoxine
4. Anticholinergic drugs are contraindicated in patients who have which of the following conditions?
   - A. Parkinsonism
   - B. glaucoma
   - C. hypocalcemia
   - D. cataracts
5. Dopaminergic drugs should be used cautiously during pregnancy because they are included in which of the following pregnancy categories?
   - A. D
   - B. C
   - C. B
   - D. A
6. Which of the following brain chemicals, necessary for forming memories, is decreased in Alzheimer's disease?
   - A. dopamine
   - B. epinephrine
   - C. melatonin
   - D. acetylcholine
7. Which of the following agents is used in Alzheimer's disease?
   - A. bromocriptine (Parlodel)
   - B. amantadine (Symmetrel)
   - C. tacrine (Cognex)
   - D. ropinirole (Requip)
8. The Alzheimer's patient is given tacrine. Which of the following adverse effects is a major consideration?
   - A. weight loss
   - B. liver toxicity
   - C. extrapyramidal side effects
   - D. myalgia
9. Cholinesterase inhibitors are used to treat which of the following conditions associated with Alzheimer's disease?
   - A. depression
   - B. dementia
   - C. urinary incontinence
   - D. peripheral paralysis

10. Which of the following is an adverse effect of gingko (an herbal substance used for Alzheimer's disease)?
    A. insomnia and dizziness
    B. tremors
    C. gastrointestinal upset and headache
    D. an inability to speak normally

Fill in the Blank

1. Parkinson's disease causes dysfunction and changes in the ______________ of the brain.
2. Parkinson's disease usually develops after age ______________.
3. Anti-parkinsonism drugs are given to restore the balance of dopamine and ______________.
4. Acetylcholinesterase inhibitors are used in the treatment of mild dementia for ______________.
5. Agents used for Alzheimer's disease are classified as ______________ inhibitors.
6. There is a significant risk of liver damage from using ______________, one of the acetylcholinesterase inhibitors.
7. Levodopa should be avoided in patients with ______________, those receiving an MAO inhibitor (MAOI), and during lactation.
8. Cholinergic blockers are used as adjunctive therapy to relieve ______________ symptoms.
9. Dopamine is a precursor of norepinephrine and ______________.
10. Patients taking levodopa should avoid foods and medications containing substantial amounts of vitamin ______________.
11. There is no specific test for ______________, and a definitive diagnosis is possible only upon autopsy.
12. Levodopa is considered the drug of choice for ______________.

Critical Thinking

A 72-year-old female is diagnosed with Parkinson's disease. In her past medical history, she has had chronic hepatitis C and hypertension.

1. Which drug is considered the drug of choice for Parkinson's disease?
2. With the history of hepatitis C, what precautions should be taken if the physician ordered this drug of choice?
3. If the patient is suffering from narrow-angle glaucoma, can this drug of choice still be used for this patient?

Drug Therapy for Seizures

CHAPTER 8

OUTLINE

OBJECTIVES

After completing this chapter, the reader should be able to:

1. Distinguish between partial and generalized seizures.
2. Classify generalized seizures.
3. Explain tonic-clonic (grand mal) seizure.
4. Discuss the most commonly used anti-seizure drugs.
5. Discuss indications and major adverse effects of phenytoin.
6. Explain the mechanism of action of succinimides and their indications.
7. Recognize major phenytoin-like drugs.
8. Discuss treatment of status epilepticus.
9. Explain the type of seizures which are common in children.
10. List the drugs that may increase the toxicity of valproic acid.

GLOSSARY

Absence seizure – generalized seizure that does not involve motor convulsions; also referred to as "petit mal"

Anticonvulsant – a drug that prevents or stops a convulsive seizure

Convulsions – abnormal motor movements

Electrical threshold – an individual's balance between excitatory and inhibitory forces in the brain; also known as "seizure threshold"

Epilepsy – condition characterized by periodic or recurrent seizures or convulsions

Generalized seizure – seizure originating and involving both cerebral hemispheres

Grand mal – generalized seizure characterized by full-body tonic and clonic motor convulsions

Partial seizure – seizure originating in one area of the brain that may spread to other areas

Seizure – abnormal discharge of brain neurons that causes alteration of behavior and/or motor activity

Status epilepticus – an emergency situation characterized by continual seizure activity with no interruptions (another term for seizure)

Tonic-clonic seizure – an alternate contraction (tonic phase) and relaxation (clonic phase) of muscles, a loss of consciousness, and abnormal behavior

Overview

Today, nearly 2.3 million people in the United States have been diagnosed with **epilepsy** (a disorder characterized by **seizures**) in one of its many forms, according to the National Institute of Neurological Disorders and Stroke (NINDS). Epilepsy is the old term for recurrent seizures, rarely used today because of the stigma once attached to patients suffering from this disorder. *Seizure* is a term for all epileptic events, while **convulsion** relates to abnormal motor movements. NINDS statistics report that 75% to 90% of seizure patients have their first seizure before age 20. Fortunately, scientific discoveries about how the brain works have enabled about 80% of those diagnosed with epilepsy to benefit from modern medicines, and implantable devices regulated by the FDA can help many patients to live productive lives. Anti-seizure drugs prevent or stop a convulsive seizure.

Classifications of Seizures

Seizures are a group of disorders that are characterized by hyperexcitability of neurons in the brain. The abnormal stimuli can produce many symptoms, from short periods of unconsciousness to violent convulsions. Seizures are usually brief, with a beginning and an end. The activity may be localized or generalized. Seizures may result acutely from any of a number of neurological disorders, as well as from metabolic disturbances, trauma, and exposure to certain toxins. Each seizure lasts for a few seconds or minutes, and the excessive activity of the neurons then ceases spontaneously. The altered pattern of electrical activity, or brain waves, during a seizure can be demonstrated on the electroencephalogram (EEG), indicating the type of seizure. Patients may experience post-seizure impairment.

Seizure disorders are classified by their location in the brain and their clinical features, including characteristic EEG patterns during and between seizures. The international classification of seizures is summarized in Table 8-1.

TABLE 8-1 Classifications of Seizures

Partial Seizures (focal)	Generalized Seizures
A. Simple	A. Tonic-clonic (grand mal)
1. Motor (includes Jacksonian)	B. Absence (petit mal)
2. Sensory (e.g., visual, auditory)	C. Myoclonic
3. Autonomic	D. Infantile spasms
4. Psychic	E. Atonic (akinetic)
B. Complex (impaired consciousness)	
1. Psychomotor	

Medical Terminology Review

encephalogram
electro = electronic
encephalo = brain
gram = x-ray
electronic x-ray of the brain

Key Concept

Absence seizures *(generalized seizures that do not involve motor convulsions; also referred to as "petit mal"), which are common in children, may decrease or be replaced by tonic-clonic or psychomotor seizures.*

This is a commonly accepted classification that incorporates current terminology and divides seizures into two basic categories: generalized and partial.

Generalized seizures have multiple foci that may cause loss of consciousness, whereas **partial seizures** have a single or focal origin, often in the cerebral cortex (Figure 8-1). Partial seizures may or may not involve altered consciousness. However, partial seizures may progress to generalized seizures. The terms *epilepsy*, *convulsions*, and *seizures* are commonly used interchangeably, although they each have a slightly different medical meaning.

Complications may arise from generalized **tonic-clonic (grand mal)** seizures that are severe and frequent. Injuries may occur during a seizure. Recurrent or continuous seizures without recovery of consciousness are termed **status epilepticus**. This condition may lead to serious consequences if not treated promptly, and it is always an emergency condition.

Anti-Seizure Drugs

Several major groups of medications are used to treat seizure disorders. The choice of medication varies according to individual patient conditions and physician preference. In treatment of epilepsy, it takes weeks to establish drug plasma levels and to determine the adequacy of therapeutic improvement. Usually the most effective drug with the least adverse effects is used initially. Drug treatment is not always necessary for the lifetime of the patient. Medications for seizures include barbiturates and benzodiazepines, which are the most useful **anticonvulsants** (drugs that stop a seizure). Other medications include hydantoins, phenytoin-like agents, and succinimides, which are detailed below.

Barbiturates

Barbiturates are chemical derivatives of barbituric acid. They are classified into four groups: ultra-short-acting, short-acting, intermediate-acting, and long-acting. They are also classified as either Schedule II or III medications. More than 2,500 barbiturates have been synthesized, but only about 50 have been approved for clinical use in the United States, and fewer than a dozen are commonly used. Barbiturates were discussed in detail in Chapter 5. Specific barbiturates used solely in the treatment of seizures are summarized in Table 8-2.

TABLE 8-2 Summary of Barbiturates Used in Seizure Disorders

Generic Name	Trade Name	Route of Administration	Average Adult Dosage
phenobarbital	Barbital®, Solfoton®	PO	50–100 mg b.i.d.-t.i.d.
phenobarbital sodium	Luminal®	IM, IV	30–320 mg; may repeat in 6 h

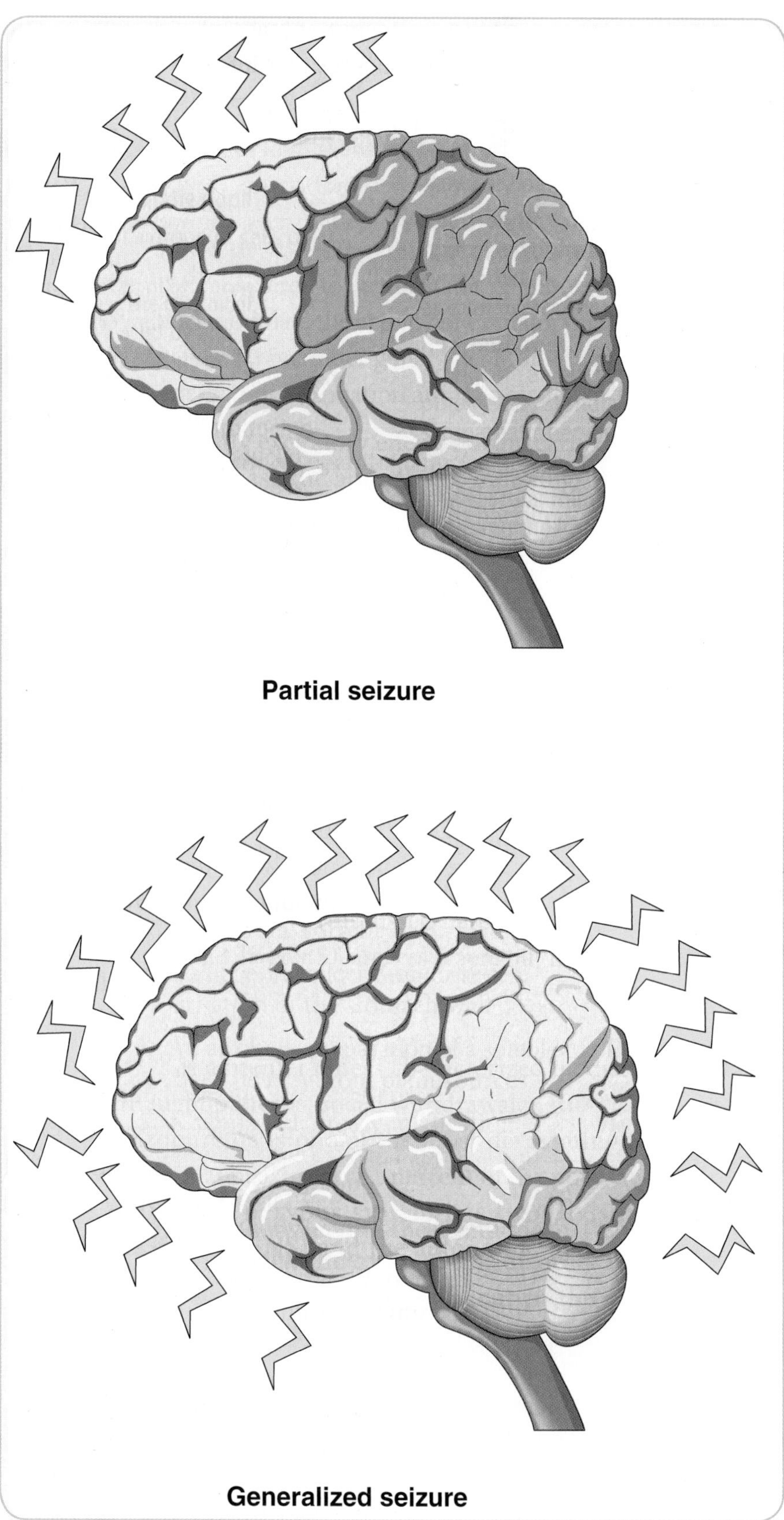

Figure 8-1 A partial seizure is characterized by chaotic firing occurring in one portion of the brain, while a generalized seizure is characterized by chaotic firing all over the brain.

TABLE 8-3 Benzodiazepines Used in Seizure Disorders

Generic Name	Trade Name	Indications	Average Adult Dosage
clonazepam	Klonopin®	Seizure disorders	0.5–1.5 mg/day in divided doses
clorazepate dipotassium	Tranxene®	Partial seizures	15–60 mg/day in divided doses
diazepam	Valium®	Status epilepticus	2–10 mg b.i.d. – q.i.d.

Benzodiazepines

Benzodiazepines are one of the most widely prescribed classes of drugs. They are used not only to control seizures but also for the treatment of anxiety, skeletal muscle spasms, and alcohol withdrawal symptoms. Benzodiazepines are drugs of choice to treat anxiety and are used for hypnosis because of their great margin of safety. Benzodiazepines were discussed in detail in Chapter 5. Specific benzodiazepines used in the treatment of seizures are listed in Table 8-3.

> ***Medical Terminology Review***
>
> **hypnosis**
> *hypno = sleep*
> *sis = condition*
> a sleep-like state

Hydantoins

The most recognizable and used drug in the hydantoin class is phenytoin, and fosphenytoin is the newest. Phenytoin is a potent broad-spectrum anti-seizure medication. Fosphenytoin is used parenterally when substitution for oral anti-seizure medications is necessary, such as after surgery (see Table 8-4).

> ***Key Concept***
>
> *Phenytoin is administered orally and fosphenytoin is administered intravenously.*

Mechanism of Action

Hydantoins act by desensitizing sodium channels in the CNS responsible for neuronal responsiveness. This desensitization prevents the spread of disruptive electrical charges in the brain that cause seizures.

> ***Medical Terminology Review***
>
> **hyperplasia**
> *hyper = over; above; beyond*
> *plasia = growth; development*
> overgrowth
>
> **hyperglycemia**
> *hyper = over; above; beyond*
> *glyc/o = sugar, sweet*
> *emia = blood condition*
> overproduction of sugar in the blood

Indications

Phenytoin is used for tonic-clonic seizures, psychomotor seizures, and seizures after head trauma. Fosphenytoin is converted to phenytoin in the body and is parenterally used for control of status epilepticus; it is a short-term substitute for oral phenytoin.

Adverse Effects

Adverse effects of phenytoin are related to plasma concentrations and include inability to coordinate muscle activity, mental confusion, dizziness, inability to sleep, headache, uncontrollable rhythmic movement of the eyes, gingival hyperplasia, toxic hepatitis, and reduction of the blood cells. Phenytoin may also cause dysrhythmias such as slow heart rate or ventricular fibrillation, abnormally low blood pressure, and hyperglycemia (excess blood glucose).

> ***Key Concept***
>
> *Gingival hyperplasia is one of the major adverse effects of long-term use of phenytoin (Dilantin). Patients who use this agent should be periodically examined for an excessive growth of gum tissue.*

TABLE 8-4 Hydantoins, Phenytoin-Like Drugs, and Succinimides

Generic Name	Trade Name	Route of Administration	Average Adult Dosage
Hydantoins			
fosphenytoin sodium	Cerebyx®	IV	Initial dose: 15–20 mg/kg at 100–150 mg/min, then 4–6 mg/kg/day
phenytoin sodium	Dilantin®	PO	15–18 mg/kg or 1 g initial dose, then 300 mg/day in 1–3 div. doses; may be gradually increased 100 mg/week
Phenytoin-Like Drugs			
carbamazepine	Tegretol®	PO	200 mg b.i.d., gradually increased to 800–1200 mg/day in 3–4 div. doses
felbamate	Felbatol®	PO	Initial: 1200 mg/day in 3–4 div. doses; may increase by 600 mg/day q2 weeks (max: 3600 mg/day)
lamotrigine	Lamictal®	PO	50 mg/day for 2 weeks, then 50 mg b.i.d. for 2 weeks; may increase gradually to 300–500 mg/day in 2 div. doses (max: 700 mg/day)
pregabalin	Lyrica®	PO	100 mg/day in 3 divided doses
primidone	Mysoline®	PO	Up to 500 mg q.i.d.
tiagabine hydrochloride	Gabitril®	PO	4–56 mg/day
topiramate	Topamax®	PO	200–400 mg/day in divided doses
valproic acid	Depakene® Depakote®	PO, IV	15 mg/kg/day in div. doses when total is >250 mg/day; increase 5–10 mg q week (max: 60 mg/kg/day)
zonisamide	Zonegran®	PO	100–600 mg/day
Succinimides			
ethosuximide	Zarontin®	PO	250 mg b.i.d., increased q4–7 days (max: 1.5 g/day)
methsuximide	Celontin®	PO	300 mg/day, may increase q4–7 days (max: 1.2 g/day in div. doses)

Contraindications and Precautions

Hydantoin products are contraindicated in patients with known hypersensitivity to these drugs. Hydantoin products are also contraindicated in patients with rash, seizures due to low blood glucose, pregnancy (category D), and lactation.

Hydantoin products should be used cautiously in older adults and in patients with impaired liver or kidney function, alcoholism, blood dyscrasias, hypotension, bradycardia, severe myocardial insufficiency, pancreatic adenoma, and diabetes mellitus.

Drug Interactions

Phenytoin has increased pharmacologic effects with chloramphenicol, cimetidine, isoniazid, and sulfonamides. Complex drug interactions and effects occur when phenytoin and valproic acid are given together. Severe hypotension may occur when phenytoin is given intravenously with dopamine. Alcohol decreases fosphenytoin effects. This drug may decrease absorption and increase metabolism of oral anticoagulants.

Phenytoin-Like Agents

Several commonly used drugs are classified as phenytoin-like drugs, including carbamazepine and valproic acid. Newer anti-seizure drugs, which have more limited uses, include zonisamide, felbamate, and lamotrigine, which are categorized as phenytoin-like drugs (see Table 8-4).

Mechanism of Action

In general, the mechanisms of action of phenytoin-like agents are not known, but resemble the mechanism of action of phenytoin.

Indications

Phenytoin-like drugs are useful for a wide range of seizure types, including absence seizures and mixed types of seizures. Valproic acid is used for prevention of migraine headaches and treatment of bipolar disorder.

Adverse Effects

Phenytoin-like drugs may result in adverse effects such as drowsiness, sedation, GI upsets, and prolonged bleeding time. Other adverse effects are visual disturbances, muscle weakness, bone marrow suppression, rash, fatal liver toxicity, weight gain, loss of hair, and abdominal pain.

Contraindications and Precautions

Phenytoin-like drugs are contraindicated in patients with known hypersensitivity to these agents, and in cardiac, hepatic, or renal disease. These drugs are also contraindicated in pregnancy (category D) and lactation. Carbamazepine should be used with caution in older adults and those with a history of cardiac disease. Valproic acid is used cautiously in patients with a history of kidney disease or renal impairment. This drug should be used with caution in patients with severe epilepsy and hypoalbuminemia.

Medical Terminology Review

hypoalbuminemia

hypo = *low; under; beneath*
albumin = *plasma protein*
emia = *blood condition*
low albumin in the blood plasma

Drug Interactions

Valproic acid interacts with many drugs. For example, chlorpromazine, felbamate, erythomycin, cimetidine, and aspirin may increase valproic acid toxicity. Lamotrigine, phenytoin, and rifampin lower valproic acid levels.

Succinimides

Succinimide drugs are another class of anti-convulsant drugs. Ethosuximide is generally considered to be the safest of the succinimide drugs, and is the most commonly prescribed drug in this class. The succinimide drugs are also listed in Table 8-4.

Mechanism of Action

Succinimides delay the entry of calcium into neurons by blocking calcium channels. Simply, anti-seizure drugs of this group increase the **electrical threshold**. Succinimides suppress the EEG pattern associated with lapses of consciousness in absence (petit mal) seizures. Its mechanism of action is not understood, but it may act to inhibit neuronal systems.

Medical Terminology Review

myocolonic
myo = muscle
clonic = contraction and relaxation
contraction and relaxation of the muscles

Indications

Succinimide drugs are used to control absence seizures and myoclonic seizures. They may be given in combination with other anticonvulsants.

Adverse Effects

Adverse effects of succinimides include ataxia, dizziness, nervousness, headache, and blurred vision. Behavioral changes are more prominent in patients with a history of psychiatric illness. Ethosuximide can also cause abnormal reduction of all circulating blood cells, vaginal bleeding, gingival hyperplasia, muscle weakness, and abnormal liver and kidney function tests.

Contraindications and Precautions

Succinimide drugs are contraindicated in patients with known hypersensitivity to these agents. Succinimides are also contraindicated in patients with bone marrow depression, or with hepatic or renal dysfunction. Ethosuximide should be used cautiously in pregnancy (category C) and lactation.

Key Concept

The FDA approved a deep brain stimulator in 1997. This implanted device delivers electrical stimulations to the brain to reduce seizures in people who do not respond well to medication.

Serious injury or death can occur in patients with implanted neurologic stimulators who undergo magnetic resonance imaging (MRI) procedures.

Drug Interactions

Drug interactions include ethosuximide, which increases phenytoin serum levels. Valproic acid causes ethosuximide serum levels to fluctuate (decrease or increase).

Summary

Seizures are a group of disorders that are characterized by hyperexcitability of neurons in the brain. Nearly 2.3 million people in the United States have seizure disorders. *Seizure* is a term for all epileptic events, while *convulsion* relates to abnormal motor movements.

Seizure disorders are classified into two basic categories: generalized and partial. Generalized seizures include tonic-clonic (grand mal), absence (petit mal), myoclonic, infantile spasms, and atonic (akinetic). Partial seizures (focal) may be divided into two categories: simple or complex (psychomotor).

Anti-seizure drugs are classified into five groups, which include: barbiturates, benzodiazepines, hydantoins, phenytoin-like agents, and succinimides. Phenytoin is the most recognizable and most used drug in the class of hydantoins. The newest drug in this class is fosphenytoin. Phenytoin is used for tonic-clonic and psychomotor seizures. Fosphenytoin is used for control of status epilepticus. Phenytoin-like drugs are useful for a wide range of seizure types, including absence seizures and mixed types of seizures.

Exploring the Web

Visit ***http://professionals.epilepsy.com***

- Under the heading diagnosis and treatment, look for additional information on drug therapies used to treat epilepsy.

Visit ***www.brainexplorer.org***

- Click on the link to "focus on brain disorders," then click on the link to epilepsy. Read more about this disorder and how the brain is affected.

Visit ***www.coolnurse.com***

- Search for "benzodiazepines" or "seizures" review for additional information on these topics.

Visit ***www.emedicine.com***

- Click on the specialty of neurology, then click on the link "seizures and epilepsy." Choose articles related to this topic to read for a greater understanding of the disorder and methods used to treat it.

Visit ***www.mayoclinic.com***

- Under Diseases and Condition center click on "nervous system" and then "seizures." Review the additional information available on this topic.

Visit *www.nlm.nih.gov*

- Click on Medline Plus and search for information related to seizures and epilepsy.

Review Questions

Multiple Choice

1. Which of the following adverse effects can be caused by ethosuximide (Zarontin)?
   A. tremors
   B. depression
   C. gingival hyperplasia
   D. hyperplasia of the prostate
2. Which of the following seizures is characterized by alternating contractions and relaxation of the muscles?
   A. febrile
   B. absence
   C. psychomotor
   D. tonic-clonic
3. Which of the following anti-seizure drugs increases phenytoin serum levels?
   A. carbamazepine (Tegretol)
   B. valproic acid (Depakene)
   C. ethosuximide (Zarontin)
   D. felbamate (Felbatol)
4. Which of the following seizures is classified as a simple seizure?
   A. infantile spasms
   B. absence (petit mal)
   C. psychic
   D. tonic-clonic (grand mal)
5. Which of the following seizures is the most dangerous, and requires prompt treatment?
   A. status epilepticus
   B. Jacksonian
   C. psychomotor
   D. absence
6. The newest drugs in the group of hydantoins is:
   A. phenytoin (Dilantin)
   B. fosphenytoin (Cerebyx)
   C. felbamate (Felbatol)
   D. valproic acid (Depakene)

7. Most anti-seizure drugs should be used cautiously in pregnancy because they are in which of the following categories?
   A. A
   B. B
   C. C
   D. D

8. Which of the following is the trade name for ethosuximide?
   A. Milontin
   B. Celontin
   C. Zarontin
   D. Zonegran

9. A specific barbiturate used solely in the treatment of seizures is known as:
   A. clonazepam
   B. clorazepate
   C. phenobarbital
   D. diazepam

10. Which of the following hydantoins is used for tonic-clonic, psychomotor, and head trauma–related seizures?
    A. carbamazepine
    B. phenytoin
    C. valproic acid
    D. fosphenytoin

11. Diazepam (Valium) is indicated for which type of seizure disorder?
    A. partial
    B. tonic-clonic
    C. absence
    D. status epilepticus

12. The most recognizable and most used drug in the category of hydantoins is:
    A. ethosuximide
    B. valproic acid
    C. phenytoin
    D. carbamazepine

13. Ethosuximide delays the entry of which of the following minerals into neurons by blocking its channels?
    A. calcium
    B. sodium
    C. potassium
    D. chloride

14. Which of the following agents is the drug of choice for absence seizures?
    A. valproic acid (Depakene)
    B. ethosuximide (Zarontin)
    C. felbamate (Felbatol)
    D. phenytoin (Dilantin)

15. Which of the following agents is the trade name of primidone?
    A. Gabitril
    B. Mysoline
    C. Lyrica
    D. Topamax

Fill in the Blank

1. The trade name of valproic acid is ______________.
2. The choice of drugs to treat seizure disorders depends on patient conditions and ______________ preference.
3. Tonic-clonic seizures are classified as ______________ seizures.
4. An example of a complex seizure which impairs consciousness is a ______________ seizure.
5. Fosphenytoin is the newest drug of the hydantoin group and is converted to ______________ in the body.
6. Absence seizures are also known as ______________.
7. Examples of phenytoin-like drugs include: carbamazepine, felbamate, lamotrigine, ______________, and ______________.

Critical Thinking

A 36-year-old female has been suffering from migraine headaches for almost two years. Her physician orders an anti-seizure, phenytoin-like medication for prevention of migraines.

1. Can you name which of the phenytoin-like drugs is used for the prevention of migraines?
2. If this patient were suffering from absence seizures, what phenytoin-like drugs may be prescribed?
3. If this patient is taking phenytoin-like drugs, name the most dangerous adverse effects.

Anesthetic Drugs

CHAPTER

9

OUTLINE

OBJECTIVES

After completing this chapter, the reader should be able to:

1. List the stages of anesthesia.
2. Define the importance of preanesthesia.
3. Outline the effects of general anesthetics.
4. Explain the mechanism of action of local anesthetics.
5. List the problems associated with the use of local anesthetics.
6. Describe the common local anesthetics and their uses.
7. Compare and contrast the five major routes for administering local anesthetics.
8. Define malignant hyperthermia.
9. Explain a malignant hyperthermia kit.
10. Define balanced anesthesia.

GLOSSARY

Anesthesia – a loss of feeling or sensation

Anesthetic – an agent that partially or completely numbs or eliminates sensitivity with or without loss of consciousness

Epidural anesthesia – injection of an anesthetic into the space immediately outside of the dura mater that contains a supporting cushion of fat and other connective tissues

General anesthesia – provision of a pain-free state for the entire body

Hypermetabolic – burning energy and nutrients at a higher rate than normal

Local anesthesia – provision of a pain-free state in a specific area of the body

Infiltration anesthesia – anesthesia produced by injecting a local anesthetic drug into tissues

Lipophilic – able to dissolve much more easily in lipids than in water

Malignant hyperthermia – a rare, genetic hypermetabolic condition that is characterized by severe overproduction of body heat with rigidity of skeletal muscles

Nystagmus – rhythmical oscillation of the eyeballs

Preanesthetic medications – drugs given before the administration of anesthesia

Spinal anesthesia – a type of regional anesthesia produced by injecting a local anesthetic drug into the subarachnoid space of the spinal cord

Volatile liquids – liquids that evaporate upon exposure to the air

Overview

For several centuries, opiates and alcohol were the mainstays of **anesthetics** (substances used to reduce sensation of pain) in the control of pain. These substances had limited success, but were probably better than nothing. It was not until the 1840s that surgical **anesthesia** (reduction or elimination of pain) became possible, with the introduction of three agents: chloroform, ether, and nitrous oxide. These three substances, upon inhalation, quickly lead to a state of unconsciousness in which pain is not felt. Nitrous oxide is still one of the most widely used gaseous anesthetics, and diethyl ether is still occasionally used. Chloroform is rarely used today because of its toxicity, but other, newer halogenated hydrocarbons, such as halothane, are extremely common.

Gaseous anesthetics are the principal agents used in the maintenance of anesthesia, but agents given by other routes are still used in the induction of anesthesia. Anesthesia is basically characterized by four reversible actions: unconsciousness, analgesia, immobility, and amnesia. The critical factor is that there should be no significant impairment of cardiovascular or respiratory functions, especially those supplying the brain and other vital organs with adequate blood, nutrients, and gases.

Medical Terminology Review

epidural

epi = on; upon; at; near; among
dural = dura mater; the outermost layer of the meninges
near the outermost layer of the meninges

General anesthetics are used to produce loss of consciousness before and during surgery. **Local anesthetics** numb small areas of the body tissue where a minor procedure is to be done, and are commonly used in dentistry for minor surgery. Regional anesthesia affects a larger (but still limited) part of the body, but does not make the person unconscious. Spinal and epidural anesthesia are examples of regional anesthesia.

Preanesthetic Medications

Preanesthetic medications are used prior to the administration of an anesthetic to facilitate induction of anesthesia and to relieve anxiety and pain. They may also be used to minimize some of the undesirable effects of anesthetics, such as excessive salivation, bradycardia, and vomiting.

Key Concept

Preanesthetic drugs may not be used in patients over 60 years of age because many of the medical conditions or disorders for which these drugs are contraindicated occur in this age group.

To accomplish these objectives, several drugs are often used at the same time. The following medications are commonly used as preoperative drugs:

- Sedative-hypnotics such as hydroxyzine, promethazine (Chapter 5)
- Antianxiety agents such as diazepam, droperidol (Chapter 5)
- Opioid analgesics such as morphine, meperidine, fentanyl (Chapter 21)
- Anticholinergics such as atropine, scopolamine (Chapter 6)

Stages and Planes of Anesthesia

Before patients reach surgical anesthesia, they go through several stages. The use of these stages and planes of anesthesia helps to describe the levels and progression of anesthesia produced by anesthetics. There are four stages of general anesthesia:

Stage I: This stage begins when the agent is administered and lasts until loss of consciousness. Stage I is characterized by:

- Analgesia
- Euphoria
- Perceptual distortions
- Amnesia

Stage II: Delirium begins with loss of consciousness and extends to the beginning of surgical anesthesia. There may be excitement and involuntary muscular activity. The skeletal muscle tone increases and breathing is irregular. At this stage, hypertension and tachycardia may occur. It is important that the passage from Stage I to Stage III be attained as quickly as possible. Sudden death can occur during Stage II.

Stage III: Surgical anesthesia lasts until spontaneous respiration ceases. It is further divided into four planes based on:

- Respiration
- The size of the pupils
- Reflex characteristics
- Eyeball movements

This stage is characterized by progressive muscular relaxation. Muscle relaxation is important during many surgical procedures as reflex movements can occur when a scalpel slices through the tissues.

Key Concept

In the induction of anesthesia with intravenous anesthetic agents, Stages I and III merge so quickly into one another that they are not apparent.

Stage IV: Medullary paralysis begins with respiratory failure and can lead to circulatory collapse. Through careful monitoring, this stage is avoided.

General Anesthetics

General anesthetics are drugs that immediately produce unconsciousness and complete analgesia. These agents are generally administered by intravenous or inhalation routes. Preanesthetic and adjunct drugs are given before, during, and after surgery.

Inhalation Anesthetics

Certain drugs that are gases or **volatile liquids** at room temperature are administered by inhalation in combination with air or oxygen. The only gas used routinely for anesthesia is nitrous oxide, commonly called laughing gas. It is usually administered in combination with oxygen. Nitrous oxide provides analgesia equivalent to 10 mg of morphine sulfate but may cause occasional episodes of nausea and vomiting. Volatile liquids are converted into a vapor and inhaled to produce their anesthetic effects. Commonly administered volatile agents are halothane, enflurane, and isoflurane. The most potent of these is halothane (see Table 9-1).

Medical Terminology Review

lipophilic
lipo = lipids (fats)
philic = having an affinity for
having an affinity for fats

Mechanism of Action

Inhaled general anesthetics are all very **lipophilic** (able to dissolve much more easily in lipids than in water). When the lipophilic anesthetic enters the lipid membrane, the whole membrane is slightly distorted and closes

TABLE 9-1 Inhaled General Anesthetics

Generic Name	Trade Name	Uses
Gas		
nitrous oxide	(generic only)	Used alone in dentistry, obstetrics, and short medical procedures Used in combination with more potent inhaled anesthetics
Volatile Liquids		
desflurane	Suprane®	Induction and maintenance of general anesthesia
enflurane	Ethrane®	Induction and maintenance of general anesthesia
halothane	Fluothane®	Induction and maintenance of general anesthesia; since safer agents have become available, its use has declined
isoflurane	Forane®	Induction and maintenance of general anesthesia; it is the most widely used inhalation anesthetic
methoxyflurane	Penthrane®	Used during labor; it does not suppress uterine contractions as greatly as other agents
sevoflurane	Ultane®	Induction and maintenance of general anesthesia

the sodium channels, causing a marginal blockage, which prevents neural conduction.

Indications

Volatile anesthetics are rarely used as the sole agents for both induction and maintenance of anesthesia. Most commonly, they are combined with intravenous agents in regimens of so-called balanced anesthesia. Of the inhaled anesthetics, nitrous oxide, desflurane, and sevoflurane are the most commonly used in the United States.

Adverse Effects

Nitrous oxide at higher doses causes anxiety, excitement, and aggressiveness. It also produces nausea, vomiting, and difficulty in breathing. Volatile anesthetics may cause headache, shivering, muscle pain, mental or mood changes, sore throat, and nightmares.

Contraindications and Precautions

Inhaled general anesthetics are contraindicated in patients with known hypersensitivity to these agents. They are also contraindicated in patients who have received monoamine oxidase inhibitors (MAOIs) within the previous 14 days (refer to Chapter 4). They should not be used by those who are intolerant to benzodiazepines, or have myasthenia gravis, acute narrow-angle glaucoma, acute alcohol intoxication, status asthmaticus, and acute intermittent porphyria.

Inhaled general anesthetics should be used cautiously during pregnancy, and in children younger than 12.

Drug Interactions

Inhaled general anesthetic drugs may interact with levodopa and increase the level of dopamine in the CNS. Skeletal muscle weakness, respiratory depression, or apnea may occur if halothane is administered with polymyxins, lincomycin, or aminoglycosides.

Injectable General Anesthetics

Intravenous anesthetics are often administered with inhaled general anesthetics. Administration of intravenous and inhaled anesthetics together allows the dose of the inhaled drug to be reduced, resulting in a decreased probability of serious side effects. They also provide more analgesia and muscle relaxation than is provided by an inhaled anesthetic alone. Drugs used as intravenous anesthetics include opioids, barbiturates, and benzodiazepines (see Table 9-2).

TABLE 9-2 Intravenous Anesthetics

Generic Name	Trade Name	Comments
Barbiturates and Barbiturate-Like Agents		
etomidate	Amidate®	For induction of anesthesia and for short medical procedures
methohexital sodium	Brevital®	Ultra–short-acting; for induction of anesthesia and as a supplement to other anesthetics
propofol	Diprivan®	For induction and maintenance of general anesthesia, and for short medical procedures
thiopental sodium	Pentothal®	Ultra–short-acting; for induction of anesthesia and as a supplement to other anesthetics
Benzodiazepines		
diazepam	Valium®	For induction of anesthesia; the prototype benzodiazepine
lorazepam	Ativan®	For induction of anesthesia, to produce conscious sedation, and for short medical procedures or surgery
midazolam hydrochloride	Versed®	For induction of anesthesia; to produce conscious sedation, and for short diagnostic procedures
Opioids		
alfentanil hydrochloride	Alfenta®	Rapid onset and short onset of action; for induction of anesthesia; used as a supplement to other anesthetics
fentanyl citrate	Sublimaze®, others	Short-acting; used during operative and perioperative periods; to supplement both general and regional anesthesia
remifentanil hydrochloride	Ultiva®	Short-acting; for induction and maintenance of general anesthesia
sufentanil citrate	Sufenta®	For induction and maintenance of anesthesia; approximately 7 times as potent as fentanyl with more rapid onset and duration of action
Others		
ketamine hydrochloride	Ketalar®	For sedation, amnesia, analgesia in short diagnostic, therapeutic, or surgical procedures; most often used in children

LOCAL ANESTHETICS

Local anesthetics are drugs that block the transmission of nerve impulses between the peripheral nervous system and the central nervous system. Their main purpose is to prevent pain impulses from pain receptors reaching the higher centers. They are mainly used in minor surgical procedures and are especially common in dentistry. Many minor surgical procedures such as suturing, excision of superficial growths, and removal of cataracts are commonly performed using a local anesthetic injected intradermally or subcutaneously. Even deeper-excision operations such as hernias are performed occasionally using local anesthetics. Local anesthesia is more accurately called surface anesthesia or regional anesthesia.

Classification of Local Anesthetics

The two major groups of local anesthetics are esters and amides (see Table 9-3). The ester-type anesthetics, represented by procaine, contain an

TABLE 9-3 Common Local Anesthetics

Generic Name	Trade Name	Use	Comments
Esters			
benzocaine	Americaine®, Solarcaine®	Topical	For earache, hemorrhoids, sore throat, sunburn, and minor skin conditions
chloroprocaine	Nesacaine®	Epidural, infiltration, and nerve block	Short duration
cocaine	(generic only)	Topical	For ear, nose, and throat procedures
procaine hydrochloride	Novocain®	Epidural, infiltration, nerve block, and spinal	Short duration
tetracaine	Pontocaine®	Spinal and topical	Long duration
Amides			
bupivacaine hydrochloride	Marcaine®	Epidural and infiltration	Long duration
dibucaine	Nupercainal®	Spinal and topical	Long duration
etidocaine hydrochloride	Duranest®	Epidural, infiltration, and nerve block	Long duration
lidocaine hydrochloride	Xylocaine®	Epidural, infiltration, nerve block, spinal, and topical	May be combined with prilocaine (EMLA cream) for topical application
mepivacaine	Carbocaine®	Epidural, infiltration, and nerve block	Intermediate duration
prilocaine	Citanest®	Epidural, infiltration, and nerve block	Intermediate duration
ropivacaine	Naropin®	Epidural, infiltration, and nerve block	Long duration
Miscellaneous Agents			
dyclonine	Dyclone®	Topical	For ear, nose, and throat procedures
pramoxine	Tronolane®	Topical	For minor medical procedures

ester linkage in their chemical structure. In contrast, the amide-type drugs, represented by lidocaine, contain an amide linkage.

The amides have several advantages over the esters. Hypersensitivity to amide local anesthetics is rare. Most of the local anesthetics in common use today belong to the amide class.

Ester-type local anesthetics have been in use longer than amides. They tend to have a rapid onset and short duration of activity (except tetracaine). Esters are associated with a higher incidence of allergic reactions due to one of their metabolites, para-amino benzoic acid (PABA). PABA is structurally similar to methylparaben.

Mechanism of Action

Local anesthetics stop nerve conduction by inhibiting movement of sodium through channels in the membrane of a neuron. Therefore, neurons cannot fire because these agents block sodium channels.

Medical Terminology Review

endoscopy
endo = inside
scopy = looking
procedure for looking inside the body

Indications

Local anesthetics are used for minor surgery, dental procedures, suturing small wounds, or making an incision into a small area for removing a superficial tissue sample for biopsy. Local anesthetics may also be used for obstetrics during labor and delivery, for diagnostic procedures such as gastrointestinal endoscopy, wart treatment, vasectomy, and neonatal circumcision.

Adverse Effects

True allergic reactions to local anesthetics are rare, and usually involve ester agents. Toxic effects are usually dose-related. Adverse effects include restlessness, dizziness, disorientation, light-headedness, **nystagmus** (rhythmical oscillation of the eyeballs), and psychosis. Slurred speech and tremors often precede seizures. Slower-than-normal heart rate, an abnormally low blood pressure, and cardiac arrest may occur.

Contraindications and Precautions

Local anesthetics are contraindicated in patients with known hypersensitivity, in the elderly, severe hemorrhage, hypotension, and shock. These agents are also contraindicated in patients with cerebrospinal deformities, blood dyscrasias, and hypertension.

Drug Interactions

Barbiturates may decrease activity of lidocaine. Increased effects of lidocaine may occur if taken with beta blockers, cimetidine, and quinidine. If lidocaine is used on a regular basis, its effectiveness may diminish when used with other medications.

Routes of Administration of Local Anesthetics

There are five major routes for applying local anesthetics (see Figure 9-1). These routes are summarized as follows:

1. Topical
2. Nerve block
3. Infiltration
4. Spinal
5. Epidural

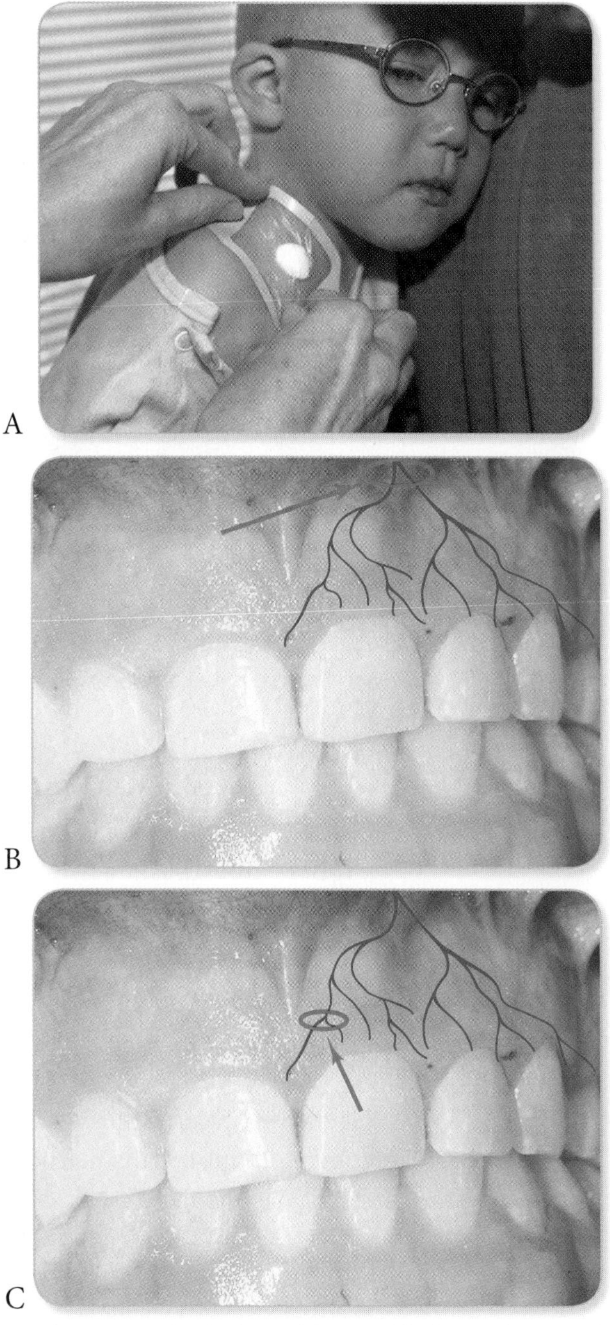

Figure 9-1 (A) Tegaderm topical anesthetic (B) nerve block anesthesia (C) local infiltration anesthesia.

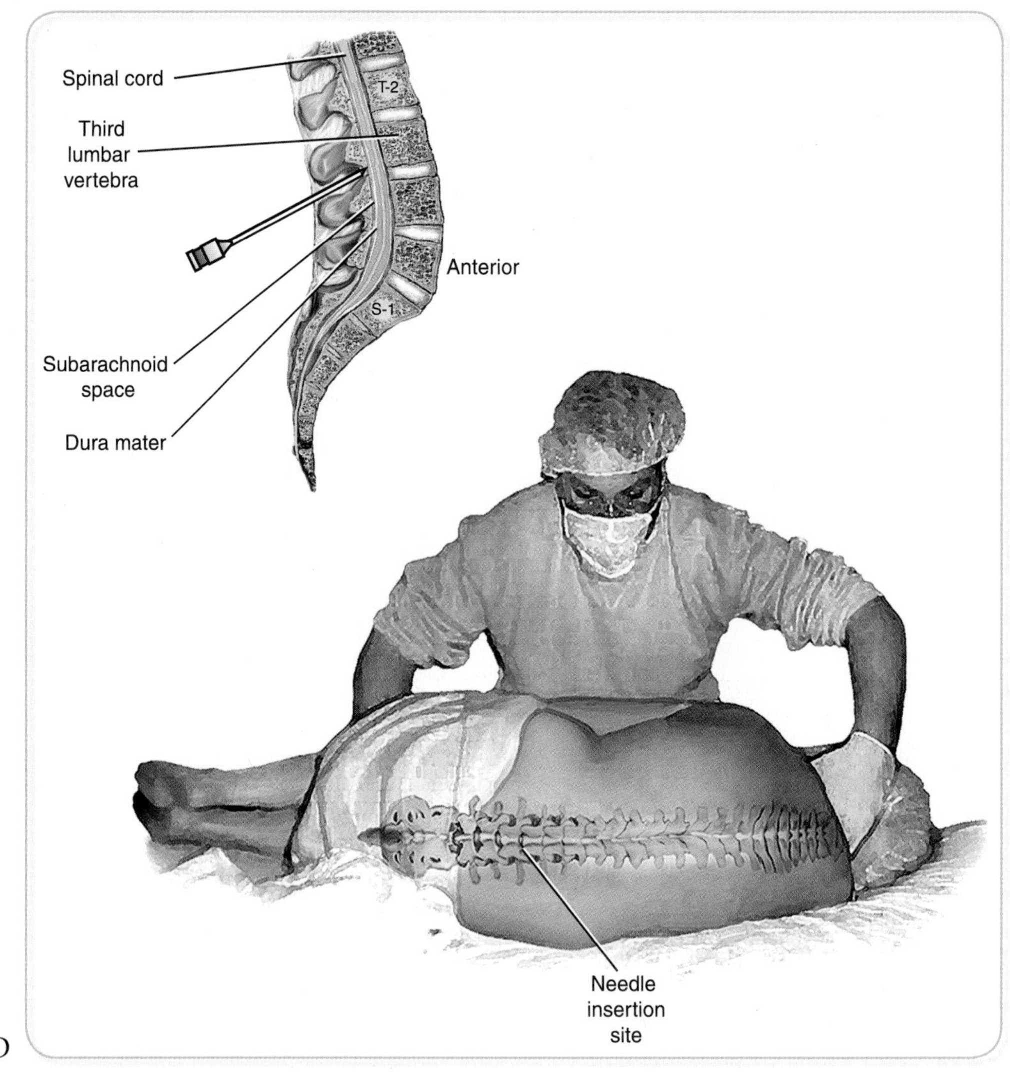

Figure 9-1 (D) spinal or epidural anesthesia (B and C courtesy of Dr. Gary Shellerud).

Topical Anesthesia

Topical anesthesia acts as a nerve conduction—blocking agent on the skin or mucus membranes. This procedure can provide anesthesia on skin and the mucus membranes of the rectum, urethra, and vagina. Lidocaine is an example of a topical anesthetic agent.

Nerve Block Anesthesia

Nerve block anesthesia affects the bundle of nerves serving the area to be operated upon. This method is used to block sensation in a limb or large area such as the face.

Local Infiltration Anesthesia

Local **infiltration anesthesia** blocks a specific group of nerves in a small area very close to the area to be operated on. Local infiltration is probably the most common route used to administer local anesthetics, and is the simplest form of regional anesthesia. Lidocaine is a popular choice for infiltration anesthesia, but bupivacaine is used for longer procedures.

Spinal Anesthesia

During **spinal anesthesia**, an anesthetic agent is injected into the subarachnoid space (beneath the arachnoid membrane or between the arachnoid and pia mater, and filled with cerebrospinal fluid) through a spinal needle. Drugs injected in this manner affect large regional areas such as the lower abdomen and legs.

Epidural Anesthesia

Medical Terminology Review

arachnoid
arach = spider
noid = like
spider-like

Epidural anesthesia involves injection of the local anesthetic into the epidural (lumbar or caudal) space via a catheter that allows repeated infusions. After injection, the anesthetic agent is very slowly absorbed into the cerebrospinal fluid. This method is most commonly used in obstetrics during labor and delivery.

Malignant Hyperthermia

Malignant hyperthermia is a rare, genetic **hypermetabolic** condition that is characterized by severe overproduction of body heat with rigidity of skeletal muscles. It is a serious adverse effect of anesthesia (relating to inhalation anesthetics) that must be treated immediately. Treatment includes administration of large doses of dantrolene sodium and 100% oxygen, followed by immediate cooling, cessation of surgery, and correction of hyperkalemia. Dantrolene has a very short shelf life and must be restocked regularly so that, when needed, its action will be potent. Malignant hyperthermia may cause the death of the patient due to brain damage, cardiac arrest, internal bleeding, or damage to other body systems. A malignant hyperthermia kit must include:

Medical Terminology Review

hyperkalemia
hyper = over; above; beyond
kalemia = condition of potassium ions in the blood
increased number of potassium ions in the blood

- Dantrolene
- Furosemide
- Glucose
- Procainamide
- Sodium bicarbonate (7.5%)
- Sterile water

Key Concept

Patients susceptible to malignant hyperthermia must be informed of the condition and potentially susceptible relatives of the patient should also be screened.

Summary

Preanesthetic drugs are used to facilitate induction of anesthesia and to relieve anxiety and pain. There are four stages of anesthesia. Stage I is characterized by analgesia, euphoria, and amnesia. Stage II increases the skeletal muscle tone and breathing is irregular. It is important that the passage from Stage I to Stage III be attained as quickly as possible. Stage III is called surgical anesthesia, which produces muscular relaxation. Stage IV causes medullary paralysis, and this stage should be avoided.

General anesthesia is a reversible stage of unconsciousness as a result of medication. It can be induced by inhalation or by injection of drugs. The combination of injectable anesthetics with inhaled general anesthetics together allows a decreased probability of serious side effects.

The two major groups of local anesthetics are esters and amides. The amides have several advantages over the esters. Local anesthetics are used for minor surgery, dental procedures, suturing small wounds, or removing a superficial tissue sample for biopsy.

Exploring the Web

Visit ***www.emedicine.com***

- Click on the specialty "Emergency Medicine," then click on toxicology and look for information related to the drugs covered in this chapter.

Visit ***www.healthline.com***

- Search by "anesthesia," and review information that related to this topic.

Visit ***www.mayoclinic.com***

- Search by "anesthesia," and review information that related to this topic.

Review Questions

Multiple Choice

1. The main purpose of local anesthetics is to prevent which of the following?

   A. falling asleep and muscle contraction
   B. allergic reaction and anaphylactic shock
   C. pain impulses from pain receptors reaching the lower limbs
   D. pain impulses from pain receptors reaching the higher centers

2. The ester-type anesthetics are represented by which of the following substances?

   A. procaine
   B. prolactin
   C. pro-hormone
   D. pro-vitamin

3. Which of the following is the most common route used to administer local anesthetics?

   A. epidural
   B. topical
   C. local infiltration
   D. nerve block

4. Which of the following stages of anesthesia must be avoided?

   A. Stage I
   B. Stage II
   C. Stage III
   D. Stage IV

5. Which of the following preanesthetic medications relieve anxiety?

   A. scopolamine
   B. promethazine
   C. diazepam
   D. atropine

6. Which of the following stages of anesthesia is characterized by euphoria and perceptual distortions?

   A. Stage I
   B. Stage II
   C. Stage III
   D. Stage IV

7. Which of the following is the only gas that is routinely used for anesthesia?

   A. chloroform
   B. ether
   C. nitrous oxide
   D. halothane

8. Which of the following volatile agents is the most potent?

   A. isoflurane
   B. halothane
   C. sevoflurane
   D. enflurane

9. All of the following agents are used as inhaled anesthetics, except:

   A. desflurane
   B. nitrous oxide
   C. halothane
   D. sevoflurane

10. Local anesthesia is more accurately called:
    A. surface anesthesia
    B. preanesthetic medication
    C. maintenance of anesthesia
    D. surgical anesthesia

11. Which of the following agents is in the local anesthetic amide group?
    A. procaine (Novocain)
    B. lidocaine (Xylocaine)
    C. tetracaine (Pontocaine)
    D. benzocaine (Americaine)

12. Which of the following is the stage of surgical anesthesia?
    A. Stage I
    B. Stage IV
    C. Stage II
    D. Stage III

Matching

Generic Names	Trade Names
_____ 1. sevoflurane	A. Penthrane
_____ 2. isoflurane	B. Suprane
_____ 3. halothane	C. Fluothane
_____ 4. enflurane	D. Ethrane
_____ 5. desflurane	E. Forane
_____ 6. methoxyflurane	F. Ultane

Fill in the Blank

1. A woman in labor will most likely receive _______________.
2. Anticholinergics used to minimize some of the undesirable after effects of anesthetics, such as excessive salvation, vomiting, and bradycardia, include _______________ and _______________.
3. Nitrous oxide is also called _______________.
4. Hypersensitivity to amide local anesthetics is _______________.

Critical Thinking

A 65-year-old man is going under local anesthesia for two dental implants. His medical history is satisfactory, but he is taking three different medications: Zocor® 10 mg and niacin 1,000 mg (for hypercholesterolemia), and Allegra® 180 mg (for allergies).

1. What would be the best type of local anesthesia for this patient?
2. If his dentist is using the preferred local anesthesia for this procedure, would there be any drug interactions with the medications that the patient is taking?
3. What may be the adverse effects for local anesthesia used in this procedure?

Drug Therapy for the Musculoskeletal System

CHAPTER 10

OUTLINE

OBJECTIVES

After completing this chapter, the reader should be able to:

1. Discuss skeletal muscle relaxants.
2. Discuss neuromuscular blocking agents.
3. Explain the goals of pharmacotherapy with skeletal muscle relaxants.
4. Define centrally acting skeletal muscle relaxants.
5. Explain the major side effect of dantrolene (direct-acting skeletal muscle relaxant).
6. Discuss drugs used to treat gout.
7. Explain the mechanism of action of corticosteroids.
8. Explain gold compounds and their indications.
9. Define drugs for gouty arthritis and drugs commonly used for treatment.

GLOSSARY

Articular – related to the joints of the body

Contusion – an injury to body part or tissue without a break in the skin

Exfoliative dermatitis – a skin disorder characterized by reddening and scaling of 100% of the skin; erythroderma

Gout – a disease caused by a congenital disorder of uric acid metabolism; metabolic arthritis

Hematoma – blood that has seeped from a blood vessel and collects in tissue, organs, or space

Laceration – cut or break in the skin

Periosteum – a thick, fibrous membrane covering the entire surface of a bone except its articular cartilage and where it attaches to tendons and ligaments

Osteoarthritis (OA) – arthritis characterized by erosion of articular cartilage that mainly affects weight-bearing joints in older adults

Rheumatoid arthritis (RA) – a chronic and progressive condition that affects more women than men, focusing mainly on the joints of the hands and feet, and leading to deformity and disability

Spasticity – a type of increase in muscle tone at rest, characterized by increase resistance of the muscles to stretching

Sprain – injury to supporting ligaments of a joint

Strain – injury resulting from overstretching a muscle, results in tear of muscle or muscle and tendon

Synapse – a specialized junction at which a nerve cell communicates with a target cell

OVERVIEW

Muscle spasms, spasticity, and joint disorders are some of the most common disorders in humans of any age. Medications used to treat these conditions may be classified in two broad categories: skeletal muscle relaxants and nonsteroidal anti-inflammatory drugs (NSAIDs). In this chapter, we will focus on drugs such as skeletal muscle relaxants (for disorders such as muscular spasticity due to neurological disorders), gold salts (for arthritis), and agents used to treat gout. NSAIDs will be discussed with more depth in Chapter 21.

ANATOMY REVIEW

- The musculoskeletal system consists of several separate body systems: the skeletal system, the muscular system, and the articular system (Figure 10-1).

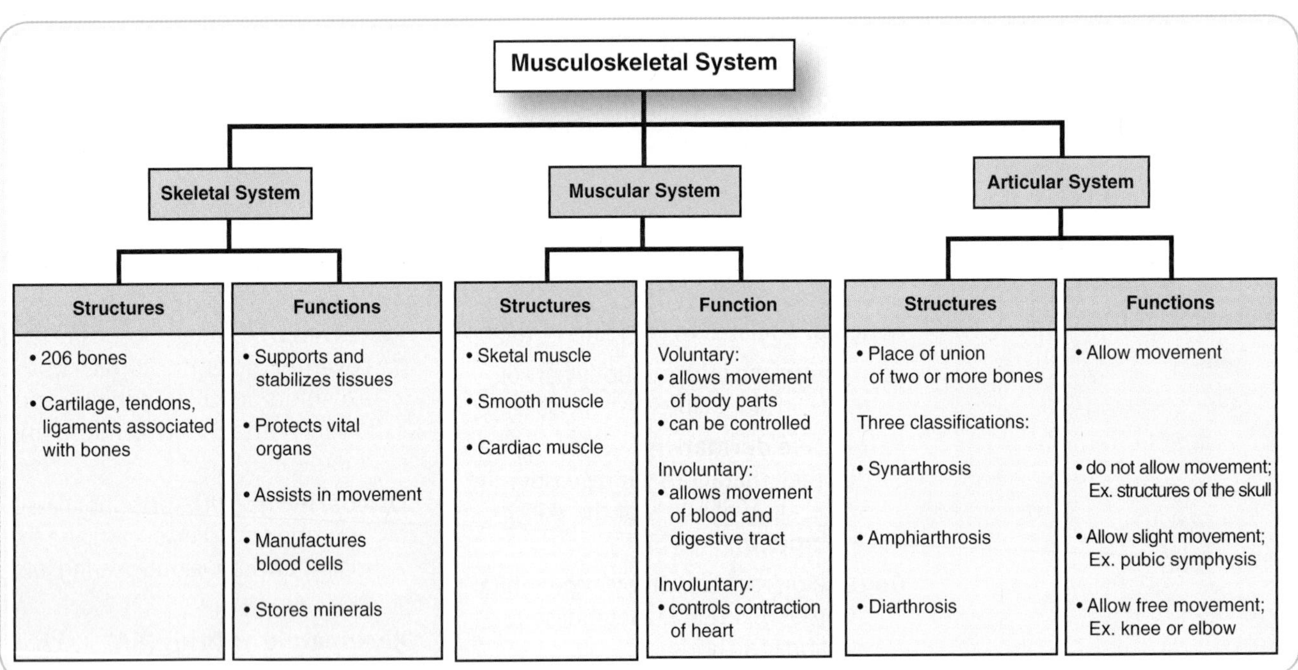

Figure 10-1 The musculoskeletal system.

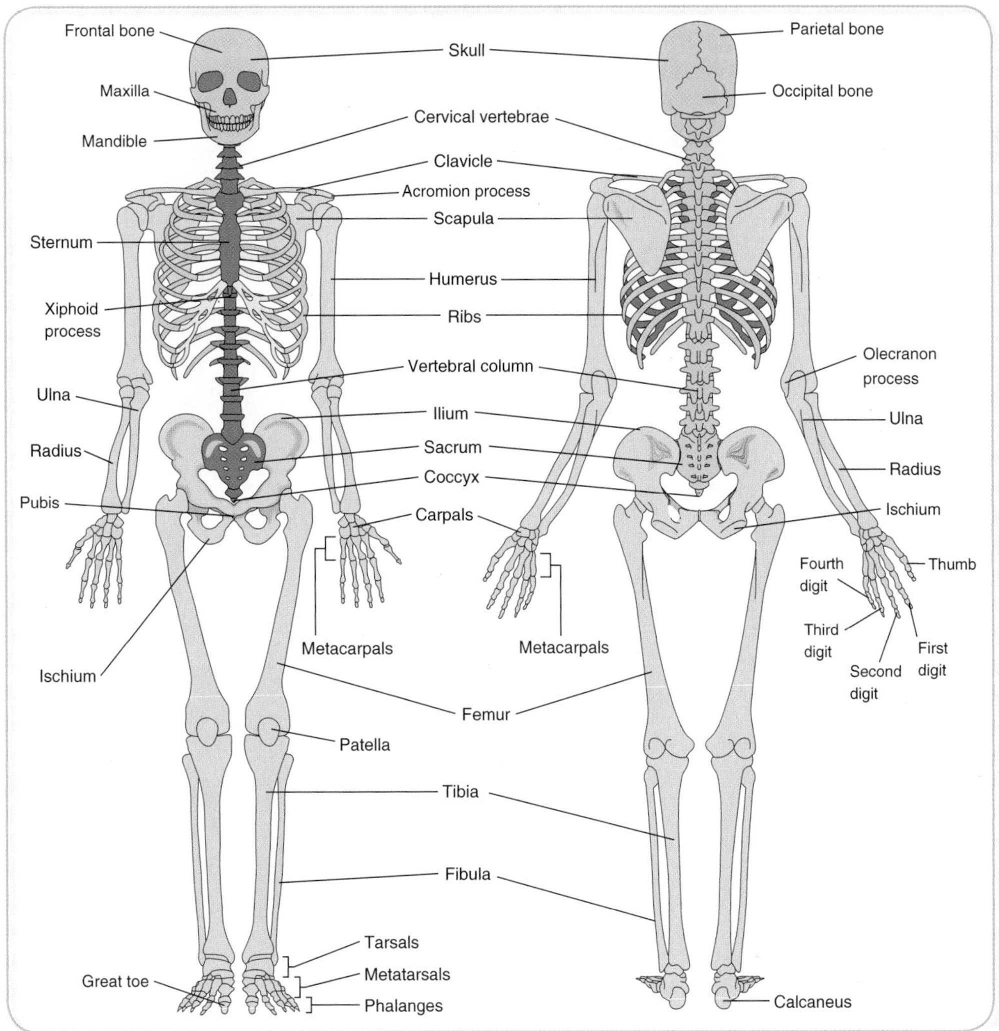

Figure 10-2 The bones of the human body.

- The skeletal system consists of 206 bones as well as the cartilage, ligaments, and tendons associated with the bones (Figure 10-2).
- Functions of the skeletal system include: support and stabilization, protection of organs, assistance with movement, manufacture of blood cells, and storage of minerals.

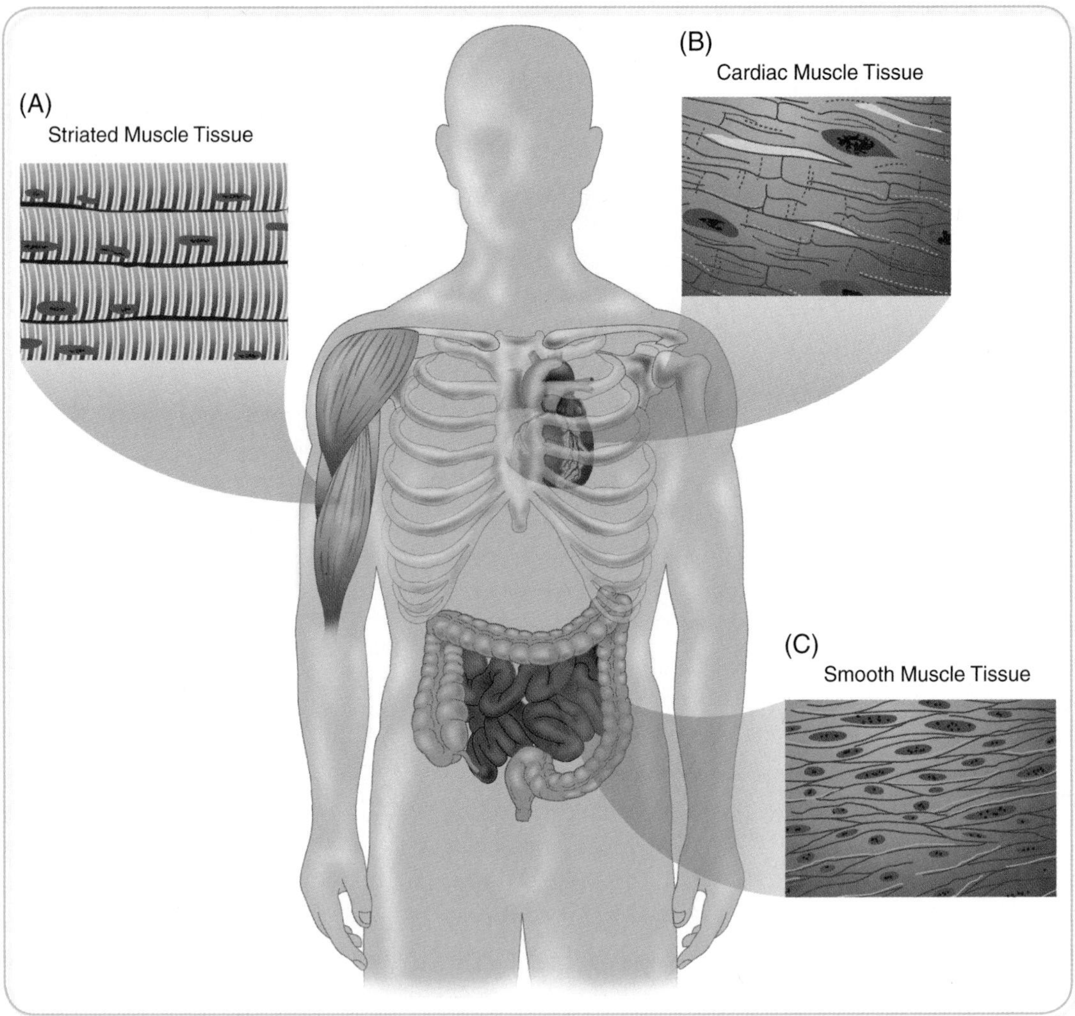

Figure 10-3 Types of muscle (A) skeletal (striated) muscle (B) cardiac muscle (C) smooth muscle.

- The muscular system consists of three types of muscle: skeletal, smooth, and cardiac (Figure 10-3).
- Skeletal muscle allows voluntary movement such as flexion and extension of the legs. Smooth muscle allows involuntary movement in particular body organs such as movement of the nutrients through the digestive tract. Cardiac muscle is found only in the heart and controls the involuntary contractions of the heart.
- The **articular** system consists of three types of joints: synarthrosis, amphiarthrosis, and diarthrosis (Figure 10-4).
- Synarthrosis joints, such as the sutures in the skull, do not allow movement.
- Amphiarthrosis joints such as the pubic symphysis allow slight movement.
- Diarthrosis joints allow free range of motion such as the movements around the shoulder girdle.

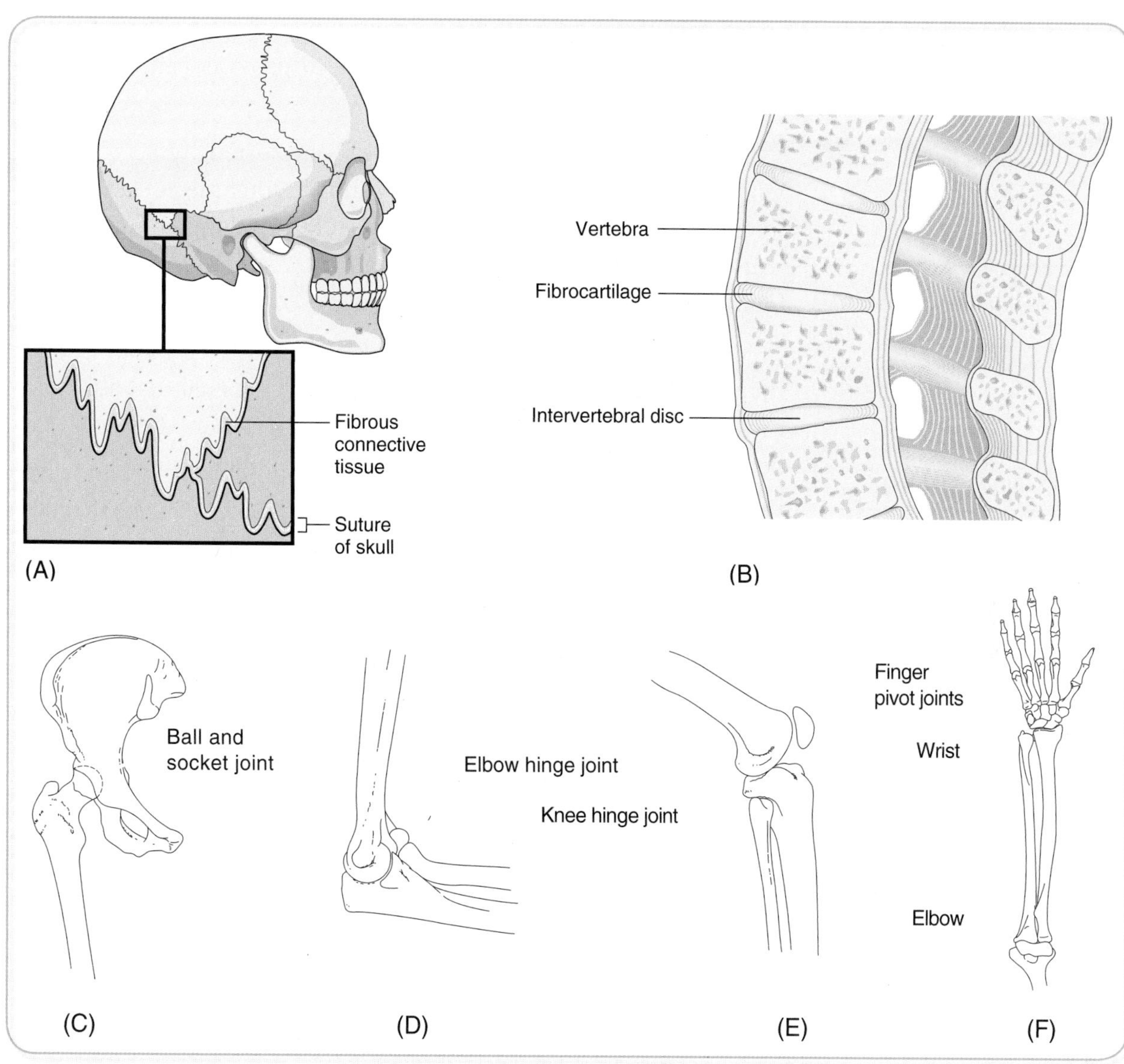

Figure 10-4 Types of joints: (A) synarthrosis (B) amphiarthrosis (C–F) diarthrosis.

Musculoskeletal Disorders

The musculoskeletal system is subject to a large number of disorders. These disorders affect persons of all age groups and occupations. They are a major cause of pain and disability.

Injury and Trauma of the Musculoskeletal System

A broad spectrum of musculoskeletal injuries results from numerous physical forces, including blunt tissue trauma, disruption of tendons and ligaments, and fractures of bony structures. Many of the forces that cause injury to the musculoskeletal system are typical for a particular environmental setting, activity, or age group. Trauma resulting from high-speed motor accidents is a common cause of injury in adults younger than 45. The most common causes of childhood injuries are falls, bicycle-related injuries, and sports injuries. Falls are the most common causes of injury in people 65 years and older, with fractures of the hip and proximal humerus particularly common in this age group.

Most skeletal injuries are accompanied by soft tissue (muscle, tendon, or ligament) injuries. These injuries include **contusions** (injuries of body parts without a break in the skin), **hematomas** (blood that has seeped from the blood vessels to become trapped in an organ, space, or tissue), and **lacerations** (a cut or break in the skin).

Medical Terminology Review

periosteum
peri- = *around*
oste- = *bone*
-um = *suffix identifying a singular noun*
structure around the bone

Joints are sites where two or more bones meet. Joints are supported by tough bundles of collagenous fibers called ligaments that attach to the joint capsule and bind the articular ends of bones together. They are also supported by tendons that join muscles to the periosteum of an articulating bone. Joint injuries involve mechanical overloading or forcible twisting or stretching.

Sprains and strains are both musculoskeletal injuries, but they differ in terms of the tissue that is affected. **Sprains** involve the supporting ligaments of a joint. A complete tear in a muscle or tendon is described as a rupture. A **strain** is a stretching or a partial tear in a muscle or a muscle-tendon unit. Strains commonly result from the sudden stretching of a muscle that is actively contracting. Strains can occur at any age, but are more common in middle-aged and older adults. Muscle strains are usually characterized by pain, stiffness, swelling, and local tenderness. Pain is increased with stretching of the muscle group.

Rheumatoid Arthritis

Rheumatoid arthritis (RA) is a systemic inflammatory disease that attacks joints by producing inflammation of the synovial membranes that leads to the destruction of the articular cartilage and underlying bone. Women are affected by this condition two to three times more frequently than men. Although the disease occurs in all age groups, its prevalence increases with age. The peak incidence among women is between the ages of 40 and 60 years, with the onset at 30 to 50 years of age.

The cause of RA has not been established. However, evidence points to a genetic predisposition and the development of joint inflammation that is immunologically mediated.

Joint involvement usually is systemic and involves more than one joint. The patient may complain of joint pain and stiffness that lasts for 30 minutes or longer, and frequently for several hours. The most commonly affected joints initially are the fingers, hands, wrists, knees, and feet. Later, other joints may become involved. Spinal involvement usually is limited to the cervical region.

Gout

Gout is actually a group of diseases known as the gout syndrome. It includes acute gouty arthritis with recurrent attacks of severe joint inflammation, and the accumulation of crystalline deposits in joint surfaces, bones, soft tissue, and cartilage. Gout also may cause gouty nephropathy or renal impairment, and uric acid kidney stones.

Uric acid is a waste product of purine metabolism, normally excreted through the kidneys. A sudden increase in serum uric acid levels usually precipitates an attack of gout. Gout often affects a single joint, such as in the big toe. When acute inflammation develops from uric acid deposits, the joint cartilage is damaged. The inflammation causes redness and swelling of the joint, accompanied by severe pain.

Osteoarthritis

Osteoarthritis is by far the most common form of arthritis among the elderly. It is the greatest cause of disability and limitation of activity in older adults. It has been suggested that osteoarthritis begins at a very young age, expressing itself in the elderly only after a long period of latency. Osteoarthritis presents a major management problem, but there is much that can be done to help lessen its effects. Self-control, by maintaining a positive attitude and a sense of self-esteem, is a frequent coping strategy. Treatment of osteoarthritis in the elderly focuses on relief of pain and improvement of functional status.

Skeletal Muscle Relaxants

Most muscle strains and spasms are self-limited and respond to rest, physical therapy, and short-term use of aspirin and other analgesics. However, **spasticity** (a form of muscular contraction), as the result of closed head injuries, stroke, cerebral palsy, multiple sclerosis, spinal cord injury, and other neurologic conditions, requires long-term use of muscle relaxants. The skeletal muscles are voluntary muscles. They are under control of the central nervous system (CNS). Skeletal muscle relaxants work by blocking somatic motor nerve impulses through depression of the neurons within the CNS. Transmission of an impulse from the motor nerve to each muscle cell occurs across a space known as the neuromuscular junction (see Figure 10-5). This space is sensitive to chemical changes in its immediate environment. Therefore, the somatic motor nerve impulses cannot be generated. This mechanism may also decrease the availability of calcium ions to the myofibrillar contractile system. Discontinuity of certain afferent reflex pathways by local anesthesia may also effect relaxation of limited muscle groups; local anesthetic block of efferent somatic motor outflow also is used occasionally to relieve localized skeletal muscle spasms.

> ***Medical Terminology Review***
>
> **neuromuscular**
> *neuro = of the nerves or nervous system*
> *muscular = of the muscles or muscular system*
> nerves affecting the muscles of the body

Neuromuscular Blocking Agents

Neuromuscular blocking agents are chemical substances that interfere locally with the transmission or reception of impulses from motor nerves to skeletal muscles. Table 10-1 shows some popular neuromuscular blocking agents.

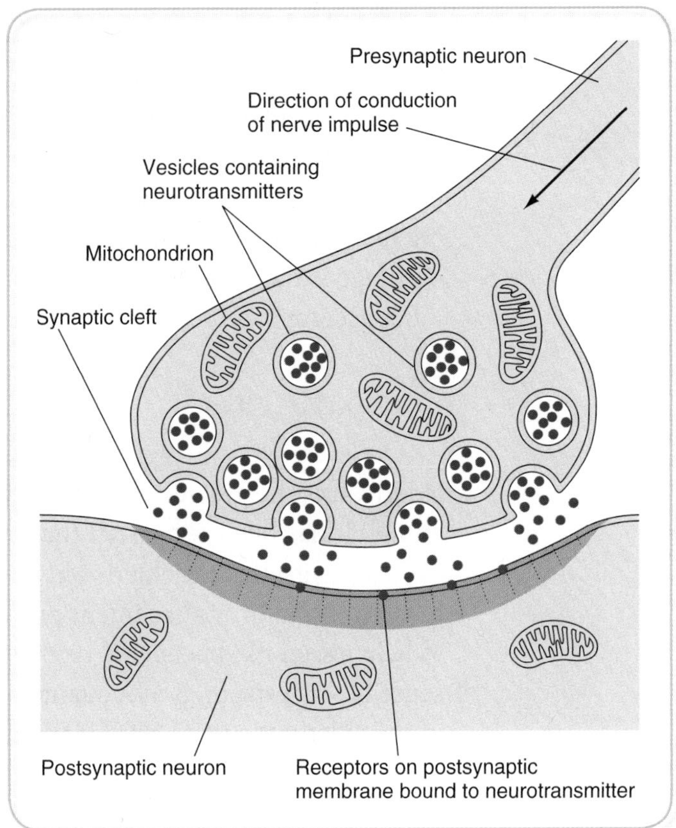

Figure 10-5 The neuromuscular junction.

TABLE 10-1 Neuromuscular Blocking Agents

Generic Name	Trade Name	Route of Administration	Average Adult Dosage
Short Duration			
succinylcholine chloride	Anectine®, Quelicin®	IM, IV	IV: 0.3–1.1 mg/kg; IM: 2.5–4 mg/kg
Intermediate Duration			
atracurium besylate	Tracrium®	IV	0.4–0.5 mg/kg initial; then 0.08–0.1 mg/kg
cisatracurium besylate	Nimbex®	IV	0.15–0.20 mg/kg
rocuronium bromide	Zemuron®	IV	0.6 mg/kg
Extended Duration			
doxacurium chloride	Nuromax®	IV	0.025–0.05 mg/kg initial; then 0.005–0.01 mg/kg
mivacurium chloride	Mivacron®	IV	0.15–0.25 mg/kg
pancuronium bromide	Pavulon®	IV	0.06–0.1 mg/kg

Mechanism of Action

Neuromuscular blocking agents prevent somatic motor nerve impulses, which affect the skeletal muscles. Some agents occupy receptor sites on the motor end plate and are able to block the action of acetylcholine. These agents are called competitive neuromuscular blocking agents. The action of other neuromuscular blocking agents resembles that of acetylcholine by depolarizing the muscle fiber. These agents are not immediately destroyed by cholinesterase. Therefore, their action is more prolonged than that of acetylcholine. Examples of these agents include succinylcholine, atracurium, and doxacurium.

Indications

The principal use of neuromuscular blocking drugs is to provide adequate skeletal muscular relaxation during surgery, controlled respiration, and orthopedic manipulations. The short-acting drugs are used to relax the laryngeal muscles during endotracheal intubation and bronchoscopy. They may also be used to decrease the severity of muscle contractions during electroconvulsive treatment. Neuromuscular blocking agents have been used in the management of tetanus and for various spastic disorders, but the results usually have been dissatisfying. Neuromuscular blocking agents are not effective for rigidity and spasticity of muscles caused by neurological disease or trauma.

Adverse Effects

The most commonly reported adverse effects of neuromuscular blocking agents include drowsiness, increased occurrence of seizures in patients with epilepsy, dry mouth, loss of strength, hypotension, muscle weakness, occasional hepatitis, and cardiac arrhythmias.

Contraindications and Precautions

Neuromuscular blocking agents are contraindicated in patients with hypersensitivity to these drugs or a family history of malignant hyperthermia. Atracurium is contraindicated in patients with myasthenia gravis. Neuromuscular blocking drugs are not safe during pregnancy (category C), lactation, or in children younger than two years.

These agents should be used cautiously in infants and patients with asthma, significant cardiovascular disease, impaired pulmonary function, dehydration, acid-base imbalance, and lactation.

Drug Interactions

Neuromuscular blocking agents play an important role in severe adverse reactions occurring during anesthesia. Most reactions to these agents are of immunological origin, and tests for possible hypersensitivity to these drugs must be conducted before administration of anesthesia. Neuromuscular blocking agents should not be used with muscle relaxants such as succinylcholine, volatile, intravenous, or local anesthetics, antibiotics,

TABLE 10-2 Centrally Acting Skeletal Muscle Relaxants

Generic Name	Trade Name	Route of Administration	Average Adult Dosage
baclofen	Lioresal®	PO	5 mg tid
carisoprodol	Soma®, Rela®	PO	350 mg tid
chlorphenesin carbamate	Maolate®	PO	800 mg tid until effective; reduce to 400 mg qid or less
chlorzoxazone	Paraflex®, Parafon Forte®	PO	250–500 mg tid
cyclobenzaprine hydrochloride	Flexeril®, Cycoflex®	PO	10–15 mg tid
diazepam	Valium®, Valrelease®	PO, IM, IV	PO: 2–10 mg bid-qid; IM/IV: 5–10 mg up to 30 mg
methocarbamol	Robaxin®	PO	1.5 g qid for 2–3 days then reduce to 1 g qid
orphenadrine citrate	Norflex®, Banflex®, Myolin®	PO, IM, IV	PO: 100 mg bid; IM/IV: 60 mg

anticonvulsants, magnesium, diuretics, corticosteroids, or acetylcholine esterase inhibitors (reversal drugs).

Centrally Acting Skeletal Muscle Relaxants

Skeletal muscles are voluntarily controlled by impulses originating in the CNS. Impulses are conducted through the spinal cord in somatic neurons that eventually **synapse** with the muscle in a neuromuscular junction. Table 10-2 shows some examples of the centrally acting skeletal muscle relaxants.

Mechanism of Action

The exact mechanism of centrally acting muscle relaxants is unknown. The neurotransmitter acetylcholine (ACh) is released to combine with ACh receptors on the muscle cell membrane. When an adequate number of ACh receptors are bound, the cell then experiences sodium ion influx, causing an impulse to travel over the cell, which causes a contraction. Relaxation occurs when ACh is broken down by acetylcholinesterase. They may act in the CNS at various levels to depress polysynaptic reflexes; sedative effects may be responsible for relaxation of muscle spasms.

Indications

Use of the centrally acting muscle relaxants is uncertain, owing to their limited selectivity. Involuntary movement of skeletal muscles, such as that which is seen in palsies, chorea, or Parkinsonism, is mostly the result of impairment of feedback control within the brain. These agents may be used to reduce muscle spasms in patients with cerebral palsy, multiple sclerosis, and spinal cord injury.

Adverse Effects

Common adverse effects of centrally acting agents include weakness, fatigue, drowsiness, and dizziness. Baclofen is often the drug of first choice because of its wide safety margin.

Contraindications and Precautions

Centrally acting skeletal muscle relaxants are contraindicated in patients with hypersensitivity to these agents. Cyclobenzaprine should be avoided in the acute recovery phase of myocardial infarction, cardiac arrhythmias, and hyperthyroidism. Centrally acting skeletal muscle relaxants are contraindicated during pregnancy (category B or C), lactation, and in children younger than five years.

These agents should be used cautiously in patients with liver or kidney impairment, bipolar disorder, seizure disorders, stroke, cerebral palsy, depression, head trauma, and diabetes mellitus.

Medical Terminology Review

hyperpyretic
hyper = over, excessive
pyr/o = fire, heat
tic = pertaining to
pertaining to overheating

Drug Interactions

Alcohol, phenothiazines, or CNS depressants may cause additive sedation if they are used with centrally acting skeletal muscle relaxants. Cyclobenzaprine should not be used within two weeks of an MAOI because hyperpyretic crisis and convulsions may occur.

Medical Terminology Review

spastic
spas = spasms
tic = condition of
the presence of spasms

Direct-Acting Skeletal Muscle Relaxants

These agents directly relax the spastic muscle. Direct-acting skeletal muscle relaxants produce about a 50% decrease in contractility of skeletal muscles, but they have no effect on smooth or cardiac muscles. Examples of direct-acting antispasmodic drugs are botulinum toxin type A and B, dantrolene, and quinine sulfate (see Table 10-3).

TABLE 10-3 Direct-Acting Antispasmodic Agents

Generic Name	Trade Name	Route of Administration	Average Adult Dosage
botulinum toxin type A	Botox®, Dysport®	IM	20–50 units injected directly into target muscle
botulinum toxin type B	Myoblock®	IM	2,500–5,000 units / dose injected directly into target muscle
dantrolene sodium	Dantrium®	PO	25 mg / day; increased to 25 mg bid-qid; may increase q4–7 days up to 100 mg bid-tid
quinine sulfate	Quinamm®, Quiphile®	PO	260–300 mg at bedtime

Mechanism of Action

Direct-acting skeletal muscle relaxants do not interfere with neuromuscular transmission or the electrical excitability of muscles. They inhibit the release of calcium ions from storage areas inside skeletal muscle cells. This action makes the muscle less responsive to nerve impulses. Dantrolene is an example of a direct-acting skeletal muscle relaxant that will be discussed in detail.

Indications

Dantrolene is used to treat spasticity resulting from upper motor neuron lesions such as those in spinal cord injury, stroke, multiple sclerosis, and cerebral palsy, but not spasticity resulting from musculoskeletal injury, lumbago, or rheumatoid disorders. The drug is also used to treat malignant hyperthermia.

Key Concept

Quinine sulfate is an antimalarial drug that is used for nocturnal leg cramps or congenital tonic spasms.

Adverse Effects

The major adverse effects of dantrolene include muscle weakness, drowsiness, dizziness, nausea, diarrhea, seizures, tachycardia, erratic blood pressure, and pericarditis.

Contraindications and Precautions

Dantrolene is contraindicated in patients with liver disease and respiratory muscle weakness. It may color the urine orange to red. Safe use during pregnancy (category C), lactation, or in children younger than five years is not established.

Dantrolene should be used cautiously in patients with impaired cardiac or pulmonary function, or in patients younger than 35 years (especially women).

Drug Interactions

The use of dantrolene with alcohol and other CNS depressants causes increased CNS depression. Estrogen increases the risk of hepatotoxicity in women younger than 35 years. The use of intravenous dantrolene with verapamil and other calcium channel blockers increases the risk of ventricular fibrillation and cardiovascular collapse.

Slow-Acting Anti-Rheumatic Drugs

Slow-acting anti-rheumatic drugs may be prescribed for patients with rheumatoid arthritis that progresses to deformity, requiring more than an anti-inflammatory agent. Altering the disease course is attempted initially with methotrexate, gold compounds, penicillamine, sulfasalazine, and hydroxychloroquine. Table 10-4 shows second-line agents for rheumatoid arthritis.

Medical Terminology Review

arthritis
arthr = joint
itis = inflammation
inflammation of the joint

Mechanism of Action

Gold compounds (auranofin and gold sodium thiomalate) suppress or prevent inflammation in the acute forms of arthritis, but do not cure the disease. The exact mechanisms of action of slow-acting anti-rheumatic drugs are not known.

TABLE 10-4 Second-Line Agents for Rheumatoid Arthritis

Generic Name	Trade Name	Route of Administration	Average Adult Dosage
auranofin	Ridaura®	PO	3 mg bid
gold sodium thiomalate	Aurolate®	IM	10 mg week 1; 1.25 mg week 2; then 25–50 mg/wk
methotrexate sodium	Mexate®	PO	15–30 mg/day for 5 days, repeat each 12 wk for 3–5 courses
hydrochloroquine	Plaquenil®	PO	200–600 mg/day
penicillamine	Depen®	PO	125–250 mg/day, may increase after several months
sulfasalazine	Azulfidine®	PO	1–3 g/day

Penicillamine is a chelating drug that is a metabolite of penicillin. It is also classified as an anti-inflammatory drug. The mechanism of action of penicillamine and hydrochloroquine is unknown.

Indications

Slow-acting anti-rheumatic drugs may be prescribed for advanced states of some rheumatoid disorders. The oral gold compound is available as auranofin, whereas the parenteral preparations are aurothioglucose and gold sodium thiomalate. Gold compounds that retard destruction of bone and joints by an unknown mechanism are long-latency drugs used in more advanced stages of some rheumatoid diseases. Gold sodium thiomalate is administered intramuscularly, and auranofin is administered orally.

Corticosteroids are used in severe, progressive rheumatoid arthritis. Prednisone may afford some degree of control, but corticosteroids are usually recognized as agents of last resort. Corticosteroids do not alter the course of rheumatoid arthritis. They may be occasionally used for elderly patients as alternatives to avoid the risks of second-line agents, for patients who cannot tolerate NSAIDs, and for patients with significant systemic manifestations of rheumatoid arthritis.

Adverse Effects

Common adverse effects of gold compounds and penicillamine include GI disturbances, dermatitis, and lesions of mucous membranes. Less common side effects include aplastic anemia and nephritic syndrome. It is important to note that, except for diarrhea, serious toxicity occurs most commonly when parenteral therapy is used. If toxicity occurs gold therapy should be stopped immediately.

Long-term administration of corticosteroids may cause GI bleeding, poor wound healing, hyperglycemia, hypertension, and osteoporosis.

Medical Terminology Review

corticosteroids
cortico = (adrenal) cortex
steroids = hormones
hormones produced in the adrenal cortex

Contraindications and Precautions

These preparations are contraindicated in patients with a history of gold-induced necrotizing enterocolitis, renal disease, **exfoliative dermatitis**, or bone marrow aplasia, in patients who have recently received radiation therapy, and in those with a history of severe toxicity from previous exposure to gold or other heavy metals. Safety during pregnancy (various categories) or lactation and in children is not established.

These agents must be used with caution in patients who have inflammatory bowel disease, rash, liver disease, a history of bone marrow depression, diabetes mellitus, congestive heart failure, and in older adults.

Drug Interactions

Gold compounds may have drug interactions with antimalarials and immunosuppressants. Penicillamine and phenylbutazone increase the risk of blood dyscrasias. Methotrexate with alcohol, azathioprine, and sulfasalazine increase risk of hepatotoxicity. Chloramphenicol, salicylates, NSAIDs, sulfonamides, phenylbutazone, phenytoin, tetracyclines, penicillin, and probenecid may increase methotrexate levels with increased toxicity. Folic acid may alter response to methotrexate.

The combination of penicillamine with antimalarials and gold therapy may potentiate hematological and renal adverse effects. Iron may decrease penicillamine absorption. Iron and antibiotics may alter sulfasalazine absorption.

Drugs for Gouty Arthritis

There are two types of clinical gouty arthritis: acute and chronic. The initial attack for acute gout is abrupt, usually occurring at night or in the early morning as synovial fluid is reabsorbed. The most common site of the initial attack is the big toe. Other sites that may be affected include the ankle, heel, knee, wrist, elbow, and fingers. There are two choices for therapy: general therapeutic drugs and specific drugs. In acute gout, immobilization of the affected joint is essential. Anti-inflammatory drug therapy should begin immediately, and urate-lowering drugs should not be given until the acute attack is controlled. Specific drugs include colchicines, NSAIDs (see Chapter 21), and corticosteroids. Colchicine and allopurinol are detailed below selectively.

> ***Medical Terminology Review***
>
> **antimitotic**
> *anti = opposing*
> *mitotic = development of chromosomes*
> development of chromosomes in opposition to one another

Colchicine

Colchicine is a gout suppressant with antimitotic and indirect anti-inflammatory properties.

Mechanism of Action

Colchicine is not an analgesic, and its precise mechanism of action is not known. The drug is well-absorbed after oral administration. It is often combined with probenecid to improve prophylactic therapy of chronic gouty arthritis. Both urinary and fecal routes eliminate colchicine.

Indications

Colchicine is the traditional drug of choice for relieving pain and inflammation and ending the acute gout attack. It is most effective when initiated 12 to 36 hours after symptoms begin. It is also used in combination with either phenylbutazone or allopurinol in the management of acute gout.

Adverse Effects

The drug is very toxic, and it should be stopped at the first symptom of toxicity, such as nausea, vomiting, diarrhea, and abdominal pain. Adverse effects of oral colchicine include nausea, abdominal cramps, and diarrhea.

Contraindications and Precautions

Colchicine is contraindicated in patients with peptic ulcers. Local pain and necrosis can occur with administration of intravenous colchicines.

Medical Terminology Review

uricosuric
urico = related to uric acid
suric = increasing excretion
increased excretion of uric acid

Drug Interactions

Colchicine may decrease intestinal absorption of vitamin B_{12}.

Allopurinol

Allopurinol is a xanthine oxidase inhibitor uricosuric agent.

Mechanism of Action

This drug is not analgesic, but it relieves gouty pain because it blocks the formation of or enhances the excretion of uric acid.

Indications

Allopurinol is used in the treatment of gout, primary or secondary uric acid nephropathy, uric acid stone formation, and renal calculi.

Adverse Effects

Adverse effects of allopurinol include: drowsiness, headache, vertigo, nausea, vomiting, diarrhea, abdominal discomfort, indigestion, malaise, thrombocytopenia, urticaria or pruritus, pruritic maculopapular rash, toxic epidermal necrolysis, hepatotoxicity, and renal insufficiency. In rare cases, allopurinol may cause agranulocytosis, aplastic anemia, and bone marrow depression.

Medical Terminology Review

hyperuricemia
hyper = over; above; beyond
uric = uric acid
emia = blood condition
excessive uric acid in the blood

Contraindications and Precautions

Allopurinol is contraindicated in children, except those with hyperuricemia secondary to cancer. It should not be used by nursing mothers, or by patients who develop a severe reaction to the drug.

Drug Interactions

Alcohol may inhibit renal excretion of uric acid. Ampicillin and amoxicillin increase the risk of skin rash. Allopurinol enhances anticoagulant effects of warfarin. Toxicity from azathioprine, mercaptopurine, cyclophosphamide, and cyclosporin increase with allopurinol.

Summary

Skeletal muscle relaxants and non-narcotic analgesics may be classified in two broad categories: skeletal muscle relaxants and NSAIDs (discussed in Chapter 21). Most muscle strains and spasms are self-limited and respond to rest, physical therapy, and aspirin. Spasticity resulting from closed head injuries, stroke, cerebral palsy, and others require long-term use of muscle relaxants. Neuromuscular blocking agents prevent somatic motor nerve impulses which affect the skeletal muscles. Gold compounds can suppress or prevent inflammation in acute forms of rheumatoid arthritis. The drug of choice for acute gouty arthritis is colchicine.

Exploring the Web

Visit ***www.drugs.com***

- Search for "skeletal muscle relaxants." Review the material presented to gain a better understanding of the drugs that fall within this category.

Visit ***www.medicinenet.com*** or ***www.nlm.nih.gov***

- Search by the disorders or drugs discussed in this chapter to enhance your understanding of the reading.

Review Questions

Multiple Choice

1. The type of muscle which attaches to bones and joints by connective tissue is which of the following?

A. smooth
B. skeletal
C. myocardium
D. tendon

2. Which of the following refers to disease of the joints?

A. bursa
B. osteoporosis
C. arthritis
D. connective

3. Skeletal muscles are voluntary muscles which are under the control of the

A. central nervous system
B. peripheral nervous system
C. environment
D. calcium ions

4. One of the principal uses of neuromuscular blocking agents is to provide adequate skeletal muscular relaxation during
   A. surgery
   B. rest
   C. epileptic seizures
   D. exercise

5. The abbreviation ACh stands for
   A. ache
   B. aluminum chloride
   C. acetylcholine
   D. acetaminophen

6. A centrally acting skeletal muscle relaxant commonly used to alleviate signs and symptoms of spasticity from multiple sclerosis is
   A. carisoprodol
   B. baclofen
   C. barbiturate
   D. codeine

7. Which of the following drugs may cause urine discoloration from orange to purple-red?
   A. dantrolene
   B. diazepam
   C. chlorzoxazone
   D. cortisol

8. A muscle relaxant which may worsen schizophrenic symptoms when mixed with propoxyphene is
   A. opium
   B. orphenadrine
   C. dantrolene sodium
   D. calcium

9. Pain-relieving drugs are also known as
   A. anaphylactics
   B. antiemetics
   C. analgesics
   D. antitoxins

10. Which of the following is a xanthine oxidase inhibitor agent?
   A. auranofin
   B. allopurinol
   C. acetaminophen
   D. colchicine

11. Gold compounds are indicated in which of the following?
   A. exfoliative dermatitis
   B. rheumatoid arthritis
   C. bone marrow aplasia
   D. exposure to heavy metals

12. The trade name of botulinum toxin type B is
    A. Botox
    B. Dantrium
    C. Dysport
    D. Myobloc
13. Allopurinol is used in the treatment of all of the following disorders, except
    A. temporary relief of mild to moderate pain
    B. secondary uric acid nephropathy
    C. uric acid stone formation
    D. gout
14. Which of the following is an example of a direct-acting antispasmodic drug?
    A. Soma
    B. Robaxin
    C. Dantrium
    D. Flexeril
15. Slow-acting antirheumatic drugs may be prescribed for patients with rheumatoid arthritis that
    A. causes muscle cramps
    B. causes numbness
    C. exists along with palpitations
    D. progresses to deformity

Fill in the Blank

1. Skeletal muscle relaxants work by blocking ______________ nerve impulses.
2. Neuromuscular blocking drugs are not safe during pregnancy because they are in category ______________.
3. Baclofen is often the drug of first choice as a centrally acting skeletal muscle relaxant because of its wide ______________.
4. Name three anti-inflammatory drugs that are classified as slow-acting anti-rheumatic drugs:
    A. ______________
    B. ______________
    C. ______________
5. Name five adverse effects of long-term administration of corticosteroids:
    A. ______________
    B. ______________
    C. ______________
    D. ______________
    E. ______________

6. The precise mechanism of action of *colchicine* is ________________.

7. The most common site of the initial attack of gout is the ________________ metatarsophalangeal ________________.

Critical Thinking

A 48-year-old woman has been diagnosed with gouty arthritis. She also has a history of hypertension and a chronic peptic ulcer.

1. Though it should be used cautiously, which of the medications for gouty arthritis discussed in this chapter should be prescribed?
2. What would be the treatment choices for acute gouty arthritis?
3. If she received the drug of choice for acute gouty arthritis, what would be the most common adverse effects?

CHAPTER 11 Drug Therapy for Cardiovascular Disorders

OBJECTIVES

After completing this chapter, the reader should be able to:

1. Describe normal cardiac function related to contractility and blood flow.
2. Explain the pathophysiology of angina pectoris.
3. Explain the different types of coronary vasodilators.
4. Explain the common adverse effects associated with each antianginal drug class.
5. Identify the various types of antiarrhythmics and their adverse effects.
6. Describe myocardial infarction and three steps that should be taken to limit myocardial necrosis.
7. List medications that are used in congestive heart failure.
8. Describe vasoconstrictors and their purpose.
9. Discuss the action of digitalis and its side effects.
10. Explain the consequences of congestive heart failure to the cardiovascular system.

GLOSSARY

Angina pectoris – an episodic, reversible oxygen insufficiency

Arrhythmias – deviations from the normal pattern of the heartbeat; also called "dysrhythmias"

Arteriosclerosis – degenerative changes in small arteries, commonly occurring in older individuals and diabetics; walls of arteries lose elasticity and become thick and hard

Atherosclerosis – disease of the arteries characterized by the presence of atheromas (plaques consisting of lipids, cells, and cell debris, often with attached thrombi, which form inside the walls of large arteries)

Atheromas – plaques consisting of lipids, cells, and cell debris, often with attached thrombi, which form inside the walls of large arteries

Beta-adrenergic blockers – drugs used to reverse sympathetic heart action caused by exercise, stress, or physical exertion

OUTLINE

(continues)

OUTLINE (continued)

Calcium channel blockers – drugs used to treat stable angina

Congestive heart failure (CHF) – condition in which the heart is not able to pump enough blood to meet the body's metabolic demands

Coronary arterial bypass graft (CABG) – a procedure wherein a vein graft is surgically implanted to bypass the part of the occlusion in the coronary artery

Coronary artery disease (CAD) – a condition in which there is an insufficient supply of oxygen to the myocardium (cardiac muscle); also referred to as "coronary heart disease" and "ischemic heart disease"

Myocardial infarction (MI) – an area of dead cardiac muscle tissue, with or without hemorrhage

Nitrates – drugs used for the treatment of angina

Percutaneous transluminal coronary angioplasty (PTCA) – reduces obstruction by means of invasive procedures requiring cardiac catheterization; the catheter contains an inflatable balloon that flattens the obstruction

Silent angina – a condition that occurs in the absence of angina pain

Vasospastic angina – decubitus angina; characterized by periodic attacks of cardiac pain that occur when a person is lying down

OVERVIEW

Cardiovascular disorders are among the most common causes of death in the United States. There are many factors that contribute to heart disease, such as age, genetics, and lifestyle. Proper diet, exercise, avoiding cigarette smoking, and getting enough rest can do a lot to keep the heart functioning for a long time. Heart disease may also be caused by other conditions or disorders such as high blood pressure, high blood cholesterol levels, obesity, and diabetes. A pharmacy technician should be familiar with the most common disorders of the cardiovascular system and the most effective agents used in the treatment of each of them.

ANATOMY REVIEW

- The cardiovascular system consists of the heart, blood vessels, blood, and lymph (Figure 11-1).
- The heart is a hollow muscular organ consisting of the myocardium, pericardium, and endocardium. Four valves control blood flow into and out of the heart (Figure 11-2).
- Coronary arteries provide blood flow and nutrients to the heart muscle itself (Figure 11-3).
- The largest of the blood vessels are the arteries, which carry oxygenated blood away from the heart to the capillaries. The pulmonary arteries are the exceptions; they carry deoxygenated blood from the heart to the lungs.

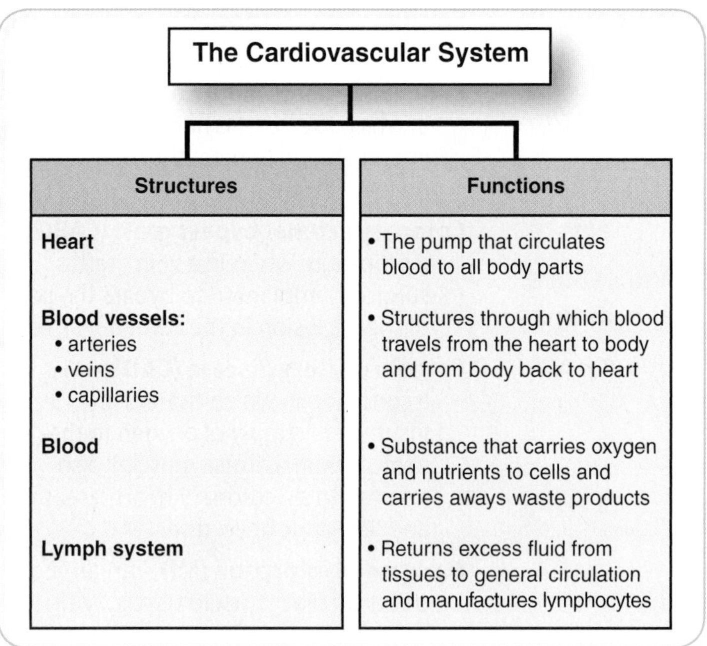
The Cardiovascular System

Structures	Functions
Heart	• The pump that circulates blood to all body parts
Blood vessels: • arteries • veins • capillaries	• Structures through which blood travels from the heart to body and from body back to heart
Blood	• Substance that carries oxygen and nutrients to cells and carries aways waste products
Lymph system	• Returns excess fluid from tissues to general circulation and manufactures lymphocytes

Figure 11-1 The cardiovascular system.

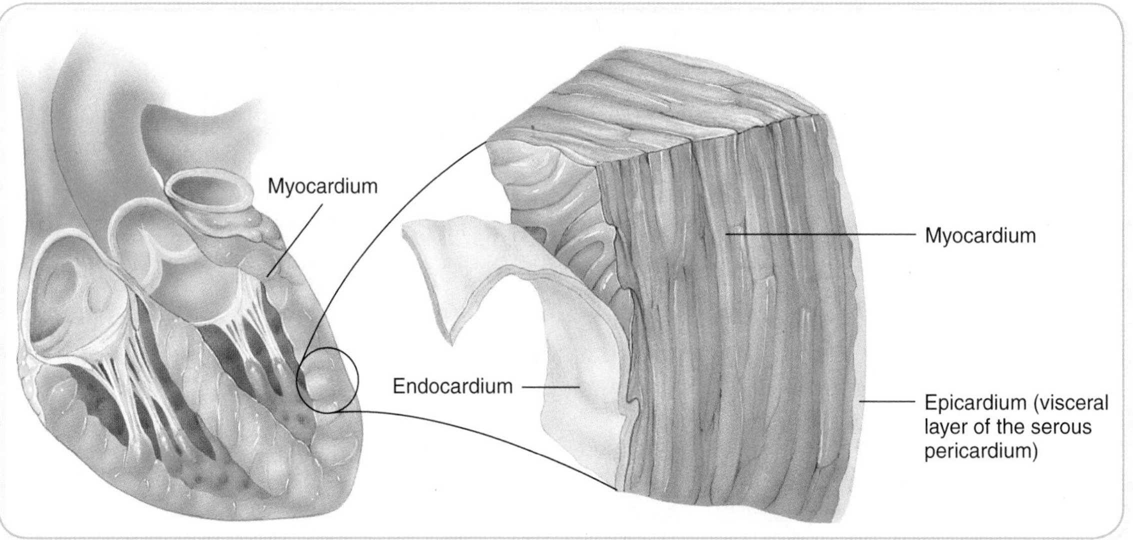

Figure 11-2 The walls and valves of the heart.

- The capillaries are the smallest of the blood vessels. They are the sites of oxygen and nutrient exchange between the blood and the organs of the body.
- The veins carry deoxygenated blood away from the capillaries to the heart.
- There are two circuits for blood flow: the left side of the heart pumps blood to the systemic circuit, while the right side of the heart pumps blood through the pulmonary circuit (Figure 11-4).

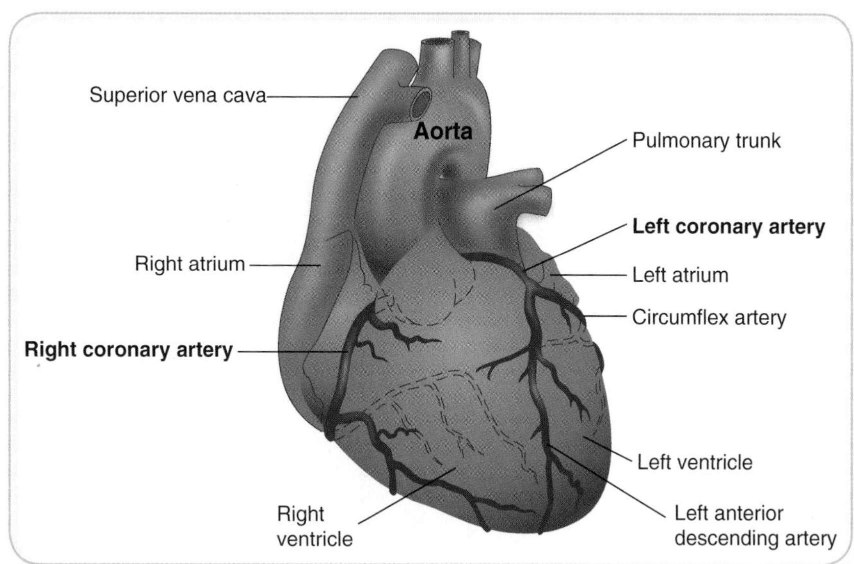

Figure 11-3 The coronary arteries.

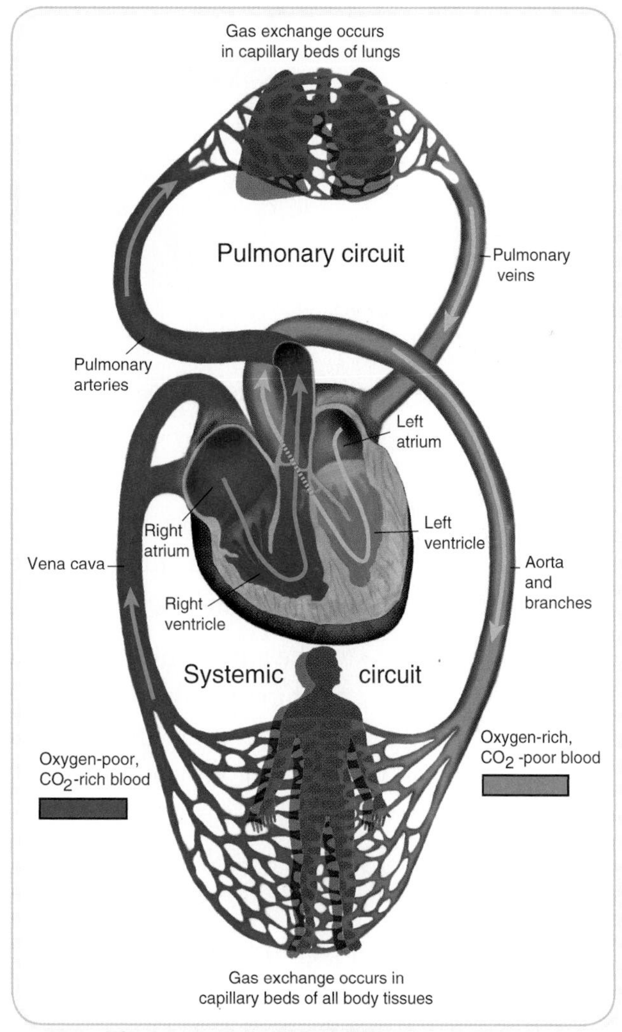

Figure 11-4 The left side of the heart pumps blood to the entire systemic circuit, while the right side pumps blood to the pulmonary circuit.

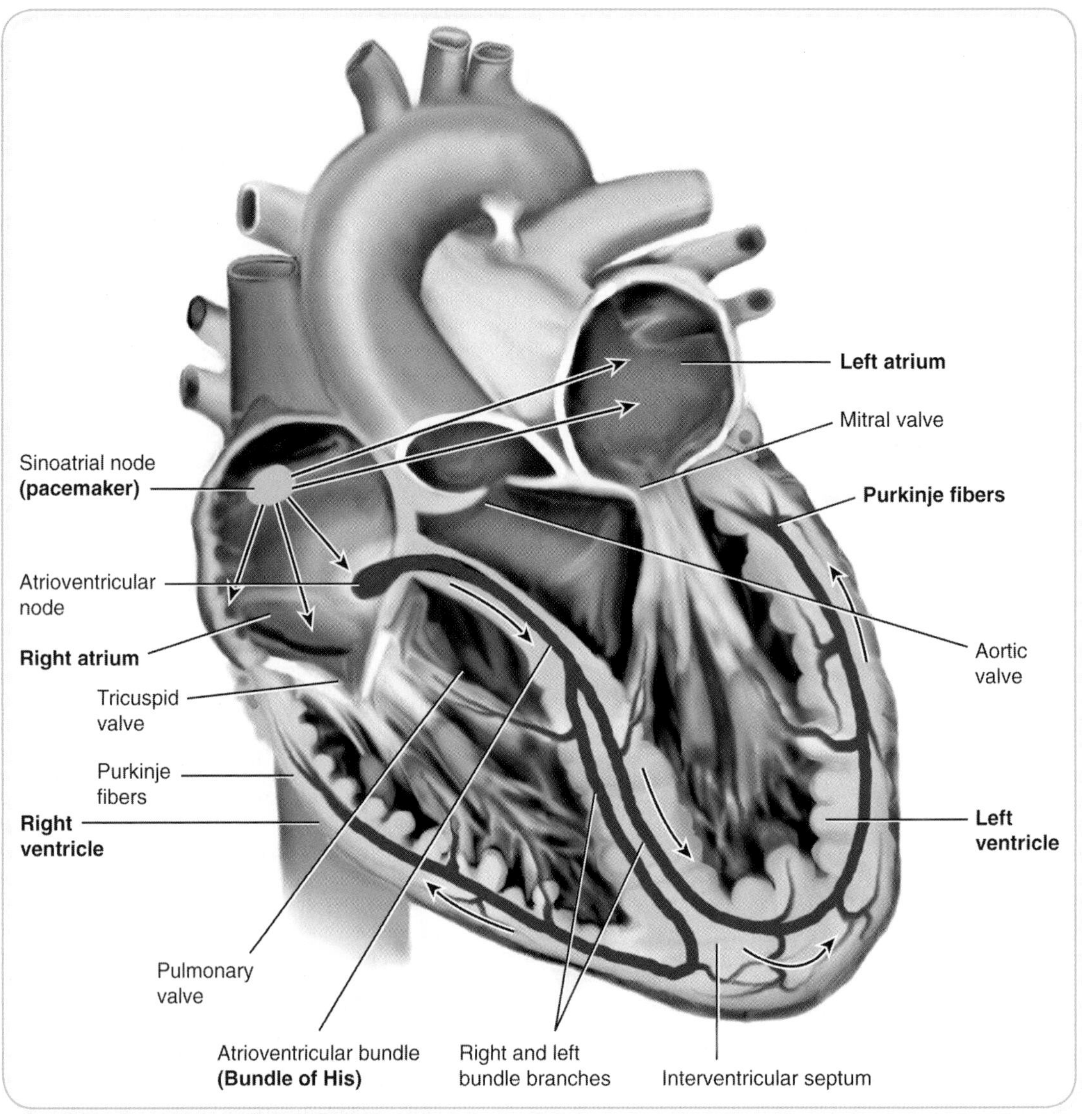

Figure 11-5 The heart's conduction system.

- The myocardium conducts its own electrical impulse, which serves to regulate the heartbeat (Figure 11-5).
- The autonomic nervous system (ANS) and the drugs that stimulate or inhibit it influence heart contractions. The sympathetic nervous system and the drugs that stimulate it *increase* heart rate, whereas the parasympathetic nervous system and the drugs that stimulate it *decrease* heart rate.

Ischemic Heart Disease

In **ischemic heart disease (IHD)**—[most commonly called **coronary artery disease** (including angina pectoris), and also referred to as **coronary heart disease (CHD)** or **myocardial infarction** (heart attack)]—, part of the heart muscle is damaged because of obstruction in an artery. The basic problem is insufficient oxygen for the needs of the heart muscle.

A common cause of disability and death, coronary artery disease may ultimately lead to heart failure, serious arrhythmias, or sudden death. There are several factors that may affect functions that control myocardial oxygen demand (see Table 11-1). It is the leading cause of death in men and women in the United States.

Medical Terminology Review

myocardial
my/o- = *muscle*
cardi/a = *heart*
-al = *pertaining to*
the heart muscle

Key Concept

Every health care professional should be certified in CPR because heart disease is the number-one cause of death in the United States. It is vital that CPR be applied correctly to patients with suspected heart attacks in order to save their lives.

TABLE 11-1 Factors Affecting Cardiac Parameters that Control Myocardial Oxygen Demand

Factors	Heart Rate	Blood Pressure
β-Blockers	Decrease	Decrease
Cold	Increase	Increase
Exercise	Increase	Increase
Nitroglycerin	Increase	Decrease
Smoking	Increase	Increase

Medical Terminology Review

arteriosclerosis
arteri/o = *artery*
sclera/o = *hard*
-sis = *condition*
hardening of the arteries

Key Concept

Having a buildup of calcium plaque in the arteries means an increased risk of heart attacks and death in multiple ethnic groups, according to recent research.

Arteriosclerosis and Atherosclerosis

Arteriosclerosis is the term used to describe degenerative changes in small arteries, commonly occurring in older individuals and diabetics. Elasticity is lost, and the walls become thick and hard. The lumen gradually narrows and may become obscured. This leads to diffuse ischemia and death in various tissues, such as those of the heart, kidneys, or brain.

Atherosclerosis is differentiated by the presence of **atheromas** (plaques consisting of lipids, cells, and cell debris, often with attached thrombi, which form inside the walls of large arteries). Atheromas form primarily in large arteries such as the aorta and the coronary arteries. Figure 11-6 illustrates accumulation of lipids in blood vessels causing occlusion.

Angina Pectoris

Angina pectoris is an episodic, reversible oxygen insufficiency. This condition is the most common form of IHD. Angina pectoris is applied to varying forms of transient chest pain that are attributable to insufficient myocardial oxygen. Atherosclerotic lesions that produce a narrowing of the coronary arteries are the major cause of angina. However, tachycardia (increased heart rate), anemia, hyperthyroidism, and hypotension can cause an oxygen imbalance. According to the American Heart Association, angina occurs more commonly in women than men. There are several types of angina: stable (classic), unstable, decubitus (nocturnal), and silent angina. The most common form is classic angina that may occur, with predictable frequency, from exertion (often from exercising), emotional stress, or a heavy meal. Classic angina is relieved by rest, nitroglycerin, or both.

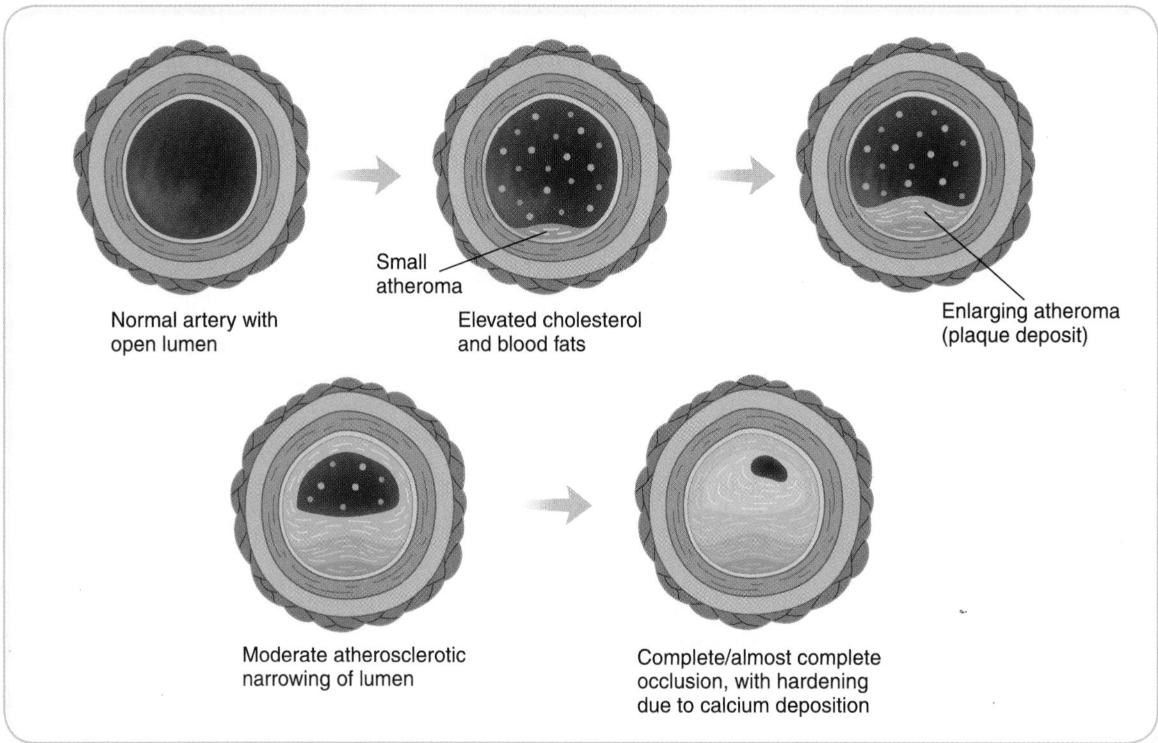

Figure 11-6 Atherosclerosis showing narrowing of the arteries from plaque buildup.

Unstable angina is a medical emergency, and the patient must be treated in a hospital. It typically has a sudden onset, sudden worsening, and stuttering reoccurrence over days and weeks, and carries a more severe short-term prognosis than stable chronic angina. Unstable angina occurs during periods of rest. Signs of unstable angina include changes in blood pressure, transient heart murmur, and arrhythmias.

Decubitus angina is a condition characterized by periodic attacks of cardiac pain that occur when a person is lying down. It is also known as **vasospastic angina**. Decubitus angina occurs when the decreased myocardial blood flow is caused by spasms of the coronary arteries.

Silent angina is a condition that occurs in the absence of angina pain. One or more coronary arteries are occluded, but the individual remains asymptomatic.

Nocturnal angina is caused by coronary artery spasms and can be treated by calcium channel blockers and nitrates. It occurs during the REM period of sleep.

> ***Medical Terminology Review***
>
> **angioplasty**
> ***angio*** *= blood and lymph vessel*
> ***plasty*** *= molding or forming surgically*
> a procedure involving the molding or forming of a blood vessel surgically

Treatment goals for angina include:

- Reducing the risk of sudden death
- Preventing myocardial infarction (MI)
- Increasing myocardial oxygen supply
- Reducing pain and anxiety associated with an angina attack

Key Concept

According to a recent study, aggressive drug therapy now appears to be just as effective as angioplasty for patients with stable heart disease.

Treatment for angina includes surgery and drug therapy. If the coronary arteries are significantly occluded or blocked, **coronary arterial bypass graft (CABG)** or **percutaneous transluminal coronary angioplasty (PTCA)** are performed. CABG is a procedure wherein a vein graft is surgically implanted to bypass the part of the occlusion in the coronary artery. PTCA reduces obstruction by means of invasive procedures requiring cardiac catheterization. The catheter contains an inflatable balloon that flattens the obstruction. Newer techniques use laser angioplasty.

Antianginal Drug Therapy

There are three groups of medications that may meet the treatment goals for angina pectoris.

1. Nitrates
2. β-Adrenergic Blockers
3. Calcium Channel Blockers

Nitrates

Nitrates were the first agents used to relieve angina. This group of drugs reduces myocardial ischemia, but may cause hypotension. Nitrates are still an important part of antianginal therapy. Table 11-2 shows nitrates commonly used in the treatment of angina.

TABLE 11-2 Commonly Used Combination Drugs for Angina and Myocardial Infarction

Generic Name	Trade Name	Route of Administration	Average Adult Dosage
Beta-adrenergic blockers			
atenolol	Tenormin®	PO	25–50 mg/day (max: 100 mg/day)
metoprolol tartrate	Lopressor®, Toprol-XL®	PO	100 mg bid (max: 400 mg/day)
propranolol hydrochloride	Inderal®, Inderal LA®	PO	10–20 mg bid-tid (max: 320 mg/day)
timolol maleate	Betimol®, Blocadren®	PO	15–45 mg tid (max: 60 mg/day)
Calcium channel blockers			
amlodipine	Norvasc®	PO	5–10 mg/day (max: 10 mg/day)
bepridil	Vascor®	PO	200 mg/day (max: 360 mg/day)

(*continues*)

TABLE 11-2 Commonly Used Combination Drugs for Angina and Myocardial Infarction—*continued*

Generic Name	Trade Name	Route of Administration	Average Adult Dosage
diltiazem hydrochloride	Cardizem®, Dilacor XR®	PO	30 mg qid (max: 360 mg/day)
nicardipine hydrochloride	Cardene®	PO	20–40 mg tid or 30–60 mg SR bid (max: 120 mg/day)
nifedipine	Adalat®, Procardia®	PO	10–20 mg tid (max: 180 mg/day)
verapamil hydrochloride	Calan®, Covera-HS®	PO	80 mg tid-qid (max: 480 mg/day) taken at bedtime
Organic nitrates			
amyl nitrate	(generic only)	Inhalation	1 ampule (0.18–0.3 mL) PRN
isosorbide dinitrate	Iso-Bid®, Isordil®	PO	2.5–30 mg qid
isosorbide mononitrate	Imdur®, ISMO®	PO	20 mg bid
nitroglycerin	Nitrostat®, Nitrocap®,	SL	1 tablet (0.3–0.6 mg) or 1 spray (0.4–0.8 mg) q3–5 min (max: 3 doses in 15 min)
	Nitro-Dur®	Topical	applied transdermally daily

Mechanism of Action

Nitrates primarily are effective in the venous circulation by relaxing vascular smooth muscle and reducing the left ventricle's work. These agents are administered to dilate the blood vessels and stop attacks of angina (see Figure 11-7).

Indications

Nitrates are used in the treatment of angina as coronary vasodilators. Nitrate preparations should be based on onset of action, duration of action, and patient compliance. Nitrate preparations are available in sublingual tablets, nitroglycerin spray bottles, topical nitroglycerin ointments, and transdermal patches. The sublingual route is the most common route of administration for nitroglycerin. This agent begins to work rapidly and lasts for about an hour. This is an ideal preparation for acute anginal pain. Administration should begin as soon as the pain begins, and should not be delayed until the pain is severe. If one tablet is not sufficient, one or two additional tablets should be taken at five-minute intervals. For persistent pain, the patient should see a physician, because he or she may have signs of a myocardial infarction. The shelf life of nitroglycerin is longer in a dark, tightly closed container. After the container is opened, the drug is effective

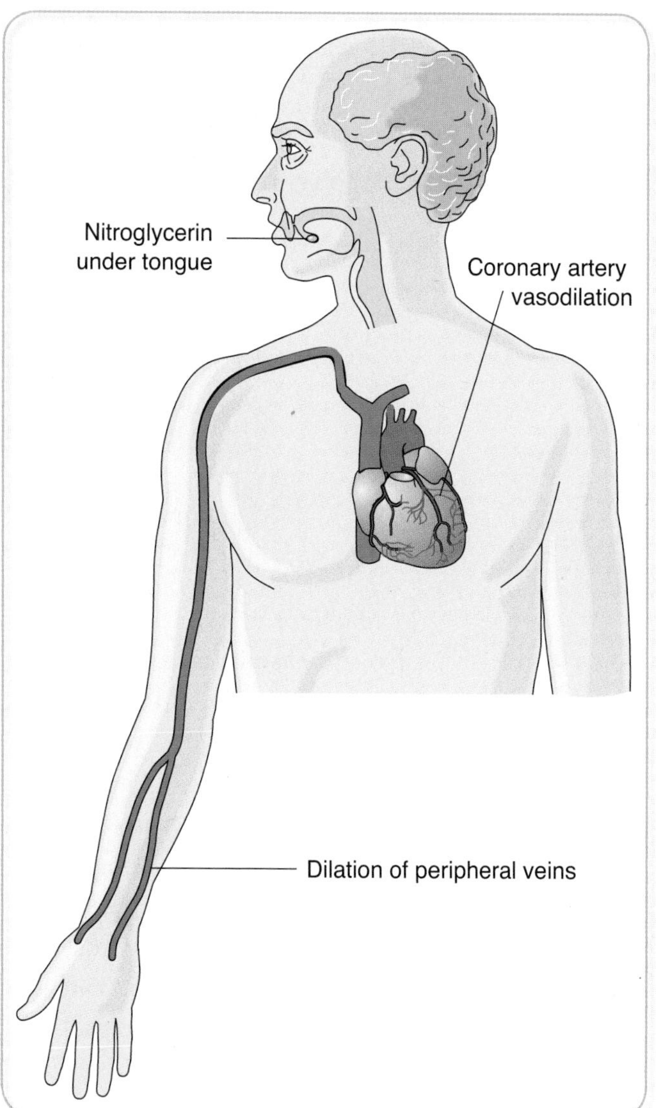

Figure 11-7 Mechanism of action of nitroglycerin.

for approximately 30 days, and the date on which it was opened should be written on the container. Thirty days after the container is opened, the medication should be discarded and replaced with a new bottle.

Transdermal patches contain a reservoir of nitroglycerin. This agent is slowly released for absorption through the skin (see Figure 11-8). The patches are slow in onset and are not effective for an ongoing anginal attack. The application site of the patch should be rotated daily to prevent irritation.

Topical ointment can also be used on the skin by using an applicator, and covering it with plastic wrap held in place with adhesive tape. The sites should be rotated to prevent local irritation.

Adverse Effects

Abrupt discontinuation of long-acting nitroglycerin preparations may cause angina. Vasodilation can lead to orthostatic hypotension, tachycardia, headache, dizziness, weakness, syncope, and blushing. Nitrate-induced

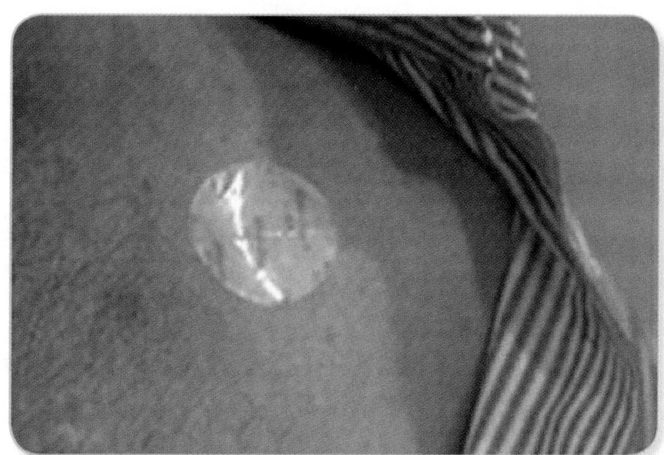

Figure 11-8 Transdermal nitroglycerin patch (Courtesy of 3M Pharmaceuticals, St. Paul, MN).

headache is a result of the dilation of cerebral blood vessels. Nitrates may also increase intraocular and intracranial pressure. Continuous exposure to nitrates may lead to tolerance. Large doses of nitrate drugs can produce methemoglobinemia (the presence of methemoglobin in the blood).

> ***Medical Terminology Review***
>
> **hyperthyroidism**
> ***hyper*** = *over; above; beyond*
> ***thyroid*** = *the thyroid gland*
> ***ism*** = *action; process; practice*
> overactive thyroid gland

Contraindications and Precautions

These agents are contraindicated in patients with hypersensitivity to nitrates, severe anemia, head trauma, and increased intracranial pressure. Nitrates are also contraindicated in glaucoma, hypotension, hyperthyroidism, and alcoholism. Safety during pregnancy (category C) and lactation is not established. Nitrate drugs should also be used cautiously in severe liver or kidney disease.

Drug Interactions

A combination of nitrates and sildenafil (Viagra) can cause prolonged and potentially life-threatening hypotension. Sildenafil therapy should therefore be contraindicated in patients who use nitrates. Beta-blockers, calcium channel blockers, vasodilators, and alcohol can enhance the hypotensive effect of nitrates. IV nitroglycerin may antagonize the effects of heparin.

Beta-adrenergic Blockers

Beta-adrenergic blockers *(β-blockers)* block the beta 1 receptor site. Beta-blockers decrease the effects of the sympathetic nervous system by blocking the release of the catecholamines epinephrine and norepinephrine, thereby decreasing the heart rate and blood pressure. (They are listed in both Tables 11-2 and 11-4.)

Mechanism of Action

Beta blockers reduce oxygen demand, both at rest and during exertion, in the myocardium, and prevent myocardial infarction (IM).

Medical Terminology Review

hypoglycemia
hypo = under; beneath; down
glyc = carbohydrate and especially sugar
emia = condition of having
low blood sugar levels

bronchospasm
broncho = windpipe; bronchial (tube)
spasm = an involuntary and abnormal muscular contraction
abnormal muscular contractions of the windpipe

Indications

The beta-blockers reduce the frequency and severity of exertional angina that is not controlled by nitrates. Therefore, these are an important part of therapy for angina pectoris. Combined therapy with nitrates is often preferred in the treatment of angina pectoris, because of a decrease in the side effects of both agents.

Adverse Effects

Beta-blockers have few adverse effects on the respiratory and cardiovascular systems. Common adverse effects of these drugs include dyspnea, bronchospasm, hypotension, bradycardia, and hypoglycemia. These agents may also cause insomnia and depression.

Contraindications and Precautions

β-blockers are contraindicated in patients with a known hypersensitivity to these agents. β-blockers are also contraindicated for use in patients with asthma, congestive heart failure, heart block, bradycardia, and diabetes mellitus. These drugs should be avoided in patients with cardiogenic shock, pulmonary edema, and peripheral vascular disease.

β-adrenergic blockers should be used with caution in patients prone to non-allergenic bronchospasm (e.g., chronic bronchitis, emphysema), major surgery, stroke, renal disease, or hepatic disease. β-blockers are used cautiously in elderly patients, patients with diabetes mellitus, and in patients prone to hypoglycemia.

Drug Interactions

These agents may interact with atropine and other anticholinergics, NSAIDs, insulin, sulfonylureas, lidocaine, verapamil, prazosin, and terazosin.

Calcium Channel Blockers

Calcium channel blockers are considered third-choice agents in the treatment of stable angina, certain dysrhythmias, and hypertension. Calcium channel blockers are also listed in Table 11-2.

Mechanism of Action

Calcium channel blockers are a type of drug that block the entry of calcium into smooth muscle cells as well as myocytes. They produce arterial vasodilation and thereby reduce arterial blood pressure. They also reduce myocardial contractility, resulting in reduction of myocardial oxygen consumption.

Indications

Calcium channel blockers are used to treat exertional angina that is not controlled by nitrates, and in combination with beta-blockers. This combination provides the most effective therapy. They are considered the drug of choice in the treatment of angina at rest. Diltiazem and verapamil will reduce the heart rate. Nifedipine, amlodipine, and felodipine are among the most potent calcium-blocking agents. β-blockers are recommended as the first-line treatment of angina pectoris, but if they are not tolerated, calcium channel blockers can be administered. Diltiazem and verapamil can be used, but they have the disadvantage of depressing contractility more than dihydropyridines do. The therapeutic goal in medication use is to reduce the frequency and intensity of anginal attacks without suppressing the cardiac action too much.

Adverse Effects

Common adverse effects related to the use of calcium channel blockers include: flushing, headaches, dizziness, hypotension, ankle edema, constipation, and palpitations. Combinations of nitrates, β-blockers, and calcium channel blockers are often preferred for treatment of angina pectoris, because these agents have fewer adverse effects.

Contraindications and Precautions

Calcium channel blockers are contraindicated in patients with a history of hypersensitivity to these drugs, hypotension, or cardiogenic shock. The major contraindications to combination therapy are associated with the use of β-blockers and calcium channel blockers, which may cause excessive cardiac depression. Calcium channel blockers should be used with caution during pregnancy (category C) and lactation, and in patients with congestive heart failure, hepatic or renal dysfunction, and hypotension.

Drug Interactions

Calcium channel blockers increase risk of orthostatic hypotension with prazosin. Increased blood pressure may occur with aspirin, bismuth subsalicylate, or magnesium salicylate. Some calcium channel blockers increase serum levels and toxicity of cyclosporine.

Myocardial Infarction

Myocardial infarction (MI) is an area of dead cardiac muscle tissue, with or without hemorrhage. Myocardial infarction is produced by an obstruction of the coronary artery, which results in a lack of oxygen to the tissue. Coronary heart disease is the primary cause of death in American males and females as well as a major cause of disability. For those who survive an MI, there is a notably greater risk of a second MI, congestive heart failure, or a stroke occurring within a short time.

A myocardial infarction, or heart attack, occurs when a coronary artery is totally obstructed, leading to prolonged ischemia (reduction of blood supply to the heart) and cell death, or infarction, of the heart wall (see Figure 11-9).

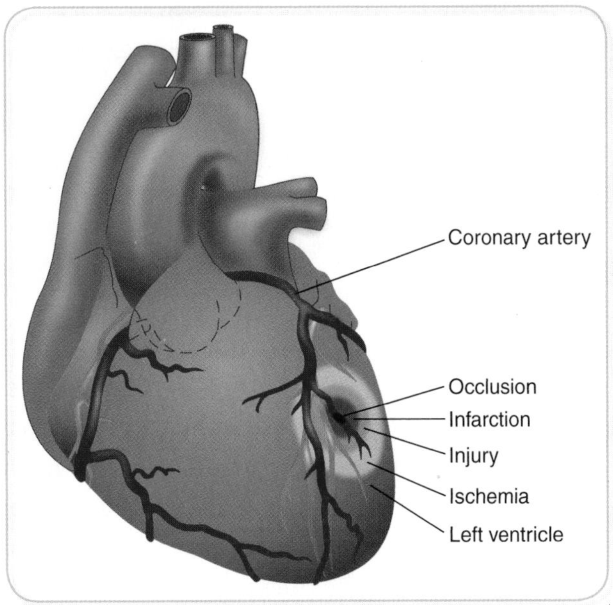

Figure 11-9 Myocardial infarction.

After myocardial infarction, there are three goals that should be achieved expeditiously and simultaneously to limit myocardial necrosis and mortality:

- Relief of pain
- Confirmation of diagnosis by electrocardiogram (ECG) and measurements of serum markers
- Assessment and treatment of hemodynamic abnormalities

Pain relief is best achieved with oxygen (2 L/min by nasal cannula), nitroglycerin, and morphine sulfate. The rationale for reperfusion therapy (thrombolytic therapy) is based on the high prevalence of occlusive thrombus in early treatment. The greatest benefit is seen when this therapy is performed within the first four hours of the onset of pain. Antithrombotic agents should be considered for all patients with an acute myocardial infarction. Antithrombotic medications include: unfractionated heparin, low molecular weight heparin, warfarin, aspirin, and antiplatelets (see Chapter 13).

Key Concept

During acute myocardial infarction, women are less likely to experience chest pain than men. Common acute symptoms in women include dyspnea, weakness, fatigue, nausea or vomiting, palpitations, and indigestion.

Cardiac Arrhythmias

Arrhythmias (dysrhythmias) are deviations from the normal cardiac rate or rhythm. They may result from damage to the heart's conduction system or from systemic causes such as electrolyte abnormalities, fever, hypoxia, stress, and drug toxicity.

TABLE 11-3 Various Cardiac Arrhythmias

Type of Arrhythmia	Beats per Minute
Bradycardia	Less than 60
Tachycardia	150 to 250
Atrial flutter	200 to 350
Atrial fibrillation	More than 350
Ventricular fibrillation	Variable
Premature atrial contraction	Variable
Premature ventricular contraction	Variable

Medical Terminology Review

dysrhythmia
dys = abnormal
rhythm = regular recurrence of action
ia = pathological condition
abnormal heart rhythm

Key Concept

According to a recent study, patients who are diagnosed for the first time with atrial fibrillation have a significantly greater early risk of dying compared with those who do not have this condition. Factors that are strongly associated with death in atrial fibrillation patients include a faster heart rate at diagnosis, being thin, a history of chronic kidney disease, and malignancy.

Arrhythmias reduce the efficiency of the heart's pumping cycle. A slight increase in heart rate increases cardiac output, but a very rapid heart rate prevents adequate filling during diastole, reducing cardiac output. A very slow heart rate also reduces output to the tissues, including the brain and the heart itself. Irregular contractions are inefficient because they interfere with the normal filling and emptying cycle. Table 11-3 summarizes various cardiac arrhythmias.

Antiarrhythmic Drugs

Antiarrhythmic agents do not cure the dysrhythmia, but the goal of treatment is to restore normal cardiac function. These agents are classified in four distinct groups, according to their effects: Class I (sodium channel blockers), which are subclassified into three groups, Class IA, IB, and IC (see Table 11-4); Class II (β-adrenergic blockers); Class III (which interfere with potassium outflow); and Class IV (calcium channel blockers). There are also other agents that may be used for the treatment of arrhythmias, such as digoxin, atropine, and magnesium.

Mechanism of Action

Class I – Fast (sodium) channel blockers decrease the fast sodium influx to the cardiac cells. These drugs decrease conduction velocity in the cardiac tissue, suppress automaticity, and increase recovery time (repolarization). There are three subgroups of fast channel blockers: IA slows conduction and prolongs repolarization (e.g., quinidine, procainamide, disopyramide); IB slows conduction and shortens repolarization (e.g., lidocaine, mexiletine, tocainide); and IC prolongs conduction with little to no effect on repolarization (e.g., flecainide).

Class II – Beta-adrenergic blockers inhibit adrenergic stimulation of the heart, and depress myocardial excitability and contractility. Therefore, they decrease conduction velocity in cardiac tissue. Major beta-adrenergic blockers are listed in Tables 11-2 and 11-4.

TABLE 11-4 Classifications of Antiarrhythmic Drugs

Generic Name	Trade Name	Route of Administration	Average Adult Dosage
Class IA (sodium channel blockers)			
disopyramide phosphate	Norpace®	PO	100–200 mg q6h or 300 mg sust. release cap. q12h
procainamide hydrochloride	Procan®, Procanbid, Pronestyl®	PO, IM, IV	PO: 50 mg/kg/day in divided doses; IM: 0.5–1g q4–8h; IV: 100 mg q5 min at a rate of 25–50 mg/min until arrhythmia is controlled
quinidine gluconate	Quinaglute®	PO	200–300 mg q3–4h for 4 or more doses until arrhythmia terminates
Class IB			
lidocaine hydrochloride	Xylocaine®	IV	50–100 mg bolus at 20–50 mg/min, may repeat in 5 min, then start infusion of 1–4 mg/min immed. after 1st bolus
mexiletine	Mexitil®	PO	200–300 mg q8h (max: 1200 mg/day)
phenytoin	Dilantin®	IV	50–100 mg q10–15 min until dysrhythmia is terminated
Class IC			
flecainide acetate	Tambocor®	PO	100 mg q12h, may increase 50 mg bid q4d (max: 400 mg/day)
moricizine hydrochloride	Ethmozine®	PO	600–900 mg/day
propafenone	Rythmol®	PO	150–300 mg/tid; increase dosage slowly, prn, (max: 900 mg/day)
Class II (β-adrenergic blockers)			
acebutolol	Sectral®	PO	200–600 mg bid increased to 1200 mg/day
atenolol	Tenormin®	PO	25–50 mg/day, may increase to 100 mg/day
esmolol hydrochloride	Brevibloc®	IV	50 mcg/kg/min (max: 200 mcg/kg/min)
nadolol	Corgard®	PO	40 mg once/day, increase to 240–320 mg/day in 1–2 div. doses
propranolol hydrochloride	Inderal®	PO	10–30 mg tid or qid

(*continues*)

TABLE 11-4 Classifications of Antiarrhythmic Drugs—*continued*

Generic Name	Trade Name	Route of Administration	Average Adult Dosage
Class III (potassium channel blockers)			
amiodarone hydrochloride	Cordarone®	PO	PO: 400–1600 mg/day in 1–3 div. doses
bretylium tosylate	Bretylol®	IV	Rapid injection (5–10 mg/kg), or 1–2 mg/min as continuous infusion
dofetilide	Tikosyn®	PO	125–500 mcg bid
ibutilide fumarate	Corvert®	IV	1 mg infused over 10 min
Class IV (calcium channel blockers)			
diltiazem	Cardizem®	IV	0.25–15 mg/kg bolus over 2 min, may repeat in 15 min with 0.35 mg/kg
verapamil hydrochloride	Calan®	IV	2.5–5 mg initial dose, then 5–10 mg after 15–30 min
Others			
atropine	Atropisol®	IM, IV	0.5–1 mg q1–2h prn (max: 2 mg)
digoxin	Lanoxin®	PO, IV	PO: 0.75–1.5 mg/kg; IV: 0.5–1 mg/kg

Class III – Antiarrhythmics interfere with potassium outflow during repolarization. They prolong the action potential duration and effective refractory period. The prolonged period decreases the frequency of heart rate. Amiodarone decreases automaticity, prolongs atrioventricular conduction, and may even block the exchange of sodium and potassium.

Class IV – Antiarrhythmics selectively block slow calcium channels. Therefore, these agents can prolong nodal conduction and effective refractory period. These calcium antagonists may also decrease the ability of the heart to produce forceful contractions, leading to congestive heart failure. These drugs also relax smooth muscle and cause vasodilation. Verapamil works on the SA node to decrease its activity, thus decreasing the heart rate. It also decreases AV node conduction and is used for AV node dysrhythmias.

Indications

Quinidine is used to treat supraventricular arrhythmias, such as atrial flutter and atrial fibrillation, acute ventricular dysrhythmias, and life-threatening ventricular dysrhythmias. This agent also exhibits antimalarial, antipyretic, and oxytocic actions. Procainamide is safer to use intravenously and has fewer gastrointestinal (GI) adverse effects. Disopyramide has been approved for the treatment of ventricular arrhythmias. Generally, it is reserved for patients who are intolerant of quinidine or procainamide. Lidocaine doses must be adjusted in patients with congestive heart failure or hepatic disease. Mexiletine is used primarily for chronic treatment of ventricular arrhythmias associated with previous myocardial infarction. Tocainide is useful for the treatment of ventricular tachyarrhythmias. Phenytoin is an antiepileptic drug that has proved to be useful in treating digitalis-induced tachyarrhythmias. β-adrenergic blockers are useful for treating tachyarrhythmias due to increased sympathetic activity, and also are used for a variety of other arrhythmias, atrial flutter, and atrial fibrillation. These are sometimes used for digitalis toxicity. Propranolol is the most common β-blocker that is used as an antiarrhythmic. Amiodarone is useful for severe refractory supraventricular and ventricular tachyarrhythmias. Amiodarone also possesses antianginal effects. Calcium channel blockers are useful for angina and for hypertension. Verapamil is useful for reentrant supraventricular tachycardia. Digitalis drugs are the principal medications for the treatment of congestive heart failure and certain arrhythmias. Digoxin is the drug most often prescribed because it can be administered orally and parenterally. It has an intermediate duration of action. The process of establishing the correct therapeutic dose of digitalis for maintaining optimal functioning of the heart without toxic effects is referred to as digitalization. The margin between effective therapy and dangerous toxicity is very narrow. Careful monitoring of the cardiac rate and rhythm with an ECG, cardiac function, adverse effects, and the blood digitalis level is required to determine the therapeutic maintenance dose.

Adverse Effects

Quinidine can lead to skeletal muscle weakness, especially in patients with myasthenia gravis. Rapid infusion of quinidine may cause severe hypotension and shock. It can produce ringing of the ears, dizziness, diarrhea, thrombocytopenia, and ventricular arrhythmias.

A high incidence of adverse reactions to procainamide is seen with chronic use. Severe or irreversible heart failure has been produced more frequently by procainamide than by quinidine. Procainamide also often causes drug-induced lupus syndrome.

Disopyramide drug may cause dry mouth, blurred vision, constipation, and urinary retention.

High doses of lidocaine can cause cardiovascular depression, confusion, and light-headedness. Otherwise, there is a low level of cardiotoxicity with the use of lidocaine. The most common side effects are neurologic, in contrast to quinidine and procainamide. Lidocaine has little effect on the autonomic nervous system. The common adverse effects of phenytoin use are nystagmus, blurred vision, vertigo, and hyperplasia of the gums.

Adverse effects of the use of beta-adrenergic blockers include bronchospasm. Bradycardia and myocardial depression may occur. Atropine

Medical Terminology Review

bradycardia
brady = slow
cardia = heart action
slow heart rate

or isoproterenol may be used to alleviate bradycardia. The most frequent cardiovascular adverse effects due to the use of propranolol are hypertension and bradycardia. It may also cause mental confusion and skin rashes.

Contraindications and Precautions

Class I antidysrhythmic agents are contraindicated in patients with hypersensitivity to these drugs, pregnancy (category B or C), and lactation. They should be avoided in patients with complete AV block, thyrotoxicosis, acute rheumatic fever, extensive myocardial damage, hypotensive states, myasthenia gravis, and digitalis intoxication. Quinidine should be used cautiously in patients with incomplete heart block, impaired kidney or liver function, bronchial asthma, myasthenia gravis, and potassium imbalance. Procainamide is used with caution in patients with hypotension, cardiac enlargement, congestive heart failure, heart attack, coronary occlusion, and hepatic or renal insufficiency.

Class II antidysrhythmic drugs (e.g., propranolol and others) are contraindicated in patients with congestive heart failure, right ventricular failure secondary to pulmonary hypertension, ventricular dysfunction, sinus bradycardia, bronchial asthma or bronchospasm, pulmonary edema, and allergic rhinitis during pollen season. Beta-adrenergic blockers are used cautiously in elderly patients and patients prone to non-allergic bronchospasm (e.g., chronic bronchitis, emphysema), stroke, major surgery, renal or hepatic disease, and diabetes mellitus.

Class III antiarrhythmic drugs (e.g., bretylium) have no contraindications for use in life-threatening ventricular arrhythmias. Safety during pregnancy (category C), lactation, or in children is not established. Amiodarone is contraindicated in patients with hypersensitivity to this agent. Amiodarone should be avoided in cardiogenic shock, severe sinus bradycardia, severe liver disease, and children. Safety during pregnancy (category D) or lactation is not established. Amiodarone is given to patients cautiously if they have cirrhosis of the liver, goiter, hypersensitivity to iodine, electrolyte imbalance, hypokalemia, hypovolemia, and open-heart surgery. It also must be used with caution in elderly patients. Bretylium is used with caution in patients with severe aortic stenosis or severe pulmonary hypertension, and angina pectoris.

Class IV antiarrythmic drugs (calcium channel blockers) are contraindicated in patients with severe hypotension, cardiogenic shock, cardiomegaly, digitalis toxicity, atrial flutter and fibrillation, and severe CHF. Safe use of these agents during pregnancy (category C) or lactation, and in children, is not established. Calcium channel blockers are used cautiously in those individuals with hepatic and renal impairment, heart attack by coronary occlusion, and aortic stenosis.

Drug Interactions

Two antiarrhythmic agents may cause additive effects and may increase the risk for drug toxicity. If quinidine and procainamide are given with digitalis, the risk of digitalis toxicity may be increased. Quinidine may interact with cimetidine or barbiturates, with quinidine blood levels being increased. Quinidine that is given concurrently with verapamil increases the risk of hypotension. Lidocaine and procainamide may interact and cause additive cardiodepressant effects. Inderal may also increase the risk of lidocaine toxicity.

Congestive Heart Failure

Congestive heart failure (CHF) is one of the most common cardiovascular disorders. This condition occurs when the heart is not able to pump enough blood to meet the body's metabolic demands. Heart failure may be caused by any disorder that affects the heart's ability to receive or eject blood.

Because there is no cure for heart failure, the treatment goals are to prevent, treat, or remove the underlying causes when possible. Drugs can relieve the symptoms of heart failure by a number of different mechanisms, including slowing the heart rate, increasing contractility, and reducing its workload. Drugs used for heart failure include ACE inhibitors, diuretics, vasodilators, and cardiac glycosides. In this section, cardiac glycosides will be discussed in detail. The other drugs also used for heart failure are discussed in Chapter 12.

Cardiac Glycosides

Cardiac glycosides are one of the oldest drugs used in the treatment of heart diseases (over 2,000 years). A number of plants contain cardiac glycosides. Digoxin is extracted from the leaves of the purple foxglove (*Digitalis purpurea*). In fact, the generic term digitalis is often used to represent all cardiac glycosides used in the clinical setting.

Cardiac glycosides increase the speed of myocardial contractions in both normal and failing hearts. Under normal cardiac conditions, digitalis treatment results in an increase in systemic vascular resistance and the constriction of smooth muscles in veins (cardiac output may decrease). In heart failure, digitalis increases the force of myocardial contractions, slows the heart rate, and slows the conduction of electrical impulses. The increased force of contractions improves the efficiency of the heart without increasing oxygen consumption. Normal blood circulation is restored and the kidney function is increased. The most common cardiac glycosides are digoxin and digitoxin. The major active ingredients found in digitalis plants are collectively referred to as digitalis. Cardiac glycosides are able to affect the congested heartbeats more forcefully within a shorter period of time. This force increases the amount of blood pumped from the heart and improves blood circulation, thus decreasing the congestion found with heart failure.

Digitalis drugs are principal medications for the treatment of congestive heart failure and certain arrhythmias (atrial fibrillation, flutter, and paroxysmal atrial tachycardias). Digoxin is prescribed the most frequently

Key Concept

Patients should never stop taking digoxin without first consulting a physician. A sudden absence of this drug can cause a serious change in heart function. Digoxin is usually required to be taken for a long time, sometimes throughout life.

because it can be administered orally and parenterally. It has an intermediate duration of action. The process of establishing the correct therapeutic dose of digitalis for maintaining optimal functioning of the heart without toxic effects is referred to as digitalization. There is a very narrow margin between effective therapy and dangerous toxicity. Careful monitoring of the cardiac rate and rhythm with an ECG, cardiac function, side effects, and blood digitalis level is required to determine the therapeutic maintenance dose.

Mechanism of Action

Cardiac glycosides act by increasing the force and velocity of myocardial systolic contraction (positive inotropic effect). They also decrease conduction velocity through the atrioventricular node.

Indications

Cardiac glycosides are used principally in the prophylactic management and treatment of heart failure, and to control the ventricular rate in patients with atrial fibrillation or flutter. These drugs are also used to treat and prevent recurrent atrial tachycardia, cardiogenic shock, and angina pectoris.

Since individual cardiac glycosides have similar pharmacologic and therapeutic properties, the choice of a preparation depends on the onset of action required, desired route of administration, and duration of action. Digoxin is the most commonly used cardiac glycoside, primarily because it may be administered by various routes, and it has an intermediate duration of action.

Adverse Effects

The most dangerous adverse effect of digoxin is its ability to cause dysrhythmias, particularly in patients who have hypokalemia. Common adverse effects of digoxin therapy include nausea, vomiting, anorexia, and abnormalities of the nervous system such as headache, blurred vision (yellow-green halos), diplopia, photophobia, drowsiness, fatigue, and confusion.

Contraindications and Precautions

Cardiac glycosides are contraindicated in patients with known hypersensitivity to these agents, ventricular tachycardia, and ventricular failure, and in the presence of digitalis toxicity.

Cardiotonics are used cautiously in patients with renal insufficiency, hypokalemia, advanced heart disease, acute MI, severe lung disease, hypothyroidism, pregnancy (category A), and lactation. Fetal toxicity and neonatal death have been reported from maternal digoxin overdosage.

Drug Interactions

Cardiotonics react with many different drugs, including antacids, cholestyramine, and diuretics. Colestipol decreases digoxin absorption.

Summary

Diseases of the cardiovascular system are among the leading causes of death in the United States. There are varieties of medications, some of which are effective on the myocardium itself, while some others affect the blood vessels of the vascular system. Vasodilators, such as nitrates, increase the size of blood vessels to improve circulation of the blood for the management of angina pectoris. Cardiac glycosides come from digitalis and are used to increase the force of myocardial contractions in congestive heart failure. Antidysrhythmics are used to treat disorders of the cardiac rhythm. These disorders may occur from coronary artery disease, electrolyte imbalances, cardiac conduction abnormalities, or even from endocrine disease (thyroid disorders).

Exploring the Web

Visit ***www.intelihealth.com***

- Search for "cardiac drugs." Read some of the related articles on disorders of the heart and cardiovascular system and the drug therapies used to treat them.

Visit ***www.americanheart.org***

- Research the diseases and conditions discussed within this chapter for further understanding of them.

Review Questions

Multiple Choice

1. Which of the following antianginal drugs are also used as antihypertensives and antiarrhythmics?

A. nitrates
B. vasoconstrictors
C. diuretics
D. beta-adrenergic blockers

2. Which of the following drugs is the class of calcium channel blockers?

A. propranolol
B. isosorbid
C. verapamil
D. atenolol

3. Early signs of toxicity of digitalis include:

A. mental disorders
B. nausea and vomiting
C. tachycardia
D. seizures

4. Which of the following medications is not used for dysrhythmia?
   A. beta-adrenergic blockers
   B. digoxin
   C. heparin
   D. atropine
5. A combination of nitrates and sildenafil (Viagra) can cause:
   A. stroke
   B. hypotension
   C. heart murmur
   D. hypertension
6. An example of a class II antidysrhythmic drug is:
   A. propranolol
   B. digoxin
   C. bretylium
   D. quinidine
7. Which of the following are common adverse effects of antidysrhythmic drugs?
   A. fatigue, diarrhea, hypertension
   B. dizziness, hypotension, and weakness
   C. anorexia, fatigue, and constipation
   D. fatigue, hypertension, and headache
8. An antidysrhythmic drug may cause:
   A. increased hepatic insufficiency
   B. decreased cardiac output
   C. increased cardiac output
   D. increased renal insufficiency
9. Which of the following administration routes for nitroglycerin is the most common?
   A. sublingual
   B. transdermal patch
   C. topical ointment
   D. parenteral
10. Combined therapy with nitrates is often preferred in treatment of angina pectoris because it results in which of the following?
    A. better toleration
    B. less adverse effects
    C. less expense
    D. increased blood volume

Fill in the Blank

1. Beta-blockers reduce the frequency and severity of exertional angina that is not controlled by ______________.
2. Class I antiarrhythmic drugs are also called ______________.
3. Calcium channel blockers are in Class ______________ of the antiarrhythmic drugs.

4. Common side effects of phenytoin use are ____________, ____________, ____________, and ____________.

5. Cardiac glycosides act by increasing the force and velocity of ____________.

Matching

_____ 1. Subclass IA (fast channel blockers)	A. verapamil (Calan)
_____ 2. Subclass IB	B. lidocaine (Xylocaine)
_____ 3. Subclass IC	C. bretylium (Bretylol)
_____ 4. Class III (agents that interfere with potassium outflow)	D. procainamide (Pronestyl)
_____ 5. Class IV (calcium channel blockers)	E. flecainide (Tambocor)

Critical Thinking

A man who is 57 years old is experiencing severe chest pains. He arrives at the emergency room of his local hospital with cool and clammy skin, blood pressure of 92/60, and a weak, irregular pulse of 90. He is given oxygen and an ECG machine is set up to monitor him. After blood tests, he is initially diagnosed with MI of the left ventricle. His wife tells the doctors that he is a heavy cigarette smoker, loves fried foods and meat, and often complains of indigestion and stomach pain. He is very busy at work and often feels fatigued at night. His father died of a heart attack, and he is fearful of the same thing happening to him. The doctors suspect generalized atherosclerosis.

1. List the elements of this patient's history that are high-risk factors for atherosclerosis.
2. How does atherosclerosis cause an MI?
3. If his reported indigestion was actually angina, explain how this pain might have occurred.

Websites:

www.americanheart.org

www.cardiologychannel.com/angina/index.shtml

CHAPTER 12

Antihypertensive Agents and Hyperlipidemia

OBJECTIVES

After completing this chapter, the reader should be able to:

1. Describe the major physiological factors that regulate blood pressure.
2. Define the three forms of hypertension.
3. Describe the effects of cardiac output, peripheral resistance, and blood volume on blood pressure.
4. Identify the major risk factor associated with hypertension.
5. Explain the role of the kidneys and renin-angiotensin-aldosterone system in blood pressure regulation.
6. Describe the classification of antihypertensives.
7. Identify different types of diuretics.
8. Describe the mechanisms of action of all drug groups used in the treatment of hypertension.
9. State common adverse effects of the antihypertensive drug groups.
10. Discuss the angiotensin-converting enzyme (ACE).
11. Describe hyperlipidemia and the importance of cholesterol and triglycerides.
12. Describe combination drug therapy for hyperlipidemia.

GLOSSARY

Angiotensin-converting enzyme inhibitors – drugs that competitively inhibit conversion of angiotensin I to angiotensin II, a potent vasoconstrictor, through the angiotensin-converting enzyme activity, with resultant lower levels of angiotensin II

Angiotensin II receptor antagonists – drugs that block the binding of angiotensin II to the angiotensin II type 1 receptor

OUTLINE

Blood Pressure

Hypertension

Antihypertensive Therapy

- Angiotensin-converting Enzyme Inhibitors
- Angiotensin II Receptor Antagonists
- Adrenergic Blockers, Centrally and Peripherally Acting Blockers (Sympatholytics)
- Peripheral Vasodilators
- Diuretics

Hyperlipidemia

Antihyperlipidemic Drugs

- HMG-CoA Reductase (The Stains)
- Bile Acid Sequestrants
- Fibric Acid Derivatives
- Niacin
- Combination Drug Therapy

Cardiac output – the amount of blood the heart pumps to the body in one minute

Diastolic blood pressure – the pressure measured at the moment the ventricles relax

Diuretics – drugs that increase sodium excretion and lower blood volume

Essential hypertension – idiopathic (occurring spontaneously from an unknown cause); also known as primary hypertension

Hyperlipidemia – an increase in triglycerides and cholesterol

Hypertension – an abnormal increase in arterial blood pressure

Lipoprotein – a class of blood chemicals whose molecules are comprised of a lipid portion and a protein portion

Malignant hypertension – an uncontrollable, severe, and rapidly progressive form of hypertension with many complications

Niacin – vitamin B_3, nicotinic acid

Primary hypertension – idiopathic (occurring spontaneously from an unknown cause); also known as essential hypertension

Rhabdomyolysis – a potentially fatal destruction of skeletal muscle, characterized by the presence of myoglobin in the urine; it is also associated with acute renal failure in heatstroke

Sclerotic – hardening, toughening

Secondary hypertension – results from renal (e.g., nephrosclerosis) or endocrine (e.g., hyperaldosteronism) disease, or pheochromocytoma, a benign tumor of the adrenal medulla; in this type of hypertension, the underlying problem must be resolved

Statins – a class of drugs that inhibits the activity of an enzyme that forms cholesterol in the body; so named because all of their generic names end with "-statin" (e.g., lovastatin)

Steatorrhea – elimination of large amounts of fat in the stool

Stroke volume – the volume of blood pumped with each heartbeat

Sympatholytic drugs – a group of drugs that blocks or inhibits the effects of epinephrine or norepinephrine on the cells that normally react to them

Systolic blood pressure – the pressure measured at the moment the heart contracts

Vasodilators – drugs used to relax or dilate vessels throughout the body

Overview

Hypertension (high blood pressure) is the most common cardiovascular disease. The prevalence varies with age, race, education, and many other variables. Sustained arterial hypertension damages blood vessels in the kidneys, heart, and brain, leading to an increased incidence of cardiac failure, coronary diseases, stroke, and renal failure. Effective pharmacologic lowering of blood pressure has been shown to prevent damage to blood vessels and to substantially reduce morbidity and mortality rates.

A number of metabolic disorders that involve elevation in levels of any of the **lipoproteins** (a class of blood chemicals whose molecules are comprised of a lipid portion and a protein portion) are termed **hyperlipidemias**. The term *hyperlipidemia* denotes increased levels of triglycerides and cholesterol in the plasma. Analysis of serum lipids includes assessment of all of the

Medical Terminology Review

hyperlipidemia
hyper = over; above; beyond
lipid = fat
emia = blood condition
condition in which there are increased levels of fat in the blood

subgroups (total cholesterol, triglycerides, low-density lipoproteins, and high-density lipoproteins), because the proportions in which these groups are found in the blood indicate the risk factors for the individual. The danger of elevated cholesterol levels is that cholesterol collects on blood vessel walls and calcifies. This hardening of the arteries causes the vessels to narrow, lose resiliency, and become rough enough to damage passing blood cells. Damaged blood cells trigger clotting, which can result in stroke or myocardial infarction.

Blood Pressure

Blood pressure is a measurement of the pressure exerted on the walls of arteries as the heart pumps. The pressure measured at the moment the heart contracts is called **systolic blood pressure**. The pressure measured at the moment the ventricles relax is called **diastolic blood pressure**. The arteries closest to the heart maintain the highest pressures. Pressure decreases in the arteries the farther the arteries are from the heart.

Key Concept

The main factors determining blood pressure are cardiac output and systemic vascular resistance (the total amount of resistance the blood has to overcome to travel throughout the body). Blood pressure is regulated by an interaction between the nervous, humoral, and renal systems.

Blood pressure is determined by **cardiac output** and **stroke volume**. The amount of blood the heart pumps to the body in one minute is the cardiac output. The stroke volume is the volume of the blood pumped with each heart beat. Cardiac output is dependent upon stroke volume and the rate at which the heart beats. Therefore, cardiac output can be increased by increasing the heart rate, increasing the stroke volume, or increasing both factors.

Hypertension

Hypertension is defined as an abnormal increase in arterial blood pressure, the incidence of which increases with age. According to the American Heart Association, in approximately 90% of cases, the cause is unknown, and more than a third of those affected have no idea that they have hypertension. Risk factors for hypertension include family history, stress, obesity, smoking, lifestyle, diabetes mellitus, and excessive lipid blood levels. Hypertension must be diagnosed in early stages (see Table 12-1). When it is not properly treated, the risk of stroke, coronary artery disease, congestive heart failure, and renal failure increases.

There are three classifications of hypertension:

1. **Primary** or **essential hypertension** is idiopathic (occurring spontaneously from an unknown cause) and is the form discussed in this section.
2. **Secondary hypertension** results from renal (e.g., nephrosclerosis) or endocrine (e.g., hyperaldosteronism) disease, or pheochromocytoma,

TABLE 12-1 Blood Pressure and Hypertension

Classification	Systolic (mm Hg)	Diastolic (mm Hg)
Normal	Less than 120	Less than 80
Prehypertension	120–139	80–89
Stage I hypertension	140–159	90–99
Stage II hypertension	160 or higher	100 or higher

a benign tumor of the adrenal medulla. In this type of hypertension, the underlying problem must be resolved.

3. **Malignant hypertension**, the third type, is an uncontrollable, severe, and rapidly progressive form of hypertension with many complications.

Hypertension is sometimes classified as systolic or diastolic depending on the measurement that is elevated. For example, elderly persons with loss of elasticity in the arteries frequently have high systolic pressure and a low diastolic value.

Essential hypertension develops when the blood pressure is consistently above 140/90. This figure may be adjusted for the individual's age. The diastolic pressure is important because it indicates the degree of peripheral resistance and the increased workload of the left ventricle. The condition may be mild, moderate, or severe.

In essential hypertension, there is an increase in arteriolar vasoconstriction, which is attributed variously to increased susceptibility to stimuli or increased stimulation, or perhaps a combination of factors. A very slight decrease in the diameter of the arterioles causes a major increase in peripheral resistance, reduces the capacity of the system, and increases the diastolic pressure. Frequently, vasoconstriction leads to decreased blood flow through the kidneys, leading to increased renin, angiotensin, and aldosterone secretion. These substances increase vasoconstriction and blood volume, further increasing blood pressure. Figure 12-1 illustrates the development of hypertension. If this cycle is not broken, blood pressure can continue to increase. Renal failure is increased during hypertension because the flow of the blood through the kidneys is reduced. Kidneys are very important in maintaining electrolyte balances, especially those of sodium and water.

The increased blood pressure causes damage to the arterial walls, which become hard and thick (**sclerotic**), narrowing the lumen. Blood supply to the involved area is reduced, leading to ischemia and necrosis with loss of function. The areas most commonly damaged are the kidneys, brain, and retinas.

Key Concept

Atherosclerosis, myocardial infarction, heart failure, renal failure, stroke, impaired mobility, and generalized edema are all associated with chronic hypertension.

Medical Terminology Review

vasoconstriction
vaso = blood vessel
constriction = narrowing
narrowing of the blood vessels

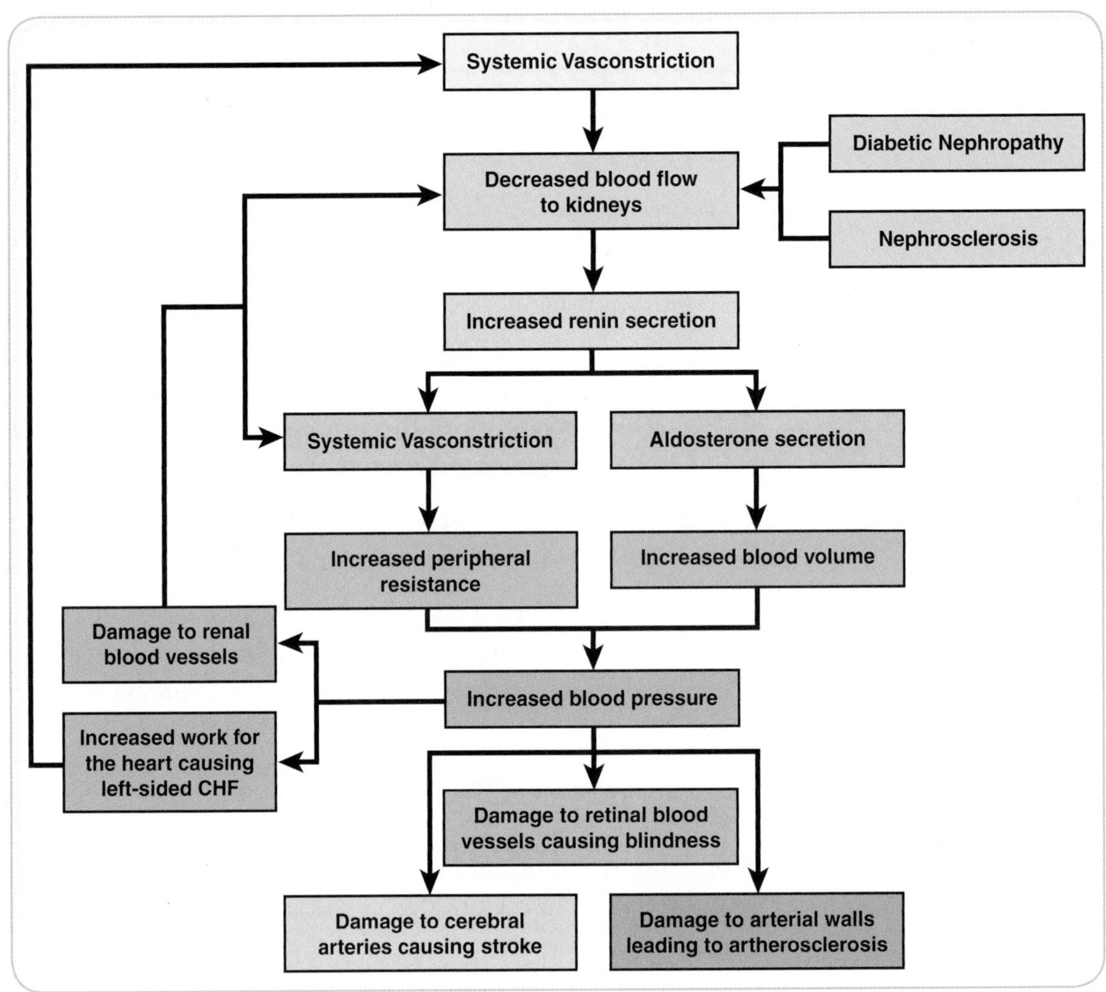

Figure 12-1 Development of hypertension.

Antihypertensive Therapy

In primary hypertension, long-term therapy is necessary to prevent the morbidity and mortality associated with uncontrolled hypertension. Treatment primarily aims to lower the blood pressure toward "normal" with minimal side effects, and to prevent or reverse organ damage. Antihypertensive drugs do not cure hypertension. They only control it. After withdrawal of the drug, the blood pressure will return to levels similar to those before treatment with medication, if all other factors remain the same. There are numerous antihypertensive drugs in the treatment and management of all degrees of hypertension. In mild cases of hypertension, the initial treatment regimen usually includes diet modification (reducing salt), weight reduction, mild exercise programs, smoking cessation, and stress reduction. Drugs prescribed to lower blood pressure act in various ways. The drug of choice varies according to the degree of hypertension (mild, moderate, or severe). Antihypertensives are sometimes combined for greater effectiveness and to reduce side effects. There are five groups

Key Concept

Drugs that primarily lower systemic vascular resistance include ACE inhibitors, α-antagonists, and peripheral vasodilators.

of drugs which act to lower blood pressure in the following manner: (1) angiotensin-converting enzyme inhibitors, (2) angiotensin II receptor antagonists, (3) adrenergic blockers, centrally and peripherally acting blockers (sympatholytics), (4) peripheral vasodilators, and (5) diuretics. They are explained below in more detail.

Angiotensin-converting Enzyme Inhibitors

Angiotensin-converting enzyme inhibitors (ACE inhibitors) competitively inhibit conversion of angiotensin I to angiotensin II, a potent vasoconstrictor, through the angiotensin-converting enzyme activity, with resultant lower levels of angiotensin II. Lower angiotensin II levels increase plasma renin activity and reduce aldosterone secretion.

Mechanism of Action

Angiotensin-converting enzyme (ACE) inhibitors slow the formation of angiotensin II, which reduces vascular resistance, blood volume, and blood pressure. Renin is an enzyme that is released by the kidneys in response to reduced renal blood circulation or hyponatremia. This enzyme acts in the plasma angiotensinogen to produce angiotensin I. Then, angiotensin I is converted to angiotensin II, mostly in the lungs. Angiotensin II is a vasoconstricting agent. It causes sodium retention via the release of aldosterone. In the adrenal gland, angiotensin II is converted to angiotensin III. Both angiotensin II and III stimulate the release of aldosterone. Angiotensin I is inactive in the cardiovascular system. Angiotensin II has several cardiovascular-renal actions. The most important site of the angiotensin-converting enzyme (ACE) is in the lungs, but ACE also is found in the kidneys, central nervous system, and elsewhere. Figure 12-2 shows the renin-angiotensin system. Examples of ACE inhibitors are shown in Table 12-2.

Key Concept

Blood pressure reduction is done in a step-wise approach, often beginning with non-pharmacologic methods that include weight loss, dietary, and lifestyle modifications.

Indications

ACE inhibitors are becoming the drugs of choice in the first-line treatment of essential hypertension.

Adverse Effects

Although ACE inhibitors as a group are relatively free of side effects or toxicities in most patients, they do occur, and some can be life-threatening. The adverse effects of ACE inhibitors may include: dizziness, angioedema, loss of taste, photosensitivity, severe hypotension, dry cough, hyperkalemia, blood dyscrasias, and renal impairment.

Contraindications and Precautions

ACE inhibitors are contraindicated in patients with hypersensitivity to these agents, kidney damage, heart failure, hepatic impairment, and diabetes mellitus. ACE inhibitors are avoided during pregnancy (category D). Safety during lactation or in children is not established.

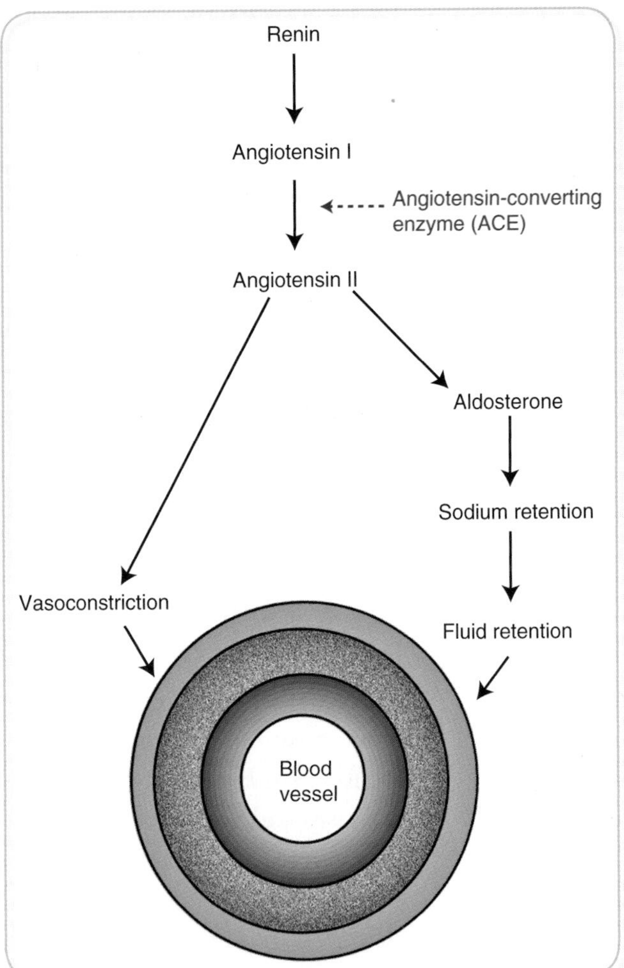

Figure 12-2 Renin-angiotensin system.

ACE inhibitors should be used cautiously in patients with renal impairment or hypovolemia, or who are receiving diuretics or undergoing dialysis. These drugs are used with caution in patients with congestive heart failure, hepatic impairment, and diabetes mellitus.

Drug Interactions

ACE inhibitors increase risk of hypersensitivity reactions with allopurinol. They decrease antihypertensive effects with indomethacin. ACE inhibitors also increase captopril effects with probenecid. Some ACE inhibitors may increase coughing if combined with capsaicin. Fosinopril increases the risk of potassium levels if taken with potassium-sparing diuretics. Quinapril may increase digoxin levels and decrease tetracycline absorption.

Angiotensin II Receptor Antagonists

Angiotensin II receptor antagonists block the binding of angiotensin II to the angiotensin I receptor. Angiotensin II receptor antagonists have

TABLE 12-2 Examples of ACE Inhibitors

Generic Name	Trade Name	Route of Administration	Average Adult Dosage
benazepril hydrochloride	Lotensin®	PO	10–40 mg/day in 1–2 divided doses
captopril	Capoten®	PO	6.25–25 mg t.i.d.; may increase to 50 mg t.i.d.
enalapril maleate	Vasotec®	PO	5–40 mg/day
fosinopril	Monopril®	PO	5–40 mg/day (max: 80 mg/day)
lisinopril	Prinivil®, Zestril®	PO	10–40 mg/day (max: 80 mg/day)
moexipril hydrochloride	Univase®	PO	7.5–30 mg/day
perindopril erbumine	Aceon®	PO	4 mg once per day; may increase to 8 mg/day
quinapril hydrochloride	Accupril®	PO	10–20 mg q.d., may increase up to 80 mg/day in 1–2 div. doses
trandolapril	Mavik®	PO	1–4 mg/day
ramipril	Altace®	PO	2.5–5 mg/day

beneficial effects on the symptoms and hemodynamics of patients with congestive heart failure.

Mechanism of Action

Angiotensin II receptor antagonist drugs work by blocking the binding of angiotensin II to the angiotensin I receptors. By blocking the receptor site, these agents inhibit the vasoconstrictor effects of angiotensin II as well as preventing the release of aldosterone due to angiotensin II from the adrenal glands.

Indications

This class of drugs has been one of the most rapidly growing groups of drugs for the treatment of hypertension. Currently, six agents are available and include candesartan cilexetil, eprosartan, irbesartan, losartan, telmisartan, and valsartan (see Table 12-3).

Key Concept

Postural hypotension is a common adverse effect of antihypertensive drugs. Abrupt withdrawal of treatment may lead to rebound hypertension.

Adverse Effects

Angiotensin receptor blockers should not be used in special hypertensive populations, such as diabetics with nephropathy or congestive heart failure, unless the patient cannot tolerate an ACE inhibitor.

TABLE 12-3 Angiotensin II Receptor Antagonists

Generic Name	Trade Name	Route of Administration	Average Adult Dosage
candesartan cilexetil	Atacand®	PO	8–32 mg/day
eprosartan mesylate	Teveten®	PO	400–800 mg/day
irbesartan	Avapro®	PO	150–300 mg/day
losartan potassium	Cozaar®	PO	25–50 mg/day
olmesartan medoxomil	Benicar®	PO	20–40 mg/day
telmisartan	Micardis®	PO	40–80 mg/day
valsartan	Diovan®	PO	80–160 mg/day

Contraindications and Precautions

Angiotensin II receptor antagonists are contraindicated in patients with a known hypersensitivity to these agents. These drugs are also contraindicated in pregnancy (category C, first trimester; category D, second and third trimesters) and lactation.

Angiotensin II receptor antagonists are used cautiously in patients with concurrent administration of high-dose diuretics, potassium-sparing diuretics, or potassium salt substitutes, and in diabetes or lactation. Angiotensin II receptor antagonists should be used with caution in patients with hepatic or renal impairment, or in elderly patients.

Drug Interactions

Some of these drugs, such as losartan, decrease serum levels and effectiveness if taken concurrently with phenobarbital. Losartan is converted to an active metabolite by cytochrome P450, which may decrease the antihypertensive effects of losartan. Telmisartan increases serum levels and risk of toxicity of digoxin if combined.

Key Concept

The beta-blockers, calcium channel antagonists, angiotensin II antagonists, combined α- and β-antagonists, and centrally acting sympathetic depressants lower both cardiac output and systemic vascular resistance.

Adrenergic Blockers, Centrally and Peripherally Acting Blockers (Sympatholytics)

The **sympatholytic** drugs include groups of medications beta-adrenergic blocking agents, centrally acting alpha-antagonists, postganglionic adrenergic blockers, and alpha-adrenergic blocking agents. These drugs are summarized in Table 12-4.

Mechanism of Action

Beta blockers reduce peripheral resistance and inhibit cardiac function. They also block renin secretion. Centrally acting antiadrenergic blockers act

TABLE 12-4 Sympatholytic Agents

Generic Name	Trade Name	Route of Administration	Average Adult Dosage
α/β-Blockers			
labetalol hydrochloride	Trandate®	PO, IV	Initial: 100 mg b.i.d.; maint: 200–400 mg b.i.d., IV 20 mg slowly over 2 min with 40–80 mg over 10 min if needed
β-Blockers			
acebutolol hydrochloride	Sectral®	PO	200–800 mg/day in 2 div. doses
atenolol	Tenormin®	PO	25–100 mg once/day
betaxolol hydrochloride	Kerlone®	PO	5–10 mg/day (max: 20 mg/day)
bisoprolol fumarate	Zebeta®	PO	2.5–20 mg/day
carteolol hydrochloride	Cartrol®	PO	2.5–10 mg/day
metoprolol tartrate	Lopressor®	PO, IV	PO: 50–450 mg/day; IV: 40–320 mg/day
nadolol	Corgard®	PO	40 mg once per day; may increase to 240–320 mg/day
penbutolol	Levatol®	PO	10–20 mg/day; may increase to 40–80 mg/day
propranolol hydrochloride	Inderal®	PO	40–60 mg b.i.d.; usually requires 160–480 mg/day
timolol maleate	Blocadren®	PO	10 mg b.i.d.; may increase to 60 mg/day
Centrally Acting Blockers			
clonidine hydrochloride	Catapres®	PO or Transdermal system	Initial: 0.1 mg b.i.d.; maint: 0.1–0.2 mg/day
guanabenz acetate	Wytensin®	PO	Initial: 4 mg b.i.d.; max. 32 mg b.i.d.
guanfacine hydrochloride	Tenex®	PO	1–3 mg/day
methyldopa	Aldomet®	PO, IV	Initial: 250 mg b.i.d.; maint: 500 mg to 3 g/day in 2–4 doses

(continues)

TABLE 12-4 Sympatholytic Agents—*continued*

Generic Name	Trade Name	Route of Administration	Average Adult Dosage
Peripherally Acting Blockers			
doxazosin mesylate	Cardura®	PO	Initial: 1 mg/day; maint: 2–16 mg qd
guanadrel	Hylorel®	PO	Initial: 10 mg/day; most require 20–75 mg/day
guanethidine	Ismelin®	PO	Initial: 10 mg/day; average 25–50 mg/day
prazosin hydrochloride	Minipress®	PO	First dose limited to 1 mg h.s.; then 1 mg b.i.d.-t.i.d.; may increase to 20 mg/day
reserpine	Serpalan/Serpasil®	PO	0.1–0.25 mg/day
terazosin	Hytrin®	PO	Initial: 1 mg h.s., then 1–5 mg/day

primarily within the central nervous system on alpha 2 receptors to decrease sympathetic outflow to the cardiovascular system. Methyldopa decreases total peripheral resistance while having little effect on cardiac output or heart rate (except in older patients). Clonidine stimulates alpha 2 receptors centrally, and decreases vasomotor tone and heart rate. Guanabenz and guanfacine are centrally acting alpha2-adrenergic agonists that have actions similar to clonidine.

Peripherally acting adrenergic inhibitors are powerful antihypertensives that may interfere with the release of norepinephrine from nerve endings or may block receptors in the vascular smooth muscle. This class of antihypertensive drug is best avoided unless it is necessary to treat severe hypertension that is unresponsive to all other medications, because agents in this class are poorly tolerated by most patients. Guanethidine is one of the most potent antihypertensive drugs currently in clinical use. Guanethidine acts in peripheral neurons, where it first produces a sympathetic blockade. Guanadrel is chemically and pharmacologically similar to guanethidine.

Indications

Beta-blockers are used for the initial treatment of hypertension. These medications can be used for angina, acute myocardial infarctions, and hypertension. Propranolol was the first beta-blocking agent shown to block both beta 1 and beta 2 receptors. It is available as both a fast-acting product and a long-acting product. Nadolol was the first beta-blocker that allowed once-daily dosing.

It blocks both beta 1 and 2 receptors. Timolol was the first beta-blocker shown to be effective after an acute myocardial infarction to prevent sudden death.

Alpha and beta blockers are drugs available for hypertensive patients who have not responded to initial antihypertensive therapy. These agents are similar to beta-blockers.

Centrally acting antiadrenergic drugs have been used in the past as alternatives to initial antihypertensives, but their use in mild to moderate hypertension has been reduced primarily due to other available drugs. Clonidine is effective in patients with renal impairment, although they may require a reduced dose or a longer dosing interval. Clonidine is also available as a transdermal patch (Clonidine-TTS), which releases the drug slowly over seven days. Guanabenz and guanfacine are recommended as adjunctive therapy with other antihypertensives for additive effects when initial therapy has failed.

Key Concept

The control of malignant hypertension is usually achieved using direct-acting peripheral vasodilators, in particular, sodium nitroprusside.

Adverse Effects

Beta-blockers are not totally safe in patients with bronchospastic diseases such as asthma and chronic obstructive pulmonary disease (COPD). Suddenly stopping beta-blocker therapy puts the patient at risk for a withdrawal syndrome.

The adverse effects of alpha and beta blockers include postural hypotension, nausea, dizziness, headache, and bronchospasm.

The use of methyldopa is limited because it may produce sedation and must be administered 2 to 4 times daily. Other less common adverse effects include hemolytic anemia, hypotension and drowsiness, nausea, vomiting, sore tongue, sexual dysfunction, nasal congestion, and hepatic dysfunction. Sedation and dry mouth are common with use of clonidine but usually disappear with continued therapy. Clonidine has a tendency to cause or worsen depression. Its action is apparent within 30 to 60 minutes after administration of an oral dose. Adverse effects of guanabenz and guanfacine include sedation, dry mouth, dizziness, and reduced heart rate.

Reserpine is derived from the *Rauwolfia serpentina* plant. Because of the high incidence of adverse effects, other drugs are usually chosen first. When used, reserpine is given in low doses and in conjunction with other antihypertensive agents. Common adverse effects include drowsiness, dizziness, weakness, lethargy, memory impairment, sleep disturbances, and weight gain. Postural and exercise hypotension, fluid retention, and sexual dysfunction are common side effects when using guanethidine. Guanadrel should be avoided in patients with congestive heart failure, angina, and stroke. Adverse effects include fainting, orthostatic hypotension, and diarrhea.

Contraindications and Precautions

Beta-blockers are contraindicated in patients with a known hypersensitivity to the individual agents. Use of beta-blockers should be avoided in patients with uncompensated heart failure, cardiogenic shock, hypotension, and pulmonary edema. Safety of these drugs during pregnancy (category B) or lactation is not established.

Alpha/beta blockers are contraindicated in bronchial asthma, uncontrolled cardiac failure, cardiogenic shock, and severe bradycardia. Safe use during pregnancy (category C), lactation, or in children is not established. Centrally acting blockers (e.g., clonidine patch) are contraindicated in patients with collagen diseases (such as systemic lupus erythematosus) and during pregnancy (category C).

Beta-blockers should be used with caution in patients with hepatic or renal impairment, diabetes mellitus, and bronchospastic disease (asthma, emphysema), and patients undergoing major surgery involving general anesthesia. Abrupt withdrawal of beta blockers should be avoided, since sudden withdrawal may result in rebound hypertension, angina, and heart attack. This drug dose should be tapered over several weeks.

Drug Interactions

Patients taking guanethidine should avoid over-the-counter preparations that contain adrenergic substances such as cold medicines, because the combination may potentiate an acute hypertensive effect.

Peripheral Vasodilators

Medical Terminology Review

vasodilator
vaso = blood vessel
dilator = agent that causes expansion
a substance that causes dilation of the blood vessel

Vasodilators are used to relax or dilate vessels throughout the body. Some work on either veins or arteries; others work on both. Vasodilators are prescribed as second-line agents to initial therapy in patients taking diuretics, beta-blockers, ACE inhibitors, calcium-channel blockers, alpha-adrenergic blockers, or alpha/beta-adrenergic blockers.

Mechanism of Action

Vasodilators block the movement of calcium into the smooth muscle of the blood vessels to cause relaxation of the smooth muscle, and dilation of the resistance vessels.

Indications

Vasodilator agents are reducers of hypertension. A peripheral vasodilator is frequently used in the treatment of moderate to severe hypertension.

Key Concept

All vasodilators should be discontinued slowly to avoid paradoxical hypertensive effects.

Hydralazine and minoxidil may be used in the treatment of moderate essential or early malignant hypertension and hypertensive emergencies, virtually always in conjunction with other antihypertensive drugs. However, mainly because of side effects, they are generally not used until other, safer therapy has failed. Because they increase renal blood flow, they are often used to treat toxemia of pregnancy. They are sometimes

TABLE 12-5 Vasodilators

Generic Name	Trade Name	Route of Administration	Average Adult Dosage
diazoxide	Hyperstat®, Proglycem®	IV	1–3 mg/kg up to 150 mg, repeat at 5–15 min intervals p.r.n.
fenoldopam mesylate	Corlopam®	IV	0.025–0.3 mcg/kg/min by continuous infusion for up to 48 hours
hydralazine hydrochloride	Apresoline®	PO, IM, IV	PO: 10–50 mg q.i.d.; IM: 10–50 mg q4–6h; IV: 10–20 mg q4–6h, may increase to 40 mg
minoxidil	Rogaine®	PO	5 mg/day, increased q3–5 days up to 40 mg/day in single or div. doses p.r.n. (max: 100 mg/day)
nitroprusside sodium	Nipride®, Nitropress®	IV	0.3–0.5 mcg/kg/min (max: 10 mcg/kg/min)
prazosin hydrochloride	Minipress®	PO	1 mg b.i.d.-t.i.d. up to 20 mg/day

used in acute congestive heart failure or after myocardial infarction (see Table 12-5).

Adverse Effects

Toxic effects of hydralazine are syndromes resembling rheumatoid arthritis or lupus erythematosus, the appearance of which necessitates the withdrawal of the drug. Common adverse effects of vasodilator drugs include headache, dizziness, tachycardia, palpitations, anxiety, nausea, vomiting, disorientation, depression, edema, impotence, and allergic reactions.

Medical Terminology Review

hyponatremia
hypo = below; beneath; under
natr = sodium
emia = blood condition
low sodium levels in the blood

Contraindications and Precautions

Vasodilators are contraindicated in patients with coronary artery disease, mitral valvular rheumatic heart disease, atriovenous shunt, and myocardial infarction. Safe use of vasodilators during pregnancy (category C) or lactation is not established.

TABLE 12-6 Diuretics Used to Treat Hypertension

Generic Name	Trade Name	Route of Administration	Average Adult Dosage
amiloride hydrochloride	Midamor®	PO	5 mg/day; may increase to 20 mg/day in 1–2 divided doses
chlorothiazide sodium	Diuril®	PO	250-500 mg–1 g in 1–2 div. doses
chlorthalidone	Thalitone®, Hygroton®	PO	12.5–25 mg/day (max: 100 mg/day)
furosemide	Lasix®	PO	20–80 mg b.i.d. (max: 600 mg/day)
hydrochlorothiazide	HydroDIURIL®, HCTZ®	PO	12.5–100 mg in 1–2 div. doses
indapamide	Lozol®	PO	2.5 mg once per day; may increase to 5 mg/day
spironolactone	Aldactone®	PO	25–100 mg/day
torsemide	Demadex®	PO, IV	10–20 mg/day, up to 200 mg/day
triamterene	Dyrenium®	PO	100 mg b.i.d. (max: 300 mg/day)

Vasodilators are used cautiously in patients with stroke, hepatic insufficiency, advanced renal impairment, hyponatremia, and in the elderly.

Key Concept

Sodium nitroprusside and diazoxide can be administered only parenterally. Hydralazine and minoxidil are orally administered agents, most suitable for effective long-term outpatient therapy.

Drug Interactions

Hydralazine should be used with caution in patients receiving MAOIs. Profound hypotensive episodes may occur when hydralazine is used along with diazoxide injections.

Diuretics

Diuretics increase sodium excretion and lower blood volume. Diuretics are divided into four categories according to their action: thiazide diuretics, loop diuretics, potassium-sparing diuretics, and osmotic diuretics. The type of diuretic used is determined by the condition being treated. For example, carbonic anhydrase inhibitors, such as acetazolamide (Diamox) are used to lower intraocular pressure. This agent is known as a diuretic compound. The most common diuretics that are used for hypertension are listed in Table 12-6.

Mechanism of Action

Thiazide agents are the most commonly used type of diuretic, increasing excretion of water, sodium, chloride, and potassium.

Loop diuretics inhibit sodium and chloride reabsorption. They are the most effective diuretics available. Potent diuretics such as furosemide (Lasix), bumetanide (Bumex), and ethacrynic acid (Edecrin) are not thiazides but act in a similar way to increase excretion of water, sodium, chloride, and potassium. Their action is more rapid and effective than that of thiazides, with a greater diuresis.

Potassium-sparing diuretics achieve their diuretic effects differently and less potently than the thiazides and loop diuretics. Their most pertinent shared feature is that they promote potassium retention.

Traditionally, substances that increase urine formation, where the excess appears in the urine accompanied by an increased volume of water, are called osmotic diuretics.

Indications

Thiazides may be prescribed for the treatment of edema caused by heart failure or cirrhosis, as well as hypertension.

Loop diuretics are not prescribed routinely for hypertension, but are used when diuresis is required. Loop diuretics are used in the treatment of edema associated with impaired renal kidney function or liver disease. They are also commonly prescribed for the treatment of congestive heart failure, pulmonary edema, and ascites caused by malignancy or cirrhosis. If thiazides are ineffective in the treatment of hypertension, loop diuretics such as furosemide or ethacrynic acid are sometimes used in combination with other antihypertensives.

Potassium-sparing diuretics include spironolactone, triamterene, and amiloride, and are sometimes administered under conditions in which potassium depletion can be dangerous. Spironolactone is a specific competitive inhibitor of aldosterone at the receptor site level. It is effective only when aldosterone is present. Triamterene and amiloride exert their effect independent of the presence or absence of aldosterone. The potassium-sparing agents are used in the management of edema associated with congestive heart failure, hepatic cirrhosis with ascites, the nephrotic syndrome, and idiopathic edema. Because these diuretics have little antihypertensive action of their own they are used mainly in combination with other drugs in the management of hypertension, and to correct hypokalemia often caused by other diuretic agents. Spironolactone also is used in primary hyperaldosteronism.

Mannitol has been shown to increase renal plasma flow and glomerular hydrostatic pressure. Mannitol and urea are most commonly used to reduce intracranial or intraocular pressure. Mannitol has also been used to prevent and treat acute renal failure or during certain cardiovascular surgery. Mannitol is also used alone or with other diuretics to promote excretions of toxins in cases of drug poisoning.

Medical Terminology Review

hyperuricemia
hyper = *over; above; beyond*
uric = *relating to uric acid or urine*
emia = *blood condition*
excess blood in the urine

Adverse Effects

Adverse effects of thiazides include: hypokalemia, hypochloremia, muscle weakness (spasm), postural hypotension, vertigo, headache, fatigue, lethargy, hyperuricemia, and hyperglycemia.

Adverse effects of loop diuretics include fluid and electrolyte imbalance with dehydration, hypotension, collapse, hypokalemia, nausea, vomiting, anorexia, diarrhea, hyperglycemia, blurred vision, and hearing impairment.

Adverse effects resulting from use of potassium-sparing diuretics are hyperkalemia (which may lead to cardiac arrhythmias), dehydration, weakness, fatigue, lethargy, weight loss, nausea, vomiting, diarrhea, and hypotension. Gynecomastia and carcinoma of the breast have been reported after using spironolactone.

The major toxic effect of osmotic diuretics is related to the amount of solute administered and its effect on the volume and distribution of body fluids. Adverse effects include: fluid and electrolyte imbalance, headache, mental confusion, nausea, vomiting, tachycardia, hypertension, hypotension, allergic reactions, and severe pulmonary edema.

Contraindications and Precautions

Thiazide diuretics are contraindicated for patients with diabetes, severe renal failure, impaired liver function, and a history of gout.

Loop diuretics should be avoided in patients with liver disease, kidney impairment, diabetes, pregnancy (category C), and lactation. Loop diuretics are also contraindicated in dehydrated patients and children under 18 years of age.

Potassium-sparing diuretics are contraindicated in patients with anuria, acute renal insufficiency, impaired renal function, or hyperkalemia.

Osmotic diuretics are contraindicated in kidney failure, severe pulmonary edema, pregnancy, lactation, and cardiovascular disease.

Diuretics are used cautiously in patients with hepatic or renal dysfunction, electrolyte imbalance, diabetes, pregnant women, lactation, and in children. ACE inhibitors should be used with caution in patients with sodium depletion, hypovolemia, and coronary insufficiency.

Drug Interactions

Many drugs can interact with the antihypertensive agents and decrease their effectiveness. These drugs include: antidepressants, antihistamines, and beta-adrenergic bronchodilators. Absorption of the ACE inhibitors may be decreased when given with antacids. The effect of angiotensin II receptor agonists may be decreased if NSAIDs or phenobarbital are given with them.

HYPERLIPIDEMIA

Lipids or fats, which are usually transported in various combinations with proteins (lipoproteins), play a key role in cardiovascular disorders. Lipids, including cholesterol and triglycerides, are essential elements in the body. They are synthesized in the liver; therefore, they can never be eliminated from the body.

Dietary or drug therapy of elevated plasma cholesterol levels can reduce the risk of atherosclerosis, and subsequent cardiovascular disease. A patient with high serum cholesterol and increased low-density lipoprotein (LDL) is at risk of atherosclerotic coronary disease and myocardial infarction. Atherosclerosis is a disorder in which lipid subgroups [total cholesterol, triglycerides, low-density lipoproteins (LDL), and high-density lipoproteins (HDL)] in various proportions indicate risk factors for the individual. Comparison of HDL and LDL is shown in Figure 12-3. Table 12-7 shows an analysis of cholesterol and triglycerides.

> **Medical Terminology Review**
>
> **atherosclerosis**
> *athero = deposit*
> *sclero = hard or hardened*
> *sis = state or condition*
> a condition of hardened deposits in the arteries

Analysis of serum lipids includes assessment of all the deposits that accumulate on the lining of the blood vessels, resulting in degenerative changes and obstruction of blood flow (see Figure 12-4). Obstructions may be partial or complete, and emboli are common. Factors such as genetic conditions, high cholesterol diet, elevated serum LDL levels, and elevated blood pressure predispose patients to development of this condition.

> **Medical Terminology Review**
>
> **hyperlipidemia**
> *hyper = over; above; beyond*
> *lipid = fat*
> *emia = blood condition*
> excess fat in the blood

Diseases of plasma lipids can be manifested as an elevation in triglycerides (hyperlipidemia), or as an elevation in cholesterol. Elevated triglycerides can produce life-threatening pancreatitis.

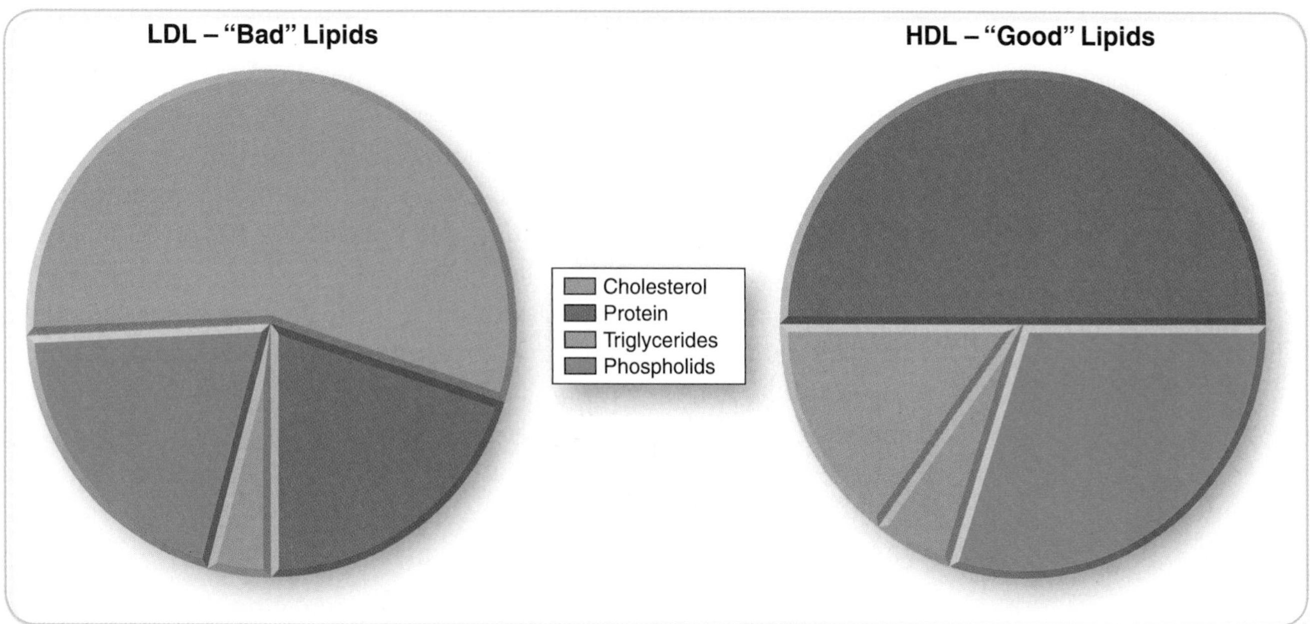

Figure 12-3 Comparison of HDL to LDL.

TABLE 12-7 Normal Values of Cholesterol and Triglyceride Levels

Cholesterol Level	Cholesterol Category
Less than 200 mg/dL	Desirable
200–239 mg/dL	Borderline
> 240 mg/dL	High
HDL Cholesterol Level	**HDL Cholesterol Category**
Less than 40 mg/dL (for men) and less than 50 mg/dL (for women)	Low HDL cholesterol. A major risk factor for heart disease.
60 mg/dL and above	High HDL cholesterol. An HDL of 60 mg/dL and above is considered protective against heart disease.
LDL Cholesterol Level	**LDL Cholesterol Category**
Less than 100 mg/dL	Optimal
100–129 mg/dL	Above optimal
130–159 mg/dL	Borderline high
160–189 mg/dL	High
≥ 190 mg/dL	Very high
Triglyceride Level	**Triglyceride Category**
Less than 150 mg/dL	Normal
150–199 mg/dL	Borderline high
200–499 mg/dL	High
500 mg/dL and above	Very high

Antihyperlipidemic Drugs

Medications are not the first line of treatment for hyperlipidemia. Antihyperlipidemic drugs are used only if diet modification and exercise programs fail to lower LDL to normal levels. When medications are started, diet therapy must continue. Antihyperlipidemics are the group of drugs prescribed in adjuvant therapy to reduce elevated cholesterol levels in patients with high cholesterol and LDL levels in the blood. These medications are used to decrease the risk of arteriosclerosis. The major drugs for reduction of LDL cholesterol levels are bile acid sequestrants and nicotinic acid. The fibric acid derivatives and clofibrate (Atromid-S) are less effective in reducing LDL cholesterol. The most effective agents for reducing plasma LDL levels are the statins. Table 12-8 lists the drugs commonly used to lower lipid levels.

Key Concept

Torcetrafib is a new drug that, when combined with Lipitor, raises HDL ("good cholesterol") levels.

HMG-CoA Reductase (The Statins)

Statins have become the mainstay of LDL-reducing therapy, and they are the most effective agents for reducing plasma LDL levels. The statins

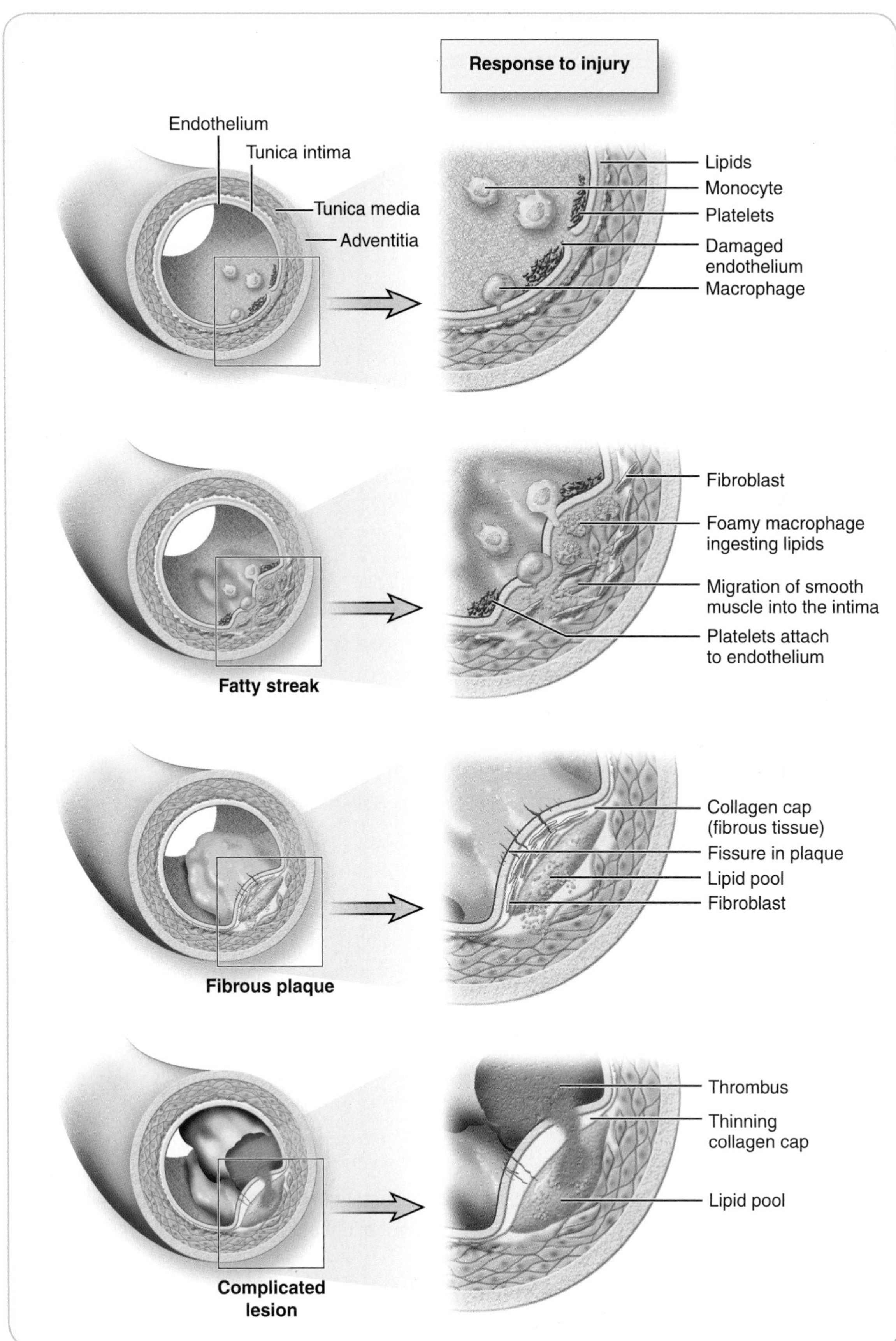

Figure 12-4 Development of atherosclerosis.

TABLE 12-8 Lipid-lowering Drugs

Generic Name	Trade Name	Route of Administration	Average Adult Dosage
HMG-CoA Reductase Inhibitors (Statins)			
atorvastatin calcium	Lipitor®	PO	10–80 mg/day
fluvastatin sodium	Lescol®, Lescol XL®	PO	20 mg h.s.; may increase to 80 mg/day in 1–2 divided doses
lovastatin	Mevacor®, Altoprev®	PO	20–40 mg 1–2 times per day
pravastatin sodium	Pravachol®	PO	10–80 mg/day
rosuvastatin calcium	Crestor®	PO	5–40 mg/day
simvastatin	Zocor®	PO	10–80 mg/day
Bile Acid Sequestrant (binding) Agents			
cholestyramine resin	Questran®, LoCHOLEST®, Prevalite®	PO	4–24 g b.i.d.-q.i.d.
colesevelam hydrochloride	Welchol®	PO	3 tablets b.i.d. with meals or 6 tablets q.d. with a meal
colestipol hydrochloride	Colestid®	PO	15–30 g b.i.d.
Fibric Acid Derivatives			
clofibrate	Atromid-S®	PO	2 g/day in div. doses
dextrothyroxine sodium	Choloxin®	PO	4–8 mg/day
fenofibrate	Tricor®	PO	54–160 mg/day
gemfibrozil	Lopid®	PO	600 mg b.i.d.
Miscellaneous Preparations			
niacin (nicotinic acid)	Niaspan®, Niac®	PO	1–3 g in div. doses or extended release: 500–2000 mg/day

include: atorvastatin, fluvastatin, lovastatin, pravastatin, and simvastatin. These statins are extremely effective and well-tolerated.

Mechanism of Action

Statins inhibit HMG co-enzyme A, the enzyme that catalyzes the first step in the cholesterol synthesis pathway, resulting in a decrease in serum cholesterol and serum LDLs.

Key Concept

HMG-CoA reductase inhibitors are usually well-tolerated. A rare but serious adverse effect is ***rhabdomyolysis*** *(destruction of skeletal muscle).*

Indications

The statin drugs are used as adjuncts to diet in treatment of elevated total cholesterol, serum triglycerides, and LDL cholesterol in patients with primary hypercholesterolemia.

Adverse Effects

HMG-CoA reductase inhibitors may cause headache, flatulence, abdominal pain, cramps, constipation, nausea, and heartburn. They have an impressively low frequency of serious adverse effects. The most important side effects are transaminase elevation and acute myositis.

Contraindications and Precautions

HMG-CoA reductase inhibitors are contraindicated in patients with hypersensitivity to these agents, serious liver disorders, and during pregnancy (category X) and lactation. HMG-CoA reductase inhibitors should be used with caution in patients with acute infection, visual disturbances, hypotension, endocrine disorders, and a history of alcoholism.

Drug Interactions

HMG-CoA reductase inhibitors may have decreased effects if taken with rifamycin. There is possible severe myopathy (disorders of the striated muscles) or rhabdomyolysis if taken with cyclosporine, erythromycin, gemfibrozil, niacin, and other statins. When the HMG-CoA reductase inhibitors are given with oral anticoagulants, the effect of the anticoagulants will be increased.

Bile Acid Sequestrants

Bile acid sequestrants are a group of drugs that chemically combine with bile acids in the intestine, causing these bile acids to be eliminated from the body. Bile acid sequestrants are prescribed to lower blood cholesterol and other blood lipid levels. Cholestyramine (Questran) and colestipol (Colestid) are examples of bile acid sequestrants.

Mechanism of Action

Bile acid sequestrant drugs bind to bile acids to form an insoluble substance that cannot be absorbed by the intestine. Therefore, it is excreted in the feces. This action increases loss of bile acids, and the liver uses cholesterol to manufacture more bile. This leads to lowered serum cholesterol levels.

Indications

Bile acid sequestrants are used as adjuncts to diet therapy in management of patients with primary hypercholesterolemia with a significant risk of atherosclerotic heart disease and MI. These agents may also be prescribed to relieve pruritus associated with partial biliary obstruction.

Adverse Effects

Constipation is a common problem associated with bile acid sequestrants. Other adverse effects are fecal impaction, hemorrhoids, nausea, and abdominal pain. Additional adverse effects include weight loss or gain, vitamin A, D, and K deficiencies (from poor absorption), and bleeding tendencies caused by depletion of vitamin K.

Contraindications and Precautions

Bile acid sequestrants are contraindicated in patients with a known hypersensitivity to the medications. Bile acid sequestrants are avoided in those with complete biliary obstruction, pregnancy (category C), and lactation. Safe use of these drugs in children younger than 16 years is not established.

Bile acid sequestrants should be used cautiously in patients with bleeding disorders, hemorrhoids, peptic ulcer, and malabsorption states (e.g., **steatorrhea**). These agents are used with caution in patients with a liver or kidney impairment, and during pregnancy or lactation.

Drug Interactions

Bile acid sequestrants decrease the absorption of oral anticoagulants, digoxin, tetracyclines, penicillins, and phenobarbital. Therefore, bile acid sequestrants should be given alone and other drugs administered at least 1 hour before or 4 hours later.

Fibric Acid Derivatives

These agents reduce hepatic synthesis of cholesterol and result in a reduction in the plasma concentration of very-low-density lipoprotein (VLDL) and triglycerides. Because more successful medications are on the market, clofibrate is no longer the hypolipidemic drug of choice, although it is still used for patients who may not respond to other medications.

Mechanism of Action

Fibric acid derivatives stimulate the liver to increase breakdown of VLDL to LDL, and decrease liver synthesis of VLDL by inhibiting cholesterol formation.

Indications

Primary indication of clofibrate is for hyperlipidemia that does not respond to diet. Clofibrate is also prescribed for patients with very high serum triglycerides with abdominal pain and pancreatitis that does not respond to diet.

Adverse Effects

Adverse effects of fibric acid derivatives include angina, arrhythmias, swelling, phlebitis, and pulmonary emboli. These agents also cause nausea, vomiting, diarrhea, flatulence, gastritis, and gall stones (with long-term therapy). Clofibrate may produce impotence, dysuria, hematuria, leukopenia, and anemia.

Contraindications and Precautions

Fibric acid derivatives are contraindicated in patients with hypersensitivity to these agents, impaired renal or hepatic function, primary biliary cirrhosis, pregnancy (category C), and lactation. Safe use of fibric acid derivatives in children younger than 14 years is not established.

Fibric acid derivatives are used cautiously in patients with a history of jaundice or hepatic disease, gallstones, peptic ulcer, hypothyroidism, and cardiovascular disease.

Drug Interactions

Fibric acid derivatives may increase anticoagulant effects by lowering plasma protein binding. They increase the effect of antidiabetics, and exaggerate diuretic response to furosemide. Clofibrate increases the effects of insulin. With probenecid, the therapeutic and toxic effects of clofibrate are increased. With ursodiol, there is increased risk of gallstone formation.

Niacin

Niacin (vitamin B_3, nicotinic acid) can exert cholesterol- and triglyceride-lowering effects at high concentrations, resulting in a decrease of LDL and VLDL levels, and an increase in HDL levels, but its use is limited by its side effects.

Mechanism of Action

Nicotinic acid may partially inhibit the release of free fatty acids from adipose tissue and increase lipoprotein activity, which could increase the rate of triglyceride removal from plasma. These actions reduce the total LDL (bad cholesterol) and triglycerides, resulting in increased HDL (good cholesterol).

Indications

Niacin may be prescribed as an adjunct to diet for treatment of adults with very high serum triglyceride levels who present a risk of pancreatitis, and who do not respond adequately to dietary control.

Adverse Effects

Nicotinic acid may cause headache, anxiety, hypotension, flushing or burning feelings in the skin, dry skin, peptic ulcer, or abnormal liver function tests. Other adverse effects of this agent include hyperuricemia, glucose intolerance, nausea, vomiting, diarrhea, hyperglycemia, and elevated plasma uric acid.

Contraindications and Precautions

Niacin is contraindicated in patients with hypersensitivity to this agent, hepatic impairment, severe hypotension, or arterial bleeding. Niacin also is contraindicated in patients with active peptic ulcer, pregnancy (category C), lactation, and children younger than 16 years.

Niacin is used cautiously in individuals with history of gallbladder disease, liver impairment, and peptic ulcer. This agent should be used with caution in glaucoma, angina, coronary artery disease, and diabetes mellitus.

Drug Interactions

Niacin can increase the effectiveness of antihypertensives or vasoactive drugs. It also increases the risk of bleeding with anticoagulants. Niacin decreases absorption with bile acid sequestrants and separate doses must be at least 4 to 6 hours apart.

Combination Drug Therapy

Certain combinations of medications can be useful in treating markedly elevated LDL cholesterol levels. Combination therapy can maximize the reduction in LDL levels. It can also allow the limiting of dosages of individual LDL-reducing drugs, thus limiting side effects. For patients with elevations in both triglycerides and LDL, the addition of nicotinic acid or a fibric acid derivative to control triglyceride levels can allow the use of a bile acid sequestrant to help reduce LDL levels. The following are the most effective combinations for lowering LDL:

- A statin plus a bile acid sequestrant
- A statin plus nicotinic acid
- Nicotinic acid plus a bile acid sequestrant
- A statin plus a bile acid sequestrant plus nicotinic acid

The combination of a fibric acid derivative with a statin should usually be avoided because of an increased risk of myopathy.

SUMMARY

Antihypertensive drugs include diuretics (to lower blood volume), ACE inhibitors, beta-blockers, and vasodilators. In some cases, calcium channel blockers must be used with care for the elderly. Medications are used only when lifestyle changes have not adequately lowered elevated blood pressure.

To reduce the circulating hyperlipidemia, medications may be required. The statins reduce the enzyme necessary for cholesterol production. Nicotinic acid reduces LDL and VLDL levels. The fibric acid derivatives decrease triglyceride and VLDL levels while raising HDL levels. These medications for hyperlipidemia are long-term therapy.

EXPLORING THE WEB

Visit ***http://www.americanheart.org***

- Search for information on management of hypertension and hyperlipidemia.

Visit ***http://www.hearthealthywomen.org***

- What are some of the challenges related to managing cardiovascular health for women that are different than for men?

Visit ***www.cvphysiology.com***

- Click on "hypertension" and review additional information to further your understanding of hypertension.

Visit ***www.hypertension-facts.org***

- For additional resources and information on hypertension.

Visit ***www.medicinenet.com*** or ***www.nlm.nih.gov/medlineplus***

- Search for the disorders or drugs discussed in this chapter. What additional information can you find?

REVIEW QUESTIONS

Multiple Choice

1. Which of the following antianginal drugs are also used as antihypertensives?

A. nitrates
B. vasoconstrictors
C. diuretics
D. beta-adrenergic blockers

2. Thiazides are contraindicated in all of the following patients, except those with:

   A. impaired liver function
   B. edema caused by heart failure
   C. diabetes
   D. a history of gout

3. Hydralazine (Apresoline) is a(n):

   A. vasodilator
   B. vasoconstrictor
   C. anticoagulant
   D. antiarrhythmic

4. An example of a angiotensin-converting enzyme (ACE) inhibitor is:

   A. captopril (Capoten)
   B. acebutolol (Sectral)
   C. lidocaine (Xylocaine)
   D. procainamide (Pronestyl)

5. Hypertension with an unknown etiology is referred to as:

   A. secondary hypertension
   B. malignant hypertension
   C. familial hypertension
   D. primary hypertension

6. The trade names of clonidine include which of the following?

   A. Corgard
   B. Catapres
   C. Aldomet
   D. Lopressor

7. Which of the following agents have become the mainstay of LDL-reducing therapy?

   A. calcium channel blockers
   B. cardiac glycosides
   C. angiotensin II receptor antagonists
   D. HMG-CoA reductase inhibitors

8. Which of the following is the initial treatment of hypertension?

   A. beta-blockers
   B. antiarrhythmic drugs
   C. antihyperlipidemic drugs
   D. cardiac glycosides

9. Which of the following is the generic name of Aramine?

   A. dopamine
   B. metaraminol
   C. ephedrine
   D. epinephrine

10. Which of the following may be caused as a result of ACE inhibitor therapy?

A. hyperglycemia
B. hypercalcemia
C. hyperkalemia
D. hypernatremia

11. Which of the following type of antihypertensive drugs may affect the renin-angiotensin system to increase urine?

A. vasodilators
B. ACE inhibitors
C. direct-acting vasodilators
D. adrenergic blockers

12. An example of a potassium-sparing diuretic is:

A. chlorothiazide (Diuril)
B. acetazolamide (Diamox)
C. furosemide (Lasix)
D. spironolactone (Aldactone)

13. Which of the following is a common adverse effect of a bile acid sequestrant?

A. double vision
B. constipation
C. insomnia
D. hypotension

14. Which of the following is the first drug of choice to lower hyperlipidemia?

A. statins
B. fibric acids
C. bile acids
D. nicotinic acids

15. Which of the following is a potent vasoconstrictor?

A. renin
B. angiotensin I
C. angiotensin II
D. aldosterone

Matching

Generic Name	Trade Name
_____ **1.** simvastatin	**A.** Welchol
_____ **2.** gemfibrozil	**B.** Lipitor
_____ **3.** fenofibrate	**C.** Pravachol
_____ **4.** pravastatin	**D.** Tricor
_____ **5.** cholestyramine	**E.** Questran
_____ **6.** atorvastatin	**F.** Lopid
_____ **7.** colesevelam	**G.** Zocor

Critical Thinking

A 48-year-old woman who was diagnosed with essential hypertension 5 years ago has avoided taking her medication for the last 4 months because she claims that she feels fine without it. She has decreased her regular exercise due to taking care of her new home business, and has noticed occasional nosebleeds, blurred vision, dizziness, and overall tiredness. Her doctor examines her and finds her blood pressure to be 185/115. He also hears crackling noises (rales) when he listens to her lungs, and notices that she has ruptures in the capillaries of the retinas in her eyes. He prescribes blood pressure medication, urinary tests to check her kidneys, rest and relaxation, and instructs her to see a nutritionist.

1. What is the pathophysiology of essential hypertension?
2. Since the patient has high diastolic pressure, what possible problems may be associated with her condition?
3. The doctor suspects mild congestive heart failure. Explain how this can develop as a result of hypertension.

Anticoagulant Drugs

CHAPTER 13

OUTLINE

Blood Coagulation

Coagulation Disorders

Anticoagulant Drugs
- Heparin
- Warfarin

Antiplatelet Drugs
- Mechanism of Action
- Indications
- Adverse Effects
- Contraindications and Precautions
- Drug Interactions

Thrombolytic Drugs
- Mechanism of Action
- Indications
- Adverse Effects
- Contraindications and Precautions
- Drug Interactions

OBJECTIVES

After completing this chapter, the reader should be able to:

1. Explain the terms *hemostasis*, *aggregation*, and *thrombophlebitis*.
2. Describe the mechanism of action of heparin.
3. Discuss the uses and adverse effects of anticoagulant.
4. Explain factors that usually predispose the development of a thrombus.
5. List three common coagulation disorders.
6. Describe the mechanism of action of thrombolytic drugs.
7. Explain the indications of antiplatelet drugs.
8. Identify oral anticoagulant agents and their indications.
9. Explain thrombocytopenia and thrombolytics.
10. Discuss the role of vitamin K in the process of clotting.

GLOSSARY

Aggregation – the clumping together of platelets to form a clot

Alopecia – loss of hair from anywhere on the body, sometimes until complete baldness is reached

Anticoagulants – agents used to prevent the formation of a blood clot

Antiplatelet agents – drugs that inhibit normal platelet function, usually by reducing their ability to aggregate and inappropriately form blood clots

Blood coagulation – the process by which blood clots

Embolism – obstruction or occlusion of a vessel

Fibrin – gel-like threads

Fibrinogen – a plasma protein

Fibrinolysis – the breakdown of fibrin

Hemostasis – a process that stops bleeding in a blood vessel

Heparin – a potent anticoagulant naturally obtained from the liver and lungs of domestic animals; in humans, it is usually found in basophils or mast cells

Mast cells – large cells found in connective tissue that contain many biochemicals, including histamine; mast cells are involved in inflammation secondary to injuries and infections, and are sometimes implicated in allergic reactions

Phlebothrombosis – clotting in a vein without primary inflammation

Placebo – an inert substance given to a patient instead of an active medicine

Prothrombin – a glycoprotein formed and stored in the parenchymal cells of the liver and present in the blood; a deficiency of prothrombin leads to impaired blood coagulation

Thrombin – enzyme occurring in blood during the clotting process

Thrombocytopenia – decrease in the number of platelets in circulating blood

Thrombogenic – substances causing blood clots

Thrombolytics – drugs designed to dissolve blood clots that have already formed within a blood vessel

Thrombophlebitis – venous inflammation with thrombus formation

Thromboplastin – substance to cause clotting

Thrombosis – the formation of a clot

Thrombus – a clot in the cardiovascular system formed during life from constituents of blood

Venous stasis – injury to the veins causing loss of proper function of the vein and impairing the ability of blood flow to return to the heart

Overview

The ability of blood to clot in response to injury is essential to protection of the body from unnecessary blood loss. Clotting disorders impair this ability of the body to protect itself. Excessive blood loss can lead to shock and ultimately death if left untreated. In this circumstance, drugs may be administered to aid the clotting process.

There are other instances in which clots may form and travel through the venous system, becoming lodged in a vessel and causing a blockage of blood flow. This can cause tissue damage and may also cause the death of the individual if the blockage occurs in the vessels of the lungs or the heart. Drugs that can dissolve or prevent clots from forming may be given to alleviate or prevent this type of event.

Blood Coagulation

Blood coagulation (clotting) is of the utmost importance in the protection of the body from undue blood loss. It is well known that people with blood-clotting disorders, such as hemophilia, lead precarious lives, which can be terminated abruptly by a minor injury, such as slight bruising. In a healthy person, such injuries would often pass unnoticed.

On the other end of the spectrum, many individuals suffer from problems of intravascular clots (thrombi) being formed. This can lead to blockage of the smaller blood vessels in the body and, consequently, tissue ischemia. A common cause of this is **venous stasis** (injury to the veins causing loss of proper function of the vein and impairing the ability of blood flow to return to the heart), due to inactivity such as that which can occur in prolonged bedrest.

Key Concept

Not all emboli are blood clots. They can be derived from various materials, such as fat, amniotic fluid, and even air.

Related to a **thrombus** is a blood embolus, which is a fragment of a blood clot that occludes a vessel. The clot may have been formed due to procedures such as surgery. In this case, a fragment of a natural clot escapes into the circulation and blocks a major vessel. For example, blockage of one of the pulmonary arteries results in a pulmonary embolism.

Medical Terminology Review

hemostasis
hemo = blood
stasis = stable state
maintaining a stable state of blood flow in the body

Hemostasis is the spontaneous arrest of bleeding from a damaged blood vessel. The normal vascular endothelial cells and circulating blood platelets are not **thrombogenic** (causing blood clots) unless blood vessels or platelets are damaged by cuts or injury. Hemostasis or blood clotting occurs as a result of the following steps:

- The immediate response of a blood vessel to injury is vasoconstriction or vascular spasm due to the release of serotonin. In small blood vessels, this decreases blood flow and allows a platelet plug to form.
- Blood platelets release **thromboplastin** (substance to cause clotting) at the site of the injury. Thromboplastin and calcium react with **prothrombin** (a plasma protein produced by the liver) to create **thrombin**.
- The thrombin then changes **fibrinogen** (a plasma protein) into **fibrin** (gel-like threads) which layers over the site of the injury like mesh. This fibrin sheath traps blood cells and plasma and forms a clot (Figure 13-1).

Key Concept

The circulating clotting factors are produced primarily in the liver. Vitamin K, a fat-soluble vitamin, is required for the synthesis of most clotting factors. Calcium ions are essential for many steps in the clotting process.

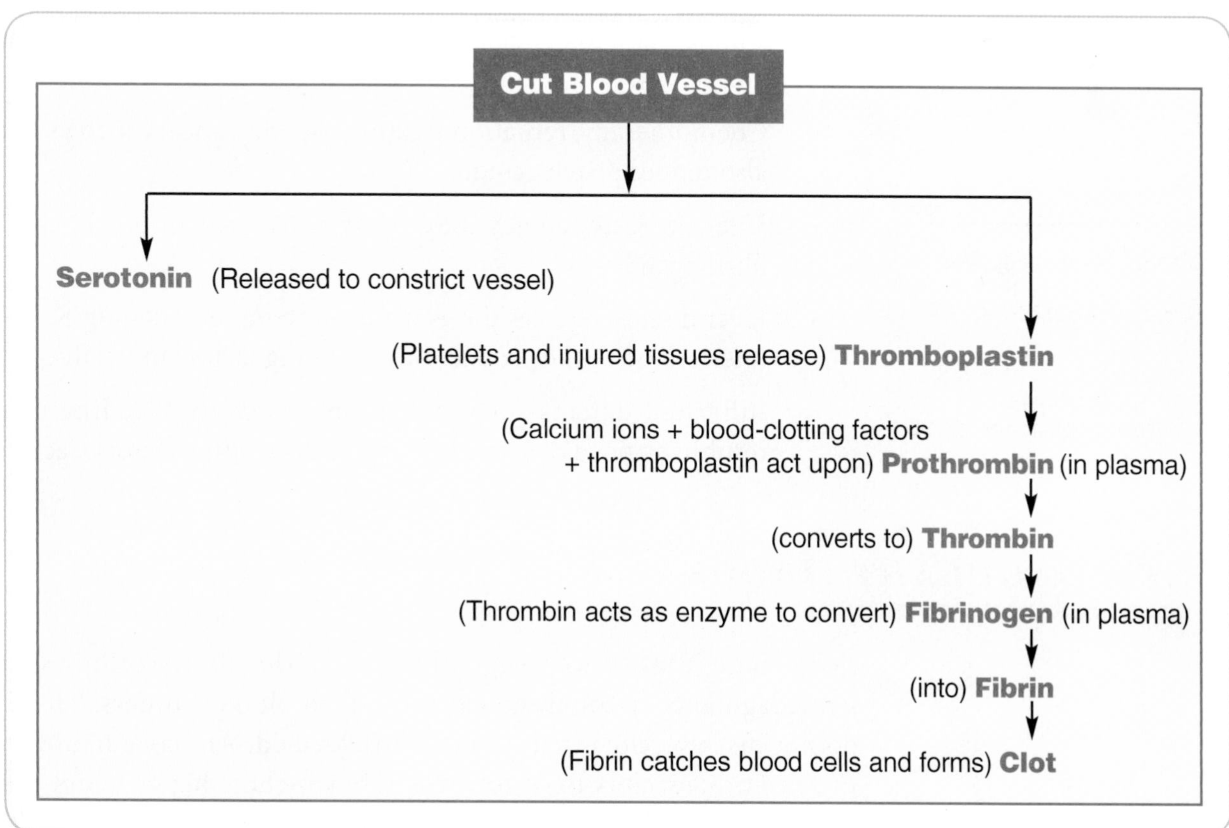

Figure 13-1 Blood clotting process.

Coagulation Disorders

Thrombophlebitis refers to the development of a thrombus in a vein where inflammation is present. The platelets adhere to the inflamed site, and a thrombus develops. In **phlebothrombosis**, a thrombus forms spontaneously in a vein without prior inflammation, although inflammation may develop secondarily in response to **thrombosis**. The clot is less firmly attached in this case, and its development is asymptomatic or silent. Several factors usually predispose the development of a thrombus:

- The first group of factors involves stasis of blood or sluggish blood flow, which is often present in people who are immobile.
- The endothelial lining of the blood vessels is injured, which may have arisen from trauma, chemical injury, intravenous injection, or inflammation.
- The third factor involves increased blood coagulability, which may result from dehydration, cancer, pregnancy, or increased platelet adhesion.

> ***Medical Terminology Review***
>
> **thrombophlebitis**
> *thrombo = blood clot; blood clotting*
> *phleb = vein*
> *itis = inflammation; disease of*
> blood clot within the vein resulting from inflammation
>
> **phlebothrombosis**
> *phlebo = vein*
> *thromb = blood clot; blood clotting*
> *osis = diseased or abnormal condition*
> abnormal formation of a blood clot within a vein

Spontaneous bleeding or excessive bleeding following minor tissue trauma often indicates a blood-clotting disorder. Excessive bleeding has many causes:

- **Thrombocytopenia** may be caused by acute viral infections in children and in adults when platelets are destroyed by HIV infection and certain drugs.
- Chemotherapy, radiation treatments, and cancers such as leukemia also reduce platelet count.
- Vitamin K deficiency may cause a decrease in prothrombin and fibrinogen levels.
- Liver disease reduces the available proteins and vitamin K, and thus, interferes with the production of clotting factors in the liver.
- Inherited defects such as hemophilia cause bleeding disorders resulting from a deficiency of one of the clotting factors (factor VIII).

> ***Medical Terminology Review***
>
> **thrombocytopenia**
> *thrombo = blood clot; blood clotting*
> *cyto = cell*
> *penia = lack; deficiency*
> lack of blood-clotting platelets

Anticoagulant Drugs

Anticoagulants are drugs that reduce the ability of blood to clot. Anticoagulants are often mistakenly called blood thinners. These drugs do not dissolve clots that have already formed. Anticoagulants are used to prevent new clots from forming. They include heparin and warfarin. Heparin may be administered intravenously to patients at risk for thrombus formation and warfarin is given orally.

Medical Terminology Review

anticoagulant
anti = opposite; not
coagulant = agent that causes clotting
agent that will prevent clotting

TABLE 13-1 Anticoagulants

Generic Name	Trade Name	Route of Administration	Average Adult Dosage
anisindione	Miradon®	PO	25–250 mg/day
argatroban	Acova®, Novastan®	IV	2–10 mcg/kg/min
bivalirudin	Angiomax®	IV	0.75 mg/kg bolus followed by 1.75 mg/kg/hr for 4h
heparin sodium	Hep-Lock®	IV	Infusion 5,000–40,000 units/day subcutaneously; 15,000–20,000 units/b.i.d.
lepirudin	Refludan®	IV	0.4 mg/kg bolus followed by 0.15–16.5 mg/kg/hr for 2–10 days
pentoxifylline	Trental®	PO	400 mg t.i.d.
warfarin sodium	Coumadin®	PO, IV	Usual dose: 2–10 mg/day
Low molecular weight (fractionated) heparins (lmwhs)			
dalteparin sodium	Fragmin®	SC	For the first 30 days, give 200 units/kg once daily (max: 18,000 units/day); Months 2–6: give 150 units/kg once daily
enoxaparin	Lovenox®	SC	30 mg b.i.d. for 10–14 days
tinzaparin sodium	Innohep®	SC	175 units/kg daily for at least 6 days

Heparin

Heparin is a potent anticoagulant naturally obtained from the liver and lungs of domestic animals. In humans, it is usually found in basophils or **mast cells**. Heparin preparations are available as heparin sodium and the low- and high-molecular weight heparins (fractionated heparins). Examples of anticoagulants are listed in Table 13-1.

Mechanism of Action

Heparin prevents the conversion of fibrinogen to fibrin, and inactivates several of the factors needed for blood clotting. Heparin can be inactivated by hydrochloric acid in the stomach, and must not be administered orally. Therefore, it is given either subcutaneously or through IV infusion. The onset of action for IV heparin is immediate, whereas subcutaneous heparin may take up to an hour for maximum therapeutic effect.

Indications

Heparin and heparin substitutes are used prophylactically for deep vein thrombosis, pulmonary embolism, or atrial embolism. Heparin is also indicated in patients with atrial fibrillation and heart valve replacement surgery. Low molecular weight heparins (LMWHs) have become the drugs of choice for many clotting disorders such as coronary occlusion, acute myocardial infarction, and peripheral arterial embolism. After the initiation of anticoagulant therapy with heparin, oral anticoagulants can be started immediately. After about 48 hours, the heparin can be withdrawn, as the oral anticoagulants take this time to exert their effect.

Adverse Effects

Spontaneous bleeding is the major complication of heparin administration. Skin rashes, pruritus, burning sensations of the feet, hypertension, fever, chills, headache, and chest pain are seen in some patients. Hypersensitivity reactions may cause bronchospasms and an anaphylactic reaction. The LMWHs may produce fewer adverse effects than other types of heparin.

Contraindications and Precautions

Heparin preparations are contraindicated in patients with a history of hypersensitivity to this agent, active bleeding hemophilia, open wounds, or severe thrombocytopenia. LMWHs should be avoided in patients with a hypersensitivity to the drug and in those patients with thrombocytopenia or active bleeding. Heparin preparations are used with caution in patients with alcoholism or history of allergy (asthma, hives, hay fever, eczema); during menstruation, pregnancy (category C), especially the last trimester, and the immediate postpartum period. Heparin therapy requires caution in the elderly, patients in hazardous occupations, and those with cerebral embolism.

Drug Interactions

Use of heparin with other anticoagulants may increase anticoagulant effects to a dangerous level. Use with caution with salicylates such as aspirin.

Warfarin

Warfarin is the mainstay of long-term anticoagulant therapy, and is one of the original drugs of the coumarin group.

Mechanism of Action

Warfarin is structurally similar to vitamin K, which is involved in the synthesis of prothrombin in the liver. Therefore, warfarin indirectly interferes with blood clotting by depressing hepatic synthesis of vitamin K-dependant coagulation factors II, VII, IX, and X.

Indications

Warfarin is used as a prophylaxis and for the treatment of deep vein thrombosis, pulmonary embolism, treatment of atrial fibrillation with embolism. Warfarin is also prescribed as an adjunct in the treatment of coronary occlusion, cerebral transient ischemic attacks (TIAs), and as a prophylactic in patients with prosthetic cardiac valves.

Adverse Effects

In the correct and individualized dosage, warfarin is almost devoid of adverse effects not related to its anticoagulant action. **Alopecia** and sustained erection are the only ones of any consequence, but these are rare. Adverse effects such as nausea and dizziness occur with similar frequency to those caused by a **placebo**.

Contraindications and Precautions

Warfarin is contraindicated in patients with a known hypersensitivity to this drug, bleeding tendencies, vitamin C or K deficiency, hemophilia, clotting factor deficiency, active bleeding, open wounds and active peptic ulcer. Warfarin should be avoided in patients with severe hepatic and renal disease, pericarditis with acute myocardial infarction, recent surgery of brain, spinal cord, or eye.

Warfarin is used cautiously in debilitated patients, older adults, and patients with alcoholism, allergic disorders, or psychosis. Warfarin should be used with caution in patients with hepatic and renal insufficiency, diarrhea, fever, and pancreatic disorders.

Drug Interactions

Cholestyramine can decrease warfarin absorption, thus reducing its effects. Colestipol and sucralfate have also been reported to interfere with warfarin absorption, but only to a minor degree.

Acetohexamide, acetaminophen, and allopurinol may enhance the anticoagulant effects of warfarin.

Antiplatelet Drugs

Platelets play a key role in hemostasis and thrombus formation. Platelets adhere to thrombin, collagen, and various other substances. Antiplatelet agents are prescribed to suppress aggregation (clumping) of platelets. A number of drugs may be used for stopping thrombi in arteries rather than anticoagulants in veins. The most commonly used antiplatelet drug is aspirin. It has been proven effective for preventing myocardial infarctions and strokes. Other medications may be used as antiplatelet drugs, including glycoprotein antagonists, ticlopidine, and abciximab (Table 13-2).

TABLE 13-2 Antiplatelet Drugs

Generic Name	Trade Name	Route of Administration	Average Adult Dosage
aspirin	ASA®(acetylsalicylic acid)	PO	80 mg daily–650 mg b.i.d.
dipyridamole	Persantine®	PO	75–100 mg/q.i.d.
ADP receptor blockers			
clopidogrel bisulfate	Plavix®	PO	75 mg daily
ticlopidine	Ticlid®	PO	250 mg b.i.d.
Glycoprotein IIB/IIIA receptor blockers			
abciximab	ReoPro®	IV	0.25 mg/kg initial bolus over 5 min; then 10 mcg/min for 12 hours
eptifibatide	Integrilin®	IV	180 mcg/kg initial bolus over 1–2 min; then 2 mcg/kg/min for 24–72 hours
tirofiban hydrochloride	Aggrastat®	IV	0.4 mcg/kg/min for 30 min; then 0.1 mcg/kg/min for 12–24 hours

Mechanism of Action

Eptifibatide and tirofiban are two of the newest glycoprotein antagonists used to delay clotting by altering platelet aggregation that have received approval by the Food and Drug Administration. These agents are prescribed in conjunction with heparin and aspirin. Other antiplatelet agents have the same mechanism of action as these new drugs.

Indications

Ticlopidine prevents platelet aggregation, which reduces risk of thrombotic stroke in patients who have experienced stroke precursors. Abciximab is an antiplatelet drug used with heparin and aspirin to prevent coronary vessel occlusion in patients undergoing percutaneous transluminal coronary angioplasty or atherectomy. Clopidogrel is an antiplatelet agent used in patients who have recently had myocardial infarction or stroke.

Key Concept

Garlic is an herb that has been shown to decrease the aggregation (stickiness) of platelets, thus producing an anticoagulant effect.

Adverse Effects

The primary side effects associated with glycoprotein antagonists are bleeding and thrombocytopenia (a decrease in blood platelet levels). Adverse effects of ticlopidine include neutropenia (a decrease in white blood cells), thrombocytopenia, and bleeding. The adverse effects of clopidogral include fatigue, arthralgic pain, headache, dizziness, hypertension, edema, and risk of bleeding.

Contraindications and Precautions

Antiplatelet drugs are contraindicated in patients with hypersensitivity to these drugs or those who have neutropenia, thrombocytopenia, bleeding ulcer, and uncontrolled hypertension. Antiplatelets should be avoided in patients with recent major surgery or trauma, intracranial bleeding within six months, renal dialysis, and aneurysm.

Antiplatelet drugs are used cautiously in patients with severe liver and renal impairment. These agents should be given with caution to patients at risk for bleeding from trauma, surgery, or GI bleeding, and pregnancy (category B).

Drug Interactions

Aspirin has drug interactions with anticoagulants, hypoglycemic agents, uricosuric agents, spironolactone, alcohol, corticosteroids, pyrazolone derivatives, NSAIDs, urinary alkalinizers, phenobarbital, phenytoin, and propranolol. Ticlopidine potentiates the effect of aspirin and NSAIDs; it also should not be used along with antacids, cimetidine, digoxin, theophylline, phenobarbital, phenytoin, or propranolol. There is no direct drug information as yet available about eptifibatide, however, its adverse effects on the body are well documented. Tirofiban, when used in combination with heparin and aspirin, has been associated with an increase in bleeding. Formal drug interaction studies with abciximab have not been conducted, although an increase in bleeding when abciximab is used concurrently with heparin, other anticoagulants, thrombolytics, and antiplatelet agents has been documented. Use of clopidogrel with NSAIDs has caused increased GI blood loss, and it should be used with aspirin, heparin, or warfarin with caution.

Thrombolytic Drugs

Thrombolytics are agents that dissolve existing clots. Administration of thrombolytic agents such as tissue plasminogen activator, urokinase, or streptokinase is capable of dissolving an arterial clot, such as a clot in a coronary artery in a patient with an acute myocardial infarction. These agents are able to dissolve clots in various access devices.

The body normally regulates **fibrinolysis** such that unwanted fibrin clots are removed, whereas fibrin present in wounds is left to maintain hemostasis. The steps of fibrinolysis are shown in Figure 13-2.

Mechanism of Action

Thrombolytic agents break down fibrin clots by converting plasminogen to plasmin (fibrinolysis). Plasmin is an enzyme that breaks down the fibrin of a blood clot.

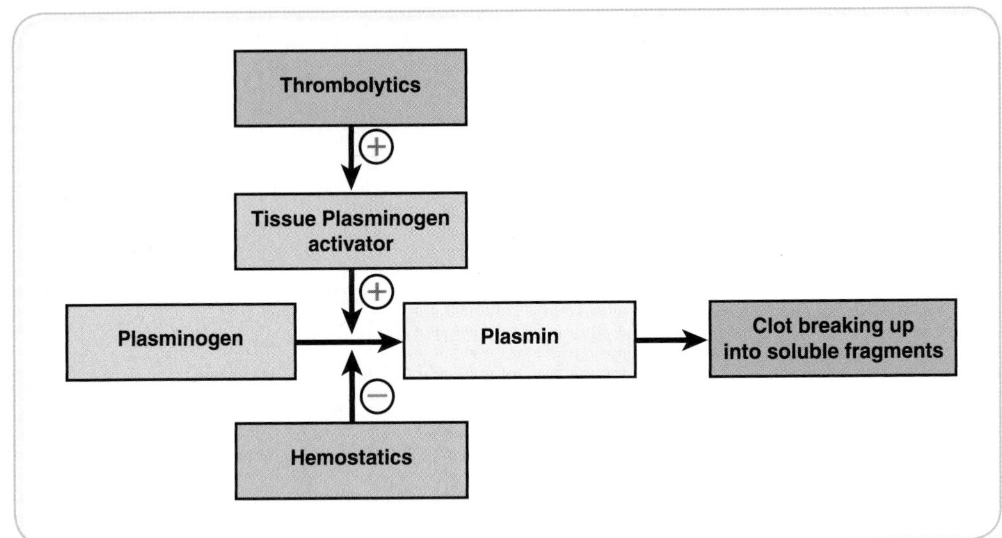

Figure 13-2 Process of fibrinolysis.

Indications

Thrombolytic drugs are used to treat acute myocardial infarction, pulmonary embolism, acute ischemic cerebrovascular accident (CVA), deep vein thrombosis, and coronary thrombosis, and to clear clots in arteriovenous cannulas and blocked IV catheters. Table 13-3 lists the major thrombolytic drugs.

Adverse Effects

Bleeding is the most common adverse effect of thrombolytic drugs, often because of percutaneous trauma or spontaneous bleeding from GI

TABLE 13-3 Thrombolytic Drugs

Generic Name	Trade Name	Route of Administration	Average Adult Dosage
alteplase recombinant	Activase®	IV	Begin with 60 mg and then infuse 20 mg/hour over next 2 hours
anistreplase	Eminase®	IV	30 units over 2–5 min
reteplase recombinant	Retavase®	IV	10 units over 2 min; repeat dose in 30 min
streptokinase	Streptase®	IV	250,000–1.5 million units over a short period of time
tenecteplase	TNKase®	IV	30–50 mg infused over 5sec
urokinase	Abbokinase®	IV	4,400–6,000 units administered over several minutes to 12 hours

tract. Other adverse effects include unstable blood pressure, ventricular dysrhythmias, itching, and nausea.

Contraindications and Precautions

Thrombolytic drugs are contraindicated in patients with a known hypersensitivity, active bleeding, a history of recent trauma, recent intracranial surgery, and a history of stroke. The patient must be monitored carefully for signs of bleeding every 15 minutes for the first hour of therapy and every 30 minutes thereafter.

Thrombolytic drugs should be used cautiously in patients who have recently undergone major surgery, or those who have hypertension and diabetic retinopathy. Thrombolytic drugs are used with caution in pregnancy (category C) with the exception of urokinase (category B).

Key Concept

Alteplase with herbal supplements (ginkgo) may increase thrombolytic effects.

Drug Interactions

Thrombolytic drugs along with aspirin, dipyridamole, or an anticoagulant may increase the risk of bleeding.

Summary

Anticoagulants are used to treat deep venous thrombosis by disrupting the coagulation process and the formation of fibrin. The most potent anticoagulants include heparin and warfarin. Antiplatelet agents suppress clumping of platelets to stop thrombi from forming in arteries. Thrombolytics dissolve existing clots by breaking down fibrin and converting plasminogen to plasmin. All of these agents are important to help avoid blood clotting problems in the body, which can lead to a variety of conditions, including tissue ischemia, various embolisms, and stroke.

Exploring the Web

Visit ***www.americanheart.org***

- Search for "anticoagulants" review-related articles to further enhance your understanding of these drugs.

Visit ***www.medicinenet.com***

- Choose a disorder or drug type discussed in this chapter, and search for it. What additional information or research is available related to this topic?

Visit ***www.webmd.com***

- From the health A-Z index choose Heart Disease, then click on "All Heat Disease topics." Look for articles related to the topics covered in this chapter. What additional information is available?

Review Questions

Multiple Choice

1. Anticoagulants are used prophylactically for all of the following conditions or disorders, except

A. prevention of thrombus in pulmonary embolus
B. hypothyroidism
C. deep vein thrombosis
D. atrial fibrillation

2. Which of the following is an antagonist of warfarin?

A. vitamin D
B. vitamin A
C. vitamin K
D. niacin

3. The spontaneous arrest of bleeding from a damaged blood vessel is called
   A. hematoma
   B. hemosiderosis
   C. hemostasis
   D. hemostatic

4. The onset of action for intravenous heparin is
   A. immediate
   B. an hour
   C. three days
   D. one week

5. Which of the following is a major complication of heparin administration?
   A. hypertension
   B. hypersensitivity reaction
   C. bronchospasms
   D. bleeding

6. Ticlid (ticlopidine) is a drug that includes which of the following groups of drugs?
   A. thrombolytics
   B. anticoagulants
   C. antiplatelets
   D. hemostatics

7. Which of the following anticoagulants have become the drugs of choice for many clotting disorders?
   A. low molecular weight heparins
   B. high molecular weight heparins
   C. warfarins
   D. vitamin K

8. Which of the following agents is used to suppress aggregation of platelets?
   A. heparin
   B. aspirin
   C. warfarin
   D. protamine sulfate

9. Which of the following is an example of thrombolytic drugs?
   A. protamine sulfate
   B. plasminogen activator
   C. warfarin
   D. heparin

10. Which of the following is the most common adverse effect of thrombolytics?
   A. constipation
   B. hypertension
   C. vomiting
   D. bleeding

Fill in the Blank

1. Thrombophlebitis refers to the development of a clot in a vein where ______________.
2. Anticoagulants are drugs that reduce the ability of ______________.
3. After initiation of anticoagulant therapy with heparin, ______________ can be started immediately.
4. The major complication for heparin administration is ______________.
5. Warfarin is structurally similar to ______________.
6. The most commonly used antiplatelet drug is ______________.

Matching

Match the first column (generic names) of LMWHs with the second column (trade names):

____ 1. tinzaparin	A. Normiflo
____ 2. danaparoid	B. Fragmin
____ 3. dalteparin	C. Orgaran
____ 4. adeparin	D. Innohep

Critical Thinking

George is 99 years old. He has had multiple disorders and taken many different medications in his life. His skin is very thin, and only a little pressure to his skin can cause bleeding. Some of his regular medications include antidepressants, antihypertensive drugs, and baby aspirin for his heart condition.

1. What do you think are the causes of bleeding from the skin?
2. What can George's physician suggest to prevent his bleeding?
3. What medications should George stop taking because they may increase the likelihood of bleeding?

Drug Therapy for Allergies and Respiratory Disorders

CHAPTER 14

OUTLINE

(continues)

OBJECTIVES

After completing this chapter, the reader should be able to:

1. Identify basic anatomical structures of the respiratory system.
2. Compare histamines and antihistamines.
3. Be able to list three popular asthma medications.
4. Discuss the uses and general drug actions of the bronchodilators in asthma.
5. Discuss different types of mucolytics and expectorants.
6. Explain how decongestants work and identify serious adverse effects.
7. Identify the chemical mediators that are important in asthma.
8. Discuss drugs used for smoking cessation.
9. Explain the indication of mast cell stabilizers and the mechanism of action.
10. Discuss chemical mediators.

GLOSSARY

Allergic rhinitis – inflammation of the nasal mucosa that is due to the sensitivity of the nasal tissue to an allergen

Allergy – a state of hypersensitivity induced by exposure to a particular antigen

Anaphylactic shock – a severe and sometimes fatal allergic reaction

Antigen – a substance that is introduced into the body and induces the formation of antibodies

Antihistamines – drugs that counteract the action of histamine

Antitussives – agents that relieve or prevent coughing

Asthma – a chronic inflammatory disorder of the airways of the respiratory system

Bronchiectasis – a destruction and widening of the large airways

Bronchodilators – agents that relax the smooth muscle of the bronchial tubes

OUTLINE *(continued)*

Chemical mediators – substances released by mast cells and platelets into interstitial fluid and blood; these substances include histamines, leukotrienes, serotonin, and prostaglandins

Chronic obstructive pulmonary disease (COPD) – a group of common chronic respiratory disorders that are characterized by progressive tissue damage and obstruction in the airways of the lungs

Cystic fibrosis – a genetic disorder affecting the exocrine glands, causing thick mucus to obstruct the bronchioles in the lungs

Dry powder inhaler (DPI) – a device used to deliver medication in the form of micronized powder into the lungs

Emphysema – the destruction of the alveolar walls and septae, which leads to large, permanently inflated alveolar air space

Expectorants – agents that promote the removal of mucus secretions from the lung, bronchi, and trachea, usually by coughing

Glucocorticoids – the most potent and consistently effective anti-inflammatory agents that are currently available for relief of respiratory conditions

Histamine – a chemical substance naturally found in all body tissues that protects the body from factors in the environment that produce allergic and inflammatory reactions

Leukotriene modifiers – a relatively new class of drugs designed to prevent asthma and allergic reactions before they occur by either inhibiting leukotriene production, or preventing leukotrienes from binding to cellular receptors

Leukotrienes – substances that contribute to the inflammation associated with asthma

Mast cell stabilizers – substances that work to prevent allergy cells (called mast cells) from breaking open and releasing chemicals that help cause inflammation; they work slowly over time

Metered dose inhaler (MDI) – a hand-held pressurized device used to deliver medications for inhalations

Mucolytic – destroying or dissolving the active agents that make up mucus

Septae – walls of the bronchioles

Xanthine derivatives – a substance that is effective for relief of bronchospasm in asthma, chronic bronchitis, and emphysema

OVERVIEW

The respiratory system provides the mechanisms for transporting oxygen from the air into the blood, and for removing carbon dioxide from the blood. Oxygen is essential for cell metabolism, and the respiratory system is the only means of acquiring oxygen. Carbon dioxide is a waste material resulting from cell metabolism.

The respiratory system consists of two anatomic areas: the upper and lower respiratory tracts. In addition, the pulmonary circulation, the muscles required for ventilation, and the nervous system (which plays a role in controlling respiratory function) are integral to the function of the respiratory system.

Anatomy Review

- The upper respiratory system consists of the nasal cavity, sinuses, and pharynx. The lower respiratory system consists of the larynx, trachea, bronchi, bronchioles, alveoli, and lungs (Figure 14-1).
- The respiratory system exchanges oxygen and carbon dioxide in the body through respiration.
- There are three types of respiration: external respiration is breathing or ventilation, internal respiration is the exchange of oxygen and carbon dioxide between the cells and lymph, and cellular respiration is the use of oxygen to release energy stored in nutrient molecules (Figure 14-2).
- Figure 14-3 outlines the functions of each of the structures that make up the respiratory system.

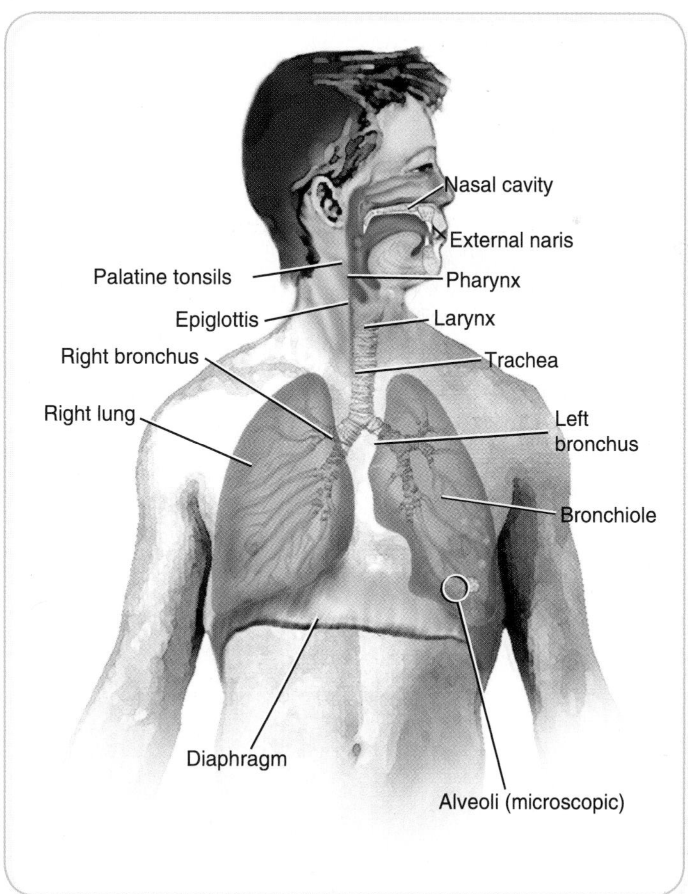

Figure 14-1 The structures of the upper and lower airways.

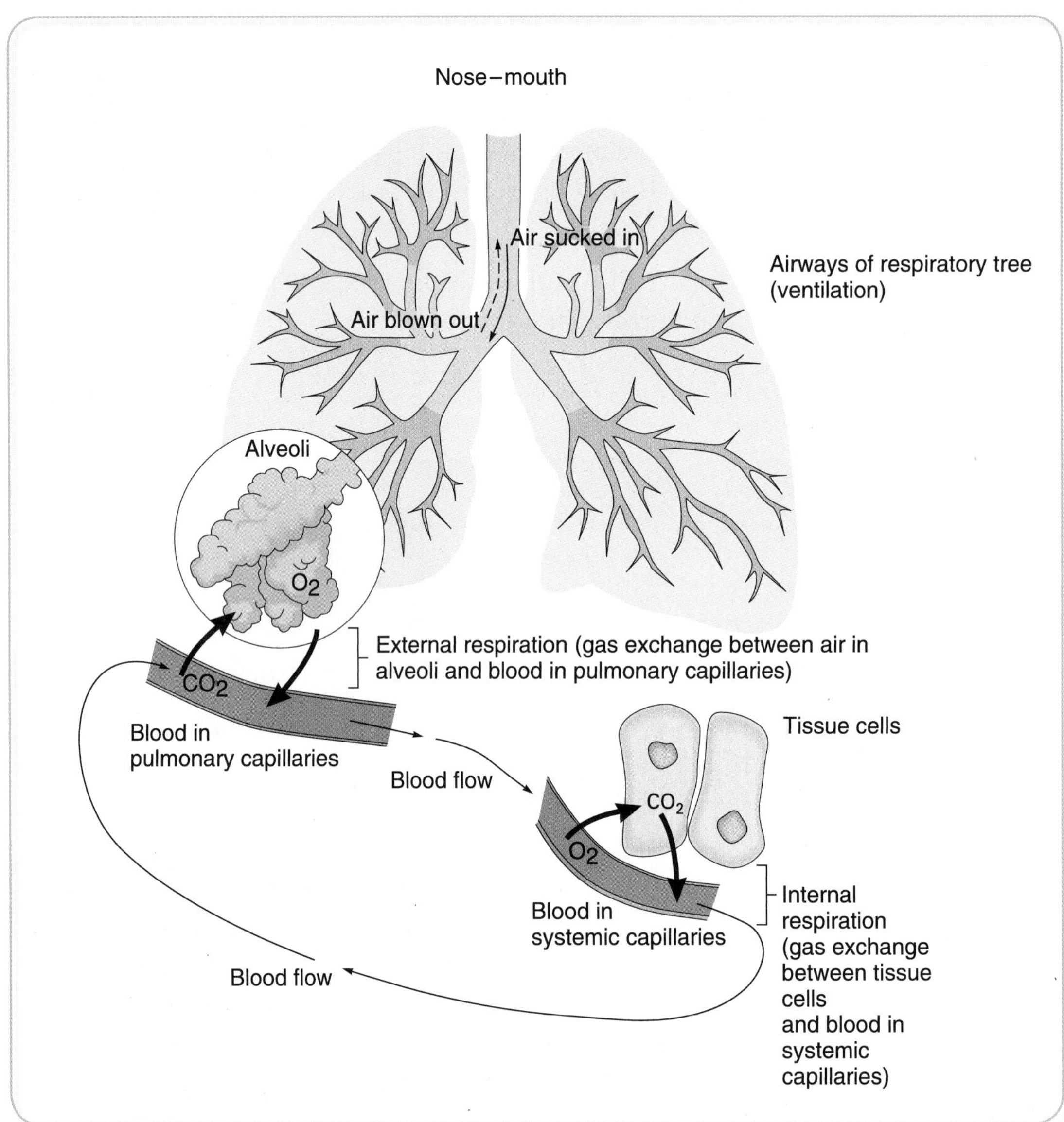

Figure 14-2 Respiration.

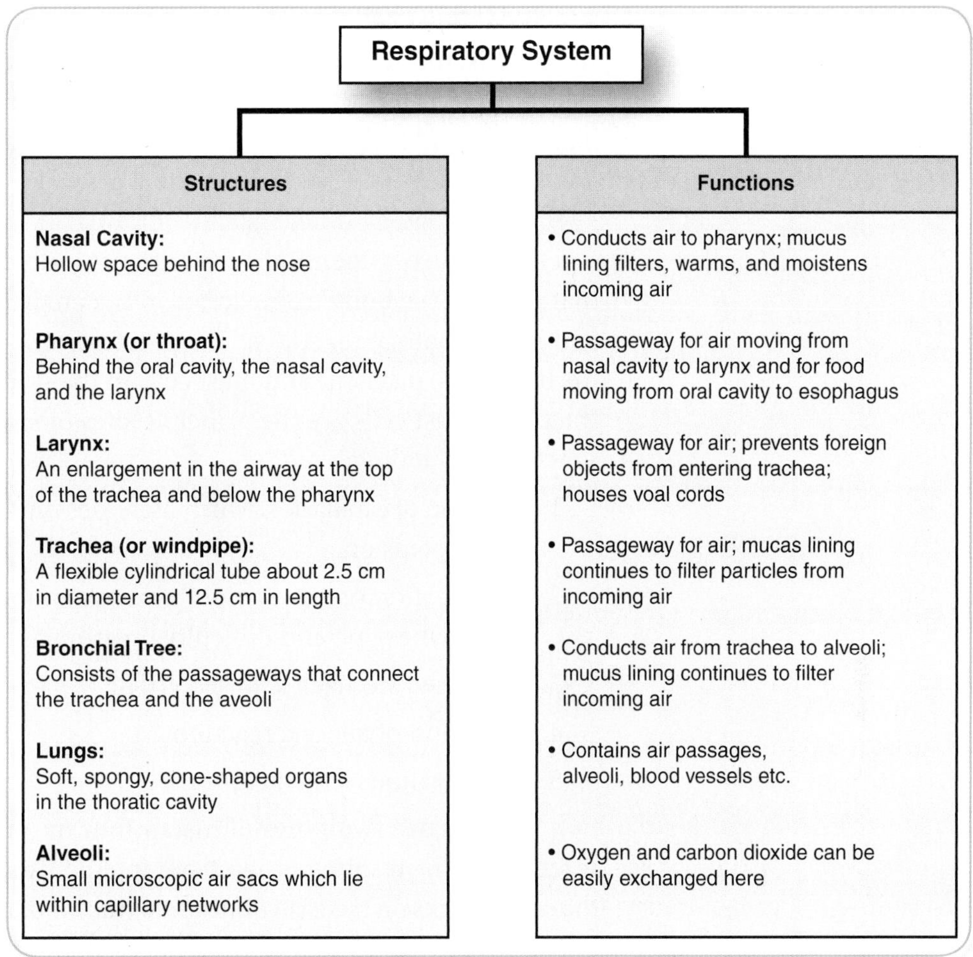

Figure 14-3 The respiratory system.

Allergies

An **allergy** is a state of hypersensitivity induced by exposure to a particular **antigen** (a substance that is introduced into the body and induces the formation of antibodies), resulting in harmful immunologic reactions on subsequent exposures. The term is usually used to refer to hypersensitivity to an environmental antigen. There are varieties of allergic reactions such as allergic rhinitis, allergic conjunctivitis, allergic asthma, and allergic dermatitis. This chapter focuses on respiratory disorders and drug therapy, with allergic rhinitis and allergic asthma being discussed.

Chemical Mediators

Allergies result in an inflammatory process in the nasal passages and airways. The inflammatory process is basically the same regardless of the cause of the allergic response. The severity of the inflammation may vary with the specific situation. The inflammation may result in tissue injury, which damages cells. Mast cells and platelets release **chemical mediators**, such as histamines and leukotrienes into the interstitial fluid and blood. The chemical mediators that are mostly involved with allergies and asthma include histamines and leukotrienes, which are discussed below.

Histamines

Histamine is a chemical substance naturally found in all the body tissues that protects the body from factors in the environment that produce allergic and inflammatory reactions. The greatest concentration of histamine is in the basophils, platelets, and mast cells in the skin, lungs, and gastrointestinal tract. The mast cells are the principle sites of storage. Histamine has several functions, including:

1. Dilation of capillaries, which increases capillary permeability and results in hypotension.
2. Contraction of most smooth muscle of the bronchial tree, which may cause wheezing and difficulty breathing.
3. Increased stomach acid secretion.
4. Initiation of allergic reactions.
5. Acceleration of the heart rate.

There are two types of histamines in our body. One causes allergic reactions in the respiratory tract and interacts with H_1 receptors on cells, and the other works on the gastrointestinal tract and interacts with H_2 receptors on cells (see Chapter 15). Histamine causes dilation and increased permeability of capillaries. It is one of the first mediators of an inflammatory response. Antihistamine drugs inhibit this immediate, transient response. Both H_1 and H_2 receptors mediate the contraction of vascular smooth muscle. Histamine has also been postulated to be a neurotransmitter in the central nervous system. The H_1 receptor may be blocked with antihistamine drugs.

Leukotrienes

Leukotrienes contribute to the inflammation associated with asthma. They are broncho-constrictive substances released during asthma and inflammation. Leukotrienes (slow-reacting substances of anaphylaxis [SRS-A]) are substances that produce effects similar to those of histamine. These substances cause smooth muscle contraction and increased vascular permeability. Leukotrienes appear to be important in the later stages of the inflammation associated with asthma. They stimulate slower and more prolonged responses than do histamines.

Allergic Reaction

An allergic reaction occurs when the immune system reacts to a foreign substance. The body attempts to get rid of the substance, be it an allergen from the environment or a medication. In the case of an allergic reaction to a medication, the body's response is harmful and may cause serious symptoms. Common allergic reactions include nausea, diarrhea, vomiting, headache, and lightheadedness. Other symptoms include anxiety, hives, palpitations, shortness of breath, rash, swelling, and wheezing. The most common allergies caused by natural environmental allergies include dust, pollen, and pet dander. The most common medications that cause allergic reactions include anticonvulsants, barbiturates, iodine, anesthetics, and antibiotics (including sulfa medications).

Anaphylactic Shock

Anaphylactic shock is an allergic reaction that may be life threatening. Its onset is sudden, severe, and involves the entire body. Anaphylactic shock causes a massive release of histamine and other substances, which cause airway constriction (making breathing very difficult), abdominal cramping, vomiting, and diarrhea. Common causes of anaphylactic shock include foods, medications, insect stings, and allergies to latex. Foods which are most likely to cause this condition include nuts, fish, milk, and eggs. Individuals who have food allergies or asthma are believed to be more likely to develop anaphylactic reactions. The most common insect stings in the United States include bees, yellow jackets, hornets, wasps, and ants. Anaphylactic reactions often begin with tingling sensations, itching, metallic taste sensation, hives, sensation of warmth, symptoms of asthma, swelling of the mouth and throat, a drop in blood pressure, or loss of consciousness. These types of reactions are usually treated with epinephrine, followed by antihistamines and steroids.

Allergic Rhinitis

Allergic rhinitis is the inflammation of the mucus membranes in the nose, throat, and airways that is due to the sensitivity of the tissue to an antigen, also called an allergen. The nasal mucosa is rich with mast cells (large cells that contain a wide variety of biochemicals, including histamine). These cells, along with basophils (a type of white blood cell), recognize environmental agents as they try to enter the body. Individuals with allergic rhinitis contain numerous mast cells. Allergic rhinitis is usually associated with watery nasal discharge and itching of the nose and eyes, caused by a localized sensitivity reaction to house dust, animal dander, or an antigen, commonly pollen. The condition may be seasonal. It is commonly known as "hay fever." Allergic rhinitis is caused by histamine release, while non-allergic rhinitis is often a symptom of the common cold.

Medical Terminology Review

rhinitis
rhin = nose
itis = inflammation
inflammation of the nose

ANTI-ALLERGIC AGENTS

The therapeutic goals of treating allergic rhinitis are to prevent its occurrence and to relieve symptoms. Drugs used to prevent or treat allergic rhinitis include antihistamines (H_1-receptor antagonists), intranasal steroids, and mast cell stabilizers. Antihistamines and common OTC antihistamine

TABLE 14-1 First- and Second-generation H_1-receptor Antagonists

Generic Name	Trade Name	Route of Administration	Average Adult Dosage
First-generation Agents			
azatadine	Optimine®	PO	1–2 mg b.i.d.-t.i.d. prn
azelastine hydrochloride	Astelin®	Intranasal	2 sprays per nostril b.i.d.
brompheniramine maleate	Veltane®	PO	4–8 mg t.i.d.-q.i.d. (max: 40 mg/day)
chlorpheniramine maleate	Chlor-Trimeton®	PO	2–4 mg t.i.d.-q.i.d. (max: 24 mg/day)
clemastine fumarate	Tavist®	PO	1.34 mg b.i.d. (max: 8.04 mg/day)
cyproheptadine hydrochloride	Periactin®	PO	4 mg t.i.d. or q.i.d. (max: 0.5 mg/kg/day)
dexbrompheniramine maleate	Drixoral®	PO	6 mg b.i.d.
dexchlorpheniramine maleate	Dexchlor®	PO	2 mg q4–6 h (max: 12 mg/day)
diphenhydramine hydrochloride	Benadryl(R)	PO	25–50 mg 3–4 times/day (max: 300 mg/day)
promethazine hydrochloride	Phenergan®	PO	12.5 mg/day (max: 50 mg/day)
tripelennamine hydrochloride	PBZ-SR®	PO	25–50 mg q4–6 h (max: 600 mg/day)
triprolidine hydrochloride	Actidil®	PO	2.5 mg b.i.d. or t.i.d.
Second-generation Agents			
cetirizine hydrochloride	Zyrtec®	PO	5–10 mg/day
desloratadine	Clarinex®	PO	5 mg/day
fexofenadine hydrochloride	Allegra®	PO	60 mg b.i.d. or 180 mg once per day
loratadine	Claritin®	PO	10 mg/day

combinations will be focused on here. Mast cell stabilizers and steroids are discussed later in this chapter.

H_1-receptor Antagonists

H_1-receptor antagonists (**antihistamines**) are commonly used for the treatment of allergies. These drugs relieve the symptoms of runny nose, sneezing, and itching of the eyes, nose, and throat as seen in allergic rhinitis. Table 14-1 shows various H_1-receptor antagonists. Antihistamines are

TABLE 14-2 OTC Combination Antihistamine Drugs

Antihistamine	Decongestant	Trade Name
chlorpheniramine	phenylephrine	Actifed® Cold and Allergy tablets
chlorpheniramine	pseudoephedrine	Actifed® Cold and Sinus caplets
diphenhydramine	phenylephrine	Benadryl® Allergy/Cold caplets
chlorpheniramine	pseudoephedrine	Chlor-Trimeton® Allergy-Decongestant tablets
brompheniramine	phenylephrine	Dimetapp® Cold and Allergy Elixir
dexbrompheniramine	pseudoephedrine	Drixoral® Allergy and Sinus Extended Release tablets
chlorpheniramine	pseudoephedrine	Sinutab® Sinus Allergy tablets
diphenhydramine	phenylephrine	Sudafed® PE Nighttime
chlorpheniramine	pseudoephedrine	Triaminic® Cold/Allergy
chlorpheniramine	pseudoephedrine	Tylenol® Allergy Sinus caplets

often combined with decongestants and antitussives in OTC sinus and cold medicines. Table 14-2 shows examples of combination OTC drugs.

Mechanism of Action

The primary action of antihistamines is to block the effect of histamine at H_1-receptors, thus blocking histamine release.

Indications

H_1-receptor antagonists are used to treat minor symptoms of various allergic conditions and the common cold, such as runny nose, sneezing, and for the prevention of motion sickness, vertigo, and reactions to blood or plasma in susceptible patients.

Adverse Effects

Common adverse effects of H_1-receptor antagonists include dry mouth, dizziness, headache, urinary retention, nausea, vomiting, sedation, hypotension, and a decrease in the number of white blood cells.

Contraindications and Precautions

H_1-receptor antagonists are contraindicated in patients with hypersensitivity to these agents, prostatic hypertrophy, glaucoma, and GI obstructions. H_1-receptor antagonists should be used cautiously in patients with asthma or hyperthyroidism.

Drug Interactions

Use of H_1-receptor antagonists with CNS depressants such as opioids or alcohol will cause increased sedation. Some OTC cold preparations (for example, diphenhydramine) may increase anticholinergic adverse effects. MAOIs may cause a hypertensive crisis.

Asthma

Asthma is defined as a chronic inflammatory disorder of the airways of the respiratory system (see Figure 14-4). It is a condition with wheezing and shortness of breath due to constriction of the bronchioles. Asthma is most commonly classified as allergic, exercise-induced, or caused by infections of the respiratory tract. Symptoms include breathlessness, cough, wheezing, and chest tightness. The airway becomes inflamed with edema and mucus plugs, and hyperactivity of the bronchial tree adds to the symptoms.

During asthmatic attacks, when bronchiole constriction and increased secretions are present, bronchodilators are used for relief. Anti-inflammatory drugs, such as glucocorticoids, leukotriene inhibitors, and cromolyn, may be

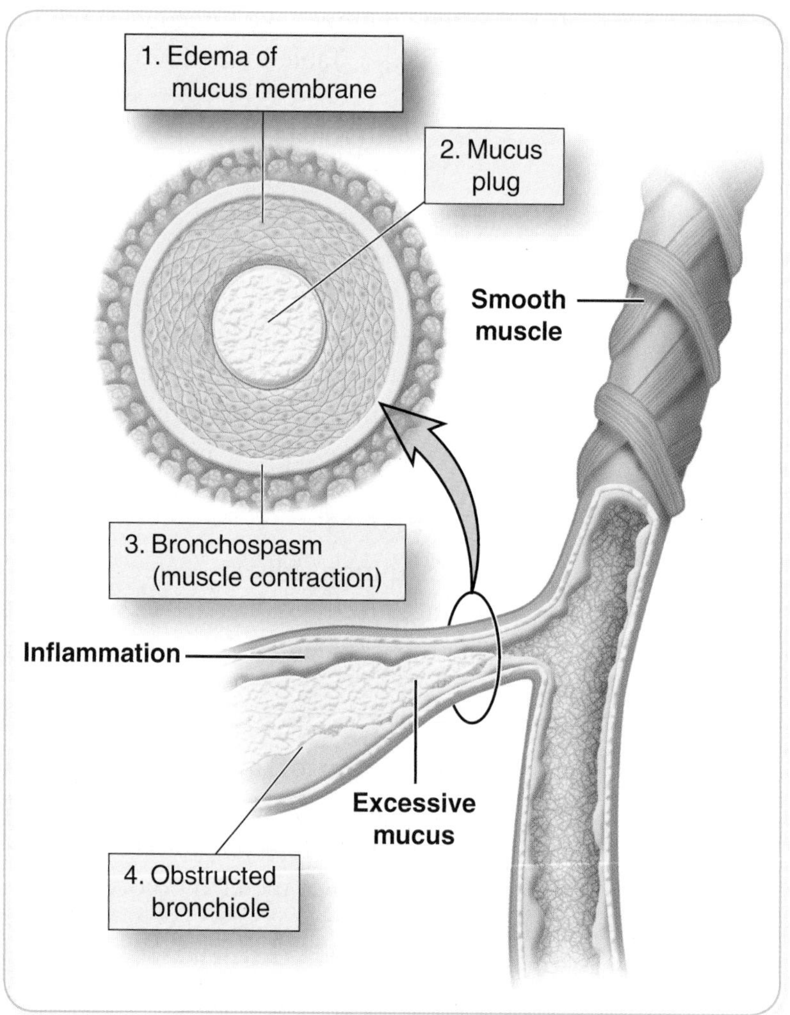

Figure 14-4 Acute asthmatic episode.

prescribed for relief of symptoms. The majority of medications for asthma are administered by inhalation. Anti-asthma medications can be divided into two categories: long-term control and quick-relief medications.

For safety, asthmatic patients should learn how to manage their disease and its complications, as well as limit exposure to irritants that will trigger asthma attacks. Since symptoms alone are not always sufficient to measure respiratory status, patients learn how to use peak flow meters. These meters measure the peak expiratory flow rate (PEFR) from a patient's lungs. They should be used two times per day with the results of each usage written down so that results over time can be discussed with the patient's physician.

Medical Terminology Review

bronchiole
bronchi = air tube
ole = small; little; minute
small tube in the airway

Anti-asthma Agents

There are various groups of medications used in the treatment of asthma, including bronchodilators, anti-inflammatory drugs, leukotriene modifiers (antagonists), and mast cell stabilizers.

Bronchodilators

Bronchodilators are agents that widen the diameter of the bronchial tubes, and are used to rapidly relieve the acute bronchospasm of asthmatic attack. Bronchodilators include beta-adrenergic agonists and xanthenes (theophylline). Beta-adrenergic drugs are the most commonly prescribed bronchodilators. Table 14-3 lists bronchodilators for asthma.

Beta-adrenergic Drugs

Beta-adrenergic drugs work as both cardiac and respiratory agonists. They are commonly referred to simply as beta-blockers. These drugs or hormones act through the sympathetic nervous system. Their effects include

TABLE 14-3 Drugs Used as Bronchodilators to Treat Asthma

Generic Name	Trade Name	Route of Administration	Average Adult Dosage
Anticholinergics			
ipratropium bromide	Atroven®	PO	2 inhalations by MDI q.i.d. (max: 12 inhalations/day)
ipratropium bromide and albuterol sulfate	Combivent®	PO	2 inhalations q6 h (max: 12 inhalations/day)
tiotropium bromide	Spiriva®	PO	1 capsule inhaled/day by Handihaler device
Beta-Agonists/Sympathomimetics			
albuterol	Proventil®, Ventolin®	PO	2–4 mg t.i.d.-q.i.d.

(continues)

TABLE 14-3 Drugs Used as Bronchodilators to Treat Asthma—*continued*

Generic Name	Trade Name	Route of Administration	Average Adult Dosage
bitolterol mesylate	Tornalate®	PO	2 inhalations by MDI t.i.d.-q.i.d.
epinephrine bitartrate	AsthmaHaler®, Bronkaid Mist suspension®	PO	0.1–0.5 mL or 1:1000 q20 by MDI min-4 h inhalation prn
formoterol fumarate	Foradil®	PO	1–2 inhalations by DPI q4 h up to 5 days
isoproterenol hydrochloride	Isuprel®	PO, IV	0.01–0.02 mg prn
levalbuterol hydrochloride	Xopenex®	Nebulizer	0.63 mg t.i.d.-q.i.d.
metaproterenol sulfate	Alupent®	PO	MDI: 2–3 inhalations q3–4 h (max: 12 inhalations/day); PO: 20 mg q6–8 h
pirbuterol acetate	Maxair®	PO	2 inhalations by MDI q.i.d. (max: 12 inhalations/day)
salmeterol xinafoate	Serevent®	PO	2 inhalations of aerosol by MDI b.i.d.
terbutaline sulfate	Brethaire®, Brethine®	PO	2.5–5 mg t.i.d. (2 inhalations by MDI q4–6 h)
Methylxanthines			
aminophylline	Truphylline®	IV	6 mg/kg over 30 minutes
theophylline	Elixophyllin®	PO, IV	PO: 5 mg/kg in divided doses, q6 h; IV: Loading dose: 5 mg/kg

increased heart rate, dilation of bronchial tubes in the lungs, and reduction of the force and rate of uterine contractions during labor.

Drugs with primary beta-1 agonist activity act mainly on the heart, increasing heart rate and raising blood pressure. The primary beta-2 agonist activity acts mainly on the lungs and uterus. Consequently, drugs that stimulate the beta-2 receptors produce bronchodilation. They are used to treat asthma and premature labor. Epinephrine (which is normally secreted from the adrenal gland) and isoproterenol are two potent beta-receptor stimulators.

Mechanism of Action. The main action is on the smooth muscle of the bronchial tree and on the heart. A typical medication is isoproterenol, which may be taken orally or by injection. Beta-2 receptor drugs are the most effective medications to reduce acute bronchospasms and exercise-induced asthma. These agents provide bronchodilation by stimulating the beta-2 receptors in the smooth muscle of the lung. Epinephrine and ephedrine are nonselective adrenergic agents, and naturally occurring catecholamine may be obtained from animal adrenal glands or prepared synthetically.

Medical Terminology Review

bronchospasm
broncho = air tube
spasm = narrowing; contraction
narrowing of the bronchioles or airways

Indications. Epinephrine is used for the temporary relief of bronchospasm. These agents are used in acute asthmatic attacks and congestion. Salmeterol is preferred for prophylaxis and maintenance therapy for asthma or bronchospasm. Salmeterol is the only agent of this class available in the U.S., and is indicated for long-term prevention of asthma symptoms and the prevention of exercise-induced bronchospasm. Salmeterol should not be used in place of anti-inflammatory therapy or to treat acute bronchospasm.

Adverse Effects. Adverse effects of beta-2 agonists include dizziness, headache, tremor, palpitations, and sinus tachycardia. Common adverse effects of epinephrine and ephedrine include insomnia, tachycardia, nervousness, and anorexia. The cardiotoxic effects have led to the discovery and use of more specific respiratory agents that do not cause tachycardia or nervousness.

Contraindications and Precautions. Beta-2 adrenergic agents are contraindicated in patients with hypersensitivity to these drugs, or during pregnancy (category C) and lactation.

Drug Interactions. Salmeterol generally does not interact with other drugs. Other beta-2 agonists may have drug interactions with anesthetics, digitalis, ergotamine, and MAOIs.

Xanthine Derivatives

This group of drugs is chemically related to caffeine, which dilates bronchioles in the lungs. **Xanthine** derivatives are effective for the relief of bronchospasm in several diseases (see Table 14-3).

Mechanism of Action. Xanthine derivatives relax the smooth muscles of the bronchial tree and stimulate cardiac muscle and the CNS. Methylxanthine is the base of xanthine derivatives that must be converted to theophylline. Theophylline has a narrow therapeutic range, and is not used as commonly today. Instead, the beta-2 adrenergic agents are safer and more effective. Theophylline provides mild bronchodilation in asthmatics. This drug may also have important anti-inflammatory properties and enhance mucociliary clearance. Theophylline is available for oral administration in standard or sustained-release formulas with forms that last up to 24 hours. Theophylline has a small therapeutic range and beta-2 agonists are safer and more effective. Therefore, the xanthenes are not used as commonly today.

Indications. These xanthine agents are used for the prevention and treatment of bronchial asthma and for the treatment of emphysema and bronchitis.

Adverse Effects. Adverse effects include tachycardia, insomnia, nervousness, headache, and nausea. Patients with hyperthyroidism, acute pulmonary edema, convulsive disorders, and heart disease cannot use xanthine derivatives. Adverse effects of theophylline at therapeutic doses include insomnia, upset stomach, aggravation of dyspepsia, and urination difficulties in elderly men with prostatism. Dose-related toxicities are common and include nausea, vomiting, tachyarrhythmias, headache, seizures, hyperglycemia, and hypokalemia.

Key Concept

Observe and report early signs of possible toxicity from xanthine derivatives, which may include: anorexia, nausea, vomiting, dizziness, shakiness, restlessness, abdominal discomfort, and marked hypotension.

Contraindications and Precautions. Xanthine derivatives are contraindicated in individuals with known hypersensitivity, seizure disorders, uncontrolled arrhythmias, peptic ulcers, and hyperthyroidism. Xanthine derivatives should be used cautiously in patients older than 60 years or those who have cardiac disease, hypertension, congestive heart failure, hypoxemia, and liver dysfunctions. These agents are used during pregnancy (category C) and lactation with caution.

Drug Interactions. Xanthine drugs can produce drug interactions with caffeine, cimetidine, fluoroquinolones, antibiotics, rifampin, phenobarbital, and phenytoin.

Anti-inflammatory Drugs

Many anti-inflammatory agents are used to reduce the incidence of asthma attacks. Glucocorticoids, leukotriene inhibitors, and mast cell stabilizers are commonly used. See Table 14-4.

TABLE 14-4 Anti-inflammatory Medications for Treatment of Asthma

Generic Name	Trade Name	Route of Administration	Average Adult Dosage
Glucocorticoids			
beclomethasone dipropionate	Beconase AQ®, Vancenase®	PO	1–2 inhalations by MDI t.i.d.-q.i.d.
budesonide	Pulmicort Turbuhaler®	PO	1–2 inhalations by MDI (200 mcg/inhalation)
flunisolide	AeroBid®	PO	2–3 inhalations by MDI b.i.d.-t.i.d.
fluticasone propionate	Flonase®, Flovent®	PO	2 inhalations by MDI (44 mcg ea.) b.i.d.
triamcinolone acetonide	Azmacort®	PO	2 inhalations by MDI t.i.d.-q.i.d.

(continues)

TABLE 14-4 Anti-inflammatory Medications for Treatment of Asthma—*continued*

Generic Name	Trade Name	Route of Administration	Average Adult Dosage
Leukotriene Modifiers			
montelukast	Singulair®	PO	10 mg/day in the evening
zafirlukast	Accolate®	PO	20 mg b.i.d. 1 h before or 2 h after meals
zileuton	Zyflo®	PO	600 mg q.i.d.
Mast Cell Stabilizers			
cromolyn sodium	Intal®	PO	1 inhalation by MDI q.i.d.
nedocromil sodium	Tilade®	PO	2 inhalations by MDI q.i.d.

Glucocorticoids

Glucocorticoids are the most potent and consistently effective anti-inflammatories that are currently available. There are three commonly used devices for inhalation administration: metered dose inhalers, nebulizers, and dry powder inhalers. Drug administration with a **metered dose inhaler (MDI)** is often accomplished with one or two puffs from a hand-held pressurized device (See Figure 14-5).

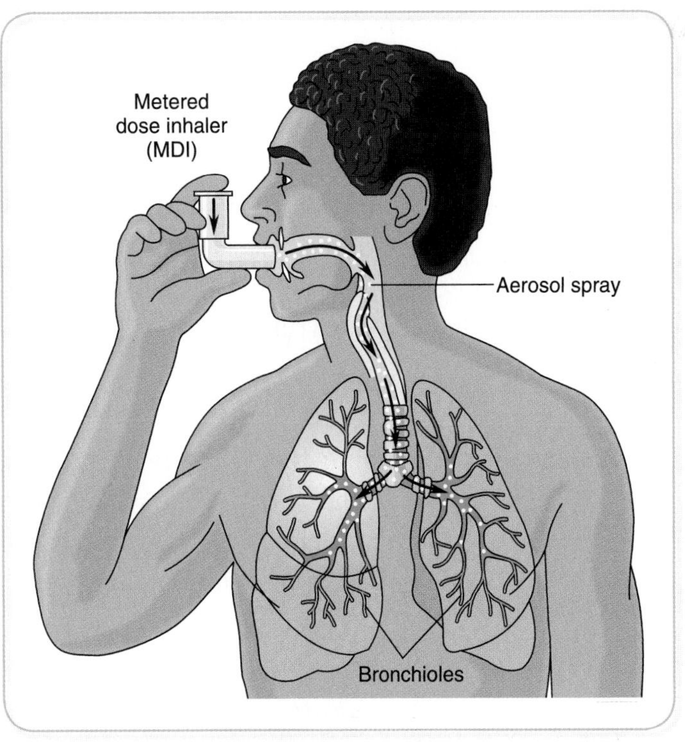

Figure 14-5 Use of metered dose inhaler.

Dry powder inhalers (DPIs) deliver medication in the form of micronized powder into the lungs. An example of a medication that is available in DPI form is albuterol. DPIs are breath-activated and are easier to use than MDIs. A nebulizer uses a small machine that converts a solution into a mist. The mist droplets are inhaled through either a facemask or a mouthpiece.

Quick-relief asthma medicines are also referred to as "rescue inhalers." They are usually given via nebulizers or MDIs. Examples of these medicines include Proventil and Atrovent. Also, certain oral steroids such as prednisone and prednisolone are utilized in rescue inhalers.

Systemic glucocorticoids are used to treat status asthmaticus and inhaled glucocorticoids are used for maintenance therapy. Inhaled glucocorticoids are the most effective means of controlling asthma. Combined preparations containing a glucocorticoid and a long-acting bronchodilator are considered useful in limiting the amount of the glucocorticoid needed to control asthma.

Mechanism of Action. They enter target cells where they have anti-inflammatory, immunosuppressive, and salt-retaining effects.

Indications. Inhaled glucocorticoids are preferred for the long-term control of asthma and are first-line agents for patients with persistent asthma. Dosages for inhaled glucocorticoids vary depending on the specific agent and delivery device. Systemic glucocorticoids are most effective for long-term asthma therapy. Long-term use of inhaled glucocorticoids in children is not recommended because these agents may suppress growth and suppress the adrenal glands for production of hormones.

Adverse Effects. Adverse reactions to corticosteroid inhalation include nasal irritation and dryness, headache, nausea, epistaxis, dizziness, hoarseness, and cough.

Contraindications and Precautions. Local (inhaled) glucocorticoids are contraindicated in patients with hypersensitivity to the drugs and lactation. These drugs should be used cautiously in patients with concomitant administration of systemic oral steroids, active tuberculosis, viral infections, and recurrent epistaxis. Glucocorticoids should be used with caution in pregnancy (category C for oral and category B for inhaled). Safety and efficacy for children younger than six years is not established.

Key Concept

Inhaled glucocorticoids may cause bronchospasm, requiring their use to be discontinued and an alternate treatment started.

Drug Interactions. Drug interactions increase the therapeutic and toxic effects of glucocorticoids if taken concurrently with troleandomycin. They decrease effects of anticholinesterases if taken concurrently with corticotropin; profound muscular depression is possible.

Leukotriene Modifiers (Antagonists)

Leukotriene modifiers are a class of biologically active compounds that occur naturally in leukocytes and produce allergic and inflammatory reactions similar to those of histamine. They are thought to play a role in the development of allergic and autoallergic diseases such as asthma, rheumatoid arthritis, inflammatory bowel disease, and psoriasis.

Mechanism of Action. Leukotriene antagonists such as zafirlukast (Accolate) block the bronchoconstriction, mucus production, and inflammation that occur with asthma. Zafirlukast was the first medication in this new anti-inflammatory class. A newer drug is called zileuton (Zyflo). It is rapidly absorbed via oral administration. Montelukast (Singulair) is the latest addition to this class of drugs. Montelukast acts as a bronchodilator, respiratory stimulant, and leukotriene receptor antagonist. This medication should be given at night for maximum effectiveness.

Indications. Leukotriene modifiers are used for prophylaxis and chronic asthma in adults and children older than 12 years. Zafirlukast is prescribed as maintenance therapy for patients with chronic asthma. Montelukast is prescribed prophylactically for asthma attacks (see Table 14-4).

Adverse Effects. Zafirlukast is a safer drug and has few adverse effects. Adverse effects of zileuton include liver toxicity and dyspepsia. The main adverse effects of montelukast are headaches and GI symptoms.

Contraindications and Precautions. The leukotriene modifiers are contraindicated in patients with history of hypersensitivity to these medications. Montelukast is contraindicated in severe asthma attacks, bronchoconstriction due to asthma, or status asthmaticus. Montelukast should be avoided during lactation. Zileuton and zafirlukast are contraindicated in patients with active liver disease and during lactation and pregnancy. The leukotriene modifiers should be used cautiously in hepatic insufficiency. Safety and effectiveness in children younger than 12 years are not established.

Drug Interactions. Leukotriene modifiers may double theophylline levels and increase toxicity. They increase the hypoprothrombinemic effects of warfarin. These agents may increase levels of beta-blockers (especially propranolol) and lead to hypotension and bradycardia.

Mast Cell Stabilizers

The two mast cell inhibitors that are available for the prophylaxis of asthma include cromolyn sodium and nedocromil. They are used to prevent asthma symptoms and improve airway function in patients with mild persistent asthma or exercise-induced asthma (see Table 14-4).

Mechanism of Action. Mast cell stabilizers suppress the release of substances that cause bronchoconstriction and inflammation from the mast cells in the respiratory tract.

Indications. Cromolyn is the drug of choice as a prophylactic for moderate allergic asthma, especially in children, because of its safety and efficacy. It is also used to reduce the symptoms of seasonal allergic attacks. Mast cell stabilizers are used in combination with other drugs in the treatment of allergic disorders and in the prevention of exercise-induced bronchospasm.

Adverse Effects. Adverse effects of mast cell stabilizers include nausea, fatigue, headache, dizziness, hypotension, and an unpleasant taste.

Contraindications and Precautions. Mast cell stabilizers are contraindicated in patients with a known hypersensitivity, coronary artery disease or history of arrhythmias, dyspnea, and acute asthma, and during pregnancy (category B) and lactation. Safe use in children younger than six years is not determined. Mast cell stabilizers should be used cautiously in patients with renal or hepatic dysfunction.

Drug Interactions. There are no clinically important drug interactions with cromolyn.

DECONGESTANTS

Key Concept

Chicken soup may actually help you fight off a cold. The heat, fluid, and salt found in chicken soup may help you fight off the viral infection that is a cold.

The common cold generally involves a runny nose, sneezing, nasal congestion, coughing, sore throat, headache, and many other symptoms. There are over one billion colds in the U.S. every year. Colds occur mostly during the winter or during rainy seasons. People are most contagious during the first two to three days of the cold, and usually not contagious at all by days seven to ten. Certain cold viruses can also cause the patient to experience muscle aches, postnasal drip, and decreased appetite. Complications of the common cold include: bronchitis, pneumonia, ear infection, sinusitis, and aggravation of asthma.

Nasal congestion and a runny nose are primarily associated with the first stage of inflammation, vasodilation, and increased capillary permeability. Decongestants cause vasoconstriction of nasal mucosa and reduce congestion or swelling. These agents are available in both oral and nasal preparations. Table 14-5 shows decongestant agents.

Mechanism of Action

The most effective way of alleviating the symptoms of nasal congestion is to induce vasoconstriction through stimulation of alpha-receptors of the sympathetic nervous system that is affiliated with the nasal vasculature. Therefore, decongestants are alpha agonists.

Indications

The most common uses for decongestants are the relief of nasal congestion due to infection or allergy, and inflammation in the eyes. They are also used to relieve respiratory distress of bronchial asthma, chronic bronchitis, and emphysema.

Adverse Effects

Decongestants should only be used by order of a physician for those patients with glaucoma, prostate cancer, and heart disease. Decongestants may increase blood sugar levels in patients with diabetes mellitus. Warnings

TABLE 14-5 Drugs Used to Treat Nasal Congestion

Generic Name	Trade Name	Route of Administration	Average Adult Dosage
Anticholinergic			
ipratropium bromide	Atrovent®	Nasal	2 sprays in each nostril 3–4 times/day for only 4 days
Sympathomimetics			
ephedrine hydrochloride	Efedron®	Intranasal	2–4 drops t.i.d.-q.i.d.
naphazoline hydrochloride	Privine®	Intranasal	2 drops q3–6 h
oxymetazoline	Afrin®, Neo-Synephrine®	Intranasal	2–3 sprays b.i.d. for up to 3–5 days
pseudoephedrine hydrochloride	Sudafed®	PO	60 mg q4–6 h
tetrahydrozoline hydrochloride	Tyzine®	Intranasal	2–4 drops or sprays q3 h
xylometazoline	Otrivin®	Intranasal	1–2 sprays b.i.d.

on the labels of OTC preparations instruct patients with hypertension, diabetes mellitus, ischemic heart disease, and hyperthyroidism about possible adverse effects involved in the use of decongestants. They may cause tachycardia, insomnia, nervousness, restlessness, blurred vision, and nausea or vomiting. Ephedrine is on the way out of the market due to its toxicities. It is still legal in many applications except dietary supplements. The purchasing of ephedrine or pseudoephedrine is currently limited and monitored, and regulations vary between states.

Contraindications and Precautions

Decongestants are contraindicated in patients with hypersensitivity to these agents, glaucoma, hypertrophy of prostate, certain types of heart disease, or diabetes mellitus. Decongestants should be avoided in patients with hyperthyroidism and hemorrhagic stroke.

Decongestants are used cautiously in patients with ischemic heart disease. The safe use of decongestants during pregnancy (category C) and lactation is not established.

Drug Interactions

Nasal decongestants such as ephedrine or pseudoephedrine may cause severe hypertension with MAOIs such as furazolidone. They may also decrease vasopressor response with reserpine, methyldopa, and urinary acidifiers.

Antitussives, Expectorants, and Mucolytics

Antitussives suppress coughing. Coughing is a reflex response to irritation of the bronchial mucosal layer, such as that seen in inflammatory conditions. The cough reflex has an important role in clearing the lungs of excessive mucus and other secretions. **Expectorants** are agents that promote the removal of mucus secretions from the lungs, bronchi, and trachea, usually by coughing. These medications are available OTC and by prescription. Expectorant and mucolytic drugs include acetylcysteine, guaifenesin, and dornase alfa (see Table 14-6).

Mechanism of Action

> **Medical Terminology Review**
>
> **mucolytic**
> *muco = mucus*
> *lytic = breaking down*
> agent to break down mucus

Expectorants are also **mucolytic** (destroying or dissolving the active agents which make up mucus). In many cases, expectorants are added to other drugs, such as antitussives, decongestants, and antihistamines, to help remove mucus. Acetylcysteine is a mucolytic agent that decreases the viscosity of mucus. It is also an antidote to acetaminophen hepatotoxicity. Guaifenesin is safer and more effective.

Indications

There are specific expectorants indicated for the treatment of cystic fibrosis, including acetylcysteine and dornase alfa. These agents are able to

TABLE 14-6 Antitussive, Expectorant, and Mucolytic Drugs

Generic Name	Trade Name	Route of Administration	Average Adult Dosage
Opioid Antitussives			
codeine	(generic only)	PO	10–20 mg q4–6 h p.r.n. (max: 120 mg/24 h)
hydrocodone bitartrate	Hycodan®, others	PO	5–10 mg q4–6 h p.r.n. (max: 15 mg/dose)
Nonopioid Antitussives			
benzonatate	Tessalon®	PO	100 mg t.i.d. p.r.n. up to 600 mg/day
dextromethorphan	Benylin®	PO	10–20 mg q4 h or 30 mg q6–8h
Expectorant			
guaifenesin	Robitussin®, others	PO	200–400 mg q4 h (max: 2.4g/day)
Mucolytic			
acetylcysteine	Mucomyst®	PO	Inhalation by MDI: 1–10 mL of 20% solution q4–6 h or 2–20 mL of 10% solution q4–6 h

reduce the risk of respiratory infections. The drug works within 3 to 7 days of starting the medication.

Adverse Effects

The common adverse effects of antitussives include dizziness, drowsiness, nausea, and vomiting. Acetylcysteine may cause bronchospasm and a burning sensation in the upper respiratory passage.

Contraindications and Precautions

The contraindications and precautions for these agents are not significant.

Drug Interactions

By inhibiting platelet function, guaifenesin may increase the risk of hemorrhage in patients receiving heparin therapy. There are no significant drug interactions listed for acetylcysteine or dornase alfa.

Chronic Obstructive Pulmonary Disease

Chronic obstructive pulmonary disease (COPD) is a group of common chronic respiratory disorders that are characterized by progressive tissue damage and obstruction in the airways of the lungs. Emphysema, chronic bronchitis, and chronic asthma are some examples. Other conditions, such as **cystic fibrosis** (a genetic disorder affecting the exocrine glands, causing thick mucus to obstruct the bronchioles in the lungs), and **bronchiectasis** may lead to similar obstructive effects. Table 14-7 compares the characteristics of emphysema and chronic bronchitis.

Emphysema

Emphysema is the destruction of the alveolar walls and **septae**, which leads to large, permanently inflated alveolar air space (see Figure 14-6). Cigarette

TABLE 14-7 Comparisons between Emphysema and Chronic Bronchitis

Characteristic	Emphysema	Chronic Bronchitis
Etiology (cause)	Smoking, genetics	Smoking, air pollution
Location	Alveoli	Bronchi
Cough and Dyspnea	Some coughing, marked dyspnea	Early, constant cough; some dyspnea
Cyanosis (bluish skin)	No	Yes
Sputum	Little	Large amounts

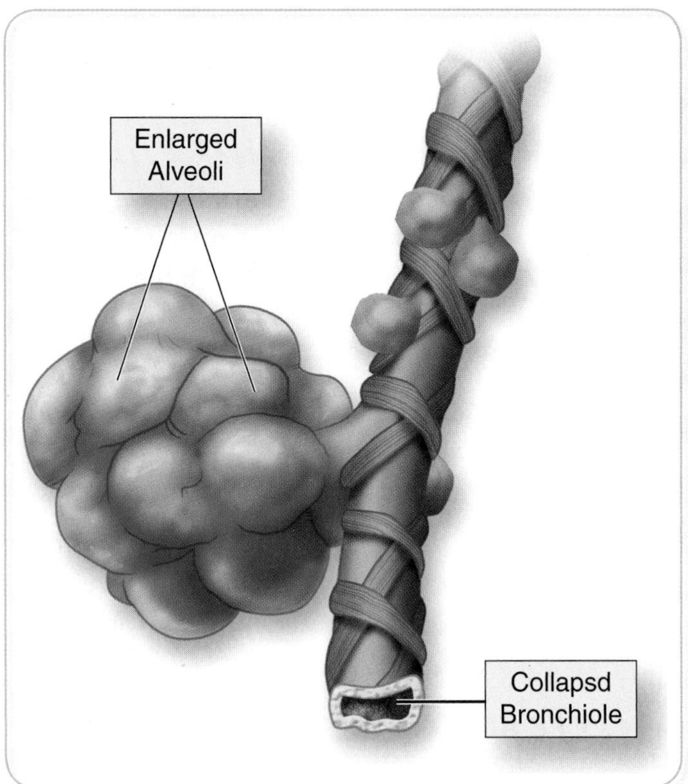

Figure 14-6 Alveoli and bronchioles affected by emphysema.

smoking is implicated in most cases of emphysema. However, a genetic factor contributes to the early development of the disease in non-smokers.

Avoidance of respiratory irritants and cessation of smoking may slow the progress of emphysema. Immunization against influenza and pneumonia is essential.

Chronic Bronchitis

Chronic bronchitis involves significant changes in the bronchi resulting from constant irritation from smoking or exposure to industrial pollution. The effects are irreversible and progressive.

Individuals with chronic bronchitis usually have a history of cigarette smoking or of living in an urban or industrial area, particularly in geographic locations where smog is common. In some cases, asthma is an associated condition.

Drugs for Smoking Cessation

Cigarettes contains chemical compounds that affect most of the organs of the human body. Cigarette smoking causes cancers of the mouth, pharynx, larynx, lungs, esophagus, pancreas, kidney, bladder, and cervix. It also may

TABLE 14-8 Drugs for the Stoppage of Smoking Tobacco

Generic Name	Trade Name	Route of Administration	Average Adult Dosage
bupropion hydrochloride	Zyban®	PO	75–100 mg t.i.d.
nicotine polacrilex	Nicorette Gum®	PO	2–4 mg q1–2 h p.r.n. (max: 24 pieces/day)
nicotine polacrilex	Nicotrol Inhaler®	Nasal	Inhalation: 4 mg p.r.n. (max: 64 mg/day)
nicotine polacrilex	Commit lozenge®	PO	4 mg q1–2 h p.r.n.
nicotine polacrilex	Nicotrol NS®	Nasal	1–2 sprays per nostril/h (max: 40 sprays per nostril/ day)
nicotine polacrilex	Nicotrol®, Nicoderm CQ®	Topical	7–21 mg/day (transdermal patch)

Key Concept

Cigarette smoking, along with the aging process, can reduce the strength of the immune system in elderly individuals, which is a predisposing factor for various conditions or infections.

cause leukemia and may increase the risk of heart disease, lung disease, or stroke. Cigarette smoking can cause the lungs to develop emphysema, chronic bronchitis, and bacterial pneumonia.

The benefits of smoking cessation include better health and a longer life. The most commonly used drugs for smoking cessation are listed in Table 14-8.

Bupropion is an antidepressant for which the dosage form for smoking cessation varies. For example, bupropion (Zyban) is used as a tablet. Habitrol, Nicoderm, Nicotrol, and Prostep are available as transdermal patches. Nicorette is used as a gum, and Nicotrol NS must be used as a spray. Zyban is the first non-nicotine drug for smoking cessation. It can be used alone or with the nicotine patch. Some nicotine inhalers may be used in combination with fluoxetine for smoking cessation. It is suspected that certain antidepressants such as fluoxetine, when added to nicotine replacement therapy (NRT), might improve abstinence rates. NRT products are intended to help patients stop smoking while dealing with withdrawal symptoms and cravings that result from ceasing the habit. NRT is thought to be useful and beneficial for tobacco users who want to quit their addiction. For most people, it is considered to be completely safe. According to the Cochrane review, former smokers using nicotine replacement therapy are 1.5 to 2 times more likely to stop smoking than patients who try to stop using any other methods.

Mechanism of Action

The neurochemical mechanism of the antidepressant effect of bupropion is not understood; it is chemically unrelated to other antidepressant agents. It is a weak blocker of neuronal uptake of serotonin and norepinephrine, and inhibits the reuptake of dopamine to some extent.

Indications

Bupropion is used for treatment of depression. It also aids in smoking cessation.

Adverse Effects

Adverse effects of nicotine, nicotine polacrilex, and nicotine transdermal systems include headache, dizziness, lightheadedness, insomnia, irritability, tachycardia, palpitations, hypertension, nausea, salivation, vomiting, cough, hiccups, and hoarseness.

Contraindications and Precautions

Products containing nicotine are contraindicated during pregnancy or lactation, in patients with known hypersensitivity, heart or blood vessel disease, high blood pressure, diabetes, overactive thyroid, skin rash or irritation, stomach ulcers, pheochromocytoma, dental problems, mouth sores, sore throat, jaw pain, or temporomandibular joint disorder. Precautions include the regular monitoring of the patient's health by his or her physician during use of smoking cessation drugs, and keeping these products away from children and pets because they can cause severe harm if ingested.

Drug Interactions

Bupropion may increase the risk of adverse effects with levodopa and toxicity with MAOIs. It also increases the risk of seizures with drugs that lower seizure threshold, including alcohol.

Summary

The exchange of oxygen and carbon dioxide in the lungs is one of the most important tasks of physiology, as it supplies oxygen at the cell level in body tissue. Oxygen is essential to sustain life. Therefore, the respiratory tract is necessary for the inspiration of oxygen and the expiration of carbon dioxide. Respiratory system disorders such as allergic asthma and chronic obstructive pulmonary disease (COPD) are common in the U.S. Antihistamines are used to relieve allergic reactions throughout the body, but they are also used commonly in patients with respiratory tract disorders to relieve rhinorrhea and allergic bronchitis. Cough-suppressing preparations are indicated for nonproductive coughs. If the cough is productive, suppression is not available, and an expectorant may be used to assist in expelling the secretions.

Bronchodilators induce smooth muscle relaxation, which eases breathing. They are used to treat asthma, COPD, and chronic bronchitis. Epinephrine and beta-2 agonists are indicated in acute asthma. Leukotriene agonists (new on the market), such as albuterol and mast cell stabilizer (cromolyn), are used for exercise-induced asthma. Glucocorticoids are administered by inhalation.

Exploring the Web

Visit ***http://familydoctor.org***

- Search for "decongestants." What information is available to further aid in your understanding of this type of drug?

Visit ***www.aafa.org***, ***www.nhlbi.nih.gov***, and ***www.lumgusa.com***

- Review information on the different types of asthma and allergies. Do a search for some of the other disorders covered in this chapter at the American Lung Association Web site. Bookmark these sites for future reference.

Review Questions

Multiple Choice

1. Which of the following substances may cause allergic rhinitis?

A. epinephrine
B. chlorpheniramine
C. hydrocodone
D. histamine

2. Adverse reactions to corticosteroid inhalation include:

A. cough, hoarseness, and headache
B. cough, diarrhea, and dyspepsia

C. pulmonary edema, convulsive disorders, and hypothyroidism
D. pulmonary edema, convulsive disorders, and hyperthyroidism

3. Which of the following drugs is an expectorant?
   A. ephedrine
   B. adrenaline
   C. acetylcysteine
   D. bupropion
4. The trade name for guaifenesin is:
   A. Tussionex
   B. Robitussin
   C. Benadryl
   D. Tessalon
5. Which of the following is indicated for cessation of smoking tobacco?
   A. bupropion
   B. diazepam
   C. salmeterol
   D. albuterol
6. Which of the following is the brand name of bupropion?
   A. Habitrol
   B. Zyban
   C. Nicotrol
   D. Prostep
7. Dextromethorphan is classified as:
   A. an opioid cough suppressant
   B. a xanthine derivative
   C. a non-steroid contraceptive
   D. a nonopioid cough suppressant
8. Another name for allergic rhinitis is:
   A. contact dermatitis
   B. hay fever
   C. yellow fever
   D. photosensitivity
9. Which of the following is/are considered to be the drug(s) of choice for chronic asthma?
   A. theophylline
   B. albuterol
   C. antihistamines
   D. glucocorticoids
10. The initial stimulus for cough probably arises from which of the following parts of the respiratory system?
    A. bronchial mucosa
    B. pharynx
    C. mouth
    D. nasal cavities

11. The trade name of fluticasone includes which of the following?
    A. Flonase
    B. Pulmicort
    C. Singulair
    D. Tilade

12. Which of the following agents is known as an opioid?
    A. guaifenesin
    B. hydrocodone
    C. albuterol
    D. aminophylline

13. Leukotrienes are part of a class of biologically active compounds that occur naturally in which of the following body cells?
    A. white blood cells
    B. red blood cells
    C. platelets
    D. mast cells

14. Which of the following agents would increase bronchial secretions?
    A. theophylline
    B. cromolyn
    C. hydrocodone
    D. acetylcysteine

Fill in the Blank

1. Cromolyn is one of the mast cell stabilizers and the drug of choice as a prophylactic for moderate ______________, especially in ______________.

2. The leukotriene modifiers are used for prophylaxis and chronic asthma in ______________.

3. Xanthine derivatives are indicated for treatment of:
   a. ______________
   b. ______________
   c. ______________

4. Zileuton is one of the leukotriene modifiers that may cause ______________.

5. Anaphylactic shock causes a massive release of ______________.

Matching

Generic Name	Trade Name
____ 1. terbutaline	A. Serevent
____ 2. pirbuterol	B. AsthmaHaler
____ 3. ephedrine bitartrate	C. Proventil
____ 4. albuterol	D. Maxair
____ 5. salmeterol	E. Brethaire

Critical Thinking

A 75-year-old man went to the emergency room for shortness of breath, coughing, sputum production, and fever. The E.R. physician ordered a chest x-ray and blood tests. The patient had a history of cigarette smoking for 30 years. After the various tests, the physician diagnosed this patient with emphysema and pneumonia.

1. Name the major predisposing factors for emphysema and pneumonia at this patient's age.
2. With this patient's history of cigarette smoking, what other complications may this patient have?
3. If the patient was advised to stop smoking, name the available drugs that help a person to stop smoking.

Drug Therapy for Gastrointestinal Disorders

CHAPTER 15

OUTLINE

(*continues*)

OBJECTIVES

After completing this chapter, the reader should be able to:

1. Explain the mechanisms of action and therapeutic effects of antacids.
2. Identify the major classes of drugs used to treat peptic ulcers.
3. Describe the use of H_2-receptor antagonists in the treatment of peptic ulcers.
4. Define proton pump inhibitor agents and their indications.
5. Explain the treatment for the bacterium *Helicobacter pylori*.
6. Identify the common adverse effects of major laxative, antidiarrheal, and antiemetic drugs.
7. Name the five major classifications of laxatives.
8. Identify the most effective antidiarrheal agents.
9. Explain adsorbent agents and their indications.
10. Describe the mechanism of action of bulk-forming agents.

GLOSSARY

Adsorbent agents – drugs with the ability to adsorb gases, toxins, and bacteria

Antacids – neutralize hydrochloric acid and raise gastric pH, thus inhibiting pepsin (a gastric enzyme)

Antiemetic – a drug that stops vomiting

Bulk-forming laxatives – natural or synthetic polysaccharide derivatives that absorb water to soften the stool and increase bulk to stimulate peristalsis

Calcium carbonate – a substance that causes acid rebound, which may delay ulcer-related pain relief and ulcer healing

Chemical digestion – the alteration of food into different forms through chemicals and enzymes

Emetic – a drug that induces vomiting

Emollient laxatives – substances that act as surfactants by allowing absorption of water into the stool

OUTLINE (continued)

Helicobacter pylori – a bacterial species that is associated with several gastroduodenal diseases

Histamine H_2-receptor antagonists – drugs that block the action of histamine on parietal cells in the stomach, decreasing acid production

Lubricant laxative – a substance, such as mineral oil, that works by increasing water retention in the stool to soften it

Mechanical digestion – the breakdown of large food particles into smaller pieces by physical means

Peptic ulcer – a lesion located in either the stomach (gastric ulcer) or in the duodenum (small intestine)

Saline laxatives – substances that create an osmotic effect to increase water content and stool volume

Stimulant laxatives – substances that stimulate bowel mobility and increase secretion of fluids in the bowel

Stool softeners – substances that decrease the consistency of stool by reducing surface tension

Zollinger-Ellison syndrome – peptic ulceration with gastric hypersecretion and tumor of the pancreatic islets

OVERVIEW

The digestive system, sometimes called the gastrointestinal tract, alimentary tract, or gut, consists of a long hollow tubule. The digestive tract secretes substances used in the process of digestion into the canal. The growth of the body depends upon the consumption, absorption, and metabolism of food. This system also involves the elimination of waste. The digestive system is subject to many disorders, some of which are very common. Numerous drugs are used to treat these varying conditions.

ANATOMY REVIEW

- The digestive system consists of the mouth, pharynx, esophagus, stomach, small intestine, large intestine, rectum, and anus (Figures 15-1 and 15-2).
- There are several accessory organs of the digestive system these include the salivary glands, liver, gallbladder, and pancreas (Figure 15-1).
- The role of the digestive tract is to change food into forms the body can use and to eliminate waste.
- There are two forms of digestion: **Mechanical digestion** breaks large food particles into smaller pieces such as by chewing. **Chemical digestion** is the alteration of the smaller food particles by substances such as digestive enzymes, bile, and acids.
- Nutrients from the digestive tract are absorbed into the blood stream by moving across the lining of the digestive tract.

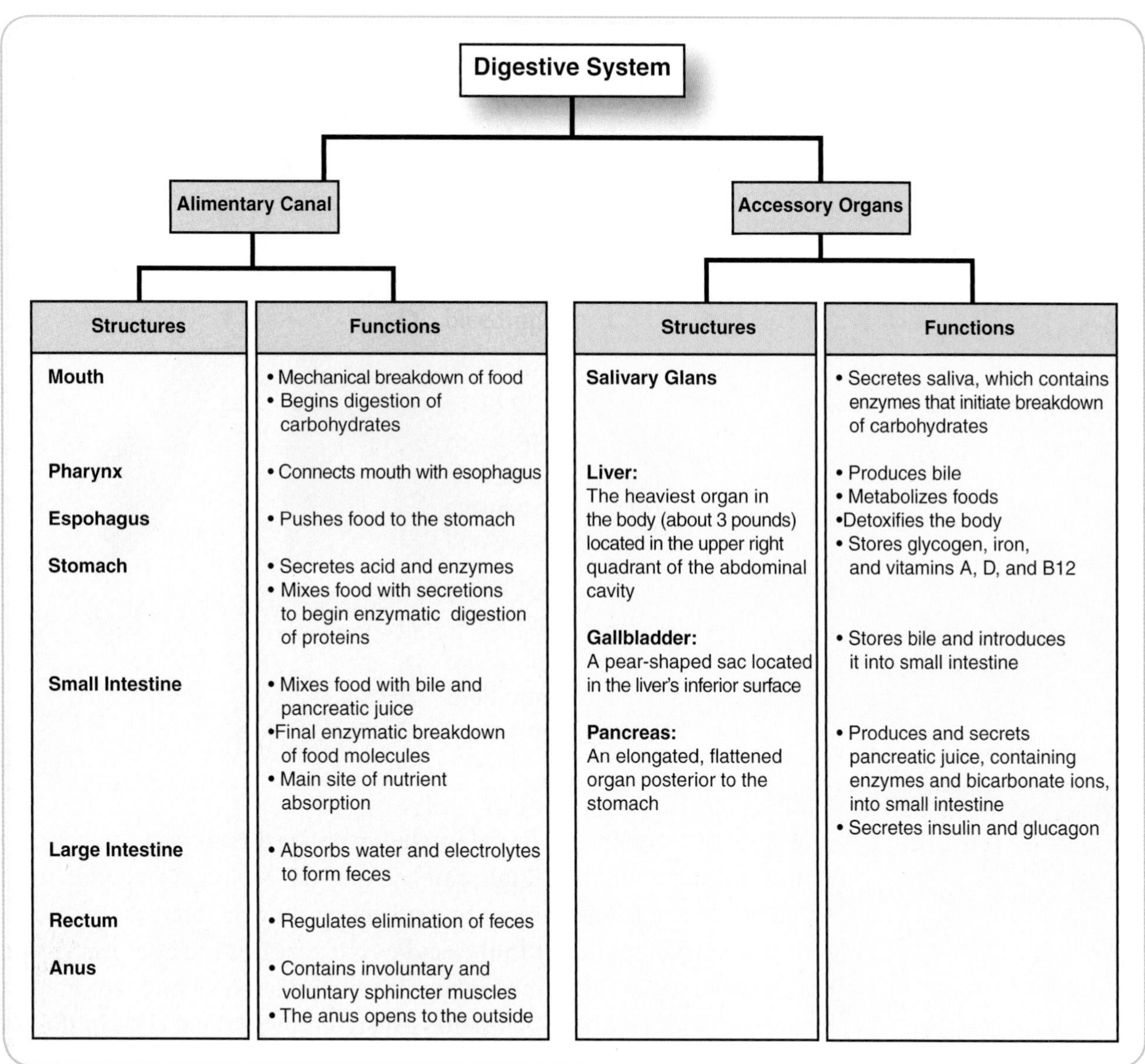

Figure 15-1 The digestive system.

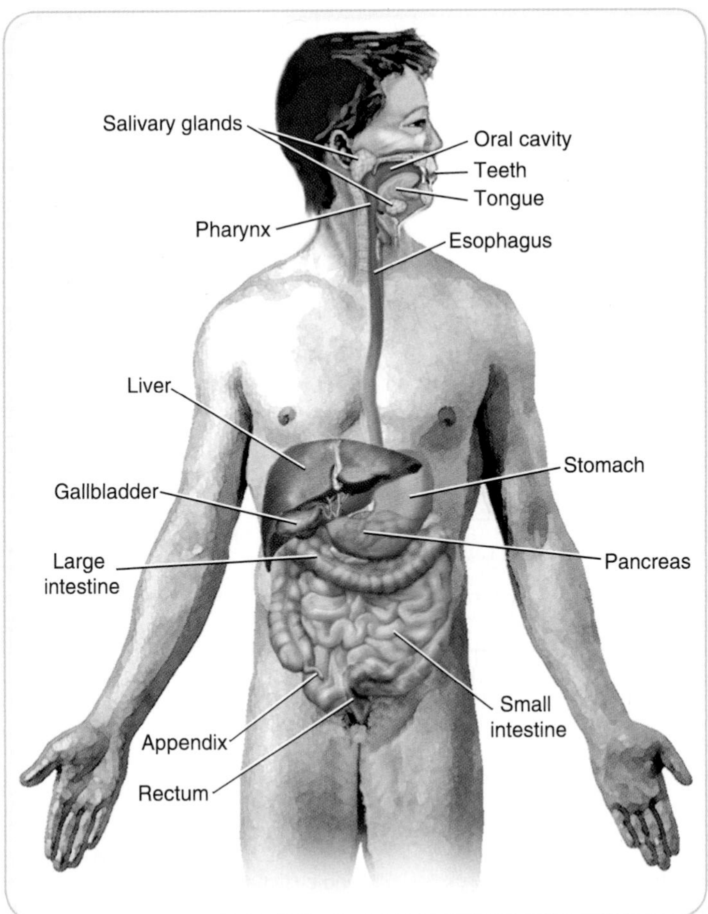

Figure 15-2 Structures of the digestive system.

Acid Peptic Diseases

Peptic ulcer refers to a lesion located in either the stomach (gastric ulcer) or in the duodenum (small intestine) (Figure 15-3). In general, ulcers occur whenever there is an increase in acid secretion or a decrease in mucosal resistance. Mucosal injury in the acid peptic diseases includes gastric ulcer, duodenal ulcer, and gastroesophageal reflux disease, which are mediated by gastric acid. Hydrochloric acid is secreted by parietal cells in the body of the stomach. It is regulated by adjacent endocrines, such as gastrin, or by histamine, somatostatin, and prostaglandin E_2. Gastrin is a relatively weak stimulant of the parietal cells. It acts primarily to cause the release of histamine, which is the most potent stimulus of acid secretion, and acts as the common mediator. Histamine antagonists inhibit acid secretion that is stimulated by gastrin and acetylcholine, as well as histamine. There are a number of causes of peptic ulcer, including:

- Family history
- Smoking tobacco
- Alcohol

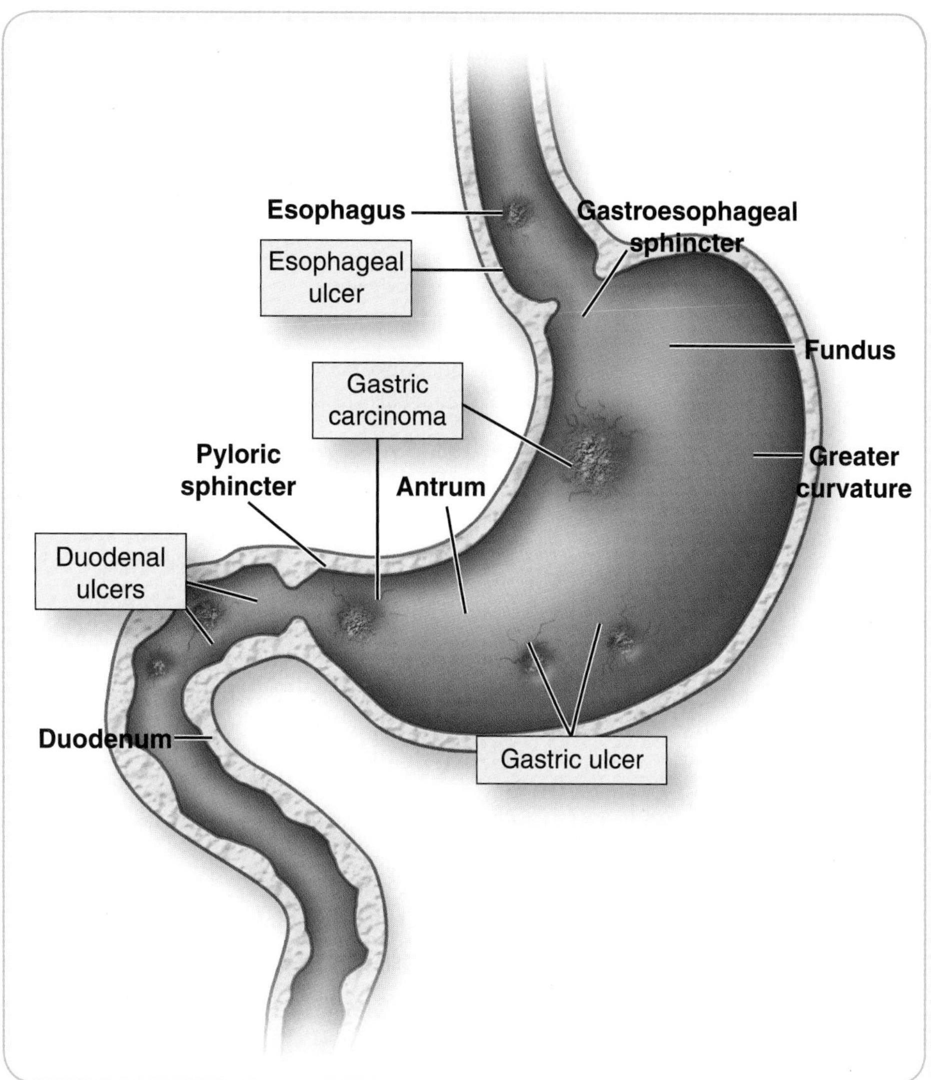

Figure 15-3 Sites of peptic ulcers.

- Coffee
- Stress
- Infection with *Helicobacter pylori* (H. pylori)
- Blood group O
- Anti-inflammatory drugs (aspirin, NSAIDs, and glucocorticoids)

A wide variety of prescription and OTC medications are available for the treatment of peptic ulcer. These drugs include: antacids, H_2-receptor antagonists, proton pump inhibitors, and antibiotics. Antibiotics treat peptic ulcers caused by *Helicobacter pylori.*

Antacids

There are differences in the types of **antacids**, in terms of their contents, neutralizing capacity, duration of action, side effects, and cost. These must be considered when choosing an antacid for therapeutic use. Antacids are

TABLE 15-1 Common Antacids

Generic Name	Trade Name	Route of Administration	Average Adult Dosage
aluminum hydroxide	Amphojel®	PO	600 mg t.i.d.-q.i.d.
calcium carbonate	Tums®	PO	0.5–2 g b.i.d.-t.i.d.
calcium carbonate with magnesium hydroxide	Mylanta Gel-caps®, Rolaids®	PO	2–4 capsules or tablets p.r.n.
magnesium hydroxide and aluminum hydroxide	Maalox®, Mylanta	PO	5–15 mL liquid or 2–4 tablets
magaldrate	Riopan®	PO	480–1080 mg (5–10 mL) or 1–2 tablets daily
sodium bicarbonate (baking soda); aspirin, and citric acid	Alka Seltzer®	PO	300 mg–2 g/day

OTC drugs. The most common antacids are shown in Table 15-1. The most widely used antacids are sodium bicarbonate, **calcium carbonate**, aluminum hydroxide, and magnesium hydroxide.

Mechanism of Action

Antacids neutralize hydrochloric acid and raise gastric pH, thus inhibiting pepsin (a gastric enzyme). Antacids reduce the concentration and total load of acid in the gastric contents. By increasing gastric pH, antacids also inhibit pepsin activity. In addition, they strengthen the gastric mucosal barrier.

Indications

These agents are used widely for the relief of heartburn, dyspepsia, and medical treatment of peptic ulcer. The primary role of antacids in the management of acid-peptic disorders is the relief of pain. Nonsystemic antacids (magnesium or aluminum substances) are preferred to systemic antacids such as sodium bicarbonate for intensive ulcer therapy because they avoid the risk of alkalosis. Liquid antacid forms have a greater buffering capacity than tablets. However, tablets are more convenient to carry. Antacid mixtures such as aluminum hydroxide with magnesium hydroxide provide more even, sustained action than single-agent antacids, and permit a lower dosage of each compound.

Medical Terminology Review

hypophosphatemia
hypo = under, below, less than normal
phosphat = phosphate
emia = blood condition
having lower than normal phosphate levels in the blood

osteomalacia
osteo = bone
malacia = softening
softening of the bone

hypercalcemia
hyper = over, above, more than normal
calc = calcium
emia = blood condition
having excess amounts of calcium in the blood

Adverse Effects

Constipation can occur in patients using calcium carbonate and aluminum-containing antacids. Diarrhea is a common adverse effect of magnesium- and sodium-containing antacids. If diarrhea occurs, the patient may alternate the antacid mixture with aluminum hydroxide. Hypophosphatemia and osteomalacia can occur with long-term use of aluminum hydroxide, but these conditions can also occur with short-term use in severely malnourished patients, such as alcoholics. Calcium carbonate usually is avoided because it causes acid rebound, hypercalcemia, vomiting, metabolic alkalosis, confusion, and renal calculi. It may also delay pain relief and ulcer healing.

Contraindications and Precautions

Antacids are contraindicated in patients with severe abdominal pain of unknown cause, and during lactation. Sodium bicarbonate is contraindicated in patients with hypertension, congestive heart failure (CHF), severe renal disease, and edema. It should not be used for ulcer therapy. All antacids should be used cautiously in elderly patients and renally impaired patients. Chronic administration of calcium carbonate-containing antacids should be avoided because of hypercalcemia. Calcium carbonate and magnesium-containing antacids should be used cautiously in patients with severe renal disease.

Drug Interactions

Because antacids alter gastric pH and affect absorption of ingested substances, they have a high potential for drug interactions. To ensure consistent absorption and therapeutic efficacy, orally administered drugs should be given 30 to 60 minutes before antacids. These agents bind with tetracycline and inhibit its absorption, reducing its therapeutic efficacy. Antacids may destroy the coating of enteric-coated drugs, leading to premature drug dissolution in the stomach. Antacids may interfere with the absorption of many drugs, including cimetidine, ranitidine, digoxin, isoniazid, iron products, anticholinergics, and phenothiazines.

Histamine H_2-Receptor Antagonists

There are two types of histamine receptors: histamine (H_1) and histamine (H_2). The second of these mediates the acid secretion from gastric parietal cells and is inhibited by the H_2-receptor-blocking drugs. These drugs may be preferred to other antiulcer agents because of their convenience and lack of effect on GI motility. H_2-receptor antagonists are listed in Table 15-2.

Mechanism of Action

Cimetidine was the first H_2-receptor antagonist approved for clinical use. It blocks the H_2 receptor on the parietal cells of the stomach, thus decreasing gastric acid secretion.

Indications

H_2-receptor antagonists are used to promote healing of gastric and duodenal ulcers, and hypersecretory states such as **Zollinger-Ellison syndrome**. Prototypes of H_2-receptor antagonists include cimetidine, famotidine, nizatidine, and ranitidine. They are a remarkably safe group of drugs.

TABLE 15-2 H_2-receptor Antagonists

Generic Name	Trade Name	Route of Administration	Average Adult Dosage
cimetidine	Tagamet®	PO	300–400 mg 1 to 2 times per day
famotidine	Pepcid®, Pepcid AC®	PO	40 mg at bedtime
nizatidine	Axid®, Axid AR®	PO	150 mg b.i.d. or 300 mg h.s.
ranitidine hydrochloride	Zantac®	PO, IV	PO: 100–150 mg b.i.d. or 300 mg at bedtime; IV: 50 mg q6–8 h; 150–300 mg/24 h by continuous infusion

Cimetidine is available OTC for the treatment of acute gastric ulcer, duodenal ulcer, and gastroesophageal reflux. It is also used in the treatment of Zollinger-Ellison syndrome.

Famotidine is the most potent H_2-receptor antagonist. After a 40-mg dose, mean nocturnal gastric acid secretion is reduced by 94 percent for up to 10 hours. It is recommended for the short-term treatment of mucosal ulcers of the GI tract. Famotidine is absorbed incompletely. It should be used in a lower dosage and at longer dosing intervals in patients with severe renal insufficiency.

The newest H_2-receptor antagonist, nizatidine, may be used to treat and prevent recurrence of duodenal ulcers. It is also used for gastric ulcers, and gastroesophageal reflux. More than 90 percent of an oral dose is excreted in the urine within 12 hours, and 60 percent as unchanged drug. Therefore, it should be used in reduced dosage in patients with severe renal insufficiency.

Ranitidine is a more potent drug. It is five to ten times more potent than cimetidine. Ranitidine requires a less frequent dosing schedule than cimetidine. It is an H_2-receptor antagonist indicated for the short-term treatment of duodenal ulcers and the management of hypersecretory conditions such as Zollinger-Ellison syndrome. The pharmacokinetic profile of ranitidine is similar to that of cimetidine.

Adverse Effects

The list of adverse reactions is long, but the incidence is low. Among the adverse effects associated with all four drugs are headache, dizziness, malaise, myalgia, nausea, diarrhea, constipation, rashes, pruritus, and impotence. Adverse effects, such as unusual bleeding, fever, sore throat, hallucinations, or skin rash should be reported promptly, and the therapy must be discontinued.

Contraindications and Precautions

Histamine H_2 antagonists should be avoided in patients with a known hypersensitivity, and during lactation or pregnancy. These agents are used cautiously in patients with hepatic or renal dysfunction. Cimetidine is used with caution in patients with diabetes mellitus. Histamine H_2 antagonists are used cautiously in elderly patients because they may cause confusion, and a dosage reduction may be needed. Cimetidine, famotidine, and ranitidine are pregnancy category B drugs, while nizatidine is a pregnancy category C drug. All of these drugs should be used cautiously during pregnancy and lactation.

Drug Interactions

Cimetidine increases the risk of decreased white blood cell counts with antimetabolites and alkylating agents. It also increases serum levels and risk of toxicity of warfarin-type anticoagulants, phenytoin, beta-adrenergic blocking agents, alcohol, quinidine, lidocaine, theophylline, chloroquine, and diazepam.

Nizatidine increases serum salicylate levels with aspirin. Ranitidine also increases the effects of warfarin and toxicity of lidocaine. Ranitidine decreases the effectiveness of diazepam and its clearance.

Proton Pump Inhibitors

The final common pathway in gastric acid secretion is the proton pump adenosine triphosphatase. The physiological essence of this enzyme is the exchange of hydrogen ions for potassium ions. Thus, hydrogen is secreted by the parietal cell into the gastric lumen in exchange for potassium. Proton pump inhibitors should be taken prior to meals, because these drugs are more potent when taken orally prior to meals. They are also absorbed more effectively in the morning.

Mechanism of Action

Proton pump inhibitors or gastric pump inhibitors inhibit H^+ and K^+ ions, which generate gastric acids.

Indications

Proton pump inhibitors are widely used in the short-term therapy of duodenal and gastric ulcers. Proton pump inhibitor agents are also used in the treatment of gastroesophageal reflux disease, gastric ulcer, and for long-term treatment of pathologic hypersecretory conditions such as Zollinger-Ellison syndrome. Examples of proton pump inhibitors are shown in Table 15-3.

Key Concept

Goals of drug therapy for peptic ulcer include the relief of symptoms, promotion of ulcer healing, and prevention of reoccurrences.

Omeprazole is used in the treatment of acid peptic disorders. It is approved for the short-term treatment of duodenal ulcers, severe gastroesophageal reflux, and hypersecretory conditions. It is also effective in the prevention of NSAID ulcers and their complications. The antisecretory effect of omeprazole occurs within one hour, with maximum effect occurring within two hours.

Lansoprazole suppresses gastric acid formation in the stomach. Lansoprazole is indicated for the short-term treatment of acute duodenal ulcer, gastric ulcer, and erosive esophagitis. It is most effective given 30 to 60 minutes prior to a meal. Like other proton pump inhibitors, it is very effective in healing acid peptic disease.

TABLE 15-3 Proton Pump Inhibitors

Generic Name	Trade Name	Route of Administration	Average Adult Dosage
esomeprazole magnesium	Nexium®	PO	20–40 mg/day
lansoprazole	Prevacid®	PO	15–60 mg/day for 4 weeks
omeprazole	Prilosec®	PO	20 mg once per day for 4–8 weeks
pantoprazole sodium	Protonix®	PO	40 mg/day
rabeprazole sodium	AcipHex®	PO	20 mg/day for 4 weeks

Adverse Effects

There are numerous adverse effects of the proton pump inhibitors, but they occur infrequently. Headache, diarrhea, abdominal pain, dizziness, rash, and constipation are seen with nearly the same frequency as is seen with the H_2-blockers.

Adverse reactions to omeprazole include headache, diarrhea, abdominal pain, nausea, dizziness, vomiting, and constipation. It is contraindicated for long-term use in patients with gastroesophageal reflux disease, duodenal ulcers, and in lactating women.

Adverse effects of lansoprazole are fatigue, dizziness, headache, nausea, diarrhea, constipation, anorexia, or increased appetite.

Contraindications and Precautions

Proton pump inhibitors are contraindicated in long-term use for gastroesophageal reflux disease (GERD) and duodenal ulcers. They are also contraindicated in patients with hypersensitivity to these agents and children younger than two years, and during pregnancy (categories B and C). Lansoprazole should be avoided in patients with severe hepatic impairment.

Key Concept

Gastroesophageal reflux disease (GERD) involves the periodic flow of gastric contents into the esophagus.

Proton pump inhibitors are used with caution in patients with dysphasia, metabolic or respiratory alkalosis, and hepatic disease, and during pregnancy. Safety and efficacy in children under the age of 18 years are not established.

Drug Interactions

Omeprazole increases serum levels and potentially increases the toxicity of benzodiazepines, phenytoin, and warfarin. This agent shows decreased absorption with sucralfate (these drugs should be given at least 30 minutes apart).

Lansoprazole decreases serum levels if taken concurrently with sucralfate. It decreases serum levels of ketoconazole and theophylline.

Rabeprazole increases serum levels and potentially increases the toxicity of benzodiazepines when taken concurrently.

Treatment for *Helicobacter pylori* with Ulcer

Peptic ulcer disease is believed to be caused by high gastric secretion. *Helicobacter pylori* is found in 75 percent of duodenal ulcers. In chronic peptic ulcer, it has been found that eradication of the bacterium prevents ulcer relapse in about 95 percent of the cases. There is also a relationship between *Helicobacter* infection and adenocarcinoma of the stomach. Treatments for peptic ulcer patients usually include antacids, H_2-receptor antagonists, or proton pump inhibitors, but other drugs are added as necessary. For the eradication of *H. pylori* and healing of duodenal and gastric ulcers in drug therapy, special antibiotics must be added. These antibiotics include amoxicillin (Amoxil), clarithromycin (Biaxin), tetracycline (Achromycin), and metronidazole (Flagyl). Bismuth products must also be added, such as bismuth subsalicylate (Pepto-Bismol) and ranitidine bismuth citrate. Bismuth compounds are highly effective when combined with proton pump inhibitors and/or antibiotics. Eradication rates with these combinations are greater than 80 percent. Adverse effects of bismuth products include neurotoxicity, dark stools and tongue, headache, diarrhea, and abdominal pain. For the treatment of *Helicobacter pylori* with ulcer, antisecretory agents (proton pump inhibitors) should be included. Therefore, combination drugs for *H. pylori* infections should be used as follows:

Helidac (bismuth, metronidazole, tetracycline)

Prevpac (amoxicillin, clarithromycin, lansoprazole)

Tritec (bismuth, ranitidine)

Key Concept

Peptic ulcers are most commonly caused by the use of NSAIDs or are due to a Helicobacter pylori infection.

The goals of treatment of active *H. pylori*–associated ulcers are to relieve dyspeptic symptoms, to promote ulcer healing, and to eradicate *H. pylori* infection.

Pancreatic Disorders

The pancreas plays an extremely important role in digestion and secretes digestive enzymes. The main pancreatic enzymes include lipase, amylase, chymotrypin, and trypsin. These enzymes aid in the digestion of fats, carbohydrates, and proteins. Fat digestion is compromised if pancreatic enzyme secretions are insufficient. The most common cause of pancreatic insufficiency is chronic pancreatitis.

Pancreatic Enzyme Replacement Therapy

Pancreatic enzyme replacements include pancreatin and pancrelipase (see Table 15-4). These agents may be obtained from beef or pork pancreas, which

TABLE 15-4 Pancreatic Enzyme Replacements

Generic Name	Trade Name	Route of Administration	Average Adult Dosage
pancreatin	Entozyme®	PO	1–3 capsules w/each meal, and 1 capsule w/each snack as directed by physician; may be swallowed whole w/ or without fluid, or contents may be sprinkled into food or drink
pancrelipase	Cotazym®, Pancrease®, Viokase®	PO	1–3 capsules or tablets, or 1–2 packets of powder 1–2 h before, during, or 1 h after meals, w/ an extra dose taken w/ any food eaten between meals

contains the necessary enzymes to digest fats, proteins, and carbohydrates. Pancrelipase is preferred because it has more enzyme activity.

Mechanism of Action

Pancreatic enzyme replacement therapy works similarly to the way pancreatin and pancrelipase work normally in the body. These enzymes hydrolyze triglycerides to fatty acids and glycerol, proteins to oligopeptides, and starches to oligosaccharides and maltose.

Indications

Pancrelipase is used as replacement therapy in the symptomatic treatment of malabsorption syndrome due to cystic fibrosis, chronic pancreatitis, pancreatectomy, GI bypass surgery, and cancer of the pancreas.

Adverse Effects

In the recommended dosage, pancrelipase is free of adverse effects. Serious adverse effects of replacement therapy of pancreatic enzymes are rare. Common adverse effects include nausea, vomiting, anorexia, diarrhea, cramping, and hyperuricemia.

Contraindications and Precautions

Pancreatic enzyme replacement therapy is contraindicated in patients with a known history of allergy to hog protein or enzymes. These agents should be avoided in patients suffering from esophageal strictures, in those with pancreatitis, and during pregnancy (category C). Pancreatic enzyme replacement therapy should be used in lactating women with caution.

Drug Interactions

Pancreatic enzyme replacement therapy may decrease the absorption of iron.

Gallstone-solubilizing Agents

The gallbladder is a hollow organ located next to the liver that acts as the storage place for bile. Bile is formed in the liver to aid in digestion. The bile is then stored in the gallbladder to be released into the intestines as food passes.

A gallstone is a solid mass that forms in the gallbladder or the bile duct (Figure 15-4). Gallstones are usually formed by the combination of cholesterol and calcium compounds. They can produce intense pain when they block the bile duct. Gallstone-solubilizing agents include ursodiol and chenodiol. Only ursodiol is sold in the U.S.

Mechanism of Action

Ursodiol is a naturally occurring bile acid that is made by the liver and secreted in bile. It blocks the liver enzyme that produces cholesterol, and thereby decreases production of cholesterol by the liver and the amount of cholesterol in bile. It also reduces the absorption of cholesterol from the intestine. By decreasing the concentration of cholesterol in bile, it prevents the formation and promotes the dissolution of cholesterol-containing gallstones.

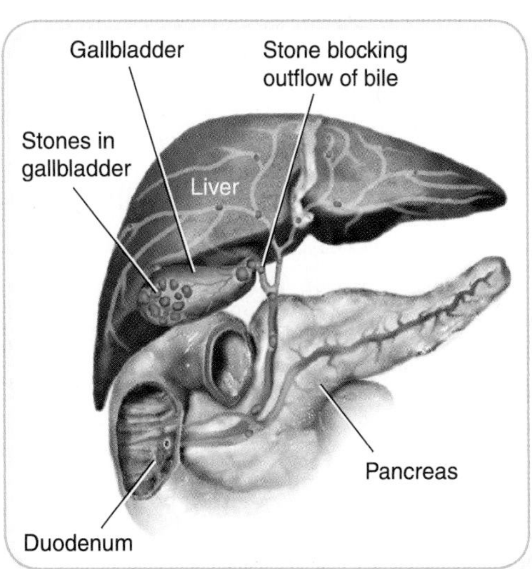

Figure 15-4 Gallstones.

Indications

Ursodiol is used to prevent cholesterol gallstones from forming during rapid loss of weight. It is also used to dissolve cholesterol gallstones that do not contain calcium and are less than 2 cm in diameter. It is also used to treat primary biliary cirrhosis.

Adverse Effects

The most common adverse effects are rash, itching, nausea, vomiting, stomach pain, back pain, constipation, and diarrhea.

Contraindications and Precautions

Contraindications include hypersensitivity to ursodiol, bile acids, or any component of the formulation, high cholesterol, radiopaque substances, bile pigment stones, stones greater than 20 mm in diameter, and allergy to bile acids.

Gallstone-solubilizing agents should be used with caution in patients with a non-visualizing gallbladder and those with chronic liver disease. Ursodiol is not recommended for use in children.

Drug Interactions

Aluminum-containing antacids, cholestyramine, and colestipol reduce the absorption of ursodiol and therefore reduce its action.

DIARRHEA

Diarrhea is the manifestation of many illnesses. Its etiology includes infections (bacterial, viral, fungal, and parasitic), irritable bowel syndrome, inflammatory bowel disease (ulcerative colitis and Crohn's disease), toxins (food poisoning), drugs, and other causes. Treatment should be directed to the underlying cause.

Antidiarrheals

It is occasionally necessary to use antidiarrheals for convenience, or for conditions for which there is no primary treatment. The most commonly used antidiarrheals are anticholinergics, opioid narcotics, meperidine congeners (diphenoxylate), and loperamide. Opioid antidiarrheals are the most effective drugs for controlling diarrhea. Selected agents used to treat diarrhea are shown in Table 15-5.

Mechanism of Action

The mechanism of action for anticholinergics and opioid narcotics is discussed in Chapters 6 and 21.

TABLE 15-5 Drugs Used to Treat Diarrhea

Generic Name	Trade Name	Route of Administration	Average Adult Dosage
bismuth subsalicylate	Pepto-Bismol®	PO	2 tablets q.i.d. with 2 additional antibiotics for 10–14 days
camphorated opium tincture (schedule iii)	Paregoric®	PO	5–10 mL after loose stool, q2 h up to q.i.d. prn
difenoxin with atropine	Motofen®	PO	1–8 mg/day
diphenoxylate with atropine	Lomotil®	PO	1–2 tablets or 5–10 mL t.i.d.-q.i.d.
loperamide	Imodium®	PO	4 mg as a single dose, then 2 mg after each diarrhea episode

Indications

Antidiarrheal agents are used to treat diarrhea, a symptom of bowel disorders, and not the disorder itself. The management of diarrhea depends on finding the underlying cause, replacing water and electrolytes as needed, reducing cramping, and reducing the passage of stools. Diarrhea is usually self-limiting and resolves without further effects. Diarrhea in children may become a medical emergency in as little as 24 hours because of the loss of electrolytes.

Adverse Effects

Adverse effects of antidiarrheal drugs commonly include nausea, vomiting, anorexia, constipation, drowsiness, sedation, euphoria, headache, dizziness, drowsiness, and rash. Diphenoxylate is a narcotic-related agent that has no analgesic activity, but causes sedation and euphoria. Generally, this drug is combined with atropine (an anticholinergic drug), which may produce dry mouth.

Contraindications and Precautions

Antidiarrheal drugs are contraindicated in patients with pseudomembranous colitis, abdominal pain of unknown origin, or obstructive jaundice. These agents should be avoided in children younger than two years.

Antidiarrheals are used with caution in patients with severe liver impairment or inflammatory bowel disease. They should be used cautiously in pregnant women (category B).

Drug Interactions

Concurrent use of antidiarrheals with an MAOI increases the risk of a hypertensive crisis. Antidiarrheals may cause an additive CNS depression when given with antihistamines, sedatives, hypnotics, alcohol, and narcotics.

Gas Retention

The production of excessive gas necessitates relief of gastric and intestinal distention. Gas retention is caused by air swallowing, peptic ulcer, dyspepsia, irritable bowel disease, and diverticulitis. Other factors for production of gas in the GI tract include gas-forming foods such as beans, onions, and cabbage, or after gastroscopy, and bowel radiography.

Antiflatulents

Medications for excessive gas, or to prevent formation of gas in the GI tract, include some antacids or carminatives (substances which stimulate the expulsion of gas from the GI tract, and also increase muscle tone, thereby stimulating peristalsis), that are available as OTC drugs. Simethicone is the most common active ingredient used, in such trade names as Phazyme, Mylanta, and Gas-X. Simethicone disperses in the GI tract, and prevents the formation of gas pockets in the GI tract.

Mechanism of Action

The actual mechanism of action for antiflatulents is unknown, but the predominant theory is that these agents reduce the surface tension of small air bubbles trapped in the GI tract. This allows them to coalesce into larger bubbles, which are more easily eliminated than the smaller ones.

Indications

Antiflatulents are used to prevent the formation of gas in the GI tract. Gas retention is a problem in conditions of air swallowing, diverticulitis (inflammation of the colon), peptic ulcer, irritable bowel disease, and dyspepsia. Another use of antiflatulents is to relieve gas following gastroscopy and bowel radiography.

Adverse Effects

Antiflatulents are generally safe and have no side effects.

Contraindications and Precautions

Antiflatulents are contraindicated in patients with a known hypersensitivity to any component of these drugs. Charcoal should be used in pregnant women with caution (category C).

Drug Interactions

There are no reported drug interactions with antiflatulents.

CONSTIPATION

Constipation is the difficult or infrequent passage of stool. Normal stool frequency ranges from two to three times daily to two to three times per week. Since constipation is a symptom rather than a disease, medical evaluation should be undertaken in patients who develop constipation.

Laxatives

Laxatives are drugs that either accelerate fecal passage or decrease fecal consistency. They work by promoting one or more of the mechanisms that cause diarrhea. Because of the wide availability and marketing of OTC laxatives, there is a potential that an appropriate diagnosis will not be sought. Table 15-6 shows the most commonly used laxatives.

TABLE 15-6 Commonly Used Laxatives

Generic Name	Trade Name	Route of Administration	Average Adult Dosage
Bulk Forming:			
methylcellulose	Citrucel®	PO	500–6000 mg/day
polycarbophil	Equalactin®, FiberNorm®	PO	1 g q.i.d. prn (max: 6 g/day)
psyllium hydrophilic muciloid	Metamucil®, Perdiem Plain®	PO	1–2 tsp in 8 oz water up to q.i.d.
Fecal Softeners:			
docusate sodium	Colace®, Dialose®, Modane®, Regutol®, Surfak®	PO	50–500 mg/day
Salines and Osmotics:			
glycerin	Fleet Babylax®, Glycerol®	Rectal	1 suppository or 5–15 mL enema (inserted high into rectum and retained for 15 min)
lactulose	Cephulac®	PO	30–60 mL/day prn
magnesium citrate	Citrate of Magnesia®	PO	1000–6000 mg/day
magnesium hydroxide	Phillips' Milk of Magnesia®	PO	15 mL h.s.

(continues)

TABLE 15-6 Commonly Used Laxatives—*continued*

Generic Name	Trade Name	Route of Administration	Average Adult Dosage
Hydroxidemagnesium:			
magnesium sodium phosphate	Fleet Enema®	Rectal	133 mL/day
sorbitol	Sorbitol®	PO, Rectal	30–150 mL/day
Stimulants:			
bisacodyl	Dulcolax®	PO, Rectal	PO: 5–15 mg prn; Rectal: 1 suppository
castor oil	Emulsoil®, Purge®	PO	15–60 mL/day p.r.n.
cascara sagrada	Cascara Sagrada® (fluid extract)	PO	0.5–1.5 mL/day
Lubricants:			
mineral oil	Kondremul®	PO	2–15 teaspoonfuls/day
Stool Softeners:			
docusate calcium	Surfak®	PO, Rectal	50–500 mg/day; Rectal: 50–100 mg added to enema fluid
docusate potassium	Dialose®	PO, Rectal	PO: 1–3 caps/day; Rectal: 1 suppository
docusate sodium	Colace®	PO, Rectal	1–4 tabs or capsules/day

Mechanism of Action

Laxatives are divided into several categories as a function of their mechanisms of action, including: bulk-forming, saline, stimulant, emollient, and lubricant laxatives. Laxatives should not be taken if nausea, vomiting, or abdominal pain is present.

Key Concept

All bulk-forming agents must be given with at least eight ounces of water to minimize the possible constipation experienced by some patients.

Bulk-forming laxatives are natural or synthetic polysaccharide derivatives that absorb water to soften the stool and increase bulk, which stimulates peristalsis. Bulk-forming laxatives work in both the small and large intestines. The onset of action of these agents is slow, usually occurring between 12 and 72 hours.

Saline laxatives work by creating an osmotic effect that increases the water content and volume of the stool. This increased volume results in distention of the intestinal lumen, causing increased peristalsis and bowel motility. The onset of action varies depending on the effect and dosage form. Rectal formulations such as enemas or suppositories have an onset of action of 5 to 30 minutes, whereas oral preparations work within 3 to 6 hours.

Stimulant laxatives work in the small and large intestine to stimulate bowel motility and increase the secretion of fluids into the bowel. The oral preparations usually have an onset of action within 6 to 10 hours. Rectal preparations usually have an onset of action within 30 to 60 minutes.

Emollient laxatives act as surfactants by allowing absorption of water into the stool, which makes the softened stool easier to pass. Emollient laxatives have a slow onset of action (24 to 72 hours), which is why they are not considered the drugs of choice for severe acute constipation. They are more useful for preventing constipation.

Mineral oil, which is a **lubricant laxative**, works in the colon to increase water retention and soften the stool. Mineral oil has an onset of action of between 6 and 8 hours.

Stool softeners decrease the consistency of stools by reducing the surface tension. Stool softeners permit easier penetration and mixing of fats and fluids with the fecal mass. This results in a softer, more easily passed stool. Docusate (Colace) acts as a detergent and stool softener. It usually takes 1 to 3 days to be effective. Stool softeners have a wide margin of safety and few potential adverse reactions. Stool softeners are combined with laxatives in such medications as Peri-Colace and Doxidan to soften stools while enhancing stool evacuation (see Table 15-6).

Indications

Laxatives are used prophylactically in patients who should avoid straining during defecation, and for treatment of constipation associated with hard, dry stools. They are prescribed for short-term relief of constipation. Certain laxatives are indicated to empty the large intestine for rectal and bowel examinations. Laxatives are particularly useful in patients who must avoid straining to pass hard stools, such as those patients who recently had a myocardial infarction or rectal surgery.

Adverse Effects

Stool softeners have a wide margin of safety and few potential adverse reactions. High doses or prolonged use of laxatives may cause diarrhea and a loss of water and electrolytes. Serious adverse effects include abdominal pain, perianal irritation, fainting, and weakness.

Contraindications and Precautions

Laxatives are contraindicated in patients with a known hypersensitivity, acute appendicitis, intestinal obstruction, fecal impaction, and acute hepatitis. Laxatives should be used cautiously in patients with rectal bleeding, in pregnant women (category C), and during lactation. Magnesium hydroxide is used with caution in patients with renal impairment.

Drug Interactions

Mineral oil may impair GI tract absorption of fat-soluble vitamins (A, D, E, and K).

VOMITING

The causes of vomiting include infectious diseases that can directly irritate vomiting centers to inhibit impulses going to the stomach. Certain drugs, radiation, and chemotherapy may irritate the GI tract or stimulate the chemoreceptor trigger zone and vomiting center in the brain (medulla). After surgery, particularly abdominal surgery, nausea and vomiting are common. The main neurotransmitters that produce nausea and vomiting include dopamine, serotonin, and acetylcholine. Persistent vomiting may cause dehydration, imbalance of electrolytes, metabolic alkalosis, and arrhythmias, which in turn, may precipitate further vomiting.

Emetics

An **emetic** is a drug that induces vomiting. Emetics (such as apomorphine, morphine, and digitalis) may act directly by stimulation of the medulla oblongata, or they may act reflexively by irritant action on the GI tract (such as copper sulfate, mustard, sodium chloride, and zinc sulfate).

Key Concept

A nasogastric tube is a safer and more efficient tool for emptying the stomach than the use of emetics.

Mechanism of Action

The emetic known as ipecac induces vomiting by stimulating the chemoreceptors of the vomiting reflex, and by the irritation of the gastric mucosal. Approximately 80 to 90 percent of people taking the medication begin vomiting within 20 to 30 minutes.

Key Concept

The administration of ipecac should be followed by a full eight-ounce glass of water to promote vomiting. If vomiting does not occur in 30 minutes, another dose may be given.

In most cases, ipecac is not absorbed because it is removed in vomitus. The effects of ipecac are stopped with activated charcoal.

Key Concept

The misuse of ipecac syrup has occurred in persons with eating disorders, such as bulimia, which may result in ipecac toxicity (muscle weakness and cardiotoxic effects).

Indications

Emetics are drugs used to promote vomiting, usually used in cases of poisoning or drug overdose. The nearest poison control center should be called prior to using these medications. Syrup of ipecac is the OTC drug used to bring about vomiting and should be included in any home emergency kit.

Adverse Effects

There are no serious adverse effects to ipecac. The only problem with any emetic is the aspiration of stomach contents.

Contraindications and Precautions

Emetics should not be used in patients who are unconscious or semicomatose, or in whom coma is expected imminently. These agents should not be used in patients with severe heart disease or advanced pregnancy. They are contraindicated in poisoning caused by corrosive or petroleum products. Safe use in pregnancy has not been established (category C).

Drug Interactions

Drug interactions with emetic drugs are rare. Other medications should not be taken with syrup of ipecac, as the rapid onset of vomiting will not allow enough time for the other medications to be absorbed.

Antiemetics

Antiemetics are used to prevent or relieve nausea and vomiting that are associated with many different disorders. Table 15-7 shows the most commonly used antiemetics.

TABLE 15-7 Common Antiemetic Agents

Generic Name	Trade Name	Route of Administration	Average Adult Dosage
Antihistamines and Anticholinergics:			
cyclizine hydrocholoride	Marezine®	PO	50 mg q4–6 h
dimenhydrinate	Calm-x®, Dramamine®	PO	50–100 mg q4–6 h
meclizine hydrochloride	Antrizine®, Bonamine®	PO	25–50 mg/day
scopolamine	Transderm-Scop®, Transderm-V®	Transdermal	1 patch q72 h starting 12 h before anticipated travel
Corticosteroids:			
dexamethasone	Decadron®	PO	0.25–4 mg b.i.d.-q.i.d.
methylprednisolone sodium succinate	Solu-Medrol®	PO	2–60 mg/day in div. doses
Dopamine Antagonists:			
droperidol	Inapsine®	IM, IV	2.5 mg; additional doses of 1.25 may be given
metoclopramide hydrochloride	Reglan®	IM, IV	10–20 mg near end of surgery
promethazine hydrochloride	Phenergan®, Prometh	PO, IM, IV	12.5–25 mg q4-6 h prn

(continues)

TABLE 15-7 Common Antiemetic Agents—*continued*

Generic Name	Trade Name	Route of Administration	Average Adult Dosage
Sedatives:			
diazepam	Diastat®, Valium®	PO, IM, IV	2–30 mg/day
lorazepam	Ativan	IV	1–1.5 mg prior to chemotherapy
Serotonin Receptor Antagonists:			
dolasetron mesylate	Anzemet®	PO	100 mg/day one hour prior to chemotherapy
granisetron	Kytril®	IV	10 mcg/kg 30 min prior to chemotherapy
ondansetron hydrochloride	Zofran®	PO	4 mg t.i.d p.r.n. 0.25 mg 30 min prior to chemotherapy
palonosetron	Aloxi®	IV	0.25 mg infused over 30 seconds (30 minutes prior to chemotherapy)
Neurokinin Receptor Antagonist:			
aprepitant	Emend®	PO	125 mg one hour prior to chemotherapy

Mechanism of Action

The mechanism of action of antiemetics is largely unknown, except that they help to relax the portion of the brain that controls muscles that cause vomiting. Some of these agents, such as prochlorperazine, depress the center of vomiting in the medulla.

Indications

There are several classes of drugs used as antiemetics, which will be discussed in various chapters. These agents are used for the treatment of drug overdose and for certain poisonings. They are also prescribed for certain conditions that are associated with vomiting, such as postchemotherapy, motion sickness, pregnancy, and other conditions.

Phenothiazines are the largest group of drugs used for severe nausea and vomiting. Prochlorperazine is the most commonly prescribed antiemetic medication in this group.

Adverse Effects

Since drowsiness is common to most of the antiemetics, patients should be cautioned not to drive or operate hazardous machinery while taking these drugs. Dose-related anticholinergics adverse effects, such as dry mouth, constipation, and tachycardia, are common.

Contraindications and Precautions

Key Concept

Transdermal scopolamine is a 72-hour patch that is placed behind the ear.

Antiemetics are contraindicated in patients with hypersensitivity to these drugs. They are also contraindicated in children younger than two years of age, and during pregnancy (category C). Antiemetics are used with caution in children, pregnant women, and dehydrated patients.

Drug Interactions

Antiemetics may have differing drug interactions based on their types. For example, serotonin antagonists usually have no drug interactions, while dopamine is affected by antiemetics, which are antagonistic. Prochlorperazine interacts with alcohol to increase CNS depression. Antacids and antidiarrheals inhibit absorption of this agent.

ADSORBENTS

Adsorbent agents have the ability to adsorb gases, toxins, and bacteria. Only certain materials that possess chemical adsorptive properties lend themselves effectively to detoxification and to the adsorption of gases resulting from abnormal intestinal fermentation. Such substances are kaolin and activated charcoal. Many of the nonsystemic antacids may serve as internal protectives and adsorbents. Antacids commonly are combined with kaolin or other adsorbents.

Mechanism of Action

These agents adsorb bacterial toxins that might be implicated in causing diarrhea or adsorb toxic substances swallowed into the GI tract by inhibiting GI adsorption. Adsorbents work by increasing the viscosity of the gut contents, and forming sludge.

Indications

Adsorbents are used for acute treatment of poisoning, primarily as an emergency antidote in many forms of poisoning. It is the emergency treatment of choice for virtually all drugs and chemicals. Charcoal capsules are also used for the relief of flatulence and the discomfort of abdominal gas.

Adverse Effects

Adverse effects include vomiting (related to rapid ingestion of high doses), constipation, diarrhea, and black stools.

Contraindications and Precautions

Adsorbents are contraindicated in patients with suspected obstructive bowel lesion, and pseudomembranous colitis. These agents should not be used for more than two days without medical direction. Safety during pregnancy (category C) or lactation is not established. Adsorbents should be used cautiously in infants or children younger than three years, and in elderly patients.

Drug Interactions

Adsorbents can inactivate syrup of ipecac and laxatives with activated charcoal. Adsorbents decrease the effectiveness of other medications.

Summary

The functions of the GI tract include digestion, storage, food absorption, and waste elimination. There are varieties of drugs that are used to treat disorders of the gastrointestinal system, including antacids, H_2-receptor antagonists, proton pump inhibitors, antidiarrheals, laxatives, antiemetics, and adsorbents. Gastric ulcer, duodenal ulcer, and gastroesophageal reflux disease are accompanied with increased secretion of hydrochloric acid, for which antacids, H_2-receptor antagonists, and proton pump inhibitors should be used. Peptic ulcer, which may be caused by *Helicobacter pylori* bacteria, should be treated with the combination of special antibiotics, bismuth products, and proton pump inhibitor drugs. There are several different laxative drugs that either accelerate fecal passage or decrease fecal consistency. Antiemetics are used to prevent or relieve nausea and vomiting. Adsorbents are used primarily as emergency antidotes in many forms of poisoning.

Exploring the Web

Visit ***http://digestive.niddk.nih.gov***

- Search for additional information about the digestive diseases and disorders discussed in this chapter. Enhance your understanding of the function of the digestive system and the drug therapies used to treat disorders of the digestive system.

Visit ***http://familydoctor.org***

- Search for OTC remedies to relieve gastrointestinal symptoms.

Visit ***www.medicalnewstoday.com***

- Search for the various types of drugs discussed in this chapter. Is there new information about or research being done on these types of drugs?

Review Questions

Multiple Choice

1. Gastrin hormones are released from the stomach and act primarily to release:

A. histamine
B. pepsin
C. pancreatic enzymes
D. all of the above

2. The generic name of Amphojel is:

A. magaldrate
B. sodium bicarbonate
C. aluminum hydroxide
D. calcium carbonate

3. Sodium bicarbonate is contraindicated in patients with:

A. congestive heart failure
B. severe renal disease
C. hypertension
D. all of the above

4. Which of the following H_2-receptor antagonists was the first drug approved for clinical use?

A. famotidine
B. nizatidine
C. ranitidine
D. cimetidine

5. The generic name of Axid is:

A. cimetidine
B. nizatidine
C. famotidine
D. ranitidine

6. Which of the following laxatives is particularly useful in patients who recently had a rectal surgery to avoid straining to pass hard stools?

A. lubricant
B. emollient
C. saline
D. stimulant

7. Which of the following is the generic name of Dulcolax?

A. bisacodyl
B. docusate
C. senna
D. cascara sagrada

8. For eradication of *Helicobacter pylori* with ulcer, you should combine:

A. bismuth products and proton pump inhibitors
B. antibiotics, bismuth, and proton pump inhibitors
C. proton pump inhibitors and antibiotics
D. antibiotics and bismuth products

9. The generic name of Tagamet is:

A. ranitidine
B. nizatidine
C. famotidine
D. cimetidine

10. Chronic administration of calcium carbonate–containing antacids may cause:

A. hyperparathyroidism
B. hypercalcemia
C. hypertension
D. hyperglycemia

11. Which of the following is the purpose of the therapeutic uses of activated charcoal?

A. decreased effectiveness of other medications
B. decreased blood sugar level
C. relief of vomiting and diarrhea
D. relief of flatulence and the discomfort of abdominal gas

12. Which of the following agents is used for treatment of vomiting after chemotherapy?

A. mineral oil
B. scopolamine patch
C. senna
D. magnesium citrate

13. The trade name of diphenoxylate with atropine is:

A. Imodium
B. Furoxone
C. Lomotil
D. Motofen

14. Which of the following is an adverse effect of antiflatulents?

A. coma
B. vomiting
C. headache
D. generally none

Matching

_____ **1.** lansoprazole	**A.** Pepcid
_____ **2.** cimetidine	**B.** Axid
_____ **3.** omeprazole	**C.** AcipHex
_____ **4.** ranitidine	**D.** Tagamet
_____ **5.** rabeprazole sodium	**E.** Prevacid
_____ **6.** famotidine	**F.** Zantac
_____ **7.** nizatidine	**G.** Prilosec

Fill in the Blank

1. What are the indications for antacids?

____

____

____

2. What is the mechanism of action of H_2-receptor antagonists?

____

____

____

3. What are the most serious adverse effects of mineral oil laxatives?

____

____

____

Critical Thinking

A 45-year-old male patient was diagnosed with gastritis caused by *H. pylori*. He exhibited symptoms of this disorder for more than 15 months, and did not take any medications or see any physicians before this visit.

1. List medications that may be used to treat this disorder.
2. If this disorder remains untreated, what would the probable consequences be?
3. Explain why *H. pylori* can grow even in the extremely acidic conditions of the stomach.

Hormonal Therapy for Endocrine Gland Disorders

CHAPTER 16

OUTLINE

(continues)

OBJECTIVES

After completing this chapter, the reader should be able to:

1. Explain the location of the major endocrine glands and their hormone secretion.
2. Describe the effect of thyroxine on the body organs.
3. Compare and contrast the roles of calcitonin hormone and parathyroid hormone.
4. Compare and contrast the functions of the pancreatic hormones.
5. Explain diabetes mellitus.
6. Name some risk factors for development of diabetes mellitus in older adults.
7. Identify the different types of insulin.
8. Explain the primary functions of the adrenal cortex.
9. Define the term "hormone" and then list the hormones that are secreted from the anterior pituitary gland.
10. Describe parathyroid hormone and its main functions.

GLOSSARY

Acromegaly – overdevelopment of the bones of the head, face, and feet

Adrenocorticotropic hormone (ACTH) – another hormone from the anterior pituitary gland that stimulates the growth of the adrenal gland cortex and the secretion of corticosteroids

Adrenogenital syndrome – congenital adrenal hyperplasia; a group of disorders involving steroid hormone production in the adrenal glands, leading to a deficiency of cortisol

Androgen – the generic term for any natural or synthetic compound, usually a steroid hormone, that stimulates or controls the development of masculine characteristics by binding to androgen receptors

Antidiuretic hormone (ADH) – released when the body is low on water, and causes the kidneys to conserve water, but not salt, by concentrating the urine and reducing urine volume

Antithyroid drug – a chemical agent that lowers the basal metabolic rate by

OUTLINE (*continued*)

interfering with the formation, release, or action of thyroid hormones

Calcitonin (CT) – produced primarily by the parafollicular cells of the thyroid gland

Conn's syndrome – a disease of the adrenal glands involving excess production of the hormone *aldosterone*

Cushing's syndrome – a disease caused by the excessive body production of cortisol; it can also be caused by excessive use of cortisol or other steroid hormones

Diabetes mellitus – a complex disorder of carbohydrate, fat, and protein metabolism caused by lack of or inefficient use of insulin in the body; classified as type I (insulin-dependent diabetes mellitus [IDDM]), or type II (non-insulin-dependent diabetes mellitus [NIDDM])

Dwarfism – a condition of lack of growth of the arms and legs in proportion to the head and trunk; it may be caused by over 200 different other conditions, including achondroplasia, kidney disease, genetic conditions, and problems with hormones or metabolism

Epinephrine (adrenaline) – produced by the medulla of adrenal glands, and is a "fight or flight" hormone that is released when danger threatens

Epiphyses – the ends of long bones that are originally separated from the main bone by a layer of cartilage, becoming unified through ossification

Follicle-stimulating hormone (FSH) – a gonadotropin that stimulates the growth and maturation of follicles in the ovary in females and promotes spermatogenesis (the process by which male gametes develop into mature spermatozoa) in males

Gigantism – condition produces excessive growth (a "giant") if the hypersecretion of GH occurs before puberty

Glucagon – an important hormone in carbohydrate metabolism

Glucocorticoids – steroid hormones that can bind with the cortisol receptor and trigger similar effects

Graves' disease – an autoimmune disorder that involves overactivity of the thyroid gland (hyperthyroidism)

Growth hormone (GH) – secreted by the anterior pituitary gland in response to growth hormone-releasing hormone (GHRH)

Hirsuitism – excessive hair growth on the face, abdomen, breasts, and back

Hormone – a chemical messenger that serves as a signal to target cells; are produced by nearly every organ system and type of tissue

Hyperactive – abnormally and easily excitable or exuberant

Hypercalcemia – an excessive amount of calcium in the blood

Hyperpituitarism – a condition that results in the excess secretion of hormones that are secreted from the pituitary gland

Hyperthyroidism – a condition of excessive amounts of thyroxine

Hypoactive – abnormally inactive

Hypothalamus – the part of the brain that lies below the thalamus; it regulates body temperature, certain metabolic processes, and other autonomic activities

Hypothyroidism – a deficiency disease that causes cretinism (mental and physical retardation) in children

Insulin – a hormone secreted by the pancreas that regulates carbohydrate and fat metabolism, especially the conversion of glucose to glycogen

Lugol's solution – Lugol's iodine; a solution of iodine often used as an antiseptic, disinfectant, or starch indicator, to replenish iodine deficiency, to protect the thyroid from radioactive materials, and for emergency disinfection of drinking water

Luteinizing hormone (LH) – secreted by the anterior lobe of the pituitary gland that is necessary for proper reproductive function

Mineralocorticoids – steroid hormones that influence salt and water balance; they are released from the adrenal cortex

Myxedema – condition of thyroid insufficiency or resistance to thyroid hormone

Negative feedback system – method by which regulation of hormones is achieved; released in response to concentration in the blood

Norepinephrine (noradrenaline) – released from the medulla of the adrenal glands, and is also a central nervous system and sympathetic nervous system neurotransmitter

Oxytocin (OT) – also acts as a neurotransmitter in the brain; in women, it is released during labor and lactation

Parathyroid hormone (PTH) – also called parathormone, is secreted by the parathyroid glands and increases the levels of calcium in the blood

Prolactin (PRL) – a hormone that is primarily associated with lactation; it is secreted from the anterior pituitary gland

Spermatogenesis – the process by which male gametes develop into mature spermatozoa

Steroids – numerous naturally occurring or synthetic fat-soluble organic compounds that include sterols, bile acids, adrenal hormones, sex hormones, digitalis compounds, and certain vitamin precursors

Thyroid-stimulating hormone (TSH) – a substance secreted by the anterior lobe of the pituitary gland that controls the release of thyroid hormone and is necessary for the growth and function of the thyroid gland

Thyroxine (T_4) – the major hormone secreted by the follicular cells of the thyroid gland

Tremors – involuntary tremblings or quiverings

Overview

The endocrine system consists of specialized cell clusters, glands, hormones, and target tissues. The glands and cell clusters secrete hormones and chemical transmitters in response to stimulation from the nervous system and other sites. Together with the nervous system, the endocrine system regulates and integrates the body's metabolic activities, and maintains internal homeostasis. Each target tissue has receptors for specific hormones. Hormones connect with the receptors, and the resulting hormone-receptor complex triggers the target cell's response.

The overactivity or underactivity of a gland is the malfunction that most commonly causes endocrine disease. If a gland secretes an excessive amount of its hormone, it is **hyperactive**. When a gland fails to secrete its hormone or secretes an inadequate amount, it is **hypoactive**.

Anatomy Review

- The major glands of the endocrine system include: pituitary, pineal, thyroid, parathyroid, thymus, adrenals, pancreas, and the gonads (Figure 16-1).
- Endocrine glands secrete **hormones**, or chemical messengers, directly into the bloodstream. These hormones coordinate and direct activities of specific target cells or organs.
- Each gland releases a specific hormone or hormones and generates specific effects (Table 16-1).

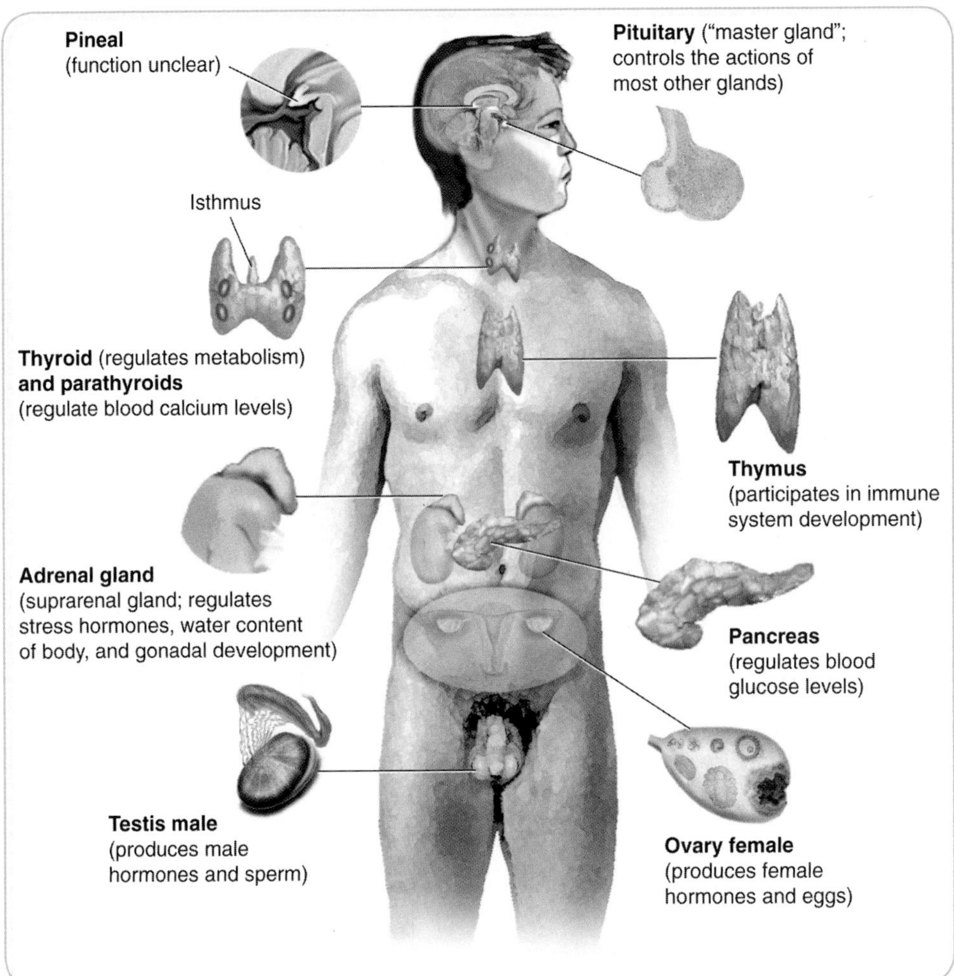

Figure 16-1 Location of the endocrine glands.

TABLE 16-1 Sources and Effects of Major Hormones

Source	Hormone	Primary Effects
Hypothalamus	Hypothalamic-releasing hormones	Stimuli to anterior pituitary to release specific hormone; decrease release of specific hormone by anterior pituitary
Pituitary – anterior lobe (adenohypophysis)	Growth hormone (GH, somatotropin)	Stimulates synthesis of protein
	Adrenocorticotropic hormone (ACTH)	Stimulates secretion of (primarily) cortisol from adrenal cortex
	Thyroid-stimulating hormone (TSH)	Stimulates the thyroid gland
	Follicle-stimulating hormone (FSH)	In women: stimulates ovarian follicle growth and estrogen secretion; in men: stimulates sperm production
	Luteinizing hormone (LH)	In women: stimulates ovum maturation and ovulation; in men: stimulates testosterone secretion

(*continues*)

TABLE 16-1 Sources and Effects of Major Hormones—*continued*

Source	Hormone	Primary Effects
Pituitary – posterior lobe (neurohypophysis)	Prolactin (PRL)	Stimulates milk production during lactation
	Antidiuretic hormone (ADH, or vasopressin)	Increases kidney reabsorption of water
	Oxytocin	Stimulates uterine contractions after delivery; stimulates milk ejection during lactation
Pancreas – beta cells of islets of Langerhans	Insulin	Transports glucose and other substances into cells; lowers blood glucose levels
Pancreas – alpha cells	Glucagon	Increases blood glucose level; glycogenolysis in the liver
Parathyroid gland	Parathyroid hormone (PTH)	Increases blood calcium levels by stimulating bone demineralization; increases absorption of serum calcium in kidneys and digestive tract
Thyroid gland	Calcitonin	Decreases calcium release from bones to lower blood calcium levels
	Thyroxine (T_4) and triiodothyronine (T_3)	Increase cellular metabolic rates
Adrenal cortex	Aldosterone	Increases water and sodium kidney reabsorption
	Cortisol	Decreases immune response; is anti-inflammatory; has a catabolic effect on tissues; stress response
Adrenal medulla	Norepinephrine	Generalized vasoconstriction
	Epinephrine	Stress response; increases force and rate of heart contraction; bronchodilation; vasodilation in skeletal muscle; visceral and cutaneous vasoconstriction

Hormonal Regulation

Hormones are secreted only as needed by the body and organs. When the concentration of a particular hormone in the body reaches a particular level, the gland that secretes the hormone will stop secretion of the hormone until the concentration of the hormone in the body drops below a particular level and it is triggered to release more. For example, insulin is secreted when the blood glucose level rises. This type of control is called a **negative feedback system**.

Role of the Hypothalamus in the Endocrine System

The **hypothalamus** of the brain is the main integrative center for the endocrine and autonomic nervous systems. The hypothalamus helps control some endocrine glands by neural and hormonal pathways. Neural pathways connect the hypothalamus to the posterior pituitary gland. Neural stimulation of the posterior pituitary causes the secretion of two effector hormones: antidiuretic hormone (also known as vasopressin) and oxytocin.

> ***Medical Terminology Review***
>
> **hypothalamus**
> *hypo* = low; under; beneath
> *thalamus* = gray matter deeply situated in the forebrain
> structure deep to the gray matter of the forebrain
>
> **corticotrophin**
> *cortico* = stimulating the cortex
> *tropin* = hormone
> a hormone that stimulates the cortex

The hypothalamus also exerts hormonal control at the anterior pituitary gland, by releasing and inhibiting hormones and factors, which arrive by a portal system. Hypothalamic hormones stimulate the pituitary glands to synthesize and release trophic hormones. These hormones include corticotropin (also called adreno-corticotropic hormone), thyroid-stimulating hormone, and gonadotropins, such as luteinizing hormone and follicle-stimulating hormone. Secretion of trophic hormones stimulates the adrenal cortex, thyroid gland, and gonads. Hypothalamic hormones also stimulate the pituitary gland to release or inhibit the release of effector hormones, such as growth hormone and prolactin (Figure 16-2).

Hormones

Hormones are natural chemical substances secreted into the bloodstream from the endocrine glands that regulate and control the activity of an organ or tissues in another part of the body. The synthesis and secretion of many hormones are controlled by other hormones or changes in the concentration of essential chemicals or electrolytes in the blood. Drugs and diseases can modify hormone secretion as well as specific hormone effects at target organs. Some hormones affect nearly all the tissues of the body, but the action of others is restricted to a few tissues or organs. The majority of hormones, such as thyroxine, epinephrine, parathyroid hormone, insulin, and glucagon, are proteins. Several other groups of hormones, such as those produced by the adrenal cortex and the gonads, are **steroids**. A list of major hormones and endocrine glands is provided in Table 16-1. Hormones from the various endocrine glands work together to regulate vital processes of the body that include the following:

1. Secretions in the digestive tract
2. Energy production
3. Composition and volume of extracellular fluid
4. Adaptation and immunity
5. Growth and development
6. Reproduction and lactation

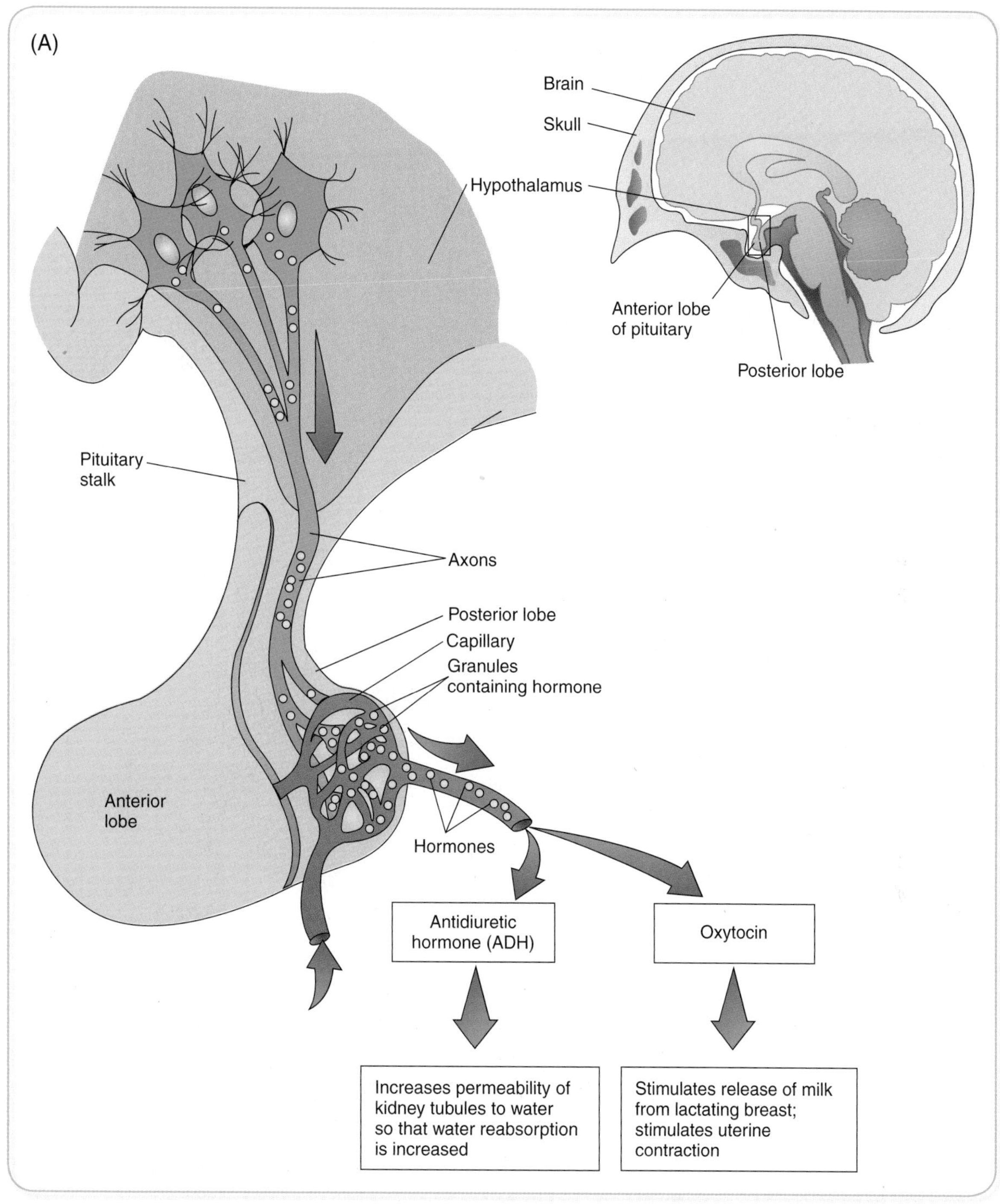

Figure 16-2A The relationship between the hypothalamus and the (A) posterior lobe of the pituitary gland (B) anterior lobe of the pituitary gland.

The inactivation of hormones occurs enzymatically in the blood, liver, kidneys, or target tissues. Hormones are secreted primarily via the urine and, to a lesser extent, via the bile. In medicine, hormones generally are used in three ways: (1) for replacement therapy; (2) for pharmacologic effects beyond replacement; and (3) for endocrine diagnostic testing.

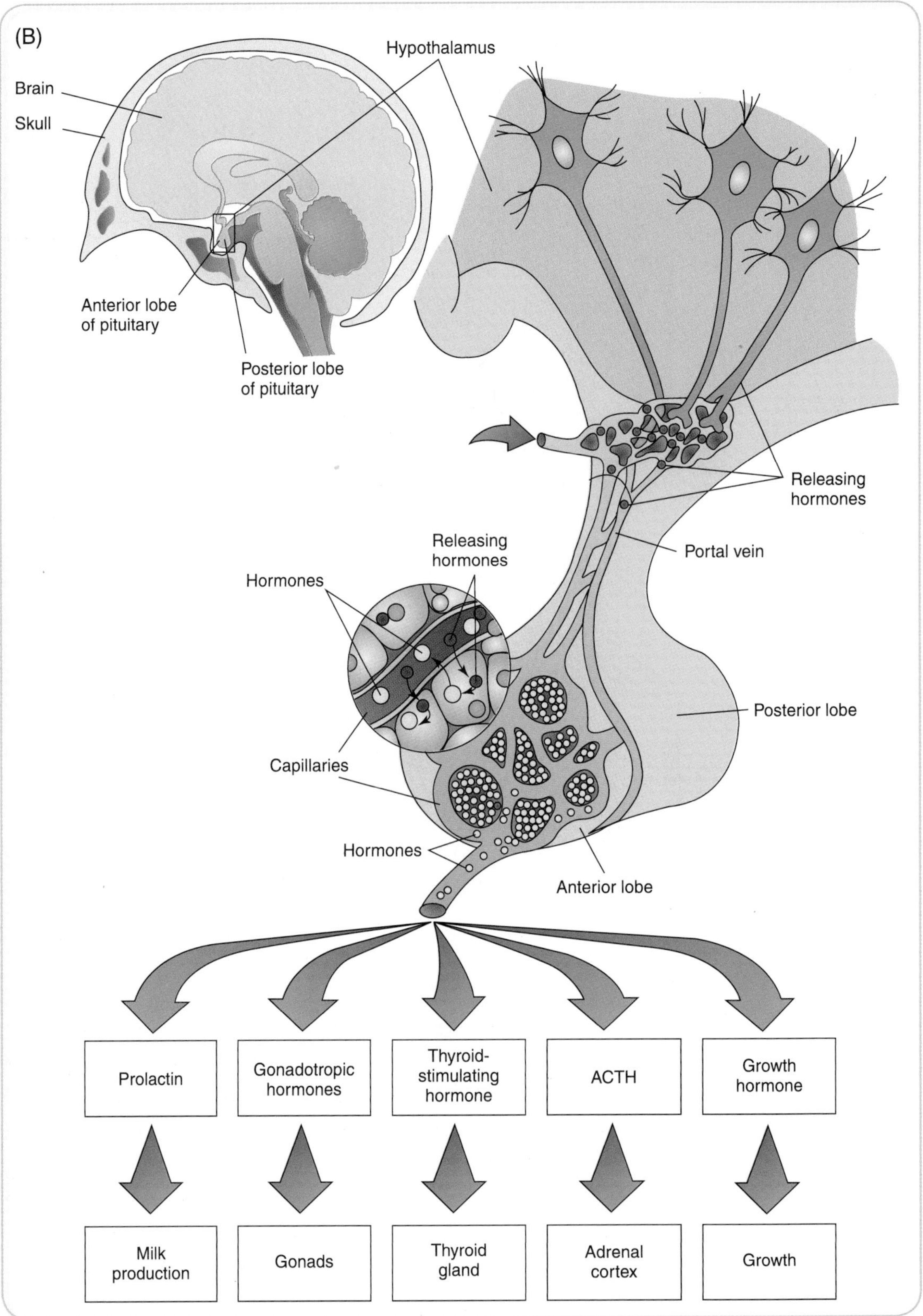

Figure 16-2B The relationship between the hypothalamus and the (A) posterior lobe of the pituitary gland (B) anterior lobe of the pituitary gland.

Growth Hormone

Growth hormone (GH) is secreted by the anterior pituitary gland in response to growth hormone-releasing hormone (GHRH). Its secretion is controlled in part by the hypothalamus. GH promotes protein synthesis in all cells, increases fat mobilization, and the use of fatty acids for energy. Growth effects depend on the presence of thyroid hormone, insulin, and carbohydrates. It is prescribed for **dwarfism**, a condition in which the growth of long bones is abnormally decreased by an inadequate production of growth hormone.

Adrenocorticotropic Hormone

Adrenocorticotropic hormone (ACTH) is another hormone from the anterior pituitary gland that stimulates the growth of the adrenal gland cortex and the secretion of corticosteroids. Under normal conditions, a diurnal rhythm occurs in ACTH secretion, with an increase beginning after the first few hours of sleep and reaching a peak at the time a person awakens. ACTH is used generally for diagnostic testing, and not for therapeutic purposes. The adverse effects include insomnia, delayed wound healing, increased susceptibility to infection, and acne.

Thyroid-stimulating Hormone

Key Concept

Many of the drugs used to alter pituitary function are proteins that cannot be administered orally. They must be injected, although some may be administered intranasally.

Thyroid-stimulating hormone (TSH) is a substance secreted by the anterior lobe of the pituitary gland that controls the release of thyroid hormone and is necessary for the growth and function of the thyroid gland. TSH stimulates the thyroid gland to increase the uptake of iodine and increase the synthesis and release of thyroid hormones. It is prescribed for hypothyroidism and diagnostic tests.

Follicle-stimulating Hormone

Follicle-stimulating hormone (FSH) is a gonadotropin that stimulates the growth and maturation of follicles in the ovary and promotes **spermatogenesis** (the process by which male gametes develop into mature spermatozoa) in the male. It is secreted by the anterior pituitary gland. The ovarian follicle produces estrogen, which reaches a high level before ovulation and suppresses release of FSH. In males, FSH maintains the integrity of the seminiferous tubules and influences all the stages of sperm production. It may be used to treat some conditions. One form is derived from the urine of postmenopausal women.

Medical Terminology Review

gonadotropin
gonado = sex
tropin = hormone
sex hormone

Luteinizing Hormone

Luteinizing hormone (LH) is secreted by the anterior lobe of the pituitary gland and is necessary for proper reproductive function. In females, an acute rise of LH triggers ovulation. In males, where LH is also called Interstitial Cell Stimulating Hormone (ICSH), it stimulates the production of testosterone.

Prolactin

Prolactin (PRL) is a hormone that is primarily associated with lactation. It is secreted from the anterior pituitary gland. Prolactin release is stimulated by thyrotropin-releasing factor.

Antidiuretic Hormone

Antidiuretic hormone (ADH) is released when the body is low on water, and causes the kidneys to conserve water, but not salt, by concentrating the urine and reducing urine volume. It also raises blood pressure by inducing vasoconstriction. ADH is released from the hypothalamus and stored in the posterior lobe of the pituitary gland.

Oxytocin

Oxytocin (OT) also acts as a neurotransmitter in the brain. In women, it is released during labor and lactation. It is also released by both sexes during orgasm. Oxytocin is mostly manufactured by the hypothalamus.

Thyroxine

Thyroxine (T_4) is the major hormone secreted by the follicular cells of the thyroid gland. It is involved in controlling metabolic body processes and influencing physical development.

Calcitonin

Calcitonin (CT) is produced primarily by the parafollicular cells of the thyroid gland. Calcitonin participates in calcium and phosphorus metabolism. In many ways, it counteracts the effects of parathyroid hormone.

Parathyroid Hormone

Parathyroid hormone (PTH), also called parathormone, is secreted by the parathyroid glands and increases the levels of calcium in the blood. Parathyroid hormone reduces the uptake of phosphate in the proximal tubules of the kidney, meaning that more phosphate is excreted through the urine.

Medical Terminology Review

glucocorticoids
gluco = glucose; glucagon; sugar
corticoids = steroid hormones
steroid hormones released in response to sugar levels in the blood

Glucocorticoids

Glucocorticoids are steroid hormones that can bind with the cortisol receptor and trigger similar effects. They are released from the adrenal cortex. Cortisol (hydrocortisone) is the most important human glucocorticoid. It regulates or supports a variety of important cardiovascular, metabolic, immunologic, and homeostatic functions.

Mineralocorticoids

Mineralocorticoids are steroid hormones that influence salt and water balance. They are released from the adrenal cortex. The primary endogenous mineralocorticoid is aldosterone, which acts on the kidneys to provide active reabsorption of sodium and passive reabsorption of water. This eventually results in an increase of blood pressure and blood volume.

Androgens

Androgen is the generic term for any natural or synthetic compound, usually a steroid hormone, which stimulates or controls the development of masculine characteristics by binding to androgen receptors. They are released from the adrenal cortex. Androgens are also the original anabolic steroids. The primary and most well-known androgen is testosterone.

Epinephrine

Epinephrine (adrenaline) is produced by the medulla of adrenal glands, and is a "fight or flight" hormone that is released when danger threatens. It increases heart rate and stroke volume, dilates the pupils, constricts arterioles in the skin and gut, and dilates arterioles in the leg muscles. It is commonly used to treat cardiac arrest and other cardiac dysrhythmias.

Norepinephrine

Norepinephrine (noradrenaline) is released from the medulla of the adrenal glands, and is also a central nervous system and sympathetic nervous system neurotransmitter. It supports the "fight or flight" response, increasing heart rate, triggering the release of glucose, and increasing skeletal muscle readiness.

Glucagon

Glucagon is a hormone that is very important for carbohydrate metabolism. It is synthesized and secreted by the alpha cells of the pancreas. Glucagon helps maintain the level of glucose in the blood by causing the liver to release glucose through a process known as glycogenolysis. This release prevents the development of hypoglycemia.

Insulin

Insulin is a hormone that regulates carbohydrate and fat metabolism. It is synthesized and released by the beta cells of the pancreas. Insulin is used medically to treat some forms of diabetes mellitus. Most insulin produced each day is produced during the digestion of meals. Insulin therapy often requires frequent blood glucose checking by the patient.

Insulin may be administered via syringes, injection pens, insulin pumps, and inhalers. Inhalation insulin uses only short-acting insulin, and is used in combination with a long-acting insulin to treat type 1 diabetes. Short, intermediate, mixed, and long-acting insulins may be injected using syringes and injection pens. Lantus insulin (insulin glargine) is a newer, ultra-long-acting type of insulin, administered by injection once per day. Its activity begins in a little more than one hour, and lasts for about 24 hours, without any peaks in its effectiveness.

ALTERATIONS IN THE FUNCTION OF THE PITUITARY GLAND

Hyperpituitarism can result from damage to the anterior lobe of the pituitary gland or from inadequate secretion of hormones. The most noticeable result of hyperpituitarism is the effect of excessive amounts of GH. The condition produces excessive growth (a "giant") if the hypersecretion of GH occurs before puberty, which is called **gigantism**. If the excessive production of GH occurs after puberty, it can result in **acromegaly** (overdevelopment of the bones of the head, face, and feet). Treatment of these two conditions includes surgery, radiation, and medication therapy. Growth hormone insufficiency during childhood causes **dwarfism**.

Key Concept

Regular monitoring of height, weight, and blood glucose levels is essential for a patient taking somatotropin.

Medical Terminology Review

somatotropin
somato = body
tropin = hormone
hormones involved in regulating body functions

Diabetes insipidus is a disease that results from a deficiency of ADH. In the absence of ADH, water is not reabsorbed by the kidneys and is excreted in the urine. Excessive water loss can quickly lead to dehydration. Whenever possible, the underlying cause of diabetes insipidus must be corrected. ADH is used in the treatment of diabetes insipidus.

Growth Hormone Replacement

Growth hormone replacement therapy may be used to treat many different conditions, including Turner syndrome, chronic renal failure, intrauterine growth retardation, and severe idiopathic short stature, to maintain muscle mass in AIDS patients, and for patients with short bowel syndrome.

Mechanism of Action

Although still widely debated, it is believed that the mechanism of action of GH is similar to that of tryptophan, which is released by increased levels of serotonin at night.

Indications

The main indication for replacement of GH is growth failure in children. Treatment is prolonged and may cause a six-inch growth in height. Special agents used for hormone therapy of the pituitary gland are listed in Table 16-2.

TABLE 16-2 Drugs used for Hormone Therapy of the Pituitary Gland

Generic Name	Trade Name	Route of Administration	Average Adult Dosage
Anterior Pituitary Gland			
Growth Hormone			
sermorelin	Geref®	SC	30 mcg/kg/day
somatropin	Humatrope®	SC	0.006 mg/kg/day (0.018 IU/kg/day)
somatrem	Protropin®	IM, SC	0.18 mg/kg/wk, divided into equal doses
Growth Hormone Inhibitor			
octreotide	Sandostatin®	SC, IV	Initial: 50 mcg; 100–600 mcg/day in 2–4 divided doses
Adrenocortical Hormones			
corticotropin	Acthar®, ACTH-80®	IM, SC	IM: 80–120 units/day; SC: 10–25 units in 500 mL D_5W infused over 8 h
cosyntropin	Cortrosyn®	IM, IV (diagnostic agent)	0.25 mg
Posterior Pituitary Gland			
desmopressin acetate	DDAVP®, Stimate®	PO, IV, SC, Nasal spray	PO: 0.2–0.4 mg/day; IV/SC: 0.3 mcg/kg/min pre-op, may repeat in 48 h p.r.n.; Nasal spray: 10 mcg b.i.d.
vasopressin	Pitressin®	IM, SC	5–10 units b.i.d. – t.i.d.

Adverse Effects

The side effects of GH therapy include headache, increased blood glucose levels, and muscle weakness. Other adverse effects include swelling at the injection site, myalgia, hypercalciuria, and hyperglycemia.

Contraindications and Precautions

Growth hormones such as somatrem and somatropin are contraindicated in patients with closed **epiphyses** (the ends of long bones that are originally separated from the main bone by a layer of cartilage, becoming unified through ossification), underlying progressive intracranial tumor, and diabetic retinopathy. These hormones should be avoided in patients during chemotherapy, radiation therapy, untreated hypothyroidism, and obesity.

Growth hormones are also contraindicated in pregnancy (category B or category C, depending on the brand).

Growth hormones should be used cautiously in patients with diabetes mellitus or family history of the disease, sleep apnea, lactation, and hypothyroidism.

Drug Interactions

Depending on dosage, anabolic steroids, androgens, estrogens, and thyroid hormones may interact with growth hormones.

ALTERATIONS IN THE FUNCTION OF THE THYROID GLAND

Hypothyroidism is a deficiency disease that causes cretinism (mental and physical retardation) in children. It is usually due to a deficiency of iodine in the mother's diet during pregnancy. Hypothyroidism in adults results from hypothalamic pituitary or thyroid insufficiency or resistance to thyroid hormone, which is called **myxedema.** The disorder can progress to hyposecretion of thyroid hormone. Hypothyroidism is more common in women than in men in the U.S. Hyposecretion of thyroid hormones may also be caused by lack of iodine in the diet, surgical removal of the thyroid, or radiation therapy to the thyroid. It may also be due to pituitary dysfunction. Thyroid hormones are approved for supplement or replacement needs of hypothyroidism. Thyroid hormones are usually initiated in small doses until adequate response is reached. Long-term use of thyroxine may cause osteoporosis or progressive loss of bone mass in postmenopausal women. Thyroxine is contraindicated in patients who have had a myocardial infarction. Table 16-3 shows common drugs used for disorders of the thyroid gland.

TABLE 16-3 Selected Medications Used as Drugs for the Thyroid Gland

Generic Name	Trade Name	Route of Administration	Average Adult Dosage
Natural thyroid replacement			
desiccated thyroid (T_3, T_4)	Armour® Thyroid	PO	None–it is based on natural production of the hormone per patient
Synthetic thyroid replacement			
levothyroxine sodium (T_4)	Levothroid®, Synthroid®	PO	100–400 mcg/day
liothyronine sodium (T_3)	Cytomel®	PO	25–75 mcg/day

(continues)

TABLE 16-3 Selected Medications Used as Drugs for the Thyroid Gland—*continued*

Generic Name	Trade Name	Route of Administration	Average Adult Dosage
liotrix (T_3, T_4)	Thyrolar®	PO	12.5–30 mcg/day
Antithyroid preparations			
potassium iodide	Pima®, Lugol's Solution®	PO	50–250 mg t.i.d. for 10–14 days before surgery
methimazole	Tapazole®	PO	5–15 mg t.i.d.
propylthiouracil (PTU)	generic only	PO	300–450 mg/day divided q8h
Calcitonin			
calcitonin (salmon)	Fortical®, Calcimar®	IM/SC, Nasal spray	IM/SC: 100 IU/day, may decrease to 50–100 IU/day; Nasal spray: 200 IU/day

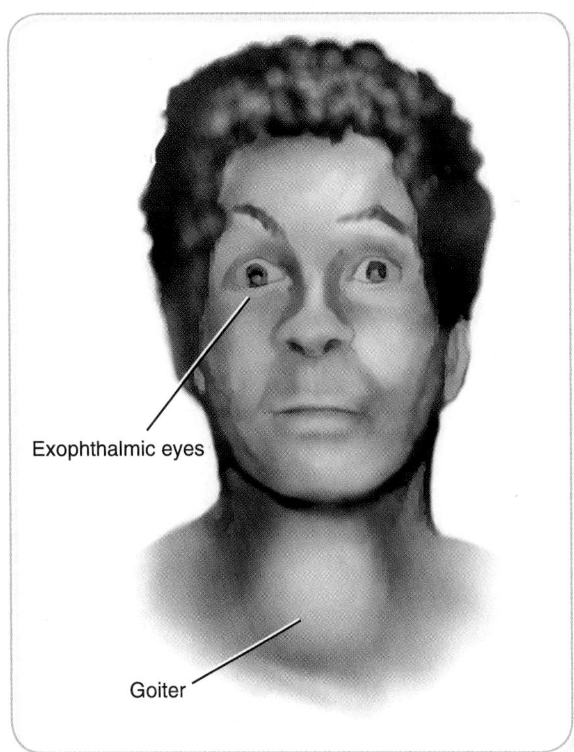

Figure 16-3 Hyperthyroidism.

Hyperthyroidism is a condition of excessive amounts of thyroxine (Figure 16-3). This condition stimulates cellular metabolism and increases respiration and body temperature. Hyperthyroidism causes nervousness and tremors (a shakiness of the hands).

Graves' disease is an example of hyperthyroidism. This disease is far more common in women than in men, and usually affects young women. Graves' disease can sometimes be treated with medication that inhibits the synthesis of thyroxine or by administration of radioactive iodine, which destroys the thyroid gland. Removal of the thyroid gland, however, may be necessary. If the gland is removed, hormonal supplements must be given. With partial removal of the thyroid gland, the remaining portion still secretes hormones.

Antithyroid Agents

An **antithyroid drug** is a chemical agent that lowers the basal metabolic rate by interfering with the formation, release, or action of thyroid hormones. A variety of compounds are known as antithyroid drugs. Iodine thyroid products (iodide ions), radioactive iodine, methimazole, and propylthiouracil are the drugs of choice for antithyroid therapy. These medications can cross the placenta and stop fetal thyroid development. They also pass through breast milk to affect the infant. Selected medication used as drugs for the thyroid gland are shown in Table 16-3.

Radioactive Iodine

Radioactive iodine is a radioactive isotope of iodine used in diagnostic radiology and radiotherapy. It is used particularly for the treatment of some thyroid conditions. Most radioactive iodine is excreted in urine, but small amounts may be found in sputum, perspiration, feces, and vomitus.

Mechanism of Action. Destructive radiation (beta rays) is emitted by the trapped isotope, which effectively destroys thyroid cells without appreciably damaging surrounding tissue.

Indications. Radioactive isotopes of iodine, particularly sodium iodide I^{131} are commonly used for the diagnosis and treatment of hyperthyroidism. When administered orally or intravenously, I^{131} is rapidly taken up and stored by the thyroid gland.

Adverse Effects. The extent of thyroid damage can be predetermined by carefully selecting the proper dose of isotope. Low doses are used diagnostically and pose a minimal risk to thyroid tissue, although high doses can effectively destroy all thyroid function, resulting in hypothyroidism.

Contraindications and Precautions. The antithyroid drugs are contraindicated in the last trimester of pregnancy (category D) and during lactation. These agents are also contraindicated with concurrent administration of sulfonamides or coal tar derivatives such as aminopyrine or antipyrine. Antithyroid agents must be used with caution in patients with infection, bone marrow depression, and impaired liver function. These drugs are also used cautiously in patients with concomitant administration of anticoagulants or other drugs known to cause agranulocytosis.

Drug Interactions. Iodine interacts with selenium and possibly with vanadium. Amiodarone, potassium iodide, or sodium iodide can reverse the efficacy of thyroid hormones.

Iodine Thyroid Products

These drugs have been shown to be useful in treatment of mild hyperthyroidism, particularly in young patients. Prior to the introduction of the thioamides in the 1940s, iodides were major antithyroid agents; today, they are rarely used as sole therapies.

Mechanism of Action. Iodine ion (**Lugol's solution**) inhibits the synthesis of the active thyroid hormones T_3 and T_4 and inhibits the release of these hormones into blood circulation.

Indications. Iodides may be used in several different forms. The most popular are Lugol's solution (strong iodine solution), which contains 5 percent iodine and 10 percent potassium iodide, and saturated solution of potassium iodide (SSKI). Iodides are used as adjunctive therapy with antithyroid drugs in preparation for thyroidectomy, treatment of thyrotoxic crisis, or neonatal thyrotoxicosis.

Adverse Effects. Lugol's solution may cause hypothyroidism, hyperthyroidism, goiter (enlargement of the thyroid), rashes, and swelling of the salivary glands.

Contraindications and Precautions. Potassium iodide is contraindicated in patients with hypersensitivity to iodine. This agent should be avoided in patients with hyperthyroidism, hyperkalemia, and acute bronchitis, and during pregnancy (category D) and lactation.

Potassium iodide should be used cautiously in patients with renal impairment, cardiac disease, pulmonary tuberculosis, and Addison's disease.

Drug Interactions. Lugol's solution can increase the risk of hypothyroidism if taken concurrently with lithium. Potassium-sparing diuretics, potassium supplements, and ACE inhibitors increase the risk of hyperkalemia.

Methimazole

Methimazole is an antithyroid agent that is about ten times more potent than propylthiouracil.

Mechanism of Action. Methimazole inhibits the synthesis of thyroid hormones by the coupling of iodine. This agent crosses the placental barrier and is concentrated by the fetal thyroid.

Indications. Methimazole has emerged as an effective drug for controlling hyperthyroidism. It is also used prior to surgery or radiotherapy of the thyroid.

Adverse Effects. Observation of patients using methimazole has shown that adverse effects are not common. Some patients may develop a mild skin rash, and agranulocytosis has developed in a small number of patients. In very rare instances, methimazole may affect the central nervous system, causing headache, depression, drowsiness, vertigo, and neuritis.

Contraindications and Precautions. Methimazole is contraindicated during lactation and pregnancy (category D). This drug should be used cautiously with other drugs known to cause agranulocytosis.

Drug Interactions. Methimazole increases theophylline clearance and decreases effectiveness if given to hyperthyroid patients. This agent alters the effects of oral anticoagulants. It increases the therapeutic effects and toxicity of digitalis glycoside, metroprolol, and propranolol when hyperthyroid patients become euthyroid.

Propylthiouracil

Propylthiouracil (PTU) is a chemically related antithyroid drug, and is a major drug for the treatment of thyrotoxicosis.

Mechanism of Action. PTU inhibits the synthesis of thyroid hormones, partially inhibiting the peripheral conversion of T_4 to T_3.

Indications. PTU is used for treatment of hyperthyroidism, iodine-induced thyrotoxicosis, and hyperthyroidism associated with thyroiditis. Propylthiouracil is also used to establish euthyroidism prior to surgery or radioactive iodine treatment.

> ***Medical Terminology Review***
>
> **thyroiditis**
> *thyroid = thyroid gland*
> *itis = inflammation; disease of*
> inflammation of the thyroid gland

> ***Key Concept***
>
> *The cross-sensitivity between propylthiouracil and methimazole is about 50 percent; therefore, switching drugs in patients with severe reactions is not recommended.*

Adverse Effects. PTU may cause neuritis, vertigo, drowsiness, depression, and headache. Other adverse effects of this agent include skin rash, skin pigmentation, loss of hair, nausea, vomiting, loss of taste, hepatitis, or nephritis. The most dangerous complication of propylthiouracil is agranulocytosis, an infrequent but potentially fatal adverse effect.

Contraindications and Precautions. PTU is contraindicated in the last trimester of pregnancy (category D) and during lactation. PTU should be avoided with concurrent administration of sulfonamides or coal tar derivatives such as aminopyrine or antipyrine. PTU is used cautiously in patients with infection, liver dysfunction, and bone marrow depression.

Drug Interactions. PTU increases risk of oral bleeding. The other side effects of PTU are similar to methimazole.

Alterations in Function of the Parathyroid Gland

A deficiency of PTH may occur in some patients for a variety of reasons, ranging from a congenital absence of the parathyroid glands to surgery involving the thyroid gland. Such a deficiency results in a reduction of serum calcium levels, elevated phosphate levels, and a wide array of symptoms, including increased neuromuscular irritability and psychiatric disorders.

The treatment of hypoparathyroidism focuses on the replenishment of calcium stores to reverse the patient's hypocalcemia. Therefore, administration of calcium salts, particularly calcium chloride and calcium gluconate, is indicated.

Vitamin D is also commonly used in patients with hypoparathyroidism to promote calcium absorption from the gastrointestinal tract and to further stabilize a patient's condition.

An overactive parathyroid gland secretes too much PTH, which raises the level of circulating calcium above normal. This condition is called **hypercalcemia**. Much of the calcium comes from bone resorption and increased absorption of calcium by the kidneys and the gastrointestinal system. As the calcium level rises, the phosphate level falls.

With the loss of calcium bones are weakened. They tend to bend, become deformed, and fracture spontaneously. Excessive amounts of calcium cause the development of kidney stones because calcium forms insoluble compounds. Calcium deposited within the walls of the blood vessels makes them hard. Calcium deposits may also be found in the stomach and lungs.

Therapy for hyperparathyroidism often includes surgery. However, phosphate supplementation and/or potent diuretics, such as furosemide (Lasix), may be administered to promote an increase in the excretion of excess calcium. Calcitonin may also be used for treating hypercalcemia.

Alterations in Function of the Adrenal Glands

Overactivity of the adrenal cortex can take different forms, depending on which group of hormones is secreted in excess. **Cushing's syndrome** develops from an excess of glucocorticoids, the hormones that raise the blood sugar level. In excess, they cause hyperglycemia. The patient with Cushing's syndrome retains salt and water, resulting in hypertension and atherosclerosis, which develops as a result of excess circulating lipids.

Conn's syndrome is another form of hyperadrenalism. In this disease, aldosterone is secreted in excess. This causes retention of sodium and water and an abnormal loss of potassium in the urine. Hypertension develops as a result of the salt imbalance and water retention. Muscles become weak to the point of paralysis.

Adrenogenital syndrome is another form of hyperadrenalism, also called adrenal virilism. In this condition, androgens (male hormones) are secreted in excess. If this excessive secretion occurs in children, it stimulates premature sexual development. The sex organs of a male child greatly enlarge, and in a female, the clitoris enlarges, a male distribution of hair develops, and the voice deepens.

> ***Medical Terminology Review***
>
> **virilism**
>
> *viril(e) = having male characteristics*
> *ism = state; condition; quality*
> a condition in which male characteristics develop

Excessive androgen secretion in a woman causes masculinization (adrenal virilism). Hair develops on the face, a condition called **hirsuitism**, and the hairline recedes. The breasts diminish in size, the clitoris enlarges, and ovulation and menstruation cease.

Addison's disease results when the adrenal glands fail to produce corticosteroids and aldosterone. The adrenal glands may be destroyed by cancer or infection, or inhibited by chronic use of steroid hormones, such as prednisone.

With aldosterone deficiency, the patient is unable to retain salt and water. The kidneys are unable to concentrate urine, and eventually dehydration ensues. Severe dehydration can ultimately lead to shock. Cortisol deficiency leads to low blood glucose levels, impaired protein and carbohydrate metabolism, and generalized weakness.

Treatment with Glucocorticoids

Prolonged use of glucocorticoids may suppress the pituitary gland, and the body will not produce its own hormone. If these hormones are used for extended periods of time, they cannot be stopped abruptly, and a step-down dosage should be used to taper gradually the amount of drug the patient is receiving.

Mechanism of Action

Cortisone enters target cells, where it has anti-inflammatory and immunosuppressive effects.

Indications

Adrenal corticosteroids are used for replacement therapy in patients with adrenal insufficiency, such as Addison's disease. In this condition, administration of both mineralocorticoids and glucocorticoids may be required. Glucocorticoids are also used to treat rheumatic, inflammatory, allergic, neoplastic, and other disorders as supportive therapy with other medications. These agents are of value in decreasing some cerebral edemas. Certain skin conditions are often markedly improved with the use of topical or systemic glucocorticoids. Probably the most use of these agents is treatment of arthritic and rheumatic disorders. Table 16-4 lists some steroids and adrenal corticosteroids.

Adverse Effects

Certain side effects may appear during the first week of treatment with glucocorticoids. They include euphoria, suicidal depression, psychoses, anorexia, hyperglycemia, increased susceptibility to infections, and acne. Chronic glucocorticoid therapy may cause additional side effects such as diabetes mellitus, glaucoma, cataracts, osteoporosis, and edema.

Glucocorticoids must be used cautiously in congestive heart failure, hypertension, liver failure, and renal failure.

TABLE 16-4 Steroids and Adrenal Corticosteroids

Generic Name	Trade Name	Route of Administration	Average Adult Dosage
Glucosteroids			
betamethasone acetate	Celestrone®	PO, IM, IV, Topical	PO: 0.6–7.2 mg/day; IM/IV: 0.5–9 mg/day as sodium phosphate; Topical: Apply thin film b.i.d.
cortisone acetate	Cortone®	PO, IM	20–300 mg/day in 1 or more div. doses, try to reduce periodically by 10–25 mg/day to lowest effective dose
dexamethasone	Decadron®, Maxidex®	PO, IM	PO: 0.25–4 mg b.i.d. to q.i.d.; IM: 8–16 mg q1–3wk or 0.8–1.6 mg intralesional q1–3 wk
methylprednisolone	Medrol®	PO	5–60 mg/day in single or divided doses
prednisone	Prelone® Aristocort®	PO	0.1–0.15 mg/kg/day
triamcinolone	Kenacort®	PO, IM, SC	4–48 mg 1–2 times/day

Contraindications and Precautions

Glucocorticoids are contraindicated in patients with emotional instability or psychotic tendencies, hyperlipidemia, diabetes mellitus, hypothyroidism, osteoporosis, and peptic ulcer.

Drug Interactions

Drug interactions include the increased therapeutic and toxic effects of cortisone if taken concurrently with troleandomycin. Cortisone also decreases the effects of anticholinesterases if taken concurrently with corticotropin, and profound muscular depression is possible. Steroid blood levels are decreased if cortisone is taken concurrently with phenytoin, phenobarbital, or rifampin. Decreased serum levels of salicylates are seen if it is taken concurrently with cortisone.

Key Concept

Addison's disease is a deficiency of all the hormones that are secreted from the adrenal cortex, which include cortisol, aldosterone, and androgens.

Treatment with Mineralocorticoids

Treatment with the primary mineralocorticoid (aldosterone) corrects the metabolism of sodium and potassium on renal tubular mineralocorticoid retention. This causes sodium reabsorption and potassium loss. Aldosterone is utilized in treating Addison's disease, which is a deficiency of adrenocortical secretions.

Treatment with Androgens

Androgen therapy is used for a variety of conditions, depending on gender. Androgens are primarily used to treat prostate cancer, breast cancer, and menopausal conditions. They are also often used illegally to build muscle mass.

Alterations in the Function of the Pancreas

The most important disease involving the endocrine pancreas is **diabetes mellitus**, a disorder of carbohydrate metabolism that involves either an insulin deficiency, insulin resistance, or both. Diabetes, if untreated or uncontrolled, leads to hyperglycemia. Severe hyperglycemia and ketoacidosis may produce diabetic coma or unconsciousness, which requires much higher doses of insulin.

Diabetes mellitus is a complex disorder of carbohydrate, fat, and protein metabolism caused by lack of or inefficient use of insulin in the body. The two general classifications for diabetes mellitus are type I, or insulin-dependent diabetes mellitus (IDDM), and type II, or non-insulin-dependent diabetes mellitus (NIDDM). Table 16-5 compares type I and type II diabetes.

Treatment with Insulin

Normally, insulin is used for the treatment of type I diabetics if the pancreas does not produce enough insulin. Insulin needs may vary every

TABLE 16-5 General Differences of Type I and Type II Diabetes

	Type I	Type II
Age at onset	Pre-adolescence (juvenile onset)	After age 30 years (adult onset)
Onset	Acute	Insidious
Body weight	Thin	Obese
Hereditary factors	Family history	Present in immediate family
Treatment	Insulin replacement	Diet or oral hypoglycemic agents or insulin replacement
Hypoglycemia or ketoacidosis	Often	Less common

TABLE 16-6 Insulin Preparations

Preparation	Trade Name	Onset of Action	Duration of Action
Short-acting Insulin			
Insulin (regular)	Novolin®, Humulin R®	30–60 min 15 min	6–8 hrs 6–8 hrs
Prompt insulin zinc suspension	Semilente®	60–90 min	12–16 hrs
Intermediate-acting Insulin			
Isophane insulin (NPH)	Novolin N®, Humulin N®	2 hrs, 2 hrs	18–24 hrs, 18–24 hrs
Insulin zinc suspension (lente)	Humulin L®, Novolin L®	60–150 min 60–150 min	18–24 hrs 18–24 hrs
Long-acting Insulin			
Protamine zinc insulin suspension	PZI®	4–8 hrs	36 hrs
Extended insulin zinc suspension	Ultralente®, Humulin U®	4–8 hrs	36 hrs

6 to 8 hours. Normal fasting insulin levels range from 80 to 100 mg/dL. Insulin preparations are available from three different species, including cows, pigs, and humans. Human insulin now is produced by chemical conversion from porcine insulin and by *Escherichia coli*, into which the human genes for insulin have been inserted. The recombinant product has the same physiological properties as insulin from beef or pork but is much less likely to cause allergic reactions. Insulins are classified based on their time of pharmacological action as short-acting, intermediate-acting, and long-acting. Most diabetic patients require a combination of short- and long-acting insulin. Table 16-6 shows varieties of insulins and their properties.

Key Concept

The most diagnostic sign of type I diabetes is sustained hyperglycemia. Fasting blood glucose levels of 126 mg/dL or greater on at least two separate occasions is diagnostic for diabetes.

Special Consideration

Patients who will be using insulin must be instructed on the rotation method of taking their medication. Insulin is absorbed more rapidly in the arm or thigh, especially with exercise. The abdomen is used for a more consistent absorption. Glucose levels should be checked per physician instructions. All insulin should be checked for expiration date and clearness. Insulin should not be given if it appears cloudy. Vials should not be shaken but rotated in between the hands to mix contents.

Key Concept

Hypoglycemic reactions may occur at any time, but most commonly occur when insulin is at its peak activity.

If regular insulin is to be mixed with NPH or lente insulin, the regular insulin should be drawn into the syringe first. Unopened vials should be stored in the refrigerator and freezing should be avoided. The vial in use can be stored at room temperature. Vials should not be put in glove compartments, suitcases, or trunks. It is imperative that the physician be called if any adverse reactions to the medications are observed.

Mechanism of Action

The primary action of insulin is to promote the entry of glucose into cells.

> ***Medical Terminology Review***
>
> **ketoacidosis**
>
> *keto = ketone; ketone group*
> *acid = having a pH below 7.0*
> *osis = condition; process; action*
>
> a condition of metabolic acidosis caused by high concentrations of ketone bodies

Indications

Insulin is used to control hyperglycemia in the diabetic patient, and for the emergency treatment of acute ketoacidosis. It may be administered intravenously or subcutaneously. Regular insulin is also available as Humulin 70/30 (a mixture of 70 percent isophane insulin and 30 percent regular insulin) or as Humulin 50/50 (a mixture of 50 percent of both isophane and regular insulin).

Adverse Effects

The most dangerous adverse effect of insulin therapy is hypoglycemia. The other adverse effects include tachycardia, sweating, drowsiness, and confusion. If severe hypoglycemia is not immediately treated with glucose, convulsions, coma, and death may occur.

Contraindications and Precautions

Insulin is contraindicated in patients with hypersensitivity to insulin animal protein. It is also contraindicated during episodes of hypoglycemia. Insulin should be used with caution in patients with insulin-resistant hyperthyroidism or hypothyroidism, during lactation, in older adults, during pregnancy (category B), and in those with renal or hepatic impairment.

Drug Interactions

Alcohol, anabolic steroids, MAOIs, and salicylates may potentiate hypoglycemic effects. Dextrothyroxine, corticosteroids, and epinephrine may antagonize hypoglycemic effects. Herbals such as garlic and ginseng may potentiate the hypoglycemic effects of insulin.

Oral Antidiabetic Agents

Type II diabetic patients are treated with the oral antidiabetics (oral hypoglycemic medications) and diet. The five classes of oral hypoglycemic medications given for type II diabetes are sulfonylureas, alpha-glucosidase inhibitors, biguanides, meglitinides, and thiazolidinediones. Table 16-7 shows some examples of oral hypoglycemic agents and their duration of action.

TABLE 16-7 Oral Hypoglycemic Agents

Generic Name	Trade Name	Route of Administration	Average Adult Dosage
Sulfonylureas First-generation			
acetohexamide	Dymelor®	PO	250 mg–1.5 g/day
chlorpropamide	Diabinese®	PO	100–250 mg/day (with breakfast)
tolazamide	Tolinase®	PO	100–1000 mg q.d.–b.i.d.
tolbutamide	Orinase®	PO	250 mg to 3 g/day in 1–2 div. doses
Second-generation			
glimepiride	Amaryl®	PO	Initial: 1–2 mg/day with breakfast; may increase to maint. dose of 1–4 mg q.d. (max: 8 mg/day)
glipizide	Glucotrol®, Glucotrol XL®	PO	2.5–5 mg 1–2 times/day
glyburide	DiaBeta®, Glynase®	PO	1.25–5 mg with breakfast
Alpha-glucosidase Inhibitors			
acarbose	Precose®	PO	Start with 25 mg t.i.d. (with meals)
miglitol	Glyset®	PO	25 mg t.i.d. at the start of each meal
Biguanides			
metformin hydrochloride	Glucophage®	PO	500–850 mg/day
Meglitinides			
nateglinide	Starlix®	PO	60–120 mg t.i.d.
repaglinide	Prandin®	PO	0.5–4.0 mg b.i.d.-q.i.d.
Thiazolidinediones			
pioglitazone hydrochloride	Actos®	PO	15–30 mg/day
rosiglitazone maleate	Avandia®	PO	2–4 mg q.d.-b.i.d.
Combination Drugs			
glipizide/metformin	Metaglip	PO	2.5 mg glipizide/250 mg metaformin per day
glyburide/metformin	Glucovance®	PO	1.25 to 5 mg glyburide/250 to 500 mg metformin per dayq. d.-b.i.d.
rosiglitazone maleate/ metformin	Avandamet®	PO	1 to 4 mg rosiglitazone maleate/500 mg metformin per day

Mechanism of Action

Oral hypoglycemic agents stimulate the pancreas to secrete more insulin and increase the sensitivity of insulin receptors in target tissues.

Indications

The advantages of using the second-generation agents are that they have a long duration of action and have fewer side effects. First generation drugs are rarely used today. Of the first-generation agents, tolazamide also has advantages similar to those of the second-generation drugs. Oral hypoglycemic agents are indicated for the treatment of uncomplicated type II diabetes in patients whose diabetes cannot be controlled by diet or exercise only.

Adverse Effects

Adverse effects include nausea, vomiting, headache, blurred vision, sedation, confusion, anxiety, nightmares, and tachycardia.

Contraindications and Precautions

Oral hypoglycemic agents are contraindicated in patients who are receiving sulfonamide or thiazide-type diuretics, who are hypersensitive to the agents, and who have acidosis, severe burns, or severe diarrhea. These agents should be used cautiously in patients with high fevers, severe infections, hyperthyroidism, or kidney function impairment.

Drug Interactions

Oral hypoglycemic medications have the potential to interact with a number of drugs; thus, the patient should always consult with a health care practitioner before adding a new medication or herbal supplement. Ingestion of alcohol will result in distressing symptoms that include headache, nausea, abdominal pain, and flushing.

Behavior Modification for Diabetes

Because diabetes is a lifelong disorder, education of the patient and the family is probably the most important obligation of the physician who provides initial care. This disease is markedly affected on a daily basis by fluctuations in environmental stress, exercise, diet, and the presence of infections. Therefore, the best persons to monitor and manage the disease are the patients themselves and their families.

SUMMARY

The endocrine system provides a means of chemical communication between body parts. The anterior pituitary gland controls activities of the thyroid, adrenals, and sex glands. It also stimulates growth, development, and tissue repair. The pituitary is called the master gland for these reasons. Pituitary activity is governed by the hypothalamus in the brain.

Hyperpituitarism causes an excess of growth hormone. This condition, if present before puberty, results in gigantism. In an adult, excessive production of growth hormone leads to acromegaly.

Severe hypopituitarism impedes growth and development in a child, causing dwarfism. Glands that depend on stimulation by the anterior pituitary are the thyroid, adrenal, and sex glands. The posterior pituitary gland releases vasopressin, also called antidiuretic hormone (ADH), and oxytocin. Insufficiency of ADH causes diabetes insipidus.

The rate of metabolism is controlled by the thyroid gland. An enlargement of this gland is called a goiter. Hyperthyroidism, which is an excess of thyroxine, accelerates heart and respiratory activity, increases metabolic rate, and raises body temperature. A congenital lack of thyroxine results in cretinism (mental and physical retardation). Myxedema is a disease of severe hypothyroidism in an adult.

Hormones of the adrenal cortex are essential to life. Aldosterone regulates salt balance and cortisol affects the metabolism of nutrients. The sex hormones estrogen and androgen are also produced by this gland. Hypoactivity of the adrenal cortex is called Addison's disease.

Hyperactivity of the adrenal cortex causes different diseases, depending on which hormones are in excess amounts. Cushing's syndrome results from an excess of cortisol, and Conn's syndrome results from excessive aldosterone. Precocious puberty and adrenal virilism develop from too much androgen secretion.

PTH regulates the level of circulating calcium and phosphate. Hyperactivity of the parathyroid glands causes hypercalcemia. The high level of calcium comes primarily from bone resorption that weakens the bones. Hypoparathyroidism reduces the level of calcium in the blood, which results in tetany. Hormones of the pancreas, insulin, and glucagon control blood sugar level. Lack of insulin causes an increase in blood glucose levels, the condition called diabetes mellitus.

Hypoglycemia, an abnormally low blood glucose level, results from excess insulin. This condition can develop in the diabetic patient from an overdosage of insulin.

With the loss of calcium, the bones are weakened. They tend to bend, become deformed, and fracture spontaneously. Excessive calcium causes the formation of kidney stones because calcium forms insoluble compounds. Calcium deposited within the walls of the blood vessels makes them hard. It may also be found in the stomach and lungs.

The therapy for hyperparathyroidism often includes surgery. However, phosphate supplementation and/or potent diuretics, such as furosemide (Lasix), may be administered to promote an increase in the excretion of excess calcium. Calcitonin may also be used to treat hypercalcemia.

Exploring the Web

Visit *www.endocrineweb.com*

- Look for additional readings and information of the various endocrine glands and the disorders that may occur when they malfunction.

Visit *www.nlm.nih.gov/medlineplus*

- Search for articles related to the topics addressed in this chapter.

Visit *www.pituitary.org*

- Review the FAQs and disorders discussed at this site to further your understanding of the function of the pituitary gland.

Review Questions

Multiple Choice

1. Which of the following is secreted from the pancreas?

A. prolactin
B. growth hormone
C. glucagon
D. calcitonin

2. Another name for vasopressin is:

A. testosterone
B. cortisol
C. prolactin
D. antidiuretic hormone

3. FSH and LH are released from which of the following organs?

A. hypothalamus
B. pituitary
C. ovaries
D. pancreas

4. Which of the following is a protein?
   A. testosterone
   B. androgen
   C. growth hormone
   D. cortisol

5. Which of the following hormones is stored in posterior parts of the pituitary gland?
   A. oxytocin
   B. growth hormone
   C. prolactin
   D. cortisol

6. The glucocorticoid hormones are under the control of:
   A. LH
   B. TSH
   C. ACTH
   D. FSH

7. Which of the following is a side effect of corticosteroids?
   A. delayed healing with infection
   B. hypotension
   C. weight loss
   D. hypertrophy of the adrenal cortex

8. Which of the following is the trade name of methimazole?
   A. Cytomel
   B. Tapazole
   C. Propyl-Thyracil
   D. Celestrone

9. Glucophage is the trade name of:
   A. metformin
   B. miglitol
   C. glimepiride
   D. glipizide

10. Which of the following agents is used for the diagnosis and treatment of hyperthyroidism?
    A. thyroxin
    B. sodium iodide
    C. parathyroid hormone
    D. phenytoin

11. Propylthiouracil (PTU) is chemically related to which of the following drugs?
    A. antineoplastic
    B. antithyroid
    C. antiparathyroid
    D. antidiuretic

12. The mechanism of action of oral hypoglycemic medications is to:
    - **A.** increase insulin production in the pancreas
    - **B.** decrease insulin secretion from the pancreas
    - **C.** release insulin into the bloodstream
    - **D.** stimulate insulin release from the pancreas
13. All of the following include intermediate-acting insulin, except:
    - **A.** NPH (Humulin)
    - **B.** Lente L
    - **C.** Humulin N
    - **D.** Crystalline zinc
14. Which of the following is the trade name of chlorpropamide?
    - **A.** Diabinese
    - **B.** Dymelor
    - **C.** Tolinase
    - **D.** Glucotrol
15. Which of the following is the most serious adverse effect of insulin?
    - **A.** hyperthermia
    - **B.** hyperthyroidism
    - **C.** hyperglycemia
    - **D.** hypoglycemia

Matching

_____ **1.** Adrenal cortex	**A.** Prolactin
_____ **2.** Thyroid	**B.** Glucagon
_____ **3.** Neurohypophysis	**C.** Norepinephrine
_____ **4.** Beta cells of pancreas	**D.** Aldosterone
_____ **5.** Alpha cells of pancreas	**E.** Insulin
_____ **6.** Adrenal medulla	**F.** Oxytocin
_____ **7.** Anterior lobe of pituitary	**G.** Calcitonin

Critical Thinking

A 43-year-old woman is experiencing chills, weight gain, and a general feeling of weakness, as well as an enlarged thyroid gland. Her physician diagnoses her with *hypothyroidism*.

1. List the most common causes of hypothyroidism.
2. Explain the common treatments for this condition.
3. If the patient were to refuse treatment, what would be the consequence?

Hormones of the Reproductive System and Contraceptives

CHAPTER 17

OUTLINE

(continues)

OBJECTIVES

After completing this chapter, the reader should be able to:

1. Explain the relationship between the anterior pituitary gland and the ovaries.
2. Describe the classes of sex hormones in both males and females.
3. Describe four indications for prescribing estrogens.
4. Discuss common adverse effects accompanying the use of estrogens.
5. Describe four indications for progestational drugs.
6. Explain four indications of androgens.
7. Discuss the therapeutic uses of anabolic drugs.
8. Explain the regulation of the menstrual cycle.
9. Describe the contraindications and precautions of oral contraceptives.
10. List five common sexually transmitted diseases and define them.

GLOSSARY

Amenorrhea – the absence of a menstrual period in a woman of reproductive age

Depot-medroxyprogesterone acetate (Depo-Provera®) – a long-acting progestin

Estrogen – substances capable of producing sexual receptivity in female individuals

Follicle-stimulating hormone (FSH) – a hormone synthesized and secreted by gonadotropes in the anterior pituitary gland; in females, it stimulates the maturation of Graafian follicles; in males, it is critical for spermatogenesis

Gonadotropes – cells in the anterior pituitary gland that produce the gonadotropins known as luteinizing hormone and follicle-stimulating hormone

Gonadotropin-releasing hormone (GnRH) – stimulates the release of FSH and LH from the anterior pituitary gland

Graafian follicles – matured and grown ovarian follicles; these egg-containing tubes grown and develop between puberty, sexual maturation, and menopause

OUTLINE *(continued)*

Hypogonadism – a condition of little or no production of sex hormones, usually due to poor function or inactivity of either the testes or the ovaries

Hypoprothrombinemic – the amount of prothrombin factor II in the circulating blood

Progesterone – secreted primarily by the ovarian cells in the corpus luteum at the time of ovulation during the female reproductive years

Testosterone – stimulates the development of the male secondary sex characteristics, initiates the production of sperm, and enhances the functional capacity of the penis and accessory sex organs

Overview

The female and male reproductive systems are controlled by a small number of hormones, particularly those secreted by the hypothalamus and the anterior pituitary glands. These hormones can be produced with natural or synthetic hormones to achieve therapeutic goals ranging from the prevention of pregnancy to milk production or even replacement therapy.

Anatomy Review

- The female reproductive system is composed of two ovaries, two fallopian tubes, the uterus, and the vagina (Figure 17-1).
- The male reproductive system is composed of two testes, seminal ducts, glands, and the penis (Figure 17-2).
- The functions of the reproductive system are to create new life through reproduction and to manufacture hormones responsible for the development of reproductive organs and secondary sex characteristics (Figure 17-3).

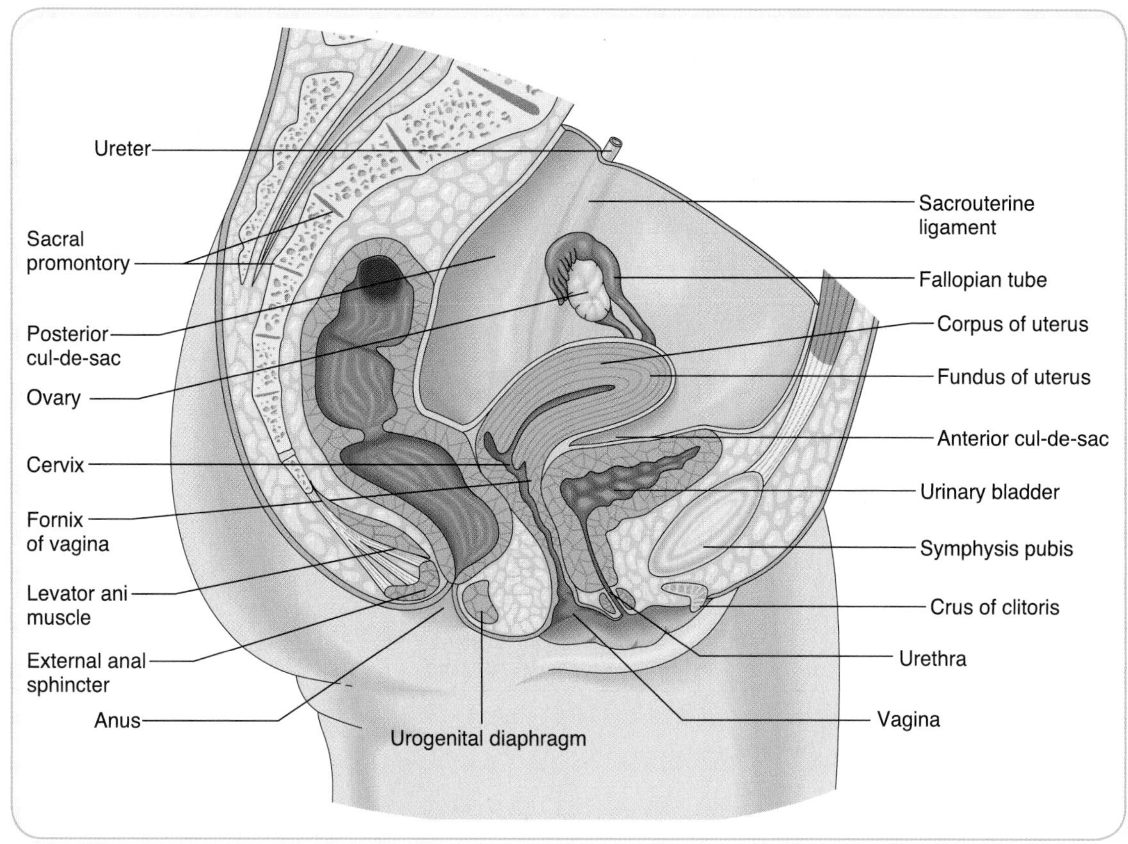

Figure 17-1 The female reproductive system.

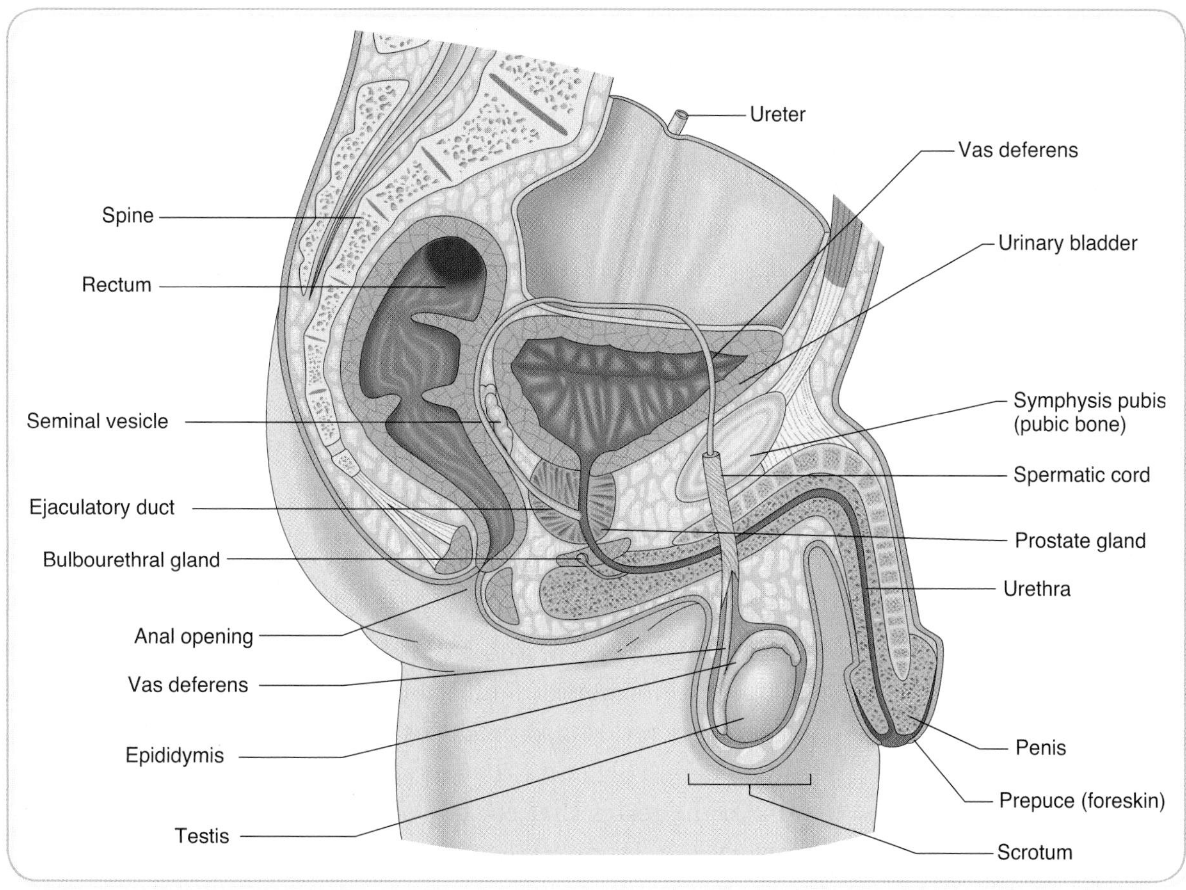

Figure 17-2 The male reproductive system.

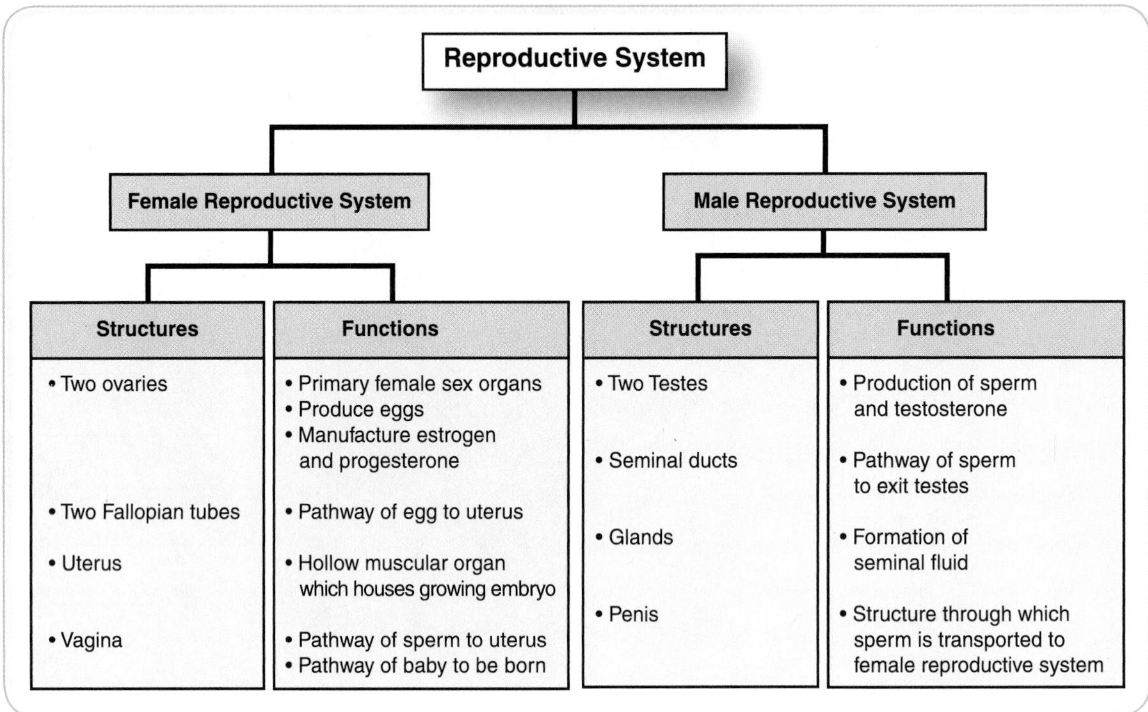

Figure 17-3 The reproductive system.

Gonadal Hormones

Three main classes of steroid hormones are produced by gonadal tissues: estrogenic, progestational, and androgenic. The ovary is the primary site for synthesis and secretion of **estrogen** and **progesterone** hormones in women. The menstrual cycle is regulated by the production of hypothalamic **gonadotropin-releasing hormone (GnRH)** that stimulates the release of FSH and LH from the anterior pituitary gland (Figure 17-4).

FSH stands for **follicle-stimulating hormone**, a hormone synthesized and secreted by **gonadotropes** (cells that produce protein hormones) in the anterior pituitary gland. In women, FSH stimulates the maturation of the **Graafian follicles** (maturing ovarian follicles, which are actually egg-containing tubes). In men, it is critical for spermatogenesis. In men and postmenopausal women, the principal source of estrogen is adipose tissue, in which the level of estrogens is regulated in part by the availability of androgenic precursors from the adrenal cortex. The most important androgenic hormone produced by the testes in men is **testosterone**, although the adrenal cortex also produces some androgenic hormones in both men and women. FSH and LH also regulate testosterone production by specific cells in the testes that control spermatogenesis and the development of primary and secondary sexual characteristics in men.

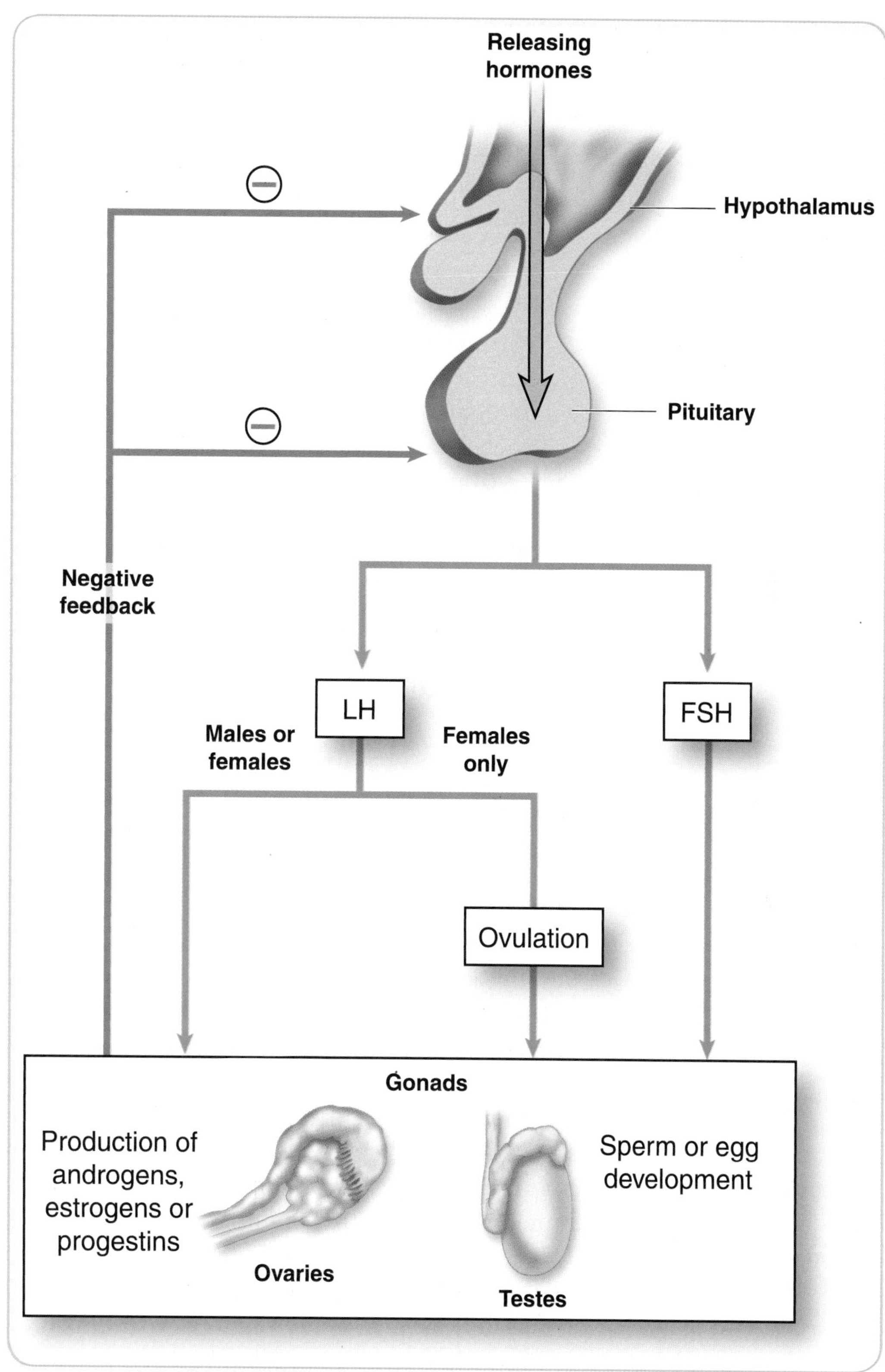

Figure 17-4 Regulation of the hormones of the reproductive system.

Oral Contraceptives

Oral contraceptives are hormone medications for the prevention of pregnancy. An oral contraceptive is commonly referred to as "the pill." Oral contraceptives include a number of estrogens and progestins, or a combination of them, to prevent ovulation.

Estrogens

Estrogens are substances capable of producing sexual receptivity in female individuals. Estrogen is involved in the development and maintenance of the female reproductive system and secondary sex characteristics. Naturally occurring estrogens include estrone, estradiol, and estriol. They are found in the blood of both males and females. Most naturally occurring estrogens are not effective when administered orally, because they are rapidly inactivated by the liver. Chemical derivatives of the natural estrogens, such as ethinyl estradiol and mestranol, are only slowly inactivated by the liver and may be administered orally. The natural estrogens and their derivatives may be administered by the intramuscular or subcutaneous route.

Mechanism of Action

Estrogen binds to intracellular receptors that stimulate DNA and RNA to synthesize proteins responsible for effects of estrogen.

Indications

Estrogens can be used for a variety of conditions. They are used for the treatment of **amenorrhea**, dysfunctional uterine bleeding, and hirsuitism, as well as the palliative treatment of breast cancer and prostate cancer. They are sometimes used for the relief of menopausal symptoms and for the prevention of osteoporosis. The beneficial effects of estrogen therapy on irritability, depression, anxiety, memory, and insomnia are more unpredictable. It is not clear whether estrogen administration can prevent arteriosclerotic cardiovascular disease. There is a choice of compounds for estrogenic therapy. Major estrogens are listed in Table 17-1. Recently, they have been of value in maintaining healthy cardiac status of women during menopause. Estrogens are also used in primary ovarian failure, atrophic vaginitis, **hypogonadism**, atrophic urethritis, and prostate cancer.

Medical Terminology Review

amenorrhea
a(-) = absence; lack; not
menorrhea = normal flow of blood during menstruation
absence of blood flow during menstruation

hypogonadism
hypo = slow, under developer
gonad = sexual organs
ism = condition
condition of underdeveloped sexual organs

Adverse Effects

The most common adverse effects are nausea, vomiting, breast swelling, fluid retention (weight gain), hypertension, and thromboembolic disorders. Other adverse effects include leg cramps, intolerance to contact lenses, spotting, changes in menstrual flow, dysmenorrhea, and amenorrhea.

Medical Terminology Review

thromboembolic
thrombo = blood clot
embolic = condition of a mass in the bloodstream
a blood clot in the bloodstream

TABLE 17-1 Major Estrogens

Generic Name	Trade Name	Route of Administration	Average Adult Dosage
estradiol	Estraderm®, Estrace®	PO, Transdermal patch	Estraderm: 0.45–2 mg twice weekly 0.45–2 mg q.d. in a cyclic regimen (21 days on, 7 days off)
estrogen, conjugated	Premarin®	PO	0.3–1.25 mg q.d. in a cyclic regimen (21 days on, 7 days off)
estropipate	Ogen®, Ortho-Est®	PO	0.75–6 mg q.d. in a cyclic regimen (21 days on, 7 days off)
estradiol cypionate	Dep-Gynogen®, Depogen®	IM	1–5 mg q3–4 weeks
estradiol valerate	Delestrogen®, Duragen-10®, Valergen®	PO	0.45–2 mg/day in a cyclic regimen (21 days on, 7 days off)
ethinyl estradiol	Estinyl®, Feminone®	PO	0.02–0.05 mg q.d. in a cyclic regimen (21 days on, 7 days off)

Contraindications and Precautions

Estrogens should not be used in patients who have a sensitivity to any of the ingredients, are pregnant, or have breast cancer, undiagnosed abnormal uterine bleeding, thrombophlebitis, and thromboembolic disorders.

Drug Interactions

Barbiturates, phenytoin, and rifampin decrease estrogen effects by increasing estrogen metabolism. Oral anticoagulants may decrease **hypoprothrombinemic** (the amount of prothrombin factor II in the circulating blood) effects due to interaction with estrogen. Estrogen may also interfere with the effects of bromocriptine and cause toxicity of cyclosporine.

Progesterone

Progesterone is secreted primarily by the ovarian cells in the corpus luteum at the time of ovulation during the female reproductive years. The corpus luteum secretes progesterone only during the last two weeks of the menstrual cycle. The greatest amount is secreted during the week after ovulation has taken place. Progesterone is responsible for the changes in the uterine endometrium during the second half of the menstrual cycle, the development of the maternal placenta after implantation, and the development of the mammary glands. Progesterone also causes an increase in the viscosity of cervical secretions, which impedes the movement of sperm. Progesterone in high doses suppresses the pituitary release of LH and the hypothalamic release of GnRH, thus preventing ovulation. Progesterone also decreases uterine motility. A synthetic form of progesterone produced by a chemical modification is needed because the natural type of hormone would be inactivated by the liver. These synthetic preparations are called progestins.

Mechanism of Action

Progesterone changes the uterine lining (endometrium) from a proliferative structure to a secretory one. If fertilization does not take place, the corpus luteum diminishes in size, progesterone and estrogen production drop, and menstruation follows.

Indications

Progesterone is used in irregular uterine bleeding and is combined with estrogen for the treatment of amenorrhea. It is also used in cases of infertility and threatened or habitual abortion. Progesterone is indicated in the treatment of endometriosis and premenstrual syndrome.

Key Concept

Progesterone can cause changes in vision, ptosis, diplopia, and retinal vascular lesions.

Adverse Effects

Common adverse effects include migraine headache, dizziness, lethargy, mental depression, and insomnia. Thromboembolic disorder and pulmonary embolism may occur with administration of progesterone.

Contraindications and Precautions

Progesterone is contraindicated in patients with thrombophlebitis, liver disease, breast cancer, reproductive organ cancer, undiagnosed vaginal bleeding, missed periods, and a hypersensitivity to the medication or any of its ingredients. Use during pregnancy and breastfeeding is not recommended. Progesterone should be used cautiously in patients who suffer from anemia and diabetes mellitus, or have a history of psychic depression. Progesterone should be used with caution in patients with asthma, seizure disorders, and cardiac or kidney dysfunction. This agent must be used cautiously in patients with impaired liver function, previous ectopic pregnancy, venereal disease, and unresolved abnormal Pap smear. Table 17-2 shows the most commonly used progestins.

Drug Interactions

Ketoconazole may inhibit progesterone metabolism. Barbiturates, carbamazepine, phenytoin, and rifampin may alter contraceptive effectiveness.

Estrogen and Progesterone Combinations

Combinations of estrogens and progestins may be used as oral contraceptives in women. This method is nearly 100 percent effective in preventing pregnancy when used as directed. Oral contraceptives contain various amounts of estrogen and progestins. The estrogen inhibits ovulation

TABLE 17-2 Most Commonly Used Progestins

Generic Name	Trade Name	Route of Administration	Average Adult Dosage
medroxyprogesterone acetate	Provera®, Depo-Provera®	PO, SC	PO: 5–10 mg/day; SC: one injection every 3 months
norethindrone	Norlutin®	PO	5–20 mg on day 5 through day 25 of menstrual cycle
progesterone	Gesterol®	PO, IM	PO: 400 mg h.s. x 10 days; IM: 5–10 mg for 6–8 consecutive days

by suppressing the normal secretion of FSH. The progestin inhibits pituitary secretion of LH, causes changes in the cervical mucus that makes it unfavorable to penetration by the sperm, and alters the nature of the endometrium.

Mechanism of Action

Fixed combinations of estrogen and progestin produce contraception by preventing ovulation and rendering reproductive tract structures hostile to sperm penetration and zygote implantation.

Indications

The use of estrogen-progestin combinations in a cyclic fashion generally results in the inhibition of conception without preventing menstruation. Most oral contraceptives are taken daily for 20 to 21 days, starting on the fifth day after menstrual bleeding begins. Also available are oral contraceptives with 28-day pill cycles, wherein a pill is taken every day of the cycle so that once started, the pill is not stopped. In the 28-day pill cycle, an inactive pill is taken during the week of menstruation, whereas with the 20- to 21-day pill there is a week without medication, and this is when menstruation takes place. The use of oral contraceptives containing only a progestin has been advocated as a means of reducing some of the risk associated with their use. These products, which are sometimes referred to as "minipills," are generally taken continuously rather than cyclically. Because they contain no estrogen, they do not suppress ovulation. Table 17-3 shows the most commonly used contraceptive agents.

Depot-medroxyprogesterone acetate (Depo-Provera) is a long-acting progestin. It is the injectable long-acting progestin which is approved for contraceptive use in the U.S. There has been extensive worldwide experience with this method over the past three decades. The medication is given as a deep intramuscular injection of 150 mg every three months and has a contraceptive efficacy of 99.7 percent. It has been proven safe and relatively inexpensive. Many women find this method more convenient than the daily oral contraceptives.

TABLE 17-3 Commonly Used Contraceptive Agents

Generic Name	Trade Name	Route of Administration	Average Adult Dosage
Monophasic Agents			
ethinyl estradiol/ drospirenone	Yasmin®	PO	0.03 mg ethinyl estradiol with 3 mg drospirenone taken cyclically (as above)
ethinyl estradiol/ ethynodiol	Zovia®, Demulen®	PO	0.035 mg or 0.05 mg ethynyl estradiol with 1 mg ethynodiol diacetate taken cyclically (as above)
ethinyl estradiol/ levonorgestrel	Alesse®, Nordette®	PO	0.02 mg ethinyl estradiol with 0.10 mg levonorgestrel taken cyclically (as above)
ethinyl estradiol/ norelgestromin	Ortho-Evra®	Transdermal patch	0.75 mg ethinyl estradiol with 6 mg norelgestromin; apply 1 patch for 21 days followed by a 7 day interval with no patch
ethinyl estradiol/ norethindrone (various strengths)	Ovcon®, Loestrin®,	PO	0.035 mg ethinyl estradiol with varying amounts of norethindrone taken cyclically (21 days on, 7 days off)
mestranol/ norethindrone	Necon 1/50®, Ortho-Novum 1/50®	PO	0.05 mg mestranol with 1 mg norethindrone taken cyclically (as above)
Biphasic Agents			
ethinyl estradiol/ norethindrone	Ortho-Novum 10/11®, Nelova 10/11®	PO	First 10 tablets contain 0.035 mg ethinyl estradiol and 0.5 mg norethindrone; the next 11 pills contain 0.035 mg ethinyl estradiol and 1 mg norethindrone; taken cyclically (as above)
Triphasic Agents			
ethinyl estradiol/ levonorgestrel	Triphasil®, Tri-Levlen®	PO	First 6 tablets contain 0.03 mg ethinyl estradiol and 0.05 mg levonorgestrel; the next 5 tablets contain 0.04 mg ethinyl estradiol and 0.075 mg levonorgestrel; the final 10 tablets contain 0.03 mg ethinyl estradiol and 0.125 mg levonorgestrel; taken cyclically (as above)
ethinyl estradiol/ norgestimate	Ortho Tri-cyclin®	PO	In this product, the amount of ethinyl estradiol remains constant at 0.035 mg per tablet, while the norgestimate increases from 0.18 mg per tablet to 0.25 mg; taken cyclically (as above)

(continues)

TABLE 17-3 Commonly Used Contraceptive Agents—*continued*

Generic Name	Trade Name	Route of Administration	Average Adult Dosage
Estrophasic Agents			
ethinyl estradiol/ norethindrone acetate	Estrostep®	PO	In this product, the amount of ethinyl estradiol changes from 0.02 to 0.03 and then to 0.035 mg per tablet, while the norethindrone acetate remains constant at 1 mg per tablet; taken cyclically (as above)
Progestin-only Agents			
norethindrone	Micronor®, Nor-QD®	PO	1 tablet of 0.35 mg/day (each package lasts 28 days with no stoppage in between packages)
norgestrel	Ovrette®	PO	0.75 mg/day
Long-acting Agents			
intrauterine progesterone contraceptive system	Progestasert®	IUD	38 mg IUD inserted by a healthcare professional – lasts for 12 months
medroxyprogesterone	Depo-Provera®	IM	150 mg/mL q13 weeks
medroxyprogesterone with estradiol	Lunelle®	IM	0.5 mL/month; first injection given during first 5 days of menstruation; follow-up injections every 28 to 33 days

Adverse Effects

The classic adverse effects associated with birth control drugs are nausea, weight gain, and breast tenderness, which result from the progesterone they contain. Other adverse effects include fluid retention, irregular vaginal bleeding, and skin discoloration. The most serious adverse effects of oral contraceptives include heart attack, stroke, hypertension, or other forms of thromboembolic disease. Table 17-4 summarizes the dose-related effects of oral contraceptives.

Contraindications and Precautions

Contraceptives are contraindicated in pregnancy (category X), lactation, and missed abortion. These agents should be avoided in individuals with familial or personal history of or existence of breast cancer. Patients with diabetes mellitus, hypertension, or hypercholesterolemia (increased blood cholesterol levels) should not take contraceptive agents. Before the use of any hormonal type of contraception, the patient should have a complete history and physical examination performed. The patient should be informed of the precautions, warnings, and adverse effects.

TABLE 17-4 Dose Related Adverse Effects of Oral Contraceptives

Estrogen excess	Progestin excess
Nausea	Increased appetite
Hypertension	Weight gain
Breast tenderness	Fatigue
Edema	Acne
Migraine headache	Hair loss
	Depression
Estrogen deficiency	**Progestin deficiency**
Early or mid-cycle bleeding	Late breakthrough bleeding
Increased spotting	Amenorrhea
Hypomenorrhea	Hypermenorrhea

Smoking increases the risk of serious adverse effects on the heart and blood vessels from oral contraceptive use. The risk increases with age and heavy smoking (15 or more cigarettes per day), and is quite marked in women older than 35 years of age.

Drug Interactions

Several drugs interact with oral contraceptive agents. Some commonly prescribed drugs in this category are phenytoin, phenobarbital (and other barbiturates), primidone, carbamazepine, and rifampin. Women taking these drugs should use another means of contraception for maximum safety.

Drugs Used During Labor and Delivery

Generally, two types of medications are used during labor and delivery: uterine stimulants and uterine relaxants.

Uterine Stimulants

Uterine stimulants cause contractions of the myometrium during labor and delivery. Many agents are capable of stimulating the smooth muscle of the uterus, but a few are selective, to be used for the myometrium. These agents are known as oxytocic substances.

Mechanism of Action

Oxytocin injection, by direct action on the myometrium, produces phasic contractions characteristic of normal delivery. It also promotes milk ejection (letdown) reflex in nursing mothers, thereby increasing flow (not volume) of milk.

Indications

Oxytocic agents are used to initiate or improve uterine contraction at term only in carefully selected patients and only after the cervix is dilated and presentation of the fetus has occurred. These agents are also indicated to relieve pain from breast engorgement and control of postpartum hemorrhage and promotion of postpartum uterine involution. Oxytocic agents are often used to induce labor in cases of maternal diabetes, pre-eclampsia, and eclampsia.

Adverse Effects

Oxytocic agents may stimulate contractions of the uterus and cause fetal trauma from rapid pushing (forward) through the pelvis. This can result in fetal death. Adverse effects of these agents may result in anaphylactic reactions, postpartum hemorrhage, edema, fetal bradycardia, maternal cardiac arrhythmias, and hypertensive episodes.

Contraindications and Precautions

Oxytocic agents are contraindicated in patients with hypersensitivity to them. These agents should be avoided in unfavorable fetal position or presentations that are undeliverable without conversion before delivery, and fetal distress in which delivery is not imminent, prematurity, placenta previa, and previous surgery of uterus or cesarean section. Oxytocic drugs should be used with caution in concomitant use of cyclopropane anesthesia or vasoconstrictive drugs.

Key Concept

Herbals such as ephedra and mahuang may interact with oxytocic drugs, causing hypertension.

Drug Interactions

Oxytocic drugs may interact with vasoconstrictors and cause severe hypertension. Oxytocic agents with clopropane anesthesia cause hypotension, maternal bradycardia, and other types of arrhythmias.

Uterine Relaxants

Uterine relaxants are prescribed in the management of preterm labor. These agents decrease uterine contraction and prolong the pregnancy for developing the fetus in full term. Two agents are currently used as uterine relaxants: ritodrine (Yutopar) and terbutaline (Brethine).

Mechanism of Action

Uterine relaxants preferentially stimulate β_2-receptors in uterine smooth muscle, reducing intensity and frequency of uterine contractions.

Indications

Uterine relaxants are used to delay preterm labor in pregnancies of greater than 20 weeks' gestation.

Adverse Effects

Uterine relaxants often alter fetal and maternal heart rates and maternal blood pressure. Common adverse effects of these drugs include nausea, vomiting, nervousness, restlessness, headache, and palpitations.

Contraindications and Precautions

Uterine relaxants are contraindicated in patients with hypersensitivity, and those with antepartum hemorrhage, eclampsia, asthma, and in pregnancies of less than 20 weeks' gestation. Uterine relaxants should be used cautiously in concomitant use of potassium-depleting diuretics and in patients with cardiac disease.

Drug Interactions

Uterine relaxants interact with corticosteroids and may precipitate pulmonary edema. These agents are able to decrease effectiveness when given with a β-adrenergic blocking drug such as propranolol.

Drugs Used in the Treatment of Sexually Transmitted Diseases

Sexually transmitted diseases (STDs) commonly include gonorrhea, chlamydia, syphilis, genital herpes and warts, and trichomoniasis. All of these diseases are spread by sexual contact. Overall, STDs are on the increase, attributable to more people engaging in premarital sex, higher divorce

TABLE 17-5 Common Sexually Transmitted Diseases

Infection	Cause	Cure or Treatment
Chlamydia	Chlamydia C. trachomatis	Antimicrobial therapy such as azithromycin; to eradicate, retesting is necessary
Genital Herpes	Virus Herpes simplex 2 (HSV-2)	No cure; treatment with antiviral drugs such as oral acyclovir, which reduces activity and shedding
Genital Warts	Virus Human papillomavirus (HPV)	Rarely cured; warts can be removed
Gonorrhea	Bacterium N. gonorrhoeae	Antibacterial drugs such as penicillin or ceftriaxone plus doxycycline; there are some drug-resistant strains; to eradicate, retesting is necessary
Syphilis	Bacterium T. pallidum	Penicillin G (long-acting); to eradicate, retesting is necessary
Trichomoniasis	Protozoa T. vaginalis	Antimicrobial drugs such as metronidazole

rates, and increased numbers of sexual partners. The avoidance of using contraceptive devices is a common factor that leads to STDs being transmitted. Other infections, such as hepatitis B and HIV, can also be spread through sexual contact.

Many STDs are asymptomatic, and a person may be unaware that they are carrying a disease. In addition, certain infections may be transmitted from an infected woman to her fetus or newborn. Recurrent infections due to a lack of immunity to many STDs occur frequently, and an individual may have more than one STD at a given time. See Table 17-5 for a list of common STD infections, their causes, and their treatments.

Male Sex Hormones

The hypothalamus, anterior pituitary gland, and testes secrete hormones that control the reproductive functions of males. These hormones initiate and maintain the production of sperm cells, and oversee the development and maintenance of male secondary sex characteristics.

The hypothalamus secretes gonadotropin-releasing hormone, which enters blood vessels that lead to the anterior pituitary gland. LH and FSH are then released. Luteinizing hormone (LH) in males, also called interstitial cell-stimulating hormone (ICSH), promotes development of testicular interstitial cells, which in turn secrete male sex hormones. FSH stimulates the supporting cells of the seminiferous tubules to respond to the effects of the male sex hormone testosterone.

Androgens are secreted mainly in the interstitial tissue of the testes in the male, and secondarily in the adrenal glands of both sexes. Androgens include testosterone and androsterone. Inadequate production of androgens in the male may be due to pituitary malfunction. Testosterone stimulates the development of the male secondary sex characteristics, initiates the production of sperm, and enhances the functional capacity of the penis and accessory sex organs.

Mechanism of Action

Synthetic steroid compound with both androgenic and anabolic activity controls development and maintenance of secondary sexual characteristics (Table 17-6).

Indications

Male sex hormones are used for replacement therapy in androgen deficiency, for the treatment of hypogonadism and cryptorchidism, and for palliative treatment of certain metastatic breast carcinomas in women.

TABLE 17-6 Male Hormones

Generic Name	Trade Name	Route of Administration	Average Adult Dosage
Androgens			
fluoxymesterone	Halotestin®	PO	Males: hypogonadism 2.5–20 mg/day; females: breast cancer, 10–40 mg/day in div. doses
methyltestosterone	Android®	PO	Males: 10–50 mg/day or via buccal tablets, 5–25 mg/day; Females: 50–200 mg/day or via buccal tablets, 25–100 mg/day
testosterone cypionate (in oil)	Depo-Testosterone®	IM	Males: 50–200 mg/dose; Females: 200–400 mg/dose
testosterone enanthate	Delatest®	IM	50–400 mg q2–4 wk
testosterone gel	Androgel®	Topical	5–10 mg/day applied to any area of skin
testosterone transdermal system	Androderm®	Transdermal	One system applied/day
Anabolic Steroids			
nandrolone decanoate	(generic only)	IM	50–200 mg q1–4 wks
oxandrolone	Oxandrin®	PO	2.5 mg b.i.d. – q.i.d. up to 4 weeks (max: 20 mg/day)
oxymetholone	Anadrol-50®	PO	1–5 mg/kg/day
stanozolol	Winstrol®	PO	2 mg t.i.d. to 4 mg q.i.d. for 5 days; may reduce to 2 mg q.d. or q.o.d.
Androgen Hormone Inhibitor			
finasteride	Proscar®	PO	5 mg/day

Adverse Effects

Adverse effects of male hormones in males include gynecomastia, excessive frequency and duration of penile erection, oligospermia, hirsuitism, male pattern baldness, acne, increased or decreased libido, headache, anxiety, and depression. In females, adverse effects include amenorrhea, menstrual irregularities, inhibition of gonadotropin secretion, and virilization (deepening of the voice, clitoral enlargement, increased growth of facial and body hair, and male type baldness).

Contraindications and Precautions

Male hormones are contraindicated in patients with known hypersensitivity to any of its ingredients, in women during pregnancy and lactation, and in men with cancer of the breast or suspected cancer of the prostate. These agents are also contraindicated in patients with pituitary insufficiency, a history of myocardial infarction, hypercalcemia, prostatic hyperplasia, hepatic dysfunction, nephrosis, and in infants and young children. They should be used with caution in elderly patients, in diabetic patients, in those who have hypertension, coronary artery disease, renal disease, hypercholesterolemia and gynecomastia, and in prepubertal males.

Drug Interactions

Testosterone may decrease insulin requirements, and it may interact with oral anticoagulants and potentiate hypoprothrombinemia.

Anabolic Steroids

A number of compounds derived from or closely related to testosterone may exhibit considerable anabolic effects without causing significant androgenic effects. The anabolic agents, or steroids, are employed to promote weight gain in underweight individuals.

Key Concept

The use of anabolic steroids by young athletic individuals to promote an increase in muscle mass and strength is a real and dangerous problem. The abuse of anabolic steroids has caused death in young, healthy persons.

Mechanism of Action

The anabolic steroids are synthetic agents chemically similar to the androgens. These drugs promote tissue-building processes.

Indications

The anabolic steroids are prescribed for management of anemia of renal insufficiency and control of metastatic breast cancer in women.

Adverse Effects

Common adverse effects of anabolic steroids include muscle cramps, nausea, vomiting, diarrhea, anorexia, and abdominal fullness. Jaundice, hepatocellular neoplasms, an increased risk of atherosclerosis, excitation, and insomnia are the most serious adverse effects with prolonged use. Virilization in women is also the most common reaction associated with the use of anabolic steroids, especially when higher doses are used. Acne occurs often in all age groups in both sexes.

Contraindications and Precautions

Anabolic steroids are contraindicated in patients with a known hypersensitivity, serious cardiac disorder, liver impairment, and in men with prostate cancer or enlargement. These agents should not be used during pregnancy (category X) and lactation. Anabolic steroids should be used cautiously in benign prostatic hypertrophy and in patients with a history of myocardial infarction.

Drug Interactions

Anabolic steroids may interact with anticoagulants and increase their effects. These agents may decrease insulin and sulfonylurea requirements.

Androgen Hormone Inhibitors

Androgen hormone inhibitors such as finasteride (Propecia, Proscar) are synthetic substitutes that are known as antiandrogens.

Mechanism of Action

Finasteride prevents the conversion of testosterone into the potent steroid 5-alpha dihydrotestosterone in the prostate gland.

Indications

Finasteride is used in the treatment of benign prostatic hypertrophy. Androgen inhibitors are also used for the prevention of male pattern baldness in men with early signs of hair loss.

Adverse Effects

The adverse effects of finasteride are usually mild. In some patients, the adverse effects may be impotence, decreased libido, and a decreased volume of ejaculate.

Contraindications and Precautions

Finasteride is contraindicated in patients with hypersensitivity to these agents, in pregnant women (Category X), and during lactation. These agents should be used cautiously in patients with liver dysfunction.

Drug Interactions

Finasteride may antagonize the GI motility effects of metoclopramide.

Summary

In females, the ovaries are the primary sites for synthesis and secretion of estrogen and progesterone hormones in women. These two hormones are under the influence of FSH and LH from the anterior pituitary gland and the hypothalamus. They produce ova and form endocrine secretions that initiate and maintain the secondary female sex characteristics. Estrogens can be used for the treatment of amenorrhea, dysfunctional uterine bleeding, hirsuitism, palliative treatment of breast cancer and prostate cancer, for relief of menopausal symptoms, and for the prevention of osteoporosis. Progesterone is used in irregular uterine bleeding, infertility, threatened or habitual abortion, endometriosis, premenstrual syndrome, and combined with estrogen for the treatment of amenorrhea.

The hypothalamus, anterior pituitary gland, and testes secrete hormones that control the reproductive functions of males. Male sex hormones include testosterone and androsterone. Male sex hormones are used for replacement therapy in androgen deficiency, for the treatment of hypogonadism and cryptorchidism, and for palliative treatment of certain metastatic breast carcinomas in women.

Exploring the Web

Visit *www.ahealthyme.com*

- Search for information on drugs used during labor.

Visit *www.healthline.com*

- Search for additional information on sex hormones.

Visit *www.healthywomen.org*

- From the health topics menu choose topics discussed in this chapter and research additional information to further your understanding of the chapter topics.

Visit *www.menopause-online.com*

- Click on treatments and look for additional information on pharmacological treatments used in the treatment of menopause.

Visit *www.nlm.nih.gov/medlineplus*

- Search for information on anabolic steroids and/or oral contraceptives. What additional information can you find on these topics?

Review Questions

Multiple Choice

1. FSH and LH are released from which of the following organs?
   A. hypothalamus
   B. pituitary
   C. ovaries
   D. pancreas
2. Which of the following is the trade name of medroxyprogesterone?
   A. Gesterol
   B. Provera
   C. Norlutate
   D. Norlutin
3. Progesterone is produced in the corpus luteum, which is located in the:
   A. kidneys
   B. ovaries
   C. uterus
   D. testes
4. Which of the following agents is used for the treatment of amenorrhea, dysfunctional uterine bleeding, and hirsuitism?
   A. progesterone
   B. testosterone
   C. oxytocin
   D. estrogen
5. Which of the following hormones is a uterine stimulant?
   A. prolactin
   B. estrogens
   C. oxytocin
   D. insulin
6. Estrogen is contraindicated in which of the following conditions or diseases?
   A. breast cancer
   B. amenorrhea
   C. hirsuitism
   D. prostate cancer
7. Which of the following is the most serious adverse effect of progesterone?
   A. lethargy
   B. mental depression
   C. diplopia
   D. pulmonary embolism
8. All of the following are adverse effects of testosterone in males, except:
   A. penile erection
   B. gynecomastia

C. gigantism
D. oligospermia

9. Which of the following is an indication of anabolic steroids?
   A. pernicious anemia
   B. megaloblastic anemia
   C. renal insufficiency anemia
   D. prostatic hypertrophy

10. Which of the following hormones is responsible for the changes in the uterine endometrium during the second half of the menstrual cycle?
    A. progesterone
    B. estrogen
    C. estrogen and progesterone
    D. testosterone

11. Which of the following is an example of androgen hormone inhibitor?
    A. medroxyprogesterone (Provera)
    B. fluoxymesterone (Halotestin)
    C. finasteride (Propecia)
    D. methyltestosterone (Virilon)

12. Gonadotropin-releasing hormone is secreted from which of the following?
    A. ovaries
    B. hypothalamus
    C. anterior pituitary
    D. posterior pituitary

13. All of the following are adverse effects of estrogens, except:
    A. weight gain
    B. deepening of the voice
    C. intolerance to contact lenses
    D. amenorrhea

14. Which of the following is a trade name of progesterone?
    A. Norlutin
    B. Norlutate
    C. Provera
    D. Gesterol

15. All of the following statements are correct about minipills, except:
    A. they contain no estrogen
    B. they are taken cyclically
    C. they do not suppress ovulation
    D. they are taken continuously

Fill in the Blank

1. Young athletes often use anabolic steroids to promote an increase in _______________.

2. Androgens are secreted mainly in the _______________ tissue of the testes in the male.

3. Inadequate production of androgens in the male may be due to ______________ malfunction.
4. The use of estrogen-progestin combinations in a cyclic fashion generally results in the inhibition of ______________ without preventing menstruation.
5. Estrogens are used for the treatment of amenorrhea, dysfunctional uterine bleeding and hirsuitism, as well as the palliative treatment of ______________ and ______________.
6. FSH is released from the ______________ and gonadotropin-releasing hormone (GnRH) is released from the ______________.
7. Depo-Provera is a long-acting ______________.

Critical Thinking

A 16-year-old male patient has been prescribed testosterone cypionate (Depo-Testosterone) to treat hypogonadism (failure of the sexual organs to develop normally).

1. Why does this patient need this hormone?
2. How should the physician explain the effects of this hormone to the patient?
3. What are the common adverse effects of male hormones such as testosterone cypionate?

Diuretics

CHAPTER 18

OUTLINE

Anatomy Review

Diuretics

- Loop Diuretics
- Thiazide and Thiazide-like Diuretics
- Potassium-sparing Diuretics
- Osmotic Diuretics
- Carbonic Anhydrase Inhibitors

OBJECTIVES

After completing this chapter, the reader should be able to:

1. Explain the main function of the urinary system.
2. Identify different sections of the nephron.
3. Describe and compare the five types of diuretics.
4. Explain the mechanisms of drug action and important adverse effects of loop diuretics.
5. Explain the contraindications of thiazide diuretics.
6. Describe the use of osmotic diuretics.
7. Identify the major diuretic groups used in the treatment of different disorders or conditions.
8. Explain the mechanisms of action of the carbonic anhydrase inhibitors.
9. Describe the most important indications for the use of loop diuretics.
10. Explain potassium-sparing diuretics.

GLOSSARY

Anuria – inability to produce urine

Diuretic – a drug that increases the secretion of urine from the kidneys

Gynecomastia – enlargement of breast tissue in males

Hyperkalemia – high blood level of potassium

Hypokalemia – low blood level of potassium

Hyponatremia – low blood level of sodium

Hypotonic – having a lesser osmotic pressure than a reference solution

Impotence – inability to achieve or maintain penile erection

Overview

The kidneys are the major organs of the body involved with water balance. They have the ability to regulate their output according to the amount of fluid ingested, and the amounts lost from the body by other routes. In conditions such as hypertension, heart failure, liver disorders, or kidney disorders, fluid may accumulate in the body's tissues and diuretics should be used.

Diuretics are mainly used to remove the excess extracellular fluid from the body that can result in edema (abnormal fluid accumulation) of the tissues, and in hypertension. These conditions occur in diseases of the heart, liver, and kidneys. In order to understand the action of diuretics, it is important to have some knowledge of the basic processes that take place in the nephron.

Anatomy Review

- The structures of the urinary system include two kidneys, two ureters, a bladder, and a urethra (Figures 18-1 and 18-2).
- The urinary system functions to remove waste materials from the body tissues and fluids, to maintain the acid-base balance, and to discharge the waste products from the body.
- The kidneys are the most important of the excretory organs. Kidney failure can result in the buildup of toxic wastes in the body and may lead to death (Figure 18-3).
- The nephron is the basic structural and functional unit of the kidney.
- The renal corpuscle is the site where the process of filtration occurs. In this process, blood pressure forces water and dissolved solutes out of the glomerular capillaries and into a chamber known as the capsular space (Figure 18-4).
- The formation of urine follows this path: blood enters the afferent arteriole → passes through the glomerulus → to Bowman's capsule → now it becomes filtrate (blood minus the red blood cells and plasma proteins) → continues through the proximal convoluted tubule → to the loop of Henle → to the distal convoluted tubule → to the collecting tubule (at this time about 99 percent of the filtrate has been reabsorbed) → approximately 1 mL of urine is formed per minute → the 1 mL of urine goes to the renal pelvis → to the ureter → to the bladder → to the urethra → to the urinary meatus.

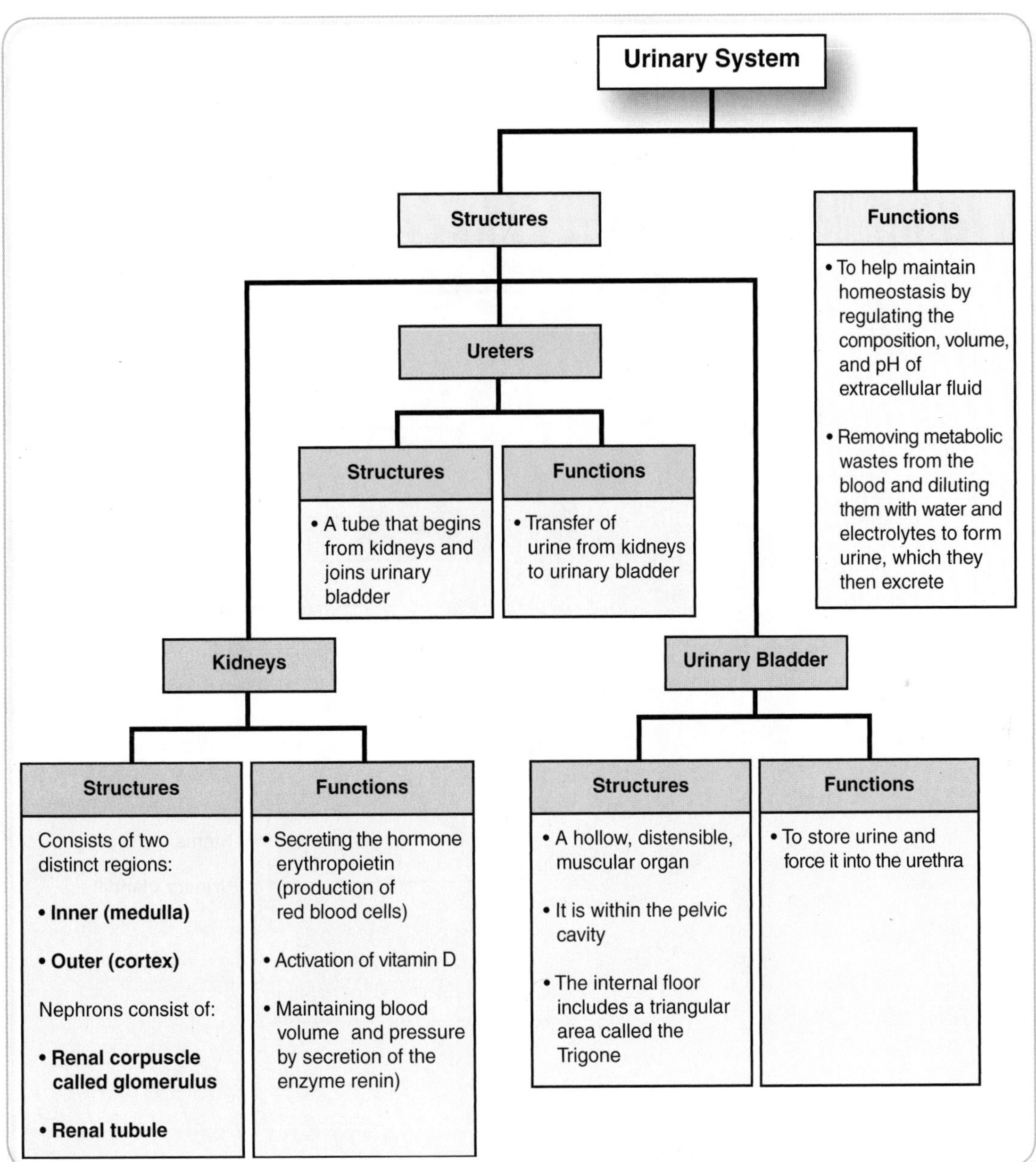

Figure 18-1 The urinary system.

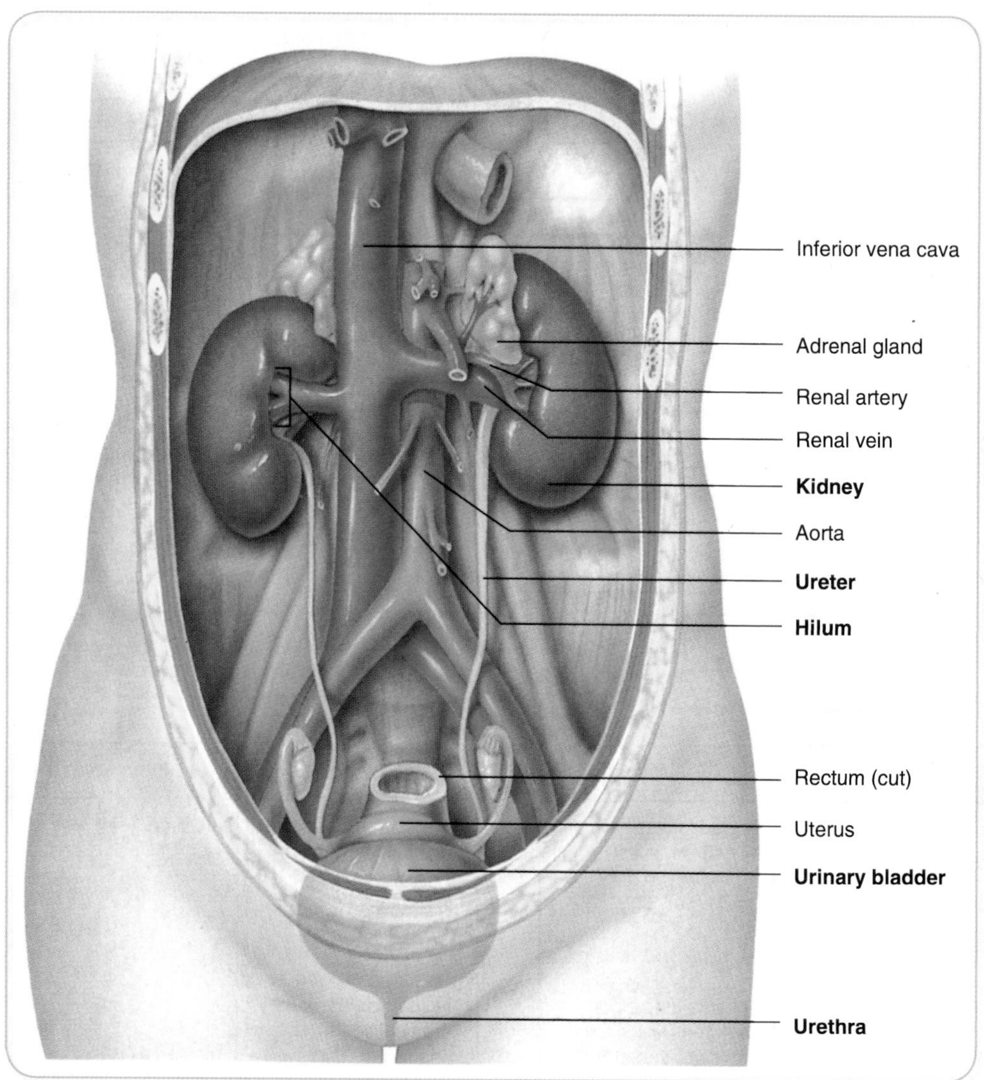

Figure 18-2 The structures of the urinary system.

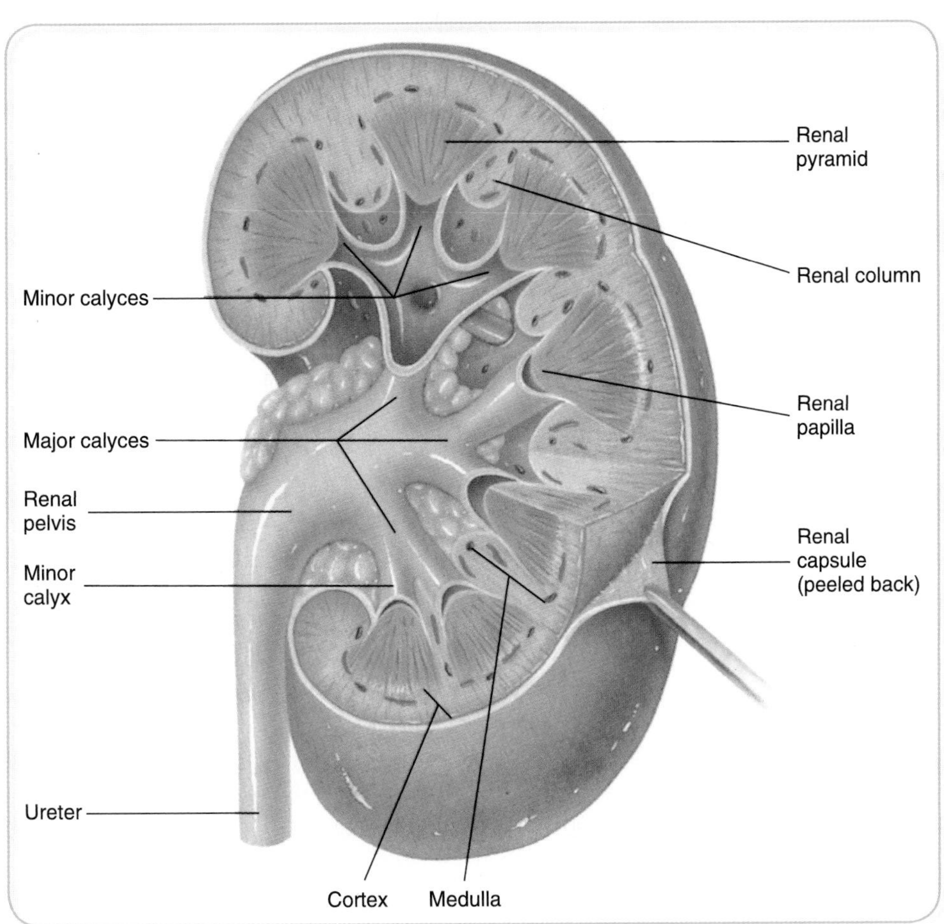

Figure 18-3 The structures of the kidney.

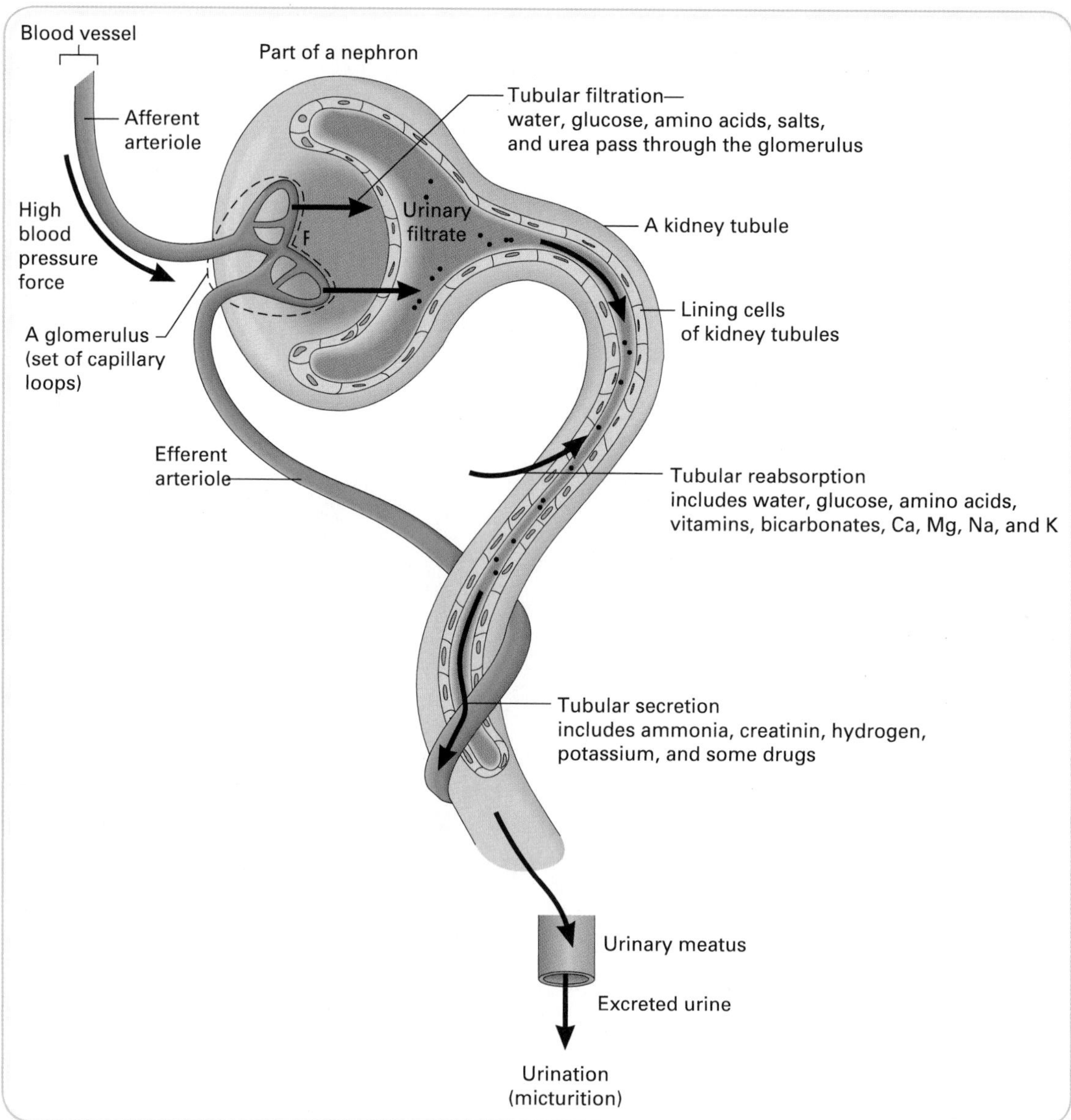

Figure 18-4 Processes and structures of the nephron.

Diuretics

Diuretics are a group of drugs that promote water loss from the body into the urine. As urine formation takes place in the kidneys, it is not surprising that diuretics have their principal action at the level of the nephron. The action of some diuretics is not confined to their action on the kidneys: they also act elsewhere in the body.

Diuretic drugs are an important part of heart failure management. In heart failure, diuretics are primarily used to clear fluid overload and to sustain normal blood volume. Diuretics are divided into five categories according to their action: loop, thiazide and thiazide-like, potassium-sparing, osmotic, and

TABLE 18-1 Loop Diuretics

Generic Name	Trade Name	Route of Administration	Average Adult Dosage
bumetanide	Bumex®	PO	0.5–2 mg/day
ethacrynic acid	Edecrin®	PO	50–100 mg once or twice/day
furosemide	Lasix®	PO	20–80 mg/day
torsemide	Demadex®	PO, IV	10–20 mg once/day

carbonic anhydrase inhibitors. The type of diuretic used is determined by the condition being treated. For example, carbonic anhydrase inhibitors, such as acetazolamide (Diamox), which is recognized as a diuretic compound, are used to lower intraocular pressure.

Loop Diuretics

Good control of water balance is achieved by alterations in the permeability of the collecting duct system of the kidney to water by the presence of antidiuretic hormone (ADH) from the posterior pituitary gland. This is one of the major control systems for water balance, and slight interference here will completely upset the normal function of the kidney and result in a variation in urine output (Table 18-1).

Mechanism of Action

Key Concept

Loop diuretics are the most efficacious diuretic agents available and are rapidly absorbed.

Loop diuretics act on the medullary part of the ascending limb of the loop (loop of Henle) of the nephron. These drugs inhibit the reabsorption of chloride and sodium ions from the loop into the interstitial fluid. The result is that the interstitial fluid becomes relatively **hypotonic** (having a lower osmotic pressure than water).

Indications

Key Concept

Routine administration of loop diuretics, and probably all diuretics, should be done before late afternoon to avoid severe nocturnal enuresis (bedwetting).

Loop diuretics are used in patients with edematous states and can be given intravenously for immediate action. The most important indications for the use of loop diuretics include acute pulmonary edema, other edematous conditions, and acute hypercalcemia. These agents can also be used in patients with hypertension, but other types of diuretics are probably better in most of these patients. In renal failure, they can also be effective in helping to normalize urine output. Loop diuretics, such as furosemide, are potent but relatively short-acting diuretics used in the management of severe chronic heart failure. They are also useful in the treatment of acute heart failure.

Adverse Effects

> **Medical Terminology Review**
>
> **hypokalemia**
> *hypo = low*
> *kalemia = blood levels of potassium*
> low levels of potassium in the blood

A major problem of loop diuretics is the loss of electrolytes from the body. Potassium and sodium are the main ions affected. Potassium loss often leads to hypokalemia, which can result in abnormal cardiac rhythms and even death. Other electrolyte changes can occur, especially with high doses of loop diuretics, and the periodic assessment of blood calcium and magnesium levels is required. Uric acid levels may rise during loop diuretic therapy, which can be problematic for people with gout.

Contraindications and Precautions

Loop diuretics are contraindicated in patients with known hypersensitivity to these drugs. Loop diuretics should be avoided in patients with **anuria** (inability to produce urine), hepatic coma, severe electrolyte deficiency, and during lactation or pregnancy (category C).

Loop diuretics should be used with caution in older adults, cardiac patients, and patients with hepatic cirrhosis, diabetes mellitus, history of gout, and pulmonary edema associated with acute myocardial infarction.

Drug Interactions

Loop diuretics may increase the effectiveness of the anticoagulants or the thrombolytics. Loop diuretics may increase the risk of glycoside toxicity and ototoxicity if taken with an aminoglycoside. Plasma levels of propranolol can increase when the drug is given with furosemide.

Thiazide and Thiazide-like Diuretics

Thiazide diuretics are a group of drugs that are chemically similar and the most commonly prescribed class of diuretics. All of the thiazide diuretics have equivalent effectiveness (Table 18-2).

Mechanism of Action

Thiazide drugs act on the cortical segment of the ascending loop and the distal convoluted tubules of the nephron, and decrease sodium reabsorption. This results in a more concentrated fluid entering the collecting ducts, and therefore decreases water reabsorption and results in a diuresis. Thiazide diuretics have an effect on the peripheral arterioles, which results in vasodilation. This, combined with their diuretic effects, makes them particularly suitable in hypertensive patients (see Chapter 13). This action of these drugs is not completely understood.

> **Key Concept**
>
> *The optimum therapeutic effects of thiazide are seen in 15 to 30 minutes when given intravenously. When given orally, thiazide diuretics may take as long as four weeks to be effective.*

Indications

Thiazide diuretics are still considered to be in the front line for the treatment of mild to moderate hypertension either on their own or combined,

TABLE 18-2 Thiazide and Thiazide-like Diuretics

Generic Name	Trade Name	Route of Administration	Average Adult Dosage
Thiazide Diuretics			
bendroflumethiazide	Naturetin®	PO	2.5–20 mg, 1–2 times/day
chlorothiazide sodium	Diuril®	PO	250 mg–1 g, 1–2 times/day
hydrochlorothiazide	Esidrix®, HCTZ®	PO	12.5–100 mg, 1–3 times/day
hydroflumethiazide	Diucardin®, Saluron®	PO	25–100 mg, 1–2 times/day
methyclothiazide	Aquatensin®, Enduron®	PO	2.5–10 mg/day
metolazone	Mykrox®	PO	5–20 mg/day
polythiazide	Renese®	PO	1–4 mg/day
trichlormethiazide	Diurese®, Metahydrin®	PO	1–4 mg, 1–2 times/day
Thiazide-like Diuretics			
chlorthalidone	Thalitone®, Hygroton®	PO	50–100 mg/day
indapamide	Lozol®	PO	2.5–5 mg/day

usually with a β-blocker. These drugs are also used to treat edema due to heart failure, liver disease, and corticosteroid or estrogen therapy.

Adverse Effects

Adverse effects of thiazide diuretics, as with loop diuretics, include potassium and sodium loss. Thiazide occasionally causes a rise in blood uric acid levels, which can be problematic in those predisposed to gout. Thiazide can also cause hyperglycemia, which is potentially dangerous in diabetics. Lactation can be suppressed, and thiazides have been used for this purpose. **Impotence** in men can also occur.

Other adverse effects of thiazide diuretics are dehydration, electrolyte imbalances, loss of appetite, dizziness, hypotension, increased sensitivity to sun exposure, and pruritus.

Contraindications and Precautions

Thiazide diuretics are contraindicated in patients with known hypersensitivity to these agents. These drugs are also contraindicated in patients with electrolyte imbalances, anuria, hepatic coma, and renal impairment. Thiazide diuretics should be given with caution during pregnancy (category C) and lactation, in children, and with liver or kidney impairment.

Drug Interactions

If thiazides are used with alcohol, nitrates, or other antihypertensive drugs, they may cause additive hypotensive effects. Anesthetic agents

TABLE 18-3 Potassium-sparing Diuretics

Generic Name	Trade Name	Route of Administration	Average Adult Dosage
amiloride hydrochloride	Midamor®	PO	5 mg/day
spironolactone	Aldactone®	PO	25–200 mg, 1–2 times/day
triamterene	Dyrenium®	PO	100 mg b.i.d.

may increase the effects of thiazides. The effects of anticoagulants may be decreased when given with thiazide diuretics.

Potassium-sparing Diuretics

There are two types of potassium-sparing diuretics, the aldosterone antagonists and those independent of aldosterone. The best-known aldosterone antagonist is spironolactone. These agents are not very powerful as diuretics (see Table 18-3).

Mechanism of Action

Key Concept

Overall, spironolactone has a rather slow onset of action, requiring several days before full therapeutic effect is achieved.

Potassium-sparing diuretics (such as spironolactone) inhibit the action of aldosterone on the distal convoluted tubule of the nephron. Aldosterone is the sodium-retaining hormone secreted from the adrenal cortex. If it acts on the distal tubule, the body retains more sodium ions, and water is passively conserved at the same time. When sodium is retained by the nephron at this site, potassium is lost. Therefore, if aldosterone is blocked, potassium is retained and sodium is lost along with a slight increase in diuresis.

Indications

Potassium-sparing diuretics are not usually required for patients who are on loop or thiazide diuretics. Spironolactone has proved to be of tremendous value in the treatment of congestive heart failure.

Adverse Effects

Adverse effects that occur with this type of diuretic are related to their mode of action, and include **hyperkalemia**, acute renal failure, kidney stones, and **hyponatremia**. In men, spironolactone can produce **gynecomastia** due to its estrogenic effect.

Contraindications and Precautions

Potassium-sparing diuretics are contraindicated in patients with hypersensitivity to these drugs, anuria, acute renal insufficiency, and hyperkalemia,

TABLE 18-4 Osmotic Diuretics

Generic Name	Trade Name	Route of Administration	Average Adult Dosage
glycerin	Glycerol®, Osmoglyn®	PO	1–1.8 g/kg given 1–1.5 h before ocular surgery
mannitol	Osmitrol®	IV	100 g as a 10–20% solution over 2–6 h
urea	Ureaphil®	IV	1–1.5 g/kg of 30% solution infused slowly over 1 to 2.5 h

and during pregnancy (category D) or lactation. Potassium-sparing diuretics should be used cautiously in patients with impaired kidney or liver function, history of gouty arthritis, diabetes mellitus, or history of kidney stones.

Drug Interactions

Alcohol, nitrate, and other antihypertensive agents may have increased hypotensive effects when a potassium-sparing diuretic is given. Potassium-sparing diuretics may cause severe hyperkalemia when potassium preparations are also given.

Osmotic Diuretics

Osmotic diuretic drugs are capable of being filtered by the glomerulus, but have a limited capability of being reabsorbed into the bloodstream (see Table 18-4).

Mechanism of Action

Osmotic diuretics work by directly interfering with osmosis. Any substance that enters the body in large enough quantities and is excreted via the kidneys will lead to water being kept in the renal tubules, leading to water loss. This is due to maintenance of a high osmotic pressure in the tubules.

Indications

Osmotic diuretics can be used to reduce increased intracranial pressure and to promote prompt removal of renal toxins. These agents can be used to maintain urine volume and to prevent anuria.

Adverse Effects

Adverse effects of osmotic diuretics include electrolyte imbalance and the potential for dehydration. This potential for dehydration is similar to that which would occur from the drinking of seawater.

Contraindications and Precautions

Osmotic diuretics are contraindicated in patients with known hypersensitivity to these drugs. Osmotic diuretics should be avoided in patients with severe dehydration, anuria, and electrolyte imbalances. Mannitol is contraindicated in patients with intracranial bleeding.

Osmotic diuretics should be used with caution in patients with electrolyte imbalances or renal impairment. Osmotic diuretics must be given cautiously to pregnant women (category C) and during lactation.

Drug Interactions

Osmotic diuretics increase urinary excretion of lithium, salicylates, barbiturates, potassium, and imipramine.

Carbonic Anhydrase Inhibitors

When a patient is taking carbonic anhydrase inhibitors, it is important that their fluid input, fluid output, glucose levels, and electrolyte levels be monitored. See Table 18-5 for these agents.

Mechanism of Action

Carbonic anhydrase is an enzyme that speeds up the conversion of carbon dioxide into bicarbonate ions and vice versa, according to the following equation:

$$CO_2 + H_2O \leftrightarrow H_2CO_3 \leftrightarrow H^+ + HCO_3^-$$

This reaction occurs in the kidney as well as in other parts of the body. In the kidney, the reaction occurs mainly in the proximal tubule and, as it involves bicarbonate loss, is concerned with acid-base balance. The tubular cells are not very permeable to bicarbonate ions or carbonic acid, but are very permeable to carbon dioxide. Under normal circumstances, carbonic anhydrase in the tubular cell converts the carbonic acid into carbon dioxide and water, which are promptly reabsorbed. If the enzyme is inhibited, there will be a net loss of bicarbonate from the body with a consequent loss of

TABLE 18-5 Carbonic Anhydrase Inhibitors

Generic Name	Trade Name	Route of Administration	Average Adult Dosage
acetazolamide	Diamox®	PO, IM, IV	For glaucoma: PO: 250 mg 1–4 times/day, 500 mg sustained release b.i.d.; IM/IV: 500 mg, may repeat in 2–4 h; For edema: PO: 250–375 mg every AM (5 mg/kg)
dichlorphenamide	Daranide®, Oratrol®	PO	100–200 mg, 1–2 times/day
methazolamide	Neptazane®	PO	50–100 mg b.i.d.-tid

water. The drug acetazolamide is a non-competitive inhibitor of this enzyme, and has been used as a diuretic.

Indications

The carbonic anhydrase inhibitors are used in the treatment of open-angle glaucoma, secondary glaucoma, and preoperative treatment of acute closed-angle glaucoma. These agents are also prescribed in the treatment of edema resulting from congestive heart failure, and drug-induced edema.

Adverse Effects

Carbonic anhydrase inhibitors may cause acidosis (a clinical state where the pH of the blood drops significantly, below 7.35), renal stones, hypokalemia, drowsiness (following large doses), and hypersensitivity reactions.

Contraindications and Precautions

Carbonic anhydrase inhibitors are contraindicated in patients with known hypersensitivity, anuria, severe renal or liver impairment, and imbalance of electrolytes.

Carbonic anhydrase inhibitors should be used cautiously in patients with kidney impairment, and during lactation and pregnancy (category C).

These drugs need to be given with caution in patients with respiratory acidosis, emphysema, or chronic respiratory disease as diuresis can be diminished in the presence of acidotic conditions.

Drug Interactions

Carbonic anhydrase inhibitors interact with renal excretion of amphetamines, ephedrine, quinidine, and procainamide. Carbonic anhydrase inhibitors may decrease the effects of tricyclic antidepressants, thereby enhancing or prolonging their effects. These diuretics also decrease the renal excretion of lithium.

Summary

Diuretics have their principal action at the level of the kidneys' nephrons. These drugs are mainly used to remove the excess extracellular fluid from the body that can result in edema of the tissues and in hypertension. The urinary system has three major functions: excretion, elimination, and homeostatic regulation of the volume of blood plasma.

Diuretic drugs are an important part of heart failure, hypertension, and edema management. These agents are divided into five categories according to their action: loops, thiazide and thiazide-like, potassium-sparing, osmotic, and carbonic anhydrase inhibitors.

Loop diuretics are major controllers for water balance and result in a variation in urine output. Thiazide and thiazide-like diuretics are the most commonly prescribed types of diuretics. The best-known potassium-sparing diuretic is spironolactone, which is an aldosterone antagonist. Osmotic diuretics work by directly interfering with osmosis, which leads the kidneys to keeping water in the renal tubules, resulting in water loss. Carbonic anhydrase is an enzyme that speeds up the conversion of carbon dioxide into bicarbonate ions and vice versa. If the enzyme is inhibited, there will be a net loss of bicarbonate from the body with a consequent loss of water.

Exploring the Web

Visit ***http://nephron.com***

- Explore articles related to the types of diuretics discussed in this chapter.

Visit ***www.mayoclinic.com*** and ***www.medicinenet.com***

- Look for information related to diuretics.

Review Questions

Multiple Choice

1. Thiazides are contraindicated in patients with all of the following conditions, except:

   A. impaired liver function
   B. edema caused by heart failure
   C. diabetes
   D. a history of gout

2. Which of the following substances may alter the permeability of the collecting duct of the nephron to water?

   A. antidiuretic hormone
   B. insulin
   C. vitamin C
   D. calcitonin

3. Which of the following is the major problem with the loop diuretics?

   A. decrease of uric acid
   B. hyperkalemia
   C. loss of glucose from the kidneys
   D. loss of electrolytes from the body

4. Thiazide drugs act on which of the following segments of the nephron?

   A. descending loop
   B. ascending loop
   C. proximal convoluted tubule
   D. collecting duct

5. Which of the following is an aldosterone antagonist?

   A. mannitol
   B. furosemide
   C. spironolactone
   D. acetazolamide

6. Which of the following is a trade name of acetazolamide?

   A. Osmitrol®
   B. Diamox®
   C. Ureaphil®
   D. Aldactone®

7. Diuretics are mainly used in which of the following?

   A. diabetes
   B. encephalitis
   C. hepatitis B
   D. hypertension

8. Which of the following diuretics are used in the treatment of open-angle glaucoma?

   A. carbonic anhydrase inhibitors
   B. potassium-sparing diuretics
   C. thiazide and thiazide-like diuretics
   D. loop diuretics

9. Which of the following time periods are required for optimum therapeutic effects of orally administered thiazides?

   A. 15 to 30 minutes
   B. 2 to 4 days
   C. 1 to 2 weeks
   D. 3 to 4 weeks

10. The most commonly used osmotic drug is:
    A. ethacrynic acid
    B. furosemide
    C. mannitol
    D. torsemide

11. Carbonic anhydrase inhibitors must be used with caution in pregnant women and are classified as:
    A. category D
    B. category C
    C. category B
    D. category A

12. The mechanism of action of mannitol (a carbonic anhydrase inhibitor) affects which of the following parts of the nephron?
    A. proximal tubule
    B. ascending loop
    C. distal tubule
    D. collecting duct

13. The generic name of Osmoglyn® is which of the following?
    A. isosorbide
    B. mannitol
    C. glycerin
    D. acetazolamide

14. Which of the following organs temporarily stores urine?
    A. kidney
    B. ureter
    C. urethra
    D. bladder

15. A capillary network of renal corpuscles is called:
    A. Bowman's capsule
    B. Henle tubule
    C. proximal convoluted tubule
    D. glomerulus

Matching

_____ 1. acetazolamide	A. Lasix
_____ 2. mannitol	B. Aldactone
_____ 3. indapamide	C. Hygroton
_____ 4. ethacrynic acid	D. Edecrin
_____ 5. chlorthalidone	E. Osmitrol
_____ 6. furosemide	F. Lozol
_____ 7. spironolactone	G. Diamox

Critical Thinking

A 25-year-old male patient is admitted to the intensive care unit (ICU) following a car-train collision. The patient sustained a depressed skull fracture and is on a ventilator. Two days after surgery, there are obvious signs of increasing intracranial pressure. The nurse administers mannitol (Osmitrol®) intravenously over 30 minutes. The patient's wife asks his physician to explain why her husband needs this drug.

1. What explanation should the physician offer?
2. If the patient shows symptoms of intracranial bleeding, what would be the explanation that the physician should give for discontinuing the drug?

SECTION III

PHARMACOLOGY FOR DISORDERS AFFECTING MULTI-BODY SYSTEMS

CHAPTER 19

Vitamins, Minerals, and Nutritional Supplements

OBJECTIVES

After completing this chapter, the reader should be able to:

1. Identify characteristics that differentiate vitamins from other nutrients.
2. Describe the functions of common vitamins and minerals.
3. Classify vitamins and minerals.
4. Explain trace elements and their major effects on the body.
5. Describe the role of vitamin and mineral therapies in the treatment of deficiency disorders.
6. Define pharma food.
7. Explain the rationale behind food labeling.
8. Describe the purposes of additives in foods and supplements.
9. Explain the major complication of total parenteral nutrition therapy.
10. Define pernicious anemia, keratomalacia, osteomalacia, and cheilosis.

OUTLINE

Vitamins
- Fat-soluble Vitamins
- Water-soluble Vitamins

Minerals and Electrolytes
- Major Minerals
- Trace Elements

Food Labeling

Food Additives

Nutritional Care
- Enteral Nutrition
- Hyperalimentation

Pharma Food

GLOSSARY

Ascorbic acid – a water-soluble vitamin that is essential for the formation of collagen and fibroid tissue for teeth, bones, cartilage, connective tissue, and skin; also known as vitamin C

Ataxia – loss of the ability to coordinate muscular movement

Beriberi – a deficiency caused by deficiency of thiamine, characterized by neurological symptoms, cardiovascular abnormalities, and edema

Biotin – a water-soluble B complex vitamin that aids in fatty acid production, and in the oxidation of fatty acids and carbohydrates; also known as vitamin B_7

Cachexia – weight loss, wasting of muscle, loss of appetite, and general debility that can occur during a chronic disease

Calciferol – a fat-soluble vitamin chemically related to steroids; calciferol is essential for the normal formation of bones and teeth and important for the absorption of calcium and phosphorus from the GI tract; also known as vitamin D;

Calcium (Ca) – the fifth-most abundant element in the human body, present mainly in the bones

Carotenoids – any of a class of yellow to red pigments, including the carotenes and xanthophylls

Cheilosis – fissures on the lips caused by deficiency of riboflavin

Chloride (Cl) – involved in the maintenance of fluid and the body's acid-base balance

Copper (Cu) – important for the synthesis of hemoglobin because it is part of a co-enzyme involved in its synthesis; also a component of several important enzymes in the body, and essential to good health

Cretinism – arrested physical and mental development with dystrophy of bones and soft tissues due to congenital lack of thyroid secretion

Cyanocobalamin – a water-soluble substance that is the common pharmaceutic form of vitamin B_{12}; involved in the metabolism of protein, fats, and carbohydrates, and also in normal blood formation and neural function

Electrolytes – compounds, particularly salts, that when dissolved in water or another solvent, dissociate into ions and are able to conduct an electric current

Enteral nutrition (EN) – feeding by tube directly into the patient's digestive tract

Fluorine – a chemical element that is used as a diagnostic aid in various tissue scans

Folic acid – essential for cell growth and the reproduction of red blood cells; also known as vitamin B_9

Food additive – any substance that becomes part of a food product

Hemolysis – the destruction or dissolution of red blood cells, with release of hemoglobin

Hypervitaminosis – an abnormal condition resulting from excessive intake of toxic amounts of one or more vitamins, especially over a long period

Hydroxocobalamin – is involved in the metabolism of protein, fats, and carbohydrates, aids in hemoglobin synthesis, is essential for normal functioning of all cells, and is important in energy metabolism; also known as vitamin B_{12}

Hyperalimentation (total parenteral nutrition) – also known as "TPN", this treatment is used to supply complete nutrition to patients when the enteral route cannot be used; all needed nutrients are injected into the body intravenously

Hypomagnesemia – an abnormally low level of magnesium in the blood

Hypovitaminosis – a condition related to the deficiency of one or more vitamins

Intrinsic factor – a substance that is secreted by the gastric mucus membrane and is essential for the absorption of vitamin B_{12} in the intestines

Iodine – an essential micronutrient of the thyroid hormone (thyroxine)

Iron (Fe) – a common metallic element essential for the formation of hemoglobin and myoglobin, as well as the transfer of oxygen to the body tissues

Keratomalacia – a condition, usually in children with vitamin A deficiency, characterized by softening, ulceration, and perforation of the cornea

Magnesium – an important ion for the function of many enzyme systems, and is the second most abundant action of the intracellular fluids in the body

Menadione – a water-soluble injectable form of the product of vitamin K_3

Minerals – inorganic substances occurring naturally in the earth's crust having characteristic chemical compositions

Niacin – contains parts of two enzymes that regulate energy metabolism and is essential for a healthy skin, tongue, and digestive system; also known as vitamin B_3 or nicotinic acid

Nicotinic acid – contains parts of two enzymes that regulate energy metabolism and is essential for a healthy skin, tongue, and digestive system; also known as niacin or vitamin B_3

Osteomalacia – a disease in which the bone softens and becomes brittle

Pantothenic acid – a member of the vitamin B complex widely distributed in plant and animal tissues and that may be an important element in human nutrition; also known as vitamin B_5

Pellagra – a disease caused by a deficiency of niacin and protein in the diet, characterized by skin eruptions, digestive and nervous system disturbances, and eventual mental deterioration

Pharma food – a system of receiving nourishment by breathing in nutritional microparticles

Phosphorus – is essential for the metabolism of protein, calcium, and glucose, aids in building strong bones and teeth, and helps in the regulation of the body's acid-base balance

Potassium – the major electrolyte in intracellular fluids, helping to regulate neuromuscular excitability and muscle contraction

Pyridoxine – a water-soluble vitamin that is part of the B complex and acts as a co-enzyme essential for the synthesis and breakdown of amino acids; also known as vitamin B_6

Retinol – a fat-soluble vitamin essential for skeletal growth, maintenance of normal mucosal epithelium, reproduction, and visual acuity; also known as vitamin A

Riboflavin – one of the heat-stable components of the B complex, it is involved as a co-enzyme in the oxidative processes of carbohydrates, fats, and proteins; also known as vitamin B_2

Rickets – a deficiency disease resulting from a lack of vitamin D or calcium and from insufficient exposure to sunlight, characterized by defective bone growth and occurring mostly in children

Sodium – one of the most important elements in the body; sodium ions are involved in acid-base balance, water balance, transmission of nerve impulses, and contraction of muscles

Sulfur – necessary to all body tissues and is found in all body cells

Thiamine – a water-soluble, crystalline compound of the B complex, essential for normal metabolism and health of the cardiovascular and nervous systems; also known as vitamin B_1

Tocopherol – a fat-soluble vitamin essential for normal reproduction, muscle development, resistance of erythrocytes to hemolysis, and various other biochemical functions; also known as vitamin E

Xerophthalmia – extreme dryness of the conjunctiva resulting from an eye disease or from a systemic deficiency of vitamin A

Vitamins – organic compounds essential in small quantities for physiologic and metabolic functioning of the body

Vitamin A – a fat-soluble vitamin essential for skeletal growth, maintenance of normal mucosal epithelium, reproduction, and visual acuity; also known as retinol

Vitamin B_1 – a water-soluble, crystalline compound of the B complex, essential for normal metabolism and health of the cardiovascular and nervous systems; also known as thiamine

Vitamin B_2 – one of the heat-stable components of the B complex, it is involved as a co-enzyme in the oxidative processes of carbohydrates, fats, and proteins; also known as riboflavin

Vitamin B_3 – contains parts of two enzymes that regulate energy metabolism and is essential for a healthy skin, tongue, and digestive system; also known as niacin or nicotinic acid

Vitamin B_5 – a member of the vitamin B complex widely distributed in plant and animal tissues and that may be an important element in human nutrition; also known as pantothenic acid

Vitamin B_6 – a water-soluble vitamin that is part of the B complex and acts as a co-enzyme essential for the synthesis and breakdown of amino acids; also known as pyridoxine

Vitamin B_7 – a water-soluble B complex vitamin that aids in fatty acid production, and in the oxidation of fatty acids and carbohydrates; also known as biotin

Vitamin B_9 – essential for cell growth and the reproduction of red blood cells; also known as folic acid

Vitamin B_{12} – is involved in the metabolism of protein, fats, and carbohydrates, aids in hemoglobin synthesis, is essential for normal functioning of all cells, and is important in energy metabolism; also known as cyanocobalamin

Vitamin B complex – a pharmaceutical term applied to drug products containing a mixture of the B vitamins, usually B_1 (thiamine), B_2 (riboflavin), B_3 (nicotinamide), and B_6 (pyridoxine)

Vitamin C – a water-soluble vitamin that is essential for the formation of collagen and fibroid tissue for teeth, bones, cartilage, connective tissue, and skin; also known as ascorbic acid

Vitamin D – a fat-soluble vitamin chemically related to steroids that is essential for the normal formation of bones and teeth and important for the absorption of calcium and phosphorus from the GI tract; also known as calciferol

Vitamin E – a fat-soluble vitamin essential for normal reproduction, muscle development, resistance of erythrocytes to hemolysis, and various other biochemical functions; also known as tocopherol

Vitamin K – essential for the synthesis of prothrombin in the liver

Zinc (Zn) – a trace element that is essential several body enzymes, growth, glucose tolerance, wound healing, and taste acuity

Overview

Vitamins and minerals are required for maintaining normal function and, more important, they are essential for life. The body cannot synthesize vitamins and minerals, and relies on outside sources to provide daily requirements. The vitamins and minerals the body needs come either from the foods we eat or from supplements. Vitamins are considered "natural substances" and food additives rather than drugs. However, niacin and vitamin K are indicated as drugs to affect cholesterol reduction and blood clotting. The vitamin, mineral, and supplement business is a multimillion-dollar industry in the U.S. Some conditions that affect a patient's health are greatly benefited by the use of nutritional supplements. Pharmacy technicians are asked many questions about foods and nutrition, including specific questions about which products or supplements a client may be considering for purchase, and what amount of product to ingest.

Vitamins

Vitamins are organic compounds essential in small quantities for physiologic and metabolic functioning of the body. With few exceptions, vitamins cannot be synthesized by the body and must be obtained from the diet or dietary supplements. No one food contains all the vitamins. Vitamin deficiency diseases produce specific symptoms that are usually alleviated by the administration of the appropriate vitamin. Vitamins are classified according to their fat or water solubility, their physiological effects, or their chemical structures. They are designated by alphabetic letters and chemical or other specific names. The fat-soluble vitamins are A, D, E, and K; the B complex and C vitamins are water-soluble.

An abnormal condition resulting from excessive intake of toxic amounts of one or more vitamins, especially over a long period, is called **hypervitaminosis**. Serious effects may result from overdoses of fat-soluble vitamins A, D, E, or K, but adverse reactions are less likely with the water-soluble B and C vitamins, except when taken in megadoses. **Hypovitaminosis** may occur due to a deficiency of one or more vitamins. Examples of diseases or conditions caused by hypovitaminosis include avitaminosis, **beriberi**, malnutrition, scurvy, rickets, scorbutus, and moon blindness.

Fat-soluble Vitamins

Each of the fat-soluble vitamins A, D, E, and K has a distinct and separate physiological role. For the most part, they are absorbed with other lipids, and efficient absorption requires the presence of bile and pancreatic juice. They are transported to the liver, and stored in various body tissues. They are not normally excreted in the urine. Table 19-1 provides a summary of the fat-soluble vitamins, sources, functions, and deficiencies or toxicities.

TABLE 19-1 Fat-soluble Vitamins

Name	Food Sources	Functions	Deficiency/ Toxicity
Fat-soluble vitamins			
Vitamin A (retinol)	**Animal**	Maintenance of vision in dim light	**Deficiency**
	• Liver	Maintenance of mucous membranes and healthy skin	Night blindness
	• Whole milk	Growth and development of bones	Xerophthalmia
	• Butter	Reproduction	Respiratory infections
	• Cream	Healthy immune system	Bone growth ceases
	• Cod liver oil		
	Plants		**Toxicity**
	• Dark green leafy vegetables		Birth defects Bone pain
	• Deep yellow or orange fruit		Anorexia
	• Fortified margarine		Enlargement of liver
Vitamin D (calciferol)	**Animal**	Regulation of absorption of calcium and phosphorus	**Deficiency**
	• Eggs	Building and maintenance of normal bones and teeth	Rickets
	• Liver	Prevention of tetany	Osteomalacia
	• Fortified milk		Osteoporosis
	• Fortified margarine		Poorly developed teeth and bones
	• Oily fish		Muscle spasms
	Plants		**Toxicity**
	• None		Kidney stones
	Sunlight		Calcification of soft tissues

(continues)

TABLE 19-1 Fat-soluble Vitamins—*continued*

Name	Food Sources	Functions	Deficiency/ Toxicity
Vitamin E (tocopherol)	**Animal**	Antioxidant	**Deficiency**
	• None	Considered essential for protection of cell structure, especially of red blood cells	Destruction of red blood cells
	Plants		**Toxicity**
	• Green and leafy vegetables		No toxicity has been reported
	• Margarines		
	• Salad dressing		
	• Wheat germ and wheat germ oils		
	• Vegetable oils		
	• Nuts		

Vitamin A

Vitamin A (retinol) is one of the fat-soluble vitamins and is essential for skeletal growth, maintenance of normal mucosal epithelium, and visual acuity. Normal stores can last up to one year but are rapidly depleted by stress. Vitamin A has essential roles in the development of vision, bone growth, the maintenance of epithelial tissue, the immunological process, and normal reproduction. Retinol is not found in plant products but fortunately most plants contain a substance called **carotenoids**, which act as provitamins and can be converted into retinol in the intestinal wall and liver. The principal carotenoid in plants is beta-carotene, which gets its name from carrots. Deficiency leads to atrophy of epithelial tissue, resulting in **keratomalacia**, **xerophthalmia**, night blindness, growth retardation (in children), and lessened resistance to infection of the mucous membranes. Plasma vitamin A concentrations are reduced in patients with cystic fibrosis, alcohol-related cirrhosis, hepatic disease, and proteinuria. Plasma vitamin A concentrations are elevated in patients with chronic renal disease.

Medical Terminology Review

xerophthalmia
xer = *dry*
ophthalm = *related to the eye or eyeball*
ia = *condition*
excessive dryness of the conjunctiva and cornea

Key Concept

Xerophthalmia is the major cause of blindness among young children in most developing countries.

Toxicity can result from taking only ten times the recommended daily allowance (RDA) for several months. Symptoms of toxicity are varied, and can include excessive peeling of the skin, hyperlipidemia, hypercalcemia, and hepatotoxicity. Ultimately, death can result. An acute dose of about 200 mg can cause immediate toxicity, resulting in increased cerebrospinal pressure. This can cause severe headache, blurring of vision, and the bulging of the fontanelles in infants. The use of vitamin A is contraindicated in hypervitaminosis A, oral use in malabsorption syndrome, hypersensitivity, and intravenous use.

Vitamin D

Vitamin D (calciferol) is another fat-soluble vitamin that is chemically related to steroids and essential for the normal formation of bones and teeth and for the absorption of calcium and phosphorus from the GI tract. Ultraviolet rays activate a form of cholesterol in an oil of the skin and convert it to a form of the vitamin, which is then absorbed. Vitamin D is considered a hormone. It is used for the prophylaxis and treatment of **rickets**, **osteomalacia**, and other hypocalcemic disorders (tetany) and hypoparathyroidism. Vitamin D_3 is the predominant form of vitamin D of animal origin. It is found in most fish-liver oils, butter, bran, and egg yolks. It is formed in skin exposed to sunlight or ultraviolet rays. Deficiency of the vitamin results in rickets in children, the destruction of bony tissue, and osteoporosis. Hypervitaminosis D produces a toxicity syndrome that may result in hypercalcemia, malabsorption (which can lead to constipation), kidney stones, and calcium deposits on bones. Vitamin D therapy is contraindicated in hypercalcemia, malabsorption syndrome, and renal dysfunction, or if an individual has evidence of vitamin D toxicity or abnormal sensitivity to the effects of vitamin D. Vitamin D_2 is also called ergocalciferol.

Medical Terminology Review

osteoporosis
osteo = bone
poro = cavity; porousness
sis = state; condition
porous state of bones

Key Concept

Inadequate exposure to sunlight and low dietary intake are usually necessary for the development of clinical vitamin D deficiency.

Vitamin E

Vitamin E (tocopherol) is a fat-soluble vitamin that is essential for normal reproduction, muscle development, and resistance of erythrocytes to **hemolysis**. It is an intracellular antioxidant and acts to maintain the stability of polyunsaturated fatty acids.

Deficiency of vitamin E is rare, but can lead to anemia in babies, especially if premature. In adults, erythrocytes may have a shortened lifespan, which may result in muscle degeneration of vascular system abnormalities and kidney damage.

Vitamin E is relatively non-toxic, and may cause problems only in the large-dosage range of about 300 mg per day (RDA is only 10 mg per day). At this range, interference with thyroid function and a prolonging of blood clotting time may occur. Sources of vitamin E include vegetable oils such as soybean, corn, cottonseed, and safflower, as well as nuts, seeds, and wheat germ.

Vitamin K

Vitamin K is essential for the synthesis of prothrombin in the liver. The naturally occurring forms, also called quinones, are vitamin K_1 (phylloquinone), which occurs in green plants, and vitamin K_2 (menaquinone), which is formed as the result of bacterial action in the intestinal tract. Water-soluble forms of vitamins K_1 and K_2 are also available. The fat-soluble synthetic compound, **menadione** (vitamin K_3), is about twice as potent biologically as the naturally occurring vitamins K_1 and K_2, on a weight basis.

In healthy adults, primary vitamin K deficiency is uncommon. Adults are protected from a lack of vitamin K because it is widely distributed in plant and animal tissues, the vitamin K cycle conserves the vitamin, and the microbiologic flora of the normal gut forms menaquinone. However, vitamin K deficiency can occur in adults with marginal dietary intake if they undergo trauma or extensive surgery. Persons with biliary obstruction, malabsorption, or liver disease also have a higher risk of vitamin K deficiency. Certain drugs, including anticonvulsants, anticoagulants, some antibiotics (particularly cephalosporins), salicylates, and megadoses of vitamin A or E can cause vulnerability to vitamin K-related bleeding disease. Vitamin K is used for coagulation disorder and vitamin K deficiency.

Key Concept

The coumarin group of drugs, such as warfarin, is vitamin K antagonists.

It is given prophylactically to infants to prevent hemorrhagic disease of the newborn. Natural vitamin K is stored in the body and is not toxic.

Water-soluble Vitamins

Most of the water-soluble vitamins are components of essential enzyme systems. Many are involved in the reactions supporting energy metabolism. These vitamins are not normally stored in the body in appreciable amounts and are usually excreted in small quantities in the urine; thus, a daily supply is desirable to avoid depletion and interruption of normal physiologic functions.

Vitamin B Complex

Vitamin B complex is a group of water-soluble vitamins that differ from each other structurally and in their biologic effects. Heat and prolonged cooking, especially cooking with water, can destroy B vitamins.

Key Concept

Thiamine malabsorption commonly occurs in patients with alcoholism, cirrhosis, or gastrointestinal disease.

Alcohol is well-known for its ability to inhibit the absorption of thiamine and folic acid. Alcohol abuse is the most common cause of thiamine deficiency in the U.S.

Vitamin B_1. **Vitamin B_1 (thiamine)** is a water-soluble component of the B vitamin complex that is essential for normal metabolism and the health of the cardiovascular and nervous systems. Thiamine plays a key role in the metabolic breakdown of carbohydrates. It is not stored in the body and must be supplied daily. Rich sources of vitamin B_1 are pork, organ meats, green leafy vegetables, legumes, sweet corn, egg yolks, corn meal, brown rice, yeast, and nuts. Deficiency of thiamine leads to the disease called beriberi, which has neurologic, cardiovascular, and GI symptoms. Thiamine is found in fortified breads, pasta, cereals, whole grains (especially wheat germ), lean meats (especially pork), fish, dried beans, peas, and soybeans. Thiamine toxicity can occur if very large doses are taken for long periods, and this can result in hepatotoxicity.

Vitamin B_2. **Vitamin B_2 (riboflavin)** is one of the heat-stable components of the B vitamin complex. It is essential for certain enzyme systems in the metabolism of fats and proteins. It is sensitive to light. It plays an important role in preventing some visual disorders, especially cataracts.

Riboflavin deficiency is associated with inadequate consumption of milk and other animal products. It is common in patients with chronic diarrhea, liver disease, and chronic alcoholism. Deficiency of riboflavin produces **cheilosis** (fissures on the lips); glossitis (inflammation of the tongue); and seborrheic dermatitis (mainly of the face).

Vitamin B_3. **Vitamin B_3 (niacin or nicotinic acid)** contains parts of two enzymes that regulate energy metabolism. It is essential for a healthy skin, tongue, and digestive system. Severe deficiency results in **pellagra**, mental disturbances, various skin eruptions, and GI disturbances. Pellagra may also occur during prolonged isoniazid therapy, and in cancer patients. Major sources of vitamin B_3 include: lean meats, chicken, eggs, fish, cooked dried beans and peas, liver, nonfat or low-fat milk and cheese, soybeans, and nuts.

Key Concept

Pellagra is characterized by skin and mouth lesions, diarrhea, and loss of memory.

In large doses, nicotinic acid can lead to peptic ulcers, diabetes mellitus, cardiac dysrhythmias, and hepatic failure. In view of its potential adverse effects at doses of 100 mg and above, nicotinic acid is being made available only by prescription.

Vitamin B_5. **Vitamin B_5 (pantothenic acid)** is a member of the vitamin B complex. The primary role of pantothenic acid is as a constituent of co-enzyme A and as such it is essential in many areas of cellular metabolism, including fatty acid metabolism, the synthesis of sex hormones, and the functioning of the nervous system and the adrenal glands.

As pantothenic acid is available in many plant and animal sources, it is very rare for individuals to have a deficiency of this vitamin. It is available generally in multivitamin preparations, and a diet rich in fruit, vegetable, cereal, or meat sources would ensure an adequate intake of pantothenic acid.

Vitamin B_6. **Vitamin B_6 (pyridoxine)** is a coenzyme essential for the synthesis and breakdown of amino acids, the conversion of tryptophan to niacin, the breakdown of glycogen to glucose, and the production of antibodies. Therefore, vitamin B_6 is important in the metabolism of blood, CNS, and skin. It is used routinely in patients on isoniazid therapy to prevent the development of neuritis. There has been some success with its use in treating nausea of pregnancy, particularly when given parenterally, and orally in the suppression of lactation. Deficiency of pyridoxine is rare, because most foods contain vitamin B_6. However, deficiency may result from malabsorption, alcoholism, oral contraceptive use, and chemical inactivation by drugs (e.g., hydralazine and penicillamine). Vitamin B_6 deficiency may cause anemia, anorexia, neuritis, nausea, dermatitis, and depressed immunity. The ingestion of megadoses (2 to 6 g/day for 2 to 40 months) of pyridoxine may cause progressive sensory **ataxia**.

Vitamin B_7. **Vitamin B_7 (biotin)** is a water-soluble vitamin that is synthesized by intestinal flora; therefore, deficiency states are rare. Biotin functions in metabolism via biotin-dependent enzymes.

Vitamin B_9. **Vitamin B_9 (folic acid)** is essential for cell growth and the reproduction of red blood cells. It functions as a co-enzyme with vitamins B_{12} and C in the breakdown of proteins and in the formation of nucleic acid and hemoglobin. It is also essential for fetal development, particularly of the neural tube. Deficiency causes anemia that may cause spina bifida in a fetus. It is also called folacin.

Vitamin B_{12}. **Vitamin B_{12} (hydroxocobalamin)** is often found as **cyanocobalamin** in pharmaceutical preparations. It is involved in the metabolism of protein, fats, and carbohydrates. It aids in hemoglobin synthesis, is essential for normal functioning of all cells, and is important in energy metabolism. Vitamin B_{12} is available in meat and animal protein foods. Its absorption is complex; it occurs in the terminal portion of the small intestine (ileum) and requires **intrinsic factor** (a secretion of the stomach walls). Deficiency causes pernicious anemia and neurological disorders.

Vitamin B_{12} deficiency is caused by a lack of activated folic acid, which is essential for DNA synthesis and cell division. Lack of vitamin B_{12} can also affect the nervous system, causing numbness in the limbs, mood disturbances, and even hallucinations in severe deficiencies.

Patients who are suffering from vitamin B_{12} deficiency usually respond to massive doses of B_{12} every day, and then need weekly or biweekly intramuscular vitamin B_{12} injections. This vitamin B_{12} therapy must be continued for the remainder of the patient's life.

Vitamin C

Vitamin C (ascorbic acid) is essential for the formation of collagen tissue and for normal intercellular matrices in teeth, bone, cartilage, connective tissues, and skin. This is one of the most controversial vitamins, with some practitioners advocating up to 10 g or more per day. Smokers may need up to 150 mg per day. Anything over that is said merely to produce expensive urine. Ascorbic acid may protect the body against infections and help heal wounds. Therefore, ascorbic acid has multiple functions as either a coenzyme or co-factor. Its role in enhancing absorption of iron is well-recognized. Deficiency causes scurvy, lowered resistance to infections, joint tenderness, dental caries, bleeding gums, delayed wound healing, bruising, hemorrhage, and anemia.

Minerals and Electrolytes

Minerals are inorganic substances occurring naturally in the earth's crust that the body needs to help build and maintain body tissues for life functions. They are classified as major and trace elements.

Electrolytes are compounds, particularly salts, that when dissolved in water or another solvent dissociate into ions and are able to conduct an electric current. The concentrations of electrolytes differ in blood plasma and other tissues. Sodium, potassium, and chloride ions are electrolytes. Minerals help keep the body's water and electrolytes in balance.

Major Minerals

The major minerals are defined as those requiring an intake of more than 100 mg/day. The six major minerals are calcium, phosphorus, chloride, sodium, potassium, and magnesium.

Calcium (Ca) is the fifth-most abundant element in the human body and is present mainly in the bones. The body requires calcium ions for the transmission of nerve impulses, muscle contraction, blood coagulation, and cardiac functions. It is a component of extracellular fluid and of soft tissue cells.

Too much calcium will lead to cardiac failure (calcium chloride is included in the lethal injection given in judicial death sentences carried out in certain states of the U.S.). Too little calcium leads to tetany, which, if severe, can result in fatal muscular convulsions. Fortunately, both vitamin D and parathyroid hormone (PTH) can normally keep these levels constant, principally by mobilizing calcium from bone if hypocalcemia is present, and shunting it back into bone in hypercalcemia. Both hypocalcemia and hypercalcemia are due to factors involving either vitamin D or PTH. Benign hypercalcemia due to excessive absorption of calcium may result in calcification of soft tissues and renal damage.

Lack of calcium in the diet results in osteoporosis, in which bone is less dense, and therefore, brittle and weak. The following factors enhance the absorption of calcium: adequate vitamin D, calcitonin, parathyroid hormone, large quantities of calcium and phosphorus in the diet, and the presence of lactose. Abnormally high levels of ionized calcium in the extracellular fluid can produce muscle weakness, lethargy, and coma. Hypocalcemia can cause tetanic seizures and hypertension.

Phosphorus (P) is essential for the metabolism of protein, calcium, and glucose. It aids in building strong bones and teeth, and helps in the regulation of the body's acid-base balance. Nutritional sources are dairy foods, meat, egg yolks, whole grains, and nuts. A nutritional deficiency of phosphorus is rare, and is usually due to secondary factors. Phosphorus deficiency can occur when people abuse antacids containing aluminum compounds. Aluminum compounds combine with phosphates to produce aluminum complexes, which render the phosphates unavailable for absorption. Deficiency of phosphorus can cause weight loss, anemia, abnormal growth, muscular weakness, and bone pains. Anemia, **cachexia**, bronchitis, and necrosis of the mandible bone characterize chronic poisoning by phosphorus. Excessive doses of phosphorus may produce hypocalcemia in some cases.

Key Concept

Soft tissue calcification may occur with intravenous administration of phosphate ions, which is less likely to occur if the infusion is given slowly.

Chloride (Cl) is involved in the maintenance of fluid and the body's acid-base balance. The most common metal chloride is sodium chloride (table salt). Chloride ions are needed for the production of hydrochloric acid in the stomach. Chloride is normally associated with sodium and potassium, which are involved in helping to maintain pressure balances between the various body compartments.

Sodium (Na) is one of the most important elements in the body. Sodium ions are involved in acid-base balance, water balance, transmission of nerve impulses, and contraction of muscles. Major dietary sources of sodium are table salt (sodium chloride), ketchup, mustard, cured meats and fish, cheese, and potato chips. Toxic levels may cause hypertension and renal disease. The kidney is the main regulator of sodium levels in body fluids. In high temperatures and high fever, the body loses sodium through sweat. A dietary deficiency of sodium and chloride ions is unknown.

Key Concept

Drinking seawater leads to dehydration as the kidneys remove the extra salt by the excretion of essential body water.

There is a misconception that during hot weather, the intake of extra sodium as salt tablets is advisable. This may be helpful only in athletes and in people doing strenuous work. In these persons, it is probably better to encourage the consumption of low-fat milk and fruit juices, which contain sodium and potassium together in a more palatable form. Sodium chloride tablets can irritate the stomach.

Potassium (K) is the major electrolyte in intracellular fluids, helping to regulate neuromuscular excitability and muscle contraction. Sources of potassium in the diet are whole grains, meat, legumes, fruit, and vegetables. Potassium is important in glycogen formation, protein synthesis, and the correction of imbalances of acid-base metabolism, especially in association with the action of sodium and hydrogen ions. Potassium salts are very important as therapeutic agents but are extremely dangerous if used improperly. The kidney plays an important role in controlling secretion and absorption of potassium by the body tissues, especially in the muscles and the liver.

Key Concept

If possible, encouraging the patient to consume a high-potassium diet best treats diuretic-induced hypokalemia. Foods that are high in potassium are fruit juices, bananas, wholegrain cereals, and nuts.

Potassium deficiency may result from increased renal excretion, which may be caused by diuretic therapy, large doses of anionic drugs, or renal disorders. Increased GI tract excretion of potassium may occur with the loss of GI fluid through vomiting, diarrhea, surgical drainage, or chronic use of laxatives. Potassium loss through the skin is rare, but can result from perspiration during excessive exercise in a hot environment. Potassium deficiency can cause dysrhythmias, so it is important that patients taking certain diuretics also take some form of potassium supplement. Severe diarrhea can also cause hypokalemia. Potassium chloride is an irritant to the stomach mucosa, so tablets are enteric-coated. Another danger with potassium supplementation is hyperkalemia, which is just as serious as hypokalemia.

Magnesium (Mg) is an important ion for the function of many enzyme systems. Magnesium is the second-most abundant action of the intracellular fluids in the body. It helps to build strong bones and teeth, and aids in regulating the heartbeat. It is stored in the bone and is excreted mainly by the kidneys. Renal excretion of magnesium increases during diuresis induced by ammonium chloride, glucose, and organic mercurials. Magnesium affects the central nervous, neuromuscular, and cardiovascular systems. Diarrhea, steatorrhea, chronic alcoholism, and diabetes mellitus can produce **hypomagnesemia**. Hypomagnesemia is often treated with administration of parenteral fluids containing magnesium sulfate or magnesium chloride. Excess magnesium (hypermagnesemia) in the body can slow the heartbeat or cause cardiac arrest. Hypermagnesemia is usually caused by renal insufficiency and is manifested by hypotension, muscle weakness, sedation, and confused mental state.

Sulfur (S) is necessary to all body tissues and is found in all body cells. It is necessary for metabolism. Sulfur is a component of some amino acids and is therefore found in protein-rich foods.

Trace Elements

Trace elements are not less important, but occur in very small amounts in the body. They include iron, iodine, zinc, fluorine, and copper. Trace elements are generally defined as those having a required intake of less than 100 mg/day. Trace elements are equally essential for their specific vital tasks.

Iron (Fe) is a common metallic element essential for the formation of hemoglobin and myoglobin. The major role of iron is to transfer oxygen to the body tissues. Inadequate supplies of iron needed to form hemoglobin, poor absorption of iron in the digestive system, or chronic bleeding can cause iron deficiency anemia. Iron exists in two ionic states, depending on its oxidative state: the ferrous (iron II) ion, or Fe^{2+}, and the ferric (iron III) ion, or Fe^{3+}. The ferrous ion is easily oxidized to the ferric ion, and antioxidants such as ascorbic acid help in the absorption of iron from the intestines. Iron is present in most meat, legumes, shellfish, and whole grains. Replacement iron may be supplied by ferrous sulfate (Feosol), preferably the oral form. Iron dextran (Imferon) is an injectable form of iron supplement. Milk and antacids should be avoided with iron consumption.

Key Concept

Patients should be made aware that iron may turn stools black, but that this effect is harmless.

Iron preparations are best consumed on an empty stomach because this allows for maximum absorption. However, iron may be given with orange juice to assist in decreasing gastrointestinal symptoms.

Iodine (I) is an essential micronutrient of the thyroid hormone (thyroxine). Almost 80 percent of the iodine present in the body is in the thyroid gland. Iodine deficiency can result in goiter or **cretinism**. Iodine is found in seafood, iodized salt, and some dairy products. Deficiencies are common in areas away from the sea, and where water levels are inadequate. Iodine deficiency results in hypothyroidism and goiter. Excessive amounts of iodine can lead to similar conditions. Moderately high amounts of iodine in the diet can be bad for acne, so in areas where there are adequate amounts obtainable in the diet, acne sufferers should avoid iodized salt. Iodine is used as a contrast medium for blood vessels in computed tomography (CT) scans. Radioisotopes of iodine are used in radioisotope-scanning procedures and in palliative treatment of cancer of the thyroid.

Key Concept

Iodine poisoning can cause a brownish-colored staining of the mucus membranes.

Zinc (Zn) is essential for several body enzymes, growth, glucose tolerance, wound healing, and taste acuity. Nearly all functional units of the immune system are adversely affected by zinc deficiency. It is also used in numerous pharmaceutics, such as zinc acetate, zinc oxide, zinc permanganate, and zinc stearate. The best sources are protein foods. Zinc deficiency is characterized by abnormal fatigue, decreased alertness, a decrease in taste and odor sensitivity, poor appetite, retarded growth, delayed sexual maturity, prolonged healing of wounds, and susceptibility to infection and injury. Excess zinc supplementation can be dangerous as it can cause an increase in copper excretion, leading to copper deficiency. Other problems with excessive zinc intake are atherosclerosis due to a rise in cholesterol and triglyceride levels, and gastric irritation. Megadoses can result in acute toxicity and can be fatal.

Fluoride (F) is probably the most controversial of the microminerals, as it is added to many of the world's water supplies, and must therefore be consumed whether one wants to or not. There does not seem to be any doubt that, as a mineral, fluoride is an essential nutrient, not just to strengthen tooth enamel, but as a coenzyme for one or more enzyme systems. Unfortunately, many areas of the world have low fluoride concentrations in the soil and drinking water, causing people in these areas to become deficient in the element, resulting in an increase in dental caries. There is also evidence that fluoride can strengthen bones against osteoporosis.

Key Concept

The only food that contains reasonable amounts of fluoride is tea.

Flourine is the gas of which flouride is an ion. Excessive amounts of fluoride are poisonous, and cause mottling of the teeth. Fluoride can also cause warts to become cancerous.

Copper (Cu), like iron, is important for the synthesis of hemoglobin, because it is part of a co-enzyme involved in its synthesis. Copper is also a component of several important enzymes in the body, and is essential to good health. Copper is mostly concentrated in the liver, heart, brain, and kidneys. Good sources of copper are liver, shellfish, nuts, and beans. Copper deficiency is rare. Copper toxicity may be seen in individuals with Wilson's disease (a rare, inherited disorder that causes accumulation of copper in the liver), and in primary biliary cirrhosis. The build-up of copper in the tissue causes widespread tissue toxicity with multiple symptoms. The drug penicillamine (Cuprimine) can bind to copper and remove it from the tissues for excretion.

Food Labeling

Food items and supplements must be labeled in the pharmacy. By labeling these items, the technician can understand the importance of nutrition labeling regulations. Labeling of foods and supplements must be accurate and not misleading. The Nutrition Labeling and Education Act of 1990

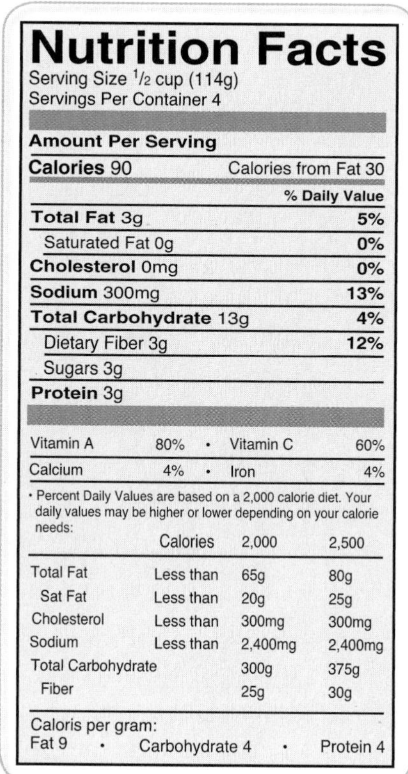

Figure 19-1 Nutrition label.

requires most packaged foods to have a list of a specified set of nutrition facts on the label. Setting of standards and enforcement for nutrition labeling are a responsibility of the Food and Drug Administration (FDA). All the nutrition information on the label is based on the stated serving size. Larger packages, such as cereal boxes, often include additional information not required by law. Figure 19-1 shows an example of a current food label with the minimum required facts.

Food Additives

Any substance that becomes part of a food product is called a **food additive**. Food additives can be added intentionally, such as when salt or cinnamon is added for flavoring, or unintentionally, such as when a pesticide used to treat crops is accidentally incorporated into the plant (or when a drug given to an animal ends up in the food product supplied by the animal). One purpose of food additives is to maintain or improve nutritional value, such as the addition of vitamins and minerals to a food product. The surge in the addition of calcium to juices and other foods is a good example of this function. Another purpose of additives is to maintain freshness in the food. Antioxidants added to foods processed with fat, such as potato chips, help to prevent the fat from becoming rancid, and preservatives help to prevent spoilage and changes in color, texture, and flavor of food. Additives also make food more appealing.

Nutritional Care

The proper intake and assimilation of nutrients, especially for the hospitalized patient, is called nutritional care. The nutritional needs of a patient depend on the patient's condition. Nutritional requirements may be provided by regular meals with menus selected from the ordered diet, by tube feeding, or by parenteral hyperalimentation.

Enteral Nutrition

Enteral nutrition (EN) is the delivery of nutrients through a GI tube, or the ingestion of food orally. Enteral tube feeding maintains the structural and functional integrity of the GI tract. It enhances the utilization of nutrients, and provides a safe and economical method of feeding. Enteral tube feedings are contraindicated in patients with the following:

- diffused peritonitis (widespread peritonitis)
- severe diarrhea
- vomiting
- intestinal obstruction that prohibits normal bowel function

Hyperalimentation (Total Parenteral Nutrition)

Hyperalimentation or **total parenteral nutrition (TPN)** is used to meet the patient's nutritional requirements when the enteral route cannot accomplish this. TPN is the treatment of choice for selected patients who are unable to tolerate and maintain adequate enteral intake. TPN is able to supply all the calories, amino acids (proteins), dextrose (carbohydrates), fats, trace elements, vitamins, and other essential nutrients needed for wound healing, immunocompetence, growth, and weight gain. The basic parenteral solution may contain amino acids, carbohydrates, lipids, vitamins, and minerals. Parenteral nutrition (PN) should be undertaken within 1 to 3 days, or in moderation if enteral support is anticipated for more than 5 to 7 days.

Pharma Food

Pharma food is a system of receiving nourishment through breathing. People constantly ingest microparticles that are suspended in the air, such as the dust in every home. The idea behind pharma food is to convert this act, the ingestion of polluting particles (which we are completely accustomed to and takes place in enclosed and outdoor urban areas), into a new form of nourishment. Pharma food is composed of a type of particle that is ingested by breathing and that has beneficial effects on the organism. These particles include (in general) vitamins, amino acids, minerals, or micronutrients, and constitute a volatile muesli that is released to be inhaled, reaching its destination by the mouth. For the particles to reach the stomach and avoid getting into the lungs, an element called saliva activator has been devised. It activates the salivary glands so that the inhaled particles adhere to saliva and are led to the stomach, where they are assimilated by the digestive system. Often, food products with pharmacological additives designed to improve health by lowering cholesterol or enhancing brain function are inhaled. Because of tough restrictions on advertising, pharma foods are not as popular as they could be, although there are continuing advances in their use. Inhaled lidocaine is now used as a treatment for asthma, which has led to a marked decline in use of steroids, the most popular type of treatment previously. Direct delivery of the lidocaine into the lungs in high concentrations results in minimal systemic exposure and toxicities, but it is not used much anymore. A similar therapy is the use of inhaled reformulated aztreonam to treat cystic fibrosis.

Summary

No single food supplies all the nutrients needed by the body. Therefore, it is important to eat a variety of foods daily to meet all the nutrient needs of the body. Vitamins and minerals are essential in small quantities for physiological and metabolic functioning of the body. Vitamins include water- or fat-soluble substances. Minerals are inorganic substances occurring naturally in the earth's crust that the body needs to help build and maintain body tissues for life functions. Deficiency and toxicity of vitamins or minerals may cause specific conditions or disorders. Pharmacy technicians must be familiar with basic nutrition dietary standards and pathological conditions. In pharmacy practice, there are many questions that clients may ask about foods and nutrition.

Exploring the Web

Visit ***http://ods.od.nih.gov***

- Explore the databases and various research that is being done on substances discussed in this chapter.

Visit ***http://win.niddk.nih.gov***

- Look at the publications that are available. Review information and recommendations related to weight loss concerns.

Visit ***www.eatright.org***

- Click on Food and Nutrition Information, and review the fact sheets related to vitamins and minerals. What foods provide the beneficial vitamins and minerals discussed in this chapter?

Visit ***www.nal.usda.gov***

- Look for information on dietary supplements. What additional information is available?

Visit ***www.nlm.nih.gov/medlineplus***

- Search for information on the vitamins and minerals discussed within this chapter.

Review Questions

Multiple Choice

1. Which of the following vitamins is used for the patient with an overdose of warfarin?

   A. vitamin D
   B. vitamin K
   C. vitamin E
   D. vitamin A

2. Physicians should prescribe vitamin B_{12} for which of the following patients?
   A. inadequate exposure to sunlight
   B. liver disease
   C. hemophilia
   D. pernicious anemia
3. Which of the following minerals should be restricted in patients who are complaining of weakness, dysrhythmias, and hypertension?
   A. magnesium
   B. aluminum
   C. sodium
   D. iron
4. The proper intake and assimilation of nutrients is known as:
   A. nutrient
   B. excretion
   C. nutritional insufficiency
   D. nutritional care
5. Severe deficiency of niacin (vitamin B_3) may result in:
   A. beriberi
   B. pellagra
   C. marasmus
   D. pernicious anemia
6. Which of the following types of feeding is more appropriate for when a patient's GI tract is not functioning?
   A. oral
   B. TPN
   C. enteral
   D. enema
7. An essential micronutrient of thyroid hormone (thyroxine) is:
   A. iron
   B. zinc
   C. iodine
   D. copper
8. Calcium deficiency may cause all of the following, except:
   A. rickets
   B. osteoporosis
   C. dwarfism
   D. osteomalacia
9. The Nutrition Labeling and Education Act of 1990 requires most packaged foods to list a specified set of:
   A. vitamin facts on the diet
   B. nutrition facts on the label
   C. mineral and vitamin facts on the diet
   D. nutritional deficiency

10. All of the following are the purposes of food additives, except:

A. to make food more appealing
B. to prevent misleading statements on the label
C. to maintain nutritional value
D. to main freshness in the food

11. A system of nourishing through breathing is known as:

A. volatile muesli
B. immune activator
C. saliva activator
D. pharma food

12. Which of the following minerals is able to help in the formation of hemoglobin and the transportation of iron to bone marrow?

A. fluoride (F)
B. copper (Cu)
C. zinc (Zn)
D. iodine (I)

13. Which of the following vitamins may protect the body against infections or help heal wounds?

A. vitamin C
B. vitamin B_{12}
C. vitamin K
D. vitamin E

14. All of the nutrition information on the label is based on which of the following?

A. the amount of cholesterol
B. the stated calories
C. the stated serving size
D. the amount of sodium

15. The purpose of food additives is:

A. to maintain nutritional value
B. to improve diets with low cholesterol
C. to improve diets with high potassium
D. all of the above

Matching

_____ **1.** vitamin B_2	**A.** folic acid
_____ **2.** vitamin B_3	**B.** nicotinamide
_____ **3.** vitamin B_5	**C.** hydroxocobalamin
_____ **4.** vitamin B_9	**D.** pantothenic acid
_____ **5.** vitamin B_{12}	**E.** riboflavin

Fill in the Blank

1. Vitamin K is an antagonist of ______________.
2. The only food that contains reasonable amounts of fluoride is ______________.
3. The drug penicillamine is able to remove ______________ from the tissues for excretion in treatment of ______________ disease.
4. Total parenteral nutrition may be administered through a(n) ______________ so that nutrition can be precisely monitored.

Critical Thinking

A pharmacy technician named John, who has been working in this position for three years, goes to Seattle to visit his grandmother whom he hasn't seen for nearly ten years. While staying at her house, he notices that she has about 15 different types of vitamins and mineral supplements on her nightstand. He asks her if she takes all of these herself, and she answers, "yes, I take all of them every day—they help me feel younger and give me more energy!" He finds out that she is also taking 3 to 4 different prescribed medications for her hypertension and diabetes.

1. What should John's advice be to his grandmother?
2. Which vitamin or mineral supplements may have potential interactions with diabetes medications?
3. If she were taking vitamin A and vitamin D in excess of the maximum daily requirements, what would be the symptoms of overdosage and toxicity from these vitamins?

Antineoplastic Agents

CHAPTER 20

OUTLINE

OBJECTIVES

After completing this chapter, the reader should be able to:

1. Identify the primary causes of cancer.
2. Explain the terms *benign, malignant,* and *neoplasm.*
3. Describe chemotherapy and the types of antineoplastic drugs.
4. Explain hormone therapy as antineoplastic drugs.
5. Describe the first group of antineoplastic agents.
6. List the classes of mitotic inhibitors (plant alkaloids).
7. Explain the mechanism of drug action of antimetabolites and antitumor antibiotics.
8. Explain toxicity of antineoplastic agents.
9. List specific side effects of certain antineoplastic agents on particular organs or systems in the body.
10. Explain different phases of the cell cycle.

GLOSSARY

Alopecia – hair loss

Antineoplastic agents – used to treat cancers or malignant neoplasms

Antimetabolites – prevent cancer cell growth by affecting its DNA production

Benign – cellular growth that is nonprogressive, and non–life-threatening

Carcinogens – any agent directly involved in or related to the promotion of cancer

Heterogeneous – consisting of a diverse range of different items

Malignant – cellular growth that is severe and becomes progressively worse, often becoming life-threatening

Metastasize – to spread from one part of the body to another

Mitotic inhibitors – drugs that block cell growth by stopping cell division

Neoplasm – a tumor; tissue that is composed of cells that grow in an abnormal way

Nitrosoureas – alkylating agents; they act by the process of alkylation to inhibit DNA repair

Palliation – treatment to relieve or reduce intensity of uncomfortable symptoms, but not to produce a cure

Radiation therapy – cancer treatment method whereby drugs are used to treat cancer either before or after surgery

Overview

Medical Terminology Review

neoplasm
neo = new
plasm = growth
new growth

metastasize
meta = changing
stasize = the state of
the process by which something undergoes change

A tumor, or **neoplasm**, arises from a single abnormal cell, which continues to divide indefinitely. The lack of growth controls, the ability to invade local tissue, and the ability to spread, or **metastasize**, are characteristics of cancer cells. These properties are not present in normal cells. Tumors are either **benign** (nonprogressive) or **malignant** (spreading). More than 100 different types of malignant neoplasms occur in man. Malignant tumors are also referred to as *cancer*, which is second only to heart disease as a cause of death in the U.S. Common sites for the development of malignant tumors are the skin, lungs, prostate, breasts, and large intestine (colon).

Cancer can be treated surgically or chemically. There are a variety of chemical treatments to consider in the treatment of cancers. The decisions for treatments may be made based upon the type of cancer being treated or the stage of the cancer when diagnosed. This chapter discusses many of the chemotherapeutic treatments used in the treatment of cancer.

Characteristics of Cancer

The proliferation of neoplastic cells leads to the formation of masses called tumors. The terms *neoplasm* and *tumor* are used synonymously. However, it is very important to note that not all neoplasms form tumors. For example, leukemia is a malignant disease of the bone marrow, but the malignant cells are in the blood circulation and thus do not form distinct masses.

Key Concept

Chromosomal changes are common in cancer cells. The Philadelphia chromosome, the first chromosomal abnormality linked to a malignant disease in humans, was found in patients with chronic myelogenous leukemia.

Causes of cancer development in humans may include exposure to chemicals, radiation, and viruses.

Cancer is the second-most common cause of death in the United States, eclipsed only by cardiovascular disease.

Most tumors can be classified clinically as either benign or malignant. Benign tumors have a limited growth potential and a good outcome, whereas malignant tumors grow uncontrollably and eventually kill the host.

Only malignant tumor cells have the capacity to metastasize. Benign tumors never metastasize and always remain localized. Metastasis involves a spread of tumor cells from a primary location to some other site in the body. The spread can occur through three main pathways:

- Through the lymphatics
- Via blood
- By seeding of the surface of body cavities

The Cell Cycle

To understand cancer treatments, normal and malignant cell replication processes should be reviewed. This cell cycle may last between 24 hours to many days. The phases of the cell cycle consist of a first growth phase (G_1), synthesis (S_1), a second growth phase (G_2), mitosis (M), and a resting phase (G_0). See Figure 20-1.

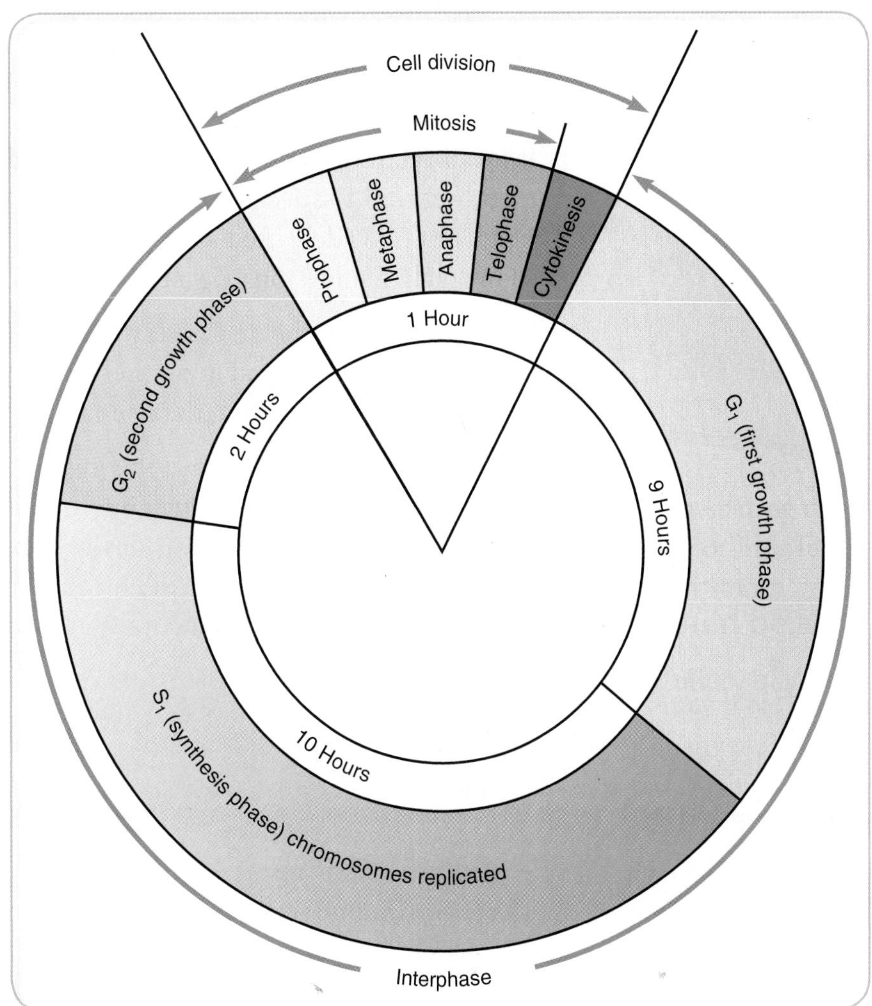

Figure 20-1 Stages of the cell cycle.

Causes of Cancer

The cause of most human cancers is unknown. Nevertheless, many potential agents (**carcinogens**) that result in the development of cancer have been identified, and the sources of many tumors have been explained (see Table 20-1).

TABLE 20-1 Exposure to Carcinogens

Causes	Cancer Sites
Sunlight (UV radiation)	Skin cancer
Human papilloma viruses	Genital warts and cervical cancer
Inhalation carcinogens (3,4-Benzpyrene); cigarette smoking	Lung cancer
Radiation	Thyroid and skin cancer
Metabolic liver carcinogens	Liver cancer
Metabolic excretory carcinogens	Bladder cancer
Metabolic carcinogens; nitrites and nitrates	Intestinal cancer

Treatment of Cancer

Cancer may be treated by using surgery, radiation therapy, and chemotherapy (drugs). Surgery is performed for the removal of a tumor that is localized in one area, or when the tumor is pressing on the airway, nerves, or other vital tissues. It remains the major form of treatment; however, irradiation is widely used as preoperative, postoperative, or primary therapy. Many malignant lesions are curable if detected in the early stage.

Radiation therapy is very effective in destroying tumor cells through non-surgical means. Radiation therapy may follow surgery to kill any cancer cells that remain following the operation.

Anticancer drugs may be given to attempt a cure, for **palliation** (treatment to relieve or reduce intensity of uncomfortable symptoms, but not to produce a cure), or occasionally, as prophylaxis to prevent cancer from occurring. Chemotherapy is often combined with surgery and radiation to increase the probability of a cure. In this chapter, the focus will be on drug therapy for cancers.

Antineoplastic Agents

Antineoplastic agents are used to treat cancers or malignant neoplasms. There are many types of drug therapies for the treatment of cancer. Antineoplastic agents are also called chemotherapeutic agents. They interrupt the development, growth, or spread of cancer cells. Antineoplastic agents are used for malignant tumors. Antineoplastic agents do not kill tumor cells directly, but interfere with cell replication (Figure 20-2). Each antineoplastic agent is effective at a specific stage in cell replication. It may inhibit DNA, RNA, and protein synthesis of cancer cells. Agents are most commonly given in combinations of two or more at a time. Many antineoplastic medications also have immunosuppressive properties that decrease the patient's ability to produce antibodies to attack infecting organisms. These medications are toxic to the body as a whole because they also destroy normal cells and decrease immunity.

The most common types of antineoplastic agents include: antimetabolites, hormonal agents, special antibiotics, alkylating agents, and mitotic inhibitors (plant alkaloids). Antineoplastic agents require the following special care and handling:

- Preparation only in restricted-access areas under biological safety cabinets
- Syringes and needles must have specialized fittings that are designed for use with these agents (for example, Luer-Lok™ fittings)
- Protective gowns must be worn during preparation

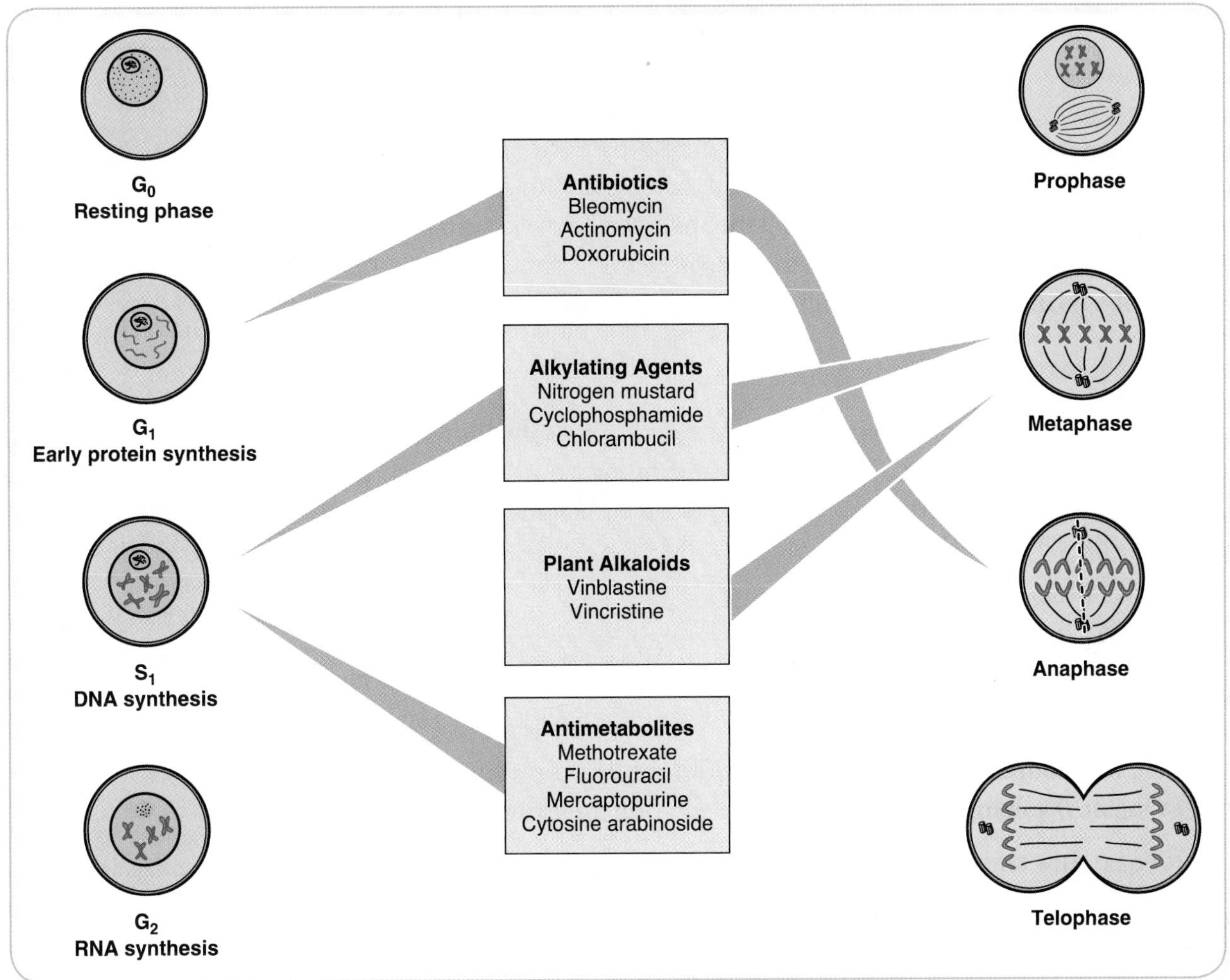

Figure 20-2 The effects of antineoplastic agents on various cell phases.

> **Medical Terminology Review**
>
> **alkylating**
> *alky(l) = free radical*
> *lating = transfer*
> the transfer of free radicals

- Two pairs of protective gloves should be worn, and periodically changed
- A plastic face shield or splash goggles should be worn
- Training classes must be attended by all workers who will be handling antineoplastic agents

Antimetabolites

Antimetabolites prevent cancer cell growth by affecting its DNA production. They are only effective against cells that are actively participating in cell metabolism. The antimetabolite drugs are listed in Table 20-2.

The classes of antimetabolites include:

1. Folic acid antagonists: methotrexate
2. Purine analogs: mercaptopurine
3. Pyrimidine analogs: fluorouracil

TABLE 20-2 Antimetabolites

Generic Name	Trade Name	Route of Administration	Average Adult Dosage
Folic Acid Antagonists			
methotrexate sodium	Amethopterin®, Mexate®	PO	15–30 mg/day for 5 days
pemetrexed	Alimta®	IV	500 mg/m^2 on day 1 of each 21 day cycle
Purine Analogs			
cladribine	Leustatin®	IV	0.09 mg/kg/day as a continuous infusion
clofarabine	Clolar®	IV	52 mg/m^2 over 2h for 5 consecutive days
fludarabine phosphate	Fludara®	IV	25 mg/m^2 daily for 5 consecutive days
mercaptopurine (6 MP)	Purinethol®	PO	2.5 mg/kg/day
nelarabine	Arranon®	IV	1500 mg/m^2 on days 1, 3, and 5; repeated every 21 days
pentostatin	Nipent®	IV	4 mg/m^2 every other week
thioguanine	Tabloid®	PO	2 mg/kg/day
Pyrimidine Analogs			
capecitabine	Xeloda®	PO	2500 mg/m^2/day for 2 weeks
cytarabine	Depo-Cyt®, Cytosar-U®	IV	200 mg/m^2 as a continuous infusion over 24 hours
floxuridine	FUDR®	Intra-arterial	0.1–0.6 mg/kg/day as a continuous infusion
fluorouracil (5 FU)	Adrucil®, Carac®	IV	12 mg/kg/day for 4 consecutive days
gemcitabine hydrochloride	Gemzar®	IV	1000 mg/m^2 q week

Mechanism of Action

Antimetabolites disrupt the metabolic functions of normal cells in the body. They interfere with the activity of enzymes and alter the DNA structure.

Indications

Antimetabolites are used in the treatment of a variety of neoplasms. Methotrexate is effective in the treatment of gestational choriocarcinoma and hydatidiform mole, as well as being immunosuppressant in kidney transplantation. Methotrexate is also used for acute and subacute leukemias and leukemic meningitis, especially in children. This drug is often indicated to treat severe psoriasis that is non-responsive to other forms of therapy.

Mercaptopurine (6-MP) is used primarily for acute lymphocytic and myelogenous leukemia. Fluorouracil (5-FU) is used systemically as a single agent and in combination with other antineoplastics for palliative treatment of carefully selected patients with inoperable neoplasms of the breast, colon or rectum, stomach, pancreas, urinary bladder, ovary, cervix, and liver.

Adverse Effects

Medical Terminology Review

leukopenia
leuko = white
penia = (blood cell) decrease
decrease in white blood cells

Antimetabolite agents may cause a wide variety of adverse effects. Common adverse effects include anorexia, nausea, vomiting, diarrhea, leukopenia, anemia, and thrombocytopenia. Some adverse effects of antimetabolites are dose-dependent, and may produce impaired liver function, hepatic necrosis, blurred vision, aphasia, and convulsions.

Contraindications and Precautions

Antimetabolite drugs are contraindicated in patients with anemia, thrombocytopenia, and poor nutrition. These agents are also contraindicated in patients with known hypersensitivity to these drugs, renal insufficiency, and during pregnancy (category D) or lactation.

Key Concept

Antimetabolite and other antineoplastic drugs in older adults may increase the risk of adverse effects. Therefore, a lower dosage is recommended for patients with renal impairment.

Antimetabolite agents should be used with caution in patients with hepatic or renal impairment, active infection, or other debilitating disorders. These drugs should be avoided in patients with peptic ulcer, ulcerative colitis, and elderly patients.

Drug Interactions

Alcohol and other CNS depressants may enhance CNS depression if taken with antimetabolites. Allopurinol may inhibit metabolism and increase toxicity of mercaptopurine.

Hormonal Agents

Hormonal agents are a class of **heterogeneous** compounds that have various effects on cells. These agents either block hormone production or block hormone action. Their action on malignant cells is highly selective. They are the least toxic of the anticancer medications. The most commonly used hormonal agents in cancer therapy are seen in Table 20-3.

Mechanism of Action

The precise action of hormones on malignant neoplasms is not known. However, these agents are able to counteract the effect of male or female hormones in hormone-dependent tumors.

TABLE 20-3 Commonly Used Hormonal Agents

Generic Name	Trade Name	Route of Administration	Average Adult Dosage
Hormones			
diethylstilbestrol	DES®, Stilbestrol®	PO	For prostate cancer: 500 mg t.i.d.; for palliation: 1–15 mg/day
ethinyl acetate	Femring®	PO	For breast cancer: 10 mg t.i.d.; for palliation of prostate cancer: 1–2 mg t.i.d.
fluoxymesterone	Halotestin®	PO	10–40 mg t.i.d.
medroxyprogesterone acetate	Provera®, Depo-Provera®	IM	400–1000 mg q week
megestrol acetate	Megace®	PO	40–160 mg b.i.d.-q.i.d.
prednisone	Deltasone®	PO	20–100 mg/m^2/day
testolactone	Teslac®	PO	250 mg q.i.d.
testosterone	Andro-Cyp®, Depo-Testosterone®	IM	200–400 mg q2–4 weeks
Hormone Antagonists			
abarelix	Plenaxis®	IM	100 mg on day 1, 15, 29 and q4 weeks thereafter
aminoglutethimide	Cytadren®	PO	250 mg b.i.d.-q.i.d.
anastrozole	Arimidex®	PO	1 mg/day
bicalutamide	Casodex®	PO	50 mg/day
exemestane	Aromasin®	PO	25 mg/day after a meal
flutamide	Eulexin®	PO	250 mg t.i.d.
goserelin acetate	Zoladex®	SC	3.6 mg q28 days
letrozole	Femara®	PO	2.5 mg/day
leuprolide acetate	Lupron®	SC, IM	SC: 1 mg/day; IM: 7.5 mg/month
nilutamide	Nilandron®	PO	300 mg/day for 30 days, then 150 mg/day
tamoxifen citrate	Nolvadex®	PO	10–20 mg b.i.d.
toremifene citrate	Fareston®	PO	60 mg/day

Indications

Hormones and their antagonists have various uses in the treatment of malignant diseases. Steroids are especially useful in treating lymphomas, leukemias, and Hodgkin's disease. They are also used in conjunction with radiation therapy to reduce nausea, weight loss, and tissue inflammation caused by other antitumor drugs. Gonadal hormones are used in carcinomas of the reproductive tract and advanced breast cancer. For example, estrogen is given to a patient with testicular cancer or carcinoma of the prostate. Estrogen may also be administered to postmenopausal women with breast cancer. Androgens (male hormones) are prescribed in premenopausal women with breast cancer. Antiestrogens, such as tamoxifen, and anti-androgens are used to inhibit hormone production in advanced stages of breast cancer.

Adverse Effects

Major adverse effects include masculization in female patients and feminization in male patient. Estrogen therapy may cause blood clots.

Contraindications and Precautions

Hormonal agents have a wide array of contraindications, including hypersensitivity to the agents. The use of hormonal agents must be avoided in patients with fungal infections, endometrial hyperplasia, thromboembolic disease, and in children. They are ranked in a variety of categories if used during pregnancy and lactation (including categories C, D, and X).

Precautions for the use of hormonal agents include patients with hypertension, gallbladder disease, diabetes mellitus, heart failure, liver or kidney dysfunction, infections, nonspecific ulcerative colitis, diverticulitis, peptic ulcer, osteoporosis, and myasthenia gravis. Hormonal agents must be used with great caution in many other conditions.

Drug Interactions

Hormonal agents may cause drug interactions with many agents, including but not limited to: carbamazepine, phenytoin, rifampin, corticosteroids, oral anticoagulants, barbiturates, amphotericin B, diuretics, ambenonium, neostigmine, and pyridostigmine. Hormonal agents may inhibit antibody response to vaccines and toxoids.

Antitumor Antibiotics

Several antibiotics of microbial origin are very effective in the treatment of certain tumors. They are used only to treat cancer, and are not used to treat infections. These antibiotics include bleomycin, doxorubicin, daunorubicin, idarubicin, mitomycin, and plicamycin (Table 20-4).

Mechanism of Action

The mechanism of action of antitumor antibiotics is the inhibition of DNA and RNA synthesis. Antitumor antibiotics attach to DNA, distorting its structure and preventing normal DNA-to-RNA synthesis.

TABLE 20-4 Antitumor Antibiotics

Generic Name	Trade Name	Route of Administration	Average Adult Dosage
bleomycin sulfate	Blenoxane®	SC, IM, IV	10–20 units/m^2 (1–2 times/week)
dactinomycin	Actinomycin D®, Cosmegan®	IV	500 mcg/day for a max. of 5 days
daunorubicin hydrochloride	Cerubidine®	IV	30–60 mg/m^2/day for 3–5 days
daunorubicin citrate liposomal	DaunoXome®	IV	40 mg/m^2 q2 weeks
doxorubicin hydrochloride	Adriamycin®, Rubex®	IV	60–75 mg/m^2 as a single dose
doxorubicin liposomal	Doxil®	IV	20 mg/m^2 q3 weeks
epirubicin hydrochloride	Ellence®	IV	100–120 mg/m^2 as a single dose
idarubicin	Idamycin PFS®	IV	8–12 mg/m^2/day for 3 days
mitomycin	Mutamycin®	IV	10–20 mg/m$^{2/}$day as a single dose
mitoxantrone hydrochloride	Novantrone®	IV	12–14 mg/m^2 q21 days
plicamycin	Mithramycin®, Mithracin®	IV	25–30 mcg/kg/day for 3–4 days
valrubicin	Valstar®	Intrabladder instillation	800 mg q week for 6 weeks

Indications

Antitumor antibiotics are used for treating a few specific types of cancer. For example, plicamycin is used only for treatment of testicular cancer. The only indication for idarubicin is acute leukemia (cancer of the blood).

Adverse Effects

The most serious adverse effects of antitumor antibiotics are low blood cell counts and congestive heart failure. Their common adverse effects include nausea, vomiting, diarrhea, fatigue, headache, and **alopecia** (hair loss). Bleomycin may cause pneumonitis, pulmonary fibrosis, and rash.

Contraindications and Precautions

Antitumor antibiotics are contraindicated in patients with known hypersensitivity, bleeding disorders, coagulation disorders, suppression of bone marrow, electrolyte imbalance, and chickenpox, herpes zoster, and other viral infections; in women of childbearing age; during pregnancy (various categories, including C and D) and lactation; and in infants less than six months of age.

Precautions for use of antitumor antibiotics include patients with compromised hepatic, renal, or pulmonary function, previous cytotoxic drug or radiation therapy, bone marrow depression, infections, gout, and obesity. There are many other precautions for these agents as well.

Drug Interactions

When bleomycin is given with cisplatin, there is an increased risk of bleomycin toxicity. Mitoxantrone, dactinomycin, mitomycin, and plicamycin increase bone marrow depression. There may be an increased risk of bleeding when plicamycin is used with aspirin, warfarin, heparin, or a nonsteroidal anti-inflammatory drug.

Alkylating Agents

Alkylating agents were the first group of antineoplastic agents. During World War I, chemical warfare was introduced using nitrogen mustard. Alkylating agents came to be used for cancer therapy as a result of observation of the effects of the mustard war gases on cell growth (Table 20-5).

TABLE 20-5 Alkylating Agents

Generic Name	Trade Name	Route of Administration	Average Adult Dosage
Nitrogen Mustards			
chlorambucil	Leukeran®	PO	Initial: 0.1–0.2 mg/kg/day; maint: 4–10 mg/day
cyclophosphamide	Cytoxan®	PO	Initial: 1–5 mg/kg/day; maint: 1–5 mg/kg q7–10 days
estramustine sodium phosphate	Emcyt®	PO	14 mg/kg t.i.d.-q.i.d.
ifosfamide	Ifex®	IV	1.2 g/m²/day for 5 days
mechlorethamine hydrochloride	Mustargen®	IV	6 mg/m² on days 1 and 8 for 28 days
melphalan	Alkeran®	PO	6 mg/day for 2–3 weeks
Nitrosoureas			
carmustine	Gliadel®	IV	150–200 mg/m² q6 weeks
lomustine	CeeNU®	PO	130 mg/m² as a single dose
streptozocin	Zanosar®	IV	500 mg/m² for 5 consecutive day

(continues)

TABLE 20-5 Alkylating Agents—*continued*

Generic Name	Trade Name	Route of Administration	Average Adult Dosage
Miscellaneous Agents			
busulfan	Myleran®	PO	4–8 mg/day
carboplatin	Paraplatin®	IV	360 mg/m^2 q4 weeks
cisplatin	Platinol®	IV	20 mg/m^2/day for 5 days
dacarbazine	DTIC-Dome®	IV	2–4.5 mg/kg/day for 10 days
oxaliplatin	Eloxatin®	IV	85 mg/m^2 infused over 120 min once q2 weeks
temozolomide	Temodar®	PO	150 mg/m^2/day for 5 consecutive days
thiotepa	Thioplex®	IV	0.3–0.4 mg/kg q1–4 week

Mechanism of Action

Most alkylating agents interact with the process of cell division of cancer cells. Antineoplastic or cytotoxic action is primarily due to cross-linking of strands of DNA and RNA as well as inhibition of protein synthesis. These drugs bind with DNA, causing breaks and preventing DNA replication.

Indications

Alkylating agents are used to treat metastatic ovarian, testicular, and bladder cancers. They are also used for the palliative treatment of other cancers. The newer drugs in this category are **nitrosoureas**, lipid-soluble drugs used in treating brain tumors and testicular or ovarian cancers.

Adverse Effects

Major adverse effects of the alkylating agents include nausea, vomiting, anorexia, diarrhea, bone marrow suppression, hepatic and renal toxicity, and dermatitis. Other adverse effects of alkylating drugs include cataracts, anxiety, fever, skin rash, hypertension, tachycardia, dizziness, and insomnia.

Contraindications and Precautions

Alkylating agents are contraindicated in patients with known hypersensitivity, impaired renal function, myelosuppression, impaired hearing, history of gout and urate renal stones, hypomagnesia, concurrent administration with loop diuretics, Raynaud syndrome, and many more conditions, and during pregnancy (various categories) and lactation. Safe use in children is not established for many of these agents.

Medical Terminology Review

myelosuppression
myelo = bone marrow
suppression = slowing of function
slowing of the production and function of the bone marrow

Precautions include use in patients with previous cytotoxic drug or radiation therapy with other ototoxic and nephrotoxic drugs, hyperuricemia,

Medical Terminology Review

hyperuricemia
hyper = more; excessive
uric = uric acid
emia = blood condition
excessive uric acid in the blood

electrolyte imbalances, hepatic impairment, and history of circulatory disorders. There are many other precautions for these agents as well.

Drug Interactions

Drug interactions with alkylating agents include aminoglycosides, amphotericin B, vancomycin, other nephrotoxic drugs, furosemide, barbiturates, phenytoin, chloral hydrate, and corticosteroids. There are other drug interactions with these various agents as well.

Mitotic Inhibitors

Mitotic inhibitors (plant alkaloids) are derived from plants. The primary plant alkaloids are vincristine and vinblastine. Teniposide is a close analog of etoposide and is active against acute leukemias in children. Topotecan is a semisynthetic plant alkaloid used for refractory ovarian cancer that may have activity against small-cell lung cancer. Examples of plant alkaloids are seen in Table 20-6.

Mechanism of Action

Mitotic inhibitors may interfere with cell division, but the antineoplastic mechanism of these agents is unclear.

TABLE 20-6 Mitotic Inhibitors and Other Plant Products

Generic Name	Trade Name	Route of Administration	Average Adult Dosage
Mitotic Inhibitors			
vinblastine sulfate	Velban®	IV	3.7–18.5 mg/m² q week
vincristine sulfate	Oncovin®	IV	1.4 mg/m² q week (max: 2 mg/m²)
vinorelbine tartrate	Navelbine®	IV	30 mg/m² q week
Taxoids			
docetaxel	Taxotere®	IV	60–100 mg/m² q3 weeks
paclitaxel	Taxol®	IV	135–175 mg/m² q3 weeks
Topoisomerase Inhibitors			
etoposide	VePesid®	IV	50–100 mg/m²/day for 5 days
irinotecan hydrochloride	Camptosar®	IV	125 mg/m² q week for 4 weeks
teniposide	Vumon®	IV	165 mg/m² q3-4 days for 4 weeks
topotecan hydrochloride	Hycamtin®	IV	1.5 mg/m²/day for 5 days

Indications

Mitotic inhibitor drugs are used in various cancers. For example, docetaxel is prescribed for breast cancer and non–small-cell lung cancer. Vinblastine is indicated for the treatment of Hodgkin's disease, lymphocytic lymphoma, testicular cancer, Kaposi's sarcoma, and breast cancer.

Vincristine is used in acute leukemia and combination therapy for various cancers. Paclitaxel is given to patients for treating ovarian and breast cancers, or for AIDS-related Kaposi's sarcoma.

Adverse Effects

Common adverse effects of mitotic inhibitors include nausea, vomiting, diarrhea, fatigue, mental depression, and alopecia. Infection and peripheral neuropathy are also considered to be unwanted effects of mitotic inhibitors.

Contraindications and Precautions

Mitotic inhibitors are contraindicated in patients with known hypersensitivity to these drugs. Mitotic inhibitors should be avoided in patients with leukopenia or bacterial infection, and during pregnancy (category D) or lactation.

Etoposide is also contraindicated in patients with severe bone marrow depression, and in severe hepatic or renal impairment. Mitotic inhibitors should be used with caution in patients who have impaired kidney or liver function, gout, obstructive jaundice, and idiopathic thrombocytopenic purpura.

Drug Interactions

Mitotic inhibitors may interact with many drugs. For example, vincristine used with asparaginase may cause increased neurotoxicity secondary to decreased liver clearance of vincristine. When mitotic inhibitors are used with calcium channel blockers, they may increase accumulation of these agents in cells.

Summary

A neoplasm is an abnormal cell division of the body. It may be benign or malignant. Only malignant tumors are capable of spreading to other organs or systems of the body. Treatment of the neoplasm depends on the progression of the tumor. Surgery, radiation therapy, chemotherapy, and immunotherapy may be indicated. There are many agents used for this purpose. Many antineoplastic medications also have immunosuppressive properties that decrease the patient's ability to produce antibodies to attack infecting organisms.

Common antineoplastic agents include antimetabolites, hormonal agents, specific antibiotics, alkylating agents, and mitotic inhibitors or plant alkaloids. In some cases, surgery and radiation therapy are also necessary. Toxicity and side effects of chemotherapy and radiation therapy are the major concerns regarding treatment of malignant tumors.

Exploring the Web

Visit the following websites for additional information on drug therapies used to treat cancer:

www.biochemweb.org

www.cancer.org

www.cancer-info.com

www.cdc.gov/niosh

www.mayoclinic.com

Review Questions

Multiple Choice

1. The cell cycle consists of several phases, such as G_0, G_1, S_1, G_2, and M. Which of the following explains the G_0 phase?
   - **A.** resting
   - **B.** synthesis
   - **C.** mitosis
   - **D.** growth
2. Which of the following agents is an antimetabolite?
   - **A.** cyclophosphamide
   - **B.** fluorouracil
   - **C.** mitomycin
   - **D.** nitrogen mustard

3. Which of the following is an example of an antitumor antibiotic?
   A. vinorelbine
   B. topotecan
   C. bleomycin
   D. mercaptopurine
4. Mitotic inhibitors (plant alkaloids) include:
   A. mercaptopurine
   B. testolactone
   C. tamoxifen
   D. vincristine
5. Mercaptopurine may have drug interactions with which of the following agents?
   A. amoxicillin
   B. alcohol
   C. allopurinol
   D. estrogen
6. An adverse effect of methotrexate includes:
   A. bone marrow aplasia
   B. arthritis
   C. hypertension
   D. hyperthyroidism
7. Busulfan has some unusual side effects in addition to its bone marrow suppressive activity. Which of the following side effects are caused by busulfan?
   A. peptic ulcer
   B. testicular cancer
   C. gynecomastia
   D. gastrointestinal bleeding
8. Which of the following is the trade name of doxorubicin?
   A. Mutamycin
   B. Adriamycin
   C. Cosmegan
   D. Blenoxane
9. The route of administration for goserelin is:
   A. oral
   B. intramuscular
   C. intravenous
   D. implant
10. Most plant alkaloids may produce:
    A. nausea and vomiting
    B. internal bleeding
    C. hypertension
    D. gout

11. Which of the following antimetabolic is useful in maintenance therapy of children with acute leukemia?
    A. fluorouracil (5-FU)
    B. methotrexate (MTX)
    C. mercaptopurine (6-MP)
    D. vincristine

12. Which of the following is the best drug that may be given to a patient with testicular cancer?
    A. tamoxifen
    B. estrogen
    C. progesterone
    D. megestrol

13. The term *metastasize* means to:
    A. arise
    B. divide
    C. spread
    D. occur

14. Hycamtin® is the trade name of which of the following agents?
    A. vincristine
    B. vinblastine
    C. vinorelbine
    D. topotecan

15. The single most active agent against breast cancer is:
    A. dactinomycin
    B. mitomycin
    C. doxorubicin
    D. bleomycin

Matching

_____ 1. Resting phase	A. G_1
_____ 2. Cell division	B. S_1
_____ 3. Synthesis	C. G_2
_____ 4. Second growth phase	D. M
_____ 5. First growth phase	E. G_0

Generic Name	Trade Name
_____ 1. vincristine	A. VePesid
_____ 2. vinblastine	B. Navelbine
_____ 3. vinorelbine	C. Oncovin
_____ 4. paclitaxel	D. Velban
_____ 5. etoposide	E. Taxol

Critical Thinking

A biopsy revealed that a 45-year-old woman had breast cancer. She underwent surgery and her left breast was removed. Her physician ordered radiation therapy and chemotherapy as adjuvant therapies to the surgery.

1. If she were to refuse radiation or chemotherapy, what would be the likely consequence?
2. List the most common adverse effects of chemotherapy.
3. If the physician diagnosed that this patient had metastasis to her bones, which types of treatment should he recommend?

Analgesics

CHAPTER 21

OUTLINE

Analgesics
- Salicylates
- Acetaminophen
- Nonsteroidal Anti-inflammatory Drugs
- Cyclooxygenase Inhibitors
- Narcotic Analgesics
- Opioid Antagonists

Migraine Headaches
- Treatment of Migraine Headaches

OBJECTIVES

After completing this chapter, the reader should be able to:

1. Differentiate salicylates from nonsalicylate nonsteroid anti-inflammatory drugs.
2. Describe the uses and adverse effects of nonsalicylate analgesics.
3. List the dangers of aspirin use.
4. Explain the contraindications of aspirin.
5. Describe the use of cyclooxygenase-2 inhibitors.
6. Explain the reason behind the use of narcotic analgesics.
7. Outline three narcotic antagonists.
8. Identify the different types of analgesics.
9. Explain the major adverse effects of narcotic analgesics.
10. Describe the opioid receptors.

GLOSSARY

Acute pain – pain that is of sudden onset and brief course; can also mean "severe"

Agonist-antagonists – agents that can initiate or resist actions

Analgesic – a compound that relieves pain by altering perception without producing anesthesia or loss of consciousness

Bradykinin – a polypeptide that mediates inflammation, increases vasodilation, and contracts smooth muscle

Chronic pain – pain that is persistent or long-term; can also mean "low-intensity"

Cyclooxygenase inhibitors – drugs that prevent the action of one of two enzymes that have an essential role in the inflammation process

Intracranial – within the cranium (skull)

Nonsteroidal anti-inflammatory drugs (NSAIDs) – drugs that have analgesic and antipyretic effects

Opioid – a natural or synthetic narcotic substance

Opioid agonists – drugs that can combine with receptors to initiate drug actions

Opioid antagonists – drugs that oppose or resist the action of others

Pain – an unpleasant sensation associated with actual or potential tissue damage

Reye syndrome – an acquired encephalopathy of young children that follows an acute febrile illness; strongly associated with aspirin use

Salicylates – salts or esters of salicylic acid

Overview

Pain is a common problem and an unpleasant sensory experience that is associated with actual damage of tissue. **Pain** is the reaction of the central nervous system to severe harmful stimuli. It may be an early warning system to prevent any further damage to the body. Pain stimuli may be caused by the process of inflammation or tissue injury. Pain may be described as mild, moderate, or severe; acute or chronic; dull or sharp; burning or piercing; and localized or generalized. **Acute pain** is severe pain with a sudden onset. **Chronic pain** lasts a long time or is marked by frequent reoccurrence. During an organ's injury or inflammation, different chemical substances are released. These substances include histamine, prostaglandins (hormone-like substances that control blood pressure, contract smooth muscle, and modulate inflammation), serotonin, and **bradykinin** (a polypeptide that mediates inflammation, increases vasodilation, and contracts smooth muscle). These chemical substances initiate an action potential along a sensory nerve fiber and/or sensitize pain receptors. This chapter provides discussion of the various medicinal products used in the relief of pain.

Analgesics

Medical Terminology Review

osteoarthritis
osteo = bone
arthr = joint
itis = inflammation
inflammation of the bones affecting the joints

Pain-relieving (**analgesic**) drugs are currently available for all levels of painful stimuli. Analgesics may be classified as **opioid** (narcotic) or nonopioid medications. Many of these agents affect pain, fever, and inflammation, depending on their properties. Nonopioid analgesics, antipyretics, and anti-inflammatory drugs are used widely for minor aches and pains, headaches, malaise, rheumatic fever, arthritis, osteoarthritis, gout, and other musculoskeletal disorders. The narcotic (opioid) analgesics are controlled substances used to treat moderate to severe pain.

Salicylates

Salicylates are the oldest of the nonopioid analgesics and nonsteroidal anti-inflammatory drugs (NSAIDs), which are discussed in detail below. They are still often used as analgesics (Table 21-1). The salicylates include aspirin (acetylsalicylic acid), which is the most commonly used. The salicylates may be combined with caffeine to increase their action. Anacin and Excedrin are examples of salicylates that are combined with caffeine. Caffeine can make some of these agents work more quickly or provide additional relief.

Mechanism of Action

The mechanism of action of salicylates is not fully understood. Major actions appear to be associated primarily with inhibiting the formation

TABLE 21-1 Salicylates and Nonsalicylates

Generic Name	Trade Name	Route of Administration	Average Adult Dosage
Salicylates			
aspirin (acetylsalicylic acid)	Bayer®, Ecotrin®	PO, Rectal	PO: 325–650 mg with up to 8 g/day in div. doses;
buffered aspirin	Ascriptin®, Asprimox®	PO, Rectal	PO: 325–650 mg with up to 8 g/day in div. doses;
choline salicylate	Arthropan®	PO	870 mg q3–4 h (max: 6 times/day)
diflusinal	Dolobid®	PO	500–1000 mg/day in 2 div. doses (max dose: 1.5 g/day)
magnesium salicylate	Doan's Pills®, Mobidin®	PO	650 mg t.i.d. or q.i.d. up to 9.6 g/day in div. doses
salsalate	Amigesic®, Artha-G®	PO	325–3000 mg/day in div. doses
sodium salicylate	(generic only)	PO	325–650 mg q4 h
sodium thiosalicylate	Rexolate®	IM	50–150 mg q4–6 h
Nonsalicylates			
acetaminophen	Tempra®, Tylenol®	PO	325–650 mg/day q4–6 h or 1 g 3–4 times/day; max. dose: 4 g/day

of prostaglandins involved in the production of inflammation, pain, and fever.

Indications

Salicylates are also prescribed as NSAIDs for rheumatoid osteoarthritis and often for other inflammatory disorders. Aspirin is absorbed rapidly from the duodenum and stomach. It is used as an antipyretic and analgesic agent in a variety of conditions. Aspirin is indicated for the relief of pain from simple headache, minor muscular aches, and fever. When drug therapy is indicated for the reduction of a fever, it is one of the most effective and safest drugs. Aspirin may be useful in the prevention of coronary thrombosis by prolonging bleeding time, and to prevent blood clots in small arteries.

> ***Medical Terminology Review***
>
> **antipyretic**
> *anti = not*
> *pyretic = producing fever*
> fever-reducing

Adverse Effects

Common adverse effects of high doses of aspirin (in 70 percent of patients) include nausea, vomiting, diarrhea or constipation, dyspepsia, epigastric pain, bleeding, and ulceration in the stomach. Intolerance is relatively common with aspirin and includes rash, bronchospasm, rhinitis, edema, or an anaphylactic reaction with shock, which may be life-threatening. Use of aspirin and other salicylates to control fever during viral infections in children and adolescents (influenza, common cold, and chicken pox), is associated with an increased incidence of **Reye syndrome**. Vomiting, hepatic disturbances, and encephalopathy characterize this illness. Salicylates that are combined with caffeine can, in very large doses, cause birth defects to a developing fetus. Caffeine, as used in some of these preparations, can make some kinds of heart disease worse.

Key Concept

Salicylates must be used cautiously in children who have fever or are dehydrated, because they are particularly prone to intoxication from relatively small doses of these drugs. An allergic sensitivity to salicylates may cause a serious problem. Patients who have asthma, nasal polyps, or allergies must be very careful when they take these drugs to avoid potentially dangerous adverse effects.

Aspirin use should be avoided in infants and young children if they have flu-like illnesses, because it may cause the development of Reye syndrome.

Contraindications and Precautions

Salicylates are contraindicated in patients with known hypersensitivity and during pregnancy (category C), but aspirin during pregnancy is category D. The salicylates should be avoided in patients with bleeding disorders or peptic ulcers, or those receiving anticoagulant or antineoplastic drugs. The salicylates, particularly aspirin, are also contraindicated in patients with chicken pox and influenza.

Drug Interactions

Salicylates increase the risk of gastrointestinal ulceration with alcohol and corticosteroids. They also increase the risk of toxicity with carbonic anhydrase inhibitors and valproic acid. Ammonium chloride and other acidifying agents decrease renal elimination and increase the risk of salicylate toxicity. Anticoagulants increase the risk of bleeding. Antacids may decrease the effects of the salicylate. In order to prevent drug interactions, patients must be instructed by their physician and pharmacist about the use of NSAIDs with other OTC analgesics.

Key Concept

Some foods, such as prunes, paprika, raisins, and tea, contain salicylates, which can increase the risk of adverse effects.

Acetaminophen

Another common nonopioid analgesic, acetaminophen is available OTC and is found in most households.

Mechanism of Action

Like aspirin, acetaminophen has analgesic and antipyretic actions. It can be used with relative safety in age groups from young children through older adults. Unlike aspirin, it does not have anti-inflammatory actions. The mechanism of action may be inhibition of prostaglandin in the peripheral nervous system, which makes the sensory neurons less likely to receive the pain signal. Acetaminophen is recommended as a substitute for children with fever of unknown etiology.

Acetaminophen does not displace other drugs from plasma proteins; it causes minimal GI irritation. Acetaminophen has little effect on platelet adhesion and aggregation. It can be substituted for aspirin to treat mild to moderate pain or fever for selected patients who:

- are intolerant to aspirin
- have a history of peptic ulcer or hemophilia

> **Medical Terminology Review**
>
> **anticoagulant**
> *anti = not*
> *coagulant = an agent that causes clotting*
> an agent that will not cause clotting of the blood

- are using anticoagulants
- are at risk (viral infection) for Reye syndrome

Indications

Acetaminophen is used for fever reduction and the temporary relief of mild to moderate pain. Acetaminophen may be used as a substitute for aspirin when the latter is not tolerated or is contraindicated.

Adverse Effects

Acute acetaminophen poisoning may produce anorexia, nausea, vomiting, dizziness, chills, abdominal pain, diarrhea, hepatotoxicity, hypoglycemia, hepatic coma, and acute renal failure (rare). Chronic ingestion of acetaminophen may cause neutropenia, pancytopenia, leukopenia, and hepatotoxicity in alcoholics, as well as renal damage.

Contraindications and Precautions

Acetaminophen is contraindicated in those with known hypersensitivity to this agent or phenacetin. Acetaminophen should not be used with alcohol.

> **Medical Terminology Review**
>
> **thrombocytopenia**
> *thrombo = clot*
> *cyto = cell (such as a platelet)*
> *penia = lack of*
> inability of the blood to clot

Precautions include use in children less than three years of age unless directed by a physician, repeated administration to patients with anemia or hepatic disease, with arthritic or rheumatoid conditions affecting children less than twelve years of age, alcoholism, malnutrition, and thrombocytopenia. Safety during pregnancy (category B) or lactation is not established.

Drug Interactions

Cholestyramine may decrease acetaminophen absorption with chronic co-administration. Barbiturates, carbamazepine, phenytoin, and rifampin may increase the potential for chronic hepatotoxicity. Chronic, excessive ingestion of alcohol will increase risk of hepatotoxicity.

Nonsteroidal Anti-inflammatory Drugs

Most of the **nonsteroidal anti-inflammatory drugs (NSAIDs)** have analgesic and antipyretic effects. Little difference is seen between the effects of different NSAIDs, but some patients may respond better to one agent than to another. Anti-inflammatory effects may develop only after several weeks of treatment. Drug selection is generally dictated by the patient's ability to tolerate adverse effects. Aspirin, other salicylates, and newer drugs with diverse structures are referred to as nonsteroidal anti-inflammatory drugs (NSAIDs) to distinguish them from the anti-inflammatory corticosteroids. The number of NSAIDs continues to increase. In addition to salicylate drugs, the NSAIDs available in the U.S. include indomethacin, meclofenamate, piroxicam, sulindac, tolmetin, celecoxib, and many more (Table 21-2).

TABLE 21-2 Nonsteroidal Anti-inflammatory Drugs (NSAIDs)

Generic Name	Trade Name	Route of Administration	Average Adult Dosage
celecoxib	Celebrex®	PO	100–200 mg b.i.d. p.r.n.
diclofenac sodium	Voltaren®	PO	Osteoarthritis: 100–150 mg/day in div. doses; Rheumatoid arthritis: 150–200 mg/day in div. doses; Ankylosing spondylitis: 100–125 mg/day in div. doses
etodolac	Lodine®, Lodine XL®	PO	Acute pain: 200–400 mg q6–8 h p.r.n.; Osteoarthritis: 600–1200 mg/day in 2–4 div. doses (max: 1200 mg/day or 20 mg/kg for patients ≤ 60 kg; Lodine XL 400–1000 mg 1x/day); Rheumatoid arthritis: 500 mg b.i.d.
fenoprofen calcium	Nalfon®	PO	Rheumatoid arthritis and osteoarthritis: 300–600 mg t.i.d.-q.i.d.; Pain: 200 mg q4–8 h
flurbiprofen	Ansaid®	PO	200–300 mg/day in div. doses
ibuprofen	Advil®, Motrin®	PO	Arthritis disorders: 400–800 mg/day in div. doses (max: 3200 mg/day); Pain: 400 mg q4–6 h; Dysmenorrhea: 400 mg q4 h
indomethacin	Indocin®	PO	Anti-inflammatory and analgesic: 25–50 mg b.i.d. -t.i.d. (max: 200 mg/day); Acute painful shoulder: 75–150 mg/day in 3–4 div. doses
ketoprofen	Oruvail®	PO	Inflammatory disease: 75 mg t.i.d. or 50 mg q.i.d. (max: 300 mg/day) or 200 mg sust. release q.d.; Pain or Dysmenorrhea: 12.5–50 mg q6–8 h
ketorolac tromethamine	Toradol®	PO, IM	PO: 10 mg q4–6 h p.r.n. (max: 40 mg/day); IM: 30–60 mg initially, followed by half of initial dose q6 h p.r.n.
meclofenamate sodium	(generic)	PO	Rheumatoid arthritis: 200–400 mg/day in 3–4 doses; Pain: 50 mg q4–6 h (max: 400 mg/day); Dysmenorrhea: 100 mg t.i.d.

(*continues*)

TABLE 21-2 Nonsteroidal Anti-inflammatory Drugs (NSAIDs)—*continued*

Generic Name	Trade Name	Route of Administration	Average Adult Dosage
mefenamic acid	Ponstel®	PO	500 mg followed by 250 mg q6 h p.r.n. (max: 1 wk of therapy)
meloxicam	Mobic®	PO	7.5–15 mg q.d.
nabumetone	Relafen®	PO	1000–2000 mg/day
naproxen sodium	Aleve®, Anaprox®	PO	Pain, primary dysmenorrhea: 500 mg initially then 250 mg q6–8 h; Arthritic disorders: 250–500 mg b.i.d.
oxaprozin	Daypro®	PO	600–1200 mg q.d.
piroxicam	Feldene®	PO	20 mg/day single dose or 10 mg b.i.d.
sulindac	Clinoril®	PO	150–200 mg b.i.d. for 1–2 wks, then reduce dose (max: 400 mg/day)
tolmetin sodium	Tolectin®	PO	400 mg b.i.d.-t.i.d. (max: 2 g / day)

Mechanism of Action

The mechanism of action of NSAIDs is unknown. It may be due to irreversible inhibition of prostaglandin (an enzyme) formation, which converts archidonic acid to prostaglandin. This action is involved in the processes of pain and inflammation. Some experts believe that NSAIDs relieve fever by central action in the hypothalamus of the brain. In low doses, baby aspirin appears to affect blood clotting by inhibiting prostaglandin formation, which prevents synthesis of platelet-aggregating substances. This can help to prevent heart attacks and strokes. NSAIDs inhibit, in varying amounts, both the COX-1 and COX-2 enzymes.

Indications

NSAIDs are used for mild to moderate pain when opioids are not indicated. Most NSAIDs are used for inflammatory conditions such as arthritis, osteoarthritis, dysmenorrhea, and dental pain. NSAIDs are available OTC in lower dosages and by prescription in larger dosages. Aspirin and ibuprofen are available as OTC drugs that are inexpensive. Ibuprofen is available in many different formulations including those designed for children.

Adverse Effects

Many NSAIDs are safe and produce adverse effects only at high doses. The most common adverse effects (at high doses) of NSAIDs are primarily GI distress, gastric ulcers, and GI bleeding. Other NSAIDs, such as the COX-2 inhibitors, are being investigated for possible adverse effects.

Contraindications and Precautions

Nonsteroidal anti-inflammatory drugs are contraindicated in patients with known hypersensitivity to any NSAIDs. These drugs are also contraindicated in patients with nasal polyps, asthma, and angioedema. NSAIDs should be avoided during pregnancy and in patients with history of peptic ulcer, or renal or hepatic impairment.

Medical Terminology Review

angioedema
angio = blood vessel
edema = swelling caused by fluid
swelling of blood vessels

Drug Interactions

NSAIDs should not be taken with any other OTC analgesics such as acetaminophen, aspirin, or other NSAIDs. NSAIDs may result in harmful drug interactions if taken with alcohol and a wide variety of other medications. Use of NSAIDs with phenobarbital, antacids, and glucocorticoids may decrease their effects. Insulin, methotrexate, phenytoin, sulfonamides, and penicillin may increase the effects of NSAIDs.

Key Concept

NSAIDs must be used cautiously with herbal supplements such as feverfew, which may increase the risk of bleeding.

Cyclooxygenase Inhibitors

The two main types of **cyclooxygenase inhibitors** (COX-1 and COX-2) have been found to have an essential role in the inflammation process. Both are present in the synovial fluid of patients with arthritis. COX-2 is more specific for prostaglandin synthesis in response to an inflammatory event. It is thought to be primarily responsible for the desired anti-inflammatory, analgesic, and antipyretic effects, whereas COX-1 has a more extensive role in the body, including protection of the GI lining.

As of May 2000, the U.S. Food and Drug Administration (FDA) has approved the COX-2 inhibitors celecoxib (Celebrex) and rofecoxib (Vioxx). Recently, rofecoxib was removed from the United States market due to problems that resulted in certain patients. A third COX-2 selective inhibitor, meloxicam (Mobic), has recently been introduced. The daily role of COX appears to be the synthesis of prostaglandins that contribute to normal homeostasis.

Key Concept

Prostaglandins are derivatives of prostanoic acid. In the body, prostaglandins are principally synthesized from arachidonic acid (lipids) by the enzyme COX.

Mechanism of Action

These agents inhibit prostaglandin synthesis by selectively targeting only the COX-2 enzymes, but they do not inhibit COX-1. The COX-2 inhibitors have similar anti-inflammatory effects without the adverse GI effects that accompany COX-1 inhibitors.

Indications

The FDA has approved celecoxib for the treatment of osteoarthritis, rheumatoid arthritis, primary dysmenorrhea, and acute pain. Rofecoxib is off the market. Meloxicam, the newest COX-2 inhibitor, has been approved by the FDA for the treatment of osteoarthritis.

Medical Terminology Review

dysmenorrhea
dys = abnormal
meno = menstrual
rrhea = flow
abnormal menstrual flow

Adverse Effects

The common adverse effects of COX-2 inhibitors include fatigue, flu-like symptoms, lower extremity swelling, and back pain. Dizziness, headache, hypertension, edema, heartburn, and nausea are also seen with the use of COX-2 inhibitors.

Contraindications and Precautions

COX-2 inhibitors are contraindicated in patients with known hypersensitivity to these agents, urticaria, asthma, or history of anaphylactic reaction after taking NSAIDs or aspirin. COX-2 inhibitors are also contraindicated in elderly patients, during pregnancy (third trimester), and in lactating women. These drugs should be avoided in patients with renal disease or hepatic dysfunction.

COX-2 inhibitors should be used cautiously in patients with congestive heart failure, fluid retention, or hypertension.

Drug Interactions

COX-2 inhibitors diminish the effectiveness of ACE inhibitors. Fluconazole increases concentrations of celecoxib. COX-2 inhibitors may increase lithium concentrations.

Narcotic Analgesics

Narcotic analgesics are agents that are derived from opium or opium-like compounds with potent analgesic effects associated with both significant alteration of mood and behavior and potential for dependence and tolerance. The analgesic compounds of opium have been known for hundreds of years. Morphine is extracted from raw opium and may be altered chemically to produce the semisynthetic narcotics, such as hydromorphone, oxymorphone, oxycodone, and heroin. Synthetic narcotics are produced in laboratories, with analgesic properties. Methadone, levorphanol, and meperidine are amongst the various narcotics listed in Table 21-3.

Key Concept

Narcotic analgesics are classified as Schedule II drugs, except for heroin, which is classified as a Schedule I drug.

Mechanism of Action

The effects of natural opium alkaloids occur by binding to opioid receptors. These receptors are located in the central nervous system (brain and spinal cord). Narcotic agonist effects are identified with three types of opioid receptors: the mu, kappa, and delta receptors. Most of the currently used opioid analgesics act primarily at mu receptors. Some other opioid analgesics act at the other types of receptors.

Indications

Narcotic analgesics are used to manage moderate to severe acute and chronic pain after non-narcotic analgesics have failed. They are also used as preanesthetic medications. Narcotic analgesics are indicated to relieve dyspnea

TABLE 21-3 Opioids

Generic Name	Trade Name	Route of Administration	Average Adult Dosage
Opioid Agonists with Moderate Effects			
codeine	(generic)	PO, SC, IM	15–60 mg q.i.d.
hydrocodone	Hycodan®, Robidone®	PO	5–10 mg q4–6 h prn (max: 15 mg/dose)
oxycodone	OxyContin®, Percolone®	PO	5–10 mg q.i.d. prn
propoxyphene	Darvon®, Darvon-N®	PO	65 mg (HCl form) or 100 mg (napsylate form) q4 h prn (max: 390 HCl/day; max: 600 mg napsylate/day)
Opioid Agonists with High Effects			
hydromorphone	Dilaudid®	PO, SC, IM, IV	PO:2–4 mg q4–6 h prn; SC/IM/IV: 0.75–2 mg q4–6 h
levorphanol	Levo-Dromoran®	PO	2–3 mg t.i.d.-q.i.d. prn
meperidine	Demerol®	PO, SC, IM, IV	50–150 mg q3–4 h prn
methadone	Dolophine®, Methadose®	PO, SC, IM, IV	PO/SC/IM: 2.5–10 mg q3–4 h prn; IV: 2.5–10 mg q8–12 h prn
morphine	Astramorph PF®, Duramorph®	PO	10–30 mg q4 h prn
oxymorphone	Numorphan®	PO, SC, IM	PO: 10–20 mg q4–6 h prn; SC/IM: 1–1.5 mg q4–6 h prn

of acute left ventricular failure and pulmonary edema and pain of myocardial infarction. These agents may be given to treat severe diarrhea, intestinal cramping (camphorated tincture of opium), and persistent cough (codeine).

Adverse Effects

The major adverse effect of opioid analgesics is respiratory depression, in which the respiratory rate and depth decrease. The most common adverse effects include sedation, anorexia, nausea, vomiting, constipation, dizziness, light-headedness, and sweating. Other adverse effects of agonist narcotic analgesics on different systems are as follows:

- Gastrointestinal: dry mouth and biliary tract spasms
- Central nervous system: euphoria, pinpoint pupils, insomnia, tremor, agitation, and impairment of mental and physical tasks
- Cardiovascular: tachycardia, bradycardia, palpitations, and peripheral circulatory collapse
- Genitourinary: spasms of the ureters and bladder sphincter, urinary retention or hesitancy

Contraindications and Precautions

Narcotic analgesics are contraindicated in patients with known hypersensitivity, acute bronchial asthma, emphysema, or upper airway obstruction. Narcotic analgesics are also contraindicated in patients with head injury, increased intracranial pressure, convulsive disorders, and severe hepatic or renal dysfunction. Narcotic analgesics should be avoided during pregnancy or labor (they are ranked as category C drugs), except oxycodone (which is ranked as a category B drug), because they prolong labor or produce respiratory depression in the neonate.

Key Concept

The use of narcotic analgesics is recommended during pregnancy only if the benefit to the mother outweighs the potential harm to the fetus.

Narcotic analgesics should be used cautiously in patients with cardiac arrhythmias, toxic psychosis, emphysema, kyphoscoliosis (deformity of the vertebral column), and severe obesity, and in very elderly patients.

Medical Terminology Review

kyphoscoliosis
kypho = hunchback
scoliosis = lateral and rotational spinal deformity
a deformity of the spinal column causing a hunchback appearance

Drug Interactions

Narcotic analgesics interact with several drugs. These drugs include CNS depressants such as alcohol, other opioids, general anesthetics, sedatives, and antidepressants such as MAOIs and tricyclics. The action of opiates is increased if used with narcotic analgesics, and the risk of severe respiratory depression (and death) is also increased.

Key Concept

Yohimbe (herbal supplements) may increase the effects of morphine.

Opioid Antagonists

Opioid antagonists are agents that prevent the effects of **opioid agonists**. The opioid antagonist drugs have an affinity for a cell receptor and compete with opioid agonists for reaching the opioid receptor site (see Table 21-4).

Mechanism of Action

Pure opioid antagonists such as naloxone are able to block both mu and kappa receptors. The mechanism of action is not clearly delineated, but it appears that its competitive binding at opioid receptor sites reduces euphoria and drug cravings without supporting addiction.

TABLE 21-4 Opioid Antagonists

Generic Name	Trade Name	Route of Administration	Average Adult Dosage
nalmefene	Revex®	SC, IM, IV	1 mg/mL concentration; nonopioid dependent: 0.5 mg/70 kg; opioid dependent: 0.1 mg/70 kg
naloxone	Narcan®	IV	0.4–2 mg, may be repeated q2–3 min up to 10 mg prn
naltrexone	ReVia®, Vivitrol®	PO	25 mg followed by another 25 mg in 1 h if no withdrawal response (max: 800 mg/day)

Indications

Opioid antagonists are used for complete or partial reversal of opioid effects in emergency conditions when acute opioid overdose is suspected. Administered intravenously, they begin to reverse opioid-initiated CNS and respiratory depression within minutes. Naloxone is the drug of choice when the nature of a depressant drug is not known and for the diagnosis of suspected acute opioid overdosage.

Adverse Effects

Opioid antagonists themselves have minimal toxicity. However, they reverse the effects of opioids and the patient may experience rapid loss of analgesia, increased blood pressure, nausea, vomiting, drowsiness, hyperventilation, and tremors.

Contraindications and Precautions

Opioid antagonists are contraindicated in respiratory depression due to nonopioid drugs. Safety during pregnancy (other than labor) (category B) or lactation is not established.

Opioid antagonist drugs should be used with caution in neonates and children, and patients with cardiac irritability and known or suspected narcotic dependence.

Drug Interactions

Opioid antagonist drug interactions include a reversal of the analgesic effects of narcotic (opiate) agonists and **agonist-antagonists**.

MIGRAINE HEADACHES

Headache is a very common type of pain. There are many categories of headache associated with different causes, and some have specific locations and characteristics. The types of headache include:

- Headaches associated with congested sinuses.
- Headaches associated with muscle spasm and tension resulting from emotional stress that causes the neck muscles to contract to a greater degree, pulling on the scalp.
- **Intracranial** headaches resulting from increased pressure inside the skull.
- Migraine headaches, which are related to abnormal changes in blood flow and metabolism in the brain. There are many precipitating factors, including atmospheric changes, stress, menstruation, hunger, and heredity. The pain of a migraine headache is usually throbbing, quite severe, and sometimes incapacitating. Characteristically, these types of headaches begin unilaterally (on one side) in the temple area, but often spread to involve the entire head. The pain is often

accompanied by dizziness, nausea, abdominal pain, fatigue, and visual disturbances. These headaches may last up to 24 hours, and there is often a prolonged recovery period.

Treatment of Migraine Headaches

Treatment is difficult, although ergotamine may be effective if administered immediately after the onset of the headache. New forms of ergotamine are available as sublingual tablets, which provide a more readily available and rapid-acting treatment. Other drugs used for migraines, and a newer group of medications, are listed in Table 21-5.

TABLE 21-5 Drugs Used to Treat Migraine Headaches

Generic Name	Trade Name	Route of Administration	Average Adult Dosage
Ergot Alkaloids			
dihydroergotamine	D.H.E. 45®, Migranal®	SC, IM, IV	1 mg repeated at 1 h intervals to a total of 3 mg IM; or 2 mg SC/IV
ergotamine	Ergomar®, Ergostat®	Sublingual	1–2 mg repeated q30 m until headache stops
ergotamine with caffeine	Cafergot®, Ercaf®	PO	1–2 mg repeated q30 m until headache stops
Triptans			
almotriptan	Axert®	PO	6.25–12.5 mg repeated in 2 h prn
electriptan	Relpax®	PO	20–40 mg repeated in 2 h prn
frovatriptan	Frova®	PO	2.5 mg repeated in 2 h prn
naratriptan	Amerge®	PO	1–2.5 mg repeated in 4 h prn
rizatriptan	Maxalt®	PO	5–10 mg repeated in 2 h prn or 5 mg with concurrent propranolol
sumatriptan	Imitrex®	PO	25 mg for 1 dose
zolmitriptan	Zomig®	PO	2.5–5 mg repeated in 2 h prn
Beta-adrenergic Blockers			
atenolol	Tenormin®	PO	25–50 mg/day
metoprolol	Lopressor®	PO	50–100 mg 1–2 times/day
propranolol	Inderal®	PO	80–240 mg/day in div. doses
timolol	Blocadren®	PO	10 mg b.i.d. up to 60 mg/day in 2 div. doses
Calcium Channel Blockers			
nifedipine	Procardia®	PO	10–20 mg t.i.d.
nimodipine	Nimotop®	PO	60 mg q4 h for 21 days, start therapy within 96 hrs of subarachnoid hemorrhage
verapamil	Isoptin®	PO	40–80 mg t.i.d.

Mechanism of Action

Anti-migraine drugs include the ergot alkaloids and the triptans, which are both serotonin agonists. Serotonergic receptors (those that are related to the neurotransmitter serotonin) are found through the CNS, GI tract, and in the cardiovascular system. These agents act by causing vasoconstriction of the cranial arteries. This vasoconstriction is moderately selective, and does not usually affect overall blood pressure.

Indications

The drugs of choice for treatment of migraine are often the triptans. Ergot alkaloids may be used to stop migraines. Prophylaxis includes various classes of drugs (such as beta blockers and calcium channel blockers) that are discussed in other chapters of this textbook.

Adverse Effects

Common adverse effects of ergot alkaloids include nausea, vomiting, abnormal pulse, weakness, and convulsive seizures. The adverse effects of triptans include warming sensations, dizziness, weakness, and tickling or prickling. The major adverse effects of triptans include: coronary artery vasospasm, heart attack, and cardiac arrest.

Contraindications and Precautions

These agents are contraindicated in patients with recent myocardial infarction, a history of angina pectoris, diabetes, and high blood pressure. Because ergot alkaloids and triptans cause vasoconstriction of blood vessels, they should be used cautiously.

Drug Interactions

Ergot alkaloids and triptans may interact with several drugs. For example, an increased effect may occur when taken with monoamine oxidase inhibitors (MAOIs) and selective serotonin reuptake inhibitors (SSRIs). Further vasoconstriction may occur.

Summary

Non-narcotic analgesics are used to relieve pain without the possibility of resulting physical dependency. Non-narcotic analgesics include the salicylates, non-salicylates (acetaminophen), and nonsteroidal anti-inflammatory drugs (NSAIDs).

Salicylates are the oldest of the nonopioid analgesics and NSAIDs. They are still commonly used as analgesics. Aspirin is the most commonly used of these agents. Some of these analgesics are also used as anti-inflammatory and antipyretic drugs.

Adverse effects of salicylate drugs are common and include heartburn, nausea, vomiting, and gastrointestinal bleeding. Acetaminophen may cause adverse reactions with chronic use or when the recommended dosage is exceeded.

New NSAIDs are available as analgesic, antipyretic, and anti-inflammatory agents. COX-2 inhibitors are more specific for prostaglandin synthesis in response to an inflammatory event. The FDA has approved the COX-2 inhibitors such as celecoxib and meloxicam.

Narcotic analgesics are controlled substances used to treat moderate to severe pain. Narcotic analgesics are classified as agonists and antagonists. One of the major adverse effects of agonist narcotic administration is respiratory depression.

Morphine is the most widely used drug in the management of chronic severe pain, and opioid antagonists are agents that prevent the effects of opioid agonists. These drugs have an affinity for a cell receptor and compete with opioid agonists for reaching the opioid receptor site.

A migraine headache is a very common type of pain. There are various agents used as anti-migraine medications. The two major drug classes used for treating migraine headaches include ergot alkaloids and triptans. Other drugs used for this purpose include beta-adrenergic blockers, calcium channel blockers, and tricyclic antidepressants.

Exploring the Web

Visit www.fda.gov

- Search for the types of drugs discussed in this chapter. Look for safety information, advisories, patient education, etc.

Visit www.healthopedia.com

- Click on "drugs and medications," and search for additional information on the drugs discussed within the chapter. You can also find drug information at www.medicinenet.com (click "medications") or www.nlm.nih.gov/medlineplus (click on "drugs and supplements").

Review Questions

Multiple Choice

1. Aspirin may be useful in the prevention of coronary thrombosis because of which of the following properties?
   - A. thrombolytic
   - B. antiarthritic
   - C. anti-inflammatory
   - D. antiplatelet
2. Celecoxib (Celebrex®) is classified as:
   - A. a COX-1 and COX-2 inhibitor
   - B. a COX-1 inhibitor
   - C. a COX-2 inhibitor
   - D. a nonselective NSAID
3. Which of the following is a main contraindication of NSAIDs?
   - A. rheumatoid arthritis
   - B. corticosteroid sensitivity
   - C. osteoarthritis
   - D. allergy to aspirin
4. Which of the following terms is used for pain-relieving drugs?
   - A. antitoxins
   - B. antiemetics
   - C. analgesics
   - D. anaphylactics
5. Examples of nonsalicylate nonsteroidal anti-inflammatory drugs include:
   - A. ibuprofen and indomethacin
   - B. mefenamic acid and magnesium sulfate
   - C. naproxen and neomycin
   - D. piroxicam and lysergic acid
6. COX-2 is more specific for synthesis of which of the following in response to an inflammatory event?
   - A. histamine
   - B. prostaglandin
   - C. heparin
   - D. epinephrine
7. Which of the following classes of drugs are *preferred* for treating migraine headaches?
   - A. tricyclic antidepressants
   - B. NSAIDs
   - C. beta-adrenergic blockers
   - D. triptans

8. Which of the following drugs is used to treat opioid dependence?
   A. hydromorphone
   B. methadone
   C. oxycodone
   D. propoxyphene

9. The main adverse effect of morphine is:
   A. diarrhea
   B. respiratory depression
   C. depression
   D. intestinal cramping

10. Narcotic analgesics are contraindicated in which of the following situations?
    A. moderate pain
    B. pulmonary edema
    C. persistent cough
    D. bronchial asthma

11. The trade name of ibuprofen is:
    A. Nalfon
    B. Advil
    C. Aleve
    D. Actron

12. Which of the following is considered an aspirin substitute?
    A. Indocin (indomethacin)
    B. Celebrex (celecoxib)
    C. Tylenol (acetaminophen)
    D. Aleve (naproxen)

13. If a patient has an allergy to aspirin, which of the following drugs may be used?
    A. sodium thiosalicylate injectable
    B. etolac
    C. acetaminophen
    D. allopurinol

14. Narcotic analgesia at the spinal level may cause which of the following?
    A. miosis and sedation
    B. physical dependence and psychosis
    C. euphoria and respiratory depression
    D. hyperventilation and tremors

15. Which of the following is an example of pure opioid antagonists?
    A. methadone
    B. oxycodone
    C. naloxone
    D. meperidine

Matching

A. morphine

B. methadone

C. oxycodone

D. hydrocodone

E. naloxone

_____ **1.** Often used with aspirin or acetaminophen.

_____ **2.** Competes with opioid agonists for reaching the opioid receptor site.

_____ **3.** More addicting than codeine.

_____ **4.** Extracted from raw opium.

_____ **5.** Used for detoxification of opioid addiction.

Critical Thinking

A 58-year-old patient with a history of a recent myocardial infarction is on beta-blocker and anticoagulant therapy. The patient has a history of peptic ulcer (which is not bothering him currently). During a recent flare-up, he began taking aspirin because it helped control the pain in his chest that he experienced.

1. What recommendation would the pharmacist have for this patient?

2. If the patient takes aspirin, what major adverse effects could occur?

3. Name a drug that the pharmacist could advise the patient to take instead of aspirin.

Anti-infectives and Systemic Antibacterial Agents

CHAPTER 22

OUTLINE

OBJECTIVES

After completing this chapter, the reader should be able to:

1. Describe the various forms of microorganisms.
2. Compare the terms *bactericidal* and *bacteriostatic.*
3. Describe various mechanisms of action of antibacterial therapy.
4. Explain the indication and contraindication of antibiotics.
5. Describe the major side effects of antibacterial agents.
6. Understand the importance of drug interactions.
7. Explain the mechanisms of action for penicillins, cephalosporins, aminoglycosides, tetracyclines, macrolides, and quinolones.
8. Compare the effectiveness of penicillins with cephalosporins.
9. Explain the first line of antituberculosis drugs.
10. Describe the significant contraindications of rifampin and ethambutol.

GLOSSARY

Antibiotics – substances that have the ability to destroy or interfere with the development of a living organism

Antimicrobial – an anti-infective drug produced from synthetic substances

Bacteria – small, one-celled microorganisms that lack a true nucleus or mechanism to provide metabolism

Bactericidal – killing bacterial growth

Bacteriostatic – suppress bacterial growth by triggering a mechanism that blocks folic acid synthesis, thereby forcing bacteria to synthesize their own folic acid

Broad-spectrum antibiotics – agent that is effective against a wide variety of both Grampositive and Gram-negative pathogenic microorganisms

Fungi – microorganisms that grow in single cells or in colonies

Gram stains – sequential procedures involving crystal violet and iodine solutions followed by alcohol that allow rapid identification of organisms as Gram-positive or Gram-negative types

Gram-negative – microorganisms that stain red or pink with Gram stain

Gram-positive – microorganisms that stain blue or purple with Gram stain

Infection – the invasion of pathogenic microorganisms that produce tissue damage within the body

OUTLINE *(continued)*

Localized infection – involve a specific area of the body such as the skin or internal organs

Mycoplasms – ultramicroscopic organisms that lack rigid cell walls and are considered to be the smallest free-living organisms

Narrow-spectrum antibiotics – antibiotics that are effective against only a few organisms

Porphyria – a group of enzyme disorders that cause skin problems (such as purple discolorations) and/or neurological complications

Protozoa – single-celled parasitic organisms with the ability to move

Rickettsia – intercellular parasites that need to be in living cells to reproduce

Red man syndrome – a rash on the upper body caused by vancomycin

Spores – bacteria in a resistant stage that can withstand an unfavorable environment

Systemic infection – impacts the whole body rather than a specific area of the body

Viruses – organisms that can live only inside cells

Overview

Pathogenic microorganisms may cause a wide spectrum of illnesses. They produce infection of different organs or systems of the body, such as upper respiratory tract infections, meningitis, pneumonia, tuberculosis, and urinary tract infections. This chapter focuses on the drugs used to treat a variety of infections.

Infections

An **infection** is described as the invasion of pathogenic microorganisms that produce tissue damage within the body. Infections may be classified primarily as either local or systemic. A **localized infection** may involve a specific area of the body such as the skin or internal organs. A localized infection can progress to a systemic infection. A **systemic infection** impacts the whole body rather than a specific area of the body. Infections are also classified as acute or chronic.

Chain of Infection

The chain of infection describes the elements of an infectious process. It is an interactive process that involves the agent, host, and environment. This process must include several essential elements or "links in the chain" for the transmission of microorganisms to occur. Figure 22-1 identifies the

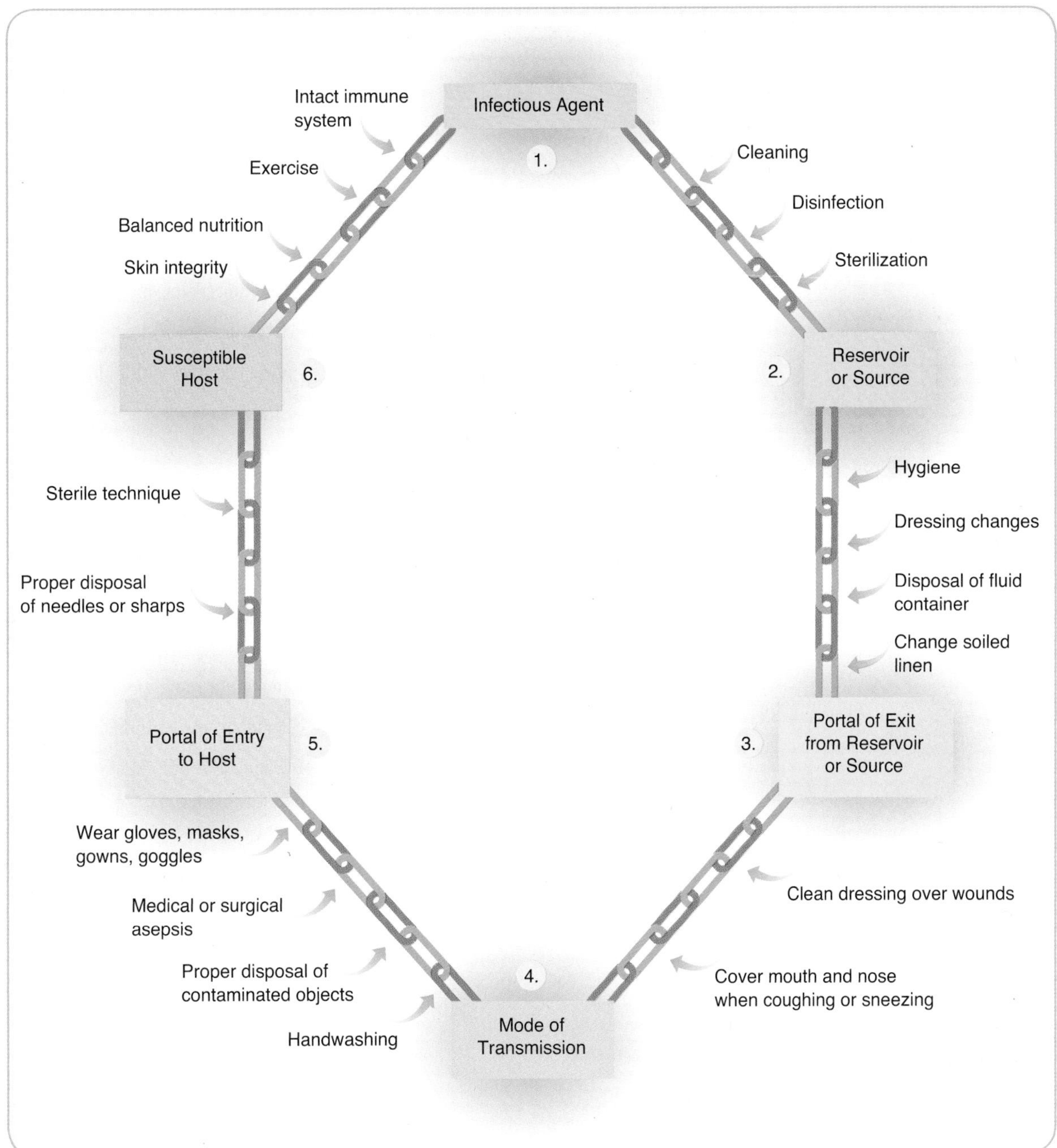

Figure 22-1 Chain of infection.

six essential links in the chain of infection. Table 22-1 summarizes modes of transmission.

Without the transmission of microorganisms, the infectious process cannot occur. Knowledge about the chain of infection facilitates control or prevention of disease by breaking the links in the chain. This is achieved by altering one or more of the interactive processes of agent, host, or environment.

TABLE 22-1 Modes of Transmission

Mode	Examples
Contact	Direct contact with infected person:
	• Touching
	• Bathing
	• Rubbing
	• Toileting (urine and feces)
	• Secretions from client
	Indirect contact with fomites:
	• Clothing
	• Bed linens
	• Dressings
	• Health care equipment
	• Instruments used in treatments
	• Specimen containers used for laboratory analysis
	• Personal belongings
	• Personal care equipment
	• Diagnostic equipment
Airborne	Inhaling microorganisms carried by moisture or dust particles in air:
	• Coughing
	• Talking
	• Sneezing
Vehicle	Contact with contaminated inanimate objects:
	• Water
	• Blood
	• Drugs
	• Food
	• Urine
Vector borne	Contact with contaminated animate hosts:
	• Animals
	• Insects

MICROORGANISMS

Microorganisms are divided into several groups: bacteria, mycoplasms, viruses, fungi, protozoa, and rickettsia. Bacteria are classified according to their shape, such as cocci, bacilli, and spirilla. They are also classified into two groups that depend upon their capacity to be stained. This staining process is called **Gram staining**. It involves sequential procedures using crystal violet and iodine solutions followed by alcohol that allow rapid identification of organisms as Gram-positive or Gram-negative types. Gram stains can identify specific types of bacteria. **Gram-negative** microorganisms stain red or rose-pink (Figure 22-2). **Gram-positive** microorganisms stain blue or purple (Figure 22-3). Fungi may also be identified by Gram staining. The culture and sensitivity tests can determine which antibiotics should be prescribed.

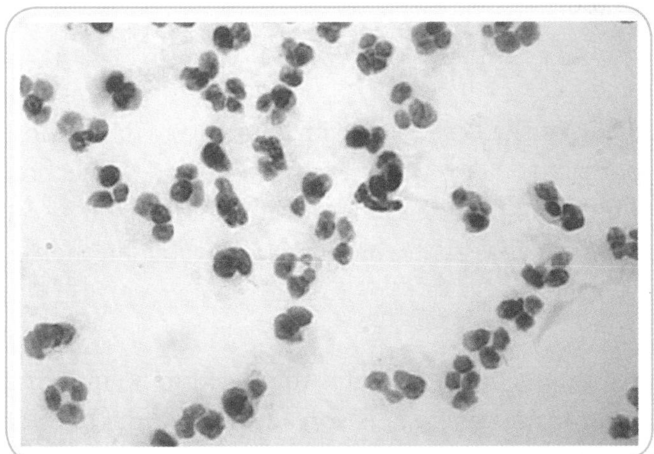

Figure 22-2 Gram-negative.

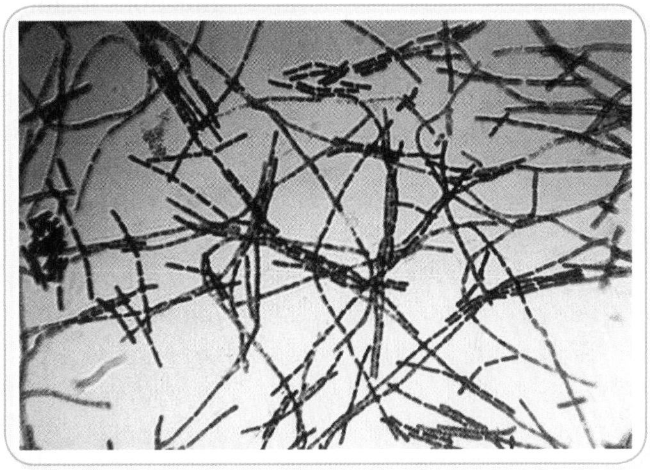

Figure 22-3 Gram-positive.

Bacteria

Bacteria are small, one-celled microorganisms that lack a true nucleus or mechanism to provide metabolism. Some forms of bacteria produce **spores**, a resistant stage that withstands an unfavorable environment. When proper environmental conditions return, spores germinate and form new cells. Spores are resistant to heat, drying, and disinfectants. Pathogenic bacteria cause a wide range of illnesses including diarrhea, pneumonia, sinusitis, urinary tract infections, and gonorrhea.

Mycoplasms

Mycoplasms are ultramicroscopic organisms that lack rigid cell walls and are considered to be the smallest free-living organisms. Some are saprophytes (a plant that lives on dead or decaying matter), some are parasites, and many are pathogens. One species is a cause of mycoplasma pneumonia, tracheobronchitis, and pharyngitis.

Viruses

Viruses are organisms that can live only inside cells. They cannot get nourishment or reproduce outside the cell. Viruses contain a core of DNA or RNA surrounded by a protein coating. Viruses damage the cell they inhabit by blocking the normal protein synthesis and by using the cell's mechanism for metabolism to reproduce themselves. Viral infections include the common cold, influenza, measles, hepatitis, genital herpes, HIV, and the West Nile virus. Treatment of viruses will be discussed in Chapter 23.

Fungi

Fungi grow in single cells as in yeast or in colonies as in molds. Fungi obtain food from living organisms or organic matter. Disease from fungi is found mainly in individuals who are immunologically impaired. Fungi can cause infections of the hair, skin, nails, and mucous membranes. Fungal infections include athlete's foot.

Protozoa

Protozoa are single-celled parasitic organisms with the ability to move. Most protozoa obtain their food from dead or decaying organic matter. Infection is spread through ingestion of contaminated food or water, or through insect bites. Common infections are malaria, gastroenteritis, and vaginal infections.

Rickettsia

Rickettsia is a group of intercellular parasites that need to be in living cells to reproduce. Infection from rickettsia is spread through the bites of fleas, ticks, mites, and lice. Common infections are Lyme disease, Rocky Mountain spotted fever, and typhus.

Principles of Anti-infective Therapy

Anti-infective agents are used to treat infection by destroying or suppressing the causative microorganisms. The goal is to suppress the causative agent sufficiently so that the body's own defenses can eliminate it. Anti-infective drugs derived from natural substances are called **antibiotics**. Those produced from synthetic substances are called **antimicrobials**. In past years, strong efforts have been made to change antibiotic usage policy rendering prescribing practices clinically stronger, but less costly. There is an emphasis on rapid conversion from parenteral to oral therapy for a variety of infectious processes. Major efforts are being taken to understand the underlying principles associated with the interaction of the antibiotics, host, and pathogens.

> ***Medical Terminology Review***
>
> **antibiotic**
>
> *anti = against; opposite; opposing; contrary*
> *biotic = a mode of living*
> suppressing the mechanism by which a microorganism lives

Selection of Agents

An anti-infective agent should be chosen on the basis of its pharmacologic properties and spectrum of activity as well as on various patient factors.

1. *Pharmacologic properties*: The drug's ability to reach the infection site and to attain a desired level of concentration in the target tissue.
2. *Spectrum of activity*: To treat an infectious disease effectively, an anti-infective agent must be effective against the causative pathogen. The effectiveness of an anti-infective drug can be confirmed by a

sensitivity test. Resistance to an anti-infective can arise by mutation in the gene that determines sensitivity/resistance to the agent.

3. *Patient factors*: There are various patient factors that determine what type of anti-infectives should be administered. These factors include: immunity of patients, age, presence of a foreign body, adverse drug reactions, pregnancy and lactation, and underlying disease. Choosing an anti-infective that doesn't offer enough protection is a common problem. Some commonly used drugs such as aminoglycosides and vancomycin are poorly absorbed and can be used to treat G.I. infections without systemic effects. Antimicrobials can be used as prophylactics for people in contact with patients with meningitis or tuberculosis; surgery to the GI, urinary tract, or dental regions; or those with rheumatoid fever. Other patient considerations in the use of anti-infective agents include:
   - diminished renal function in the elderly
   - partially developed hepatic function in neonates
   - circulation problems such as with diabetes

Duration of Anti-infective Therapy

The most important goal of anti-infective therapy is to continue it for a sufficient duration. All antibiotics should be completed through the prescribed amount of time. Treatment for chronic infection such as osteomyelitis or endocarditis may require a longer duration, for example, 4 to 6 weeks.

Antibiotic Spectrum

Effectiveness of antibiotics against different microorganisms may be divided into two groups: broad-spectrum and narrow-spectrum. **Broad-spectrum antibiotics** are effective against a wide variety of both Gram-positive and Gram-negative pathogenic microorganisms. **Narrow-spectrum antibiotics** can be effective on a few Gram-positive or Gram-negative pathogens.

Superinfections

The normal flora (nonpathogenic microorganisms within the body) may be disrupted by administration of oral antibiotics, which causes superinfection. This process of destruction of large numbers of normal flora by antibiotics can alter the chemical environment. Therefore, uncontrolled growth of bacteria or fungal microorganisms may occur. Any antibiotic that is administered for a long time, or a repeated course of therapy, may result in superinfections. A superinfection may develop suddenly and may be serious or life-threatening. Bacterial superinfections can be seen frequently with the use of oral penicillins and involve the large intestine. Pseudomembranous colitis is a common bacterial superinfection, and moniliasis is a common type of fungal superinfection.

Antibacterial Agents

Antibacterial agents are used to treat infections caused by bacteria. The major categories for antibacterial agents include: sulfonamides, penicillins, cephalosporins, aminoglycosides, macrolides, tetracyclines, fluoroquinolones, and miscellaneous antibacterial agents.

Sulfonamides

Sulfonamides are the synthetic derivatives of sulfanilamide (Table 22-2). These agents were the first drugs to prevent and cure human bacterial infection successfully. They are well-absorbed from the gastrointestinal tract. Sulfonamides readily penetrate the cerebrospinal fluid. These agents are metabolized to various degrees in the liver, and are eliminated by the kidneys. Sulfonamides were originally active against a wide range of Gram-positive and Gram-negative bacteria; however, the increasing incidence of resistance in bacteria formerly susceptible to sulfonamides has decreased the clinical usefulness of the drug. However, sulfonamides remain the drug of choice for certain infections. The major sulfonamides are generally classified as short-acting, intermediate-acting, or long-acting. Their rate of action depends on how quickly they are absorbed and eliminated.

Key Concept

Sulfonamides were the first antimicrobial agents, but their clinical use has been greatly restricted as a result of the development of resistant bacteria.

Mechanism of Action

Sulfonamides are **bacteriostatic**; they suppress bacterial growth by triggering a mechanism that blocks folic acid synthesis, thereby forcing bacteria to synthesize their own folic acid.

Medical Terminology Review

bacteriostatic
bacterio = bacteria; bacterial
static = slowing; stoppage
slowing or stopping the growth of bacteria

TABLE 22-2 Classification of Sulfonamides

Generic Name	Trade Name	Route of Administration	Common Dosage Range
Short-acting (4–8 hours)			
sulfamethizole	Thiosulfil Forte®	PO	7.5 mg–1 g
sulfasalazine	Azulfidine®	PO	1–2 g/day in 4 div. doses; may increase up to 8 g/day
sulfisoxazole	Gantrisin®	PO	2–4 g initially, followed by 1–2 g q.i.d.
Intermediate-acting (7–17 hours)			
sulfadizine	Microsulfon®	PO	2–4 g
sulfamethoxazole	Gantanol®	PO	2 g initially, followed by 1 g b.i.d.
trimethoprim-sulfamethoxazole	Bactrim®, Septra®	PO	160 mg TMP/800 mg b.i.d.
Long-acting (17+ hours)			
sulfadoxine-pyrimethamine	Fansidar®	PO	1 tablet/wk

Indications

Sulfonamides most often are used to treat urinary tract infections by *E. coli*, including acute and chronic cystitis, and chronic upper urinary tract infections. Prophylactic sulfonamide therapy has been used successfully to prevent streptococcal infections and rheumatic fever recurrences.

Adverse Effects

Key Concept

Elderly patients and patients with impairment of the kidney who are given sulfonamides have a risk for more renal damage. An increase of fluid intake up to 2,000 mL decreases the risk of crystals and stones forming in the urinary tract.

Sulfonamides may cause blood dyscrasias such as hemolytic anemia, aplastic anemia, thrombocytopenia, and agranulocytosis. Hypersensitivity reactions may occur with sulfonamide therapy. Hematuria and crystalluria are two of the major adverse effects of sulfonamide agents. Sulfonamides should be used with caution in patients with renal impairment. Life-threatening hepatitis caused by drugs is a rare adverse effect. Patients who take sulfonamides have increased susceptibility to adverse effects from sun exposure.

Contraindications and Precautions

Sulfonamides must be avoided in patients with a history of hypersensitivity to these drugs. They are contraindicated in the treatment of group A beta-hemolytic streptococcal infections or in infants less than two months of age (except in the treatment of congenital toxoplasmosis). Sulfonamides must not be used in patients with **porphyria**, advanced kidney or liver disease, intestinal obstruction, or urinary obstruction. They are contraindicated during pregnancy (if near term) and in lactating women. Sulfonamides must be used cautiously in patients with impaired kidney or liver function, severe allergy, bronchial asthma, and blood dyscrasias.

Drug Interactions

Sulfonamides may increase the effects of phenytoin, oral anticoagulants, and sulfonylureas.

Penicillins

Sir Arthur Fleming discovered the antibacterial properties of natural penicillins in 1928 while he was performing research on influenza. In 1938, British scientists realized the effects of natural penicillins on disease-causing microorganisms. In 1941, natural penicillins were used for the treatment of infections.

Natural or semisynthetic antibiotics are produced by or derived from certain species of the fungus *Penicillium*. Penicillins are the most widely used anti-infective agents; however, cephalosporin usage has increased in the last decade. Among the most important antibiotics, natural penicillins are the

Key Concept

Penicillin was the first antibiotic to be produced commercially and still assumes a position of major importance in this field.

preferred drugs in the treatment of many infectious diseases. The major cause of resistance to penicillin is due to production of beta-lactamases (penicillinases). Common organisms that are capable of producing penicillinase include *Staphylococcus aureus*, *Escherichia coli*, *Pseudomonas aeruginosa*, and species of *Bacillus*, *Proteus*, and *Bactericides*. Penicillins are available as penicillin G, penicillin V, penicillin G procaine, and penicillin G benzathine. Table 22-3 shows common types of penicillins and the route of administration.

Mechanism of Action

Penicillins are **bactericidal**. They inhibit bacterial cell wall synthesis in similar ways to the cephalosporins. Natural penicillins are highly active against Gram-positive and against some Gram-negative cocci. Penicillin G is ten times more active than penicillin V against Gram-negative organisms.

TABLE 22-3 Common Penicillins and Routes of Administration

Generic Name	Trade Name	Route of Administration	Common Dosage Range
Natural Penicillins			
penicillin G potassium	Pentids®	PO	400,000–800,000 units/day
penicillin V potassium	Pen Vee K®, Veetids®	PO	125–250 mg q.i.d.
penicillin G procaine	Crysticillin®	IM	600,000–1.2 million units/day
penicillin G benzathine	Bicillin®	IM	1.2 million units as a single dose
Penicillinase-Resistant Penicillins			
cloxacillin sodium	Cloxapen®	PO	250–500 mg q.i.d.
dicloxacillin sodium	Dycill®, Dynapen®	PO	125–500 mg q.i.d.
nafcillin sodium	Nafcil®, Unipen®	PO, IM, IV	500 mg–1 g q.i.d.
oxacillin sodium	Bactocill®	PO, IM, IV	500 mg–1 g q.i.d., IM/IV: 250 mg–1 g q4–6 h
Semisynthetic Penicillins			
amoxicillin	Amoxil®, Trimox®	PO	250–500 mg t.i.d.
amoxicillin and clavulanate potassium	Augmentin®	PO	250–500 mg q8–12 h
ampicillin	Polycillin®, Omnipen®	PO, IM, IV	250–500 mg q.i.d.
bacampicillin hydrochloride	Spectrobid®	PO	400–800 mg b.i.d.

Indications

Penicillin G is the drug of choice for all *Streptococcus pneumoniae* organisms. Penicillins G and V are highly effective against other streptococcal infections such as bacteremia, pharyngitis, otitis media, and sinusitis. Penicillin G is also the drug of choice against many gonococcal infections, post-exposure inhalational anthrax, syphilis, and gas gangrene. Penicillin G procaine is effective against syphilis and uncomplicated gonorrhea. Penicillin G benzathine is very effective against group A beta-hemolytic streptococcal infections. Penicillins G and V may be indicated for prophylactic treatment to prevent streptococcal infection, rheumatic fever, and neonatal gonorrhea ophthalmia.

Adverse Effects

Key Concept

Injection of penicillin to a patient may cause anaphylactic reactions within 30 minutes after administration. Therefore, the patient must be monitored for 30 minutes.

Hypersensitivity occurs in nearly ten percent of cases. Reactions from simple rash to anaphylaxis can be observed from within two minutes and up to three days following administration. Anaphylaxis is a life-threatening reaction that most commonly occurs with parenteral administration. Signs and symptoms include severe hypotension, bronchoconstriction, nausea, vomiting, and abdominal pain. Before penicillin therapy begins, the patient's history should be evaluated for allergy to penicillin.

Contraindications and Precautions

Penicillins must be avoided in patients with a history of hypersensitivity to penicillin or cephalosporins. Penicillins should be used cautiously in patients with kidney disease and during pregnancy (category C) and lactation. These drugs are to be used with caution in patients with bleeding disorders, gastrointestinal diseases, and asthma.

Drug Interactions

The most significant drugs that may increase or decrease the effects of penicillin include: probenecid, erythromycins, tetracyclines, and chloramphenicol. Probenecid increases blood levels of natural penicillin. On the other hand, chloramphenicol, erythromycins, and tetracyclines are antagonists with penicillin.

Penicillinase-resistant Penicillins

The penicillin resistance of many Gram-positive and Gram-negative bacteria is because of penicillin-destroying enzymes called beta-lactamases. The enzymes from *staphylococci*, *enterococci*, *meningococci*, *gonococci*, and various other bacteria were the first-known beta-lactamases and were called penicillinases.

Resistance of bacteria to penicillin cannot be explained entirely on penicillinase production because many resistant organisms produce little or no penicillinase. Nonpenicillinase-mediated resistance is called methicillin resistance.

Resistant penicillins are used predominantly for penicillinase-producing staphylococcal infections. Most staphylococci are now resistant to benzylpenillin because they produce a penicillinase. As their name suggests, penicillinase-resistant penicillins are resistant to the action of this enzyme and are therefore indicated in infections caused by penicillin-resistant *staphylococcus*. Oxacillin, cloxacillin, dicloxacillin, and nafcillin can be given orally. Methicillin is administered parenterally. Nafcillin is used parenterally for more serious infections. Penicillinase-resistant penicillins are used solely in staphylococcal infections resulting from organisms that resist natural penicillins. These agents are less potent than natural penicillins against organisms susceptible to natural penicillins. Penicillinase-resistant penicillins are the preferred choice for skin and soft tissue infections due to staphylococci. Higher doses should be used for severe infections or for infections of the lower respiratory tract. In suspension form, these agents should be taken on an empty stomach, are stable for 14 days after mixing (but refrigeration is required), and are known for having a bitter aftertaste.

Mechanism of Action

Penicillinase-resistant penicillins prevent cell wall synthesis by binding to enzymes called penicillin-binding proteins (PBPs). These enzymes are essential for the synthesis of the bacterial cell wall.

> ***Medical Terminology Review***
>
> **hypersensitivity**
> *hyper* = *over; above; beyond*
> *sensitivity* = *the quality or condition of being responsive or reactive*
> overly reactive to a particular agent
>
> **nephrotoxicity**
> *nephro* = *kidney*
> *toxicity* = *the quality or condition of being poisonous*
> poisoning of the kidney
>
> **hepatotoxicity**
> *hepato* = *liver*
> *toxicity* = *the quality or condition of being poisonous*
> poisoning of the liver

Indications

Indications of penicillinase-resistant penicillins include prevention and treatment of bacterial infections, including *streptococcus*, *enterococcus*, and *staphylococcus* strains.

Adverse Effects

The penicillinase-resistant group can also cause hypersensitivity reactions like natural penicillins. Methicillin may cause nephrotoxicity. Oxacillin can produce hepatotoxicity. They may cause nausea, vomiting, diarrhea, or skin rash.

Contraindications and Precautions

These agents are contraindicated in patients with hypersensitivity to penicillins or cephalosporins. Safe use during pregnancy (category B) is not established.

Penicillinase-resistant penicillins should be used cautiously in patients with a history of, or suspected, allergy (hives, eczema, hay fever, asthma); in premature infants and neonates; and during lactation (which may cause infant diarrhea). They also should be used with great caution in patients with renal or hepatic function impairment.

Drug Interactions

Penicillinase-resistant penicillins can inactivate aminoglycoside serum samples from patients receiving both drugs.

Semi-synthetic Penicillins (Amoxicillin/ Clavulanate Potassium)

Streptococcus pneumoniae is the most common cause of acute bacterial sinusitis (ABS) and community-acquired pneumonia (CAP). Amoxicillin/ clavulanate potassium is the first FDA-approved antibiotic for both of these infections.

Mechanism of Action

The amoxicillin component of the formulation exerts a bactericidal action against many Gram-negative and Gram-positive strains. The clavulanate potassium component protects the amoxicillin from degradation by inactivating harmful beta-lactamase enzymes.

Indications

This combination is used for the treatment of infections caused by susceptible beta-lactamase-producing organisms of upper respiratory infections such as otitis media, tonsillitis, and sinusitis. It is also used to treat lower respiratory infections such as bronchitis and pneumonia. Urinary tract, skin, and soft tissue infections are also treatable with this combination agent.

Adverse Effects

Amoxicillin/clavulanate potassium should not be used in patients with hepatic dysfunction because of the danger of transient hepatitis and cholestatic jaundice. Serious and occasionally fatal hypersensitivity reactions have been reported in patients on penicillin therapy. Diarrhea, nausea, vomiting, urticaria, and candidal vaginitis may occur.

Contraindications and Precautions

This combination should not be used in patients with hypersensitivity to penicillins, infectious mononucleosis, and during pregnancy (category B) and lactation. The combination of amoxicillin and clavulanate potassium shares the toxic potential of ampicillin.

Drug Interactions

Concurrent use of this agent with probenecid may result in increased and prolonged blood levels of amoxicillin. This agent interacts with coumarin or indandione-derivative anticoagulants, heparin, NSAIDs (especially aspirin), other platelet aggregation inhibitors or thrombolytic agents, and estrogen-containing oral contraceptives.

TABLE 22-4 Extended-spectrum Penicillins

Generic Name	Trade Name	Route of	Common Dosage Range
Carboxypenicillins			
carbenicillin	Geocillin®	PO	382–764 mg q.i.d.
ticarcillin disodium and clavulanate potassium	Timentin®	IV	>60 kg, 3.1 g q4–6 h
Ureidopenicillins			
mezlocillin	Mezlin®	IM, IV	25–50 mg/kg/day
piperacillin	Pipracil®	IM, IV	8–16 g/day

Extended-spectrum Penicillins

This group of penicillins has the widest antibacterial spectrum. Included are the carboxypenicillins and the ureidopenicillins (Table 22-4).

Mechanism of Action

Extended-spectrum penicillins are also bactericidal and inhibit bacterial cell wall synthesis.

Indications

Extended-spectrum penicillins are prescribed mainly to treat serious infections caused by Gram-negative organisms such as sepsis, pneumonia, peritonitis, osteomyelitis, and soft tissue infections.

Adverse Effects

As with other penicillins, hypersensitivity reactions may occur. Carbenicillin and ticarcillin may cause hypokalemia. The use of these two drugs may be a danger to patients with congestive heart failure because of the high sodium content of carbenicillin and ticarcillin.

Contraindications and Precautions

These agents are contraindicated in patients with hypersensitivity to penicillins and during pregnancy (category B). Safe use in children is not established.

Extended spectrum penicillins should be used cautiously in patients with a history of, or suspected, atopy or allergies, or history of allergy to cephalosporins; during lactation; in patients with impaired renal and hepatic function; and in patients on sodium restricted diets.

Drug Interactions

Extended spectrum penicillins agents may increase the risk of bleeding if used with anticoagulants. Elimination of ticarcillin is decreased by the use of probenecid.

Cephalosporins

These agents are known as beta-lactam antibiotics. Cephalosporins are semisynthetic antibiotics structurally and pharmacologically related to penicillins. Cephalosporins are usually bactericidal in action. The antibacterial activity of the cephalosporin results from inhibition of mucopeptide synthesis in the bacterial cell wall. The cephalosporins are classified into four different "generations." Particular cephalosporins may be differentiated within each group according to the bacteria that are sensitive to them (see Table 22-5).

First-generation cephalosporins are effective against most Gram-positive organisms and some Gram-negative organisms. They are used mainly for *Klebsiella* infections, and for those who have penicillin- and sulfonamide-resistant urinary tract infections. Cephapirin and cefazolin are used parenterally; others can be administered orally. Cephalosporins do not penetrate the cerebrospinal fluid (CSF).

Second-generation cephalosporins extend the spectrum of the first generation to include *Haemophilus influenzae* and some *Proteus*. Second-generation cephalosporins are used primarily in the treatment of urinary tract, bone, and soft tissue infections, and prophylactically in various surgical procedures. All are administered parenterally except for cefaclor and cefuroxime, which may be given orally.

Third-generation cephalosporins have even broader Gram-negative activity and less Gram-positive activity than do second-generation agents. High third-generation cephalosporins include cefotaxime, which is potent against *Haemophilus influenza*, *Neisseria gonorrhea*, and *Enterobacteria*. All are administered parenterally. Third-generation agents are used primarily for serious Gram-negative infections, alone or in combination with aminoglycosides. Cefixime is given orally.

Fourth-generation cephalosporins have the greatest action against Gram-negative organisms among the four generations and minimal action against Gram-positive organisms.

Mechanism of Action

The mechanism of action of cephalosporins lies in preventing cell wall synthesis as they bind to enzymes called penicillin-binding proteins (PBPs). These enzymes are essential for the synthesis of the bacterial cell wall.

Indications

Cephalosporins are used to treat community-acquired and hospital-acquired infections of the skin, soft tissue, urinary tract, and respiratory tract. Parenteral first-generation agents are used for surgical wound prophylaxis. The cephamycin group is useful for mixed aerobic/anaerobic infections of the skin and soft tissues, intra-abdominal, and gynecologic infections, as well as for surgical prophylaxis.

TABLE 22-5 Classification of Cephalosporins

Generic Name	Trade Name	Route of Administration	Common Dosage Range
First-generation			
cephradine	Velosef®	PO	250–500 mg q6 h
cephapirin	Cefadyl®	IM, IV	500 mg–1 g q4–6 h
cephalexin	Keflex®	PO	250–500 mg q.i.d.
cefadroxil	Duricef®	PO	1–2 g/day in 1–2 div. doses
cefazolin sodium	Ancef®, Zolicef®, Kefzol®	IM, IV	250 mg–2 g t.i.d.
Second-generation			
cefoxitin sodium	Mefoxin®	IM, IV	1–2 g q6–8 h
cefaclor	Ceclor®	PO	250–500 mg t.i.d.
cefuroxime sodium	Zinacef®	PO	250–500 mg b.i.d.
cefonicid	Monocid®	IM	1–2 g/day
cefprozil	Cefzil®	PO	250–500 mg, 1–2 times/day
cefmetazole	Zefazone®	IV	1–2 g q6–12 h
cefotetan	Cefotan®	IM, IV	1–2 g q12 h
Third-generation			
cefdinir	Omnicef®	PO	300 mg b.i.d.
cefditoren pivoxil	Spectracef®	PO	200 mg b.i.d.
cefpodoxime proxetil	Vantin®	PO	200 mg b.i.d.
ceftazidime	Fortaz®	IM, IV	1–2 g b.i.d.
ceftibuten	Cedax®	PO	400 mg/day
ceftizoxime sodium	Cefizox®	IM, IV	1–2 g b.i.d. or t.i.d.
cefotaxime sodium	Claforan®	IM, IV	1–2 g, 12–24 h
cefixime	Suprax®	PO	400 mg/day in 1–2 div. doses
ceftriaxone sodium	Rocephin®	IM, IV	1–2 g, 12–24 h
cefoperazone sodium	Cefobid®	IM, IV	1–2 g, q12 h
Fourth-generation			
cefepime hydrochloride	Maxipime®	IM, IV	0.5–1 g, q12 h

Adverse Effects

The kidneys eliminate all cephalosporins except cefoperazone. Doses must be adjusted for patients with renal impairment. They can cause hypersensitivity reactions similar to penicillin. The most common adverse

Key Concept

Nephrotoxicity may occur with the use of cephalosporins. A decrease in urine output is an early sign of the adverse effect on patients with kidney impairments.

effects include nausea, vomiting, diarrhea, and nephrotoxicity. Adverse effects of cephalosporins include hypoprothrombinemia and bleeding, alcohol intolerance, hypersensitivity reactions, and thrombophlebitis.

Contraindications and Precautions

Cephalosporins are contraindicated if the patient has a history of allergies to these agents or penicillins. Cephalosporins should be avoided in pregnant and lactating women. Cephalosporins are to be used cautiously in patients with renal or hepatic impairment, and in patients with bleeding disorders.

Drug Interactions

Cephalosporins have drug interactions with alcohol, diarrhea medications, birth control pills, anticoagulants, blood viscosity reducing medicines, and antiseizure medicines. Cephalosporins are contraindicated for use with alcohol, alcohol-containing medications, aminoglycosides, anticoagulants, carbenicillin by injection, dipyridamole, divalproex, heparin, pentoxifylline, plicamycin, sulfinpyrazone, ticarcillin, thrombolytic agents, valproic acid, potent diuretics, iron-iron supplements, and probenecid.

Aminoglycosides

Aminoglycosides are broad-spectrum antibiotics. The toxic potential of these drugs limits their use. Since their introduction into clinical use 50 years ago, aminoglycosides continue to play an important role in the treatment of severe infections. Major aminoglycosides include amikacin, gentamicin, kanamycin, neomycin, netilmicin, streptomycin, and tobramycin. These agents are shown in Table 22-6.

Mechanism of Action

Aminoglycosides are bactericidal; they inhibit bacterial protein synthesis, causing cell death. Their mechanism of action is not fully known.

Indications

Aminoglycosides are prescribed for a variety of disorders and infectious diseases.

- Streptomycin: This can be used to treat tularemia, acute brucellosis, bacterial endocarditis, tuberculosis, and plague.
- Amikacin, gentamycin, netilmicin, and tobramycin: These are prescribed for serious Gram-negative bacillary infections such as *Enterobacter*, *klebsiella*, bacteremia, meningitis, and peritonitis.
- Neomycin: This is used for pre-operative bowel sterilization, hepatic coma, and in topical form for burns.

TABLE 22-6 Major Aminoglycosides

Generic Name	Trade Name	Route of Administration	Common Dosage Range
amikacin sulfate	Amikin®	IM, IV	5–7.5 mg/kg/day in 2–3 divided doses
gentamicin sulfate	Garamycin®	IM, IV	1.5–2.0 mg/kg/day (standard dose)
kanamycin	Kantrex®	IM, IV	15 mg/kg each 8–12 hours for serious infections
neomycin sulfate	Mycifradin®	PO, IM, Topical	PO: 50 mg/kg in 4 div. doses for 2–3 days; IM: 1.3–2.6 mg/kg q.i.d.; Topical: apply 1–3 times/day
netilmicin	Netromycin®	IM	4 mg/kg in 2 div. doses
paromomycin sulfate	Humatin®	PO	25–35 mg/kg t.i.d.
streptomycin	generic only	IM	15 mg/kg up to 1 g/d as a single dose
tobramycin sulfate	Tobrex®	IM, IV	3 mg/kg t.i.d.

Adverse Effects

Aminoglycosides can cause serious adverse effects such as ototoxicity (including hearing loss) and nephrotoxicity. Neomycin is the most nephrotoxic aminoglycoside, and streptomycin is the least nephrotoxic. Gentamycin and tobramycin are nephrotoxic to the same degree. Aminoglycosides are also potentially neurotoxic, and these adverse effects may cause permanent damage to the organs.

Contraindications and Precautions

History of hypersensitivity or toxic reaction to an aminoglycoside antibiotic is contraindicated. Safety during pregnancy (category C) and lactation, in neonates and infants, or use for a period exceeding 14 days is not established. Aminoglycosides should be used cautiously in patients with impaired renal function, eighth cranial (auditory) nerve impairment, or in older adults. Other cautions include use in premature infants, neonates, and infants.

Drug Interactions

The risks of nephrotoxicity may increase by using an aminoglycoside with cephalosporins. If an aminoglycoside is used with loop diuretics (furosemide, ethacrynic acid, etc.), there is an increased risk of ototoxicity.

TABLE 22-7 Most Commonly Used Macrolides

Generic Name	Trade Name	Route of Administration	Common Dosage Range
erythromycin base	Eryc®, E-mycin®	PO	250–500 mg q.i.d.
erythromycin estolate	Ilosone®	PO, IM, IV	250–500 mg
erythromycin stearate	SK-Erythromycin®	PO	250–500 mg
clarithromycin	Biaxin®	PO	250–500 mg b.i.d.
azithromycin	Zithromax®, Zmax®	PO	500 mg on day 1, then 250 mg/d
dirithromycin	Dynabac®	PO	500 mg once/day

Macrolides

The macrolides include erythromycin, azithromycin, and clarithromycin. Erythromycin is produced by *Streptomyces erythreus*. They are also used as alternative agents when the patient is allergic to penicillin. Table 22-7 shows common macrolides.

Mechanism of Action

Macrolides may be bactericidal (bringing death to bacteria) or bacteriostatic (tending to restrain the development or reproduction of bacteria). They inhibit bacterial protein synthesis by binding to cell membranes. Erythromycins generally penetrate the cell wall of Gram-positive bacteria more readily than those of Gram-negative bacteria.

Indications

Macrolides are effective in the treatment of infections caused by a wide range of Gram-negative and Gram-positive microorganisms. They are the drug of choice for the treatment of *Mycoplasma pneumoniae*, campylobacteria infections, Legionnaires' disease, chlamydial infections, and pertussis. In patients with penicillin allergy, erythromycins are the best alternatives in the treatment of gonorrhea, syphilis, and pneumococcal pneumonia. Erythromycins may be given prophylactically before dental procedures to prevent bacterial endocarditis.

Adverse Effects

Macrolides rarely cause serious adverse effects. Nausea, vomiting, and diarrhea may occur with all forms of macrolides.

Contraindications and Precautions

Macrolides are contraindicated in patients with hypersensitivity, and in patients with liver diseases. These drugs should be used cautiously during pregnancy and lactation. Erythromycin and azithromycin are contraindicated in pregnancy (category B); and clarithromycin and troleandomycin are pregnancy category C drugs. Macrolides must be used with great caution in patients with liver diseases.

Drug Interactions

Macrolides inhibit the hepatic metabolism of theophylline. They may interfere with the metabolism of digoxin, corticosteroids, and cyclosporin. Use of antacids decreases the absorption of most macrolides. Chloramphenicol, clindamycin, and lincomycin are able to decrease the therapeutic activity of the macrolides if they are used concurrently.

Tetracyclines

Tetracyclines are broad-spectrum agents that are effective against certain bacterial strains that resist other antibiotics. The major tetracyclines and the administration routes are shown in Table 22-8.

Mechanism of Action

Tetracyclines are bacteriostatic (capable of slowing the multiplication of bacteria). They inhibit bacterial protein synthesis, which is a process necessary for reproduction of the microorganism.

TABLE 22-8 Major Tetracyclines and Administration Routes

Generic Name	Trade Name	Route of Administration	Common Dosage Range
demeclocycline hydrochloride	Declomycin®	PO	150 mg q.i.d. or 300 mg b.i.d.
doxycycline hyclate	Vibramycin®	PO, IV	100 mg b.i.d. on day 1, then 100 mg/day
methacycline hydrochloride	Rondomycin®	PO	600 mg/day in 2–4 div. doses
minocycline hydrochloride	Minocin®	PO	4 mg/kg/day–200 mg/day; 200 mg followed by 100 mg b.i.d.
oxytetracycline	Terramycin®	PO, IM, IV	PO: 250–500 mg b.i.d.-q.i.d.; IM: 100 mg t.i.d.; IV: 250–500 mg b.i.d.
tetracycline hydrochloride	Achromycin®, Sumycin®	PO	250–500 mg b.i.d.
tigecycline	Tygacil®	IV	100 mg followed by 50 mg q12 h

Indications

Tetracyclines are active against Gram-negative and Gram-positive organisms, spirochetes, mycoplasmal and chlamydial organisms, rickettsial species, and certain protozoa. They are the drugs of choice in rickettsial infections (such as Rocky Mountain spotted fever), chlamydial infections, amebiasis, cholera, brucellosis, and tularemia. Tetracyclines are prescribed as an alternative to penicillin in the treatment of anthrax, syphilis, gonorrhea, Lyme disease, and *Haemophilus influenzae* respiratory infections. Oral or topical tetracycline may be used as a treatment for acne. Doxycycline is highly effective in the prophylaxis of "traveler's diarrhea."

Adverse Effects

Abdominal discomfort, nausea, diarrhea, and anorexia are common adverse effects of tetracyclines. Cross-sensitivity within the tetracyclines are also common. Use of the drugs in infants has resulted in retardation of bone growth. Because tetracyclines localize in the dentin and enamel of developing teeth, use of the drugs during tooth development may cause enamel hypoplasia and permanent yellow-gray to brown discoloration of the teeth. Tetracycline can cause fetal toxicity when administered to pregnant women (e.g., retardation of skeletal development). Liver toxicity has occurred following IV administration of tetracyclines to pregnant women. Oxytetracycline is the least hepatotoxic. Phototoxicity may occur in patients when they are exposed to strong sunlight (ultraviolet), especially with demeclocycline (Declomycin). Minocycline can cause vestibular toxicity. IV administration of tetracyclines is irritating and may cause phlebitis.

Contraindications and Precautions

Key Concept

Tetracyclines should not be used during pregnancy, infancy, and childhood (up to eight years of age), or during lactation, because they cause permanent discoloration of teeth in children.

Tetracyclines are contraindicated in patients who are allergic to them, or to any ingredient used in their formulations. Tetracyclines should not be used in children younger than eight years of age unless other appropriate drugs are ineffective or are contraindicated. Tetracyclines should be avoided in patients with severe renal or hepatic impairment. They are also contraindicated in those individuals with common bile duct obstruction.

Tetracyclines should be used cautiously in patients with renal function impairment or a history of liver dysfunction. History of allergy, asthma, and undernourished patients are other factors that cause tetracyclines to be used with caution.

Drug Interactions

There are certain foods (dairy products) and agents such as iron preparations, laxatives, and antacids that contain aluminum and calcium, which may effect a reduction of tetracycline absorption. Therefore, they are recommended to be taken on an empty stomach. Barbiturates and phenytoin can decrease the effectiveness of tetracyclines.

Fluoroquinolones

Fluoroquinolones (also known as quinolones) are related to nalidixic acid and are bactericidal for growing bacteria. The most commonly used quinolones are shown in Table 22-9.

Mechanism of Action

Fluoroquinolones exert their bactericidal (bacteria-destroying) effects by interfering with an enzyme (DNA gyrase) that is required by bacteria for the synthesis of DNA. This action results in the prevention of cell reproduction and in bacterial death.

Indications

Fluoroquinolones are used in the treatment of infections caused by Gram-positive and Gram-negative microorganisms. The indications of

TABLE 22-9 Fluoroquinolones

Generic Name	Trade Name	Route of Administration	Common Dosage Range
First-generation			
nalidixic acid	NegGram®	PO	500 mg–1 g q.i.d.
Second-generation			
ciprofloxacin hydrochloride	Cipro®, Cipro XR®	PO, IV	PO: 250 mg q12h or 500 mg (Cipro XR) q.d. × 3 days; IV: 200 mg q12h, infused over 60 min
lomefloxacin hydrochloride	Maxaquin®	PO	400 mg q.d. × 10 days
norfloxacin	Noroxin®	PO	400 mg b.i.d.
ofloxacin	Floxin®	PO	400 mg for 1 dose
Third-generation			
gatifloxacin	Zymer®	PO	400 mg/day
levofloxacin	Levaquin®	PO, IV	500 mg/day
Fourth-generation			
gemifloxacin	Factive®	PO	320 mg/day
moxifloxacin hydrochloride	Avelox®, Vigamox®	PO, IV	400 mg/day
trovafloxacin	Trovan®	PO	100–300 mg/day

fluoroquinolones are primarily in the treatment of urinary tract and lower respiratory infections, skin and skin structure infections, and sexually transmitted diseases. Ciprofloxacin, norfloxacin, and ofloxacin are used in ophthalmic forms for eye infections.

Adverse Effects

Fluoroquinolone agents may produce nausea, headache, dizziness, dyspepsia, insomnia, photosensitivity, and hypoglycemia. Crystalluria can occur with high doses at alkaline pH. Therefore, fluoroquinolones should be taken with water and the patient should stay well-hydrated. These drugs may cause pain, inflammation, or rupture of a tendon (the most common tendon to be ruptured is the Achilles tendon).

Contraindications and Precautions

Fluoroquinolones are contraindicated in patients with a history of hypersensitivity, during pregnancy (category C) and lactation, and in children younger than 18 years. These agents are also contraindicated in patients who have syphilis, viral infections, tendon inflammation, and tendon pain. Fluoroquinolones should be used cautiously in patients with a history of seizures, in patients with renal dysfunction, in patients on dialysis, or in elderly adults.

Drug Interactions

Ciprofloxacin may increase theophylline levels in blood. Antacids and iron can decrease the absorption of fluoroquinolones. They may increase prothrombin times in patients receiving warfarin.

Miscellaneous Antibacterial Agents

Some antibiotics are classified as miscellaneous antibacterial agents, such as chloramphenicol, clindamycin, dapsone, spectinomycin, and vancomycin (Table 22-10). A few examples of these drugs are detailed below.

Chloramphenicol

This antibiotic is highly effective against rickettsia as well as many Gram-positive and Gram-negative organisms.

Mechanism of Action. Chloramphenicol is principally bacteriostatic but may be bactericidal against a few bacterial strains (e.g., Haemophilus influenzae) or when given in higher concentrations. Chloramphenicol inhibits protein synthesis.

Indications. Chloramphenicol is used only for specific infections that cannot be treated effectively with other antibiotics. It is particularly effective against typhoid fever, rickettsial infections in pregnant women, and meningococcal infections in cephalosporin-allergic patients. Chloramphenicol is also used for infections in patients who have a history of allergies to tetracycline.

TABLE 22-10 Miscellaneous Antibacterial Agents

Generic Name	Trade Name	Route of Administration	Average Adult Dosage
chloramphenicol	Chloromycetin®	PO, IV	50 mg/kg q.i.d.
clindamycin hydrochloride	Cleocin®	PO, IM, IV	PO: 150–450 mg q.i.d.; IM/IV: 600–1200 mg/day in div. doses
dapsone	Aczone®	PO	100 mg/day (with 6 months of rifampin at 600 mg/day for a minimum of 3 years)
ertapenem sodium	Invanz®	IM, IV	1 g/day
lincomycin hydrochloride	Lincocin®	IM, IV	IM: 600 mg every 12–24 h; IV: 600 mg–1 g b.i.d. or t.i.d.
methenamine	Mandelamine®, Hiprex®	PO	1 g b.i.d. (Hiprex) or q.i.d. (Mandelamine)
nitrofurantoin	Furadantin®, Macrobid®	PO	50–100 mg q.i.d.
spectinomycin hydrochloride	Trobicin®	IM	2 g as single dose or q12 h for 7 days until switched to an oral medication
telithromycin	Ketek®	PO	800 mg/day
vancomycin hydrochloride	Vancocin®	IV	500 mg q.i.d. or 1 g b.i.d.

Adverse Effects. Chloramphenicol can cause suppression of bone marrow (in high doses) with resulting pancytopenia. This agent can lead to aplastic anemia in rare, non–dose-related cases. Chloramphenicol therapy can also lead to gray baby syndrome in neonates.

Contraindications and Precautions. Chloramphenicol is contraindicated in patients with a history of hypersensitivity or toxic reaction to chloramphenicol. This agent should be avoided in the treatment of minor infections, for prophylactic use, in typhoid carrier state, in patients with a history or family history of drug-induced bone marrow depression, and during pregnancy (category C) and lactation.

Key Concept

Chloramphenicol may cause non–dose-related and irreversible aplastic anemia and pancytopenia (abnormal reduction in the number of all circulating blood cells).

Chloramphenicol should be given cautiously to patients with impaired hepatic or renal function. This drug may be used cautiously in premature and full-term infants and children.

Drug Interactions. Chloramphenicol may inhibit the metabolism of phenytoin, dicumarol, and tolbutamide, leading to prolonged action and increased effects of these drugs. Phenobarbital can reduce the effect of chloramphenicol therapy. Acetaminophen elevates chloramphenicol levels and may cause toxicity. Penicillins can cause antibiotic antagonism.

Clindamycin

Clindamycin is an anti-infective and antibiotic that has marked toxicity. Clindamycin should be prescribed for special infections when it has been determined to be the most effective drug to treat them.

Mechanism of Action. Clindamycin is bacteriostatic and inhibits bacterial protein synthesis. This agent is active against most Gram-positive and many anaerobic organisms.

Indications. Clindamycin is used in serious infections when less toxic alternatives are inappropriate. Clindamycin is used for joint, bone, and abdominal infections. Topical applications are used in the treatment of acne vulgaris. Vaginal applications are used in the treatment of bacterial vaginosis in non-pregnant women.

Adverse Effects. Clindamycin may cause rash, nausea, vomiting, diarrhea, and pseudomembranous colitis. Leukopenia, agranulocytosis, and thrombocytopenia may also occur.

Contraindications and Precautions. Clindamycin is contraindicated in patients with a history of hypersensitivity to clindamycin or lincomycin. This agent also should not be used in patients with a history of regional enteritis, ulcerative colitis, or antibiotic-associated colitis. Clindamycin is contraindicated in pregnancy (category B) and lactation. It must be used cautiously in patients with history of GI disease, renal or hepatic disease, eczema, asthma, and hay fever.

Drug Interactions. Clindamycin may potentiate the effects of neuromuscular blocking agents, atracurium, tubocurarine, and pancuronium. It is antagonistic to chloramphenicol and erythromycin.

Dapsone

Dapsone is the primary agent in the treatment of all forms of leprosy.

Mechanism of Action. Dapsone is bacteriostatic and bactericidal for Mycobacterium leprae by blocking folic acid synthesis, thereby forcing microorganisms to synthesize their own folic acid.

Indications. Dapsone is the drug of choice for treating leprosy. It is also used prophylactically in contacts of patients with all forms of leprosy except tuberculoid and indeterminate leprosy. Dapsone may be indicated for treatment of dermatitis herpetiformis. The topical (gel) form of dapsone is used for acne vulgaris.

Adverse Effects. Nausea, vomiting, and anorexia are common adverse effects of dapsone. This agent may cause skin rash, peripheral neuropathy, blurred vision, hepatitis, hemolysis (destruction of red blood cells), and cholestatic jaundice.

Contraindications and Precautions. Dapsone is contraindicated in patients with history of hypersensitivity to sulfones or their derivatives,

Key Concept

Dapsone is excreted in breast milk, and may cause hemolytic reactions in neonates.

advanced renal dysfunction, and anemia. Safe use of dapsone during pregnancy (category C) or lactation is not established. Dapsone may be used with caution in patients with hepatic dysfunction, anemia, severe cardiopulmonary disease, and during pregnancy.

Drug Interactions. Probenecid can elevate blood levels of dapsone that may result in toxicity. Otherwise, there are no significant drug-drug interactions associated with the use of dapsone.

Spectinomycin

Spectinomycin is a wide-spectrum antibiotic with moderate activity against both Gram-positive and Gram-negative bacteria.

Mechanism of Action. Its action is usually bacteriostatic, but it has variable activity against a wide variety of Gram-negative and Gram-positive organisms.

Indications. Spectinomycin is used clinically for only one purpose, namely, to treat or prevent acute gonorrhea when the organism is resistant to penicillin, or when the patient is allergic to penicillin. It is not as effective as ceftriaxone.

Adverse Effects. Untoward effects include frequent pain at the injection site, an infrequent headache, nausea, vomiting, insomnia, chills, fever, mild pruritus, and urticaria.

Contraindications and Precautions. Safety during pregnancy (category B) or lactation, and in infants and children age eight years or under, is not established. Spectinomycin should be used with caution in those with a history of allergies.

Drug Interactions. No clinically significant interactions with spectinomycin have been established.

Vancomycin

Vancomycin can destroy most Gram-positive organisms.

Mechanism of Action. Vancomycin is bactericidal and bacteriostatic. It inhibits bacterial cell wall synthesis. Vancomycin acts against susceptible Gram-positive bacteria.

Indications. Vancomycin usually is reserved for serious infections, especially those caused by methicillin-resistant staphylococci, or other serious Gram-positive infections that do not respond to treatment with other anti-infective agents. It is useful in patients who are allergic to penicillin or cephalosporins. Typical uses include treatment of osteomyelitis, endocarditis, and staphylococcal pneumonia.

Adverse Effects. Vancomycin (in higher doses) may cause ototoxicity and nephrotoxicity, which can lead to uremia. It may cause rash on the upper

Key Concept

IV administration of vancomycin should be over a minimum of 60 minutes for a 1 gm dose.

body, sometimes called "**Red man syndrome**." This condition can produce facial flushing and hypotension due to very rapid infusion of the drug.

Contraindications and Precautions. Vancomycin is contraindicated in patients with known hypersensitivity. This medication is used cautiously in patients with hearing impairment or renal dysfunction and during pregnancy (category C) and lactation.

Key Concept

Vancomycin may be used orally only in Clostridium difficile *colitis.*

Drug Interactions. Vancomycin may have added toxicity if used with aminoglycosides, cisplatin, polymyxin B, cyclosporine, and amphotericin B. These drugs (with vancomycin) will result in additive effects of ototoxicity and nephrotoxicity.

Antitubercular Drugs

Tuberculosis is a highly contagious infection caused by *Mycobacterium tuberculosis*. While tuberculosis most commonly affects the lungs, it can also invade any part of the body, including bone, the gastrointestinal tract, and the kidneys. Tuberculosis lesions are characterized by the death of affected tissue with sloughing of tissue and formation of cavities.

Antitubercular drugs are used to treat tuberculosis by suppressing or killing the slow-growing mycobacteria that causes this disease. Antitubercular agents fall into two main categories: primary and re-treatment agents. Because the causative organisms tend to develop resistance to any single drug, combination drug therapy has become standard in the treatment of tuberculosis. Agents chosen for therapy must eradicate mycobacterium. Drugs available include isoniazid, streptomycin, ethambutol, rifampin, pyrazinamide, and rifabutin. Combination drug therapy is essential. Agents showing the lowest incidence of resistance such as isoniazid, rifampin, and streptomycin are usually used in combination with ethambutol or pyrazinamide. Most patients are started on isoniazid, rifampin, and pyrazinamide. A fourth drug (ethambutol or streptomycin) is added with suspected resistance (see Table 22-11 for a list of antitubercular drugs). Some antitubercular drugs are discussed in detail below.

Key Concept

General treatment for any bacterial infection is the administration of a single antibiotic. For tuberculosis, as many as four different drug combinations may be required. These combinations are divided into the first- and second-line antituberculotics on the basis of their efficacy.

Primary Antitubercular Drugs

These include isoniazid, ethambutol, rifampin, pyrazinamide, and streptomycin. These drugs usually offer the greatest effectiveness with the least toxicity. In most cases, the combination of isoniazid, rifampin, and pyrazinamide is most effective. These antibiotics must be administered concurrently during the 6- to 24-month treatment period.

Isoniazid

This agent is the mainstay of antitubercular therapy and is used in all therapeutic regimens.

TABLE 22-11 Antituberculotics

Generic Name	Trade Name	Route of Administration	Average Adult Dosage
First-line agents			
ethambutol hydrochloride	Myambutol®	PO	15–25 mg/kg/day
isoniazid	INH®, Laninzid	PO, IM	5 mg/kg/day
pyrazinamide	PZA®	PO	15–35 mg/kg t.i.d.-q.i.d. (max: 2 g/day)
rifampin	Rifadin®, Rimactane®	PO, IV	600 mg/day as a single dose
rifapentine	Priftin®	PO	600 mg 2x/wk for 2 mo; then 1x/wk for 4 mo
streptomycin sulfate	Streptomycin®	IM	15 mg/kg up to 1 g/day as a single dose
Second-line agents			
amikacin sulfate	Amikin®	IM, IV	5–7.5 mg/kg loading dose; then 7.5 mg/kg b.i.d.
capreomycin	Capastat Sulfate®	IM, IV	1 g/day (not to exceed 20 mg/kg/day) for 60–120 days, then 1 g 2–3 times/wk
ciprofloxacin hydrochloride	Cipro®	PO	250–750 mg b.i.d.
cycloserine	Seromycin®	PO	250 mg q12h for 2 wk; may increase to 500 mg q12 h (max: 1 g/day)
ethionamide	Trecator ®	PO	0.5–1.0 g/day div. q8–12 h
kanamycin	Kantrex®	IM, IV	15 mg/kg b.i.d.-t.i.d.
ofloxacin	Floxin®	PO	400 mg in 1 dose
rifabutin	Mycobutin®	PO	300 mg q.i.d., may give 150 mg b.i.d. if nausea is a problem

Mechanism of Action. Isoniazid is bacteriostatic and bactericidal, but bacteriostatic for dormant mycobacteria. It is postulated to act by interfering with biosynthesis of bacterial proteins, nucleic acid, and lipids. The mechanism of action is not completely known.

Indications. Isoniazid is the most widely prescribed antitubercular drug. It should be used in combination with another antitubercular agent to prevent drug resistance in tuberculosis. In the majority of cases of tuberculosis, isoniazid should be recommended at least for six months. Its agent, though, may last from six months to two years depending on the severity of the disease. During isoniazid therapy, the patient should be given

Key Concept

Prophylactic isoniazid may be given alone for up to one year in adults or children who have a positive tuberculin test result, but lack active lesions.

pyridoxine (vitamin B6) supplements to prevent neuritis (inflammation of a nerve).

Adverse Effects. The most common adverse effects of isoniazid are fever, jaundice, peripheral neuritis, and skin rash. Hepatitis can be severe and fatal. Aplastic or hemolytic anemia and thrombocytopenia may occur. Isoniazid may increase the excretion of pyridoxine, which can lead to peripheral neuritis, particularly in poorly nourished patients.

Contraindications and Precautions. Isoniazid is contraindicated in patients with history of isoniazid-associated hypersensitivity reactions, including hepatic injury or acute liver damage (from any cause). Isoniazid should be avoided during pregnancy (category C) unless the risk is warranted.

Isoniazid should be used cautiously in chronic liver disease, renal dysfunction, and chronic alcoholism. This drug must be used cautiously in people over 35 years of age, and during lactation.

Drug Interactions. Food and antacids that contain aluminum decrease the absorption of isoniazid. Disulfiram may cause coordination difficulties or psychotic reactions. Drinking alcohol with isoniazid may increase the risk of liver damage.

Ethambutol

Ethambutol is a synthetic water-based compound. It is an anti-tuberculosis and anti-infective drug.

Mechanism of Action. Ethambutol is bacteriostatic. The actual mechanism of action is unknown, but it appears to inhibit RNA synthesis and thus arrest multiplication of tubercle bacilli. The emergence of resistant strains is delayed by administering ethambutol in combination with other antituberculosis drugs.

Indications. Ethambutol is prescribed in the treatment of pulmonary tuberculosis in conjunction with at least one other antituberculosis drug.

Adverse Effects. Ethambutol may cause optic neuritis (a decrease in visual acuity and changes in color perception), drug fever, dizziness, confusion, hallucinations, and joint pains.

Contraindications and Precautions. Ethambutol is contraindicated in patients with a history of hypersensitivity. The drug should be avoided for children under the age of six years, or in patients with optic neuritis. Ethambutol should be used with caution in patients with renal and hepatic impairment, during lactation, or pregnancy (category B). Ethambutol is given to patients with diabetic retinopathy because of the danger of optic neuritis.

Drug Interactions. Aluminum-containing antacids can decrease absorption of ethambutol.

Rifampin

Rifampin is a complex macrocyclic agent.

Mechanism of Action. Rifampin has both bacteriostatic and bactericidal actions. This agent inhibits DNA-dependent RNA polymerase activity in susceptible bacterial cells, thereby suppressing RNA synthesis.

Indications. The combination of rifampin and isoniazid is the most effective drug for treatment of tuberculosis. It should not be given alone because it may cause drug-resistance for organisms. Rifampin may be prescribed in combination with dapsone for the treatment of leprosy. Rifampin is also effective against prevention of Neisseria meningitides, and a wide range of Gram-negative and Gram-positive organisms.

Key Concept

Rifampin may change the colors of urine, tears, saliva, sweat, and feces to orange-red.

Adverse Effects. Liver damage can result from rifampin therapy. Liver function tests should be routinely checked. Headache, dizziness, fatigue, confusion, skin rash, nausea, and vomiting may occur.

Key Concept

Patients who wear soft contact lenses should be instructed that rifampin therapy may permanently stain these lenses.

Contraindications and Precautions. Rifampin is contraindicated in patients with a history of hypersensitivity, hepatic and renal impairment, meningococcal disease, and lactation. Safe use during pregnancy (category C) or in children less than five years of age is not established. Rifampin should be used cautiously in patients with hepatic disease or history of alcoholism.

Drug Interactions. Rifampin may decrease the effect of many drugs, such as warfarin, oral contraceptives, oral hypoglycemics, digitoxin, and corticosteroids. There is also a decrease in the effects of phenytoin, verapamil, and chloramphenicol. Probenecid may increase blood levels of rifampin.

Streptomycin

Streptomycin is one of the aminoglycosides that is given in combination with other antitubercular agents (see discussion of aminoglycosides).

Summary

The invasion of pathogenic microorganisms may cause either local or systemic infection. The pathogen can be present in the blood circulation causing bacteremia. Anti-infective drugs, generally called antibiotics, are used to treat infection. Selection of antibiotics depends on various factors such as pharmacologic properties and spectrum activity of the drugs, and patient factors such as immunity, age, adverse drugs reactions, and underlying diseases. Pregnancy and lactation also play a major role. There are broad classifications of anti-infective drugs that may affect specific pathogens such as bacteria viruses, fungi, protozoa, and mycoplasms. Penicillins are the most widely used anti-infective agents. However, cephalosporin usage has increased in the last decade. There are specific antibiotics that are used predominantly for penicillinase-resistant penicillins. The first drugs used successfully to prevent and treat human bacterial infections were sulfonamides.

Exploring the Web

Visit any of the following Web sites to search for information on various types of diseases caused by infectious agents or the drugs used to treat them that were discussed in this chapter.

- ***http://healthresources.caremark.com***
- ***www.cdc.gov***
- ***www.mayoclinic.com***
- ***www.nfid.org***
- To learn more about the concerns and adverse affects of using antibiotics, review the information found at ***www.tufts.edu/med/apua.***

Review Questions

Multiple Choice

1. Third-generation cephalosporins are potent against all of the following, except:

A. Neisseria gonorrhea
B. mycobacterium tuberculosis
C. Haemophilus influenzae
D. enterobacteria

2. Which of the antibiotics should not be used in children under age 18 years?

A. chloramphenicol
B. penicillins
C. isoniazid
D. ciprofloxacin

3. All of the following agents are in the class of macrolides, antibiotics, except:
   A. sulfonamide
   B. erythromycin
   C. troleandomycin
   D. clarithromycin

4. Penicillinase may be produced by:
   A. Streptococci
   B. Necesseria gonorrhea
   C. Staphylococci
   D. Haemophilus influenzae

5. Streptomycin is an aminoglycoside-like antibiotic indicated for the treatment of which of the following:
   A. tuberculosis
   B. Gram-negative bacillary septicemia
   C. penicillin-resistant gonococcal infection
   D. syphilis

6. Which of the following antibiotics may cause enamel hypoplasia and permanent yellow-gray color of the teeth in young children?
   A. isoniazid
   B. streptomycin
   C. rifampin
   D. tetracyclines

7. Which of the following antibiotics may lead to gray baby syndrome?
   A. tetracyclines
   B. chloramphenicol
   C. streptomycin
   D. metronidazole

8. A person who lacks resistance to an agent and is vulnerable to a disease is called a:
   A. compromised host
   B. susceptible host
   C. virulent host
   D. parasitic host

9. Viable bacteria which is present in the circulatory system is called:
   A. bacteremia
   B. virimia
   C. anemia
   D. hyperemia

10. The reservoir is a place where:
   A. an infectious agent leaves the body
   B. an organism invades the host
   C. an agent can be spread to others
   D. the agent can survive, colonize, and reproduce

11. Anti-infective drugs derived from natural substances are called:

A. antivirals
B. Gram stains
C. antibiotics
D. antifungals

12. A 42-year-old man has an upper respiratory infection. Four years ago, he experienced an episode of bronchospasm following penicillin V therapy. The culture now reveals a Gram-positive *Streptococcus pneumoniae* that is sensitive to all of the following drugs. Which of the following drugs would be the best choice for this patient?

A. cefaclor
B. ampicillin
C. amoxicillin/clavulanate
D. erythromycin

13. Isoniazid is a primary antitubercular agent that:

A. may be nephrotoxic and ototoxic
B. requires vitamin B_6 (pyridoxine supplementation)
C. should never be used due to hepatotoxic potential
D. causes ocular complications that are reversible if the drug is discontinued.

14. All of the following drugs are suitable oral therapy for a lower urinary tract infection due to Gram-negative bacteria, except:

A. ciprofloxacin
B. norfloxacin
C. sulfadiazine
D. cefoxitin

15. Which of the following is the drug of choice for Chlamydial organisms and rickettsial species?

A. tetracycline
B. isoniazid
C. rephampin
D. penicillin

Matching

_____ **1.** Contraindicated in children younger than eight years of age	**A.** isoniazid
_____ **2.** Causes aplastic anemia in infants	**B.** erythromycin
_____ **3.** Changes the color of urine or saliva to orange-red	**C.** sulfonamide
_____ **4.** This agent is used for preoperative bowel sterilization and hepatic coma	**D.** neomycin

_____ 5. The drug of choice for the treatment Legionnaires' disease, and pertussis — E. rifampin

_____ 6. The first drug discovered to prevent and cure human bacterial infections — F. chloramphenicol

_____ 7. The most widely prescribed antitubercular drug — G. tetracyclines

Critical Thinking

Christian is a 16-year-old who goes to a private school. He wanted to work at a local hospital as a volunteer. Therefore, they required that he had to have a tuberculin test. His physician diagnosed that his TB test was positive with a reading of 16 mm, and ordered a chest x-ray. The result of the chest x-ray was negative, so the physician recommended that Christian go to the local Health Department for tuberculosis evaluation. They determined that he had been exposed to tuberculosis, but did not have the primary form of tuberculosis himself.

1. What drug or drugs would the Health Department recommend for this patient?
2. How long do you think he will need to take the drug or drugs that he is prescribed?
3. Since Christian had been exposed to tuberculosis, will his entire family also need to receive preventative medications?

Antiviral, Antifungal, and Antiprotozoal Agents

CHAPTER 23

OUTLINE

OBJECTIVES

After completing this chapter, the reader should be able to:

1. Describe why antiviral drug treatments are limited compared with other antibacterial agents.
2. Identify viral diseases that may benefit from drug therapy.
3. Describe the expected outcomes of HIV drug therapy.
4. Define HAART and explain why it is commonly used in the drug therapy of HIV infection.
5. Explain the mechanisms of action of antiviral, antifungal, and antiprotozoal agents.
6. Explain the four commonly used antifungal agents.
7. Compare the drug therapy of superficial and systemic fungal infections.
8. Name common drugs used for malarial parasites.
9. Explain the important adverse effects of systemic antifungal and antiprotozoal drugs.
10. Name three important amebicides and their mechanisms of action.

GLOSSARY

Acquired Immunodeficiency Syndrome (AIDS) – a severe immunological disorder caused by the retrovirus HIV, resulting in a defect in cell-mediated immune response

Amebicides and trichomonacides – drugs use to treat amebic and trichomonal infections

Antimalarial agents – drugs used to treat malaria infections

Epidemic – an outbreak of a disease or infection that spreads widely and rapidly

Fungi – a distinct group of organisms that are neither plant nor animal

Human immunodeficiency virus (HIV) – a retrovirus that infects helper T cells of the immune system, leading to AIDS

Malaria – a severe generalized infection caused by the bite of an *anopheles* mosquito that is infected with a *Plasmodium* protozoon

Mycoses – fungal diseases

Pro-drug – inactive or partially active drug that is metabolically changed in the body to an active drug

Protozoa – single-celled parasitic organisms, many of which are motile (able to move spontaneously)

Replication – the process of reproduction or copying of genetic material

Superficial mycoses – involving a surface or a shallow depth of tissue

Systemic mycoses – relating to or affecting an entire body or an entire organism

Viruses – intracellular parasites that take over the metabolic machinery of host cells and use it for their own survival and replication

OVERVIEW

Many infections may be caused by viruses, fungi, and protozoa. Some of these infections may result in no permanent damage, and usually disappear within seven to ten days if the patient is otherwise healthy. Many of these infections may cause serious viral infections that may be fatal, such as HIV, and may require aggressive drug therapy. Fungal infections are seen commonly in patients with immune deficiency diseases. Fungi and protozoans are more complex than bacteria and there are fewer medications to treat these types of infections.

VIRUSES

Viruses are intracellular parasites that take over the metabolic machinery of host cells and use it for their own survival and replication, often resulting in the destruction of the infected cells. Viral diseases are the most common causes of disease in humans. Viruses result in a wide variety of diseases ranging from the common cold and the "cold sore" of herpes immune simplex to several types of cancers and AIDS.

Key Concept

Ebola virus, Dengue virus, and human immunodeficiency virus are examples of emerging viruses that threaten the public health and kill thousands of people each year.

Viruses are extremely small, and contain their genetic information in either deoxyribonucleic acid (DNA) or ribonucleic acid (RNA), which are surrounded by a protein coat (capsid). After infection, viruses usually make multiple copies of their genetic material and produce the necessary viral proteins for replication. Some animal viruses are responsible for diseases such as hemorrhagic fever (Ebola virus), influenza virus, and measles (rubeola virus).

Antiviral Drugs

Antiviral drugs are used to treat viral infections by influencing viral **replication**. Viruses are not able to independently provide their metabolic activity, and can replicate only within living host cells. Therefore, antiviral agents tend to damage the host as well as viral cells. The majority of antivirals are active against only one virus, either DNA or RNA types. These viruses may include herpes simplex virus (HSV) 1 and 2, varicella-zoster virus (VZV), cytomegalovirus (CMV), and influenza A. Table 23-1 shows

TABLE 23-1 Antiviral Drugs and Their Therapeutic Uses

Generic Name	Trade Name	Route of Administration	Common Adult Dosage
Non-HIV Antivirals			
acyclovir	Zovirax®	Topical, PO, IV	Topical: Apply 5 times/day for 4 days; PO: 400 mg t.i.d.; IV: 5 mg/kg t.i.d.
amantadine	Symmetrel®	PO	200 mg once/day
cidofovir	Vistide®	IV	5 mg/kg once weekly for 2 weeks
famciclovir	Famvir®	PO	500 mg t.i.d.
ganciclovir	Cytovene®	IV	5 mg/kg b.i.d.
rimantadine	Flumadine®	PO	100 mg b.i.d.
ribavirin	Rebetrol®, Virazole®	PO	600 mg b.i.d. for 24–48 weeks
valacyclovir	Valtrex®	PO	1 g t.i.d.
HIV Antivirals			
abacavir sulfate	Ziagen®	PO	300 mg b.i.d.
didanosine (DDI)	Videx®	PO	250 mg q.d.
indinavir sulfate	Crixivan®	PO	800 mg t.i.d.
nevirapine	Viramune®	PO	200 mg once daily
stavudine (D4T)	Zerit®	PO	40 mg b.i.d.
zidovudine (formerly azidothymidine, AZT)	Retrovir®	PO, IV	PO: 300 mg b.i.d.; IV: 1–2 mg/kg q4 h

antiviral agents that are currently approved for treatment of some viruses. The following antiviral drugs are a few examples.

Acyclovir

Acyclovir is a synthetic acyclic analog of guanosine with activity against various herpes viruses. Herpes viruses can infect neonates, children, and adults, causing a wide spectrum of diseases. Herpes simplex type 1 virus is responsible for systemic infections involving the liver and other organs, including the central nervous system, and localized infections that may involve the skin, eyes, and mouth. Other medically important herpes viruses include cytomegalovirus (CMV), varicella (Chicken Pox), and varicella-zoster (shingles). Acyclovir is available in capsules ranging from 200 to 800 mg.

Mechanism of Action. Acyclovir is taken up selectively by cells that are infected with herpes viruses. Its activity depends upon conversion to the triphosphate where it becomes incorporated into viral DNA and inhibits viral replication.

Indications. Acyclovir is most effective against HSV-1 and HSV-2. IV acyclovir is used for HSV encephalitis, neonatal HSV, and life-threatening HSV and VZV infections in immunocompromised patients. Oral acyclovir is indicated for the treatment of primary and recurrent genital herpes. Acyclovir ophthalmic ointment is effective for herpes simplex keratitis.

Adverse Effects. Acyclovir may cause nausea, vomiting, and diarrhea. The drug can precipitate in the renal tubules with excessive dosages or when it is given by rapid infusion, which may cause acute renal failure. Other adverse effects of acyclovir include headache, drowsiness, fatigue, uncontrollable rhythmic shaking, confusion, and seizures.

Contraindications and Precautions. Acyclovir is contraindicated in patients with hypersensitivity to this agent. Acyclovir should be used with caution in lactation, pregnancy (category B), dehydration, and renal insufficiency.

Drug Interactions. Amphotericin B may raise the plasma and renal concentrations of acyclovir. Probenecid decreases acyclovir elimination. Zidovudine may cause increased drowsiness and lethargy.

> ***Medical Terminology Review***
>
> **immunocompromised**
> *immuno = relating to the immune system*
> *compromised = impaired (for example, by disease or treatment)*
> impairment of the immune system
>
> **keratitis**
> *kerat = cornea (of the eye)*
> *itis = inflammation*
> inflammation of the cornea

> ***Key Concept***
>
> *The patient must be aware that a full therapeutic response to famciclovir may take several weeks.*

Famciclovir

Famciclovir is a **pro-drug** (inactive or partially active drug that is metabolically changed in the body to an active drug) of the antiviral agent penciclovir.

Mechanism of Action. Famciclovir prevents viral replication by inhibition of DNA formation.

Indications. Famciclovir is used for the management of acute herpes zoster (shingles) and recurrent genital herpes in immunocompetent patients. It is effective against HSV-1, HSV-2, and VZV.

> ***Medical Terminology Review***
>
> **immunocompetent**
> *immuno = relating to the immune system*
> *competent = normal ability to respond*
> normal functioning of the immune system

Adverse Effects. Common adverse effects resulting from famciclovir use include fatigue, nausea, diarrhea, vomiting, constipation, and anorexia. Headache is also frequently reported.

Contraindications and Precautions. Famciclovir is contraindicated in patients with known hypersensitivity to this agent and lactation. This drug should be used cautiously in patients with renal or hepatic impairment, or carcinoma, in older adults, and during pregnancy (category B). Safety of this drug in children less than 18 years is not established.

Drug Interactions. Probenecid can increase plasma concentration of penciclovir. Famciclovir may increase digoxin levels.

Amantadine

Amantadine is an antiviral and anticholinergic agent effective for viral respiratory infections such as influenza A virus (it is not effective against influenza B infections), and Parkinson's disease.

Mechanism of Action. The mechanism of the antiviral activity of amantadine is unknown. Its action appears to occur early in the course of viral infection.

Indications. Amantadine is indicated for the prophylaxis and treatment of influenza A virus infections, as well as for Parkinson's disease. Individuals who have not received vaccine prophylaxis can benefit from amantadine prophylaxis given for at least ten days after a known exposure to influenza A.

Adverse Effects. Amantadine causes mild adverse effects, including blurred vision, anxiety, insomnia, and dizziness. Urinary retention is another potential adverse effect. Serious adverse effects in patients treated for Parkinson's disease have included congestive heart failure, hypotension, peripheral edema, depression, seizures, psychosis, and leukopenia.

Contraindications and Precautions. Amantadine is contraindicated in pregnancy (category C), lactation, and in children less than one year. Amantadine should be used cautiously in patients with history of epilepsy, congestive heart failure, peripheral edema, drops in blood pressure when the patient stands up from a lying or sitting position, psychoses, and hepatic disease.

Drug Interactions. Amantadine interacts with anticholinergic drugs to produce atropine-like effects unless the dosage of the anticholinergic drug is reduced. Amantadine prophylaxis or treatment does not interfere with the immune response to influenza vaccination given concurrently.

Ganciclovir

Ganciclovir is an antiviral agent and synthetic purine nucleoside analog that is approved for the treatment of cytomegalovirus (CMV) infection.

Mechanism of Action. After conversion to ganciclovir triphosphate, ganciclovir is incorporated into viral DNA, and inhibits the replication of the DNA virus. By this mechanism, it can terminate viral replication.

Indications. Ganciclovir is prescribed for CMV retinitis, prophylaxis and treatment of systemic CMV infections in immunocompromised patients, including HIV-positive and transplant patients.

Adverse Effects. Ganciclovir has black box warnings concerning increased potential for dose-limited neutropenia, thrombocytopenia, and anemia. The FDA issues black box warnings when a serious problem concerning the use of a drug has been discovered, so that medical practitioners are aware of the problem and its resulting adverse effects. Inflammation of a vein and pain may occur at the site of infusion.

Key Concept

Ganciclovir should not be administered during pregnancy because of its carcinogenic potential.

Contraindications and Precautions. Ganciclovir is contraindicated in patients with known hypersensitivity, and during lactation. This drug should be used cautiously in patients with renal impairment, older adults, and during pregnancy (category C). Safety and efficacy in children are not established.

Drug Interactions. Probenecid may increase ganciclovir levels and possibly toxicity.

Antiretroviral Drugs for HIV-AIDS

In 1981, an **epidemic** of fatal infections first appeared in homosexual men. The spread of this illness to these groups suggested that an infectious agent, transmissible through blood and semen, caused the immunodeficiency that was common to all the patients. The term **Acquired Immunodeficiency Syndrome**, or **AIDS**, was coined to describe this illness. At the outset of the epidemic, most people with AIDS died within a year of this diagnosis. In 1983, researchers isolated the virus that causes AIDS. Today, we have learned much about AIDS since the first case reports. We now know that AIDS is caused by **human immunodeficiency virus (HIV)**, its modes of transmission, and who is at risk for HIV infection. We know that HIV kills lymphocytes (cells in the blood stream necessary to respond to bacteria, fungi, protozoa, and viruses). Antiviral medications for HIV-AIDS slow the growth of HIV in several different ways.

None of the available medications can cure the disease and, due to the rapid mutation of HIV and its resistant strains, new HIV antiviral agents are constantly being developed. The decision of exactly when to begin pharmacotherapy must be made early enough after the diagnosis is established in order to give each patient the best chance of receiving effective treatment. HIV may remain dormant for either months or years after initial exposure. It is important to begin treatment during the latent stage in order to delay acute symptoms and the onset of full-blown AIDS.

HAART Therapy

Highly Active Anti-Retroviral Therapy (HAART) has been shown to reduce viral load and increase CD4 lymphocytes in persons infected with HIV, delay onset of AIDS, and prolong survival with AIDS. The incidence and mortality of AIDS has declined substantially since 1996 due to HAART. The benefits of HAART, which involves the combination of three to four drug combinations against HIV, have been widely publicized. However, HAART presents formidable challenges, including adverse effects and the potential for the rapid spread of drug resistance. Protease inhibitors do not work as well with HIV drugs such as non-nucleoside analogues, and they should not be taken alone. If one of the drugs involved in multiple drug therapy is not well tolerated, or if a patient's HIV infection becomes resistant to it, a whole new set of drugs must be prescribed for the regimen to be effective. Currently, due to the limited number of HAART medications available in the U.S. market, only a few different drug combinations are possible. HAART regimens can also fail because of the lack of viral load response, or poor treatment adherence. Missing a single dose of HAART medication even twice a week can cause the development of drug-resistant HIV—a real danger, because adherence to the drug regimens is difficult. For each group of antiretroviral drugs for HIV-AIDS, only one selected drug will be discussed here. Table 23-2 shows antiretroviral drugs used for HIV-AIDS.

TABLE 23-2 Antiretroviral Drugs used for HIV-AIDS

Generic Name	Trade Name	Route of Administration	Common Adult Dosage
Non-Nucleoside Reverse Transcriptase Inhibitors (NNRTIs)			
delavirdine mesylate	Rescriptor®	PO	400 mg t.i.d.
efavirenz	Sustiva®	PO	600 mg/day
nevirapine	Viramune®	PO	200 mg/day x 14 days, then increase to b.i.d.
Nucleoside Reverse Transcriptase Inhibitors (NRTIs)			
abacavir sulfate	Ziagen®	PO	300 mg b.i.d.
didanosine (DDI)	Videx®	PO	400 mg q.d.
emtricitabine	Emtriva®	PO	200 mg/day
lamivudine	Epivir®	PO	300 mg/day
stavudine (D4T)	Zerit®	PO	40 mg b.i.d.
zalcitabine (DDC)	Hivid®	PO	0.75 mg t.i.d.
zidovudine (formerly AZT)	Retrovir®	PO, IV	PO: 300 mg b.i.d.; IV: 1–2 mg/kg q4 h
Protease Inhibitors (PIs)			
amprenavir	Agenerase®	PO	1200 mg b.i.d.
atazanavir	Reyataz®	PO	400 mg/day
indinavir sulfate	Crixivan®	PO	800 mg t.i.d.
nelfinavir mesylate	Viracept®	PO	750 mg t.i.d.
ritonavir	Norvir®	PO	600 mg t.i.d. w/meals
saquinavir mesylate	Invirase	PO	600 mg t.i.d.
Miscellaneous Drugs			
enfuvirtide	Fuzeon®	SC	90 mg b.i.d.
tenofovir disoproxil fumarate	Viread®	PO	300 mg once/day

Delavirdine

Delavirdine is a nonnucleoside reverse transcriptase inhibitor that prevents the replication of HIV-1 virus.

Mechanism of Actions. Delavirdine binds directly to reverse transcriptase of HIV-1 and blocks RNA- and DNA- dependent DNA polymerase activities.

Indications. Delavirdine is used in the treatment of HIV infection in combination with other antiretroviral agents.

Adverse Effects. Delavirdine may cause headache, fatigue, allergic reaction, chills, edema, and joint pain. Administration of delavirdine may also cause abnormal coordination, amnesia, anxiety, confusion, and dizziness. Common adverse effects of delavirdine include nausea, vomiting, diarrhea, abdominal cramps, and anorexia.

Contraindications and Precautions. Delavirdine is contraindicated in patients with hypersensitivity to this agent, and during lactation. Delavirdine must be used cautiously in patients with impaired liver function, pregnancy (category C). Safety and efficacy in children younger than 16 years have not been established.

Drug Interactions. Antacids and H2-receptor antagonists decrease the absorption of delavirdine. Didanosine and delavirdine should be taken one hour apart to avoid decreased delavirdine levels.

Lamivudine

Lamivudine is one example of a nucleoside reverse transcriptase inhibitor (NRTI). This agent is used in combination with other medications to treat HIV infection in patients with AIDS. It is not a cure, and may not decrease the number of HIV-related illnesses. Lamivudine does not prevent the spread of HIV to other people. It is also used to treat hepatitis B infection. It is often used in combination with zidovudine.

Mechanism of Action. Lamivudine is in a class of medications called nucleoside reverse transcriptase inhibitors (NRTIs), which work by interfering with viral reproduction by preventing the creation of new viral RNA. It should never be used alone due to resistance, which can occur very rapidly.

Indications. Lamivudine is used to treat HIV infection in combination with zidovudine. It is also used in the treatment of chronic hepatitis B. The combination of these two drugs may stop the spread of both viruses.

Adverse Effects. The most serious adverse effects of lamivudine include rash, stomach pain, vomiting or upset stomach (in children), fever, muscle pain, and a numbness, tingling, or burning sensation in the fingers or toes.

Contraindications and Precautions. Lamivudine is contraindicated in patients with hypersensitivity to this agent. Lamivudine should be avoided during lactation. This drug is used with caution in patients with renal impairment, during pregnancy (category C), and in children.

Drug Interactions. The use of lamivudine with trimethoprim/sulfamethoxazole can increase the amount of lamivudine in the body. However, it is not necessary to change the dosages of either of these agents. Lamivudine increases the risk of lactic acidosis in combination with other reverse transcriptase inhibitors and antiretroviral agents.

Ritonavir

Ritonavir is an anti-HIV drug that is a protease inhibitor. It is used to treat HIV infection when therapy is warranted.

Mechanism of Action. By interfering with the formation of essential proteins and enzymes, ritonavir blocks the maturation of the HIV virus and causes the formation of nonfunctional, immature, noninfectious virions.

Indications. Ritonavir is used to treat HIV in adults and children, in combination with other antiretroviral agents. Because it inhibits the metabolism of other protease inhibitors, it is increasingly used for boosting and maintaining plasma concentrations of protease inhibitors.

Adverse Effects. One of the more serious effects of ritonavir is potentially fatal pancreatitis. Other serious adverse effects include body fat redistribution and accumulation, increased bleeding in patients with hemophilia type A and B, hyperglycemia, hyperlipidemia, new-onset diabetes mellitus, and the exacerbation of existing diabetes mellitus.

Contraindications and Precautions. Ritonavir is contraindicated in patients with hypersensitivity to this drug. Ritonavir should not be given in patients with antimicrobial resistance to protease inhibitors, or those suffering from pancreatitis. Safety and efficacy in children less than two years are not established.

Ritonavir is used with caution in pregnancy (category B), hepatic diseases, advanced HIV disease, diabetes mellitus, hyperlipidemia, and renal insufficiency.

Drug Interactions. When ritonavir is given in combination with other protease inhibitors, the dosage of the other protease inhibitors may be reduced. Drug interactions may occur when ritonavir is administered with a wide variety of other drugs, mostly due to pharmacokinetic interactions. Concomitant use of ritonavir with lovastatin or simvastatin is not recommended. Caution should also be taken when ritonavir is used with atorvastatin, cerivastatin, St. John's wort, sildenafil, astemizole, or cisapride.

Tenofovir

Tenofovir is one of the miscellaneous agents for treatment of HIV-AIDS. This agent is an antiviral drug that is approved for the treatment of HIV infection. It is able to reduce the amount of HIV in the blood and, when used in combination with other antiviral drugs, it can help prevent or reverse damage to the immune system and reduce the risk of AIDS-related illnesses. It is also an experimental treatment for hepatitis B.

Mechanism of Action. Tenofovir is a potent inhibitor of retroviruses, including HIV-1. It may be active against nucleoside-resistant HIV strains. The active form of tenofovir persists in HIV-infected cells for prolonged periods; thus, it results in sustained inhibition of HIV replication. It reduces the viral load and CD4 counts.

Indications. Tenofovir is used in combination with other antiretrovirals for the treatment of HIV.

Adverse Effects. Tenofovir may cause asthenia, anorexia, neutropenia, increased creatine kinase, AST, ALT, serum amylase, triglycerides, or serum glucose. Nausea, vomiting, diarrhea, flatulence, abdominal pain, and anorexia are common adverse effects of tenofovir.

Contraindications and Precautions. Tenofovir is contraindicated in patients with hypersensitivity to tenofovir, hepatitis, and lactic acidosis. Tenofovir should be avoided with concurrent administration of nephrotoxic agents, in patients with renal failure, and during lactation. Tenofovir must be used cautiously in patients with hepatic dysfunction, alcoholism, renal impairment, and obesity, during pregnancy (category B), and in children.

Drug Interactions. Tenofovir may increase didanosine toxicity. Use of this agent with acyclovir, amphotericin B, cidofovir, foscarnet, ganciclovir, probenecid, valacyclovir, or valganciclovir may increase tenofovir toxicity by decreasing its renal elimination.

FUNGI

Fungi are a distinct group of organisms that are neither plant nor animal. Fungi grow in single cells, as in yeast, or in colonies, as in molds. Fungi obtain food from living organisms or organic matter. Disease from fungi is found mainly in individuals who are immunologically impaired, but is also seen (less commonly) in other patients. Fungi can cause infections of the hair, skin, nails, and mucous membranes. Fungi infections include athlete's foot, histoplasmosis, cryptococcosis, *Candida* infections, and tinea.

Antifungal Drugs

Antifungal agents are used to treat systemic, local, and topical fungal infections. As fungi are single-celled or multicellular organisms that are more complex than bacteria, most antibacterial agents are ineffective against fungi. The human body is generally resistant to infection by fungi, but patients infected with HIV may frequently exhibit fungal infections, some of which may need intensive drug therapy. Fungal diseases are called **mycoses**.

Fungal infections may be classified into two groups: **superficial mycoses** (of the skin) and **systemic mycoses**, which affect internal organs such as the lungs, digestive organs, and brain. Antifungals are used to treat systemic, local fungal, and topical fungal infections. A table of antifungal drugs can be found in Table 23-3. A selective few agents will be discussed here in detail.

TABLE 23-3 Antifungal Agents

Generic Name	Trade Name	Route of Administration	Common Dosage Range
amphotericin B	Fungizone®, Amphocin®	IV	0.25–0.3 mg/kg/day
butoconazole nitrate	Femstat 3®, Gynazole 1®	Vaginal	One full applicator h.s.
caspofungin	Cancidas®	IV	70 mg on day one; then 50 mg q.d. thereafter
clotrimazole	Mycelex®, Lotrimin®	Topical, Vaginal	Topical: 10 mg b.i.d. prn; Vaginal: 5–100 mg in applicator h.s.
econazole nitrate	Spectazole®	Topical	15–85 g prn
fluconazole	Diflucan®	PO, IV	PO: 100–200 mg/day; IV: 200 mg for 14–21 (max: 400 mg q.i.d.)
griseofulvin	Grifulvin®, Fulvicin®	PO	500 mg–1 g/day
itraconazole	Sporanox®	PO	100–400 mg/day
ketoconazole	Nizoral®	PO , Topical	200–400 mg single dose/day
miconazole nitrate	Monistat®	Topical, Vaginal	Apply cream or insert suppository into vagina h.s.
nystatin	Mycostatin®	PO, Vaginal , Topical	PO: 500,000–1,000,000 units q.i.d.; Vaginal: 1–2 times/day for 2 weeks
terbinafine hydrochloride	Lamisil®	Topical	Apply thin layer to affected area
tioconazole	Vagistat-1®	Vaginal	5 mg (one applicator) once/day
tolnaftate	Tinactin®	Topical	2 oz prn

Amphotericin B

Amphotericin B is the most effective agent available for the treatment of most systemic fungal infections.

Mechanism of Action. Amphotericin B is fungistatic, antibiotic, and may be fungicidal at higher concentrations, depending on the sensitivity of the fungus. It has a wide spectrum of activity on most of the fungi pathogenic to humans. Amphotericin B acts by binding to fungal cell membranes, causing them to become permeable.

Key Concept

Topical administration of amphotericin B is also possible, and includes the application of creams, lotions, ointment, tinctures, sprays, and powders to the surface of skin and mucous membranes.

Indications. Amphotericin B is used intravenously for a wide spectrum of potentially fatal systemic fungal (mycotic) infections, including aspergillosis, blastomycosis, coccidiomycosis, cryptococcosis, disseminated candidiasis, and histoplasmosis. Treatment may continue for several months. Unlike antibiotics, resistance to amphotericin B is not common. Topical preparations are used to treat cutaneous and mucocutaneous infections caused by *Candida (monilia).*

Key Concept

Kidney damage is the most serious adverse effect of amphotericin B. Reduction of dosage or increasing time between dosages is essential. Serum creatinine levels and blood urea nitrogen levels are checked frequently during the course of therapy to monitor kidney function.

Adverse Effects. Amphotericin B can cause many serious adverse effects. Therefore, it should be administered in a hospital. Adverse effects include fever, chills, nausea, vomiting, headache, hypotension, muscle pain, dyspnea, and tachypnea. Nephrotoxicity, anaphylactoid reactions, phlebitis, and liver damage may occur. Amphotericin B for parenteral use should only be mixed in D5W and should be protected from light. Sometimes patients may be pre-medicated with diphenhydramine IV or acetaminophen prior to administration.

Contraindications and Precautions. Amphotericin B is contraindicated in patients with a known hypersensitivity and during lactation. This agent is used cautiously in patients with severe bone marrow depression or renal function impairment. Amphotericin B should be used during pregnancy (category B) only when there is a life-threatening situation.

Drug Interactions. When amphotericin B is given with corticosteroids, severe hypokalemia may occur, and the hypokalemia increases the risk of digitalis toxicity. Aminoglycosides, colistin, furosemide, and vancomycin may interact with amphotericin B and cause the possibility of nephrotoxicity.

Griseofulvin

Griseofulvin is a drug that is deposited in the skin, and bound to keratin. It is an antifungal, antibiotic, and anti-infective agent.

Mechanism of Action. Griseofulvin is fungistatic. It inhibits fungal cell activity. This agent is active against various strains of Microsporum, Trichophyton, and Epidermophyton. Griseofulvin has no effect on other fungi, including Candida, bacteria, and yeast.

Indications. Griseofulvin is effective in mycotic infections of the nails, hair, and skin. It is available only in oral form.

Adverse Effects. Griseofulvin may produce fatigue, headache, confusion, syncope, and lethargy. It also occasionally causes leukopenia and, in rare cases, serum sickness and hepatotoxicity. Heartburn, nausea, vomiting, diarrhea, flatulence, dry mouth, and unpleasant taste are common adverse effects of griseofulvin.

Contraindications and Precautions. Griseofulvin must be avoided in patients with known hypersensitivity and severe liver disease. Griseofulvin is used cautiously during pregnancy (category C) and lactation.

Drug Interactions. Griseofulvin may increase the metabolism of anticoagulants and decrease the effects of these agents. Barbiturates can reduce absorption of griseofulvin. A decrease in the effects of an oral contraceptive may occur with the administration of griseofulvin, causing breakthrough bleeding, amenorrhea, or pregnancy. Alcohol consumption can cause flushing and tachycardia when griseofulvin is used.

Nystatin

The chemical structure of nystatin is similar to amphotericin B, and is the common topical treatment for thrush, which can show up in the mouth or on the tongue, gums, or skin. It is not considered a systemic antifungal, but acts locally. It is available in tablets or a liquid suspension, as well as a cream, ointment, and topical powder; and therapy is usually continued for two weeks to be effective.

Mechanism of Action. Nystatin is fungicidal and fungistatic. It is effective against a variety of yeasts and fungi (Candida infections).

Indications. Nystatin is prescribed primarily as a local infection of skin and mucous membranes caused by Candida albicans (e.g. vulvovaginal, orpharyngeal, and intestinal candidiasis). It is also used for candidal diaper rashes. It is often used prophylactically on the diaper area when an oral Candida infection is present.

Adverse Effects. Nystatin can temporarily affect the sense of taste, and thus decrease appetite. Other adverse effects include nausea, vomiting, diarrhea, and stomach pain. If used to treat vaginal infections, the patient should avoid using sanitary napkins and refrain from sexual contact until the infection subsides.

Contraindications and Precautions. Vaginal tablets of nystatin are contraindicated during pregnancy (category C), and with vaginal infections caused by Trichomonas species. Nystatin should be used cautiously during lactation.

Drug Interactions. There are no listed drug interactions with Nystatin.

Itraconazole

Itraconazole is an antifungal indicated in the treatment of histoplasmosis, aspergillosis, and blastomycosis. Liver function should be monitored during treatment with itraconazole.

Mechanism of Action. Itraconazole is fungistatic, and may also be fungicidal depending on the concentration. Itraconazole interferes with the formation of ergosterol, the principal sterol in the fungal cell membrane that, when depleted, interrupts membrane functions.

Indications. Itraconazole is used in the treatment of systemic fungal infections caused by blastomycosis, histoplasmosis, and aspergillosis due to dermatophytes of the toenail with or without fingernail involvement, or mouth and throat candidiasis.

Adverse Effects. Itraconazole may cause heart failure. With high doses, hypertension may occur. Other adverse effects include headache, dizziness, fatigue, euphoria, drowsiness, gynecomastia, hypokalemia (low potassium level), hypertriglyceridemia, impotence, rash, pruritus, and adrenal insufficiency.

Contraindications and Precautions. Itraconazole is contraindicated in patients with a known hypersensitivity or renal failure, and during pregnancy (category C) and lactation.

Itraconazole should be used cautiously in patients with hypochlorhydria, hepatitis, and HIV. Itraconazole also must be used with great caution in patients with pulmonary, renal, and valvular heart diseases.

Drug Interactions. Itraconazole may increase levels and toxicity of oral hypoglycemic agents. Combination with oral midazolam, pimozide, levomethadyl, or quinidine may cause severe cardiac events including cardiac arrest or sudden death. Itraconazole levels are decreased by carbamazepine, phenytoin, phenobarbital, isoniazid, and rifampin.

> ***Key Concept***
>
> *Herbal supplements such as St. John's wort and garlic may affect itraconazole levels.*

Fluconazole

Fluconazole is an antifungal for both systemic and superficial mycoses.

Mechanism of Action. Fluconazole interferes with the formation of ergosterol, resulting in decreased cell wall integrity and leakage of essential cellular components. Fluconazole is fungistatic and it may also be fungicidal, depending on the concentration used.

> ***Key Concept***
>
> *In the use of fluconazole in elderly patients or those who have renal impairments, a creatinine clearance test should be provided before administration of the drug.*

Indications. Fluconazole has been shown to be effective against meningitis, as well as oropharyngeal and systemic candidiasis, both of which are commonly seen in AIDS patients. Fluconazole is also used for vaginal candidiasis.

Adverse Effects. The most common adverse effects of fluconazole include elevated liver enzymes, gastrointestinal complaints, headache, and skin rash.

Contraindications and Precautions. Fluconazole is contraindicated in patients with known hypersensitivity and during pregnancy (category C) and lactation. Fluconazole is used cautiously in patients with renal impairment. This agent may be given during pregnancy if the benefit of the drug outweighs any possible risk to the fetus.

Drug Interactions. Fluconazole administration may increase the effect of oral hypoglycemics and decreases the metabolism of phenytoin and warfarin.

Ketoconazole

Ketoconazole is an antifungal agent effective for the treatment of candidiasis, histoplasmosis, blastomycosis, and aspergillosis.

Mechanism of Action. Ketoconazole is fungistatic and may also be fungicidal depending on the concentration used. Ketoconazole interferes with the formation of ergosterol, the principal sterol in the fungal cell wall, interrupting membrane function.

Indications. Ketoconazole is used for severe systemic fungal infections, including candidiasis (e.g., oral thrush, candiduria), chronic mucocutaneous and pulmonary candidiasis. Topical forms are available for superficial mycoses.

Adverse Effects. Ketoconazole is usually well-tolerated. In some cases, nausea, vomiting, dizziness, headache, abdominal pain, and pruritus have been reported. Most adverse effects are mild and transient. In rare cases, fatal hepatic necrosis may occur. Periodic hepatic function tests should be used to monitor for hepatic toxicity.

Contraindications and Precautions. Ketoconazole is contraindicated in patients with known hypersensitivity to ketoconazole or to any component in its formulation, as well as chronic alcoholism. Safe administration of ketoconazole during pregnancy (category C) and lactation, or in children less than two years of age is not established.

Drug Interactions. Ketoconazole increases the anticoagulant effects of warfarin and causes hepatotoxicity when administered with alcohol. The absorption of ketoconazole is decreased when this agent is given with histamine antagonists and antacids.

PROTOZOA

Protozoa are single-celled parasitic organisms, many of which are motile. Most protozoa obtain their food from dead or decaying organic matter. Infection is spread through the ingestion of contaminated food or water, or through insect bites. Some protozoa are agents of disease, and some cause infections among the most serious known to humanity. Common

TABLE 23-4 Protozoa That Cause Major Diseases and Preferred Site of Infection

Protozoan Group	Genus	Preferred Site of Infection	Disease
Amoebae	Entamoeba	Intestine	Amebiasis
Sporozoa	Plasmodium	Bloodstream, liver	Malaria
	Toxoplasma	Intestine	Toxoplasmosis
Flagellates	Trypanosoma	Blood	Trypanosomiasis
	Trichomonas	Genital tract	Trichomoniasis
	Giardia	Intestine	Giardiasis

infections caused by protozoa include amebiasis, malaria, toxoplasmosis, trypanosomiasis, trichomoniasis, and giardiasis. Although many of these diseases are rare in the United States, travelers to Africa, South America, and Asia may acquire them overseas and return home with the infection. Table 23-4 shows the characteristics of each group.

Antiprotozoal Drugs

Antiprotozoal drugs fall into two main categories: **antimalarial agents** used to treat malaria infection; and **amebicides** and **trichomonacides**, which are prescribed to treat amebic and trichomonal infections.

Amebicides and Trichomonacides

These drugs are very important in the treatment of amebiasis, giardiasis, and trichomoniasis. These drugs include metronidazole, iodoquinol, and paromomycin (Table 23-5).

Metronidazole. Metronidazole is an antitrichomonal, amebicide, and antibiotic.

Mechanism of Action. Metronidazole is a synthetic compound with direct trichomonacidal and amebicidal activity as well as antibacterial activity against anaerobic bacteria and some Gram-negative bacteria.

Indications. Metronidazole is the drug of choice in amebic dysentery, giardiasis, and trichomoniasis. It is used in asymptomatic and symptomatic dysentery, which is a gastrointestinal disorder resulting from ulcerative inflammation of the colon caused chiefly by infection with Entamoeba histolytica. Entamoeba, Giardia, toxoplasma, and trypanosomia are commonly found in Africa, Asia, and Latin America. These infections are rare in the U.S. Trichomona Vaginalis is usually transmitted through sexual contact, which is frequently seen in the United States in females and males. Metronidazole is also used in an acute intestinal amebiasis and amebic liver abscess. This agent

TABLE 23-5 Drug Effects on Protozoal Infections

Generic Name	Trade Name	Route of Administration	Common Adult Dosage
Antiprotozoals (nonmalarial)			
metronidazole	Flagyl®	PO, IV	PO: 250–500 mg t.i.d.; IV: loading dose 15 mg/kg, maintenance dose 7.5 mg/kg q6 h
pentamidine isoethionate	Nebupent®	IM, IV	4 mg/kg daily × 14–21 days: infuse over 60 min
trimetrexate	Neutrexin®	IV	45 mg/m^2 daily
Antimalarials			
atovaquone	Mepron®	PO	750 mg b.i.d. × 21 days
chloroquine phosphate	Aralen®	PO	600 mg initial dose, then 300 mg weekly
hydroxychloroquine	Plaquenil®	PO	620 mg initial dose, then 310 mg weekly
mefloquine hydrochloride	Lariam®	PO	Prevention: begin with 250 mg once a week × 4 weeks, then 250 mg every other week; Treatment: 1250 mg as a single dose
primaquine phosphate	Primaquine®	PO	30 mg/day
pyrimethamine	Daraprim®	PO	25 mg once per week × 10 weeks
quinine	Quinamm®	PO	260–650 mg t.i.d. for 3 days
Amebicides			
doxycycline	Vibramycin®	PO	100 mg/day
iodoquinol	Yodoxin®	PO	650 mg t.i.d. × 20 days (max: 2 g/day)
paromomycin sulfate	Humatin®	PO	25–35 mg/kg divided in 3 doses for 5–10 days

Key Concept

Alcohol must be avoided while a patient is taking metronidazole to prevent profound vomiting.

commonly indicates for preoperative prophylaxis in colorectal surgery, elective hysterectomy, or vaginal repair. IV metronidazole is used for the treatment of serious infections caused by susceptible anaerobic bacteria in intra-abdominal infections, skin infections, and septicemia.

Adverse Effects. Metronidazole causes nausea, vomiting, diarrhea, metallic taste or bitter taste, and, occasionally, neurologic reactions. This agent may also cause polyuria, dysuria, pyuria, incontinence, cystitis, decreased libido, and vaginal dryness.

Contraindications and Precautions. Metronidazole is contraindicated in patients with known hypersensitivity, blood dyscrasias, and active CNS disease. Metronidazole cannot be used in the first trimester of pregnancy (category B), or during lactation. This drug should be cautiously used in patients with coexistent candidiasis, alcoholism, and liver disease, and during the second and third trimesters of pregnancy.

Drug Interactions. Alcohol may elicit disulfiram reaction, which consists of flushing, a throbbing headache, nausea, vomiting, arrhythmias, and many other unpleasant effects. Metronidazole interacts with many drugs, including oral solutions of citalopram ritonavir and IV formulations of sulfamethoxazole. Trimethoprim and nitroglycerin, if used with metronidazole, may elicit disulfiram reaction due to the alcohol content of the dosage form. Phenobarbital increases metronidazole metabolism.

Antimalarial Agents

Malaria is a severe generalized infection caused by the bite of an *anopheles* mosquito that is infected with *Plasmodium* protozoa. The most important human parasite among the sporozoa is *Plasmodium*, which causes malaria. There are four different types of *Plasmodium*: *P. falciparum*, *P. malariae*, *P. vivax*, and *P. ovale*. According to Integrated Regional Information Networks (www.irinnews.org), it has been estimated that more than 100 million people are infected, and about one million die annually of malaria in Africa alone. Antimalarial drugs are selectively active during different phases of the protozoan life cycle. Antimalarial drugs include chloroquine, primaquine, quinine, and hydroxychloroquine. Agents that are employed in the prevention of malaria include mefloquine, quinacrine, and folic acid antagonists. Mefloquine is chemically related to quinine. It is used both in the prevention of malaria and in the treatment of acute malarial infections. Quinacrine was once the most popular drug for malaria prophylaxis, but the use of quinacrine has declined sharply with the development of safer and more effective agents. Folic acid antagonists such as pyrimethamine and sulfa drugs interfere with the synthesis of folic acid. They may be used alone or in combination to suppress and prevent malaria caused by susceptible strains of *Plasmodium*.

Mechanism of Action. Chloroquine and hydroxychloroquine bind to and alter the properties of *Plasmodium*. The mechanism of action of primaquine and quinine is unknown.

Indications. Chloroquine is the drug of choice to suppress malaria symptoms and treat acute malaria attacks resulting from *P. falciparum* and

P. malariae infections. Chloroquine is the most useful antimalarial agent. Hydroxychloroquine is prescribed as an alternative to chloroquine in patients that cannot tolerate chloroquine or when chloroquine is unavailable. Primaquine is used to cure relapses of *P. vivax* and *P. ovale* malaria, to prevent malaria in exposed persons, and in the prevention and treatment of chloroquine-resistant strains of *P. falciparum*. Quinine is prescribed for acute malaria caused by chloroquine-resistant strains. Quinine is always given in combination with another antimalarial agent.

Key Concept

Chloroquine may cause irreversible retinal damage in patients who are on this drug for a long-term therapy.

Key Concept

If patients experience itching, rash, fever, difficulty breathing, or vision problems, they must stop taking quinine.

Adverse Effects. Chloroquine and hydroxychloroquine can concentrate in the liver and must be used carefully in patients with liver diseases. They may cause visual disturbances, headache, and skin rash.

Primaquine may cause anemia, granulocytopenia, nausea, vomiting, and abdominal cramps.

Quinine overdose or hypersensitivity reactions may be fatal. Toxicity of quinine produces visual and hearing disturbances, headache, fever, syncope, and cardiovascular collapse.

Contraindications and Precautions. Chloroquine is contraindicated with patients with hypersensitivity to this agent and renal disease, or who are suffering from psoriasis. Chloraquine should be avoided for long-term therapy in children and during pregnancy (category C) and lactation. Safe use in women of childbearing potential has not been established.

Chloroquine should be used with caution in patients with impaired hepatic function, alcoholism, and eczema, and in infants and children.

Primaquine is contraindicated in patients with rheumatoid arthritis and lupus erythematosus. Primaquine is also contraindicated in patients with recent or concomitant use of agents capable of bone marrow depression (e.g., quinacrine). This drug is not used during pregnancy (category C) or lactation.

Quinine is contraindicated in patients with myasthenia gravis, tinnitus, and optic neuritis, and during pregnancy (category X). This drug should be avoided during lactation. Quinine is used cautiously in patients with cardiac arrhythmias.

Drug Interactions. Antacids containing aluminum and magnesium decrease chloroquine absorption. Toxicity of both primaquine and quinacrine are increased. Quinine may increase digoxin levels. Anticonvulsants, barbiturates, and rifampin increase the metabolism of quinine.

Summary

Antiretroviral drugs are undergoing constant changes as new products are added to the market. It is an area of intense research interest, and new information is being discovered every day that will help patients with immune deficiency problems. Most antiviral drugs act by inhibiting viral DNA or RNA replication in the virus, causing viral death. These agents have limited use because they are effective against only a small number of specific viral infections.

Superficial mycotic (fungal) infections occur on the surface of, or just below, the skin or nails. Deep mycotic infections develop inside the body, such as the lungs. Treatment for deep mycotic infections is often difficult and prolonged. Antiprotozoal drugs include antimalarial, antiamebia, antitrichomoniasis, and others. Diseases caused by protozoa are rare in the U.S. They are seen commonly in Africa, Asia, and Latin America.

Exploring the Web

Look for additional information on HIV and AIDS and the treatments used to combat the diseases on the following sites:

- ***www.aegis.com***
- ***www.thebodypro.com***
- ***www.unicef.com***

Review Questions

Multiple Choice

1. Amantadine is prescribed for the prophylaxis and treatment of:

A. malaria
B. *Candida* infections
C. HIV
D. influenza A

2. Which of the following antimicrobial agents is similar to amphotericin B (in its chemical structure)?

A. ribavirin
B. streptomycin
C. amantadin
D. nystatin

3. Which of the following are parasitic, minute organisms that may invade normal cells, and cause disease?

A. fungi
B. protozoa
C. viruses
D. bacteria

4. Herpes simplex virus type 2 (HSV-2) causes which of the following conditions or diseases?

   A. cold sores
   B. AIDS
   C. fever blisters
   D. genital herpes

5. Ketoconazole is contraindicated in children less than how old?

   A. 2 years
   B. 6 years
   C. 12 years
   D. 18 years

6. All of the following parasitic organisms include the classification of protozoa, except:

   A. flagellates
   B. spriochetes
   C. sporozoa
   D. amoebae

7. IV metronidazole is used for the treatment of which of the following serious infections?

   A. susceptible anaerobic bacteria
   B. trichomoniasis
   C. giardiasis
   D. amebic dysentery

8. Which of the following is the reason to decline sharply the use of quinacrine in the treatment of malaria?

   A. less safe and less effective
   B. price is higher than others
   C. discontinuation of the products
   D. none of the above

9. Which of the following agents is indicated to treat cytomegalovirus?

   A. zidovudine
   B. abacavir
   C. ganciclovir
   D. nelfinavir

10. The trade names of enfuvirtide (miscellaneous drug for treatment of HIV-AIDS) include which of the following?

    A. Fuzeon
    B. Viread
    C. Hivid
    D. Norvir

11. Which of the following antiviral drugs may be indicated for treatment of Parkinson's disease?

    A. famciclovir
    B. ritonavir
    C. acyclovir
    D. amantadine

12. All of the following diseases may be caused by protozoa, except:
    A. giardiasis
    B. aspergillosis
    C. trichomoniasis
    D. malaria
13. HAART therapy in HIV-AIDS patients has been shown to reduce viral load, resulting in which of the following?
    A. increased CD4 lymphocytes
    B. decreased length of survival with AIDS
    C. decreased CD4 lymphocytes
    D. increased risk of mortality of AIDS patients
14. The first cases of AIDS were seen in which of the following years?
    A. 1969
    B. 1975
    C. 1981
    D. 1996

Matching

Generic Name	Trade Name
_____ 1. tioconazole	A. Fulvicin
_____ 2. fluconazole	B. Monistat
_____ 3. nystatin	C. Nizoral
_____ 4. ketoconazole	D. Sporanox
_____ 5. miconazole	E. Fungizone
_____ 6. griseofulvin	F. Diflucan
_____ 7. amphotericin B	G. Mycostatin
_____ 8. itraconazole	H. Vagistat

Critical Thinking

A young female client who was recently diagnosed with insulin-dependent diabetes has been given a prescription for metronidazole (Flagyl) for a vaginal infection.

1. What would be the most important recommendations by her physician regarding this vaginal infection?
2. What foods or beverages must be avoided with this medication?

SECTION IV

PHARMACOLOGY FOR SPECIFIC POPULATIONS

CHAPTER 24 Drug Therapy During Pregnancy and Lactation

OBJECTIVES

After completing this chapter, the reader should be able to:

1. Identify how normal physiologic changes with pregnancy alter the pharmacokinetics of drug therapy.
2. Define "teratogenic effect" and its relevance in managing drug therapy in pregnant patients.
3. Differentiate the classifications of drugs for use in pregnancy.
4. Describe why adverse effects of drug therapy may be overlooked in pregnant patients.
5. Identify how drug therapy in pregnant or breast-feeding patients may vary from drugs in other groups.
6. Discuss FDA pregnancy categories.
7. Identify potential drugs that cause problems during breast-feeding.
8. Explain pharmacodynamics of drugs during pregnancy.
9. Describe the common conditions affecting pregnant patients.
10. Define *preeclampsia* and *eclampsia*.

GLOSSARY

Affinity – the force that impels certain atoms to unite with certain others

Eclampsia – the occurrence of seizures (convulsions) in a pregnant woman, usually occurring after the twentieth week of pregnancy

Floppy infant syndrome – also called "infantile hypotonia", this is a condition of abnormally low muscle tone, often with reduced muscle strength

Hemodynamic – related to blood circulation or blood flow

Hyperemesis gravidarum – pernicious vomiting during pregnancy

Lipophilic – fat-soluble

Organogenesis – from implantation to about 60 days after, the time when major fetal organs form

Preeclampsia – the development of elevated blood pressure and protein in the urine after the twentieth week of pregnancy; it may also cause swelling of the face and hands

Teratogenic – causing developmental malformations

OUTLINE

Overview

> **Medical Terminology Review**
>
> **preeclampsia**
> *pre = before*
> *eclampsia = a serious complication of pregnancy involving convulsions*
> a condition that exists prior to a more serious condition of pregnancy

A developing fetus must always be carefully considered when drugs are administered to a pregnant woman. Each drug prescribed for a woman during pregnancy must be evaluated for its utmost effectiveness while weighing this against its potential adverse effects. Practitioners must always consider the dangers these drugs may present to the fetus. There are many conditions that occur which are secondary to pregnancy, including **preeclampsia** (high blood pressure, weight gain, and protein in the urine), **eclampsia** (a seizure disorder that may follow preeclampsia), or gestational diabetes. Sometimes, fetal conditions are treated by administering drugs to the mother, who passes them to the fetus through the placenta. An example of this is digoxin, used to treat fetal congestive heart failure or tachycardia.

Pharmacokinetics During Pregnancy

> **Medical Terminology Review**
>
> **pharmacokinetic**
> *pharmaco = related to drugs*
> *kinetic = putting into motion; activity*
> the movement of drugs within the body

During pregnancy, physiologic and anatomic changes occur that can alter drug pharmacokinetics. These changes involve the endocrine, cardiovascular, circulatory, gastrointestinal (GI), and renal systems.

Absorption

The function of the gastrointestinal tract may be greatly altered by hormonal action during pregnancy. Peristalsis and gastric emptying may be slowed to such a degree as to affect the amount of drug absorbed from the gut. Gastric acid secretion is also more erratic, which can affect the degree of absorption of acidic agents. However, because of individual differences in the effects of pregnancy, the observed effects on absorption can vary greatly, and are difficult to predict. Nevertheless, an awareness of the kinds of pharmacokinetic effects that can be expected during pregnancy is valuable, even if these effects don't occur every time.

Distribution

Because of **hemodynamic** changes (those that relate to the mechanics of blood circulation), many alterations occur in a pregnant woman's body. The heart rate increases by about 10 to 15 beats per minute. The blood volume increases by 40 percent. Plasma volume increases by 50 percent throughout pregnancy. These changes alter drug transportation and distribution. Other factors that determine distribution during pregnancy include plasma protein concentration and **affinity** for the drug, body fluid levels, drug solubility, body fat content, and the tissue blood flow. Therefore, distribution of drugs in pregnant women can be altered.

The fetus receives drugs from the mother's circulatory system, which passes them through the placenta. Drugs are affected by pregnancy hormones, which can result in a larger than normal amount of free drugs in circulation, which can cross the placental membrane easily. Fat-soluble drugs especially pass through the placenta's lipid membrane with ease.

> ***Medical Terminology Review***
>
> **hemodynamic**
> *hemo = blood*
> *dynamic = properties; actions*
> the actions of blood in the body

> ***Medical Terminology Review***
>
> **lipophilic**
> *lipo = fat*
> *philic = soluble*
> ability to dissolve in fatty substances

Drugs can be distributed in a mother's breast milk, usually in low concentrations. It is important to note that drugs with increased lipid solubility and low protein binding (such as CNS agents), may be present in high concentrations in breast milk. Since breast milk contains a high percentage of fats, **lipophilic** (fat-soluble) drugs pass easily through breast milk. Other drugs that easily diffuse in breast milk include those with lower molecular weights or organic bases.

Drug levels in breast milk are not the same as drug levels in the mother's blood. This is because of the influence of factors that was discussed above. Those with poor bioavailability don't usually achieve high concentrations in a neonate's circulation. Less than 2 percent of the mother's total dose of these drugs is usually ingested by a nursing infant.

Metabolism

Drug metabolism may be altered in patients with liver disease, hepatic blood flow, conditions that affect hepatic enzyme levels, or diet in general, but drug metabolism is not altered by breast-feeding or pregnancy.

Excretion

Changes in renal plasma flow (usually 40 to 50 percent), glomerular filtration rates, and tubular reabsorption cause changes in renal function during pregnancy. Increased renal plasma flow causes greater capillary pressure and increased glomerular filtration (by approximately 50 percent). Drug excretion rates are therefore increased during pregnancy.

Pharmacodynamics

> ***Medical Terminology Review***
>
> **pharmacodynamics**
> *pharmaco = related to drugs*
> *dynamic = properties; actions*
> the actions and properties of drugs

By the 32nd week of pregnancy, a woman's cardiac output has increased by 50 percent. Her arterial blood pressure increases, beginning in the second trimester. Because of these changes, a drug's pharmacodynamics must be carefully evaluated before administration. Therefore, the mechanism of action of any drug that is used in pregnant women has important clinical applications. Knowledge of therapeutic indexes, dose-response relationships, and drug receptor interactions will help pharmacy technicians provide cautious, safe, and effective treatment during pregnancy.

Pregnancy Drug Categories

Pregnancy drug categories were developed in 1980 by the Food and Drug Administration to help classify drugs by the risks they pose to a developing fetus. See Table 24-1 for a listing of these categories.

TABLE 24-1 Pregnancy Drug Categories

Category	Explanation
A	Controlled studies in pregnant women show no risk to the fetus
B	Animal studies fail to show fetal risk, but no controlled human studies were conducted; or animal studies show fetal risk that is not confirmed in human studies
C	Animal studies show fetal risk, but no controlled human studies were conducted; or there are no animal or human studies—these drugs are given if their benefit justifies their risks
D	Controlled human studies show fetal risk; the benefit of these drugs may be acceptable, despite risks, in life-threatening situations
X	Controlled human studies show fetal risk that outweighs any possible benefit; these drugs are contraindicated for use in pregnant or potentially pregnant women

Drug manufacturers are required to state these pregnancy categories in all printed drug reference materials and package inserts. There are many stated concerns about these categories and how accurate they are in describing the dangers of various drugs. Category C in particular is being revised because it contains drugs that have undergone no human studies, but animal studies have indicated fetal harm. Animal studies do not always accurately predict human responses to the studied drug. The FDA is working to clarify the categorization of drugs with more focus on their actual fetal risks.

Adverse Effects

There are two major considerations that need to be remembered when evaluating the adverse effects of drug therapy in pregnant women. They are as follows:

- Common side effects of pregnancy
- The adverse effect that maternal drug therapy can have upon the fetus

Many of the side effects of pregnancy can mask the adverse effects of drug therapy in pregnant patients. These signs and symptoms include:

- Light-headedness or hypotension
- Constipation
- Heartburn
- Nausea and vomiting
- Heart palpitations
- Fatigue
- Frequent urination

The dose and duration of drug therapy, the type of adverse effects that may occur, and the stage of pregnancy must all be considered in determining

TABLE 24-2 Common Non-teratogenic Drugs with Adverse Fetal Effects

Non-teratogenic Drug	Adverse Fetal Effects
Acetaminophen	Renal failure
Adrenocortical hormones	Adrenocortical suppression, electrolyte imbalance
Amphetamines	Withdrawal
Cocaine	Vascular disruption, withdrawal, intrauterine growth retardation
Meperidine	Neonatal depression
Phenobarbital (if excessively used)	Neonatal bleeding, death
Cigarette smoking	Premature births, intrauterine growth retardation
Thiazide diuretics	Thrombocytopenia, salt and water depletion, possible neonatal death

Key Concept

The timing of drug exposure is critical because of the vulnerability of the fetus during constant changes in development.

drug administration and potential fetal risks. Before a fertilized ovum is implanted in the uterus, certain drugs such as alcohol can produce a hostile environment capable of preventing implantation or causing a spontaneous abortion.

Key Concept

The effects of most approved drugs on a developing human fetus are unknown.

Some drugs that are not normally **teratogenic** (causing developmental malformations) can cause a situation wherein a neonate cannot correctly adapt to life outside the uterus (see Table 24-2). Benzodiazepines can cause **floppy infant syndrome**, while nonsteroidal anti-inflammatory drugs such as aspirin or indomethacin can cause premature closing of the neonate's ductus arteriosus.

Contraindications and Precautions

Some drugs are contraindicated for use during the first trimester of pregnancy. Caution is advised for using others because certain drugs may pass through the placenta to the fetus and cause teratogenic effects. Some others should not be used at all during pregnancy and lactation. As the above categories of drugs show, the prescribing or administration of medications during pregnancy must be done cautiously.

During the period of **organogenesis** (from implantation to about 60 days after, the time when major fetal organs form), teratogenic drugs may cause serious malformations, or even spontaneous abortion, to occur (see Table 24-3). Drug therapy should be delayed until after this time if possible. The embryonic phase is completed at about 60 days, when the fetal phase begins. Effects that may occur during this phase include:

- Damage to structures or organs that were normally formed during organogenesis
- Damage to systems currently undergoing tissue development

Medical Terminology Review

organogenesis
organo = related to organs
genesis = development
development of organs

TABLE 24-3 Common Teratogenic Drugs

Drug or Drug Class	Indications
Aminopterin, methylaminopter, busulfan, cyclophosphamide, thalidomide	Antineoplastic
Androgenic hormones, diethylstilbestrol	Hormone replacement
Coumarin	Anticoagulant
Etretinate	Psoriasis
Isotretinoin	Recalcitrant cystic acne
Lithium	Antimanic
Methimazole	Antithyroid
Penicillamine	Cystinuria and rheumatoid arthritis
Phenytoin, trimethadione, valproic acid	Anticonvulsant
Tetracycline	Antibiotic

- Retardation of growth
- Fetal death or stillbirth

Key Concept

The minimum therapeutic dose should be used for as short a time as possible during pregnancy. If possible, drug therapy should be delayed until after the first trimester of pregnancy.

Combinations of drug effects may occur, with growth retardation being the most common fetal effect. For example, coumarin derivatives that are used as anticoagulants can produce eye and brain defects due to hemorrhagic accidents in the developing fetus.

Lactation Drug Categories

The American Academy of Pediatrics published a report in 2001 that identified several categories of drugs that may cause problems during breast-feeding. These categories are listed below:

- Cytotoxic drugs that can interfere with a nursing infant's cellular metabolism
- Abused drugs with reported adverse effects on nursing infants
- Radioactive agents that require the stopping of breast-feeding
- Drugs that have unknown but possibly dangerous effects on nursing infants
- Drugs that have caused harm to some nursing infants and should be given to nursing mothers only with caution
- Maternal medications that are usually compatible with breast-feeding
- Food and environmental agents that affect nursing infants

It is recommended that all drugs of abuse be avoided by lactating women, regardless of documented effects on nursing infants. Women should not breast-feed while they are taking active radioactive agents. Drugs that have unknown neonatal effects include antianxiety drugs, antidepressants, and neuroleptics and must be used with caution. Nursing mothers should be informed that these drugs may be passed to their infant, and can affect the development of the central nervous system with long-term effects. Other drugs that may have adverse effects on neonates include anti-infectives, aspirin, phenobarbital, and sulfasalazine. While most drugs that are administered to nursing mothers are safe for use, with only minimal effects, many drugs are not part of large research studies and realistically need to be further tested in order to ensure safety.

Key Concept

Drugs may be excreted into breast milk, although the total amount received by the infant is a small percentage of the maternal dose.

Common Conditions Affecting the Pregnant Patient

Pregnant patients who have pre-existing conditions requiring drug therapy have special needs. Physicians must consider how drug therapy will affect the developing fetus. Also, any adverse effects caused by pregnancy must be identified so that drug therapy may be changed if needed. If the pregnancy causes health changes that require new drug therapy, adverse effects of these new drugs upon the fetus must also be considered.

During pregnancy, special attention should be given to cardiovascular problems that may develop. The cardiovascular system changes and experiences more stress during pregnancy, possibly requiring changes in drug selection or dosage. The use of over-the-counter drugs, which can pose additional risks to the fetus, must also be assessed.

Seizure Disorders

Seizure disorders are important to consider during pregnancy. A woman with a seizure disorder who is planning to become pregnant must first discuss her condition with her physician, and seriously consider how anticonvulsant drug therapy might affect her fetus. Anticonvulsant drug therapy may adversely affect a developing fetus. Physicians must carefully assess how pregnant women with seizure disorders should be treated to avoid possible teratogenic effects to the fetus. It is believed by many experts that seizures in a pregnant woman can cause fetal hypoxia, which leads to central nervous system damage. The anticonvulsants known as trimethadione and valproic acid should be avoided in pregnant women. However, only drugs of pregnancy category X are strictly contraindicated. The decision whether to maintain therapy with category D or even category C drugs must be made based on the ratio of risks to benefits.

Depression

Though little accurate information exists, the use of antidepressants by pregnant women must be carefully controlled. Drugs such as selective serotonin reuptake inhibitors (SSRIs) do not appear to cause increased risk for fetal complications. However, high doses of fluoxetine (Prozac) have been shown to cause low birth weight.

Diabetes

According to the Food and Drug Administration approximately 9 percent of all women in the U.S. have diabetes and about one-third of these women don't know they have the disorder. Also, gestational diabetes may develop in 2 to 5 percent of all pregnancies and resolves after birth. During pregnancy, production of hormones increases thus insulin demands also increase. This can cause insulin resistance in the pregnant patient. Insulin therapy may be required to prevent hyperglycemia, which can cause congenital anomalies that can harm the fetus. Insulin is preferred over oral hypoglycemic drugs because it does not cross the placenta. After the baby is delivered, insulin therapy is usually no longer required for women who have developed gestational diabetes, because their blood sugar levels return to normal.

Women with diabetes or who acquire diabetes during their pregnancies are at risk for having babies with higher birth weights resulting in an increase in cesarean sections. These women are also at an increased risk of developing toxemia.

Hyperemesis During Pregnancy

Key Concept

When using antiemetics, especially during the first trimester, the risk for adverse fetal effects must be considered.

Hyperemesis gravidarum (pernicious vomiting during pregnancy) may require antiemetic drug therapy. This currently consists of piperazines and phenothiazines. Of these classes of antiemetic drugs, piperazines are not known to be teratogenic, while the phenothiazines are generally considered safe in low, infrequent doses.

Preeclampsia

Preeclampsia is a hypertensive condition developing usually after the twentieth gestational week. It is characterized by hypertension, cerebral edema, and proteinuria. Preeclampsia may lead to eclampsia, and the primary goal of preeclampsia treatment is to prevent this condition from developing. Treatment is aimed at decreasing central nervous system irritability and reducing maternal blood pressure. The drugs of choice for preeclampsia are magnesium sulfate (to prevent convulsions) and hydralazine (to treat hypertension). Other medications used in the treatment of hypertension in preeclampsia include diazoxide, nifedipine, and labetalol (see Chapter 12).

Eclampsia

Eclampsia is a more serious condition in which the blood pressure is higher, and kidney dysfunction is indicated by proteinuria, weight gain, and generalized edema (of the face, hands, feet, and legs). In some patients, preeclampsia may progress to eclampsia, in which the blood pressure becomes extremely high, and generalized seizures (*grand mal*) or coma develops. Immediate hospitalization is required for adequate treatment of eclampsia.

Summary

Drug therapy may be required to manage preexisting or newly developed conditions in pregnant or lactating women. However, drug therapy can adversely affect the fetus or infant. Since physiologic changes related to pregnancy can alter drug absorption, distribution, and elimination, potential risks must always be considered before administering any drug. Also, potential fetal risks must be compared with maternal benefits when drug therapy is needed. Drugs may be excreted into breast milk in varying amounts. Limiting drug use during pregnancy and lactation decreases adverse effects to both the mother and infant.

Exploring the Web

Visit ***www.aafp.org***

- Search for and read the article "Medications in the Breastfeeding Mother."

Visit the following Web sites and search by "pregnancy"; read additional articles relevant to the discussion presented in this chapter.

- ***www.drugtopics.com***
- ***www.emedicine.com***
- ***www.fda.gov***
- ***www.perinatology.com***
- ***www.uspharmacist.com***

Review Questions

Multiple Choice

1. Which of the following is a result of pharmacokinetics of orally administered drugs that may be altered by progesterone during pregnancy?
   - **A.** increased opening of the center of the iris of each eye
   - **B.** decreased volume of the respiratory system to absorb more inhaled medications
   - **C.** decreased gastric tone and motility
   - **D.** increased the time it takes the urinary bladder to empty
2. Which of the following is a true statement?
   - **A.** Drug levels in breast milk are more than the drug levels in the mother's blood.
   - **B.** Drug levels in breast milk are not the same as the drug levels in the mother's blood.

C. Drugs with increased lipid solubility and low protein binding may be present in low concentrations in breast milk.
D. Fat-soluble drugs are not able to pass easily through breast milk.

3. By the eighth month of pregnancy, a female's cardiac output has:
   A. increased by 50 percent
   B. increased by 80 percent
   C. decreased by 50 percent
   D. decreased by 80 percent

4. Which of the following pregnancy drug categories are absolutely contraindicated for use in pregnant women?
   A. category B
   B. category C
   C. category D
   D. category X

5. Women should *not* breast-feed while they are taking:
   A. tetracycline
   B. aspirin
   C. acetaminophen
   D. radioactive agents

6. Which of the following drugs is non-teratogenic and may be used during pregnancy?
   A. cocaine
   B. coumarin
   C. meperidine
   D. thiazide diuretics

7. Methimazole is a teratogenic drug that is indicated for:
   A. congestive heart failure
   B. hypertension
   C. thyroid conditions
   D. diabetes mellitus

8. Which of the following conditions during pregnancy may be accompanied by convulsions?
   A. depression
   B. diabetes
   C. preeclampsia
   D. eclampsia

9. Seizures in pregnant women can cause fetal:
   A. hypertension
   B. hypoxia
   C. pernicious vomiting
   D. all of the above

10. Administration of high doses of fluoxetine (Prozac) during pregnancy may cause which of the following in newborns?
    A. low birth weight
    B. high birth weight

C. low blood sugar
D. high blood sugar

11. Which of the following drugs may be required to prevent hyperglycemia during pregnancy?

A. oral hypoglycemics
B. insulin
C. vitamin B_6
D. none of the above

12. Which of the following medications may be used for pernicious vomiting during pregnancy?

A. vitamin C
B. vitamin B_{12}
C. piperazine
D. minocycline

13. Drug excretion rates during pregnancy are:

A. increased
B. decreased
C. not changed
D. changed only in depressed women

14. Which of the following classes of drugs are safer during pregnancy in women with severe depression?

A. monoamine oxidase inhibitors
B. tricyclic antidepressants
C. selective serotonin reuptake inhibitors
D. A and B

15. Which of the following is an adverse fetal effect of acetaminophen during pregnancy?

A. renal failure
B. heart failure
C. liver failure
D. low birth weight

16. Common teratogenic drugs include which of the following?

A. methimazole
B. coumarin
C. tetracycline
D. all of the above

17. Lithium is classified as:

A. a hormone replacement
B. an antithyroid agent
C. an antimanic agent
D. an anticonvulsant

18. Which of the following antibiotics is contraindicated during pregnancy?

A. penicillin
B. erythromycin
C. tetracycline
D. none of the above

19. Which of the following is a consequence of cigarette smoking during pregnancy?

A. premature birth
B. intracranial pressure in the newborn
C. intrauterine growth retardation
D. A and C

20. Which of the following is an appropriate treatment in women with gestational diabetes after delivery?

A. insulin injections
B. oral hypoglycemic drugs
C. tranquilizers
D. observation only

Critical Thinking

A 37-year-old woman had a root canal procedure at her local dentist's office. The dentist ordered ibuprofen to be taken every four hours for pain. This woman also had a painkiller at home, so she did not get her dentist's prescription filled. Every four hours, she took this painkiller, which was Tylenol III. Unknowingly, she continued to breast-feed her 4-month-old baby while taking Tylenol III. After several sessions of breast-feeding, the baby went into deep sleep, could not be awoken, and was rushed to the emergency unit, where the baby died.

1. What was the likely cause of the baby's death?
2. What drugs are combined in Tylenol III?
3. If she had filled her dentist's prescription and used it as instructed, would there have been any danger to her baby?

Drug Therapy for Pediatric Patients

CHAPTER 25

OUTLINE

Defining the Neonatal and Pediatric Population

Unique Characteristics of Pediatric Medication Administration

- Pharmacokinetics
- Pharmacodynamics

Fever

Childhood Respiratory Diseases

- Apnea
- Respiratory Syncytial Virus (RSV)
- Asthma
- Respiratory Distress Syndrome (RDS)
- Croup
- Epiglottis
- Pneumonia

Common Childhood Illnesses

- Otitis Media

(continues)

OBJECTIVES

After completing this chapter, the reader should be able to:

1. Recognize common childhood respiratory diseases.
2. Identify treatment of asthma in children.
3. Describe otitis media in children.
4. Understand the factors affecting pharmacokinetics and pharmacodynamics in children.
5. Identify cardiovascular and blood disorders.
6. Define sickle cell anemia.
7. List five common examples of infectious diseases in pediatrics.
8. Explain acute bacterial meningitis.
9. Describe diabetes mellitus in pediatrics.
10. Explain international classification of seizures.

GLOSSARY

Apnea – the cessation of respiration for more than 20 seconds with or without cyanosis, hypotonia, or bradycardia

Asthma – a chronic, reversible, obstruction of the bronchial airways

Bacteremia – a condition in which bacteria are recovered from blood cultures of a patient and may or may not be associated with the disease

Congestive heart failure – a disorder in which the heart cannot pump the blood returning to the right side of the heart or provide adequate circulation to meet the needs of organs and tissues in the body

Croup – a viral infection that affects the larynx and the trachea

Epiglottitis – an acute bacterial infection of the epiglottis (an appendage which closes the glottis while food or drink is passing through the pharynx) and the surrounding areas that causes airway obstruction

Eustachian tubes – tubes within the ear by which fluids drain

OUTLINE (*continued*)

Gestational age – the time measured from the first day of the mother's last menstrual cycle to the current date

Insulin-dependent diabetes mellitus – a disorder caused by complete lack of insulin secretion by the pancreas

Iron deficiency anemia – anemia characterized by low serum iron, increased serum iron-binding capacity, decreased serum ferritin, and decreased marrow iron stores

Kernicterus – yellow staining and degenerative lesions in basal ganglia associated with high levels of unconjugated bilirubin in infants; also known as "bilirubin encephalopathy"

Neonatal period – the time from birth to approximately 28 days of age

Otitis media – an inflammation of the middle ear

Patent ductus arteriosus – a condition in which the normal channel between the pulmonary artery and the aorta fails to close at birth

Pediatric period – the period from birth to approximately age 18

Pneumonia – an inflammation or infection of the pulmonary parenchyma; caused by viruses, bacteria, mycoplasmas, and aspiration of foreign substances

pneumonitis – inflammation of the lungs

Respiratory distress syndrome (RDS) – the result of the absence, deficiency, or alteration of the components of pulmonary surfactant

Respiratory syncytial virus (RSV) – the major cause of bronchiolitis and pneumonia in infants under one year of age; caused by a virus and exhibits mild cold-like symptoms

Septicemia – bacteremia associated with active disease, whether localized or systemic

Sickle cell anemia – an inherited disorder characterized by the presence of abnormal hemoglobin; hemoglobin contains hemoglobin S (HbS)

OVERVIEW

Pediatric drug therapy is a special consideration in medicine. It is problematic even for practitioners with extensive experience. To put it simply, a child's age, weight, development, and lack of information about the clinical pharmacology of specific agents for pediatric patients can all complicate drug therapy. A drug undergoes the same processes in a child as it does in an adult, but a child's body is distinctive and constantly changing, which affects how it responds to a drug. During the past few decades, drug administration, usage, and research in pediatric patients have been challenging. Children are not merely miniature adults. Therefore, knowledge about pediatric medications cannot simply be extrapolated from the adult research, literature, and clinical trials. In fact, if a label does not contain a pediatric dose, do not assume that the drug is safe for anyone less than 12 years of age. The pharmacy technician should be sure that a drug is safe for children by asking the doctor or pharmacist. Effective and safe drug therapy in newborns, infants, and children requires an understanding of maturational changes that affect drug action, metabolism, and disposition.

TABLE 25-1 Stages of Childhood Growth and Development

Age	Description
Newborn	Birth to one month
Infancy	One month to one year
Toddlerhood	One to three years
Preschool age	Three to six years
School age	Six to 12 years
Adolescence	12 to 18 years

Pediatric drug dosage must be adjusted for the characteristics of individual drugs, and for the patient's age, disease states, sex, and individual needs to prevent ineffective treatment or toxicity.

Defining the Neonatal and Pediatric Population

The **neonatal period** generally covers the time from birth to approximately 28 days of age. This general category also includes premature infants of varying gestational ages. **Gestational age** (the time measured from the first day of the mother's last menstrual cycle to the current date) will factor in dosing for various medications and may even preclude the use of some. The **pediatric period** covers a wide range of ages, from birth to approximately age 18 (see Table 25-1).

Unique Characteristics in Pediatric Medication Administration

A child's body surface area, metabolism, development, and tolerance are quite different from those of an adult. For many drugs, safe and effective use in children requires additional pharmacokinetic and pharmacodynamic data. According to the American Academy of Pediatrics, 20 percent of all medications marketed today do not have U.S. Food and Drug Administration (FDA) approved labeling for use in neonates, infants, children, and adolescents, and only 5 of the 80 drugs most often used in newborns and infants are labeled for pediatric use. The FDA has recently made regulatory changes to facilitate labeling of drugs for pediatric use.

To complicate matters even more, most drugs are not tested on children. In many instances, no one knows for sure if a given drug is safe or effective in children, or what dosage is appropriate. Only about 30 percent of FDA-approved drugs have been approved for specific pediatric indications,

Key Concept

Children younger than two years should not be given any OTC drug without a doctor's approval.

Children will respond differently to some drugs than adults. For example, certain barbiturates which make adults feel sluggish will make a child hyperactive. Amphetamines, which stimulate adults, can calm children.

and few approved drugs come in child-appropriate dosage forms, which means that health care professionals must formulate pediatric doses.

It is essential that pharmacy technicians be familiar with most common diseases and conditions of neonatal and young children, the principles of pharmacology, and the required drug therapy. The technician should also consider the four processes involved in pharmacokinetics: absorption, distribution, metabolism, and excretion.

Pharmacokinetics

Pharmacokinetics focuses on how drugs move throughout the body. This includes the processes of absorption, distribution, biotransformation, and excretion. Pharmacokinetics deals with how drugs enter the body, reach their site of action (in what concentration), and how the body eliminates them. The body's effects on drugs, or how the body handles drugs, can be described as pharmacokinetics.

Neonates, infants, and children have different pharmacokinetic processes than adults. It is important to understand the developmental differences of children in order to understand how drugs are concentrated at the site of action, how intense their effects will be, and how long their action will last.

Absorption

Absorption involves the movement of drugs from their site of administration into the bloodstream. Two factors that influence oral drug absorption are gastric emptying time and pH. In neonates and infants, gastric emptying time is slower than in adults, reaching adult values at around six months of age. Delayed gastric emptying delays drug absorption of drugs designed to be absorbed from the intestine. More complete absorption may occur for drugs that are absorbed mostly from the stomach.

In newborns, gastric pH is more alkaline, becoming more acidic at around two to three years of age. Acidic drugs are better absorbed from an acidic environment while basic (alkaline) drugs are better absorbed from an alkaline environment. During infancy, basic drugs are more easily absorbed from the stomach, while acidic drugs are less well-absorbed. This is different in comparison to older children and adults.

Topical medications are absorbed more rapidly by infants and children. This is because they have a greater ratio of body surface area (BSA) to weight. Also, their skin is thinner, and thus more permeable.

Distribution

The movement or transport of drugs throughout the body is known as distribution. In this process, drugs are made available to body tissues and fluids. Body composition, fluid distribution, blood flow to the tissues, special membrane barriers, and protein binding all influence drug distribution in the body.

Neonates, infants, and young children have more body water than adults. Premature neonates have 85 percent body water, neonates have 70 to 75 percent, and adults have only 50 to 60 percent body water. Body fat percentage is different, based on age and gender, and even differs between individual children. A neonate's body is comprised of 15 to 16 percent fat. Premature infants may have as little as 1 percent fat. Body fat percentage peaks at about nine months of age, decreasing (between one and five years) to between 8 and 12 percent, increasing again around adolescence. Girls have a higher percentage of body fat than boys.

Key Concept

Sulfonamide antimicrobials compete with serum bilirubin for binding to albumin. Drugs given to a neonate with jaundice can displace bilirubin from albumin. Because of the greater permeability of the neonatal blood-brain barrier, substantial amounts of bilirubin may enter the brain and cause **kernicterus** *(yellow staining and degenerative lesions in basal ganglia associated with high levels of unconjugated bilirubin in infants; also known as "bilirubin encephalopathy").*

Lipid-soluble drugs can be stored in body fat, and have a high affinity for adipose (fat) tissue. As a result, lower levels of drug may be left available in circulation and at the site of action. People with higher percentages of body fat need a higher mg/kg dose of lipid-soluble drugs than people who have a lower percentage of body fat.

Children under two years of age have an immature blood-brain barrier that allows a relatively easy access to their central nervous systems. Therefore, they are more sensitive to drugs that affect the brain, with increased risk of CNS toxicity. To protect young children from undesired drug effects, lower doses of certain drugs may be required.

Metabolism

Metabolism (biotransformation) involves the alteration or transformation of chemicals from their original form, aiding in the eventual excretion of the substance via the renal system. Most biotransformation of drugs happens in the liver. In infants and neonates, liver immaturity influences drug-metabolizing capacity. Hepatic enzyme activity is not mature until 1 to 2 years of age. At this stage of life, drugs metabolized by the liver have a longer half-life and there is more chance for toxicity. A drug's half-life is the time needed for 50 percent of a drug's administered dose to be eliminated.

As a result, reduction of some drug dosages and less frequent drug administration may be required. Young children have higher metabolic rates and metabolize drugs more rapidly. Between 2 and 6 years of age, this condition is more pronounced. Higher doses or more frequent administration is required, and this condition can continue until 10 to 12 years of age.

Excretion

The process involving the removal of drugs, active metabolites, and inactive metabolites from the body is known as excretion. Most drugs are excreted via the kidneys. Renal function increases rapidly during infancy, reaching adult levels by 6 to 12 months of age. During infancy, reduced renal excretion causes longer drug half-lives and the increased possibility of toxicity to drugs primarily excreted through the renal system. Especially during the neonatal period, reduced dosages are required. By three years of

Key Concept

The kidneys of infants less than 6 months of age are not very well developed. They should not be given water to drink because it will remove sodium ions and cause an increase in potassium ions in their blood. Breast milk and formula supply all of their needed fluids.

age, drugs are eliminated more rapidly because the glomerular filtration rate surpasses the adult rate. In toddlers, a drug's half-life may be shorter than in older children and adults.

Pharmacodynamics

The way drugs affect the body and how they accomplish this can be explained as pharmacodynamics. This can be further described as the biochemical and physical effects of drugs (drug effects and the responses resulting from drug action) and their mechanisms of drug action. Most drugs are believed to act at the cellular level. They do this by attaching to cell receptors where they block or mimic the action of endogenous molecules that regulate cell action.

A drug's mechanism of action is the same in all individuals. However, drug effects may be different in infants and children than in adults. This is because of immaturity of target organs and the sensitivity of receptors. As a result, an infant or child may need either a lower or higher dose of a drug than may be expected, and usually has a heightened sensitivity to drugs.

FEVER

Fever is a common reason why parents seek medical attention for their children, and approximately 30 percent of visits to pediatricians are fever-related. Parents believe that fever is a disease rather than a symptom. Fever is part of the febrile response, which includes the activation of numerous physiologic, endocrinologic, and immunologic systems. Microbes, toxins, or products of microbial origin, antigen-antibody complexes, complement (a group of proteins in the blood that assist the function of antibodies in the immune system) and other chemical agents are pyrogens that cause fever.

This evidence indicates that fever is an important defense mechanism and that treating the fever may have detrimental effects. In varicella, for example, acetaminophen prolongs the time of crusting of skin lesions. Nevertheless, many clinicians and caregivers believe that fever is harmful. A small percentage of children younger than five years may develop a seizure when they have a fever.

Acetaminophen is one of the most widely used antipyretics. Like aspirin and other nonsteroidal anti-inflammatory drugs (NSAIDs), acetaminophen blocks the conversion of arachidonic acid to prostaglandin. Current evidence still suggests that acetaminophen is the drug of choice for antipyresis in children.

Ibuprofen (Motrin) is another option as an antipyretic. This agent has been shown to provide a greater temperature decrement in febrile children and a longer duration of antipyresis than noted with acetaminophen when the two drugs were administered in equal doses (10 mg/kg). Physical methods to reduce temperature are ineffective if shivering is not prevented, and such methods do not alter the hypothalamic set point.

Childhood Respiratory Diseases

The patterns of respiratory tract diseases in childhood are modified by age, sex, race, season, geography, and environmental and socioeconomic conditions. Immediately after birth, tuberculosis can be transmitted to the newborn, presenting after several weeks of life as a severe **pneumonitis**. Lung immaturity and other events related to the perinatal period predispose to hyaline membrane disease. The incidence of respiratory tract infections also peaks during the first 2 to 3 school years. Respiratory diseases affect many children each year. Respiratory syncytial virus (RSV) and asthma are two specific problems quite often treated in the pediatric/neonatal patient population. Apnea is seen in the neonatal age group, especially in premature infants.

> ***Medical Terminology Review***
>
> *pneumonitis*
> *pneumo(n) = breathing; the lungs*
> *itis = inflammation; condition*
> inflammation of the lungs impairing breathing

> ***Medical Terminology Review***
>
> **cyanosis**
> *cyan/o = blue*
> *-osis = condition of*
> condition characterized by blue coloring of skin and membranes
>
> **hypotonia**
> *hypo- = decreasing, below*
> *-tonia = tone, tension*
> decreased tone or tension in muscles

Apnea

Apnea is the cessation of respiration for more than 20 seconds with or without cyanosis, hypotonia, or bradycardia. Apnea may be a symptom of another disorder that resolves upon treatment of the disorder. These disorders may include infection, gastroesophageal reflux, hypoglycemia, metabolic disorders, drug toxicity, hydrocephalus, or thermal instability in newborns. Immaturity of the central nervous system often accounts for apnea of the newborn, which occurs most commonly during active sleep.

Treatment for Apnea

The airway should be opened and cardio-respiratory resuscitation should be initiated when a child presents with apnea. The treatment of central apnea that is most commonly used for premature infants includes minimizing potential causes such as temperature variances and feeding intolerance. The use of xanthine medications such as caffeine and theophylline (see Chapter 14) provide CNS stimulation. Pulmonary function support may include the use of supplemental oxygen and continuous positive airway pressure at low pressures.

Respiratory Syncytial Virus (RSV)

Respiratory syncytial virus (RSV) is the major cause of bronchiolitis and pneumonia in infants younger than one year. It is the most important respiratory tract pathogen of early childhood. It causes mild cold-like symptoms in infants and most children. However, RSV can cause a more serious respiratory disease in premature infants that sometimes requires hospitalization. The at-risk group includes infants born at less than 36 weeks' gestation or those with chronic lung disease. The respiratory disease occurs because of the immaturity of the infants' lungs and because these infants have not received sufficient antiviral substances from their mothers. In most parts of the U.S., RSV infection occurs seasonally, generally from fall through spring (October through March). At-risk infants are now treated before discharge from the hospital to provide some immunoprophylaxis.

Treatments for Respiratory Syncytial Virus

Palivizumab (Synagis) is used for immunoprophylaxis against severe lower respiratory tract RSV infections. In infants with uncomplicated bronchiolitis, treatment is symptomatic. Humidified oxygen is usually indicated for hospitalized infants because most have hypoxia. Fluids should be carefully administered. Often, intravenous or tube feeding is helpful when sucking is difficult. Bronchodilators should not be routinely used. However, a course of epinephrine should be used in children with wheezing who are older than one year, and bronchodilators should be administered if found to be beneficial. The use of corticosteroids is not indicated except as a last resort in patients whose condition is critical. Sedatives are rarely necessary. The antiviral drug ribavirin, delivered by small-particle aerosol and breathed along with the required concentration of oxygen for 20 to 24 hours per day for 3 to 5 days, has a beneficial effect on the course of pneumonia caused by RSV.

Asthma

Asthma is a leading cause of chronic illness in childhood, and is responsible for a significant proportion of school days missed because of chronic illness. Asthma is a chronic, reversible obstruction of the bronchial airways. The airways become over-reactive because of this inflammation and increased mucus secretion; mucosal swelling and muscle contraction then occur. This leads to airway obstruction, chest tightness, coughing, wheezing, and, if asthma is severe, shortness of breath and low blood oxygen levels. Most children experience their first symptoms by 4 to 5 years of age. Allergies, viral respiratory infections, and airborne irritants produce the inflammation that can lead to asthma. Childhood asthma is a disease with a strong allergic component and a genetic predisposition. Approximately 75 to 80 percent of children with asthma have allergies.

Treatment for Asthma

Treatment for asthma generally involves two types of medications: quick-relief medications (also called bronchodilators), and controller medications. Controller medications get their name because they help control inflammation to make breathing easier. These medications must be taken daily to be effective. Medications in the bronchodilators and controller group are listed in Table 25-2.

TABLE 25-2 Bronchodilators and Controller Groups for Asthma

Generic Name	Trade Name	Route of Administration
Bronchodilators		
albuterol	Ventolin®, Proventil®	PO, Nasal
bitolterol mesylate	Tornalate®	Nasal
epinephrine	Adrenalin®, Primatene Mist®	SC, IM, IV, Nasal
isoproterenol hydrochloride	Isuprel®	IV
metaproterenol sulfate	Alupent®, Metaprel®	PO, Nasal
pirbuterol acetate	Maxair®	Nasal
salmeterol xinafoate	Serevent®	Nasal
terbutaline sulfate	Brethaire®	Nasal, SC
Xanthine Derivatives		
aminophylline	Truphylline®	PO, IV
theophylline	Elixophyllin®	PO, IV
Leukotriene Inhibitors		
montelukast	Singulair®	PO
zafirlukast	Accolate®	PO
Corticosteroids		
dexamethasone	Decadron®	PO, IM, IV
hydrocortisone sodium	Solu-Cortef®	PO
prednisolone	Prelone®	PO
beclomethasone sodium phosphate	Beconase AQ®	Intranasal
budesonide	Rhinocort®	Nasal
fluticasone	Flovent®	Nasal, Intranasal
Mast Cell Stabilizers		
cromolyn sodium	Intal®	Nasal
nedocromil sodium	Tilade®, Alocril®	Nasal

IM, intramuscular; IV, intravenous; SC, subcutaneous

Respiratory Distress Syndrome

Respiratory distress syndrome (RDS), or hyaline membrane disease, is the result of the absence, deficiency, or alteration of the components of pulmonary surfactant. Surfactant, a lipoprotein complex, is an ingredient of the film-like surface of each alveolus that prevents alveolar collapse. When the amount of surfactant is inadequate, alveolar collapse and hypoxia result.

> **Medical Terminology Review**
>
> **lipoprotein**
> *lipo = fats; triglycerides*
> *protein = amino acid complex*
> amino acid complex with fatty substance

The younger the infants are, the greater the incidence of RDS. However, the occurrence of RDS appears to be more dependent on lung maturity than actual gestational age. The severity of RDS is decreased in infants whose mothers received corticosteroids 24 to 48 hours before delivery. Corticosteroids are most effective when newborns are less than 34 weeks' gestational age, and they are administered for at least 24 hours, but no longer than seven days before delivery.

Treatment for Respiratory Distress Syndrome

Infants at risk for RDS, as well as infants with respiratory failure due to meconium aspiration syndrome, persistent pulmonary hypertension, or pneumonia, are treated with natural, animal-derived, or synthetic surfactant. Continuous positive airway pressure, via nasal prongs, is required to prevent volume loss during expiration or mechanical ventilation via endotracheal tube for severe hypoxemia and/or hypercapnia. Aerosol administration of bronchodilators is also prescribed.

Croup

Croup, or acute laryngo-tracheobronchitis, is a viral infection that affects the larynx and the trachea, resulting in subglottic edema with upper respiratory tract obstruction accompanied by thick secretions. Children are susceptible to airway obstruction because the diameter of the subglottic area is narrow. Croup is caused by any virus associated with upper respiratory tract infection. Spasmodic croup is a sudden attack of croup, which usually occurs during the night, and can be associated with an upper respiratory tract infection, fever, or allergies. The incidence of croup is higher in the late fall and early winter. The age range of occurrence is 6 months to 6 years. The peak age of onset is 2 years.

Treatment for Croup

When a child with suspected croup is seen at the hospital, supplemental humidified oxygen is given as indicated by the child's appearance, result of pulse oximetry, and vital signs. The child can be treated with bronchodilators, usually administered with epinephrine if humidification alone is ineffective. The use of corticosteroids is controversial. Children who receive corticosteroids need endotracheal intubation less often, and their stridor is more quickly resolved. Antibiotics are administered if secondary bacterial infection is suspected.

Epiglottitis

Epiglottitis is an acute bacterial infection of the epiglottis (an appendage that closes the glottis while food or drink is passing through the pharynx) and the surrounding areas that causes airway obstruction. The infection is caused by *Haemophilus influenzae* type B or, on rare occasions, streptococci

> **Medical Terminology Review**
>
> **epiglottitis**
> *epi = above*
> *glott = the tongue*
> *itis = inflammation; condition*
> inflammation of the tissue above the tongue in the airway

and pneumococci. The use of *H. influenzae* type B vaccine in infants has resulted in a dramatic reduction in the incidence of epiglottitis. Onset is sudden and infection progresses rapidly, causing acute respiratory difficulty. This condition requires emergency airway stabilization and medical measures because a fatal outcome can occur. Boys between ages 2 to 7 are most often affected. The incidence of epiglottitis is highest in the winter.

Treatment for Epiglottitis

Visual examination of the throat is contraindicated until a tracheostomy is performed. The child is observed in the intensive care area until swelling of the epiglottis decreases (usually by the third day). Antibiotics are given for a total of 7 to 10 days.

Pneumonia

Pneumonia is an inflammation or infection of the pulmonary parenchyma. Pneumonia is caused by viruses, bacteria, *Mycoplasma* organisms, and aspiration of foreign substances. Viral pneumonia occurs more often than bacterial pneumonia.

Treatment for Pneumonia

Medical treatment is primarily supportive and includes improving oxygenation with oxygen and respiratory treatments. Antibiotics are used to treat bacterial pneumonia based on culture and sensitivity testing. Hospitalization depends on the severity of illness, the child's age, and the suspected organism.

Common Childhood Illnesses

It is impossible to discuss all pediatric disorders and illnesses in one chapter. Therefore, some selective examples of the most common childhood illnesses will be discussed.

Otitis Media

Otitis media is an inflammation of the middle ear. Children six years of age and younger are at particular risk for otitis media because their **eustachian tubes** are shorter and more horizontal. Otitis media is the most commonly encountered diagnosis in office visits for children younger than 15 years of age in the United States. Otitis media occurs most often in children between 3 months and 3 years with peak incidences occurring between 5 to 24 months and 4 to 6 years. Boys have more ear infections than girls. Tympanic membrane rupture with discharge and short-term conductive hearing loss are common complications of otitis media.

Treatment for Otitis Media

The efficacy of steroid therapy, decongestants, and antihistamines for the resolution of otitis media has not been proven. Their use should not be encouraged. Surgical removal of tonsils or adenoids is not recommended for the treatment of otitis media with effusion in the absence of specific tonsil or adenoid pathological conditions. The first-line antibiotic medication most often prescribed is amoxicillin or ampicillin. The second-line medication regimen (to be used when an amoxicillin-resistant organism is suspected) includes amoxicillin with clavulanate, cefaclor, cotrimoxazole, erythromycin, or sulfisoxazole. In the penicillin-allergic child, erythromycin with a sulfonamide or trimethoprim-sulfamethoxazole may be used. Generic names, trades names, and routes of administration were discussed in Chapter 22. Myringotomy is the surgical procedure of inserting pressure-equalizing tubes into the tympanic membrane. This allows ventilation of the middle ear, relieves the negative pressure, and permits drainage of fluid. The tubes usually fall out after 6 to 12 months.

Diabetes Mellitus

Insulin-dependent diabetes mellitus (IDDM), or Type I (juvenile-onset) diabetes, is caused by complete lack of insulin secretion by the pancreas. Insulin is necessary for many physiological functions of the body. Insulin deficiency results in unrestricted glucose production without appropriate use, resulting in hyperglycemia and increased production of ketones in the blood. Age ranges of peak incidence are 5 to 7 years and puberty. Among children 5 to 10 years of age, the disease is more commonly diagnosed in girls. Type I diabetes usually starts with polyphagia, weight loss, polydipsia, and polyuria. Long-term effects of IDDM include failure to grow at a normal rate, neuropathy (the impairment of sensory and motor nerve functions), recurrent infection, renal microvascular disease, and ischemic heart disease.

Medical Terminology Review

polyphagia
poly = *much*
phagia = *to eat*
excessive eating

polydipsia
poly = *much*
dipsia = *thirst*
excessive thirst

polyuria
poly = *much*
uria = *urine*
excessive urine

Treatment for Insulin-dependent Diabetes Mellitus (IDDM)

As soon as hyperglycemia or glucosuria is detected, immediate medical attention is needed because of the potential for rapid deterioration of the patient's condition. The initial therapy will depend on how early the diagnosis is made, and on the state of the child. Medical management includes the regulation of serum glucose, fluid, and electrolyte levels. Once glucose levels are stabilized, the child's insulin dose is typically dictated by a sliding scale based on the serum glucose level. Regulation of nutrition and exercise is also a key factor in managing diabetes. For older children, or children who are in the midst of the adolescent growth spurt, a regimen of twice-daily injections of a mixture of preferably NPH and regular insulin before breakfast and before supper may be started immediately. Table 25-3 shows types and action of insulins (see Chapter 16).

TABLE 25-3 Types and Action of Insulin

Type and Action	Action (in hours)	
	Peak	Duration
Fast		
Regular	2–4	5–7
Semilente	2–8	8–16
Intermediate		
NPH	8–12	18–24
Lente	8–12	18–28
Slow		
Ultralente	16–18	20–36
Protamine zinc	16–20	24–36

Treatment of Diabetes in Infants

Symptomatic hyperglycemia can occur in newborn infants. These babies usually suffer from severe intrauterine malnutrition and, therefore, are small for their gestational age. They are hypoinsulinemic and their pancreas fails to release insulin in response to any of the standard body demands. They must be treated with divided doses of exogenous insulin of up to 1–2 units/kg/24 h. Insulin requirements are best established by starting a continuous intravenous insulin infusion at rates to provide at least 0.5 units/kg/24 h. Insulin treatment is simplified by using diluted insulin so that inadvertent overdoses do not occur. In most cases, pancreas function develops sometime between the age of 6 and 12 weeks. The children do well after the newborn period and do not appear to be at increased risk of developing Type I diabetes at a later age. See Chapter 16 for more information on the endocrine system, hormones, and related subjects.

Seizure Disorders

Seizure is a sudden, transient alteration in brain function as a result of abnormal neuronal activity and excessive cerebral electric discharge. The causes of seizure include perinatal factors, infectious disease (encephalitis and meningitis), febrile illness, metabolic disorders, trauma, neoplasms, toxins, circulatory disturbances, and degenerative diseases of the nervous system. Epilepsy is a disorder characterized by recurrent, unprovoked seizures, in which seizures are of primary cerebral origin, indicating underlying brain dysfunction. Epilepsy is not a disease in itself.

Medical Terminology Review

encephalitis
encephal = brain
itis = inflammation
inflammation of the brain

Treatment for Epilepsy

Antiepileptic drug therapy is the mainstay of medical management. Single-drug therapy is the most desirable, with the goal of establishing a balance between seizure control and adverse side effects. The drug of choice is based on seizure type, epileptic syndrome, and patient variables. Drug combinations may be needed to achieve seizure control. Complete control is achieved in only 50 to 75 percent of children with epilepsy. The most commonly used anticonvulsants were discussed in Chapter 8.

Cardiovascular and Blood Disorders

Medications to support cardiovascular functions in the pediatric/neonatal patient population differ little from those used with adults. Digoxin, diuretics, and, occasionally, antihypertensives are utilized. Their indications and dosage generally are the same in all groups. Discussion in this section will focus on a topic unique to the neonatal population, (patent ductus arteriosus), and the use of inotropic agents to support blood pressure. The pharmacy technician may need to recognize the medications used and prepare them for proper use.

Patent Ductus Arteriosus

During fetal life, most of the pulmonary arterial blood is shunted through the ductus arteriosus into the aorta. Functional closure of the ductus normally occurs soon after birth, but if the ductus remains patent when pulmonary vascular resistance falls, aortic blood is shunted into the pulmonary artery. **Patent ductus arteriosus** (PDA) is one of the most common congenital cardiovascular anomalies associated with maternal rubella (German measles) during early pregnancy. The entire phenomenon of transition is not completely understood, and the transition period of infants is a particularly important time. In uncomplicated PDA, the ductus closes spontaneously within the first weeks or months of life.

Treatment for Patent Ductus Arteriosus

When a large symptomatic PDA is present, general treatment may include fluid restriction, correction of anemia, digitalization, and diuretic therapy. Ductus arteriosus patency is mediated through the prostaglandins, and the ductus arteriosus in the pre-term infant with RDS can be constricted and closed by the administration of inhibitors of prostaglandin synthesis such as indomethacin. Early administration of indomethacin in the course of RDS associated with large ductal left-to-right shunts is approximately 80 percent effective in closing the ductus. Surgical closure is a safe and effective backup technique for management when indomethacin is contraindicated or indomethacin treatment has not been successful. Administration is by intravenous infusion over at least 30 minutes to minimize adverse effects on cerebral, renal, and gastrointestinal blood flow. Usually, three doses per course are given, with a maximum of two courses. Urine output must be closely monitored and if anuria (no urine output) or oliguria occurs, subsequent doses should be delayed.

Congestive Heart Failure

Congestive heart failure (CHF) occurs when the heart cannot pump the blood returning to the right side of the heart or provide adequate circulation to meet the needs of organs and tissues in the body. Causes of CHF include the following:

1. High output state, usually related to congenital heart diseases in which there is increased pulmonary blood flow, returning to the right side of the heart.
2. Low output state, related to (1) congenital heart diseases in which there are left-side heart obstructions causing the heart to pump harder to bypass the restrictive area, such as with coarctation of the aorta or aortic valve stenosis, (2) a primary heart muscle disease, such as a cardiomyopathy, or (3) rhythm disturbances (tachycardia or bradycardia). Ninety percent of infants with congenital heart defects develop CHF within the first year of life. The majority of affected infants manifest symptoms within the first few months of life.

Treatment for Congestive Heart Failure

The initial management of CHF is accomplished by the use of pharmacologic agents that act to improve the function of the heart muscle and reduce the workload on the heart. Digitalis is given to increase cardiac output by slowing conduction through the atrioventricular node to make each contraction stronger. Diuretics decrease preload volume because as their actions result in decreased extracellular fluid volume. Fluids are usually restricted to two-thirds of maintenance levels, and attention is given to nutrition and rest. Medical management continues with the plan for interventional cardiac catheterization or surgical intervention if indicated. See Chapter 11 for more information about the cardiovascular system and related subjects.

Iron Deficiency Anemia

Iron deficiency anemia is the most common anemia affecting children in North America. The full-term infant born of a well-nourished, nonanemic mother has sufficient iron stores until the birth weight is doubled, generally at 4 to 6 months. Iron deficiency anemia is generally not evident until nine months of age. After that period, iron must be available from the diet to meet the child's nutritional needs. If dietary iron intake is insufficient, iron deficiency anemia results. Pre-term infants, those with significant perinatal blood loss, or infants born to a poorly nourished mother with iron deficiency, may have inadequate iron stores. This infant would have a significantly higher risk for iron deficiency anemia before the age of six months. Iron deficiency anemia may also result from chronic blood loss. In the infant, this may be due to chronic intestinal bleeding caused by the heat-labile protein in cow's milk. Other causes of iron deficiency anemia include nutritional deficiencies such as folate (vitamin B_{12}) deficiency, sickle cell anemia, infections, and chronic inflammation.

Treatment for Iron Deficiency Anemia

Treatment efforts are focused on prevention and intervention. Prevention includes encouraging mothers to breast-feed (only until the infant is between 4 to 6 months), to eat foods that are rich in iron, and to take iron-fortified prenatal vitamins (approximately 1 mg/kg of iron supplement per day). Therapy to treat iron deficiency anemia consists of a medication regimen. Iron is administered by mouth in doses of 2 to 3 mg/kg of elemental iron. All forms of iron (ferrous sulfate, ferrous fumarate, ferrous succinate, and ferrous gluconate) are equally effective. Vitamin C must be administered simultaneously with iron (ascorbic acid increases iron absorption). Iron is best absorbed when it is taken one hour before a meal. Iron therapy should continue for a minimum of six weeks after the anemia is corrected to replenish iron stores. Injectable iron is seldom used unless small bowel malabsorption disease is present.

Sickle Cell Anemia

Sickle cell anemia is an inherited disorder. Children with sickle cell anemia have abnormal hemoglobin. Their hemoglobin contains hemoglobin S (HbS). Sickled red blood cells are crescent-shaped, have decreased oxygen-carrying capacity, and are destroyed at a higher rate than that for normal red blood cells. Sickling results in clumping of red blood cells in the vessels, decreased oxygen transport, and increased destruction of red blood cells. Ischemia and tissue death result from the obstruction of vessels and decreased blood flow. Sickle cell traits occur in 8 to 10 percent of African Americans. Most commonly, death occurs in children at 1 to 3 years of age from organ failure or thrombosis of major organs, usually the lungs and brain. With new treatments, 85 percent of affected individuals survive to the age of 20.

Treatment of Sickle Cell Anemia

Medical management focuses on pain control, oxygenation, hydration, and careful monitoring for other complications of vasoocclusion. Administration of prophylactic penicillin to prevent septicemia should be initiated at 2 to 3 months of age and continued through five years of life. Additional immunizations required are:

- pneumococcal vaccine at two years of age with a booster at 4 to 5 years
- influenza vaccine

Analgesics are used to control pain during a crisis period. The only cure is thought to be a bone marrow transplant, which also involves risks. This may be a promising treatment modality in the near future.

Infectious Diseases

Various types of infectious agents have effects on different body systems in newborns and children, which can cause infectious diseases. Discussion of the many infectious diseases that exist is beyond the scope of this text, but the following are a few examples of symptoms or complications resulting from infectious diseases that are seen more often in children.

Diarrhea

Diarrhea is one of the most common problems encountered by pediatricians. Diarrhea is defined as an increase in frequency, fluidity, and volume of feces. During the first three years of life, it is estimated that a child will experience an acute, severe episode of diarrhea one to three times. It may be caused by a variety of infectious agents such as bacteria, viruses, protozoans, and parasites. Hospitalization is usually necessary for severe diarrhea because of the possibility of bacterial disease, which should be treated there, and because hydration often requires fluid therapy.

Treatment for Diarrhea

Treatment for diarrhea is symptomatic. Antipyretic drugs are recommended for fever. Codeine, morphine, and the phenothiazine derivatives, often used for pain and vomiting but rarely needed for children, should be avoided because they may induce misleading signs and symptoms.

Medical Terminology Review

bacteremia
bacter = bacteria; bacterial
emia = blood
bacteria in the blood

septicemia
septic = presence of pathogens or toxins
emia = blood
pathogens in the blood

Bacteremia and Septicemia

The terms *bacteremia* and *septicemia* describe the presence of bacteria in the blood. In **bacteremia**, bacteria are recovered from blood cultures of a patient and may or may not be associated with the disease. **Septicemia** is bacteremia associated with active disease, whether localized or systemic. In some patients, bacteremia or septicemia may be associated with focal infection (e.g., pneumonia, osteomyelitis, endocarditis, or meningitis). Primary bacteremia, however, also occurs in normal infants and children.

Treatment for Bacteremia and Septicemia

Treatment may be initiated with ampicillin and a semisynthetic penicillinase-resistant penicillin (methicillin, oxacillin, nafcillin) administered intravenously. In some patients, the use of chloramphenicol may also be indicated.

TABLE 25-4 Most Common Infectious Agents Causing Meningitis in Different Age Groups

Age Group	Infective Causes
Neonates	Group B streptococci, *Escherichia coli*
Infants	*Haemophilus influenzae* type B, *Streptococcus pneumoniae*
Young Children	*Streptococcus pneumoniae* or *Neisseria meningitidis*

Acute Bacterial Meningitis

The incidence of bacterial meningitis (especially that caused by *Haemophilus influenzae* type B and group B *β-hemolytic streptococci*) is increasing. Mortality and morbidity are significant, but the reported number of deaths has decreased over time. Acute bacterial meningitis may be caused by several types of bacteria, depending on the age group of the child. Table 25-4 shows the most common infectious agents that cause meningitis in different age groups.

Treatment for Meningitis

Initial therapy includes immediate administration of multiple antibiotics including a third-generation cephalosporin (such as ceftriaxone or cefotaxime) after an intravenous line has been placed and blood has been drawn for cultures. Vancomycin, with or without rifampin, is usually added, as is ampicillin or gentamycin. Heparin therapy should be considered for patients with the syndrome of disseminated intravascular coagulation. Corticosteroids have been suggested as a therapeutic adjunct that may reduce cerebral edema and inflammation.

Streptococcal Infections

Streptococci are among the most common causes of bacterial infections in infancy and childhood. Group A streptococci are the most common bacteria causing acute pharyngitis.

Key Concept

For an intramuscular injection, the vastus lateralis is the preferred site. Because of underdevelopment of the gluteal muscles, they are not recommended for use in children under three years of age.

Treatment for Streptococcal Infections

Penicillin is the drug of choice for the treatment of streptococcal infections. The goal of therapy is to maintain, for at least ten days, blood and tissue levels of penicillin sufficient to kill streptococci. Various subjects related to antimicrobial infections and the agents used to treat them were covered in Chapter 22.

Human Immunodeficiency Virus and Acquired Immunodeficiency Syndrome

The cause of acquired immunodeficiency syndrome (AIDS) is the human immunodeficiency virus (HIV). This virus attaches to lymphocytes and other immunological cells, which results in a gradual destruction of T-helper lymphocytes. Therefore, HIV is able to reduce and damage immune functions of the body. The virus is transmitted only through direct contact with infected blood or blood products and body fluids through intravenous drug use, sexual contact, perinatal transmission from mother to infant, and breast-feeding. There is no evidence that HIV infection is acquired through casual contact. Zidovudine is given to pregnant HIV-infected women, which significantly reduces the probability of transmission from mother to child. Infants infected through perinatal transmission from infected mothers accounts for more than 85 percent of children with AIDS who are younger than 13 years. Infants who have been breast-fed (primarily in developing countries) and children who have received blood products (especially children with hemophilia) account for the remaining 15 percent of children with AIDS.

Treatment for AIDS

There is currently no cure for HIV infection and AIDS. Management begins with a staging evaluation to determine disease progression and the appropriate course of treatment. Zidovudine (AZT, ZDV), didanosine (DDI), zalcitabine (DDC), and lamivudine (3TC) slow down multiplication of the virus. Combination drug treatment is used, and many children are enrolled in research drug protocols. Trimethoprim-sulfamethoxazole (Septra, Bactrim) and pentamidine are used for treatment and prophylaxis of *Pneumocystis carinii* pneumonia. Monthly administration of intravenous immunoglobulin has been useful in preventing serious bacterial infections in children, as well as hypogammaglobulinemia. Immunizations are recommended for children with HIV infection, but instead of the oral poliovirus vaccine, the inactivated poliovirus vaccine is given. See Chapter 23 for more information about immunological agents and related subjects.

Summary

The administration of drugs to a growing and developing infant or child may present a unique problem to the physician, who must be constantly aware of the changes in drug dosages that are determined by alterations in processes of disposition at different ages. Underlying this approach is the concept that there are complex changes in the anatomy, physiology, biochemistry, and behavior from one stage of development to another over the time frame of growth from conception to adulthood. Drugs are double-edged swords. Although they can save lives, they can also endanger lives. Effective and safe drug therapy in neonates, infants, and children requires an understanding of the differences in drug action, metabolism, and disposition that are apparent during growth and development. Virtually all pharmacokinetic parameters change with age. Therefore, pediatric drug dosage regimens must be adjusted for age, disease state, sex, and individual needs. Failure to make such adjustments may lead to ineffective treatment or even to toxicity. Pharmacy technicians must be educated so that they have the required knowledge about, and can pay proper attention to, this important matter. It is impossible to cover each topic or aspect of pediatric diseases, conditions, and pharmacology in this chapter. Therefore, special considerations for selected diseases and their therapies were chosen for discussion.

Exploring the Web

Visit ***www.aap.org***

- Look for information on the disorders covered in this chapter. You may also find information on disorders that are not covered in this chapter. Create flashcards of the diseases and disorders and their treatments to use for preparation of exams.

Visit the following Web sites to research articles related to pediatric illnesses and treatments.

- ***www.emedicine.com***
- ***www.medscape.com***
- Visit ***www.nichd.nih.gov*** and search for the information related to the Pediatric Pharmacology Research Units (PPRU) Network. What are the goals of this network? What research is being conducted? What are the results of some of the research to date?

Review Questions

Multiple Choice

1. Which of the following factors may cause slower drug excretion and increase the risk of drug toxicity in an infant?
   A. kidney stones
   B. pyelonephritis
   C. urethritis
   D. renal immaturity
2. Complications of apnea include which of the following?
   A. sudden infant death syndrome
   B. hypertension
   C. asthma
   D. congestive heart failure
3. Palivizumab (Synagis) is used for immunoprophylaxis against which of the following infections?
   A. epiglottitis
   B. pneumonia
   C. respiratory syncytial virus
   D. asthma
4. Which of the following years of age exhibits the peak onset for croup?
   A. 1
   B. 2
   C. 4
   D. 6
5. Which of the following is the most commonly encountered diagnosis of respiratory disorders in office visits for children younger than the age of 15 in the United States?
   A. pneumonia
   B. flu
   C. epiglottitis
   D. otitis media
6. Patent ductus arteriosus is one of the most common congenital cardiovascular anomalies associated with which of the following maternal infections?
   A. hepatitis b
   B. rubella
   C. AIDS
   D. pneumonia
7. Ninety percent of infants with congenital heart defects develop which of the following complications within the first year of life?
   A. iron deficiency anemia
   B. cystic fibrosis
   C. sickle cell anemia
   D. congestive heart failure

8. The most common cause of death in children between 1 to 3 years who are suffering from sickle cell anemia is:

   A. thrombosis of major organs
   B. encephalitis
   C. kidney failure
   D. meningitis

9. The first-line antibiotic medication most often prescribed for otitis media is:

   A. tetracycline
   B. gentamycin
   C. tobramycin
   D. amoxicillin

10. Which of the following infectious diseases may be related to bacteremia?

    A. hepatitis b
    B. cystitis
    C. osteomyelitis
    D. epiglottitis

11. The goal of therapy for treatment of streptococcal infections is to:

    A. maintain for at least 10 days blood and tissue levels of penicillin sufficient to kill streptococci
    B. prevent myocarditis by using corticosteroids
    C. maintain for at least 3 days blood and tissue levels of corticosteroids to deal with stress
    D. prevent nephritic syndrome by using antineoplastic agents

12. Which of the following infectious diseases probably requires monthly administration of intravenous immunoglobulin to prevent serious bacterial infections in children?

    A. epiglottitis
    B. croup
    C. asthma
    D. AIDS

13. Which of the following types of insulins is classified as intermediate action?

    A. NPH
    B. regular
    C. ultralente
    D. protamine zinc

14. The drug of choice for epilepsy is based on which of the following factors?

    A. types of seizure
    B. pregnancy
    C. maturation of patients
    D. race and age of patients

15. Treatment for patent ductus arteriosus includes which of the following agents?
    A. oxygen
    B. morphine
    C. indomethacin
    D. acetaminophen

Fill in the Blank

1. In children, bacteremia may be associated with infections such as:
    a. ______________
    b. ______________
    c. ______________ or ______________
2. The two mainstays of treatment for congestive heart failure are ______________ and ______________.
3. The most common congenital cardiovascular anomaly is ______________, which may indicate indomethacin therapy.
4. 97 percent of all juvenile patients with newly diagnosed diabetes have insulin ______________.
5. Epiglottitis infection is commonly caused by ______________, type B.
6. Respiratory distress syndrome or hyaline membrane disease is the result of the absence of ______________.
7. The most widely used antipyretic in children is ______________.

Critical Thinking

A 15-month-old infant who has only been breast-fed without any formula or other foods is brought into the pediatrician's office. He examines her and orders blood tests, which reveal that she has severe anemia.

1. With this history of the infant, what type of anemia do you think she has?
2. What would be the way to prevent an infant from developing this type of anemia?
3. What other types of anemia can be seen in children of this age?

CHAPTER 26

Drug Therapy in Geriatrics

OBJECTIVES

After completing this chapter, the reader should be able to:

1. Identify the most popular types of drugs that elderly patients need.
2. Discuss clinical concerns of drug therapy and the way elderly patients react to certain drugs differently than younger patients.
3. Compare the way aging affects drug interaction, absorption, and distribution.
4. Understand how drug metabolism changes with age.
5. Discuss differences in renal function in elderly patients.
6. List some of the adverse effects that certain drugs have upon older patients.
7. Review some of the ways aging can be slowed with a healthy diet and exercise.
8. Identify age-related changes to the integumentary system.
9. Discuss common disorders in the elderly.
10. Describe the use of cold remedies in elderly people, and potential related consequences.

GLOSSARY

Collagen – a strong fibrous protein found in connective tissue

Dermis – a thick layer of loose connective tissue that is well-supplied with blood vessels, lymphatic vessels, nerves, and accessory organs

Elastin – an extracellular connective tissue protein

Pharmacodynamic interactions – differences in effects produced by a given plasma level of a drug

Pharmacokinetic interactions – differences in the plasma levels of a drug achieved with a given dose of that drug

Polypharmacy – the practice of prescribing multiple medicines to a single patient simultaneously

OUTLINE

(*continues*)

Overview

The phenomenon of aging is unavoidable because aging is a universal process. The difference between aging and disease is that the aging process is intrinsic and depends on genetic factors, whereas disease is intrinsic and extrinsic, depending on both genetic and environmental factors. Aging is always progressive, whereas disease may be discontinuous, and may progress, regress, or be arrested entirely. Aging is irreversible, whereas disease may be treatable and often has a known cause. The average life expectancy in the U.S. has increased largely because of improvements in sanitation, food, and water supplies, and the advent of antibiotics and vaccinations.

Aging Patients

The impact of age on medical care is substantial, and thus a significantly altered approach to treatment is needed for the older patient. As individuals age, they are more likely to be affected by many chronic disorders and disabilities. Consequently, they use more drugs than any other age group. Combined with a decrease in physiological reserve, these added burdens (if present) make the older person more vulnerable to environmental, pathologic, or pharmacologic illnesses. Understanding these facts is essential for optimal care of older patients. Aging alters pharmacodynamics and pharmacokinetics, affecting the choice, dose, and rate of administration of many drugs. In addition, pharmacotherapy may be complicated by an elderly patient's inability to purchase or obtain drugs, or to comply with drug regimens.

Many drugs benefit elderly persons. Some can save lives, such as antibiotics and thrombolytic therapy in acute illness. Oral hypoglycemic drugs can improve independence and quality of life while controlling chronic disease. Antihypertensive drugs and influenza vaccines can help prevent or decrease morbidity. Analgesics and antidepressants can control debilitating symptoms. Therefore, the appropriateness of the potential benefits in outweighing the potential risks should guide therapy. The health problems and medical management of elderly patients differs from those of younger ones in important ways, which explains the development of training in geriatrics as a medical specialty. Prescribing medications for elderly patients is always a challenge for physicians. Body functions decline dramatically in elderly patients. Safe, effective pharmacotherapy remains one of the greatest challenges in the practice of clinical geriatrics. Therefore, the normal aging process can lead to altered drug effects and the need for altered doses.

Physiologic Aging

Not all functions in the human body show age-related changes. For example, the hematocrit does not change with age. However, testosterone, cortisol, thyroxine, and insulin do show age-related declines.

It is extremely difficult to differentiate among primary age changes (physiological), secondary age changes (pathophysiological), and tertiary age changes (sociogenic and behavioral). Age-related changes may be responsible for the atypical presentation of diseases in elderly persons, which can be observed in hyperthyroidism, depression, uncontrolled diabetes mellitus, and rheumatoid arthritis. Although aging changes may lessen the severity of some diseases, they may also be responsible for more severe presentations. For example, normal human aging is associated with a progressive reduction in dopamine concentrations in the brain, which may influence the onset or severity of Parkinson's disease. Menopause clearly is related to an increase in osteoporosis and atherosclerosis. Arteriosclerosis accounts for the age-related increase in diastolic blood pressure, a major risk factor for cerebrovascular disease (stroke).

The Blood and Lymphatic Systems

The effect of the aging process on the blood results mainly from a reduced capacity to make new blood cells quickly when disease has occurred. After age 70 (approximately), the amount of bone marrow space that is occupied by tissue that produces blood cells declines progressively. This decrease in the ability to produce new blood cells when disease has occurred is a serious problem for elderly patients.

In the lymphatic system, age-related changes affect immune responses. Specific antibody responses to foreign antigens are impaired by the aging process. Elderly individuals may be more susceptible to infections and malignancies due to decreased immunity. In the elderly, infections are a leading cause of morbidity and mortality (see Table 26-1).

The Cardiovascular System

With advancing age, the heart weight increases significantly. In the myocardium (the heart muscle) fat, **collagen** (a strong fibrous protein found in connective tissue), and **elastin** (an extracellular connective tissue protein) increase. Arterial compliance in the internal and external carotid pathways significantly decrease. Fibrous plaques are present in many individuals' arteries at ages 15 to 24 years. Within another decade of life, 85 percent of blood vessels have these plaques. More than 60 percent of hearts at ages 55 to 64 years show vascular calcification. Narrowing heart vessels are also more prevalent with age, and occlusion may occur in at least one of the three major coronary arteries. See Chapter 12 for more information on the cardiovascular system.

TABLE 26-1 Common Infections in the Elderly

Disorder	Causes	Prevention or Treatment
Pneumonia	Bacterial	Vaccine and Antibiotics
Influenza	Viral	Vaccine
Urinary Tract	Bacterial	Antibiotics
Herpes zoster (shingles)	Viral	Vaccine

The Urinary System

Age-associated kidney changes can be categorized as anatomic or functional. Anatomic changes include loss of glomeruli, decreased kidney size, renal tubular changes, and renal vascular changes. Anatomic changes involving the lower urinary tract make men more susceptible to prostatic hypertrophy. Women become prone to pelvic relaxation, urinary incontinence, urinary tract infections, and the development of uterine and cervical cancers. Renal function declines progressively starting in the fifth decade, so that by age 70 normal renal function greatly declines in comparison to people at age 30. Glomerular filtration rate declines by about 1 mL/min/year. Even in the absence of cardiovascular, renal, or acute illness, the decline is more rapid in men than in women. Renal blood flow and plasma flow also decrease with age. Drug metabolism is often impaired in the elderly because of a decrease in the glomerular filtration rate, as well as reduced hepatic clearance. See Chapter 18 for more information on the urinary system.

The Endocrine System

Specific age-related disturbances in extrahepatic hormonal regulatory mechanisms have been proposed. The reduced availability of hormones results in diminished endocrine regulatory mechanisms, deficiencies in hormonal feedback mechanisms, and decreased binding affinities and receptors. Altered pancreatic and adrenal hormone concentrations decrease glucose tolerance with age. Insulin release is impaired in some older individuals, whereas others have fewer insulin receptors or exhibit postreceptor abnormalities. The peripheral glucose disposal rate is significantly lower in older than in younger persons. Production of sex hormones also decreases with age. In postmenopausal women, reduced estrogen concentrations have been linked to increased incidences of osteoporosis and cardiovascular disease. See Chapter 17 for more information on the endocrine system.

The Skeletal System

Normal age-related changes of the musculoskeletal system affect mobility in most cases. The musculoskeletal system gradually loses bone mass after age 50 because bone formation and resorption becomes unstable. The skeletal systems of elderly people are affected by a decrease in total body mass. Bone mass, density, and strength all decrease, and at the same time, bone fragility increases. Elderly skeletal system diseases and disorders are influenced by these factors. See Chapter 10 for more information on the musculoskeletal system.

The Respiratory System

Changes in the respiratory system with age have been reviewed. The diameters of the trachea and central airways increase, enlarging anatomic dead space. The volume of the alveolar ducts increases, whereas the membranous bronchioles narrow. Lung weight decreases dramatically, and chest wall compliance also decreases. These and other changes result in less elastic recoil in the lung, increased closing volume, and decreased maximal expiratory flow.

Thus, elderly persons have an increased risk for respiratory failure. Aspiration or inhalation of foreign material into the tracheobronchial tree can produce major respiratory illness, which is more likely to occur in older than younger people. Finally, asthma in elderly persons must be differentiated from other causes of airflow obstruction, such as acute bronchitis or congestive heart failure. See Chapter 14 for more information on the respiratory system.

The Gastrointestinal System

Age-associated changes in the gastrointestinal system have been reviewed. The gastrointestinal system starts with the oral cavity, where age-related changes reflect perturbation in oral health resulting from poor hygiene, disease, or disease treatment, rather than from dysfunction directly related to age. Nevertheless, oral disorders are common among elderly persons. As many as 50 percent of older people experience traumatic lesions of the oral cavity, which may be ulcerative, atrophic, or hyperplastic. These changes make the oral mucosa more susceptible to disease, a problem that can be exacerbated by corticosteroids, antibiotics, cytotoxic agents, and immunosuppressive therapy. Elderly persons may have an increased risk of local adverse drug reactions such as fixed eruptions (round or oval patches of reddened blisters on the skin), swelling, glossitis (inflammation of the tongue), and stomatitis (inflammation of the mouth).

Gastric secretion declines with age. Gastric cell function decreases and gastric pH rises. Gastric emptying is about 2.5 times faster in younger than in older persons, perhaps because it is under the control of the CNS, which may lose efficiency with advancing age. Slowing of gastric emptying also follows a reduction in gastric acid secretion. Gastric emptying is reduced by stress, lack of ambulation, gastric ulcer, intestinal obstruction, myocardial infarction, and diabetes mellitus. Emptying is delayed by fatty meals in the elderly more so than in younger people. Bleeding is a fairly common complication of ulcers in elderly persons. The normal aging process leads to a reduction in vitamin D absorption and a profound decline in the intestinal absorption of calcium. There is little existing evidence that the motility of the small intestine is altered by the aging process. Constipation is common because of alteration of motility in the large intestine.

The liver is the organ least affected by primary age changes. It continues to function in those persons not affected by disease. In general, just a small part can perform the tasks of the entire liver. Liver weight correlates with body weight, and both decrease starting in the fifth or sixth decade.

Primary aging may be responsible for decreased hepatic blood flow. Hepatic blood flow decrease probably affects the metabolic clearance of certain drugs. These functional changes are thought to be most relevant with drugs that have a high first-pass extraction ratio. Clearance is limited by the capacity of the organ, and hepatic clearance cannot exceed hepatic blood flow, which is approximately 1.5 L/min. Thus, reduced blood flow can alter drug action in the elderly. For at least some drugs, hepatic metabolism in the elderly apparently is altered.

The reduction in hepatic clearance is due to the decreased activity of microsomal enzymes and reduced hepatic perfusion with aging. The distribution of drugs is also affected. In addition, serum albumin levels decrease, especially in sick patients, so that protein binding of some drugs (such as warfarin and phenytoin) is reduced. This leaves more free (active) drugs available. Also, older individuals often have altered responses to a given serum drug level. See Chapter 15 for more information on the gastrointestinal system.

The Nervous System

With age, cellular brain mass and cerebral blood flow decrease. Sensory conduction takes longer, and the blood-brain barrier may become more permeable. These changes may decrease coordination, prolong reaction time, and impair short-term memory. Manifestations include more falls (particularly among elderly women), urinary incontinence, and confusion. Homeostatic response (the balance of the internal body systems) also declines.

In short, the brain shrinks with advancing age and loses nerve cells. The brain weighs less at 70 years of age than it weighs at age 30. Various areas of the brain lose substantial amounts of their nerve cells, although the nerve cells that control eye movement are not affected. The greatest loss of cells appears to take place in the temporal area, but the functional effect is surprisingly small. Cerebral blood flow is controlled by autoregulation, metabolic regulation, and chemical factors. Its regulation is influenced by the disease processes prevailing in old age, such as dementia, atherosclerosis, diabetes mellitus, stroke, and hypertension.

Short-term memory is significantly affected by aging, a loss that can be minimized by teaching methods of memorization to older adults. The declines in both learning facility and information retrieval, and perhaps also the loss in processing speed, appear to contribute to failing short-term memory.

Serotonin (a neurotransmitter) is widely distributed throughout the CNS. It is implicated in a variety of neural functions, such as pain, feeding, sleep, sexual behavior, cardiac regulation, and cognition. Changes in the serotonin system occur in association with healthy aging. See Chapter 4 for more information on the nervous system.

The Special Senses (Eye and Ear)

Vision impairment is one of the three most common medical problems among the elderly. Significant visual difficulties are caused by the aging process, resulting in difficulty reading or conducting daily activities independently. With aging, the size of the pupil decreases, necessitating brighter lighting in order to see. Sensitivity to glares also increases because of age-related changes in the eyes' lens opacity. As we age, color discrimination decreases and depth perception becomes altered.

Hearing impairment is the second-most common health problem seen in elderly patients. High frequencies often become inaudible by the age of 50, with a marked decline occurring after age 65. The term "hard of hearing" may relate more to high-frequency hearing loss than an overall decline in hearing perception. Therefore, it is usually easier for an elderly adult to hear voices, telephones, doorbells, and horns since they have lower tones and are of high intensity.

The Integumentary System

Cells in the epidermis, which contain melanocytes (that produce the melanin pigment), must be continuously replaced with new cells that divide, by mitosis, in the lower layers. The rate of production of these new cells decreases between ages 20 and 70. It is clear that during long periods of time, individual epidermal cells are exposed to carcinogens (cancer-causing agents), such as ultraviolet light from the sun. Furthermore, the number of melanocytes and the amount of protective melanin pigment decreases with age, making ultraviolet light more dangerous.

The **dermis** is a thick layer of loose connective tissue that is well-supplied with blood vessels, lymphatic vessels, nerves, and accessory organs. The predominant cells found in the dermis are fibroblasts, mast cells, and macrophages. Fibroblasts produce and release collagen and elastin into the extracellular matrix, which give skin its strength and elasticity, respectively.

The amount of collagen and elastin in the dermis decreases as people age, accounting for the thinning and wrinkling of the skin in elderly persons. Loss of collagen makes the skin more susceptible to wear and tear, whereas loss of elastin causes skin to lose its resiliency over time.

Perhaps the most striking age-related changes in the integumentary system are the graying, thinning, and loss of the hair. Hair color depends on varying amounts of melanin pigment within the specialized cells.

The Reproductive System

As men age, testosterone levels decrease, sperm production slows, the scrotum loses muscle tone, and the testicles lose size and firmness. With age, the prostate gland enlarges considerably. Sexual activity is still normal and possible in elderly patients if they have no major health problems.

In women, physical changes occur after menopause. The ovaries cease producing ova (eggs), and lowered estrogen levels may cause physiological symptoms. Women experience a general atrophy of the genitalia that is related to hormonal changes, including less fat, the loss of external hair, and flattening of the labia. An elderly female's uterus is about one-half the size of the uterus of a young adult female. With age, the vagina also becomes drier and narrower.

After menopause, women experience changes in breast tissue resulting in less glandular tissue, reduced elasticity, more connective tissue, and more fat. As a result, the breasts experience sagging, though the size of the breasts may not change. Many of the physiological changes in body systems are summarized in Table 26-2.

TABLE 26-2 Physiological Changes Due to Aging

System or Process	Changes
Muscular system	Strength and flexibility decline.
Metabolism	Slows down, generally causing weight gain.
Nervous system	Motor nerves deteriorate, slowing reaction time.
Skeletal system	Bones lose calcium, weakening them.
Body temperature	Ability to maintain normal temperature declines.
Bloodstream	Ability to use glucose in the bloodstream declines, increasing risk for diabetes. Good (HDL) cholesterol level lowers while bad (LDL) cholesterol level raises.
Cardiovascular system	The heart becomes less efficient, working harder to pump blood.
Digestive system	Motions of this system decrease, altering digestion. Secretions decrease, altering defecation. Mouth secretions decrease, causing greater tooth decay; speaking, swallowing, and tasting may be affected.
Urinary system	Kidney function declines. Muscles of the bladder weaken, causing loss of urine control. In men, the prostate enlarges, also causing loss of urine control.
Brain processes	Memory becomes less efficient. Reflexes become slower; coordination decreases.
Special senses	Degeneration of eye structures causes poor vision; tear production declines. Hearing ability decreases.
Integumentary system	Skin thins and dries, becoming wrinkled. Nail growth slows.
Reproductive system	The vagina narrows and becomes drier. The penis becomes less able to achieve or maintain erections.

Principles of Drug Therapy in Elderly Patients

The principal clinical concerns of drug therapy include efficacy and safety, dosage, complexity of regimen, number of drugs, cost, and patient compliance. There are several reasons for the greater incidence of adverse reactions of drugs in the elderly population.

Thus, the elderly are more sensitive to some drugs, (e.g., opioids), and less sensitive to others (e.g., β-blocking agents). Finally, the older patient with multiple chronic conditions is likely to be receiving many drugs, including non-prescribed agents. Drug doses in elderly patients must often be reduced, although dose requirements may vary considerably from person to person. In general, starting doses of about one-third to one-half the usual adult dose are indicated for drugs with a low therapeutic index.

The Physiopathology of Aging

Many of the physiological changes associated with aging can be slowed to some extent with a healthy diet and consistent regimen of moderate exercise. Many of the chronic diseases prevalent in elderly persons are either preventable or modifiable with healthy lifestyle habits. Reduction of dietary fat (especially saturated fats and cholesterol) lowers the risk of coronary artery disease and stroke, as well as breast and colon cancer. It is clear that our health and well-being depend on the degree to which our organ systems can successfully work together to maintain homeostasis (internal stability) in the body. Diminished function in one organ system is lessened by appropriate compensatory mechanisms in other systems. The aging process affects all body systems physiologically.

Common Disorders in the Elderly

Some disorders occur almost exclusively in elderly persons, and some occur in persons of all ages but are far more common in elderly persons than in other age groups. For example, multiple disorders, accidental hypothermia, and urinary incontinence are almost exclusively found in elderly persons. Some other examples include lymphoma, chronic lymphocytic leukemia, prostate cancer, degenerative osteoarthritis, dementia, falls, hip fracture, osteoporosis, Parkinsonism, hypertension, heart failure, stroke, and herpes zoster. These disorders are available for study and review in many medical textbooks. In this chapter, the most common disorders in elderly persons will be discussed selectively.

Multiple Disorders

Normal and abnormal effects of the aging process on different systems of the body in elderly persons may cause multiple disorders after middle age. A patient may suffer from several disorders, such as peptic ulcer, hypertension, and diabetes mellitus. Therefore, some patients are receiving several different medications that may cause drug interactions and side effects.

Cardiovascular Disorders

The incidence and prevalence of most cardiovascular disorders increases markedly with advancing age. Significant fat accumulations and calcifications in blood vessels of the heart (coronary arteries), brain, or peripheral arterial system are found in the majority of men and women older than 70 years of age. The combined effects of the pathological and physiological changes contribute to a high prevalence of problems, such as heart failure and cardiac arrhythmias in the elderly. There is good evidence that risk factors such as hypertension and hyperlipidemia can be successfully modified in older people, reducing the risk of ischemic vascular events. Multiple disorders are common in old age and coexistent diseases often can influence the choice of drugs for a cardiovascular condition. In addition, both pharmacokinetic and pharmacodynamic drug profiles may be altered in older subjects. These can influence both choice of drug and dosing regimen.

Ischemic Heart Disease

Aging is associated with a progressive rise in morbidity and mortality due to ischemic heart disease, which is the most common cause of death in elderly people in the United States. The three main groups of drugs used to treat angina pectoris are β-adrenergic receptor blocking agents, calcium channel blockers, and nitrates, which are discussed in Chapter 11.

Acute Myocardial Infarction

Acute myocardial infarction (AMI) is painless in many persons older than 70 years of age. The mortality from AMI is greater in older subjects than in young and middle-aged subjects. This is due to a number of factors, including increased severity of underlying coronary artery disease, a greater prevalence of previous myocardial infarction, and an associated increase in the incidence of cardiac failure. The aims of treatment are to relieve symptoms, reduce mortality, and prevent late cardiovascular disability. Pain relief is usually attempted by the use of intravenous opiates such as diamorphine. Intravenous nitrates are sometimes used to reduce opiate requirements, and may also be helpful in the treatment of associated cardiac failure; however, adverse effects, including hypotension and bradycardia, are more common in elderly subjects. When used in elderly persons, the dosage should be reduced.

Aspirin has been shown to significantly reduce mortality, reinfarction, and stroke rate after AMI in older patients. Treatment with the combination of thrombolytic agents and oral aspirin confers additional benefit.

Cardiac Failure

The incidence and prevalence of cardiac failure increase sharply with increasing age. In postmortem examinations of elderly persons, the most common underlying pathologic conditions are ischemia and hypertensive heart disease. The appropriate treatment of cardiac failure depends on accurate diagnosis including the underlying cardiac pathological conditions. Treatments for cardiac failure are discussed in Chapter 11.

Hypertension

The major causes of death and morbidity associated with hypertension are myocardial infarction and stroke. In addition, congestive heart failure is more common in elderly hypertensive patients than in their younger counterparts. Blood pressure rises with age up to about 75 years. Hypertension is perhaps best defined as the blood pressure level at which treatment is likely to be beneficial.

The best choice of antihypertensive treatment for elderly patients remains highly controversial. Drugs that are effective in younger patients also will lower blood pressure in the elderly patients. In the absence of specific contraindications, different agents seem to be tolerated equally well in elderly patients, though some patients may develop adverse reactions requiring a change of drug. Treatment of hypertension is discussed in Chapter 12.

Cerebrovascular Disease

Stroke continues to be a significant public health problem in the United States. It is estimated that every minute, one person in the United States suffers a stroke, making it the third leading cause of death and the major cause of long-term disability in adults. Because two-thirds of all patients affected by stroke are older than 65 years, this disease mostly affects the elderly population.

The most significant unmodifiable risk factor for stroke is advanced age. The risk for stroke in African Americans is much higher than in Caucasians, even after controlling for the effects of age, hypertension, and diabetes. Cigarette smoking and excessive alcohol consumption are important independent risk factors for stroke. Hypertension is by far the most important modifiable risk factor. It is a contributing factor in more than two-thirds of strokes, and lowering diastolic blood pressure significantly reduces stroke risk by 40 percent.

General therapeutic measures for stroke patients include maintaining an open airway, hydration with intravenous fluids, and judicious treatment of hypertension and hypoglycemia.

Cancer

The management of cancer with aging is an increasingly common problem as the number of elderly patients with cancer grows. Elderly persons comprise approximately 12 percent of the U.S. population. According to the

Journal of Allied Health, the number of elderly people (those aged 65 years or older) is projected to reach almost 40 million by 2010. After heart disease, cancer is the second leading cause of death in the U.S.

Malignant tumor incidence increases progressively with age, although the increase is not uniform for each type of cancer. The reason for the increased incidence of cancer with age is not fully understood. The duration of carcinogenesis (agents that cause cancers), and the prolonged exposure to chemical, physical, or biologic carcinogens may explain the association.

Cancer in older persons should be considered differently because of the physiological effects of aging. There are two important pharmacokinetic factors that occur with aging: a change in the volume of distribution, and a decrease in the concentration of serum albumin. The treatment of different cancers was discussed in Chapter 20.

Arthritis

Arthritis is the most common chronic ailment in elderly persons. Most people aged 70 years or older report having arthritis, occasionally resulting in physical limitations. After age 65, the prevalence is approximately 50 percent, and it increases every decade thereafter. The two most common forms of arthritis in elderly persons are rheumatoid arthritis (RA), and osteoarthritis (OA).

Rheumatoid Arthritis

The clinical manifestations of RA in elderly people may differ from those of the typical younger adult patient with this disease. The abrupt appearance of symptoms is more common in elderly-onset disease, whereas bone erosions and nodules are less common. A multidisciplinary treatment approach is required for elderly patients with RA. It includes physical therapy, occupational therapy, pharmacotherapy, and, occasionally, surgical intervention. The goals of therapy for elderly patients are the same as those for younger patients: to relieve symptoms, reduce inflammation, avoid joint destruction, prevent deformities, maintain functional capacity, and preserve quality of life. The pharmacotherapy of RA is similar in young and old patients. Age alone does not contraindicate the use of the first- or second-line antirheumatic drugs. The adverse effects of some drugs are more pronounced in elderly patients. Nonsteroidal anti-inflammatory drugs (NSAIDs), including aspirin and nonacetylated salicylates, are useful in treating arthritic symptoms in elderly subjects. Drug therapy must be monitored vigilantly in elderly patients because of the increased risk of complications. Anti-inflammatory complications of NSAIDs in elderly patients include cardiovascular (congestive heart failure and hypertension), CNS (confusion, dizziness, headaches, and hearing loss), gastrointestinal (gastritis, ulcers, and epigastric pain), and renal (electrolyte imbalances, fluid retention, and renal insufficiency) complications.

Osteoarthritis (OA)

The other common type of arthritis is osteoarthritis (OA), which is characterized by degeneration of cartilage, bone remodeling, and overgrowth of bone. This form of arthritis, also referred to as degenerative joint disease, is the most common form in elderly people. Radiographic evidence of OA is present in the majority of those older than age 65, yet many are asymptomatic. Pain is the primary complaint of patients with OA. Pain can be absent despite severe joint damage. Joint stiffness, pain at night, pain at rest, and crepitus (a feeling of crackling as the joint is moved) also are common symptoms. Commonly affected joints include the interphalangeal joints of the hands, knees, hips, first metatarsophalangeal joint, and the lumbar and cervical spine.

The primary goals in treating OA are to minimize joint pain, maintain functional mobility, and allow use of the affected joints. A combination of pharmacotherapy and nonpharmacological therapeutic interventions is often necessary. Resting the joints sometimes relieves pain. Joint replacement may be the treatment of choice in patients with severe OA that cannot be adequately managed with other modalities. For more information for pharmacotherapy, refer to Chapter 10.

Osteoporosis

Osteoporosis is a metabolic bone disorder in which the rate of bone reabsorption accelerates while the rate of bone formation slows down, causing a loss of bone mass. Bones affected by this disease lose calcium and phosphate salts, and thus become porous, brittle, and abnormally vulnerable to fractures. Osteoporosis may be primary or secondary to an underlying disease. Primary osteoporosis is often called postmenopausal osteoporosis because it develops more commonly in postmenopausal women. Osteoporosis is usually discovered when an elderly person bends to lift something, hears a snapping sound, then feels a sudden pain in the lower back. Osteoporosis can develop insidiously with increasing deformity, kyphosis, and loss of height. As bones weaken, spontaneous wedge fractures, pathological fractures of the neck or femur and hip, become increasingly common. Osteoporosis, often affecting older people, is a major risk factor in vertebral compression fractures and hip fractures.

The aims of treatment are to prevent additional fractures and control pain. A physical therapy program, emphasizing gentle exercise and activity, is an important part of the treatment. Hormone replacement therapy (HRT) with estrogen and progesterone may retard bone loss and prevent the occurrence of fractures. HRT decreases bone reabsorption and increases bone mass. Other medications may include alendronate (Fosamax) and calcitonin; however, adequate calcium and vitamin D intakes are needed for maximum effect. Drug therapy merely arrests osteoporosis; it does not cure it. Surgery can correct pathologic fractures. For information on pharmacotherapy, refer to Chapter 17.

Ophthalmic Disorders

One of the consequences of aging is a gradual impairment of vision. Like other tissues and organs in the body, the eye is constantly undergoing changes, both physical and functional. Changes may be a consequence of the aging process, diet, environment, or disease. Conditions that are commonly associated with age-related deterioration of ocular function include reduction in precorneal tear production; changes affecting the clarity and flexibility of the crystalline lens; an elevation in intraocular pressure, and changes in vessels supplying blood to regions in the eye.

Dry Eye Syndrome

Dry eye syndrome (xerosis) in elderly persons may be caused by a number of conditions, including trachoma, vitamin A deficiency, chemical burn, radiation, and chemotherapy. Dry eye is a common disorder affecting the elderly population, especially individuals older than 40 years. In elderly persons, a thinned conjunctiva and diminished corneal sensation add to the problem of dry eyes.

The primary treatment for dry eyes is replacement of deficient tear production with artificial tear preparations. Sterile isotonic saline preparations have been used to replace aqueous tear deficiencies, but the duration of relief is extremely short, requiring frequent dosing. Relief can be prolonged by the addition of water-soluble polymers, which increase the viscosity of the solution and provide an aqueous film over the corneal surface for an extended period.

Presbyopia

In the normal resting state, the eye can focus on an image of a distant object. However, to focus on a near object, the refractive power of the lens must increase. This is accomplished by contraction of the ciliary muscles, which causes the lens to become more spherical. This process is referred to as accommodation. The closest distance that the eye is able to accommodate (near point) is extremely short in infancy, and it progressively increases with age. When a person reaches the mid-40s, presbyopia, a condition in which the near point of accommodation moves beyond a comfortable reading distance, gradually develops. Presbyopia is presently treated using corrective eyeglasses. Bifocal or trifocal contact lenses are also available, but they have had limited acceptance.

Cataract

A cataract is defined as any opacity or loss in transparency in the crystalline lens of the eye. When a cataract interferes with transmission of light to the retina, some loss in visual acuity, and possibly complete loss of vision, may result. Cataracts are a leading cause of blindness and visual impairment worldwide.

Cataracts may be congenital or acquired (secondary). Most cataracts have no known etiology, and they usually occur in individuals older than 50 years of age. There is significant correlation between age and the occurrence of lens opacities, which are found to some degree in most people older than 60.

At present, no medical treatment will restore an opaque lens to its transparent state. Surgery remains the only effective method of treatment.

Glaucoma

Glaucoma includes a group of ocular diseases that are characterized by increased intraocular pressure, which may produce compression of the optic disk, resulting in damage to the optic nerve that leads to loss of the peripheral visual field and visual acuity.

Glaucoma is the second leading cause of blindness in the world. According to the Glaucoma Foundation, it is estimated that 67 million people worldwide have primary glaucoma. It is also a common cause of blindness in the United States.

The treatment of glaucoma centers on the reduction of the elevated intraocular pressure. Currently, this is accomplished with medical, laser, or surgical treatment.

Drug Interactions

A drug interaction occurs whenever the pharmacological action of a drug is altered by a second substance. This change may be related to **pharmacokinetic interactions** (differences in the plasma levels of a drug achieved with a given dose of that drug), and **pharmacodynamic interactions** (differences in effects produced by a given plasma level of a drug). The duration and intensity of the action of a drug are a function of the plasma level of the drug, which is related directly to the absorption, distribution, metabolism, and excretion of that drug. These rates may be altered by previous drug therapy, dietary factors, and exposure to environmental chemicals (chemicals not used for therapeutic purposes). Physical factors such as ambient temperature and effects of disease (e.g., fever) may also have an impact.

Pharmacokinetics

Pharmacokinetics is the study of the activities of drugs occurring within the body after a drug is administered, including absorption, distribution, excretion, and metabolism. It also involves the amount of time that each of these processes requires. Pharmacokinetics is also the study of the onset of action, duration of effect, biotransformation, and routes of excretion of the metabolites of the drug. It is difficult to determine the amount of drug reaching its site of action as a function of time after administration. In most cases, this is not feasible; therefore, it is the plasma concentration of the drug that is measured. This provides useful information, since the amount of drug in the tissues is related to plasma concentration. Pharmacokinetics are also greatly affected by the aging process.

Drug Absorption

Key Concept

The differences in pharmacokinetics can lead to stronger or weaker drug effects in the elderly compared with those in young adults.

Physiological changes with aging, such as changes of gastric pH, slowed gastric emptying rate, reduced cardiac output (blood flow), reductions of absorptive surfaces, and slowed gastrointestinal (GI) track motility, are factors that affect not only drug absorption but also drug distribution and metabolism. Different diseases and conditions of the GI tract are also obvious factors that affect drug absorption. Examples are peptic ulcer, diarrhea, and constipation.

Drug Distribution

Alterations in drug distribution in elderly patients depend on many factors, such as a reduction of total body water content, decreased plasma albumin concentration, reduced lean body mass, and increased body fat. Many drugs, especially acidic ones, bind to plasma proteins. Drugs can compete for plasma protein-binding sites. Plasma protein-binding sites are especially significant when a high percentage of the drug (more than 90 percent) is normally protein-bound, as with coumarin anticoagulants, sulfonamides, salicylates, indomethacin, and most other nonsteroidal anti-inflammatory agents. Lipid-soluble drugs such as lidocaine and diazepam have a large volume of distribution in elderly persons, whereas water-soluble drugs such as ethanol and acetaminophen have a smaller volume of distribution. Digoxin also has a lower volume of distribution in elderly persons, and therefore, doses must be reduced.

Drug Metabolism

The most common and most important cause for differences in the plasma levels of a drug is a change in the rate of biotransformation of the drug. Variations in a person's plasma drug levels are more common with drugs that undergo extensive GI metabolism or first-pass hepatic metabolism. The total liver blood flow declines significantly with aging because of a reduction of cardiac output. Therefore, if severe and progressive liver damage is present in an elderly person, drug metabolism would be affected. Otherwise, the decline in the ability of elderly persons to metabolize most drugs is relatively small and difficult to predict. In older persons, presystemic (first-pass) metabolism of some drugs given orally is decreased and their serum concentration and bioavailability are increased. Examples of these drugs include labetalol, propranolol, and verapamil. Consequently, initial doses of these drugs should be reduced as required. However, presystemic metabolism of other metabolized drugs such as imipramine, amitriptyline, morphine, and meperidine is not decreased. The effects of cigarette smoking, diet, and alcohol consumption may be more important than the physiological changes in the liver.

Drug Elimination

Drugs may be eliminated from the body by many routes, including urine, feces (e.g., unabsorbed drugs or those secreted in bile), saliva, sweat, tears, breast milk, and lungs (e.g., alcohols and anesthetics). Any route may be important for a given drug, but the kidney is the most important route for the elimination of the majority of drugs. Some drugs are excreted unchanged in the urine, whereas other drugs are so extensively metabolized that only a small fraction of the original chemical substance is excreted unchanged. Different responses to drug therapy may be seen in elderly individuals because of a decline in hepatic and renal function, which is often accompanied by a concurrent disease process. The rate of elimination of any drug by the kidney is reduced in elderly persons. Renal blood flow, mainly in the renal cortex, decreases significantly with aging. This physiological change causes a decrease in renal drug elimination.

Because renal function is dynamic, maintenance doses of drugs should be adjusted when a patient becomes acutely ill or dehydrated or has recently recovered from dehydration. In addition, because renal function continues to decline, the dose of drugs given long-term should be reviewed periodically. Examples of these drugs are the aminoglycosides, chlorpropamide, digoxin, and lithium carbonate. To prevent drug toxicity, renal function must be estimated, and the dosage of the drug should be adjusted. Most elderly patients do not have normal renal function, and the majority require adjustments in the dosages of drugs that are eliminated primarily by the kidneys. See Chapter 3 for more information on drug elimination and the renal system.

Pharmacodynamics

Drug action is defined as physiological changes in the body caused by a drug, or responses to the pharmacological effects of a drug. Pharmacodynamics refers to the chemical reaction of drugs in the body. This can be different in elderly persons because of physiological changes that occur with aging. Drugs can modify the way the body acts, but they do not give body organs and tissues new functions. They usually either slow down or speed up ordinary cell processes.

The most common way in which drugs display their action is by forming a chemical bond with specific receptors within the body. This binding may occur if the drug and its receptors have a compatible chemical shape. Figure 26-1 illustrates a drug-receptor interaction.

The effects of similar concentrations of drugs at the site of action may be greater or lesser in elderly persons than they are in younger persons. The difference may be due to changes in drug-receptor interactions. The increased sensitivity that occurs with aging must be considered when drugs that can have serious adverse effects are used. These drugs include morphine, pentazocine, warfarin, angiotensin-converting enzyme inhibitors, diazepam (especially when it is given parenterally), and levodopa. Some drugs whose

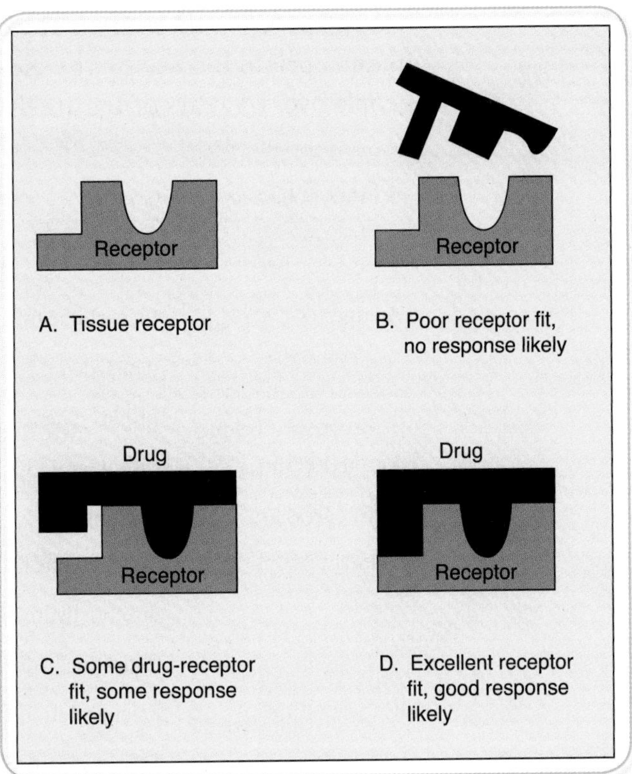

Figure 26-1 Drug-receptor interaction.

effects are reduced in elderly persons include tolbutamide, glyburide, and β-blockers, which should also be used with caution because serious dose-related toxicity can still occur, and signs of toxicity may be delayed.

Polypharmacy

Polypharmacy is the practice of prescribing multiple medicines simultaneously to a single patient. It increases costs for treatment as well as the chances for drug interactions and multiple adverse effects. Polypharmacy is more common in elderly patients because they often need several medical specialists and also may be using OTC drugs and herbal supplements. Herbal supplements must be considered to be drugs because of their potential to interact adversely with prescribed and OTC drugs.

Liver dysfunction, confusion, falls, and malnutrition may all be caused by polypharmacy. Liver dysfunction contributes to confused mental states and delirium, with perception disturbances and misinterpretations of information commonly seen.

Specific Drug Considerations for the Elderly

Several classes of drugs that are commonly prescribed for elderly persons will be selectively discussed here. They include cardiovascular drugs, central nervous system drugs, anti-inflammatory drugs, and gastrointestinal

Key Concept

Non-compliance with drug therapy in the elderly is a significant problem. The reasons for this relate to the aging process, the patient's social circumstances, prescribing patterns, and the level of communication between health professionals.

drugs. However, there are many different types of drugs that are potentially inappropriate for use by the elderly. Drugs that are dangerous if used by people over 65 years of age are listed in Table 26-3.

TABLE 26-3 Dangerous Medications for Adults over 65 Years of Age

Classification	Generic Name	Trade Name
Analgesics	meperidine hydrochloride	Demerol®
	pentazocine	Talwin®
	propoxyphene hydrochloride	Darvon, Darvocet N®
Antiarrhythmics	disopyramide	Norpace®
Antidepressants and Antipsychotics		
Antidepressants	amitriptyline hydrochloride	Enovil®
	doxepin hydrochloride	Sinequan®
	fluoxetine hydrochloride	Prozac®
Antipsychotics	haloperidol	Haldol®
	thioridazine hydrochloride	Mellaril®
Antiemetics	trimethobenzamide hydrochloride	Tigan®
Antihypertensives	clonidine hydrochloride	Catapres®
	hydrochlorothiazide	Esidrix®, HydroDIURIL®
	methyldopa	Aldomet®
	propranolol	Inderal®
	reserpine	Serpasil®
Anti-infectives and Antihistamines		
Anti-infectives	nitrofurantoin	Macrodantin®
Antihistamines	chlorpheniramine maleate	Chlor-Trimeton®
	diphenhydramine hydrochloride	Benadryl®, Tylenol PM®
	hydroxyzine pamoate	Vistaril®, Atarax®
	promethazine hydrochloride	Phenergan®
Antispasmodics	belladonna alkaloids	Donnatal® and others
	dicyclomine hydrochloride	Bentyl®
	hyoscyamine sulfate	Levsin®
	oxybutynin chloride	Ditropan®
	tolterodine tartrate	Detrol®
Decongestants	oxymetazoline	Afrin®, Dristan®, others
	phenylephrine hydrochloride	Neo-Synephrine®
	pseudoephedrine hydrochloride	Sudafed®

(*continues*)

TABLE 26-3 Dangerous Medications for Adults over 65 Years of Age—*continued*

Classification	Generic Name	Trade Name
Histamine-2 Blockers	cimetidine	Tagamet®
Iron	ferrous sulfate	Feosol® and others
Muscle Relaxants	carisoprodol	Soma®
	cyclobenzaprine hydrochloride	Flexeril®
	methocarbamol	Robaxin®
	orphenadrine	Norflex®
NSAIDs	indomethacin	Indocin®
	ketorolac tromethamine	Toradol®
	phenylbutazone	Butazolidin®
Oral Hypoglycemics	chlorpropamide	Diabinese®
Platelet Inhibitors	dipyridamole	Persantine®
Sedative-Hypnotics	alprazolam	Xanax®
	chlordiazepoxide	Librium®, Limbitrol®
	diazepam	Valium®
	flurazepam	Dalmane®
	lorazepam	Ativan®
	meprobamate	Miltown®
	oxazepam	Serax®
	temazepam	Restoril®
	triazolam	Halcion®

Cardiovascular Drugs

Almost one-third of all deaths in Western countries can be attributed to heart disease. Many cardiovascular drugs must be used cautiously in the elderly for the treatment of hypertension, congestive heart failure, myocardial infarction, and stroke, amongst other disorders and conditions.

Blood pressure increases with age, leading to serious health problems. Treatment of hypertension is effective in older patients. Antihypertensive drugs include thiazides, which are the most commonly prescribed class of diuretics. In the elderly, because of potential adverse effects, these agents should be used in lowered doses. Unfortunately, thiazides can increase the risk of worsening gout, which is a common elderly condition. Beta blockers and ACE inhibitors are prescribed less than thiazides because they may conflict with certain elderly disorders. $Alpha_1$ blockers are infrequently used for elderly patients because of their adverse effects.

The toxic effects of cardiac glycosides are particularly dangerous in elderly patients because of their increased susceptibility to arrhythmias. Renal function should be considered when dosing regimens are being contemplated. Digoxin is considered safe for older adults if there is close monitoring of serum digoxin levels, creatinine clearance tests, and monitoring of vital signs.

Because older people exhibit changes in hemodynamic reserve, treating patients in this age group who have arrhythmias (dysrhythmias) is challenging. Disopyramide should be avoided due to its major toxicities. Patients with arrhythmias should receive therapy that is designed to control their ventricular rate without conversion to normal sinus rhythm. The prevention of possible thromboembolism in chronic atrial fibrillation is an important goal.

Anticoagulants

Many elderly patients with atrial fibrillation are not given anticoagulants because physicians fear injuries and secondary bleeding due to falls. Head injuries from falling are usually of greatest concern. Given that anticoagulation can result in an annual absolute reduction in the risk of stroke, the benefits of anticoagulation outweigh the risks of falling in most instances (see Chapter 13).

Central Nervous System Drugs

Central nervous system drugs may act by blocking receptors and preventing transmitters from binding them. CNS drugs for geriatric patients include sedative-hypnotics, narcotic analgesics, antidepressants, antipsychotics, and drugs used for Alzheimer's disease.

The second most common group of drugs prescribed for (or taken OTC) by the elderly are sedatives and hypnotics. The half-lives of many of these drugs show a greatest age-related increase in people who are 60 to 70 years of age. Reduced renal function or liver disease affects the rate at which these drugs can be eliminated. Ataxia and other motor impairments should be closely watched for in older patients when they are taking these drugs, which include barbiturates and benzodiazepines.

Narcotic analgesics may cause dose-related adverse effects in the elderly. Because of the way respiratory function changes as we age, geriatric patients are often more sensitive to the respiratory effects of these drugs. Use of narcotics may cause hypotension in the elderly. Opioids are often underutilized in the elderly, though good pain management plans are easily obtained for this age group.

Antidepressants and antipsychotics have sometimes been overused in the elderly for the treatment of such disorders as schizophrenia, dementia, aggressiveness, delirium, and paranoia. Older drugs of this type, such as chlorpromazine, should be avoided in the elderly because they induce orthostatic hypotension. According to the patient's tolerance, drug doses should be gradually increased to achieve the desired therapeutic effect, with close monitoring for adverse effects.

Some phenothiazines should be started at just a fraction of the amounts used for young adults when they are being used for the elderly. Due to its clearance by the kidneys, lithium must be dosage-adjusted, and it should never be used concurrently with thiazide diuretics. Antidepressants often cause more toxicity in older adults, and those with reduced antimuscarinic effects (such as nortriptyline and desipramine) should be used. It is important to remember that major depression and senile dementia must be carefully diagnosed due to the possibility of them resembling each other.

Alzheimer's disease is characterized by progressive memory and cognitive function impairment. Cholinomimetic drugs are usually used for this condition, to decrease the release of gamma-aminobutyric acid (GABA), and increase the release of norepinephrine, dopamine, and serotonin from nerve endings. Some agents, such as donepezil, rivastigmine, and galantamine have been shown to improve cognitive activity in some Alzheimer's patients, and may even reduce morbidity from other diseases. This is important in prolonging the life of the patient. However, these agents should be used with caution in patients receiving other cytochrome P450 enzyme inhibitors.

Anti-inflammatory Drugs

About one-half of patients with cancer who are dying have severe pain. Patients perceive pain differently, depending on factors such as fatigue, insomnia, anxiety, depression, and nausea. Addressing these factors together with a supportive environment can help control pain.

The choice of analgesic depends largely on pain intensity, which can be determined only by talking with and observing the patient. All pain can be relieved by an appropriately potent drug at the right dosage, which may also produce sedation or confusion. Commonly used drugs are aspirin, acetaminophen, or NSAIDs for mild pain; codeine or oxycodone for moderate pain; and hydromorphone or morphine for severe pain. For a detailed discussion of analgesic use, see Chapter 21.

Key Concept

For the administration of drugs in elderly patients, neurological status and parameters relating to renal, liver, cardiac, and respiratory function should be noted.

Cold Remedies

Over-the-counter cold remedies often cause adverse effects in elderly people. The anticholinergic properties of many create confusion, impair bladder emptying, or cause constipation and decongestants may cause urinary hesitance or retention in men.

Gastrointestinal Drugs

Many seriously ill patients experience nausea, often without vomiting. Contributors to nausea include GI problems such as constipation and gastritis, metabolic abnormalities such as hypercalcemia and uremia (elevation of urea in blood), drug side effects, and increased intracranial pressure due to brain cancer. Treatment should be guided by the probable etiology, such as discontinuation of NSAIDs and administration of H_2-receptor blockers such as ranitidine (Zantac), famotidine (Pepcid), and cimetidine (Tagamet) in a patient with gastritis. In contrast, a patient with known or suspected brain metastasis may have nausea due to increased intracranial pressure and would best be treated with a course of corticosteroids. Metoclopramide, orally or by injection, is useful for nausea caused by gastric distension. If a reason for mild nausea is not identifiable, nonspecific treatment with phenothiazines such as promethazine or prochlorperazine before meals may be given. Anticholinergic drugs such as scopolamine and the antihistamine meclizine prevent recurrent nausea in many patients. Second-line drugs for intractable nausea include haloperidol and granisetron. Constipation is common in elderly people because of inactivity, use of opioid and anticholinergic drugs, and decreased fluid and dietary fiber intake. Laxatives help prevent fecal impaction, especially for those receiving opioids. Laxative drugs are discussed in Chapter 15.

Antimicrobial Drugs

Due to alterations in their T-lymphocyte function, many elderly patients appear to have reduced host defenses, and are more susceptible to serious infections and diseases such as cancer. It is important to remember that decreased renal function greatly affects the use of certain antimicrobial drugs, such as aminoglycosides, in the elderly. Antimicrobial drugs that are considered safe for the elderly include penicillins, cephalosporins, sulfonamides, and tetracyclines. Drug doses should be decreased if the patient has decreased renal drug clearance or the drug has a prolonged half-life.

Summary

Throughout the aging process, individuals are more likely to be affected by many chronic disorders and disabilities. Consequently, elderly persons use more drugs than any other age group. The normal function of each system and organ of the body changes during the aging process. However, some functions in the human body do not show age-related changes. There are three factors that are associated with the aging process: physiological, pathophysiological, and sociogenic or behavioral. The principles of drug therapy in elderly patients are based on efficacy and safety, dosage, complexity of regimen, number of drugs, cost, and patient compliance. Many disorders and conditions are more common in elderly men, women, or both. The most common diseases seen in elderly persons in the United States have been selectively discussed. Several classes of drugs that are commonly prescribed for elderly patients should be given special consideration because of their side effects, drug interactions, and dosages. They include anticoagulants, glaucoma medications, analgesics, antihypertensives, cold remedies, antiemetics, and benzodiazepines.

Exploring the Web

Visit the following Web sites and search for articles and information related to the body as it ages and the effects of pharmacotherapy in the elderly:

- ***www.nlm.nih.gov/medlineplus***
- ***www.postgradmed.com***
- ***http://healthlibrary.stanford.edu***
- ***www.4therapy.com/consumer/medications/item.php?uniqueid=4712&categoryid=163&***
- ***www.adaa.org/aboutADAA/newsletter/AnxietyandAging.htm***
- ***Visit www.ageworks.com***
- Look at the various online courses and continuing education courses. Choose a course you feel would enhance your understanding of the factors affecting aging and health.

Review Questions

Multiple Choice

1. Which of the following disorders is the most common cause of death in the United States?

A. cancer
B. AIDS

C. rheumatoid arthritis
D. myocardial infarction

2. The goal of treatment for osteoporosis includes:

A. stopping the aging process
B. preventing additional fractures and controlling pain
C. preventing surgery for pathologic fractures and controlling pain
D. stopping the use of hormone replacement

3. In postmenopausal women, reduced estrogen blood levels have been linked to increased incidence of which of the following conditions or diseases?

A. upper respiratory tract infections
B. rheumatoid arthritis
C. breast cancer
D. cardiovascular disease

4. Which of the following drugs requires a lower dosage in elderly persons because of reduction of renal function?

A. warfarin
B. gentamicin
C. digoxin
D. ranitidine

5. Which of the following medications in elderly patients may cause falls and hip fractures?

A. thiazides
B. diazepam
C. vitamin B_{12}
D. cimetidine

6. Physiological changes with aging may alter all of the following, except:

A. reduction of cardiac output
B. reduction of absorptive surfaces
C. increased gastric emptying rate
D. changes in gastric pH

7. All of the following are reasons for the greater incidence of adverse reactions of drugs in elderly individuals, except:

A. increased total body fluid
B. impaired drug metabolism
C. decreased serum albumin levels
D. medication errors are more likely to occur

8. Which of the following drugs has a large volume of distribution?

A. diazepam
B. acetaminophen
C. digoxin
D. ethanol

9. Which of the following body systems is the most important for elimination of the majority of drugs?
   A. digestive
   B. respiratory
   C. reproductive
   D. urinary

10. Which of the following agents can cause systemic side effects such as bradycardia, asthma, and heart failure?
    A. diazepam
    B. diphenhydramine
    C. warfarin
    D. bethanechol

11. The number of melanocytes and the amount of protective melanin ______________ in elderly people.
    A. increases
    B. decreases
    C. does not change
    D. depends on what types of medications are being taken

12. The most important route for the elimination of the majority of drugs includes which of the following?
    A. sweat
    B. saliva
    C. lungs
    D. kidneys

13. The effects of similar drug concentrations at the site of action are called:
    A. pharmacology
    B. pharmacokinetic
    C. pharmacodynamic
    D. pharmacogenetic

14. In the United States, about ______________ of persons older than 65 years take prescription and nonprescription (over-the-counter) drugs.
    A. one-half
    B. one-fourth
    C. two-thirds
    D. three-fifths

15. Primary age changes are also known as ______________ age changes.
    A. physiological
    B. pathophysiological
    C. sociogenic
    D. tertiary

Fill in the Blank

1. Anticholinergic properties of many over-the-counter cold remedies often cause adverse effects in elderly people, such as:
   a. ______________
   b. ______________
   c. ______________
   d. ______________

2. Scopolamine and the antihistamine meclizine prevent recurrent ______________ in many elderly patients.

3. Longer-acting benzodiazepines should be avoided in elderly people because ______________.

4. Many elderly patients with atrial fibrillation are not given anticoagulants because physicians fear ______________ and secondary bleeding due to ______________.

5. The most significant unmodifiable risk factor for stroke is ______________.

6. Digoxin has a lower volume of distribution in elderly patients; therefore, doses ______________.

7. Topical β-blockers can cause systemic side effects in elderly patients, such as ______________, ______________, and ______________.

Critical Thinking

A 65-year-old man has had a history of alcoholism for the past 20 years. He has been taking warfarin for the past ten days. It is known that with cirrhosis of the liver, serum albumin decreases, as does hepatic blood flow.

1. What would be the consequences of taking warfarin in his condition?

2. Explain the hepatic clearance in elderly people who are suffering from liver diseases.

3. If this patient also takes phenytoin, what would be the potential outcome?

APPENDIX

Case Studies A

1. A 4-year-old boy presents with the following symptoms. He is experiencing a fever of 101.9° F, chills, sore throat, and rash. The best recommendation for treating this child's fever is:

   A. choline salicylate, because it is in the liquid form, and therefore more easily swallowed
   B. acetaminophen, since the specific disease condition is not known
   C. pediatric aspirin, because it is flavored and will ensure patient compliance
   D. any of the above recommendations are acceptable

Questions 2–4

A 60-year-old hypertensive woman brings three prescriptions to your pharmacy. They include furosemide, enalapril, and irbesartan.

2. Which of the following is an example of an ACE inhibitor?

   A. furosemide
   B. enalapril
   C. digoxin
   D. irbesartan

3. Which of the following is the trade name of furosemide?

   A. Midamor
   B. Hygroton
   C. Aldactone
   D. Lasix

4. Irbesartan is classified as which of the following antihypertensive drugs?

   A. peripheral vasodilator
   B. angiotensin II receptor antagonist
   C. adrenergic blocker
   D. angiotensin-converting enzyme inhibitor

5. A 31-year-old woman presents with a 2-month history of depressed mood, absence of pleasure from the performance of any act, increased appetite, weight gain, and suicidal ideation. This is the patient's first episode of major depression. Which of the following agents would be most appropriate in the treatment of this patient?

   A. sertraline (Zoloft)
   B. chlorpromazine (Thorazine)
   C. thioridazine (Mellaril)
   D. ritodrine (Yutopar)

Questions 6–7

A 56-year-old man has been diagnosed with acute gouty arthritis of the right large toe.

6. Which of the following is the drug of choice for relieving pain and inflammation, and for ending the acute gout attack?

   A. mivacurium
   B. gold sodium thiomalate
   C. aspirin
   D. colchicine

7. If the traditional drug of choice is not an analgesic, which of the following agents may be used in combination in the management of pain for acute gout?

   A. succinylcholine
   B. allopurinol
   C. acetaminophen
   D. oxycodone

Questions 8–9

A 72-year-old man with advanced inoperable throat cancer is hospitalized for pain management. He is given a morphine solution (40 mg orally) every 3 hours for pain. He complains of difficulty swallowing and about the frequency with which he must take the morphine.

8. An appropriate analgesic alternative for this patient would be:
   A. intramuscular methadone
   B. controlled-release oral morphine
   C. transdermal fentanyl
   D. not another medication; simply increase the dose of the oral morphine solution

9. If there is no other analgesic alternative and the attending physician increases the oral dosage of morphine, which of the following might be the consequence?
   A. excellent pain relief
   B. worsening renal function
   C. excessive appetite
   D. overdose

Questions 10–12

A 21-year-old, previously healthy man is brought to the emergency room with a 2-week history of excessive elimination of urine, excessive thirst, and an unintentional weight loss of 25 pounds. No retinopathy is present. Laboratory values reveal high blood glucose and high glucose in the urine.

10. What is the most likely diagnosis for this patient?
    A. Type I diabetes mellitus
    B. Type II diabetes mellitus
    C. Type III diabetes mellitus
    D. diabetes insipidus

11. Which of the following is the appropriate initial therapy?
    A. intravenous fluids and a sulfonylurea agent
    B. intravenous fluids and intravenous regular insulin
    C. intravenous fluids and 10 units of subcutaneous regular insulin
    D. intravenous fluids alone

12. The patient is at risk for developing which of the following complications?
    A. coronary artery disease
    B. retinopathy
    C. hypoglycemia
    D. all of the above

Questions 13–15

A 75-year-old man with a history of cigarette smoking for 50 years is brought to the emergency room with a fever of 103°F (which he has had for 4 days), cough, chills, and chest pain. Chest x-ray reveals pneumonia with confirmation via blood tests.

13. If this patient was diagnosed with bacterial pneumonia, which of the following antibiotics is the most appropriate to administer intravenously?
    A. chloramphenicol
    B. cephradine
    C. amphotericin B
    D. rifampin

14. If the patient has an allergy to the drug of choice (which is one of the four choices in Question 13), which of the following would be the best drug of choice?
    A. chloramphenicol
    B. cephradine
    C. amphotericin B
    D. rifampin

15. The physician orders chloramphenicol 50 mg/kg/day in divided doses (every 6 hours). Which of the following is the most serious adverse effect of this drug?
    A. ototoxicity
    B. nephrotoxicity
    C. phlebitis at injection site
    D. bone marrow depression

Questions 16–17

A 25-year-old man has burns on over 75% of his body. He has been admitted for two weeks at a local hospital, where he developed Zollinger-Ellison syndrome (a hypersecretion condition of the stomach with gastric ulcers).

16. Which of the following prototypes of H_2-receptor antagonists is used in the treatment of this condition?
    A. cimetidine
    B. famotidine
    C. nizatidine
    D. ranitidine

17. Which of the following prototype H_2-receptor antagonists is the most potent?

A. ranitidine
B. cimetidine
C. famotidine
D. nizatidine

18. Erythromycin 500 mg bid × 8 days is prescribed. The pharmacy technician has only the 250 mg dose in stock. How many capsules will the technician dispense for this patient?

A. 16
B. 24
C. 32
D. 48

Questions 19–21

A 62-year-old female has been diagnosed with congestive heart failure and pulmonary edema. Her physician orders digitalis, a diuretic, ACE inhibitors, and beta-blockers.

19. Which of the following diuretics are preferred?

A. loop diuretics
B. thiazide and thiazide-like diuretics
C. potassium-sparing diuretics
D. carbonic anhydrase inhibitors

20. If the order is for thiazide or loop diuretics, which of the following is the most dangerous adverse effect?

A. hypertension
B. hyperkalemia
C. hypokalemia
D. loss of appetite

21. If the physician orders spironolactone, which of the following adverse effects may occur?

A. hyperkalemia
B. gynecomastia
C. hyponatremia
D. all of the above

22. A pediatrician orders penicillin for an 11-year-old patient without closely checking the patient's chart. While the pharmacy technician is dispensing the prescription, he notices that the computer chart indicates that the patient has an allergy to penicillin. Which of the following would be the best drug of choice in this case?

A. ciprofloxacin
B. clarithromycin
C. amikacin
D. vancomycin

23. A 75-year-old patient with advanced metastatic prostate cancer and a long history of renal failure presents with severe bone pain. He is given meperidine. Two days later, he develops a generalized seizure condition. What is the likely mechanism of this complication?

A. worsening renal failure
B. buildup of meperidine metabolite levels
C. hypercalcemia
D. brain metastasis

24. A 55-year-old patient with a history of hypertension and recent edema in her legs is treated with a thiazide diuretic. She should be monitored regularly for altered plasma levels of:

A. uric acid
B. calcium
C. glucose
D. potassium

25. A 27-year-old woman who breast-feeds her 7-month-old infant presents with chronic panic disorder. Her physician prescribes a benzodiazepine for her. All of the following properties of this drug are desirable for breastfeeding, except:

A. hepatic metabolism to inactive metabolites
B. a tendency to bind to milk proteins
C. a rapid onset of action
D. a short half-life

Answer Key

1. B	2. B	3. D	4. B	5. A	6. D
7. B	8. C	9. D	10. A	11. B	12. D
13. B	14. A	15. D	16. A	17. C	18. C
19. A	20. C	21. D	22. B	23. B	24. D
25. B					

APPENDIX

B Top 200 Drugs by Prescription

Number	Generic Name	Trade Name
1	hydrocodone w/APAP	Hydrocodone w/ APAP®
2	atorvastatin	Lipitor®
3	amoxicillin	Trimox®
4	lisinopril	Prinivil®, Zestril®
5	hydrochlorothiazide	Diaqua®, Esidrix®
6	atenolol	Tenormin®
7	azithromycin	Zithromax®
8	furosemide	Lasix®
9	alprazolam	Xanax®
10	metoprolol	Toprol XL®
11	albuterol	Proventil®
12	amlodipine	Norvasc®
13	levothyroxine	Synthroid®
14	metformin	Glucophage®, Glucophage XR®
15	sertraline	Zoloft®
16	escitalopram	Lexapro®
17	ibuprofen	Motrin®
18	cephalexin	Keflex®
19	zolpidem	Ambien®
20	prednisone	Deltasone®
21	esomeprazole magnesium	Nexium®
22	triamterene	Dyrenium®
23	propoxyphene napsylate	Darvon-N®
24	simvastatin	Zocor®
25	montelukast	Singulair®
26	lansoprazole	Prevacid®
27	metoprolol tartrate	Lopressor®
28	fluoxetine	Prozac®
29	lorazepam	Ativan®
30	clopidogrel	Plavix®

Number	Generic Name	Trade Name
31	oxycodone w/APAP	Oxycodone w/APAP®
32	salmeterol	Serevent®
33	alendronate	Fosamax®
34	venlafaxine	Effexor®, Effexor XR®
35	warfarin	Coumadin®
36	paroxetine hydrochloride	Paxil®
37	clonazepam	Klonopin®
38	cetirizine	Zyrtec®
39	pantoprazole	Protonix®
40	potassium chloride	Potassium Chloride®
41	acetaminophen/codeine	Tylenol-Codeine®
42	trimethoprim/ sulfamethoxazole	TMP-SMZ®
43	gabapentin	Neurontin®
44	conjugated estrogens	Premarin®
45	fluticasone	Flonase®
46	trazodone	Desyrel®
47	cyclobenzaprine	Flexeril®
48	amitriptyline	Elavil®, Enovil®
49	levofloxacin	Levaquin®
50	tramadol	Ultram®
51	ciprofloxacin	Cipro®
52	amlodipine/benazepril	Lotrel®
53	ranitidine	Zantac®
54	fexofenadine	Allegra®
55	levothyroxine	Levoxyl®
56	valsartan	Diovan®
57	enalapril	Vasotec®
58	diazepam	Valium®
59	naproxen	Anaprox®, Naprosyn®
60	fluconazole	Diflucan®

Number	Generic Name	Trade Name
61	lisinopril/HCTZ	Zestoretic®
62	potassium chloride	Klor-Con®
63	ramipril	Altace®
64	bupropion	Wellbutrin®, Wellbutrin XL®
65	celecoxib	Celebrex®
66	sildenafil citrate	Viagra®
67	doxycycline hyclate	Vibra-Tabs®
68	ezetimibe	Zetia®
69	rosiglitazone maleate	Avandia®
70	lovastatin	Mevacor®
71	valsartan/ hydrochlorothiazide	Diovan HCT®
72	carisoprodol	Soma®, Rela®
73	drospirenone/ ethinyl estradiol	Yasmin 28®
74	allopurinol	Alloprin®
75	clonidine	Catapres®
76	methylprednisolone	Medrol®
77	pioglitazone hydrochloride	Actos®
78	pravastatin	Pravachol®
79	risedronate sodium	Actonel®
80	norelgestromin/ ethinyl estradiol	Ortho Evra®
81	citalopram hydrobromide	Celexa®
82	verapamil	Calan®
83	isosorbide mononitrate	Ismotic®
84	penicillin V	Penicillin VK®
85	glyburide	Micronase®
86	amphetamine sulfate	Adderall®
87	mometasone furoate	Nasonex®
88	folic acid	Folacin®

Number	Generic Name	Trade Name
89	quetiapine fumarate	Seroquel®
90	losartan potassium	Cozaar®
91	fenofibrate	Tricor®
92	carvedilol	Coreg®
93	methylphenidate hydrochloride	Concerta®
94	ezetimibe	Vytorin®
95	insulin glargine	Lantus®
96	promethazine hydrochloride	Phenergan®
97	meloxicam	Mobic®
98	tamsulosin hydrochloride	Flomax®
99	rosuvastatin	Crestor®
100	glipizide	Glucotrol XL®
101	norgestimate/ ethinyl estradiol	Ortho Tri-Cyclen Lo®
102	temazepam	Restoril®
103	omeprazole	Prilosec®
104	cefdinivir	Omnicef®
105	albuterol	Ventolin®
106	risperidone	Risperdal®
107	rabeprazole sodium	AcipHex®
108	digoxin	Digitek®
109	spironolactone	Aldactone®
110	valacyclovir hydrochloride	Valtrex®
111	latanoprost	Xalatan®
112	metformin	Fortamet®
113	losartan potassium/ hydrochlorothiazide	Hyzaar®
114	quinapril	Accupril®
115	clindamycin	Cleocin®
116	metronidazole	Flagyl®
117	triamcinolone	Atolone®
118	topiramate	Topamax®

Number	Generic Name	Trade Name
119	ipratropium bromide/ albuterol sulfate	Combivent®
120	benazepril	Lotensin®
121	gemfibrozil	Lopid®
122	irbesartan	Avapro®
123	glimepiride	Amaryl®
124	norgestimate/ethinyl estradiol	Trinessa®
125	estradiol	Alora®, Climara®
126	hydroxyzine	Atarax®
127	metoclopramide	Maxolon®, Reglan®
128	fexofenadine/ pseudoephedrine	Allegra-D 12 Hour®
129	doxazosin mesylate	Cardura®
130	warfarin	Jantoven®
131	glipizide	Glucotrol®
132	diclofenac sodium	Voltaren®
133	raloxifene hydrochloride	Evista®
134	diltiazem	Cardizem®, Tiazac®
135	tolterodine tartrate	Detrol®, Detrol LA®
136	meclizine	Antivert®, Bonamine®
137	glyburide/metformin	Glucovance®
138	atomoxetine	Strattera®
139	duloxetine hydrochloride	Cymbalta®
140	nitrofurantoin	Furadantin®
141	promethazine/codeine	Phenergan with Codeine®
142	olmesartan medoxomil	Benicar®
143	mirtazapine	Remeron®
144	bisoprolol/HCTZ	Ziac®
145	desloratadine	Clarinex®
146	oxycodone	OxyContin®
147	minocycline	Arestin®, Minocin®
148	sumatriptan	Imitrex®

Number	Generic Name	Trade Name
149	nabumetone	Relafen®
150	olanzapine	Zyprexa®
151	lamotrigine	Lamictal®
152	cetirizine/ pseudoephedrine	Zyrtec-D®
153	polyethylene glycol	Glycolax®
154	acyclovir	Zovirax®
155	propranolol	Inderal®
156	triamcinolone acetonide	Nasacort AQ®
157	donepezil hydrochloride	Aricept®
158	butalbital/ acetaminophen/caffeine	Fioricet®
159	niacin	Niaspan®
160	azithromycin	Zmax®
161	divalproex sodium	Depakote®
162	buspirone	Buspar®
163	norgestimate/ethinyl estradiol	Tri-Sprintec®
164	methotrexate	Amethopterin®, MTX®
165	oxycodone	Roxicodone®
166	budesonide	Rhinocort Aqua®
167	olmesartan medoxomil hydrochlorothiazide	Benicar HCT®
168	terazosin	Hytrin®
169	metaxalone	Skelaxin®
170	clotrimazole/ betamethasone	Lotrisone®
171	tadalafil	Cialis®
172	irbesartan/ hydrochlorothiazide	Avalide®
173	fexofenadine	Telfast®
174	norgestimate/ethinyl estradiol	Ortho Tri-Cyclen®
175	bupropion hydrochloride	Wellbutrin®, Zyban®
176	benzonatate	Tessalon®

Number	Generic Name	Trade Name
177	olopatadine hydrochloride	Patanol®
178	quinine	Quinamm®, Quiphile®
179	diltiazem hydrochloride	Cartia XT®
180	insulin lispro, rDNA origin	Humalog®
181	paroxetine	Paxil CR®
182	levonorgestrel and ethinyl estradiol	Aviane®
183	digoxin	Lanoxin®
184	amphetamine	Adderall XR®
185	famotidine	Pepcid®, Pepcid AC®
186	digoxin	Lanoxicaps®
187	levothyroxine	Levothroid®
188	nifedipine	Adalat®, Procardia®

Number	Generic Name	Trade Name
189	nortriptyline	Aventyl®
190	hydrocodone polistirex/ chlorpheniramine polistirex	Tussionex®
191	nitroglycerin	NitroQuick®
192	phenytoin	Dilantin®
193	budesonide	Endocet®
194	etodolac	Lodine®, Lodine XL®
195	atenolol/chlorthalidone	Tenoretic®
196	phentermine	Fastin®
197	tramadol/ acetaminophen	Ultracet®
198	tizanidine	Zanaflex®
199	cetirizine hydrochloride/ pseudoephedrine	Virlix-D®
200	divalproex sodium	Depakote ER®

APPENDIX C Common Look-alike and Sound-alike Drugs

Generic Names	Brand Names	Possible Dangers
celecoxib citalopram hydrobromide fosphenytoin	Celebrex® Celexa® Cerebyx®	Mix-ups may cause decreased mental ability, lack of pain or seizure control, and other serious adverse events.
cisplatin carboplatin	Platinol® Paraplatin®	Though the generic names are similar, safe doses of carboplatin usually exceed the maximum safe dose of cisplatin, potentially causing toxicity and death.
clonidine clonazepam	Catapres® Klonopin®	Easily confused generic or trade names.
concentrated liquid morphines versus conventional liquid morphine concentrations	Concentrated: Roxanol®, MSIR® Conventional: morphine oral liquid	Concentrated forms can be confused with standard concentrations can lead to fatal errors due to differences in labeling or prescribing by volume versus milligrams, e.g., 10 mg versus 10 mL.
ephedrine epinephrine	Ephedrine® Adrenalin®	Similar names and clinical uses can cause these drugs to be stored close to each other; also, they are packaged in similar amber-colored vials and ampules.
fentanyl sufentanil	Sublimaze® Sufenta®	These non-interchangeable drugs have very different potencies, and can cause respiratory arrest if misused.
hydromorphone injection morphine injection	Dilaudid® Astramorph®, Duramorph®, Infumorph®	Hydromorphone is not the generic equivalent of morphine and they are not interchangeable. Due to close storage and similar concentrations, they may be easily misused, causing death because of potency differences influencing respiratory arrest.
insulin glargine insulin zinc suspension human insulin insulin lispro human insulin aspart 70% isophane insulin NPH/ 30% insulin regular 70% insulin aspart protamine suspension and 30% insulin aspart	Lantus® Lente® Humulin®, Novolin® Humalog® Novolog® Novolin 70/30® Novolog Mix 70/30®	Similar names, strengths, and concentrations can cause medication errors; also mix-ups between 100 units/mL and 500 units/mL can occur.
lipid-based: doxorubicin liposomal daunorubicin citrate liposomal conventional: daunorubicin doxorubicin	Doxil® Daunoxome® Cerubidine® Adriamycin®, Rubex®	Confusion between liposomal and conventional formulations can occur easily, but these products are not interchangeable; accidental use of liposomal forms instead of conventional forms has resulted in severe side effects and death.
nefazodone quetiapine	Serzone® Seroquel®	Similar names and available dosages, as well as use in similar clinical settings, can cause many adverse events and potentially dangerous drug interactions with other agents that may be used concurrently.

Generic Names	Brand Names	Possible Dangers
paclitaxel docetaxel	Taxol® Taxotere®	These cancer agents have different dosing recommendations and can cause serious adverse outcomes,
vinblastine vincristine	Velban® Oncovin®	Fatal errors can occur due to name similarity and wide variances in safe recommended dosages of each.
olanzapine cetirizine	Zyprexa® Zyrtec®	Name similarity can easily cause mix-ups; Zyrtec is an antihistamine, while Zyprexa is an antipsychotic; serious physical or mental injury or impairment can occur.

APPENDIX D

Classifications of Drug Schedules in the United States and Canada

Drug	U.S. Drug Schedule	Canadian Drug Schedule
alfentanil	II	I
alprazolam	IV	IV
amobarbital	II	IV
amphetamine	II	III
aprobarbital	III	IV
benzophetamine	III	III
buprenorphine	III	I
butabarbital	III	IV
butorphanol	IV	IV
chloral hydrate	IV	Not controlled
chlordiazepoxide	IV	IV
clonazepam	IV	IV
clorazepate	IV	IV
cocaine	II	I
codeine	II	I
dexmethylphenidate	II	Not available
dextroamphetamine	II	III
dextropropoxyphene (bulk) dextropropoxyphene (dosage forms)	II IV	I I
diazepam	IV	IV
diethylpropion	IV	IV
difenoxin products	V	I
diphenoxylate products	V	I
dronabinol	III	Not controlled
estazolam	IV	IV
ethchlorvynol	IV	IV
fentanyl	II	I
fluoxymesterone	III	IV
flurazepam	IV	IV

Drug	U.S. Drug Schedule	Canadian Drug Schedule
glutethimide	II	IV
halazepam	IV	IV
hydrocodone	Only available in C-III combination drugs	I
hydromorphone	II	I
ketamine	III	Not controlled
levorphanol	II	I
lorazepam	IV	IV
mazindol	IV	IV
meperidine	II	I
mephobarbital	IV	IV
meprobamate	IV	IV
methadone	II	I
methamphetamine	II	III
methandrostenalone	III	IV
methylphenidate	II	III
methyltestosterone	III	IV
midazolam	IV	IV
modafinil	IV	Not controlled
morphine	II	I
nandrolone	III	IV
opium opium products	II V	I I
oxandrolone	III	IV
oxazepam	IV	IV
oxycodone	II	I
oxymetholone	III	IV
oxymorphone	II	I
paraldehyde	IV	Not controlled
paregoric	III	I

Drug	U.S. Drug Schedule	Canadian Drug Schedule
pemoline	IV	Not controlled
pentazocine	IV	I
pentobarbital sodium PO rectal	 II III	 IV IV
phencyclidine	II	I
phendimetrazine	III	IV
phenobarbital	IV	IV
phentermine	IV	IV
prazepam	Not available	IV
quazepam	IV	IV
remifentanil	II	Not available
secobarbital	II	IV
sibutramine	IV	Not available
stanolone	III	IV
stanozolol	III	IV
sufentanil	II	I
temazepam	IV	IV
testosterone	III	IV
thiopental	III	IV
triazolam	IV	IV
zaleplon	IV	Not available
zolpidem	IV	Not available

APPENDIX

Drug Dosage Calculations E

Using Ratios and Proportions to Calculate Dosages

1. Ratios may be written as follows: 3 : 4, which means 3 parts of drug #1 to 4 parts of solution or solvent. *Ratios* are used to express the relationship between two or more quantities. Ratios are usually expressed as fractions in drug calculations, as follows:

$$\frac{\text{3 parts of drug \#1}}{\text{4 parts of a solution}} = \frac{3}{4}$$

Proportions show the relationship between two ratios, as follows:

$$\frac{\text{Dose on hand}}{\text{Quantity on hand}} = \frac{\text{Desired dose}}{\text{Desired quantity (X)}}$$

The same formula can be written as follows by using cross multiplication:

$$\text{Desired quantity (X)} = \frac{\text{Desired dose}}{\text{Dose on hand} \times \text{Quantity on hand}}$$

If the dose on hand is 200 mg, the desired dose is 400 mg, and the quantity on hand is 10 mL, what is the desired quantity (X)?

$$\frac{\text{Dose on hand (200 mg)}}{\text{Quantity on hand (10 mL)}} = \frac{\text{Desired dose (400 mg)}}{\text{Desired quantity (X)}}$$

When cross-multiplying, we find:

$$200 \times X = 10 \text{ mL} \times 400$$

$$200X = 4{,}000 \text{ mL}$$

$$X = 20 \text{ mL}$$

The dose to be administered is 20 mL.

2. The same proportion method can solve solid dosage calculations, as follows:

If the dose on hand is available as 5 mg tablets, and the desired dose is 25 mg/day, how many tablets should be administered each day?

$$\frac{\text{Dose on hand (5 mg)}}{\text{1 tablet}} = \frac{\text{Desired dose (25 mg)}}{\text{Desired quantity (X)}}$$

By cross-multiplying, it is found that:

$$5 \text{ mg} \times X = 25 \text{ mg} \times 1 \text{ tablet}$$

$$5X = 25 \text{ mg}$$

$$X = 5 \text{ tablets/day}$$

Therefore, 5 tablets should be administered daily.

Dosage Calculations by Weight

Drug dosages are often expressed as milligrams per unit of body weight (usually kilograms rather than pounds), and are commonly used in depicting pediatric doses. An example recommended dose of a drug might be 1 mg/kg/24 hours. This information can be used to calculate the dose for a specific patient, or to check that prescribed doses are correct and not significantly under or over the required doses for that patient.

Caution must always be used in converting between pounds and kilograms.
The formula that should be understood is as follows:

Body weight × (dose in mg/kg) = X mg of drug

Example: Chewable tablets for a 110-pound child are to be administered at the rate of 20 mg/kg/dose. How many tablets, if they are 500 mg each, should be administered to this patient for each dose?

First, convert the patient's weight to kilograms as follows:

$$1 \text{ kg} = 2.2 \text{ lbs}$$

$$\frac{1 \text{ kg}}{2.2 \text{ lbs}} = \frac{X \text{ kg}}{110 \text{ lbs}}$$

$$X = 50 \text{ kg}$$

Next, calculate the total daily dose as follows. For each kg of body weight, you should give 20 mg of the drug.

$$\frac{20 \text{ mg}}{1 \text{ kg}} = \frac{X \text{ mg}}{50 \text{ kg}}$$

$$X = 1{,}000 \text{ mg}$$

Finally, calculate the number of tablets needed to supply 1,000 mg per dose.

Remember that the concentration of the tablets on hand is 500 mg per tablet.

$$\frac{500 \text{ mg}}{1 \text{ tablet}} = \frac{1{,}000 \text{ mg}}{X \text{ tablets}}$$

$$X = 2 \text{ tablets per dose}$$

Calculating Dosage by Body Surface Area

Using body surface area to calculate pediatric dosages is a very accurate method. Nomograms are charts that use patient weight and height to determine body surface area in square meters (m^2). This body surface area (BSA) is then placed into a ratio with the average adult's body surface area (1.73 m^2). The following formula is then used:

$$\text{Child's dose} = \frac{\text{Child's BSA in m}^2}{1.73 \text{ m}^2} \times \text{Adult dose}$$

Nomogram scales contain metric and avoirdupois values for height and weight, enabling body surface area to be determined in pounds and inches or kilograms and centimeters without needing to make conversions. See the figure of the nomogram scale at the end of this Appendix.

WEST NOMOGRAM

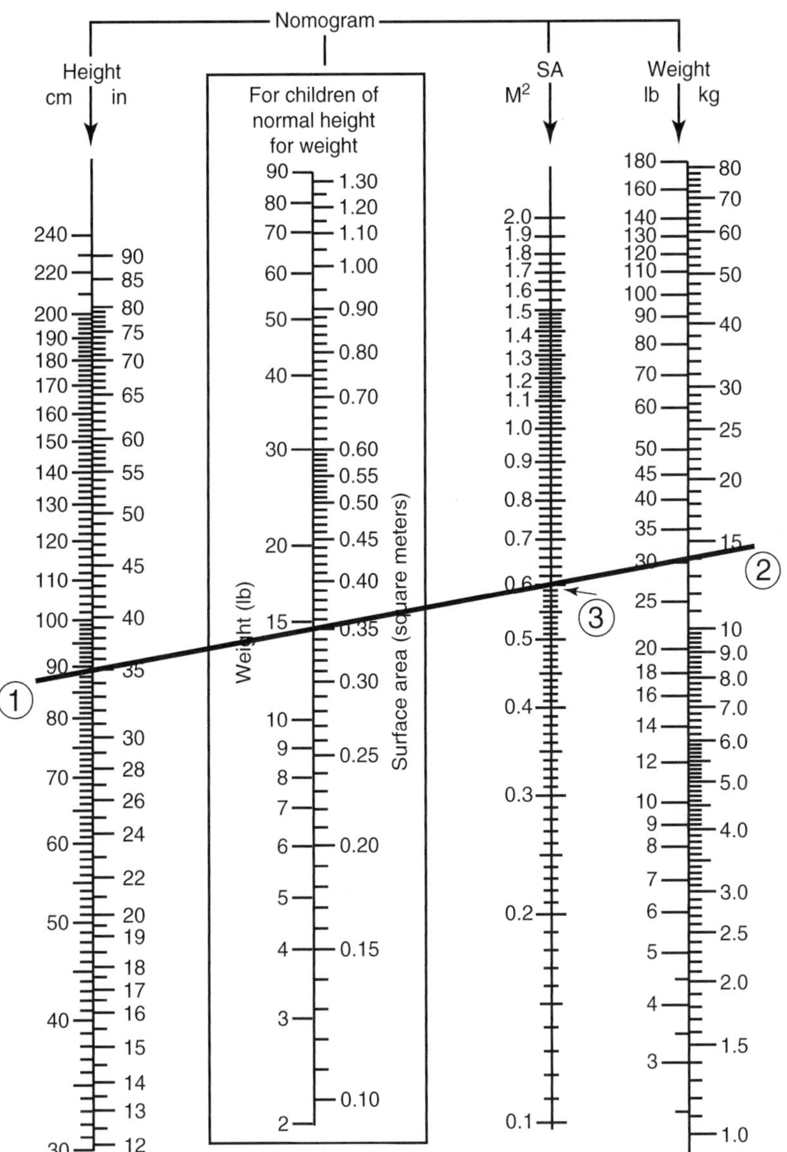

To determine BSA, a ruler or straightedge is recommended. After determining the patient's height and weight, place the ruler or straightedge on the nomogram and connect the two points on the height and weight scales that represent the patient's values. Where the ruler or straightedge crosses the center column (BSA), the corresponding reading is the value of the BSA in square meters. Substitute the BSA value in the formula to calculate the dosage for this patient. If this child's BSA is 0.52 m^2, and the adult dosage of the required drug is 500 mg, use the following formula to determine the child's dose:

$$\text{Child's dose} = \frac{0.52\ \text{m}^2}{1.73\ \text{m}^2} \times \text{Adult dose (500 mg)}$$

$$= 0.3 \times 500\ \text{mg}$$

$$= 150\ \text{mg (child's dose)}$$

Calculating IV Infusion Rates

To calculate the flow rate using the ratio and proportion method, follow these steps:

1. Determine the number of milliliters the patient will receive per hour.
2. Determine the number of milliliters the patient will receive per minute.
3. Determine the number of drops per minute that will equal the number of milliliters calculated above. The IV set's drop rate must be considered. This is expressed as a ratio of drops per milliliter (gtt/mL).

Example: The prescriber orders 3,000 mL of dextrose 5% in water (D_5W) IV over 24 hours. If the IV set delivers 15 drops per milliliter, how many drops must be administered per minute?

First, calculate mL/hr.

$$\frac{3{,}000\ \text{mL}}{24\ \text{hrs}} = \frac{X\ \text{mL}}{1\ \text{hr}}$$

$$X = 125\ \text{mL/hr or } 125\ \text{mL/60 min}$$

Next, calculate mL/min.

$$\frac{125\ \text{mL}}{60\ \text{min}} = \frac{X\ \text{mL}}{1\ \text{min}}$$

$$X = 2\ \text{mL/min}$$

Finally, calculate gtt/min using the drop rate per minute of the IV set. (IV set drop rate = 15 drops/mL)

$$\frac{15\ \text{gtt}}{1\ \text{mL}} = \frac{X\ \text{gtt}}{2\ \text{mL (amount needed/min)}}$$

$$X = 30\ \text{gtt/min}$$

APPENDIX F

Immunizations

DEPARTMENT OF HEALTH AND HUMAN SERVICES • CENTERS FOR DISEASE CONTROL AND PREVENTION

Recommended Immunization Schedule for Persons Aged 0–6 Years—UNITED STATES • 2007

<table>
<tr><th>Vaccine ▼ Age ▶</th><th>Birth</th><th>1 month</th><th>2 months</th><th>4 months</th><th>6 months</th><th>12 months</th><th>15 months</th><th>18 months</th><th>19–23 months</th><th>2–3 years</th><th>4–6 years</th></tr>
<tr><td>Hepatitis B[1]</td><td>HepB</td><td colspan="2">HepB</td><td>see footnote 1</td><td colspan="4">HepB</td><td colspan="3">HepB Series</td></tr>
<tr><td>Rotavirus[2]</td><td></td><td></td><td>Rota</td><td>Rota</td><td>Rota</td><td></td><td></td><td></td><td></td><td></td><td></td></tr>
<tr><td>Diphtheria, Tetanus, Pertussis[3]</td><td></td><td></td><td>DTaP</td><td>DTaP</td><td>DTaP</td><td></td><td colspan="2">DTaP</td><td></td><td></td><td>DTaP</td></tr>
<tr><td>Haemophilus influenzae type b[4]</td><td></td><td></td><td>Hib</td><td>Hib</td><td>Hib[4]</td><td colspan="2">Hib</td><td colspan="3">Hib</td><td></td></tr>
<tr><td>Pneumococcal[5]</td><td></td><td></td><td>PCV</td><td>PCV</td><td>PCV</td><td colspan="2">PCV</td><td></td><td></td><td colspan="2">PCV
PPV</td></tr>
<tr><td>Inactivated Poliovirus</td><td></td><td></td><td>IPV</td><td>IPV</td><td colspan="4">IPV</td><td></td><td></td><td>IPV</td></tr>
<tr><td>Influenza[6]</td><td></td><td></td><td></td><td></td><td colspan="7">Influenza (Yearly)</td></tr>
<tr><td>Measles, Mumps, Rubella[7]</td><td></td><td></td><td></td><td></td><td></td><td colspan="2">MMR</td><td></td><td></td><td></td><td>MMR</td></tr>
<tr><td>Varicella[8]</td><td></td><td></td><td></td><td></td><td></td><td colspan="2">Varicella</td><td></td><td></td><td></td><td>Varicella</td></tr>
<tr><td>Hepatitis A[9]</td><td></td><td></td><td></td><td></td><td></td><td colspan="4">HepA (2 doses)</td><td colspan="2">HepA Series</td></tr>
<tr><td>Meningococcal[10]</td><td></td><td></td><td></td><td></td><td></td><td></td><td></td><td></td><td></td><td colspan="2">MPSV4</td></tr>
</table>

Range of recommended ages

Catch-up immunization

Certain high-risk groups

This schedule indicates the recommended ages for routine administration of currently licensed childhood vaccines, as of December 1, 2006, for children aged 0–6 years. Additional information is available at http://www.cdc.gov/nip/recs/child-schedule.htm. Any dose not administered at the recommended age should be administered at any subsequent visit, when indicated and feasible. Additional vaccines may be licensed and recommended during the year. Licensed combination vaccines may be used whenever any components of the combination are indicated and other components of the vaccine are not contraindicated and if approved by the Food and Drug Administration for that dose of the series. Providers should consult the respective Advisory Committee on Immunization Practices statement for detailed recommendations. Clinically significant adverse events that follow immunization should be reported to the Vaccine Adverse Event Reporting System (VAERS). Guidance about how to obtain and complete a VAERS form is available at **http://www.vaers, hhs.gov** or by telephone, **800-822-7967**.

1. **Hepatitis B vaccine (HepB).** *(Minimum age: birth)*
   At birth:
   - Administer monovalent HepB to all newborns before hospital discharge.
   - If mother is hepatitis surface antigen (HBsAg)-positive, administer HepB and 0.5 mL of hepatitis B immune globulin (HBIG) within 12 hours of birth.
   - If mother's HBsAg status is unknown, administer HepB within 12 hours of birth. Determine the HBsAg status as soon as possible and if HBsAg-positive, administer HBIG (no later than age 1 week).
   - If mother is HBsAg-negative, the birth dose can only be delayed with physician's order and mother's negative HBsAg laboratory report documented in the infant's medical record.

   After the birth dose:
   - The HepB series should be completed with either monovalent HepB or a combination vaccine containing HepB. The second dose should be administered at age 1–2 months. The final dose should be administered at age ≥24 weeks. Infants born to HBsAg-positive mothers should be tested for HBsAg and antibody to HBsAg after completion of ≥3 doses of a licensed HepB series, at age 9–18 months (generally at the next well-child visit).

   4-month dose:
   - It is permissible to administer 4 doses of HepB when combination vaccines are administered after the birth dose. If monovalent HepB is used for doses after the birth dose, a dose at age 4 months is not needed.
2. **Rotavirus vaccine (Rota).** *(Minimum age: 6 weeks)*
   - Administer the first dose at age 6–12 weeks. Do not start the series later than age 12 weeks.
   - Administer the final dose in the series by age 32 weeks. Do not administer a dose later than age 32 weeks.
   - Data on safety and efficacy outside of these age ranges are insufficient.
3. **Diphtheria and tetanus toxoids and acellular pertussis vaccine (DTaP).** *(Minimum age: 6 weeks)*
   - The fourth dose of DTaP may be administered as early as age 12 months, provided 6 months have elapsed since the third dose.
   - Administer the final dose in the series at age 4–6 years.
4. ***Haemophilus influenzae* type b conjugate vaccine (Hib).** *(Minimum age: 6 weeks)*
   - If PRP-OMP (PedvaxHIB® or ComVax® [Merck]) is administered at ages 2 and 4 months, a dose at age 6 months is not required.
   - TriHiBit® (DTaP/Hib) combination products should not be used for primary immunization but can be used as boosters following any Hib vaccine in children aged ≥12 months.
5. **Pneumococcal vaccine.** *(Minimum age: 6 weeks for pneumococcal conjugate vaccine [PCV]; 2 years for pneumococcal polysaccharide vaccine [PPV])*
   - Administer PCV at ages 24–59 months in certain high-risk groups. Administer PPV to children aged ≥2 years in certain high-risk groups. See *MMWR* 2000;49(No. RR-9):1–35.
6. **Influenza vaccine.** *(Minimum age: 6 months for trivalent inactivated influenza vaccine [TIV]; 5 years for live, attenuated influenza vaccine [LAIV])*
   - All children aged 6–59 months and close contacts of all children aged 0–59 months are recommended to receive influenza vaccine.
   - Influenza vaccine is recommended annually for children aged ≥59 months with certain risk factors, health-care workers, and other persons (including household members) in close contact with persons in groups at high risk. See *MMWR* 2006;55(No. RR-10):1–41.
   - For healthy persons aged 5–49 years, LAIV may be used as an alternative to TIV.
   - Children receiving TIV should receive 0.25 mL if aged 6–35 months or 0.5 mL if aged ≥3 years.
   - Children aged <9 years who are receiving influenza vaccine for the first time should receive 2 doses (separated by ≥4 weeks for TIV and ≥6 weeks for LAIV).
7. **Measles, mumps, and rubella vaccine (MMR).** *(Minimum age: 12 months)*
   - Administer the second dose of MMR at age 4–6 years. MMR may be administered before age 4–6 years, provided ≥4 weeks have elapsed since the first dose and both doses are administered at age ≥12 months.
8. **Varicella vaccine.** *(Minimum age: 12 months)*
   - Administer the second dose of varicella vaccine at age 4–6 years. Varicella vaccine may be administered before age 4–6 years, provided that ≥3 months have elapsed since the first dose and both doses are administered at age ≥12 months. If second dose was administered ≥28 days following the first dose, the second dose does not need to be repeated.
9. **Hepatitis A vaccine (HepA).** *(Minimum age: 12 months)*
   - HepA is recommended for all children aged 1 year (i.e., aged 12–23 months). The 2 doses in the series should be administered at least 6 months apart.
   - Children not fully vaccinated by age 2 years can be vaccinated at subsequent visits.
   - HepA is recommended for certain other groups of children, including in areas where vaccination programs target older children. See *MMWR* 2006;55(No. RR-7):1–23.
10. **Meningococcal polysaccharide vaccine (MPSV4).** *(Minimum age: 2 years)*
    - Administer MPSV4 to children aged 2–10 years with terminal complement deficiencies or anatomic or functional asplenia and certain other high-risk groups. See *MMWR* 2005;54(No. RR-7):1–21.

The Recommended Immunization Schedules for Persons Aged 0–18 Years are approved by the Advisory Committee on Immunization Practices (http://www.cdc.gov/nip/acip), the American Academy of Pediatrics (http://www.aap.org), and the American Academy of Family Physicians (http://www.aafp.org).

SAFER • HEALTHIER • PEOPLE™

CS103164

DEPARTMENT OF HEALTH AND HUMAN SERVICES • CENTERS FOR DISEASE CONTROL AND PREVENTION

Recommended Immunization Schedule for Persons Aged 7–18 Years—UNITED STATES • 2007

Vaccine ▼ Age ▶	7–10 years	11–12 YEARS	13–14 years	15 years	16–18 years
Tetanus, Diphtheria, Pertussis[1]	see footnote 1	Tdap	Tdap		
Human Papillomavirus[2]	see footnote 2	HPV (3 doses)	HPV Series		
Meningococcal[3]	MPSV4	MCV4	MCV4[3] MCV4		
Pneumococcal[4]	PPV				
Influenza[5]	Influenza (Yearly)				
Hepatitis A[6]	HepA Series				
Hepatitis B[7]	HepB Series				
Inactivated Poliovirus[8]	IPV Series				
Measles, Mumps, Rubella[9]	MMR Series				
Varicella[10]	Varicella Series				

Range of recommended ages

Catch-up immunization

Certain high-risk groups

This schedule indicates the recommended ages for routine administration of currently licensed childhood vaccines, as of December 1, 2006, for children aged 7–18 years. Additional information is available at **http://www.cdc.gov/nip/recs/child-schedule.htm**. Any dose not administered at the recommended age should be administered at any subsequent visit, when indicated and feasible. Additional vaccines may be licensed and recommended during the year. Licensed combination vaccines may be used whenever any components of the combination are indicated and other components of the vaccine are not contraindicated and if approved by the Food and Drug Administration for that dose of the series. Providers should consult the respective Advisory Committee on Immunization Practices statement for detailed recommendations. Clinically significant adverse events that follow immunization should be reported to the Vaccine Adverse Event Reporting System (VAERS). Guidance about how to obtain and complete a VAERS form is available at **http://www.vaers.hhs.gov** or by telephone, **800-822-7967**.

1. **Tetanus and diphtheria toxoids and acellular pertussis vaccine (Tdap).**
   (Minimum age: 10 years for BOOSTRIX® and 11 years for ADACEL™)
   - Administer at age 11–12 years for those who have completed the recommended childhood DTP/DTaP vaccination series and have not received a tetanus and diphtheria toxoids vaccine (Td) booster dose.
   - Adolescents aged 13–18 years who missed the 11–12 year Td/Tdap booster dose should also receive a single dose of Tdap if they have completed the recommended childhood DTP/DTaP vaccination series.
2. **Human papillomavirus vaccine (HPV).** *(Minimum age: 9 years)*
   - Administer the first dose of the HPV vaccine series to females at age 11–12 years.
   - Administer the second dose 2 months after the first dose and the third dose 6 months after the first dose.
   - Administer the HPV vaccine series to females at age 13–18 years if not previously vaccinated.
3. **Meningococcal vaccine.** *(Minimum age: 11 years for meningococcal conjugate vaccine [MCV4]; 2 years for meningococcal polysaccharide vaccine [MPSV4])*
   - Administer MCV4 at age 11–12 years and to previously unvaccinated adolescents at high school entry (at approximately age 15 years).
   - Administer MCV4 to previously unvaccinated college freshmen living in dormitories; MPSV4 is an acceptable alternative.
   - Vaccination against invasive meningococcal disease is recommended for children and adolescents aged ≥2 years with terminal complement deficiencies or anatomic or functional asplenia and certain other high-risk groups. See *MMWR* 2005;54(No. RR-7):1–21. Use MPSV4 for children aged 2–10 years and MCV4 or MPSV4 for older children.
4. **Pneumococcal polysaccharide vaccine (PPV).** *(Minimum age: 2 years)*
   - Administer for certain high-risk groups. See *MMWR* 1997;46(No. RR-8):1–24, and *MMWR* 2000;49(No. RR-9):1–35.
5. **Influenza vaccine.** *(Minimum age: 6 months for trivalent inactivated influenza vaccine [TIV]; 5 years for live, attenuated influenza vaccine [LAIV])*
   - Influenza vaccine is recommended annually for persons with certain risk factors, health-care workers, and other persons (including household members) in close contact with persons in groups at high risk. See *MMWR* 2006;55 (No. RR-10):1–41.
   - For healthy persons aged 5–49 years, LAIV may be used as an alternative to TIV.
   - Children aged <9 years who are receiving influenza vaccine for the first time should receive 2 doses (separated by ≥4 weeks for TIV and ≥6 weeks for LAIV).
6. **Hepatitis A vaccine (HepA).** *(Minimum age: 12 months)*
   - The 2 doses in the series should be administered at least 6 months apart.
   - HepA is recommended for certain other groups of children, including in areas where vaccination programs target older children. See *MMWR* 2006;55 (No. RR-7):1–23.
7. **Hepatitis B vaccine (HepB).** *(Minimum age: birth)*
   - Administer the 3-dose series to those who were not previously vaccinated.
   - A 2-dose series of Recombivax HB® is licensed for children aged 11–15 years.
8. **Inactivated poliovirus vaccine (IPV).** *(Minimum age: 6 weeks)*
   - For children who received an all-IPV or all-oral poliovirus (OPV) series, a fourth dose is not necessary if the third dose was administered at age ≥4 years.
   - If both OPV and IPV were administered as part of a series, a total of 4 doses should be administered, regardless of the child's current age.
9. **Measles, mumps, and rubella vaccine (MMR).** *(Minimum age: 12 months)*
   - If not previously vaccinated, administer 2 doses of MMR during any visit, with ≥4 weeks between the doses.
10. **Varicella vaccine.** *(Minimum age: 12 months)*
    - Administer 2 doses of varicella vaccine to persons without evidence of immunity.
    - Administer 2 doses of varicella vaccine to persons aged <13 years at least 3 months apart. Do not repeat the second dose, if administered ≥28 days after the first dose.
    - Administer 2 doses of varicella vaccine to persons aged ≥13 years at least 4 weeks apart.

The Recommended Immunization Schedules for Persons Aged 0–18 Years are approved by the Advisory Committee on Immunization Practices (http://www.cdc.gov/nip/acip), the American Academy of Pediatrics (http://www.aap.org), and the American Academy of Family Physicians (http://www.aafp.org).

SAFER • HEALTHIER • PEOPLE™

CS100131

Catch-up Immunization Schedule

UNITED STATES • 2007

for Persons Aged 4 Months–18 Years Who Start Late or Who Are More Than 1 Month Behind

The table below provides catch-up schedules and minimum intervals between doses for children whose vaccinations have been delayed. A vaccine series does not need to be restarted, regardless of the time that has elapsed between doses. Use the section appropriate for the child's age.

Vaccine	Minimum Age for Dose 1	Minimum Interval Between Doses: Dose 1 to Dose 2	Dose 2 to Dose 3	Dose 3 to Dose 4	Dose 4 to Dose 5
CATCH-UP SCHEDULE FOR PERSONS AGED 4 MONTHS–6 YEARS					
Hepatitis B[1]	Birth	4 weeks	8 weeks (and 16 weeks after first dose)		
Rotavirus[2]	6 wks	4 weeks	4 weeks		
Diphtheria, Tetanus, Pertussis[3]	6 wks	4 weeks	4 weeks	6 months	6 months[3]
Haemophilus influenzae type b[4]	6 wks	**4 weeks** if first dose administered at age <12 months **8 weeks (as final dose)** if first dose administered at age 12-14 months **No further doses needed** if first dose administered at age ≥15 months	**4 weeks**[4] if current age <12 months **8 weeks (as final dose)**[4] if current age ≥12 months and second dose administered at age <15 months **No further doses needed** if previous dose administered at age ≥15 months	**8 weeks (as final dose)** This dose only necessary for children aged 12 months–5 years who received 3 doses before age 12 months	
Pneumococcal[5]	6 wks	**4 weeks** if first dose administered at age <12 months and current age <24 months **8 weeks (as final dose)** if first dose administered at age ≥12 months or current age 24–59 months **No further doses needed** for healthy children if first dose administered at age ≥24 months	**4 weeks** if current age <12 months **8 weeks (as final dose)** if current age ≥12 months **No further doses needed** for healthy children if previous dose administered at age ≥24 months	**8 weeks (as final dose)** This dose only necessary for children aged 12 months–5 years who received 3 doses before age 12 months	
Inactivated Poliovirus[6]	6 wks	4 weeks	4 weeks	4 weeks[6]	
Measles, Mumps, Rubella[7]	12 mos	4 weeks			
Varicella[8]	12 mos	3 months			
Hepatitis A[9]	12 mos	6 months			
CATCH-UP SCHEDULE FOR PERSONS AGED 7–18 YEARS					
Tetanus, Diphtheria/ Tetanus, Diphtheria, Pertussis[10]	7 yrs[10]	4 weeks	**8 weeks** if first dose administered at age <12 months **6 months** if first dose administered at age ≥12 months	**6 months** if first dose administered at age <12 months	
Human Papillomavirus[11]	9 yrs	4 weeks	12 weeks		
Hepatitis A[9]	12 mos	6 months			
Hepatitis B[1]	Birth	4 weeks	8 weeks (and 16 weeks after first dose)		
Inactivated Poliovirus[6]	6 wks	4 weeks	4 weeks	4 weeks[6]	
Measles, Mumps, Rubella[7]	12 mos	4 weeks			
Varicella[8]	12 mos	**4 weeks** if first dose administered at age ≥13 years **3 months** if first dose administered at age <13 years			

1. **Hepatitis B vaccine (HepB).** *(Minimum age: birth)*
   - Administer the 3-dose series to those who were not previously vaccinated.
   - A 2-dose series of Recombivax HB® is licensed for children aged 11–15 years.
2. **Rotavirus vaccine (Rota).** *(Minimum age: 6 weeks)*
   - Do not start the series later than age 12 weeks.
   - Administer the final dose in the series by age 32 weeks. Do not administer a dose later than age 32 weeks.
   - Data on safety and efficacy outside of these age ranges are insufficient.
3. **Diphtheria and tetanus toxoids and acellular pertussis vaccine (DTaP).** *(Minimum age: 6 weeks)*
   - The fifth dose is not necessary if the fourth dose was administered at age ≥4 years.
   - DTaP is not indicated for persons aged ≥7 years.
4. ***Haemophilus influenzae* type b conjugate vaccine (Hib).** *(Minimum age: 6 weeks)*
   - Vaccine is not generally recommended for children aged ≥5 years.
   - If current age <12 months and the first 2 doses were PRP-OMP (PedvaxHIB® or ComVax® [Merck]), the third (and final) dose should be administered at age 12–15 months and at least 8 weeks after the second dose.
   - If first dose was administered at age 7–11 months, administer 2 doses separated by 4 weeks plus a booster at age 12–15 months.
5. **Pneumococcal conjugate vaccine (PCV).** *(Minimum age: 6 weeks)*
   - Vaccine is not generally recommended for children aged ≥5 years.
6. **Inactivated poliovirus vaccine (IPV).** *(Minimum age: 6 weeks)*
   - For children who received an all-IPV or all-oral poliovirus (OPV) series, a fourth dose is not necessary if third dose was administered at age ≥4 years.
   - If both OPV and IPV were administered as part of a series, a total of 4 doses should be administered, regardless of the child's current age.
7. **Measles, mumps, and rubella vaccine (MMR).** *(Minimum age: 12 months)*
   - The second dose of MMR is recommended routinely at age 4–6 years but may be administered earlier if desired.
   - If not previously vaccinated, administer 2 doses of MMR during any visit with ≥4 weeks between the doses.
8. **Varicella vaccine.** *(Minimum age: 12 months)*
   - The second dose of varicella vaccine is recommended routinely at age 4–6 years but may be administered earlier if desired.
   - Do not repeat the second dose in persons aged <13 years if administered ≥28 days after the first dose.
9. **Hepatitis A vaccine (HepA).** *(Minimum age: 12 months)*
   - HepA is recommended for certain groups of children, including in areas where vaccination programs target older children. See *MMWR* 2006;55(No. RR-7):1–23.
10. **Tetanus and diphtheria toxoids vaccine (Td) and tetanus and diphtheria toxoids and acellular pertussis vaccine (Tdap).** *(Minimum ages: 7 years for Td, 10 years for BOOSTRIX®, and 11 years for ADACEL™)*
    - Tdap should be substituted for a single dose of Td in the primary catch-up series or as a booster if age appropriate; use Td for other doses.
    - A 5-year interval from the last Td dose is encouraged when Tdap is used as a booster dose. A booster (fourth) dose is needed if any of the previous doses were administered at age <12 months. Refer to ACIP recommendations for further information. See *MMWR* 2006;55(No. RR-3).
11. **Human papillomavirus vaccine (HPV).** *(Minimum age: 9 years)*
    - Administer the HPV vaccine series to females at age 13–18 years if not previously vaccinated.

Information about reporting reactions after immunization is available online at **http://www.vaers.hhs.gov** or by telephone via the 24-hour national toll-free information line 800-822-7967. Suspected cases of vaccine-preventable diseases should be reported to the state or local health department. Additional information, including precautions and contraindications for immunization, is available from the National Center for Immunization and Respiratory Diseases at **http://www.cdc.gov/nip/default.htm** or telephone, **800-CDC-INFO (800-232-4636)**.

DEPARTMENT OF HEALTH AND HUMAN SERVICES • CENTERS FOR DISEASE CONTROL AND PREVENTION • SAFER • HEALTHIER • PEOPLE

CS103164

APPENDIX

G Specific Antidotes

Poisonings account for approximately 5 million injuries per year in the United States. Of these, 5,000 people die annually. Poisonings are responsible for 9 percent of all ambulance transports, 10 percent of all hospital emergency visits, and 5 percent of all hospital inpatient admissions. In children, many poisonings result from failure to store hazardous household substances and medications in a safe place. Poisons are often classified according to the body organ they primarily affect. The following table lists the specific antidotes for toxic substances.

Toxin	Antidote (s)
Acetaminophen	acetylcysteine (Mucomyst)
Anticholinergic agents (such as tricyclic antidepressants)	physostigmine salicylate (Antilirium)
Anticholinesterase agents (such as organophosphate insecticides)	pralidoxime chloride, PAM (Protopam Chloride)
Arsenic	dimercaprol (BAL in Oil)
Benzodiazepines	flumazenil (Romazicon)
Calcium and digitalis	edentate disodium (Endrate, Sodium Versenate)
Cholinergic agents	atropine
Cyanide	amyl nitrite, sodium thiosulfate
Digoxin	digoxin immune FAB (Digibind)
Folic acid antagonists (such as methotrexate)	leucovorin calcium
Gold	dimercaprol
Heparin	protamine sulfate
Ifosfamide	mesna (Mesnex)
Insulin	glucagon
Iron	deferoxamine mesylate (Desferal Mesylate)
Lead	edentate calcium disodium (Calcium Disodium Versenate), succimer (Chemet), dimercaprol, cuprimine
Mercury	dimercaprol
Narcotics (opiates)	naloxone HCl (Narcan), nalmefene HCl (Revex)
Warfarin	vitamin K

APPENDIX H

Reporting of Medical Errors

Medical errors can potentially cause great harm to patients. Hundreds of thousands of people die each year as a result of medical errors or accidents. Some studies have shown that medication errors account for 10 to 25 percent of all medical errors. The following form is used by the FDA to document adverse events related to medications, medical devices, and other medical products.

U.S. Department of Health and Human Services

MEDWATCH

The FDA Safety Information and Adverse Event Reporting Program

For VOLUNTARY reporting of adverse events, product problems and product use errors

Page ___ of ___

Form Approved: OMB No. 0910-0291, Expires: 10/31/08
See OMB statement on reverse.

FDA USE ONLY

Triage unit sequence #

PLEASE TYPE OR USE BLACK INK

A. PATIENT INFORMATION

1. Patient Identifier ___ In confidence
2. Age at Time of Event, or Date of Birth:
3. Sex ☐ Female ☐ Male
4. Weight ___ lb or ___ kg

B. ADVERSE EVENT, PRODUCT PROBLEM OR ERROR

Check all that apply:

1. ☐ Adverse Event ☐ Product Problem (e.g., defects/malfunctions)
☐ Product Use Error ☐ Problem with Different Manufacturer of Same Medicine

2. Outcomes Attributed to Adverse Event (Check all that apply)

☐ Death: ___ (mm/dd/yyyy) ☐ Disability or Permanent Damage
☐ Life-threatening ☐ Congenital Anomaly/Birth Defect
☐ Hospitalization - initial or prolonged ☐ Other Serious (Important Medical Events)
☐ Required Intervention to Prevent Permanent Impairment/Damage (Devices)

3. Date of Event (mm/dd/yyyy)
4. Date of this Report (mm/dd/yyyy)
5. Describe Event, Problem or Product Use Error
6. Relevant Tests/Laboratory Data, Including Dates
7. Other Relevant History, Including Preexisting Medical Conditions (e.g., allergies, race, pregnancy, smoking and alcohol use, liver/kidney problems, etc.)

C. PRODUCT AVAILABILITY

Product Available for Evaluation? (Do not send product to FDA)

☐ Yes ☐ No ☐ Returned to Manufacturer on: ___ (mm/dd/yyyy)

D. SUSPECT PRODUCT(S)

1. Name, Strength, Manufacturer (from product label)
#1
#2

2.	Dose or Amount	Frequency	Route
#1			
#2			

3. Dates of Use (If unknown, give duration) from/to (or best estimate)
#1
#2

4. Diagnosis or Reason for Use (Indication)
#1
#2

5. Event Abated After Use Stopped or Dose Reduced?
#1 ☐ Yes ☐ No ☐ Doesn't Apply
#2 ☐ Yes ☐ No ☐ Doesn't Apply

6. Lot #
#1
#2

7. Expiration Date
#1
#2

8. Event Reappeared After Reintroduction?
#1 ☐ Yes ☐ No ☐ Doesn't Apply
#2 ☐ Yes ☐ No ☐ Doesn't Apply

9. NDC # or Unique ID

E. SUSPECT MEDICAL DEVICE

1. Brand Name
2. Common Device Name
3. Manufacturer Name, City and State
4. Model # / Lot # / Catalog # / Expiration Date (mm/dd/yyyy) / Serial # / Other #
5. Operator of Device ☐ Health Professional ☐ Lay User/Patient ☐ Other:
6. If Implanted, Give Date (mm/dd/yyyy)
7. If Explanted, Give Date (mm/dd/yyyy)
8. Is this a Single-use Device that was Reprocessed and Reused on a Patient? ☐ Yes ☐ No
9. If Yes to Item No. 8, Enter Name and Address of Reprocessor

F. OTHER (CONCOMITANT) MEDICAL PRODUCTS

Product names and therapy dates (exclude treatment of event)

G. REPORTER *(See confidentiality section on back)*

1. Name and Address
Phone # / E-mail
2. Health Professional? ☐ Yes ☐ No
3. Occupation
4. Also Reported to: ☐ Manufacturer ☐ User Facility ☐ Distributor/Importer
5. If you do NOT want your identity disclosed to the manufacturer, place an "X" in this box: ☐

FORM FDA 3500 (10/05) Submission of a report does not constitute an admission that medical personnel or the product caused or contributed to the event.

-Fold Here-

ADVICE ABOUT VOLUNTARY REPORTING

Detailed instructions available at: http://www.fda.gov/medwatch/report/consumer/instruct.htm

Report adverse events, product problems or product use errors with:

- Medications *(drugs or biologics)*
- Medical devices *(including in-vitro diagnostics)*
- Combination products *(medication & medical devices)*
- Human cells, tissues, and cellular and tissue-based products
- Special nutritional products *(dietary supplements, medical foods, infant formulas)*
- Cosmetics

Report product problems - quality, performance or safety concerns such as:

- Suspected counterfeit product
- Suspected contamination
- Questionable stability
- Defective components
- Poor packaging or labeling
- Therapeutic failures (product didn't work)

Report SERIOUS adverse events. An event is serious when the patient outcome is:

- Death
- Life-threatening
- Hospitalization - initial or prolonged
- Disability or permanent damage
- Congenital anomaly/birth defect
- Required intervention to prevent permanent impairment or damage
- Other serious (important medical events)

Report even if:

- You're not certain the product caused the event
- You don't have all the details

How to report:

- Just fill in the sections that apply to your report
- Use section D for all products except medical devices
- Attach additional pages if needed
- Use a separate form for each patient
- Report either to FDA or the manufacturer *(or both)*

Other methods of reporting:

- 1-800-FDA-0178 -- To FAX report
- 1-800-FDA-1088 -- To report by phone
- www.fda.gov/medwatch/report.htm -- To report online

If your report involves a serious adverse event with a device and it occurred in a facility outside a doctor's office, that facility may be legally required to report to FDA and/or the manufacturer. Please notify the person in that facility who would handle such reporting.

If your report involves a serious adverse event with a vaccine call 1-800-822-7967 to report.

Confidentiality: The patient's identity is held in strict confidence by FDA and protected to the fullest extent of the law. FDA will not disclose the reporter's identity in response to a request from the public, pursuant to the Freedom of Information Act. The reporter's identity, including the identity of a self-reporter, may be shared with the manufacturer unless requested otherwise.

-Fold Here-

The public reporting burden for this collection of information has been estimated to average 36 minutes per response, including the time for reviewing instructions, searching existing data sources, gathering and maintaining the data needed, and completing and reviewing the collection of information. Send comments regarding this burden estimate or any other aspect of this collection of information, including suggestions for reducing this burden to:

Department of Health and Human Services
Food and Drug Administration - MedWatch
10903 New Hampshire Avenue
Building 22, Mail Stop 4447
Silver Spring, MD 20993-0002

Please DO NOT RETURN this form to this address.

OMB statement:
"An agency may not conduct or sponsor, and a person is not required to respond to, a collection of information unless it displays a currently valid OMB control number."

U.S. DEPARTMENT OF HEALTH AND HUMAN SERVICES
Food and Drug Administration

FORM FDA 3500 (10/05) (Back) **Please Use Address Provided Below -- Fold in Thirds, Tape and Mail**

DEPARTMENT OF
HEALTH & HUMAN SERVICES

Public Health Service
Food and Drug Administration
Rockville, MD 20857

Official Business
Penalty for Private Use $300

BUSINESS REPLY MAIL
FIRST CLASS MAIL PERMIT NO. 946 ROCKVILLE MD

MEDWATCH
The FDA Safety Information and Adverse Event Reporting Program
Food and Drug Administration
5600 Fishers Lane
Rockville, MD 20852-9787

APPENDIX

I Drug/Food Interactions

A. DRUGS THAT SHOULD BE TAKEN WHILE FASTING

Alendronate
Ampicillin
AzoGantanol/Gantrisin
Bacampicillin
Bethanechol (may experience N&V)
Bisacodyl
Calcium carbonate
Captopril
Carbenicillin
Castor oil
Chloramphenicol
Claritin
Cyclosporine gel caps only (avoid fatty meals)
Demeclocycline (avoid high calcium foods/dairy products)
Dicloxacillin
Digoxin (avoid high fiber cereals and oatmeal)
Disopyramide
Digitalis preparations (not with high fiber foods)
Erythromycin base/estolate
Etidronate
Ferrous salts (not with tea, coffee, egg, cereals, fiber, or milk)
Fexofenadine
Flavoxate
Furosemide
Isoniazid
Isosorbide dinitrate
Ketoprofen (if GI distress occurs, may take with food)
Lansoprazole
Levodopa (not with high protein foods; meals delay absorption and peak plasma concentration; avoid caffeine)
Lisinopril
Lomustine (empty stomach will reduce nausea)
Methotrexate (milk, cream, or yogurt may decrease absorption)
Methyldopa (not with high protein foods; meals delay absorption and peak plasma concentration; avoid caffeine)
Nafcillin (inactivated by stomach acid; absorption variable with/without food)
Nalidixic acid
Naltrexone
Norfloxacin (milk, cream, or yogurt may decrease absorption)
Oxytetracycline (avoid dairy products and foods high in calcium)
Penicillamine (antacids, iron, and food decreases absorption)
Penicillin
Phenytoin (if GI distress occurs, may take with food; food effect depends on preparation)
Propantheline
Rifampicin
Sotalol
Sulfamethoxazole
Tetracycline (avoid dairy products and foods high in calcium)
Theophylline (absorption of controlled release varies by preparation)
Thyroid hormone preparations (limit foods containing goitrogens)
Terbutaline sulfate
Trientine (antacids, iron, and food reduces absorption)
Trimethoprim
Zyrtec

B. DRUGS THAT SHOULD BE TAKEN WITH FOOD

Allopurinol (after meal)
Atovaquone
Augmentin
Aspirin
Amiodarone
Baclofen
Bromocriptine
Buspirone
Carbamazepine (erratic absorption)
Carvedilol
Cefpodoxime
Chloroquine
Chlorothiazide
Cimetidine
Clofazimine
Diclofenac
Divalproex
Doxycyline
Felbamate
Fenofibrate (TriCor)
Fiorinal
Fludrocortisone
Fenoprofen
Gemfibrozil
Glyburide
Griseofulvin (high fat meals)
Hydrocortisone
Hydroxychloroquine (Plaquenil)
Indomethacin
Iron products
Isotretinoin
Itraconazole capsules
Ketorolac
Labetalol
Lithium
Lovastatin
Mebendazole
Methenamine
Methylprednisolone
Metoprolol
Metronidazole
Misoprostol
Metoprolol
Naltrexone
Naproxen
Nelfinavir (Viracept)
Niacin
Nifedipine (grapefruit juice increases bioavailability)
Nitrofurantoin
Olsalazine
Oxcarbazepine
Pentoxifylline
Pergolide
Piroxicam
Potassium salts
Prednisone
Probucol (high fat meals)

Procainamide
Propranolol
Ritonavir
Salsalate
Saquinavir
Sevelamer
Spironolactone
Sulfasalazine
Sulfinpyrazone
Sulindac
Ticlopidine
Tolmetin
Trazodone
Verapamil SR (absorption varies by manufacturer; too rapid absorption may cause heart block)

C. CONSTIPATING AGENTS

Antacids
Anticholinergic drugs
Anticonvulsants
Antihistamines
Antiparkinsonian drugs
BP meds (calcium channel blockers)
Clonidine
Corticosteroids
Diuretics
Ganglionic blocking agents
Iron supplements
Laxatives (when abused)
Lithium
MAO Inhibitors
Muscle relaxants
NSAIDs
Octreotide
Opioids
Phenothiazines
Prostaglandin synthesis inhibitors
Tranquilizers
Tricyclic antidepressants

D. DIARRHEAL AGENTS

Adrenergic neuron blockers: reserpine, guanethidine
Antacids (Mg containing)
H_2 receptor antagonists (i.e., ranitidine) PPIs (i.e, Omeprazole)
Antiarrhythmics (i.e., quinidine)
Antibiotics (especially broad spectrum agents)
Antihypertensives (beta blockers, ACE Inhibitors)
Anti-inflammatory drugs (NSAIDs, colchicine)
Chemotherapy agents
Cholinergic agonists and cholinesterase inhibitors
Glucophage
Metoclopramide
Misoprostol
Osmotic and stimulant laxatives
Theophylline

E. TYRAMINE CONTAINING FOODS

Moderate amounts of tyramine:
Banana peel
Broad beans
Cheese (all except cream cheese and cottage cheese)
Chianti, vermouth
Concentrated yeast extracts/ Brewer's yeast
Fermented cabbage products: sauerkraut, kimchee
Fermented soy products: fermented bean curd, soya bean paste, miso soup
Hydrolyzed protein extracts for sauces, soups, gravies
Imitation cheese
Liquid and powdered protein supplements
Meat extracts
Nonalcoholic beers
Prepared meats (sausage, chopped liver, pate, salami, mortadella)
Raspberries
Some non-United States brands of beer
Yeast products

Significant amounts of tyramine:
Avocado
Chocolate
Cream from fresh pasteurized milk
Distilled spirits
Peanuts
Red and white wines, port wines
Soy sauce
Yogurt

F. FOODS CONTAINING GOITROGENS

Asparagus
Brocolli
Brussels sprouts
Cabbage
Cauliflower
Kale
Lettuce
Millet
Mustard
Other leafy green vegetables
Peaches
Peanuts
Peas
Radishes
Rutabaga
Soy beans
Spinach
Strawberries
Turnip greens
Watercress

G. COUMARIN ANTICOAGULANTS AND DIETARY EFFECTS

Consumption of vitamin K-enriched foods may counteract the effects of anticoagulants since the drugs act through antagonism of vitamin K. Advise client on anticoagulants to maintain a steady, consistent intake of vitamin K-containing foods. The drug monograph for warfarin clearly lists these foods. Additionally, certain herbal teas (green tea, buckeye, horse chestnut, Woodruff, tonka beans, melitot) contain natural coumarins that can potentiate the effects of coumadin and should be avoided. Large amounts of avocado also potentiate the drug's effects. Brussels sprouts, broccoli, spinach, kale, turnip greens, and other cruciferous vegetables increase the catabolism of warfarin thereby decreasing its anticoagulant activities. Caffeinated beverages (i.e., cola, coffee, tea, hot chocolate, chocolate milk) can affect therapy. Alcohol intake of more than three drinks per day can affect clotting times. Herbal supplements can also affect bleeding time: Coenzyme Q10 is structurally similar to vitamin K, feverfew, garlic, and ginseng. Avoid herbal medications while on warfarin therapy.

H. GENERAL DRUG CLASS RECOMMENDATIONS

ACE inhibitors: Take captopril and moexipril 1 h before or 2 h after meals; food decreases absorption. Avoid high potassium foods as ACE increases K^+.

Analgesic/Antipyretic: Take on an empty stomach as food may slow the absorption.

Antacids: Take 1 h after or between meals. Avoid dairy foods as the protein in them can increase stomach acid.

Anti-anxiety agents: Caffeine may cause excitability, nervousness, and hyperactivity lessening the anti-anxiety drug effects.

Antibiotics: Penicillin generally should be taken on an empty stomach; may take with food if GI upset occurs. Do not mix with acidic foods: coffee, citrus fruits, and tomatoes; the acid interferes with absorption of penicillin, ampicillin, erythromycin and cloxacillin.

Anticoagulants: High vitamin K produces blood-clotting substance and may reduce drug effectiveness. Vitamin E >400 IU may prolong clotting time and increase bleeding risk.

Antidepressant drugs: May be taken with or without food.

Antifungals: Avoid taking with dairy products; avoid alcohol.

Antihistamines: Take on an empty stomach to increase effectiveness.

Bronchodilators with theophylline: High-fat meals may increase bio-availability while high-carbohydrate meals may decrease it. Food increases absorption of Theo-24 and Uniphyl which may cause increased N&V, headache, and irritability.

Cephalosporins: Take on an empty stomach 1 h before or 2 h after meals. May take with food if GI upset occurs.

Diuretics: Vary in interactions; some cause loss of potassium, calcium, and magnesium. Avoid salty food and natural black licorice as these increase K and Mg losses. Large doses of vitamin D can elevate blood pressure.

H_2 blockers: May take with or without regard to food.

HMG-CoA reductase inhibitors: Take lovastatin with the evening meal to enhance absorption.

Laxatives: Avoid dairy foods as calcium can decrease absorption.

Macrolides: Take on an empty stomach 1 h before or 2 h after meals. May take with food for GI upset.

MAO inhibitors: Have many dietary restrictions, so follow dietary guidelines as prescribed. Foods or alcoholic beverages containing tyramine may cause a fatal increase in BP.

Narcotic analgesics: Avoid alcohol as it may increase sedative effects.

Nitroimadazole (metronidazole): Avoid alcohol or food prepared with alcohol for at least three days after finishing the medicine. Alcohol may cause nausea, abdominal cramps, vomiting, headaches, and flushing.

NSAIDs: Take with food or milk to prevent irritation of the stomach.

Quinolones: Take on an empty stomach 1 h before or 2 h after meals. May take with food for GI upset but avoid calcium containing foods such as milk, yogurt, vitamins/minerals containing iron and antacids because they decrease drug concentrations. Caffeine containing products may lead to excitability and nervousness.

Sulfonamides: Take on an empty stomach 1 h before or 2 h after meals. May take with food if GI upset occurs.

Tetracyclines: Take on an empty stomach 1 h before or 2 h after meals. May take with food but avoid dairy products, antacids, and vitamins containing iron with tetracycline.

Reprinted from Spratto, G. and Woods, A. (2009) Delmar Nurse's Drug Handbook. Delmar, Cengage Learning: Clifton Park, NY.

APPENDIX J

Drugs That Should not Be Crushed

As a rule of thumb, any sustained-release or extended-release formulation should never be crushed. Instead, attempt to get a liquid formulation of the product so that it can be administered in that form. Coated products also should not be crushed. They were coated for a specific purpose, e.g., to prevent stomach irritation by the product, to prevent destruction of the product by stomach acid, to prevent an unwanted reaction, or to produce a prolonged or an extended effect.

These are some of the drugs that should not be crushed:

Accutane®
Aciphex®
Adalat cc SR®
Advicor ER®
Afrinol Repetab®
Allerest® capsule
Allegra D®
Aminodur Duratab®
Artane Sequel®
Arthrotec®
ASA E.C.®
ASA Enseal®
Augmentin XR®
Azulfadine Entab®
Betaphen-VK®
Biaxin XL®
Biscodyl EC®
Calan SR®
Cardizem LA, SR®
Ceclor CD®
Ceftin®
Chlortrimeton SR®
Choledyl SR®
Cipro XR®
Claritin-D®
Colace®
Colestid®
Compazine Spansule®
Concerta SR®
Creon EC®
Depakote ER®
Desyrel®
Dexedrine SR®
Diamox Sequel®
Dilacor XR®
Dimetapp SR®
Ditropan XL®
Donnatal Extentab®
Drixoral® tablet
Ecotrin® tablet
Effexor XR®
E-Mycin® tablet
Entex LA®
Erythromycin EC®
Feldene®
Feosol Spansule®
Feosol® tablet
Ferro Grad-500® tablet
Flomax®
Glucophage XR®
Glucatrol XL®
Humibid DM, LA®
Imdur SR, LA®
Indocin SR®
Isoptin SR®
Isordil® sublingual
Isordil Tembids®, Dinitrate
Kaon® tablet
K-Dur®, K-tab®
Klor-Con®
Levbid SR®
Lithobid SR®
Macrobid SR®
Mestinon Timespans®
Metadate CD, SR®
MS Contin®
Mucinex®
Nexium®
Niaspan®
Nitroglycerin® tablet
Nitrospan® capsule
Norpace CR®
Ornade Spansule®
OxyContin®
Pancrease EC, MT®
Paxil CR®
Pentosa®
Phazyme®
Plendil SR®
Prevacid®
Prilosec SR®
Procardia XL®
Protonix®
Proventil Repetabs®
Prozac weekly®
Quinaglute Duratab®
Quinidex Extenutab®
Slow K® tablet; Slow Mag®, Slow Fe®
Sorbitrate
Sudafed SA® capsule
Tegretol XR®
Teldrin® capsule
Tenuate Dospan®
Tessalon Perles®
Theobid Duracaps®
Theolair SR®
Thorazine Spansules®
Tiazac SR®
Toprol XL®
Trental SR®
Tylenol ER®
Uniphyl SR®
Verelan PM®
Volmax SR®
Voltaren EC®
Voltaren SR®
Wellbutrin SR®
Xanax SR®
Zerit XR®
Zomig ZMT®
Zyban®
Zyrtec-D®

Reprinted from Spratto, G. and Woods, A. (2009) Delmar Nurse's Drug Handbook. Delmar, Cengage Learning: Clifton Park, NY.

APPENDIX K

Drug Identification Guide

ACARBOSE
Precose
BAYER
Antidiabetic, oral; alpha-glucosidase inhibitor

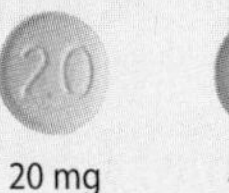

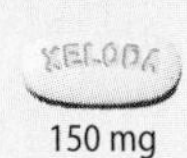

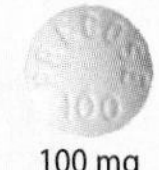
25 mg 50 mg 100 mg

ACETAMINOPHEN AND HYDROCODONE BITARTRATE
Vicodin
ABBOTT
Analgesic

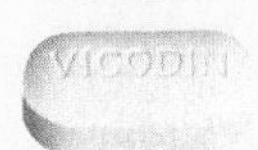

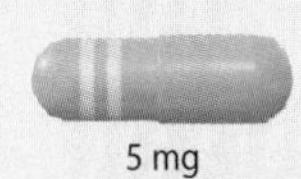

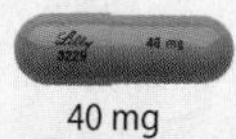

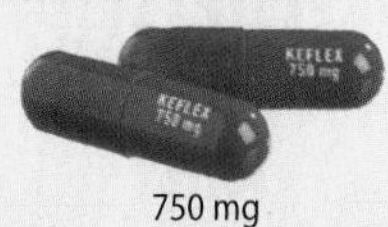

500 mg / 5 mg

Vicodin ES
ABBOTT

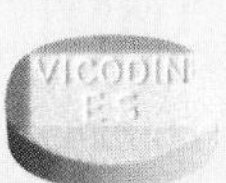

7.5 mg / 750 mg

Vicodin HP
ABBOTT

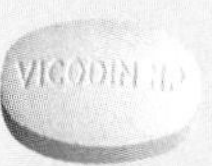

10 mg / 660 mg

ACETAMINOPHEN AND OXYCODONE HCl
Percocet
ENDO
Analgesic

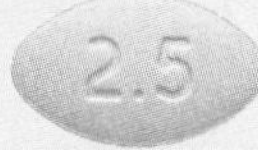

325 mg / 2.5 mg

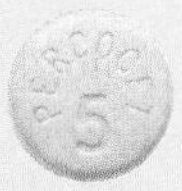

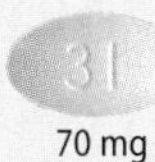

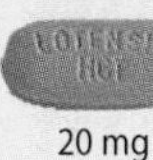

325 mg / 5 mg

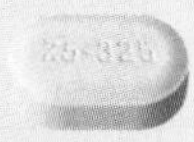
325 mg / 7.5 mg

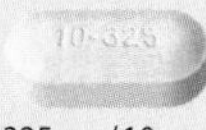

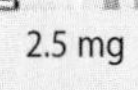
325 mg / 10 mg

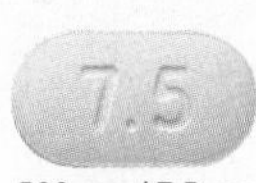

500 mg / 7.5 mg

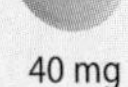

650 mg / 10 mg

ALENDRONATE SODIUM
Fosamax
MERCK
Bone growth regulator, biphosphonate

5 mg

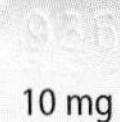
10 mg

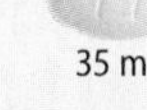

35 mg

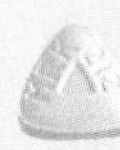

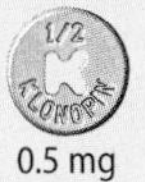
40 mg

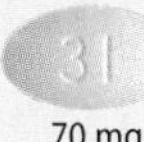
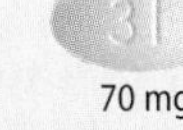

70 mg

AMLODIPINE AND BENAZEPRIL
Lotrel
NOVARTIS
Calcium channel blocker

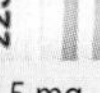

2.5 mg

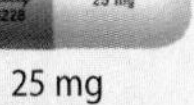

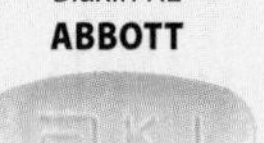
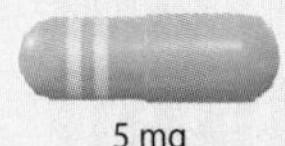
5 mg

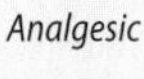

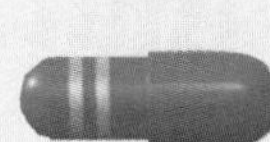

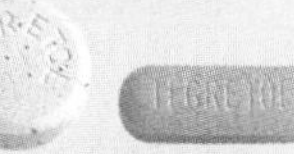
10 mg

AMPHETAMINE MIXTURES
Adderall XR
SHIRE
CNS stimulant

5 mg

ATENOLOL
Tenormin
ASTRAZENECA
Beta-adrenergic blocking agent

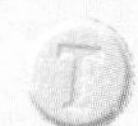
 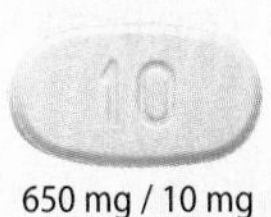 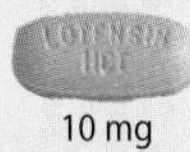

ATOMOXETINE HCl
Strattera
ELI LILLY
Antidepressant, selective serotonin reuptake inhibitor

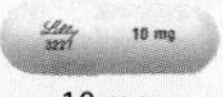

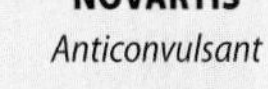
10 mg

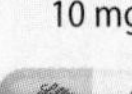

18 mg

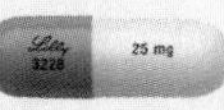
25 mg

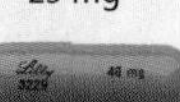

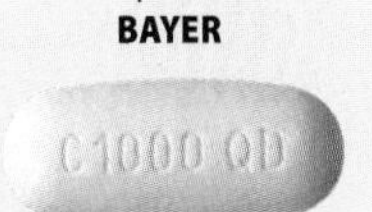
40 mg

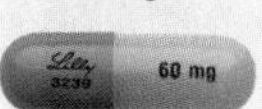

60 mg

BENAZEPRIL HCl
Lotensin
NOVARTIS
Antihypertensive, ACE inhibitor

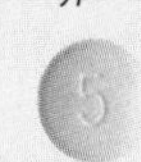

5 mg

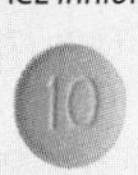
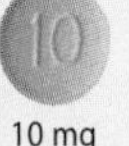
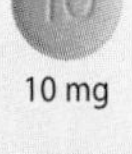

10 mg

20 mg

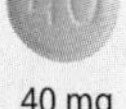

40 mg

Lotensin HCT
NOVARTIS

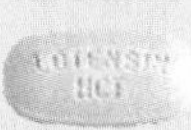
5 mg

Lotensin HCT
NOVARTIS

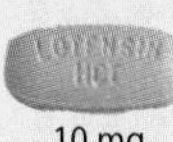

10 mg

Lotensin HCT
NOVARTIS

20 mg

BUDESONIDE
Pulmicort Respules
ASTRAZENECA
Glucocorticoid

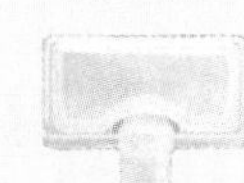
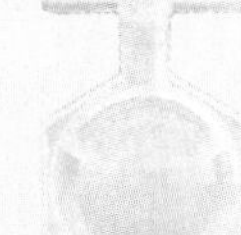

CANDESARTAN CILEXETIL
Atacand
ASTRAZENECA LP
Antihypertensive, angiotensin II receptor blocker

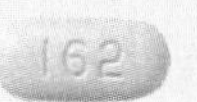
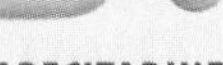

CAPECITABINE
Xeloda
LA ROCHE
Antineoplastic, antimetabolite

150 mg

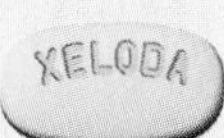

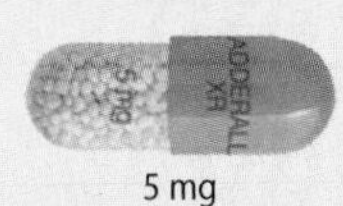

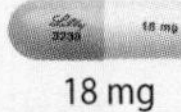

500 mg

CARBAMAZEPINE
Tegretol
NOVARTIS
Anticonvulsant

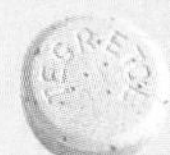
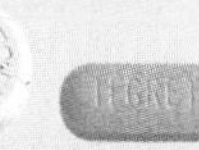
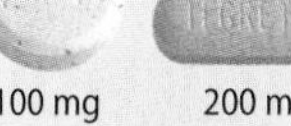
100 mg 200 mg

CEPHALEXIN HCl MONOHYDRATE
Keflex
ADVANCIS
Cephalosporin, first generation

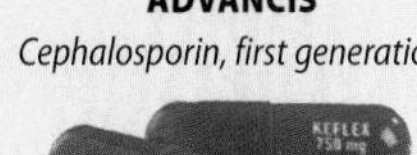
750 mg

CIPROFLOXACIN HCl
Cipro
BAYER
Antibiotic, fluoroquinolone

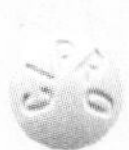

100 mg 250 mg

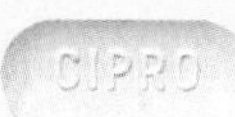

500 mg

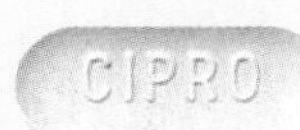

750 mg

Cipro XR
BAYER

500 mg

Cipro XR
BAYER

1000 mg

CLARITHROMYCIN
Biaxin
ABBOTT
Antibiotic, macrolide

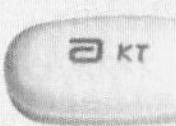
250 mg

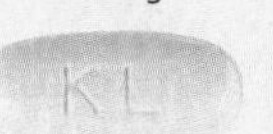

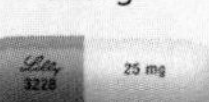

500 mg

Biaxin XL
ABBOTT

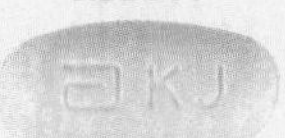

500 mg

CLONAZEPAM
Klonopin
LA ROCHE
Anticonvulsant

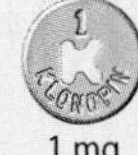
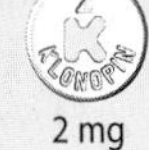
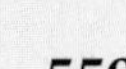
0.5 mg 1 mg 2 mg

CYCLOBENZAPRINE HCl
Flexeril
MERCK
Skeletal muscle relaxant, centrally acting

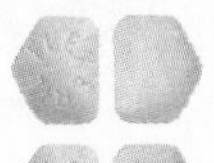

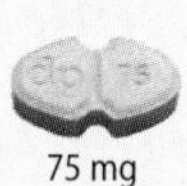

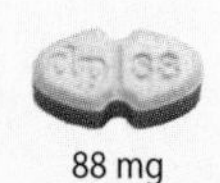

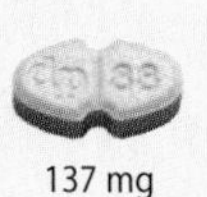

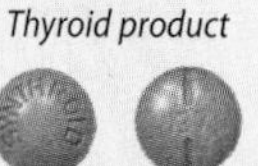
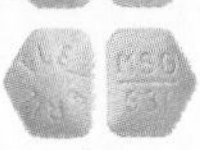

DEXMETHYLPHENIDATE HCl
Focalin
NOVARTIS
CNS stimulant

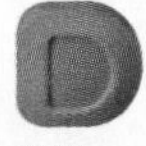

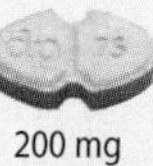
2.5 mg

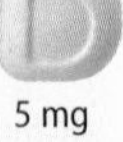

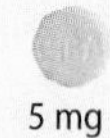
5 mg

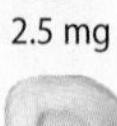

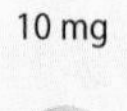

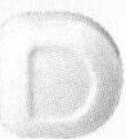
10 mg

DIAZEPAM
Valium
LA ROCHE
Antianxiety, benzodiazepine

2 mg

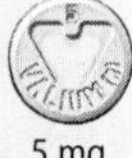
5 mg

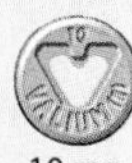
10 mg

DICLOFENAC SODIUM
Voltaren
NOVARTIS
Non steroidal anti-inflammatory

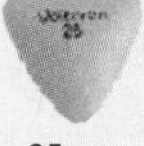
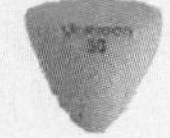

25 mg 50 mg 75 mg

ESOMEPRAZOLE MG
Nexium
ASTRAZENECA
Proton pump inhibitor

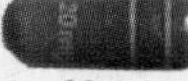
20 mg

EZETIMIBE
Zetia
MERCK
Antihyperlipidemic, HMG-CoA reductase inhibitor

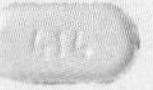
 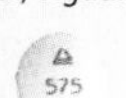

FELODIPINE
Plendil
ASTRAZENECA
Calcium channel blocker

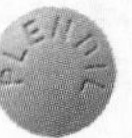
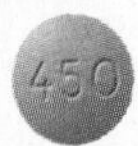

FENOFIBRATE
Tricor
ABBOTT
Antihyperlipidemic

48 mg

145 mg

FINASTERIDE
Proscar
ABBOTT
Androgen hormone inhibitor

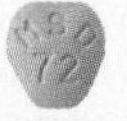
5 mg

FLUOXETINE HCl
Prozac
ELI- LILLY
Antidepressant, selective serotonin reuptake inhibitor

10 mg

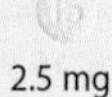

20 mg

FLUVASTATIN SODIUM
Lescol
NOVARTIS
Antihyperlipidemic, HMG-CoA reductase inhibitor

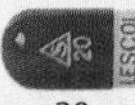
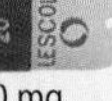
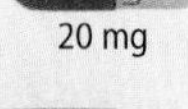
20 mg

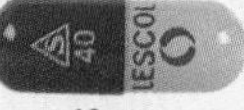
40 mg

GRANISETRON HCl
Kytril
LA ROCHE
Antiemetic, 5-HT3 receptor antagonist

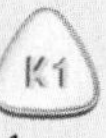
1 mg

HYDROCODONE BITARTRATE/ HOMATROPINE METHYBROMIDE
Hycodan
ENDO
Analgesic

KETOROLAC
Toradol oral
LA ROCHE
Nonsteroidal anti-inflammatory

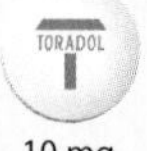
10 mg

LEVOTHYROXINE SODIUM (T4)
Levoxyl
KING
Thyroid product

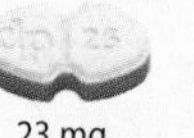
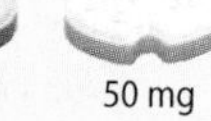
23 mg 50 mg

 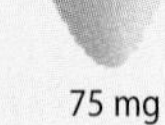
75 mg 88 mg

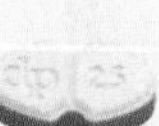

100 mg 112 mg

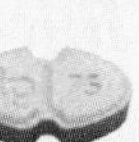

125 mg 137 mg

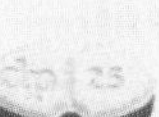
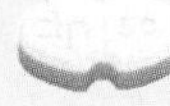
150 mg 175 mg

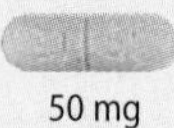

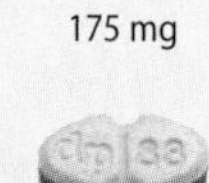

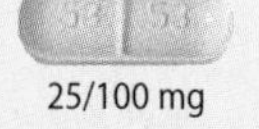
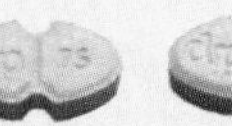

 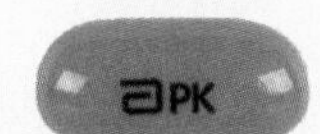
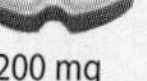
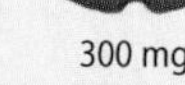
200 mg 300 mg

LEVOTHYROXINE SODIUM (T4)
Synthroid
ABBOTT
Thyroid product

 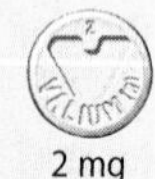

LISINOPRIL
Prinivil
MERCK
Antihypertensive, ACE inhibitor

2.5 mg

5 mg

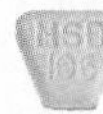
10 mg

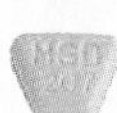
20 mg

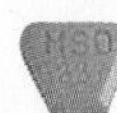
40 mg

LISINOPRIL
Zestril
ASTRAZENECA
Antihypertensive, ACE inhibitor

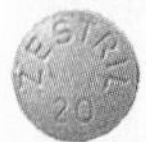
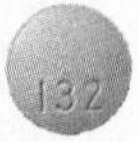

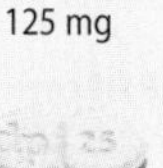

LOPINAVIR/RITONAVIR
Kaletra
ABBOTT
HIV protease inhibitor

LOSARTAN HCTZ
Hyzaar
MERCK
Angiotensin II receptor antagonist and diuretic

LOSARTAN POTASSIUM
Cozaar
MERCK
Antihypertensive, angiotensin II receptor blocker

25 mg

50 mg

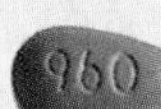
100 mg

LOVASTATIN
Mevacor
MERCK
Antihyperlipidemic, HMG-CoA reductase inhibitor

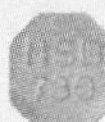

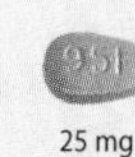
10 mg

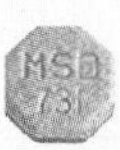
20 mg

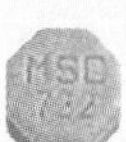
40 mg

METAXALONE
Skelaxin
KING
Muscle relaxant

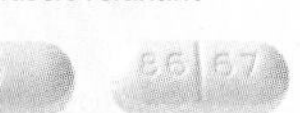

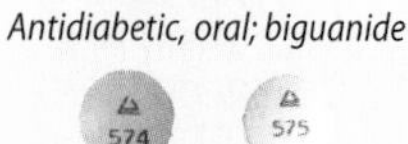

METFORMIN
Fortamet
FIRST HORIZON
Antidiabetic, oral; biguanide

 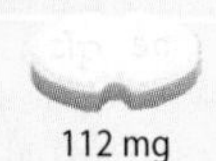

METHYLPHENIDATE HCl
Ritalin
NOVARTIS
CNS stimulant

5 mg

10 mg

20 mg

METOPROLOL SUCCINATE
Toprol
ASTRAZENECA
Beta-adrenergic blocking agent

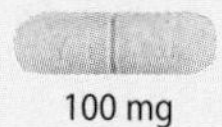

METOPROLOL TARTRATE
Lopressor
NOVARTIS
Beta-adrenergic blocking agent

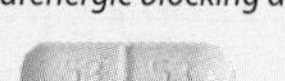
25/100 mg

50/100 mg

50 mg

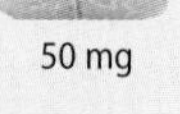

100 mg

MONTELUKAST SODIUM
Singulair
MERCK
Antiasthmatic, leukotriene receptor antagonist

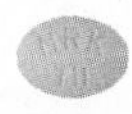
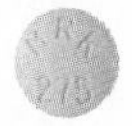

MOXIFLOXACIN HCl
Avelox
BAYER
Antibiotic, fluoroquinolone

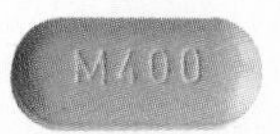

NAPROXEN
Naprosyn
LA ROCHE
Nonsteroidal anti-inflammatory

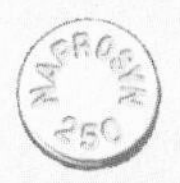
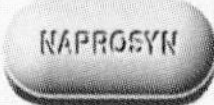 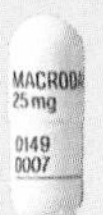

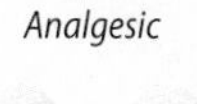

NAPROXEN SODIUM
Anaprox
LA ROCHE
Nonsteroidal anti-inflammatory

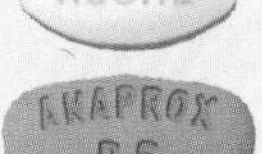

NITROFURANTOIN
Macrobid
PROCTOR AND GAMBLE
Antibiotic

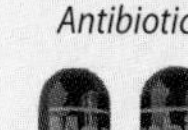
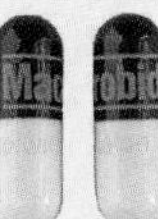 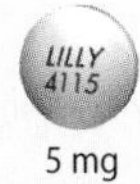

NITROFURANTOIN
Macrodantin
PROCTOR AND GAMBLE
Antibiotic

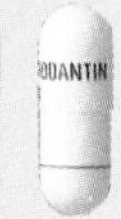
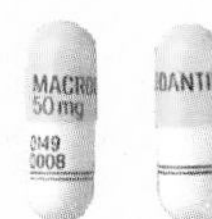
 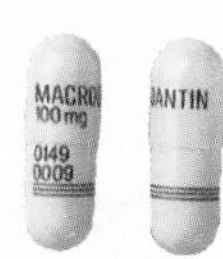

OLANZAPINE
Zyprexa
ELI LILLY
Antipsychotic

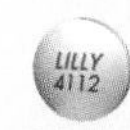

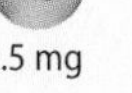

2.5 mg 5 mg

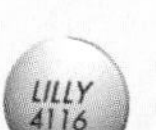
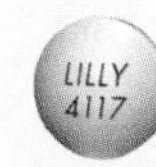

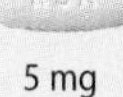

7.5 mg 10 mg

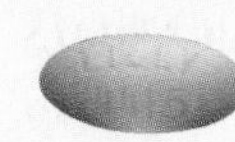

15 mg

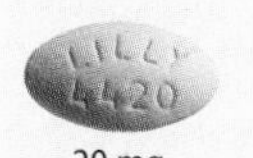

20 mg

Zyprexa Zydia
ELI LILLY

15 mg

Zyprexa Zydia
ELI LILLY

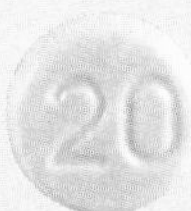

20 mg

OSELTAMIVIR PHOSPHATE
Tamiflu
LA ROCHE
Antiviral

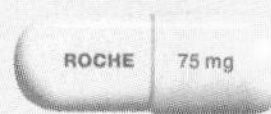

QUETIAPINE FUMARATE
Seroquel
ASTRAZENECA
Antipsychotic

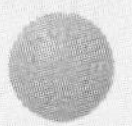

OXYCODONE AND ACETAMINOPHEN
Endocet
ENDO
Analgesic

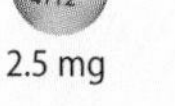

5 mg / 325 mg

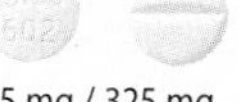
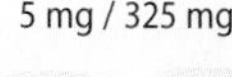

7.5 mg / 325 mg

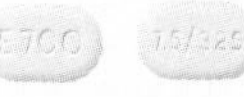

10 mg / 325 mg

7.5 mg / 500 mg

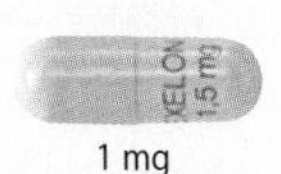

10 mg / 650 mg

POTASSIUM SALTS
Klor-con and Klor-con M20
UPSHER SMITH
Electrolyte

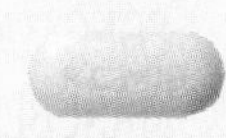
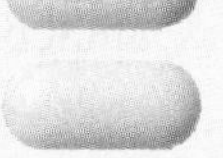

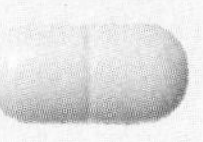

RALOXIFENE HCl
Evista
ELI LILLY
Estrogen receptor modulator

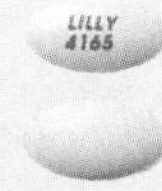

RISEDRONATE SODIUM
Actonel
PROCTOR AND GAMBLE
Bone growth regulator, biphosphonate

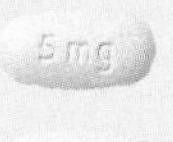

5 mg

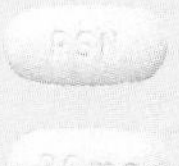

30 mg

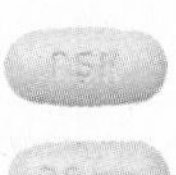
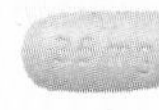

35 mg

RIVASTIGMINE TARTRATE
Exelon
NOVARTIS
Treatment of Alzheimer's Disease

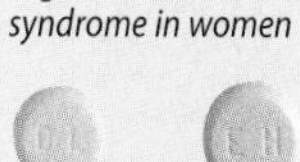

1 mg

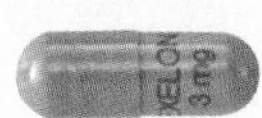

3 mg

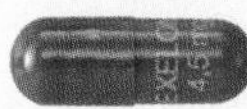

4.5 mg

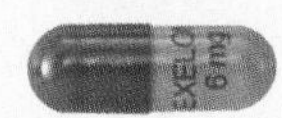

6 mg

RIZATRIPTAN BENZOATE
Maxalt
MERCK

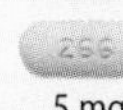

5 mg

10 mg

Maxalt MLT
MERCK

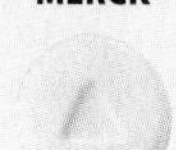

5 mg

Maxalt MLT
MERCK
Antimigraine

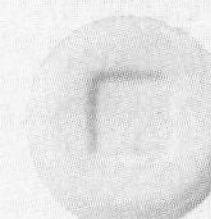

10 mg

ROFECOXIB
Vioxx
MERCK
Nonsteroidal anti-inflammatory; COX-2 inhibitor

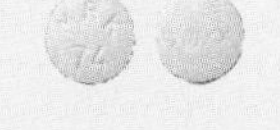

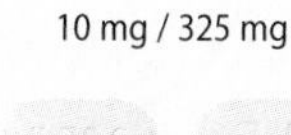

ROSUVASTATIN
Crestor
ASTRAZENECA
Antihyperlipidemic, HMG-CoA reductase inhibitor

SIMVASTATIN
Zocor
MERCK
Antihyperlipidemic, HMG-CoA reductase inhibitor

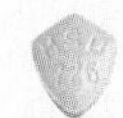

5 mg

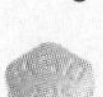

10 mg

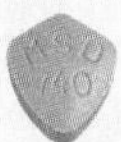

20 mg

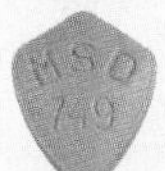

40 mg

80 mg

SPIRONOLACTONE
Aldactone
MYLAN
Diuretic, potassium-sparing

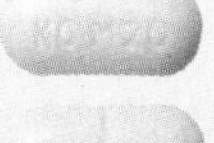

TAMOXIFEN CITRATE
Nolvadex
ASTRAZENECA
Antiestrogen

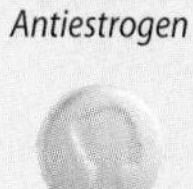

TEGASEROD MALEATE
Zelnorm
NOVARTIS
Drug for irritable bowel syndrome in women

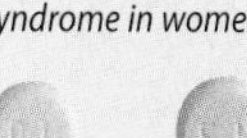

5 mg 6 mg

TEMAZEPAM

Restoril

MALLINCKRODT

Sedative-hypnotic, benzodiazepine

7.5 mg

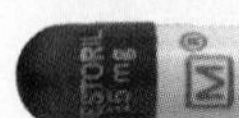

15 mg

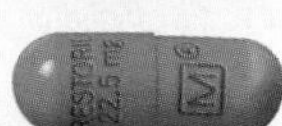

22.5 mg

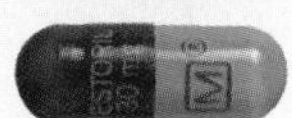

30 mg

TRIAMTERENE AND HYDROCHLOROTHIAZIDE

Maxide

MYLAN

Antihypertensive, combination drug

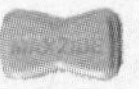

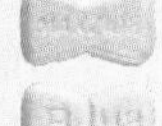

VALGANCICLOVIR HCl

Valcyte

LA ROCHE

Antiviral

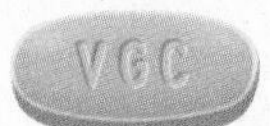

20 mg

ZAFIRLUKAST

Accolate

ASTRAZENECA

Antiasthmatic

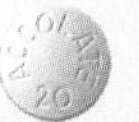

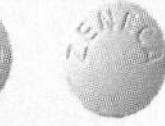

ZOLMITRIPTAN

Zomig

ASTRAZENECA

Antimigraine

Answer Keys

Chapter 1

Short Answer

1. C-II drugs have high abuse potential and accepted medical use, require a prescription, and no refills are permitted without a prescription; C-V drugs have low abuse potential and accepted medical use, and do not require a prescription for individuals 18 or older.
2. Drug Enforcement Agency (DEA) is tasked with the regulation and enforcement of laws related to drug use, sale, distribution, and manufacturing. The DEA also requires maintenance of transactions related to controlled substances.
3. The FDA is responsible for drug product development as well as general safety standards in the production of drugs, foods, and cosmetics.
4. 1906; Pure Food and Drug Act.
5. a. Regulates the manufacture, distribution, and dispensation of drugs with a potential for abuse; deals with control and enforcement.
   b. The first attempt to control and regulate the manufacture, distribution, and sale of drugs.
   c. The importation, manufacture, sale, and use of opium, codeine, and their derivatives and compounds; it was replaced by the CSA.
   d. Prescription drugs.

Multiple Choice

1. A 2. D 3. B 4. B 5. A 6. B
7. D 8. C 9. D 10. A 11. C 12. D

Matching

1. D 2. C 3. B 4. A

Answers to Critical Thinking Questions:

1. The Harrison Narcotic Act of 1914, which was replaced by the Comprehensive Drug Abuse Prevention and Control Act.
2. The FDA has the power to approve or deny new drug applications and even to conduct inspections to ensure compliance.
3. The Pure Food and Drug Act of 1906.

Chapter 2

Multiple Choice

1. B 2. A 3. C 4. D 5. B 6. B
7. D 8. D 9. A 10. C 11. D 12. A

Matching

1. J 2. I 3. H 4. E 5. F 6. C
7. D 8. B 9. G 10. A

Answers to Critical Thinking Questions:

1. It is cheaper.
2. Because generic drug formularies may be different, the inert ingredients may be somewhat different and consequently may affect the ability of the drug to reach the target cells and produce an effect.
3. He must verify that the physician did not intend to prescribe only the trade name version of the drug.

Chapter 3

Multiple Choice

1. C 2. B 3. C 4. A 5. B 6. D
7. D 8. A 9. C 10. B 11. D 12. A
13. A 14. C 15. B

Fill in the Blank

1. first-pass effect
2. efficacy
3. pharmacodynamics
4. glomerular filtration rate
5. rapidly
6. Newborns
7. placebo

Answers to Critical Thinking Questions:

1. Therapeutic Index (TI) = median lethal dose: LD_{50}

$$\frac{\text{median lethal dose: } LD_{50}}{\text{median effective dose: } ED_{50}}$$

2. Elderly patients normally lose approximately 35% of their nephrons by the age of 75; the physician should consider a dose that is much lower than the average adult dose.
3. Gentamicin can cause hearing loss (ototoxicity) and may be potentially neurotoxic.

Chapter 4

Multiple Choice

1. B	2. D	3. C	4. D	5. A	6. D
7. B	8. C	9. B	10. D		

Matching

1. E	2. D	3. A	4. C	5. B

Fill in the Blank

1. 5-HT
2. neuroleptic
3. mental illness
4. bipolar
5. manic-depressive
6. lithium
7. major depression

Answers to Critical Thinking Questions:

1. SSRIs are much safer than other types, and are the drug(s) of choice for major depression.
2. SSRIs are the newest type of antidepressants.
3. Contraindicated foods include: beer, red wines, cheese, chocolate, avocados, bananas, etc.

Chapter 5

Multiple Choice

1. B	2. C	3. D	4. A	5. D	6. B
7. A	8. A	9. D	10. C	11. D	12. D
13. A	14. C	15. D			

Fill in the Blank

1. anxiety; insomnia
2. dependence
3. GABA
4. panic attacks
5. anxiety; insomnia
6. tranquilizers
7. D

Answers to Critical Thinking Questions:

1. There are two choices: either paroxetine or sertraline hydrochloride.
2. No, both paroxetine and sertraline hydrochloride are also used for panic disorders.
3. The most severe adverse effect would be CNS and respiratory depression.

Chapter 6

Multiple Choice

1. C	2. D	3. D	4. A	5. B	6. C
7. A	8. A	9. D	10. B	11. A	12. B
13. D	14. A	15. C			

True or False

1. T	2. F	3. F	4. F	5. T	6. T
7. T	8. T	9. T	10. F		

Answers to Critical Thinking Questions:

1. Cholinergic agonists are the best class of drugs for these conditions.
2. Undesirable effects of cholinergic agonist drugs include flushing, sweating, abdominal cramps, difficulty in visual accommodation, headache, and convulsions (at high doses). Specific GI adverse effects include epigastric distress, diarrhea, involuntary defecation, nausea and vomiting, and colic.
3. The drug of choice should only be used cautiously in patients with asthma and hyperthyroidism.

Chapter 7

Multiple Choice

1. B	2. D	3. A	4. B	5. B	6. D
7. C	8. B	9. B	10. C		

Fill in the Blank

1. basal nuclei
2. 60
3. acetylcholine
4. Alzheimer's disease
5. acetylcholinesterase
6. tacrine
7. narrow-angle glaucoma
8. Parkinsonism
9. epinephrine
10. B_6
11. Alzheimer's disease
12. Parkinson's disease

Answers to Critical Thinking Questions:

1. Levodopa is the drug of choice for Parkinson's disease.
2. It should be used only with caution because of her history of hepatitis C.
3. No, levodopa should be avoided in patients with narrow-angle glaucoma.

Chapter 8

Multiple Choice

1. B	2. D	3. C	4. C	5. A	6. B
7. D	8. C	9. C	10. B	11. D	12. C
13. A	14. D	15. B			

Fill in the Blank

1. Depakene
2. physician
3. generalized
4. psychomotor
5. phenytoin
6. petit mal
7. valproic acid; zonisamide

Answers to Critical Thinking Questions:

1. The phenytoin-like drug valproic acid is used for prevention of migraines.
2. Succinimides are the type of phenytoin-like drugs used to treat absence seizures.
3. The most dangerous adverse effects of phenytoin-like drugs may be fatal liver toxicity and bone marrow suppression.

Chapter 9

Multiple Choice

1. D	2. A	3. C	4. D	5. C	6. A
7. C	8. B	9. C	10. A	11. B	12. D

Matching

1. F	2. E	3. C	4. D	5. B	6. A

Fill in the Blank

1. nerve block
2. atropine; scopolamine
3. laughing gas
4. rare

Answers to Critical Thinking Questions:

1. Local infiltration anesthesia would be the best type to use for this patient.
2. Normally there are no drug interactions between local infiltration anesthesia and these drugs.
3. The only potential adverse effect would occur if the patient has a true allergic reaction to the local anesthetic used.

Chapter 10

Multiple Choice

1. B	2. C	3. A	4. A	5. C	6. B
7. A	8. B	9. C	10. B	11. B	12. D
13. A	14. C	15. D			

Fill in the Blank

1. somatic motor
2. C

3. safety margin
4. A. gold compounds
   B. penicillamine
   C. corticosteroids
5. A. poor wound healing
   B. hyperglycemia
   C. hypertension
   D. osteoporosis
   E. GI bleeding
6. not known
7. first; joint

Answers to Critical Thinking Questions:

1. Allopurinol should be used with caution; the other choice, colchicine, is contraindicated in the presence of peptic ulcer.
2. Colchicine is the drug of choice for acute gouty arthritis.
3. The drug is very toxic, and it should be stopped at the first symptom of toxicity, such as nausea, vomiting, diarrhea, and abdominal pain. Adverse effects of oral colchicine include nausea, abdominal cramps, and diarrhea.

Chapter 11

Multiple Choice

1. D 2. C 3. B 4. C 5. B 6. A
7. B 8. C 9. A 10. B

Fill in the Blank

1. nitrates
2. fast channel blockers
3. IV
4. nystagmus, blurred vision, vertigo, and hyperplasia of the gums
5. myocardial systolic contraction

Matching

1. D 2. B 3. E 4. C 5. A

Answers to Critical Thinking Questions:

1. Cigarette smoking, fried foods and meat, and stress.
2. By narrowing the small arteries (such as the coronary artery) causing occlusion, reducing blood and oxygen supply to the myocardium.
3. With angina, the myocardium suffers from oxygen depletion, causing necrosis (death) of the muscle; this causes chest pain.

Chapter 12

Multiple Choice

1. D 2. B 3. A 4. A 5. D 6. B
7. D 8. A 9. B 10. C 11. B 12. D
13. B 14. A 15. C

Matching

1. G 2. F 3. D 4. C 5. E 6. B
7. A

Answers to Critical Thinking Questions:

1. The pathophysiology of essential (primary) hypertension is unknown.
2. Atherosclerosis or arteriosclerosis.
3. Hypertension causes the eventual weakening of the heart muscle. This results in a reduced capacity of the heart to pump blood efficiently, causing blood to collect in certain body locations (such as the lungs). The term "congestive" refers to this collection of blood.

Chapter 13

Multiple Choice

1. B 2. C 3. C 4. A 5. D 6. C
7. A 8. B 9. B 10. D

Fill in the Blank

1. inflammation is present
2. blood to clot
3. oral anticoagulants
4. spontaneous bleeding
5. vitamin K
6. aspirin

Matching

1. D 2. C 3. B 4. A

Answers to Critical Thinking Questions:

1. The aging process changes many organs in the body. Because of George's age, his skin is much thinner than when he was young. Aspirin is an anticoagulant which may cause internal or external bleeding.
2. George's physician should order blood tests to rule out blood clotting disorders and thrombocytopenia. He may also suggest that George discontinue taking the aspirin.
3. George should probably stop taking the aspirin. His other medications do not affect bleeding.

Chapter 14

Multiple Choice

1. D 2. A 3. C 4. B 5. A 6. B
7. D 8. B 9. D 10. A 11. A 12. B
13. D 14. D

Fill in the Blank

1. allergic asthma; children
2. adults and children older than 12 years
3. a. bronchial asthma
   b. emphysema
   c. bronchitis
4. liver toxicity and dyspepsia
5. histamine

Matching

1. E 2. D 3. B 4. C 5. A

Answers to Critical Thinking Questions:

1. The main predisposing factors for emphysema and pneumonia include: history of cigarette smoking, age, respiratory irritants, genetic factors, and immune deficiency.
2. Other complications may include: chronic bronchitis; heart disease; stroke; or cancers of the mouth, pharynx, larynx, lung, esophagus, pancreas, kidney, bladder, or cervix.
3. The various drugs that are available to help a person stop smoking include: bupropion and nicotine (in gum and patch forms).

Chapter 15

Multiple Choice

1. A 2. C 3. D 4. D 5. B 6. B
7. A 8. B 9. D 10. B 11. D 12. B
13. C 14. D

Matching

1. E 2. D 3. G 4. F 5. C 6. A
7. B

Fill in the Blank

1. Heartburn, dyspepsia, and peptic ulcer
2. They block the H_2 receptors in the stomach and decrease gastric acid secretion
3. They impair GI tract absorption of fat-soluble vitamins

Answers to Critical Thinking Questions:

1. A wide variety of prescriptions and OTC medications are available for the treatment of gastritis or peptic ulcer. These drugs include: antacids, H_2-receptor antagonists, proton pump inhibitors, and antibiotics.
2. If *Helicobacter* infection (that causes peptic ulcer and gastritis) remains untreated, there will be a risk of adenocarcinoma of the stomach.
3. Because of the strong acid environment of the stomach, microorganisms are usually unable to grow, except *Helicobacter pylori.*

Chapter 16

Multiple Choice

1. C 2. D 3. B 4. C 5. A 6. C
7. A 8. B 9. A 10. B 11. B 12. D
13. D 14. A 15. D

Matching

1. D 2. G 3. F 4. E 5. B 6. C
7. A

Answers to Critical Thinking Questions:

1. The most common causes of hypothyroidism in adults include: lack of iodine in the diet, surgical removal of the thyroid, or radiation therapy to the thyroid. Hypothyroidism may also be due to pituitary dysfunction.
2. Natural thyroid hormones are approved for supplement or replacement needs of hypothyroidism. Synthetic thyroid replacements include: levothyroxine, liothyronine, and liotrix.
3. Untreated hypothyroidism may result in severe myxedema, coma, and death.

Chapter 17

Multiple Choice

1. B	2. B	3. B	4. D	5. C	6. A
7. D	8. C	9. C	10. A	11. C	12. B
13. B	14. D	15. B			

Fill in the Blank

1. muscle mass
2. interstitial
3. pituitary
4. conception
5. breast cancer; prostate cancer
6. anterior pituitary gland; hypothalamus
7. progestin

Answers to Critical Thinking Questions:

1. Testosterone cypionate is used for replacement therapy in androgen deficiency.
2. This agent controls development and maintenance of secondary sexual characteristics.
3. Adverse effects of testosterone cypionate include hirsuitism, acne, gynecomastia, male pattern baldness, headache, anxiety, and depression.

Chapter 18

Multiple Choice

1. B	2. A	3. D	4. B	5. C	6. B
7. D	8. A	9. D	10. C	11. B	12. A
13. C	14. D	15. D			

Matching

1. G	2. E	3. F	4. D	5. C	6. A
7. B					

Answers to Critical Thinking Questions:

1. The physician should explain that this drug reduces intracranial pressure.
2. The physician should explain that mannitol is contraindicated during intracranial bleeding; thus, its use in this situation should be discontinued.

Chapter 19

Multiple Choice

1. B	2. D	3. A	4. A	5. B	6. B
7. C	8. C	9. B	10. B	11. D	12. B
13. C	14. C	15. A			

Matching

1. E	2. B	3. D	4. A	5. C

Fill in the Blank

1. warfarin
2. tea
3. copper; Wilson's
4. infusion pump

Answers to Critical Thinking Questions:

1. John should tell his grandmother that excessive use of certain vitamins and minerals may cause toxicity.
2. Nicotinic acid and magnesium are examples of supplements that may have potential interactions with diabetes medications.

3. Excessive amounts of vitamin A can cause the following signs and symptoms: excessive peeling of the skin, hyperlipidemia, hypercalcemia, hepatotoxicity, and can lead to death. Excessive amounts of vitamin D may lead to a toxicity syndrome that can result in hypercalcemia, malabsorption (which may lead to constipation), kidney stones, and calcium deposits on bones.

Chapter 20

Multiple Choice

1. A 2. B 3. C 4. D 5. C 6. A
7. C 8. B 9. D 10. A 11. C 12. B
13. C 14. D 15. C

Matching

1. E 2. D 3. B 4. C 5. A

Matching: Generic to Brand Names

1. C 2. D 3. B 4. E 5. A

Answers to Critical Thinking Questions:

1. The likely consequence to refusal of radiation therapy and chemotherapy after the surgery would be the development of more cancer cells.
2. The most common adverse effects of chemotherapy agents include: anorexia, nausea, vomiting, diarrhea, hair loss, leukopenia, anemia, and thrombocytopenia (fewer than normal platelets in the blood).
3. Radiation therapy and chemotherapy are initially recommended; surgery may be an option based on the progress of the metastasis.

Chapter 21

Multiple Choice

1. A 2. C 3. D 4. C 5. A 6. B
7. D 8. B 9. B 10. D 11. B 12. C
13. C 14. A 15. C

Matching

1. C 2. E 3. D 4. A 5. B

Answers to Critical Thinking Questions:

1. The pharmacist should advise the patient that aspirin is contraindicated for those individuals who have a history of peptic ulcer.
2. The major adverse effects of aspirin include epigastric pain, stomach bleeding, and stomach ulceration.
3. Since the patient has experienced chest pain, the pharmacist may advise the patient to take nitroglycerin instead of aspirin.

Chapter 22

Multiple Choice

1. B 2. D 3. A 4. C 5. A 6. D
7. B 8. B 9. A 10. D 11. C 12. D
13. B 14. D 15. A

Matching

1. G 2. F 3. E 4. D 5. B 6. C
7. A

Answers to Critical Thinking Questions:

1. For Christian's exposure to tuberculosis, he should be given only isoniazid as a prophylactic against contracting the disease.
2. Christian will need to take isoniazid for up to one year to treat his exposure.
3. Since Christian does not have tuberculosis, and was only exposed to its microorganism, his family does not need to receive preventative medications.

Chapter 23

Multiple Choice

1. D 2. D 3. C 4. D 5. A 6. B
7. A 8. A 9. C 10. A 11. D 12. B
13. A 14. C

Matching

1. H 2. F 3. G 4. C 5. B 6. A
7. E 8. D

Answers to Critical Thinking Questions:

1. Diabetic women are at higher risk of vaginal infections due to their internal body environment being more conducive to bacterial and yeast growth. The physician should recommend regular follow-ups after treatment for her infection to prevent reoccurrence.
2. Alcohol must be avoided when using Flagyl.

Chapter 24

Multiple Choice

1. C	2. B	3. A	4. D	5. D	6. B
7. C	8. D	9. B	10. A	11. B	12. C
13. A	14. C	15. A	16. D	17. C	18. C
19. D	20. D				

Answers to Critical Thinking Questions:

1. Tylenol III contains codeine, which is easily passed through the breast milk. This can cause respiratory depression and death.
2. Acetaminophen and codeine.
3. No, because ibuprofen is unlikely to cause respiratory depression when passed through breast milk to an infant.

Chapter 25

Multiple Choice

1. D	2. A	3. C	4. B	5. D	6. B
7. D	8. A	9. D	10. C	11. A	12. D
13. A	14. A	15. C			

Fill in the Blank

1. a. pneumonia
   b. osteomyelitis
   c. endocarditis or meningitis
2. digitalis; diuretics
3. patent ductus arteriosus
4. dependent diabetes mellitus
5. *Haemophilus influenzae*
6. pulmonary surfactant
7. acetaminophen

Answers to Critical Thinking Questions

1. Iron deficiency anemia.
2. After four months, it is important to add baby foods, formula, or iron supplements.
3. Sickle-cell anemia may be seen in African-American infants who have the sickle cell trait; when untreated, it usually causes death

Chapter 26

Multiple Choice

1. D	2. B	3. D	4. C	5. B	6. C
7. A	8. A	9. D	10. D	11. B	12. D
13. C	14. C	15. A			

Fill in the Blank

1. a. confusion
   b. impairment of bladder emptying
   c. decongestant activity
   d. constipation
2. nausea
3. risk of toxicity is increased
4. injuries; falls
5. advanced age
6. must be reduced
7. bradycardia, asthma, and heart failure

Answers to Critical Thinking Questions:

1. He is more likely to experience external or internal bleeding.
2. Hepatic clearance is decreased in elderly people with liver diseases, meaning that there is less blood circulation in the liver. Therefore, metabolism of drugs will decrease.
3. Since the protein binding of phenytoin would be reduced as a result of this patient's liver disease, the phenytoin may remain in the liver for a longer period, causing toxicity.

Glossary

A

Absence seizure – generalized seizure that does not involve motor convulsions; also referred to as "petit mal"

Absorption – the movement of a drug from its site of administration into the bloodstream

Acetylcholine – a neurotransmitter that plays a major role in cognitive function and memory formation as well as motor control

Acquired Immunodeficiency Syndrome (AIDS) – a severe immunological disorder caused by the retrovirus HIV, resulting in a defect in cell-mediated immune response

Acromegaly – overdevelopment of the bones of the head, face, and feet

Active transport – a process that moves particles in fluid through membranes from a region of lower concentration to a region of high concentration

Acute pain – pain that is of sudden onset and brief course; can also mean "severe"

Adrenergic blocker agents – drugs that antagonize the secretion of epinephrine and norepinephrine from sympathetic terminal neurons; also known as sympatholytics

Adrenergic receptor – receptors that mediate responses to epinephrine (adrenaline) and norepinephrine

Adrenocorticotropic hormone (ACTH) – another hormone from the anterior pituitary gland that stimulates the growth of the adrenal gland cortex and the secretion of corticosteroids

Adrenogenital syndrome – congenital adrenal hyperplasia; a group of disorders involving steroid hormone production in the adrenal glands, leading to a deficiency of cortisol

Adsorbent agents – drugs with the ability to adsorb gases, toxins, and bacteria

Affinity – the force that impels certain atoms to unite with certain others

Aggregation – the clumping together of platelets to form a clot

Agonist – the drug that produces a functional change in a cell

Agonist-antagonists – agents that can initiate or resist actions

Allergic rhinitis – inflammation of the nasal mucosa that is due to the sensitivity of the nasal tissue to an allergen

Allergy – a state of hypersensitivity induced by exposure to a particular antigen

Alopecia – loss of hair from anywhere on the body, sometimes until complete baldness is reached

Alpha-receptors – an adrenergic receptor; there are two types: $alpha_1$ and $alpha_2$

Alzheimer's disease – a disorder causing severe cognitive dysfunction in older persons in which the brain experiences atrophy (shrinkage) and exhibits senile plaques

Amebicides and trichomonacides – drugs use to treat amebic and trichomonal infections

Amenorrhea – the absence of a menstrual period in a woman of reproductive age

Analgesic – a compound that relieves pain by altering perception without producing anesthesia or loss of consciousness

Anaphylactic reaction – a severe, life-threatening allergic reaction to a drug

Anaphylactic shock – a severe and sometimes fatal allergic reaction

Androgen – the generic term for any natural or synthetic compound, usually a steroid hormone, that stimulates or controls the development of masculine characteristics by binding to androgen receptors

Anesthesia – a loss of feeling or sensation

Anesthetic – an agent that partially or completely numbs or eliminates sensitivity with or without loss of consciousness

Angina pectoris – an episodic, reversible oxygen insufficiency

Angiotensin II receptor antagonists – drugs that block the binding of angiotensin II to the angiotensin II type 1 receptor

Angiotensin-converting enzyme inhibitors – drugs that competitively inhibit conversion of angiotensin I to angiotensin II, a potent vasoconstrictor, through the angiotensin-converting enzyme activity, with resultant lower levels of angiotensin II

Anorexia nervosa – an eating disorder characterized by a psychological fear of being overweight; view of body image is distorted

Antacids – neutralize hydrochloric acid and raise gastric pH, thus inhibiting pepsin (a gastric enzyme)

Antagonist – the drug blocks a functional change in the cell

Antianxiety agents – drugs that relieve anxiety; also known as anxiolytics

Antibiotics – substances that have the ability to destroy or interfere with the development of a living organism

Anticoagulants – agents used to prevent the formation of a blood clot

Anticonvulsant – a drug that prevents or stops a convulsive seizure

Antidepressants – drugs used to treat depression

Antidiuretic hormone (ADH) – released when the body is low on water, and causes the kidneys to conserve water, but not salt, by concentrating the urine and reducing urine volume

Antiemetic – a drug that stops vomiting

Antigen – a substance that is introduced into the body and induces the formation of antibodies

Antihistamines – drugs that counteract the action of histamine

Antimalarial agents – drugs used to treat malaria infections

Antimetabolite – a substance that is produced to alter the actions of liver enzymes

Antimetabolites – prevent cancer cell growth by affecting its DNA production

Antimicrobial – an anti-infective drug produced from synthetic substances

Antineoplastic agents – used to treat cancers or malignant neoplasms

Antiplatelet agents – drugs that inhibit normal platelet function, usually by reducing their ability to aggregate and inappropriately form blood clots

Antipsychotic drugs – the major therapeutic modality for psychotic disorders; also known as neuroleptic drugs

Antithyroid drug – a chemical agent that lowers the basal metabolic rate by interfering with the formation, release, or action of thyroid hormones

Antitussives – agents that relieve or prevent coughing

Anuria – inability to produce urine

Anxiety – state of apprehension and autonomic nervous system activation resulting from exposure to a nonspecific or unknown cause

Anxiolytics – drugs that relieve anxiety; also known as antianxiety agents

Apnea – the cessation of respiration for more than 20 seconds with or without cyanosis, hypotonia, or bradycardia

Aromatic water – a mixture of distilled water with an aromatic volatile oil

Arrhythmias – deviations from the normal pattern of the heartbeat; also called dysrhythmias

Arteriosclerosis – degenerative changes in small arteries, commonly occurring in older individuals and diabetics; walls of arteries lose elasticity and become thick and hard

Articular – related to the joints of the body

Ascorbic acid – a water-soluble vitamin that is essential for the formation of collagen and fibroid tissue for teeth, bones, cartilage, connective tissue, and skin; also known as vitamin C

Asthma – a chronic inflammatory disorder of the airways of the respiratory system

Ataxia – loss of the ability to coordinate muscular movement

Atheromas – plaques consisting of lipids, cells, and cell debris, often with attached thrombi, which form inside the walls of large arteries

Atherosclerosis – disease of the arteries characterized by the presence of atheromas (plaques consisting of lipids, cells, and cell debris, often with attached thrombi, which form inside the walls of large arteries)

Atrophy – wasting away or "without development"

B

Bacteremia – a condition in which bacteria are recovered from blood cultures of a patient and may or may not be associated with the disease

Bacteria – small, one-celled microorganisms that lack a true nucleus or mechanism to provide metabolism

Bactericidal – killing bacterial growth

Bacteriostatic – suppress bacterial growth by triggering a mechanism that blocks folic acid synthesis, thereby forcing bacteria to synthesize their own folic acid

Barbiturates – drugs that depress multiple aspects of central nervous system function and can be used for sleep, seizures, and general anesthesia

Basal nuclei – clusters of nerve cells at the base of the brain; responsible for body movement and coordination

Benign – cellular growth that is nonprogressive, and non–life-threatening

Benzodiazepines – drugs of first choice for treating anxiety and insomnia

Beriberi – a deficiency caused by deficiency of thiamine, characterized by neurological symptoms, cardiovascular abnormalities, and edema

Beta-adrenergic blockers – drugs used to reverse sympathetic heart action caused by exercise, stress, or physical exertion

Beta-receptors – an adrenergic receptor; there are two types: $beta_1$ and $beta_2$

Bioavailability – measurement of the rate of absorption and total amount of drug that reaches the systemic circulation

Biotin – a water-soluble B complex vitamin that aids in fatty acid production, and in the oxidation of fatty acids and carbohydrates; also known as vitamin B_7

Biotransformation – the conversion of a drug within the body; also known as metabolism

Bipolar disorder – a type of mental illness characterized by periods of extreme excitation, or mania, and deep depression

Blood coagulation – the process by which blood clots

Bradykinesia – a decrease in spontaneity and movement, as seen in Parkinson's disease

Bradykinin – a polypeptide that mediates inflammation, increases vasodilation, and contracts smooth muscle

Broad-spectrum antibiotics – antibiotics that are used for the treatment of diseases caused by multiple organisms

Bronchiectasis – a destruction and widening of the large airways

Bronchodilators – agents that relax the smooth muscle of the bronchial tubes

Buffered tablet – a type of tablet manufactured to prevent irritation of the stomach

Bulimia nervosa – an eating disorder characterized by recurrent (at least twice a week) episodes of binge eating, during which the patient consumes large amounts of food and feels unable to stop eating

Bulk-forming laxatives – natural or synthetic polysaccharide derivatives that absorb water to soften the stool and increase bulk to stimulate peristalsis

Buspirone – an anxiolytic drug that differs significantly from the benzodiazepines

C

Cachexia – weight loss, wasting of muscle, loss of appetite, and general debility that can occur during a chronic disease

Calciferol – a fat-soluble vitamin chemically related to steroids; calciferol is essential for the normal formation of bones and teeth and important for the absorption of calcium and phosphorus from the GI tract; also known as vitamin D

Calcitonin (CT) – produced primarily by the parafollicular cells of the thyroid gland

Calcium (Ca) – the fifth-most abundant element in the human body, present mainly in the bones

Calcium carbonate – a substance that causes acid rebound, which may delay ulcer-related pain relief and ulcer healing

Calcium channel blockers – drugs used to treat stable angina

Caplet – a tablet shaped like a capsule

Capsule – a solid dosage form in which the drug is enclosed in either a hard or soft shell of soluble material

Carcinogens – any agent directly involved in or related to the promotion of cancer

Cardiac output – the amount of blood the heart pumps to the body in one minute

Carotenoids – any of a class of yellow to red pigments, including the carotenes and xanthophylls

Catecholamines – a group of chemically related compounds having a sympathomimetic action

Cheilosis – fissures on the lips caused by deficiency of riboflavin

Chemical digestion – the alteration of food into different forms through chemicals and enzymes

Chemical mediators – substances released by mast cells and platelets into interstitial fluid and blood; these substances include histamines, leukotrienes, serotonin, and prostaglandins

Chemical name – a drug's full name, that refers to its complete chemical makeup

Chloride (Cl) – involved in the maintenance of fluid and the body's acid-base balance

Cholinergic receptor – receptors that mediate responses to acetylcholine

Chronic obstructive pulmonary disease (COPD) – a group of common chronic respiratory disorders that are characterized by progressive tissue damage and obstruction in the airways of the lungs

Chronic pain – pain that is persistent or long-term; can also mean "low-intensity"

Clinical pharmacology – an area of medicine devoted to the evaluation of drugs used for human benefit

Collagen – a strong fibrous protein found in connective tissue

Compulsion – a ritualized behavior or mental act that a patient is driven to perform in response to his or her obsessions

Congenital megacolon – congenital dilation and hypertrophy of the colon due to reduction in motor neurons of the parasympathetic nervous system, resulting in extreme constipation, and if untreated, growth retardation; also known as Hirschsprung's disease

Congestive heart failure – a disorder in which the heart cannot pump the blood returning to the right side of the heart or provide adequate circulation to meet the needs of organs and tissues in the body

Congestive heart failure (CHF) – condition in which the heart is not able to pump enough blood to meet the body's metabolic demands

Conn's syndrome – a disease of the adrenal glands involving excess production of the hormone *aldosterone*

Controlled substances – drugs recognized by the Drug Enforcement Agency (DEA) as having abuse potential

Contusion – an injury to body part or tissue without a break in the skin

Convulsions – abnormal motor movements

Copper (Cu) – important for the synthesis of hemoglobin because it is part of a co-enzyme involved in its synthesis; also a component of several important enzymes in the body, and essential to good health

Coronary arterial bypass graft (CABG) – a procedure wherein a vein graft is surgically implanted to bypass the part of the occlusion in the coronary artery

Coronary artery disease (CAD) – a condition in which there is an insufficient supply of oxygen to the myocardium (cardiac muscle); also referred to as "coronary heart disease" and "ischemic heart disease"

Corpus striatum – a layer of nervous tissue within the brain

Cream – a semisolid emulsion of either the oil-in-water or the water-in-oil type, ordinarily intended for topical use

Cretinism – arrested physical and mental development with dystrophy of bones and soft tissues due to congenital lack of thyroid secretion

Croup – a viral infection that affects the larynx and the trachea

Cushing's syndrome – a disease caused by the excessive body production of cortisol; it can also be caused by excessive use of cortisol or other steroid hormones

Cyanocobalamin – a water-soluble substance that is the common pharmaceutic form of vitamin B_{12}; involved in the metabolism of protein, fats, and carbohydrates, and also in normal blood formation and neural function

Cyclooxygenase inhibitors – drugs that prevent the action of one of two enzymes that have an essential role in the inflammation process

Cycloplegia – paralysis of the ciliary muscles of the eye, resulting in loss of visual accommodation

Cystic fibrosis – a genetic disorder affecting the exocrine glands, causing thick mucus to obstruct the bronchioles in the lungs

D

Dementia – a chronic deterioration of intellectual function and other cognitive skills severe enough to interfere with the ability to perform activities of daily living

Depot-medroxyprogesteroneacetate (Depo-Provera®) – a long-acting progestin

Depression – a mood disorder

Dermis – a thick layer of loose connective tissue that is well-supplied with blood vessels, lymphatic vessels, nerves, and accessory organs

Diabetes mellitus – a complex disorder of carbohydrate, fat, and protein metabolism caused by lack of or inefficient use of insulin in the body; classified as type I (insulin-dependent diabetes mellitus [IDDM]), or type II (non-insulin-dependent diabetes mellitus [NIDDM])

Diastolic blood pressure – the pressure measured at the moment the ventricles relax

Diffusion – the process of particles in a fluid moving from an area of higher concentration to an area of lower concentration, resulting in an even distribution of the particles in the fluid

Diuretics – a drug that promotes urine formation and elimination. Sodium passing through the kidneys attract water from the circulatory system and increases the volume of urine

Dopamine – a neurotransmitter that is naturally produced in the brain, affecting motor control, memory, attention span, the ability to problem solve, motivation, pleasure, and creative thought

Dopamine receptors – an adrenergic receptor

Dose-effect relationship – the relationship between drug dose and blood, or other biological fluid concentrations

Drug clearance – elimination rate over time divided by the drug's concentration

Drug Enforcement Agency (DEA) – the government agency concerned with controlled substances that enforces laws against drug activities, including illegal drug use, dealing, and manufacturing

Dry powder inhaler (DPI) – a device used to deliver medication in the form of micronized powder into the lungs

Dwarfism – a condition of lack of growth of the arms and legs in proportion to the head and trunk; it may be caused by over 200 different other conditions, including achondroplasia, kidney disease, genetic conditions, and problems with hormones or metabolism

E

Eclampsia – the occurrence of seizures (convulsions) in a pregnant woman, usually occurring after the twentieth week of pregnancy

Elastin – an extracellular connective tissue protein

Electrical threshold – an individual's balance between excitatory and inhibitory forces in the brain; also known as seizure threshold

Electrolytes – compounds, particularly salts, that when dissolved in water or another solvent, dissociate into ions and are able to conduct an electric current

Elixir – a clear, sweetened, flavored, hydroalcoholic liquid medication intended for oral use

Embolism – obstruction or occlusion of a vessel

Emetic – a drug that induces vomiting

Emollient laxatives – substances that act as surfactants by allowing absorption of water into the stool

Emphysema – the destruction of the alveolar walls and septae, which leads to large, permanently inflated alveolar air space

Emulsion – a system containing two liquids that cannot be mixed together in which one is dispersed in the form of very small globules throughout the other

Encephalitis – inflammation of the brain's connective tissue framework

Enteral nutrition (EN) – feeding by tube directly into the patient's digestive tract

Enteric-coated tablet – a tablet covered in a special coating to protect it from stomach acid, allowing the drug to dissolve in the intestines

Epidemic – an outbreak of a disease or infection that spreads widely and rapidly

Epidural anesthesia – injection of an anesthetic into the space immediately outside of the dura mater that contains a supporting cushion of fat and other connective tissues

Epiglottitis – an acute bacterial infection of the epiglottis (an appendage which closes the glottis while food or drink is passing through the pharynx) and the surrounding areas that causes airway obstruction

Epilepsy – condition characterized by periodic or recurrent seizures or convulsions

Epinephrine – a major transmitter released by the adrenal medulla

Epinephrine (adrenaline) – produced by the medulla of adrenal glands, and is a "fight or flight" hormone that is released when danger threatens

Epiphyses – the ends of long bones that are originally separated from the main bone by a layer of cartilage, becoming unified through ossification

Essential hypertension – idiopathic (occurring spontaneously from an unknown cause); also known as primary hypertension

Estrogen – substances capable of producing sexual receptivity in female individuals

Eustachian tubes – tubes within the ear by which fluids drain

Excretion – the process whereby the undigested residue of food and waste products of metabolism are eliminated, material is removed to regulate composition of body fluids and tissues, or substances are expelled to perform functions on an exterior surface

Exfoliative dermatitis – a skin disorder characterized by reddening and scaling of 100% of the skin; erythroderma

Expectorants – agents that promote the removal of mucus secretions from the lung, bronchi, and trachea, usually by coughing

Extrapyramidal – nerves in the brain that control movement

F

Fibrin – gel-like threads

Fibrinogen – a plasma protein

Fibrinolysis – the breakdown of fibrin

Filtration – the movement of water and dissolved substances from the glomerulus to the Bowman's capsule

First-pass effect – drugs reaching the liver where they are partially metabolized before being sent to the body

Floppy infant syndrome – also called "infantile hypotonia," this is a condition of abnormally low muscle tone, often with reduced muscle strength

Fluidextract – a pharmacopoeial liquid preparation of vegetable drugs, made by filtration, containing alcohol as a solvent or as a preservative, or both

Fluorine – a chemical element that is used as a diagnostic aid in various tissue scans

Folic acid – essential for cell growth and the reproduction of red blood cells; also known as vitamin B_9

Follicle-stimulating hormone (FSH) – a gonadotropin that stimulates the growth and maturation of follicles in the ovary in females and promotes spermatogenesis (the process by which male gametes develop into mature spermatozoa) in males

Food additive – any substance that becomes part of a food product

Food and Drug Administration (FDA) – the branch of the U.S. Department of Health and Human Services that is responsible for the regulation of foods, drugs, cosmetics, and medical devices

Fungi – a distinct group of organisms that are neither plant nor animal. Fungi grow in single cells or in colonies

G

Gamma-aminobutyric acid (GABA) – a neurotransmitter distributed throughout the brain and spinal cord; now considered to be the major inhibitory neurotransmitter in the CNS, acting to modulate the activity of excitatory pathways

Gel – a jelly or the solid or semisolid phase of a colloidal solution

Gelcap – an oil-based medication that is enclosed in a soft gelatin capsule

General anesthesia – provision of a pain-free state for the entire body

Generalized anxiety disorder – difficult-to-control, excessive anxiety that lasts six months or more

Generalized seizure – seizure originating and involving both cerebral hemispheres

Generic name – a drug not protected by a trademark, but regulated by the FDA. Also called the *official name*

Genetic engineering – techniques wherein genes from one organism are spliced into the chromosomes of another organism; also known as recombinant DNA technology

Gestational age – the time measured from the first day of the mother's last menstrual cycle to the current date

Gigantism – condition produces excessive growth (a "giant") if the hypersecretion of GH occurs before puberty

Glomerular filtration rate (GFR) – the rate of filtration in the kidneys

Glucagon – an important hormone in carbohydrate metabolism

Glucocorticoids – a class of corticosteroid so named because it increase blood sugar levels. Glucocorticoids are mainly used for their anti-inflammatory effect

Glutamate – an amino acid that acts as a neurotransmitter and is a key molecule in cellular metabolism, playing an important role in the body's disposal of excess or waste nitrogen

Gonadotropes – cells in the anterior pituitary gland that produce the gonadotropins known as luteinizing hormone and follicle-stimulating hormone

Gonadotropin-releasing hormone (GnRH) – stimulates the release of FSH and LH from the anterior pituitary gland

Gout – a disease caused by a congenital disorder of uric acid metabolism; metabolic arthritis

Graafian follicles – matured and grown ovarian follicles; these egg-containing tubes grown and develop between puberty, sexual maturation, and menopause

Gram stains – sequential procedures involving crystal violet and iodine solutions followed by alcohol that allow rapid identification of organisms as Gram-positive or Gram-negative types

Gram-negative – microorganisms that stain red or pink with Gram stain

Gram-positive – microorganisms that stain blue or purple with Gram stain

Grand mal – generalized seizure characterized by full-body tonic and clonic motor convulsions

Granule – a very small pill, usually gelatin- or sugar-coated, containing a drug to be given in a small dose

Graves' disease – an autoimmune disorder that involves overactivity of the thyroid gland (hyperthyroidism)

Growth hormone (GH) – secreted by the anterior pituitary gland in response to growth hormone-releasing hormone (GHRH)

Gynecomastia – enlargement of breast tissue in males

H

Half-life – the time it takes for the plasma concentration (e.g., of a drug) to be reduced by 50 percent

Hallucinations – false or distorted sensory experiences that appear to be real perceptions

Helicobacter pylori – a bacterial species that is associated with several gastroduodenal diseases

Hematoma – blood that has seeped from a blood vessel and collects in tissue, organs, or space

Hemodynamic – related to blood circulation or blood flow

Hemolysis – the destruction or dissolution of red blood cells, with release of hemoglobin

Hemostasis – a process that stops bleeding in a blood vessel

Heparin – a potent anticoagulant naturally obtained from the liver and lungs of domestic animals; in humans, it is usually found in basophils or mast cells

Hepatic portal circulation – the circulation of blood through the liver

Heterogeneous – consisting of a diverse range of different items

Hirsuitism – excessive hair growth on the face, abdomen, breasts, and back

Histamine – a chemical substance naturally found in all body tissues that protects the body from factors in the environment that produce allergic and inflammatory reactions

Histamine H_2-receptor antagonists – drugs that block the action of histamine on parietal cells in the stomach, decreasing acid production

Hormone – a chemical messenger that serves as a signal to target cells; are produced by nearly every organ system and type of tissue

Human immunodeficiency virus (HIV) – a retrovirus that infects helper T cells of the immune system, leading to AIDS

Hydroxocobalamin – is involved in the metabolism of protein, fats, and carbohydrates, aids in hemoglobin synthesis, is essential for normal functioning of all cells, and is important in energy metabolism; also known as vitamin B_{12}

Hyperactive – abnormally and easily excitable or exuberant

Hyperalimentation (total parenteral nutrition) – Also known as "TPN," this treatment is used to supply complete nutrition to patients when the enteral route cannot be used; all needed nutrients are injected into the body intravenously

Hypercalcemia – an excessive amount of calcium in the blood

Hyperemesis gravidarum – pernicious vomiting during pregnancy

Hyperkalemia – high blood level of potassium

Hyperlipidemia – an increase in triglycerides and cholesterol

Hypermetabolic – burning energy and nutrients at a higher rate than normal

Hyperpituitarism – a condition that results in the excess secretion of hormones that are secreted from the pituitary gland

Hypertension – an abnormal increase in arterial blood pressure

Hyperthyroidism – a condition of excessive amounts of thyroxine

Hypervitaminosis – an abnormal condition resulting from excessive intake of toxic amounts of one or more vitamins, especially over a long period

Hypnotics – drugs given to promote sleep

Hypoactive – abnormally inactive

Hypogonadism – a condition of little or no production of sex hormones, usually due to poor function or inactivity of either the testes or the ovaries

Hypokalemia – low blood level of potassium

Hypomagnesemia – an abnormally low level of magnesium in the blood

Hyponatremia – low blood level of sodium

Hypoprothrombinemic – the amount of prothrombin factor II in the circulating blood

Hypothalamus – the part of the brain that lies below the thalamus; it regulates body temperature, certain metabolic processes, and other autonomic activities

Hypothyroidism – a deficiency disease that causes cretinism (mental and physical retardation) in children

Hypotonic – having a lesser osmotic pressure than a reference solution

Hypovitaminosis – a condition related to the deficiency of one or more vitamins

I

Idiosyncratic reaction – experience of a unique, strange, or unpredicted reaction to a drug

Impotence – inability to achieve or maintain penile erection

Infection – the invasion of pathogenic microorganisms that produce tissue damage within the body

Infiltration anesthesia – anesthesia produced by injecting a local anesthetic drug into tissues

Insomnia – the inability to fall asleep or stay asleep

Insulin – a hormone secreted by the pancreas that regulates carbohydrate and fat metabolism, especially the conversion of glucose to glycogen

Insulin-dependent diabetes mellitus – a disorder caused by complete lack of insulin secretion by the pancreas

Intracranial – within the cranium (skull)

Intrinsic factor – a substance that is secreted by the gastric mucus membrane and is essential for the absorption of vitamin B_{12} in the intestines

Investigational new drug (IND) application – an application for human drug testing that is submitted to the FDA once enough data has been collected on a new drug

Iodine – an essential micronutrient of the thyroid hormone (thyroxine)

Iritis – inflammation of the iris

Iron (Fe) – A common metallic element essential for the formation of hemoglobin and myoglobin, as well as the transfer of oxygen to the body tissues

Iron deficiency anemia – anemia characterized by low serum iron, increased serum iron-binding capacity, decreased serum ferritin, and decreased marrow iron stores

K

Keratomalacia – a condition, usually in children with vitamin A deficiency, characterized by softening, ulceration, and perforation of the cornea

Kernicterus – yellow staining and degenerative lesions in basal ganglia associated with high levels of unconjugated bilirubin in infants; also known as bilirubin encephalopathy

L

Laceration – cut or break in the skin

Legend drug – a prescription drug

Leukotriene modifiers – a relatively new class of drugs designed to prevent asthma and allergic reactions before they occur by either inhibiting leukotriene production, or preventing leukotrienes from binding to cellular receptors

Leukotrienes – substances that contribute to the inflammation associated with asthma

Liniment – a liquid preparation for external use, usually applied by friction to the skin

Lipid solubility – the ability to dissolve in a fatty medium

Lipophilic – able to dissolve much more easily in lipids than in water

Lipoprotein – a class of blood chemicals whose molecules are comprised of a lipid portion and a protein portion

Local anesthesia – provision of a pain-free state in a specific area of the body

Localized infection – involve a specific area of the body such as the skin or internal organs

Lozenge – a small, disk-shaped tablet composed of solidifying paste containing an astringent, an antiseptic, or an oil-based drug used for local treatment of the mouth or throat and is held in the mouth until dissolved; also known as a troche

Lubricant laxative – a substance, such as mineral oil, that works by increasing water retention in the stool to soften it

Lugol's solution – Lugol's iodine; a solution of iodine often used as an antiseptic, disinfectant, or starch indicator, to replenish iodine deficiency, to protect the thyroid from radioactive materials, and for emergency disinfection of drinking water

Luteinizing hormone (LH) – secreted by the anterior lobe of the pituitary gland that is necessary for proper reproductive function

M

Magnesium – an important ion for the function of many enzyme systems, and is the second most abundant action of the intracellular fluids in the body

Malaria – a severe generalized infection caused by the bite of an *anopheles* mosquito that is infected with a *Plasmodium* protozoon

Malignant – cellular growth that is severe and becomes progressively worse, often becoming life-threatening

Malignant hypertension – an uncontrollable, severe, and rapidly progressive form of hypertension with many complications

Malignant hyperthermia – a rare, genetic hypermetabolic condition that is characterized by severe overproduction of body heat with rigidity of skeletal muscles

Mania – a severe medical condition characterized by extremely elevated mood, energy, and unusual thought patterns; a characteristic of bipolar disorder

Mast cell stabilizers – substances that work to prevent allergy cells (called mast cells) from breaking open and releasing chemicals that help cause inflammation; they work slowly over time

Mast cells – large cells found in connective tissue that contain many biochemicals, including histamine; mast cells are involved in inflammation secondary to injuries and infections, and are sometimes implicated in allergic reactions

Mechanical digestion – the breakdown of large food particles into smaller pieces by physical means

Melatonin – an important hormone secreted from the pineal gland that is believed to induce sleep

Menadione – a water-soluble injectable form of the product of vitamin K_3

Metabolism – the conversion of a drug within the body; also known as biotransformation

Metastasize – to spread from one part of the body to another

Metered dose inhaler (MDI) – a hand-held pressurized device used to deliver medications for inhalations

Mineralocorticoids – steroid hormones that influence salt and water balance; they are released from the adrenal cortex

Minerals – inorganic substances occurring naturally in the earth's crust having characteristic chemical compositions

Miosis – contraction of the pupil of the eye

Mitotic inhibitors – drugs that block cell growth by stopping cell division

Mixture – a mutual incorporation of two or more substances, without chemical union, in which the physical characteristics of each of the components are retained

Monoamine oxidase inhibitor (MAOI) – a class of drugs effective for the treatment of depression

Mucolytic – destroying or dissolving the active agents that make up mucus

Mycoplasms – ultramicroscopic organisms that lack rigid cell walls and are considered to be the smallest free-living organisms

Mycoses – fungal diseases

Mydriasis – dilation of the pupil

Myocardial infarction (MI) – an area of dead cardiac muscle tissue, with or without hemorrhage

Myxedema – condition of thyroid insufficiency or resistance to thyroid hormone

N

Narcotics – drugs that produce a sedative or pain relieving affect

Narrow-spectrum antibiotics – antibiotics that are effective against only a few organisms

Necrosis – death of a group of cells or tissues

Negative feedback system – method by which regulation of hormones is achieved; released in response to concentration in the blood

Neonatal period – the time from birth to approximately 28 days of age

Neoplasm – a tumor; tissue that is composed of cells that grow in an abnormal way

Neuroleptic drugs – the major therapeutic modality for psychotic disorders; also known as antipsychotic drugs

Neurotransmitter – a biochemical that is formed in and released from a neuron in order to stimulate or inhibit the actions of another cell

Niacin – contains parts of two enzymes that regulate energy metabolism and is essential for a healthy skin, tongue, and digestive system; also known as vitamin B_3 or nicotinic acid

Nicotinic acid – contains parts of two enzymes that regulate energy metabolism and is essential for a healthy skin, tongue, and digestive system; also known as niacin or vitamin B_3

Nitrates – drugs used for the treatment of angina

Nitrosoureas – alkylating agents; they act by the process of alkylation to inhibit DNA repair

Nocturnal enuresis – nighttime bedwetting

Nonsteroidal anti-inflammatory drugs (NSAIDs) – drugs that have analgesic and antipyretic effects

Norepinephrine (noradrenaline) – released from the medulla of the adrenal glands, and is also a central nervous system and sympathetic nervous system neurotransmitter

Nystagmus – rhythmical oscillation of the eyeballs

O

Obsession – a recurrent, persistent thought, impulse, or mental image that is unwanted and distressing, and comes involuntarily to mind despite attempts to ignore or suppress it

Obsessive-compulsive disorder – anxiety characterized by recurrent, repetitive behaviors that interfere with normal activities or relationships

Ointment – a semisolid preparation usually containing medicinal substances and is intended for external application

Opioid – a natural or synthetic narcotic substance

Opioid agonists – drugs that can combine with receptors to initiate drug actions

Opioid antagonists – drugs that oppose or resist the action of others

Organogenesis – from implantation to about 60 days after, the time when major fetal organs form

Osteoarthritis (OA) – arthritis characterized by erosion of articular cartilage that mainly affects weight-bearing joints in older adults

Osteomalacia – a disease in which the bone softens and becomes brittle

Otitis media – an inflammation of the middle ear

Over-the-counter (OTC) – nonprescription drugs

Oxytocin (OT) – also acts as a neurotransmitter in the brain; in women, it is released during labor and lactation

P

Pain – an unpleasant sensation associated with actual or potential tissue damage

Palliation – treatment to relieve or reduce intensity of uncomfortable symptoms, but not to produce a cure

Panic attacks – of sudden onset, reaching peak intensity within ten minutes; symptoms may include trembling, shortness of breath, heart palpitations, chest pain (or chest tightness), sweating, nausea, dizziness (or slight vertigo), light-headedness, hyperventilation, paresthesias (tingling sensations), and sensations of choking or smothering

Panic disorder – anxiety characterized by intense feelings of immediate apprehension, fearfulness, and terror

Pantothenic acid – a member of the vitamin B complex widely distributed in plant and animal tissues and that may be an important element in human nutrition; also known as vitamin B_5

Parasympathomimetic – producing effects similar to those produced when a parasympathetic nerve is stimulated

Parathyroid hormone (PTH) – also called parathormone, is secreted by the parathyroid glands and increases the levels of calcium in the blood

Parkinson's disease – a neurological syndrome usually resulting from deficiency of dopamine because of degenerative, vascular, or inflammatory changes in the basal ganglia

Partial seizure – seizure originating in one area of the brain that may spread to other areas

Passive transport – the most common and important mode of traversal of drugs through membranes; diffusion

Patent ductus arteriosus – a condition in which the normal channel between the pulmonary artery and the aorta fails to close at birth

Pediatric period – the period from birth to approximately age 18

Pellagra – a disease caused by a deficiency of niacin and protein in the diet, characterized by skin eruptions, digestive and nervous system disturbances, and eventual mental deterioration

Peptic ulcer – a lesion located in either the stomach (gastric ulcer) or in the duodenum (small intestine)

Percutaneous transluminal coronary angioplasty (PTCA) – reduces obstruction by means of invasive procedures requiring cardiac catheterization; the catheter contains an inflatable balloon that flattens the obstruction

Periosteum – a thick, fibrous membrane covering the entire surface of a bone except its articular cartilage and where it attaches to tendons and ligaments

Pharma food – A system of receiving nourishment by breathing in nutritional microparticles

Pharmacodynamic interactions – differences in effects produced by a given plasma level of a drug

Pharmacodynamics – the study of the biochemical and physiological effects of drugs

Pharmacokinetic interactions – differences in the plasma levels of a drug achieved with a given dose of that drug

Pharmacokinetics – the study of the absorption, distribution, metabolism, and excretion of drugs

Pharmacology – the science concerned with drugs and their sources, appearance, chemistry, actions, and uses

Pheochromocytoma – a usually benign tumor of the adrenal medulla or the sympathetic nervous system in which the affected cells secrete increased amounts of epinephrine or norepinephrine

Phlebothrombosis – clotting in a vein without primary inflammation

Phosphorus – is essential for the metabolism of protein, calcium, and glucose, aids in building strong bones and teeth, and helps in the regulation of the body's acid-base balance

Pill – a small, globular mass of soluble material containing a medicinal substance to be swallowed

Placebo – an inert substance given to a patient instead of an active medicine

Plaster – a solid preparation that can be spread when heated and then becomes adhesive at the temperature of the body

Pneumonia – an inflammation or infection of the pulmonary parenchyma; caused by viruses, bacteria, mycoplasmas, and aspiration of foreign substances

Pneumonitis – inflammation of the lungs

Polypharmacy – the practice of prescribing multiple medicines to a single patient simultaneously

Porphyria – a group of enzyme disorders that cause skin problems (such as purple discolorations) and/or neurological complications

Post-traumatic stress disorder – anxiety characterized by a sense of helplessness and the re-experiencing of a traumatic event

Potassium – the major electrolyte in intracellular fluids, helping to regulate neuromuscular excitability and muscle contraction

Powder – a dry mass of minute separate particles of any substance

Preanesthetic medications – drugs given before the administration of anesthesia

Preeclampsia – the development of elevated blood pressure and protein in the urine after the twentieth week of pregnancy; it may also cause swelling of the face and hands

Primary hypertension – idiopathic (occurring spontaneously from an unknown cause); also known as essential hypertension

Pro-drug – inactive or partially active drug that is metabolically changed in the body to an active drug

Progesterone – secreted primarily by the ovarian cells in the corpus luteum at the time of ovulation during the female reproductive years

Prolactin (PRL) – a hormone that is primarily associated with lactation; it is secreted from the anterior pituitary gland

Prothrombin – a glycoprotein formed and stored in the parenchymal cells of the liver and present in the blood; a deficiency of prothrombin leads to impaired blood coagulation

Protozoa – single-celled parasitic organisms, many of which are motile (able to move spontaneously)

Pyridoxine – a water-soluble vitamin that is part of the B complex and acts as a co-enzyme essential for the synthesis and breakdown of amino acids; also known as vitamin B_6

R

Radiation therapy – cancer treatment method whereby drugs are used to treat cancer either before or after surgery

Reabsorption – the movement of water and selected substances from the tubules to the peritubular capillaries

Recombinant DNA technology – techniques wherein genes from one organism are spliced into the chromosomes of another organism; also known as genetic engineering

Red man syndrome – a rash on the upper body caused by vancomycin

Replication – the process of reproduction or copying of genetic material

Respiratory distress syndrome (RDS) – the result of the absence, deficiency, or alteration of the components of pulmonary surfactant

Respiratory syncytial virus (RSV) – the major cause of bronchiolitis and pneumonia in infants under one year of age; caused by a virus and exhibits mild cold-like symptoms

Retinol – a fat-soluble vitamin essential for skeletal growth, maintenance of normal mucosal epithelium, reproduction, and visual acuity; also known as vitamin A

Reye syndrome – an acquired encephalopathy of young children that follows an acute febrile illness; strongly associated with aspirin use

Rhabdomyolysis – a potentially fatal destruction of skeletal muscle, characterized by the presence of myoglobin in the urine; it is also associated with acute renal failure in heatstroke

Rheumatoid arthritis (RA) – a chronic and progressive condition that affects more women than men, focusing mainly on the joints of the hands and feet, and leading to deformity and disability

Riboflavin – one of the heat-stable components of the B complex, it is involved as a co-enzyme in the oxidative processes of carbohydrates, fats, and proteins; also known as vitamin B_2

Rickets – a deficiency disease resulting from a lack of vitamin D or calcium and from insufficient exposure to sunlight, characterized by defective bone growth and occurring mostly in children

Rickettsia – intercellular parasites that need to be in living cells to reproduce

S

Salicylates – salts or esters of salicylic acid

Saline laxatives – substances that create an osmotic effect to increase water content and stool volume

Schizophrenia – a mental illness characterized by distortion of reality, disorganized thought patterns, social withdrawal, hallucinations, and poor judgment

Sclerotic – hardening, toughening

Secondary hypertension – results from renal (e.g., nephrosclerosis) or endocrine (e.g., hyperaldosteronism) disease, or pheochromocytoma, a benign tumor of the adrenal medulla; in this type of hypertension, the underlying problem must be resolved

Sedative-hypnotics – drugs that when given in lower doses, produce a calming effect, and when given in higher doses, produce sleep

Seizure – abnormal discharge of brain neurons that causes alteration of behavior and/or motor activity

Selective serotonin reuptake inhibitor (SSRI) – a class of drugs used as antidepressants; they block resorption of serotonin in nerve cells in the brain

Septae – walls of the bronchioles

Septicemia – bacteremia associated with active disease, whether localized or systemic

Serotonin – a neurotransmitter that regulates appetite, sleep, arousal, mood, temperature, and hormone release

Serotonin syndrome – a rare condition resulting from intentional self-poisoning with serotonin, use of the drug therapeutically, or from inadvertent drug interactions characterized by progressively worsening symptoms such as: mental confusion, shivering or muscle twitching, sweating or fever, hallucinations, hypertension, tachycardia, headache, tremor, nausea, diarrhea, coma, and death; also known as serotonin toxicity

Sickle cell anemia – an inherited disorder characterized by the presence of abnormal hemoglobin; hemoglobin contains hemoglobin S (HbS)

Silent angina – a condition that occurs in the absence of angina pain

Social anxiety disorder – characterized by an intense, irrational fear of situations in which one might be scrutinized by others, or might do something that is embarrassing or humiliating; also known as social phobia

Social phobia – characterized by an intense, irrational fear of situations in which one might be scrutinized by others, or might do something that is embarrassing or humiliating; also known as social anxiety disorder

Sodium – one of the most important elements in the body; sodium ions are involved in acid-base balance, water balance, transmission of nerve impulses, and contraction of muscles

Solution – a liquid dosage form in which active ingredients are dissolved in a liquid vehicle

Somnolence – prolonged drowsiness that may last hours to days

Spasticity – a type of increase in muscle tone at rest, characterized by increase resistance of the muscles to stretching

Spermatogenesis – the process by which male gametes develop into mature spermatozoa

Spinal anesthesia – a type of regional anesthesia produced by injecting a local anesthetic drug into the subarachnoid space of the spinal cord

Spirits – alcoholic or hydroalcoholic solutions of volatile substances

Spores – bacteria in a resistant stage that can withstand an unfavorable environment

Sprain – injury to supporting ligaments of a joint

Statins – a class of drugs that inhibits the activity of an enzyme that forms cholesterol in the body; so named because all of their generic names end with "-statin" (e.g., lovastatin)

Status epilepticus – an emergency situation characterized by continual seizure activity with no interruptions (another term for seizure)

Steatorrhea – elimination of large amounts of fat in the stool

Steroids – numerous naturally occurring or synthetic fat-soluble organic compounds that include sterols, bile acids, adrenal hormones, sex hormones, digitalis compounds, and certain vitamin precursors

Stimulant laxatives – substances that stimulate bowel mobility and increase secretion of fluids in the bowel

Stool softeners – substances that decrease the consistency of stool by reducing surface tension

Strain – injury resulting from overstretching a muscle, results in tear of muscle or muscle and tendon

Stroke volume – the volume of blood pumped with each heartbeat

Substantia nigra – pigmented cells in the midbrain responsible for the production of dopamine

Sulfur – necessary to all body tissues and is found in all body cells

Superficial mycoses – involving a surface or a shallow depth of tissue

Suppository – a small, solid body shaped for ready introduction into one of the orifices of the body other than the oral cavity (e.g., rectum, urethra, or vagina), made of a substance, usually medicated, that is solid at ordinary temperature but melts at body temperature

Suspension – a liquid dosage form that contains solid drug particles floating in a liquid medium

Sustained release (SR) capsule – a capsule with a controlled release of the dosage over a special period of time

Sympatholytic – inhibiting or opposing adrenergic nerve function; sympatholytic agents are also known as adrenergic blocker agents

Sympatholytic drugs – a group of drugs that blocks or inhibits the effects of epinephrine or norepinephrine on the cells that normally react to them

Sympathomimetic – adrenergic, or producing an effect similar to that obtained by stimulation of the sympathetic nervous system

Synapse – a specialized junction at which a nerve cell communicates with a target cell

Syrup – a liquid preparation in a concentrated aqueous solution of a sugar used for medicinal purposes or to add flavor to a substance

Systemic infection – impacts the whole body rather than a specific area of the body

Systemic mycoses – relating to or affecting an entire body or an entire organism

Systolic blood pressure – the pressure measured at the moment the heart contracts

T

Tablet – a solid dosage form containing medicinal substances with or without suitable diluents

Target sites – the areas where a drug's greatest action takes place at the cellular level

Teratogenic – causing developmental malformations

Testosterone – stimulates the development of the male secondary sex characteristics, initiates the production of sperm, and enhances the functional capacity of the penis and accessory sex organs

Thiamine – a water-soluble, crystalline compound of the B complex, essential for normal metabolism and health of the cardiovascular and nervous systems; also known as vitamin B_1

Thrombin – enzyme occurring in blood during the clotting process

Thrombocytopenia – decrease in the number of platelets in circulating blood

Thrombogenic – substances causing blood clots

Thrombolytics – drugs designed to dissolve blood clots that have already formed within a blood vessel

Thrombophlebitis – venous inflammation with thrombus formation

Thromboplastin – substance to cause clotting

Thrombosis – the formation of a clot

Thrombus – a clot in the cardiovascular system formed during life from constituents of blood

Thyroid-stimulating hormone (TSH) – a substance secreted by the anterior lobe of the pituitary gland that controls the release of thyroid hormone and is necessary for the growth and function of the thyroid gland

Thyroxine (T4) – the major hormone secreted by the follicular cells of the thyroid gland

Tincture – an alcoholic solution prepared from vegetable materials or from chemical substances, used as a skin disinfectant

Tocopherol – a fat-soluble vitamin essential for normal reproduction, muscle development, resistance of erythrocytes to hemolysis, and various other biochemical functions; also known as vitamin E

Tolerance – reduced responsiveness of a drug because of adaptation to it

Tonic-clonic seizure – an alternate contraction (tonic phase) and relaxation (clonic phase) of muscles, a loss of consciousness, and abnormal behavior

Trade name – brand name given to a drug by its manufacturer (such drugs are marked with the symbol®). Trade names are also called *proprietary* or *brand* names

Tremor – repetitive, often regular, oscillatory movements caused by alternate, or synchronous, but irregular contraction of opposing muscle groups

Tricyclic antidepressant (TCA) – a class of antidepressants; they inhibit reabsorption of serotonin, norepinephrine, and dopamine in the brain

Troche – a small, disk-shaped tablet composed of solidifying paste containing an astringent, antiseptic, or oil-based drug used for local treatment of the mouth or throat and is held in the mouth until dissolved; also known as a lozenge

Tubular secretion – the active secretion of substances such as potassium from the peritubular capillaries into the tubules

U

Uveitis – inflammation of the uvea (the vascular middle layer of the eye, including the iris, ciliary body, and choroid)

V

Vasodilators – drugs used to relax or dilate vessels throughout the body

Vasospastic angina – decubitus angina; characterized by periodic attacks of cardiac pain that occur when a person is lying down

Venous stasis – injury to the veins causing loss of proper function of the vein and impairing the ability of blood flow to return to the heart

Viruses – intracellular parasites that take over the metabolic machinery of host cells and use it for their own survival and replication

Vitamin A – a fat-soluble vitamin essential for skeletal growth, maintenance of normal mucosal epithelium, reproduction, and visual acuity; also known as retinol

Vitamin B complex – a pharmaceutical term applied to drug products containing a mixture of the B vitamins, usually B_1 (thiamine), B_2 (riboflavin), B_3 (nicotinamide), and B_6 (pyridoxine)

Vitamin B_1 – a water-soluble, crystalline compound of the B complex, essential for normal metabolism and health of the cardiovascular and nervous systems; also known as thiamine

Vitamin B_{12} – is involved in the metabolism of protein, fats, and carbohydrates, aids in hemoglobin synthesis, is essential for normal functioning of all cells, and is important in energy metabolism; also known as cyanocobalamin

Vitamin B_2 – one of the heat-stable components of the B complex, it is involved as a co-enzyme in the oxidative processes of carbohydrates, fats, and proteins; also known as riboflavin

Vitamin B_3 – contains parts of two enzymes that regulate energy metabolism and is essential for a healthy skin, tongue, and digestive system; also known as niacin or nicotinic acid

Vitamin B_5 – a member of the vitamin B complex widely distributed in plant and animal tissues and that may be an important element in human nutrition; also known as pantothenic acid

Vitamin B_6 – a water-soluble vitamin that is part of the B complex and acts as a co-enzyme essential for the synthesis and breakdown of amino acids; also known as pyridoxine

Vitamin B_7 – a water-soluble B complex vitamin that aids in fatty acid production, and in the oxidation of fatty acids and carbohydrates; also known as biotin

Vitamin B_9 – essential for cell growth and the reproduction of red blood cells; also known as folic acid

Vitamin C – a water-soluble vitamin that is essential for the formation of collagen and fibroid tissue for teeth, bones, cartilage, connective tissue, and skin; also known as ascorbic acid

Vitamin D – a fat-soluble vitamin chemically related to steroids that is essential for the normal formation of bones and teeth and important for the absorption of calcium and phosphorus from the GI tract; also known as calciferol

Vitamin E – a fat-soluble vitamin essential for normal reproduction, muscle development, resistance of erythrocytes to hemolysis, and various other biochemical functions; also known as tocopherol

Vitamin K – essential for the synthesis of prothrombin in the liver

Vitamins – organic compounds essential in small quantities for physiologic and metabolic functioning of the body

Volatile liquids – liquids that evaporate upon exposure to the air

X

Xanthine derivatives – a substance that is effective for relief of bronchospasm in asthma, chronic bronchitis, and emphysema

Xerophthalmia – extreme dryness of the conjunctiva resulting from an eye disease or from a systemic deficiency of vitamin A

Z

Zinc (Zn) – A trace element that is essential for several body enzymes, growth, glucose tolerance, wound healing, and taste acuity

Zollinger-Ellison syndrome – peptic ulceration with gastric hypersecretion and tumor of the pancreatic islets

Index

B

Service Management

Operations, Strategy, and Information Technology

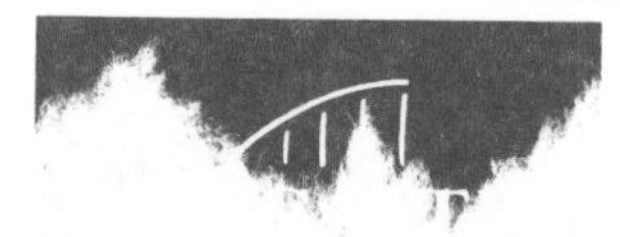

Service Management

Operations, Strategy, and Information Technology

SECOND EDITION

James A. Fitzsimmons
William H. Seay Centennial Professor of Business University of Texas at Austin

Mona J. Fitzsimmons

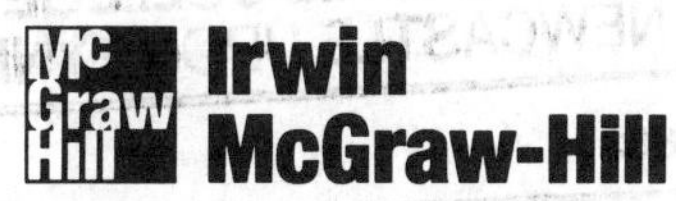

Boston, Massachusetts Burr Ridge, Illinois Dubuque, Iowa
Madison, Wisconsin New York, New York San Francisco, California St. Louis, Missouri

Irwin/McGraw-Hill

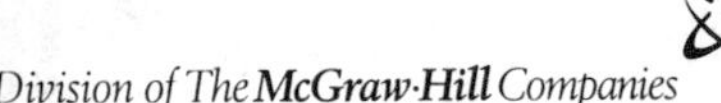

SERVICE MANAGEMENT:
Operations, Strategy, and Information Technology
International Editions 1999

10 9 8 7 6 5 4 3
20 9 8 7 6 5 4 3 2 1 0 9
PMP KKP

Library of Congress Cataloging-In-Publication Data

Fitzsimmons, James A.
Service management : operations, strategy, and information Technology / James A. Fitzsimmons, Mona J. Fitzsimmons. – 2nd ed.
p. cm.
Updated ed. of: Service management for competitive advantage. 1994
Includes bibliographical references and indexes.
ISBN 0-07-021760-2
1. Service industries - Management. I. Fitzsimmons, Mona J. II. Fitzsimmons, James A, Service management for competitive advantage. III. Title.
HD9980.5.F549 1999
658–dc21 97-8293
CIP

www.mhhe.com

When ordering this title, use ISBN 0-07-115709-3

Printed in Singapore

About the Authors

JAMES A. FITZSIMMONS is the William H. Seay Centennial Professor of Business at the University of Texas. He received a BSE in industrial engineering from the University of Michigan, an MBA from Western Michigan University, and a Ph.D. with distinction from the University of California at Los Angeles. His principal research interest is in the area of service management, and he won the Stan Hardy Award in 1983 for the best paper published in the field of operations management, on the topic of emergency ambulance location. A computer methodology that he designed, referred to as CALL, has been used by major cities worldwide to plan emergency ambulance systems. Consulting assignments include the RAND Corporation; the U.S. Air Force; the cities of Los Angeles, Denver, Austin, Melbourne, and Auckland; the state of Texas; General Motors; La Quinta Motor Inns; Greyhound; and McDonald's. Teaching experience includes faculty appointments at the University of California at Los Angeles, California State University at Northridge, the University of New Mexico, Boston University Overseas Graduate Program, California Polytechnic State University at San Luis Obispo, and recently the Helsinki School of Economics and Business. He has held positions at Corning Glass Works and Hughes Aircraft Company in the role of an industrial engineer with professional registration in the state of Michigan. He served in the U.S. Air Force as an officer in charge of base construction projects. He held the position of Ph.D. graduate adviser for eight years in the Department of Management at the University of Texas and was nominated for six teaching awards. He is a founding member and first treasurer of the Operations Management Association, former at-large vice president of the Decision Sciences Institute, and served ten years as associate editor of *Management Science.* He has contributed chapters to several books and is the author or co-author of more than forty journal articles. He is currently an associate editor for the *Journal of Operations Management* and serves on the editorial advisory board for the *International Journal of Service Industry Management.*

MONA J. FITZSIMMONS, a graduate of the University of Michigan, received her undergraduate degree in journalism with major supporting work in chemistry and psychology. Her graduate work was in geology, and she taught in public and private schools and at the university level. She has done writing and editing for the Encyclopaedia Britannica Education Corporation and for various professional journals and organizations. She edited and indexed *Service Operations Management,* written by James A. Fitzsimmons and Robert S. Sullivan and published by McGraw-Hill in 1982. Her nonprofessional activities have included volunteer work for the Red Cross aquatics program and wildlife rehabilitation. Currently, she is a free-lance consumer activist who has particular interests in the areas of responsible environmental behaviors, the responsibilities of patients and physicians in the health care equation, and relief from the health and financial burdens that tobacco use places on society.

To Our Children:
Michael, Gary, and Samantha
and Granddaughter:
Colleen

Contents

Part III
STRUCTURING THE SERVICE ENTERPRISE

6. The Supporting Facility 123

7. Service Facility Location 161

Part VI
QUANTITATIVE MODELS WITH SERVICE APPLICATIONS

Preface

This book represents a gauntlet—a challenge to those who administer, teach, and learn in our colleges and universities. The future economic, social, and environmental prosperity of the nation depends on creative management of services.

Services touch the lives of every person in this country every day: food services, communication services, and emergency services, to name only a few. Our welfare and the welfare of our economy are now based on services. The activities of manufacturing and agriculture will always be necessary, but we can eat only so much food and we can use only so many goods. Services, however, are largely experiential, and we will always have a limitless appetite for them.

Within the past decade, service operations management has been established as a field of study that embraces all service industries. For example, under the leadership of the senior author of this text, the discipline was recognized as an academic field and designated as a separate track by the Decision Sciences Institute (DSI) beginning with its 1987 Boston meeting. Next, in 1989, the *International Journal of Service Industry Management* was inaugurated. Finally, the First International Service Research Seminar in Service Management was held in France in 1990, drawing participants from the fields of operations management, marketing, and organizational behavior. This conference recognized the multidisciplinary nature of services and dropped the adjective "operations" in order to emphasize the integrative nature of service management. Following the 1996 Orlando DSI meeting, a Web site (http:soma.byu.edu) was established to support faculty and students interested in the field of service management.

In this second edition, chapters on project management and managing service inventories have been added to make the text appropriate for use in the introductory course in operations management. Now all students of business can have the opportunity of studying operations from the prospective of their future employment in a service economy. As we discuss in the first chapter, only in services are new jobs being created and many are in high-tech firms offering professional salaries. Furthermore, entrepreneurial opportunities for creative students abound in services.

The second edition has been retitled to emphasize the three themes that run throughout the book. First, this is a book devoted to the management of service *operations* from an open systems view, which means that the customer is a participant in the delivery process. Second, for services the "process is the product" and, therefore, marketing and *strategic* issues cannot be separated from operations, which in turn cannot ignore behavioral issues associated with customer contact. Finally, *information technology* is recognized as the enabler of continuous improvement in productivity and quality in services.

This book acknowledges and emphasizes the essential uniqueness of service management. These are some key features:

- The book is written in an engaging literary style, makes extensive use of examples, and is based on the research and consulting experience of the authors.
- The theme of managing services for competitive advantage is emphasized in each chapter and provides a focus for each management topic.
- The integration of marketing, operations, and human behavior is recognized as central to effective service management.
- To dispel the common belief that manufacturing management principles can be applied to services without recognizing the different operating environments, the role of services in society and the uniqueness of service delivery systems are stressed.
- Information technologies such as yield management and data envelopment analysis are included as illustrations of the strategic role of information in managing services.
- Emphasis is placed on the need for continuous improvement in quality and productivity in order to compete effectively in a global environment.
- To facilitate pedagogical flexibility, all quantitative models are contained in chapter supplements and in the final section of the book, Part VI.
- To motivate the reader, a vignette of a well-known company starts each chapter, illustrating the strategic nature of the topic to be covered.
- Each chapter has a preview, a closing summary, topics for discussion, exercises when appropriate, and one or more cases.
- The instructor's manual contains case analyses, exercise solutions, a video library list, and supplementary cases and readings. For the second edition PowerPoint lecture presentations are available on computer disks and computer software to support two in-class games.

In the second edition the following pedagogical features have been added to each chapter:

- *Learning objectives* to help students focus on the key concepts to be explored in the chapter.
- *Service Benchmarks* to illustrate an outstanding example of excellence in service.
- *Key Terms and Definitions* are listed at the conclusion of the chapter as a quick reference and reminder of the new vocabulary just presented.
- *Solved Problems* are provided before the exercises to illustrate in detail the steps to resolve a quantitative problem.

We were very fortunate to have our manuscript reviewed by several colleagues—all people of integrity, wit, and vision. Their detailed comments, insights, and thought-provoking suggestions were gratefully received and incorporated in the text in many places. Special thanks and acknowledgment go to the following people for their valuable reviews of the first edition: Mohammad Ala, California State University, Los Angeles; Joanna R. Baker, Virginia Polytechnic Institute and State University; Mark Davis, Bentley College; Maling Ebrahimpour, University of Rhode Island; Michael Gleeson, Indiana University; Ray Haynes, California Polytechnic State University at San Luis Obispo; Art Hill, the University of Minnesota; Sheryl Kimes, Cornell University; and Richard Reid, the University of New Mexico.

The second edition has benefited from the constructive comments of the following reviewers: Kimberly A. Bates, New York University; Avi Dechter, California State University, Northridge; Scott A. Dellana, East Carolina University; Sheryl Kimes, Cornell University; Larry J. LeBlanc, Vanderbilt University; Robert Lucas, Metropolitan State College of Denver; Barbara A. Osyk, University of Akron; Michael J. Showalter, Florida State University; and V. Sridharan, Clemson University; and Suresh K Tadisina, Southern Illinois University, Carbondale.

Fang Wu, Ph.D. student at the University of Texas at Austin, assisted in the development of additional exercises and preparation of the PowerPoint lecture presentations. We also wish to thank Melba L. Jett for her indexing expertise and encouragement throughout this project. The personal computer, printer, and software provided through the generosity of William H. Seay, who endowed the senior author's professorship, made the writing of this book a great pleasure.

We express special appreciation to all our friends who encouraged us and tolerated our social lapses while we produced this book. In particular, we are indebted for the support of Richard and Janice Reid, who have provided lively and stimulating conversations and activities over many years and who generously allowed us the use of their mountain retreat. The beginning of the first edition was written in the splendid isolation of their part of the Jemez Mountains of New Mexico. No authors could want for better inspiration.

James A. Fitzsimmons
Mona J. Fitzsimmons

Overview of the Book

Part I begins with a discussion of the role of services in an economy. We first look at the evolution of societies based on economic activity, beginning with agriculture and moving to industrialization and finally to service economies. Next, we consider the distinctive characteristics of the service operations which lead to an open-systems view of services. This section sets the stage and examines the environment in which services now operate.

In Part II, we begin by developing the strategic service concept followed by a discussion of the generic competitive service strategies of overall cost leadership, differentiation, and focus. The necessity of integrating marketing and operations in services is first realized when a market position is established and the competitive service strategy is formulated. For services, information technology plays a central strategic role by creating barriers to entry, generating revenue, being an asset, and being a source for productivity improvement. The competitive role of information is captured in the concept of the virtual value chain which is a new topic of the second edition.

Structuring the service enterprise to support the competitive strategy is the topic of Part III. The service delivery system is engineered through the use of a process flowcharting concept called blueprinting, which explicitly recognizes the front office, where customer contact occurs, and the behind-the-scenes back-office operations. Questions concerning the facility design and layout are next addressed from the perspective of both customer participation and operations efficiency. Using analytical models, the critical decision of where to locate the service facility is determined. Finally, a new chapter on managing service projects has been included in the second edition.

Management of day-to-day operations is addressed in Part IV. We begin with the notion of the service encounter, which describes the interaction between service provider and customer in the context of a service organization. A treatment of service quality follows naturally once we have established a customer service orientation. The question of managing waiting lines is addressed from a psychological viewpoint. A new chapter on managing facilitating goods has been included in the second edition. Because the nature of services provides a challenge in matching capacity with demand, strategies are discussed, including the concept of yield management.

In Part V, we look at strategies to achieve world-class service. The concept of continual improvement in quality and productivity is discussed in the context of the stages of service firm competitiveness. Growth and expansion strategies are explored in the second edition with new material on global service strategies.

Part VI contains a selection of quantitative decision models with important service applications. This concluding part presents models used to forecast service demand, queuing models for capacity planning, and linear programming models with applications in services illustrated with Microsoft® Excel Solver, a new feature of the second edition.

PART ONE

Services and the Economy

We begin our study of service management in Chapter 1 with an appreciation of the central role that services play in the economies of nations and in world commerce. No economy can function without the infrastructure that services provide in the form of transportation and communications and without government services such as education and health care. As an economy develops, however, services become even more important, and soon the vast majority of the population is employed in service activities.

The management of services has unique challenges that are different from those found in manufacturing, which has been the traditional focus of management research and teaching. Thus, Chapter 2 will address the nature of service operations and identify their distinctive characteristics. Perhaps the most important characteristic of service operations is the presence of the customer in the service delivery system. Focusing on the customer and serving his or her needs has always been an important daily activity for service providers.

CHAPTER 1

The Role of Services in an Economy

LEARNING OBJECTIVES

After completing this chapter, you should be able to:

1. Describe the central role of services in an economy.
2. Discuss the evolution of an economy from an agrarian society to a service society.
3. Describe the features of preindustrial, industrial, and postindustrial societies.
4. Discuss the role of service managers with respect to innovation, social trends, and management challenges.

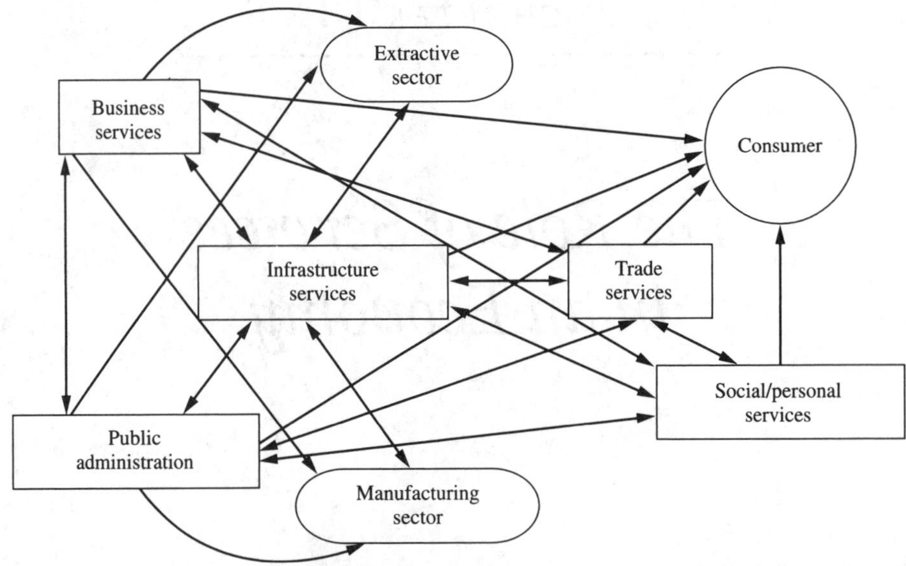

FIGURE 1.1. Interactive model of an economy.
(After Dorothy I. Riddle, Service-Led Growth, *Praeger, New York, 1986, p. 27.)*

Services lie at the very hub of economic activity in any society. Writing about the role of the service sector in world development, Dorothy Riddle formulated the economic model shown in Figure 1.1. This model shows the flow of activity among the three principal sectors of the economy: extractive (mining and farming), manufacturing, and service, which is divided into five subgroups. All activity eventually leads to the consumer. Examples of services in each of the five subgroups are:

Business services. Consulting, finance, banking

Trade services. Retailing, maintenance, repair

Infrastructure services. Communications, transportation

Social/personal services. Restaurants, health care

Public administration. Education, government

Infrastructure services, such as transportation and communications, are the essential links between all sectors of the economy, including the final consumer. In a complex economy, both infrastructure and trade services function as intermediaries between the extractive and manufacturing sectors and as the channel of distribution to the final consumer. Infrastructure services are a prerequisite for an economy to become industrialized; therefore, no advanced society can be without these services.

In an industrialized economy, specialized firms can supply business services to manufacturing firms more cheaply and efficiently than manufacturing firms can supply these services for themselves. Thus, more and more often we find advertising, consulting, financing, testing, and other business functions being provided for the manufacturing sector by service firms.

Except for basic subsistence living, where individual households are self-sufficient, service activities are absolutely necessary for the economy to function and to enhance the quality of life. Consider, for example, the importance of a banking industry to transfer funds and a transportation industry to move food products to areas that cannot produce them. Moreover, a wide variety of social and personal services, such as restaurants, lodging, cleaning, and child care, have been created to move former household functions into the economy.

Public administration plays a critical role in providing a stable environment for investment and economic growth. Services such as public education, health care, well-maintained roads, safe drinking water, clean air, and public safety are necessary for any nation's economy to survive and people to prosper.

Thus, it is imperative to recognize that services are not peripheral activities but rather integral parts of society. They are central to a functioning and healthy economy and lie at the heart of that economy. The service sector not only facilitates but also makes possible the goods-producing activities of the extractive and manufacturing sectors. Services are the crucial force for today's change toward a global economy.

CHAPTER PREVIEW

We begin with a discussion of economic evolution, finding that modern industrialized economies are dominated by employment in the service sector industries. This represents a natural evolution of economies from preindustrial to industrial and, finally, to postindustrial societies. The economic activity of a society determines the nature of how its people live and how the standard of living is measured. The nature of the service sector is explored in terms of employment opportunities, contributions to economic stability, and sources of economic leadership. Finally, the role of the service manager is discussed in terms of innovation, opportunities for new services based on demographic trends, and the many managerial challenges in an expanding service economy.

ECONOMIC EVOLUTION

In the early 1900s, only three of every ten workers in the United States were employed in the services sector. The remaining workers were active in agriculture and industry. By 1950, employment in services accounted for 50 percent of the workforce. Today, services employ about eight out of every ten workers. During the past 90 years, we have witnessed a major evolution in our society from being predominantly manufacturing-based to being predominantly service-based.

Economists studying economic growth are not surprised by these events. Colin Clark argues that as nations become industrialized, there is an inevitable shift of employment from one sector of the economy to another.[1] As productivity increases in one sector, the labor force moves into another. This observation, known as the *Clark-Fisher hypothesis*, leads to a classification of economies by noting the activity of the majority of the workforce.

[1]Colin Clark, *The Conditions of Economic Progress*, 3d ed., The Macmillan Co., London, 1957.

TABLE 1.1. Stages of Economic Activity

Primary (Extractive)	*Quaternary* (Trade and Commerce Services)
Agriculture	Transportation
Mining	Retailing
Fishing	Communication
Forestry	Finance and insurance
	Real estate
	Government
Secondary (Goods-Producing)	*Quinary* (Refining and Extending Human Capacities)
Manufacturing	Health
Processing	Education
	Research
	Recreation
	Arts
Tertiary (Domestic Services)	
Restaurants and hotels	
Barber and beauty shops	
Laundry and dry cleaning	
Maintenance and repair	

Table 1.1 describes five stages of economic activity. Many economists, including Clark, limited their analyses to only three stages, of which the tertiary stage was simply services. We have taken the suggestion of Nelson N. Foote and Paul K. Hatt and subdivided the service stage into three categories.[2]

Today, an overwhelming number of countries are still in a primary stage of development. These economies are based on extracting natural resources from the land. Their productivity is low, and income is subject to fluctuations based on the prices of commodities such as sugar and copper. In much of Africa and parts of Asia, more than 70 percent of the labor force is engaged in extractive activities.

Based on the work activity of their populations, however, many of the so-called advanced industrial nations would be better described as service economies. Table 1.2 is a partial list of industrialized countries ranked in order of the percentage of those employed in service-producing jobs. This table contains some surprises, such as finding Canada and Australia (known for their mining industries) high on the list. Several observations can be made: global economic development is progressing in unanticipated directions, successful industrial economies are built on a strong service sector, and just as it has in manufacturing, competition in services will become global. In fact, many of the largest commercial banks in the world at present are owned by the Japanese. Trade in services remains a challenge, however, because many countries erect barriers to protect domestic firms. For example, India and Mexico, among others, prohibit the sale of insurance by foreign companies.

[2]N. N. Foote and P. K. Hatt, "Social Mobility and Economic Advancement," *American Economic Review,* May 1953, pp. 364–378.

TABLE 1.2. Percent Employment in Service Jobs for Selected Industrialized Nations, 1980–1993

Country	1980	1987	1993
Canada	67.2	70.8	74.8
United States	67.1	71.0	74.3
Australia	64.7	69.7	71.8
Belgium	64.3	70.1	70.7
Israel	63.3	66.0	68.0
France	56.9	63.6	66.4
Finland	52.2	60.1	65.9
Italy	48.7	57.7	60.2
Japan	54.5	58.1	59.9
United Kingdom	60.4	67.7	NA

NA—Not available.

Source: 1993 Statistical Yearbook, Department of International Economic and Social Affairs Statistical Office, United Nations, New York, 1993, pp. 236–242.

As Figure 1.2 shows, the service sector now accounts for more than three-fourths of total employment in the United States, which continues a trend that began more than one century ago. Therefore, based on employment figures, the United States can no longer be characterized as an industrial society; instead, it is a postindustrial, or service, society.

STAGES OF ECONOMIC DEVELOPMENT

Describing where our society has been, its current condition, and its most likely future is the task of social historians. Daniel Bell, a professor of sociology at Harvard University, has written extensively on this topic, and the material that follows is based on his work.[3] To place the concept of a postindustrial society in perspective, we must compare its features with those of preindustrial and industrial societies.

Preindustrial Society

The condition of most of the world's population today is one of subsistence, or a *preindustrial society.* Life is characterized as a game against nature. Working with muscle power and tradition, the labor force is engaged in agriculture, mining, and fishing. Life is conditioned by the elements, such as the weather, the quality of the soil, and the availability of water. The rhythm of life is shaped by nature, and the pace of work varies with the seasons. Productivity is low and bears little evidence of technology. Social life revolves around the extended household, and this combination of low productivity and large population results in high rates of underemployment (workers not fully utilized). Many seek positions in

[3]Daniel Bell, *The Coming of Post-Industrial Society: A Venture in Social Forecasting,* Basic Books, Inc., New York, 1973.

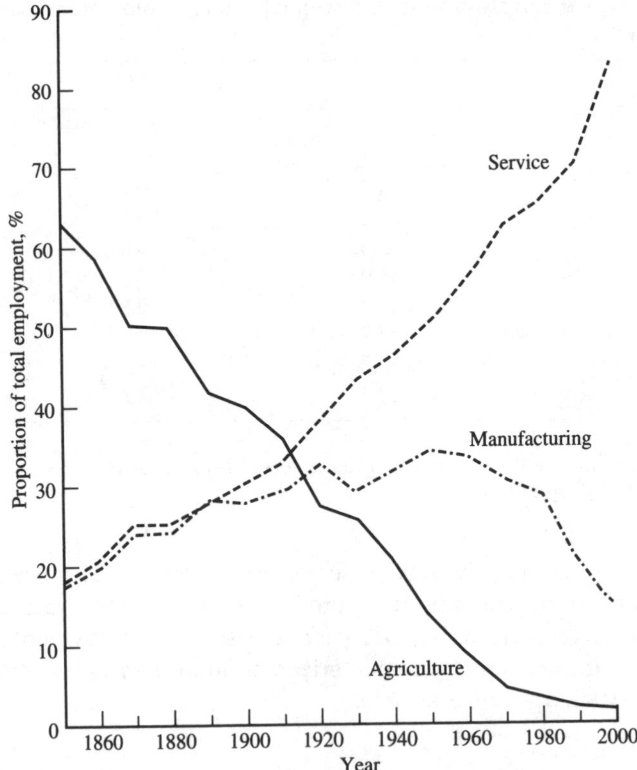

FIGURE 1.2. Trends in U.S employment by sector, 1850–2000. *(From U.S. Department of Commerce, Bureau of the Census,* Historical Statistics of the United States, *1975, p. 137, and U.S. Department of Commerce, Bureau of the Census,* Statistical Abstract of the U.S., *1995, p. 417.)*

services, but of the personal or household variety. Preindustrial societies are agrarian and structured around tradition, routine, and authority.

Industrial Society

The predominant activity in an *industrial society* is the production of goods. The focus of attention is on making more with less. Energy and machines multiply the output per labor-hour and structure the nature of work. Division of labor is the operational "law" that creates routine tasks and the notion of the semiskilled worker. Work is accomplished in the artificial environment of the factory, and people tend the machines. Life becomes a game that is played against a fabricated nature—a world of cities, factories, and tenements. The rhythm of life is machine-paced and dominated by rigid working hours and time clocks.

An industrial society is a world of schedules and acute awareness of the value of time. The standard of living becomes measured by the quantity of goods, but note that the complexity of coordinating the production and distribution of goods results in the creation of large bureaucratic and hierarchic organizations. These organizations are designed with certain roles for their members, and their operation tends to be impersonal, with persons treated as things. The individual is the unit of social life in a society that is considered to be the sum total of all the individual decisions being made in the marketplace. Of course, the unrelenting pressure of industrial life is softened by the countervailing force of labor unions.

Postindustrial Society

While an industrial society defines the standard of living by the quantity of goods, the *postindustrial society* is concerned with the quality of life, as measured by services such as health, education, and recreation. The central figure is the professional person, because rather than energy or physical strength, information is the key resource. Life now is a game played among persons. Social life becomes more difficult, because political claims and social rights multiply. Society becomes aware that the independent actions of individuals can combine to create havoc for everyone, as seen in traffic congestion and environmental pollution. The community rather than the individual becomes the social unit.

Bell suggests that the transformation from an industrial to a postindustrial society occurs in many ways. First, there is a natural development of services, such as transportation and utilities, to support industrial development. As labor-saving devices are introduced into the production process, more workers engage in nonmanufacturing activities, such as maintenance and repair. Second, growth of the population and mass consumption of goods increase wholesale and retail trade, along with banking, real estate, and insurance. Third, as income increases, the proportion spent on the necessities of food and home decreases, and the remainder creates a demand for durables and then for services.

Ernst Engel, a Prussian statistician of the nineteenth century, observed that as family incomes increase, the percentage spent on food and durables drops while consumption of services that reflect a desire for a more enriched life increases correspondingly. This phenomenon is analogous to the Maslow hierarchy of needs, which says that once the basic requirements of food and shelter are satisfied, people seek physical goods and, finally, personal development. However, a necessary condition for the "good life" is health and education. In our attempts to eliminate disease and increase the span of life, health services become a critical feature of modern society.

Higher education becomes the condition for entry into a postindustrial society, which requires professional and technical skills of its population. Also, claims for more services and social justice lead to a growth in government. Concerns for environmental protection require government intervention and illustrate the interdependent and even global character of postindustrial problems. Table 1.3 summarizes the features that characterize the preindustrial, industrial, and postindustrial stages of economic development.

NATURE OF THE SERVICE SECTOR

For many people, *service* is synonymous with *servitude* and brings to mind workers flipping hamburgers and waiting on tables. However, the service sector that has grown significantly over the past 30 years cannot be accurately described as

TABLE 1.3. Comparison of Societies

	Features						
Society	Game	Predominant Activity	Use of Human Labor	Unit of Social Life	Standard of Living Measure	Structure	Technology
Preindustrial	Against nature	Agriculture, mining	Raw muscle power	Extended household	Subsistence	Routine, traditional, authoritative	Simple hand tools
Industrial	Against fabricated nature	Goods production	Machine tending	Individual	Quantity of goods	Bureaucratic, hierarchic	Machines
Postindustrial	Among persons	Services	Artistic, creative, intellectual	Community	Quality of life in terms of health, education, recreation	Interdependent, global	Information

composed only of low-wage or low-skill jobs in department stores and fast-food restaurants. Instead, as Table 1.4 shows, the fastest-growing jobs within the service sector are in finance, insurance, real estate, miscellaneous services (e.g., health, education, professional services), and retail trade. Note that job areas whose growth rates were less than the rate of increase in total jobs (i.e., less than 31.8 percent) lost market share, even though they showed gains in their absolute numbers. The exceptions are in mining and manufacturing, which lost in absolute numbers and thus showed negative growth rates. This trend should accelerate with the end of the cold war and the subsequent downsizing of the military and defense industry.

Changes in the pattern of employment will have implications on where and how people live, on educational requirements, and, consequently, on the kinds of organizations that will be important to that society. Industrialization created the need for the semiskilled worker who could be trained in a few weeks to perform the routine machine-tending tasks. The subsequent growth in the service sector has caused a shift to white-collar occupations. In the United States, the year 1956 was a turning point. For the first time in the history of industrial society, the number of white-collar workers exceeded the number of blue-collar work-

TABLE 1.4. Rate of Growth of U.S. Jobs, January 1982–April 1996

	Nonfarm Jobs Jan. 82, in 1000's	Nonfarm Jobs Jan. 82, %	Nonfarm Jobs April 96, in 1000's	Nonfarm Jobs April 96, %	Growth of Nonfarm Jobs, %
Service-producing					
Finance, insurance, real estate	5341	6.0	7060	6.0	32.2
Miscellaneous services	19,036	21.3	33,642	28.5	76.7
State and local government	13,098	14.6	16,600	14.0	26.7
Wholesale trade	5296	5.9	6444	5.5	21.7
Retail trade	15,161	16.9	21,100	17.9	39.2
Transportation and utilities	5082	5.7	6262	5.3	23.2
Federal government	2739	3.1	2775	2.3	16.6
Total	65,753	73.5	93,883	79.5	
Goods-producing					
Construction	3905	4.4	5378	4.6	37.7
Mining	1127	1.3	574	0.5	–49.1
Manufacturing	18,781	21.0	18,187	15.4	–3.2
Total	23,813	26.7	24,139	20.5	
Total jobs	89,566		118,022	Percent increase	31.8

Source: *Economic Indicators*, prepared for the Joint Economic Committee by the Council of Economic Advisors, U.S. Government Printing Office, June 1996, p. 14.

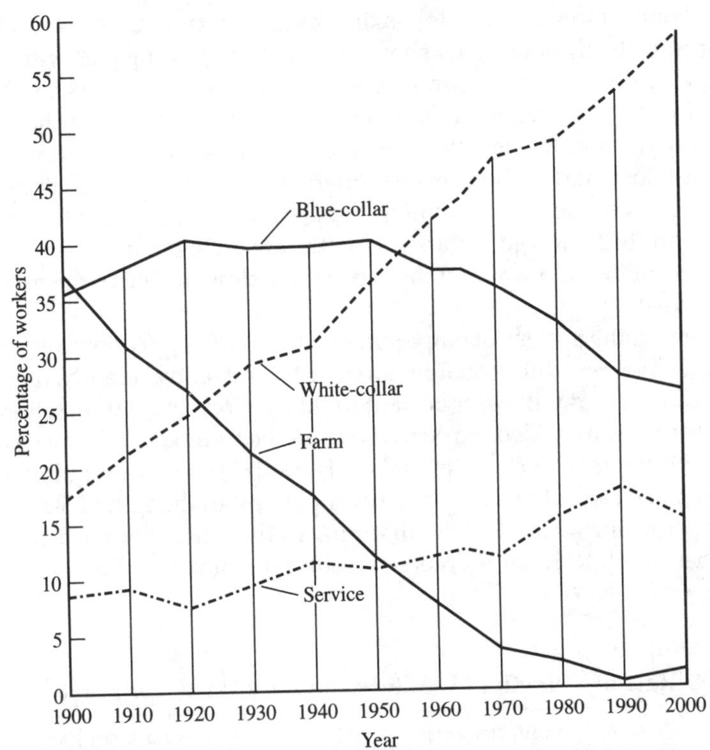

FIGURE 1.3. Occupational distribution of the U.S. labor force, 1900–2000.
(From U.S. Department of Commerce, Bureau of Census, Statistical Abstract of the U.S., 1995.)

ers, and the gap has been widening since then. The most interesting growth has been in the managerial and professional-technical fields, which are jobs that require a college education. Figure 1.3 shows the shift in employment from an industrial society of machine operators to a postindustrial society of professional and technical workers.

Today, service industries are the source of economic leadership. During the past 30 years, more than 44 million new jobs have been created in the service sector to absorb the influx of women into the workforce and to provide an alternative to the lack of job opportunities in manufacturing. The service industries now account for approximately 70 percent of the national income in the United States. Given that there is a limit to how many cars a consumer can use and how much one can eat and drink, this should not be surprising. The appetite for services, however, especially innovative ones, is insatiable. Among the services presently in demand are those that reflect an aging population, such as geriatric health care, and others that reflect a two-income family, such as day care.

The growth of the service sector has produced a less cyclic national economy.

During the past four recessions in the United States, employment by service industries has actually increased, while jobs in manufacturing have been lost. This suggests that consumers are willing to postpone the purchase of products but will not sacrifice essential services like education, telephone, banking, health care, and public services such as fire and police protection.

Several reasons can explain the recession-resistant nature of services. First, by their nature, services cannot be inventoried, as is the case for products. Because consumption and production occur simultaneously for services, the demand for them is more stable than that for manufactured goods. When the economy falters, many services continue to survive. Hospitals keep busy as usual, and, while commissions may drop in real estate, insurance, and security businesses, employees need not be laid off.

Second, during a recession, both consumers and business firms defer capital expenditures and instead fix up and make do with existing equipment. Thus, service jobs in maintenance and repair are created.

ROLE OF THE SERVICE MANAGER

Successful growth of the service sector will depend on innovation and skilled management that will promote an ethic of continuous improvement in both quality and productivity.

Innovation

The product development model that is driven by technology and engineering could be called a *push theory of innovation.* A concept for a new product germinates in the laboratory with a new scientific discovery that becomes a solution looking for a problem. The 3M experience with Post-it notes is one example of this innovation process. The laboratory discovery was a poor adhesive, which found a creative use as a glue for notes to be attached temporarily to objects without leaving a mark when removed.

Information technology provides many examples of the push theory of service innovation. The growth of the World Wide Web as a place of commerce is changing the delivery of services. People can browse the Internet for every imaginable product or service from around the world. In fact, to stay competitive, many businesses may soon be required to offer new cost-effective and convenient services for customers who have home computers equipped with modems.

For services, the Cash Management Account introduced by Merrill Lynch is an example of the *pull theory of innovation.* During the period of high interest rates in the 1980s, a need arose to finance short-term corporate cash flows, and individual investors were interested in obtaining an interest rate that was higher than those currently available on passbook bank deposits.

The French Revolution provides another view of service formation, this time based on changing demographics. Before the revolution, only two restaurants were in existence in Paris; shortly afterward, there were more than 500. The dispossessed nobility had been forced to give up their private chefs, who found that opening their own restaurants was a logical solution to their unemployment.

For a manufacturing firm, product innovation is often driven by engineering-based research, but in service firms, software engineers and programmers are the technocrats who develop new innovations. Customers interact directly in the service process; therefore, the focus on meeting customer needs drives service innovation and explains why marketing plays such a central role in service management.

The introduction of a new technology, however, does have an ancillary effect on service innovation. For example, the VCR has spawned a video rental business and created a renewed demand for old movies. Thus, the creation of an innovative service enterprise has many sources.

Service innovation also can arise from exploiting information available from other activities. For example, records of sales by auto parts stores can be used to identify frequent failure areas in particular models of cars. This information has value both for the manufacturer, who can accomplish engineering changes, and for the retailer, who can diagnose customer problems. In addition, the creative use of information can be a source of new services, or it can add value to existing services. For example, an annual summary statement of transactions furnished by one's financial institution has added value at income tax time.

Service innovators face a difficult problem in testing their service ideas. The process of product development includes building a laboratory prototype for testing before full-scale production is initiated. New services are seldom tested before they are launched in the marketplace, however, which provides a partial explanation for the observed high failure rate of service innovations, particularly in retailing and restaurants. At present, new service concepts usually must prove themselves in the field instead of in a "laboratory" setting. Methods to simulate service delivery systems before their introduction must be developed. One example of an effort in this direction is provided by Burger King, which acquired a warehouse in Miami to enclose a replica of its standard outlet. This mock restaurant was used to simulate changes in layout that would be required for the introduction of new features such as drive-through window service and a breakfast menu. The marketing concept of a "focus group," consisting of customers selected to review service proposals in a roundtable discussion, is another means of evaluating new service ideas. The difficulty in service prototyping is the need to evaluate the service delivery system in operation where technology, service providers, and customers are integrated.

Social Trends

Three social trends will have a major influence on services: the aging of the U.S. population, the growth of two-income families, and the increase in the number of single people. As the baby boom generation matures, the percentage of older people in America will increase greatly. Currently, 6.2 million Americans are older than 80 years old. By the year 2000, this figure is projected to be 8 million, and by the year 2010, the number will be 21.1 million.[4] This aging of the population will create opportunities for retired people to take part-time work, in part because of fewer young people entering the workforce. In the future, companies facing

[4]Susan B. Garland, "The Graying of America Spawns a New Crisis," *BusinessWeek,* Aug. 17, 1987, pp. 60–62.

a labor shortage may be forced to hire retired workers, at least on a temporary or part-time basis, and this trend is already apparent. For example, The Travelers' Insurance Company has developed a Retirement Job Bank of its retired employees that is used as a source of skilled labor to fill in during peak work times, absences, and vacations.[5] Also, elderly people are living longer and have more active lives, with consequent demands on health care, public transportation, and leisure services.

The two-income family is fast replacing the traditional family of the 1950s, which consisted of a husband, a housewife, and two children. The new two-income family unit has created demands for services such as day care, preschool, and "eating out" services. For two-income families, time is at a premium, and they are willing to pay for services that give them more free time. As a result, many new services have been created that focus exclusively on saving time for these individuals. Examples include home delivery services and personal shopping services for everything from gifts to clothing. Increased disposable income from two wage earners also may translate into increased demands for leisure, entertainment, and tourism services.

The number of single people in America is growing, and this trend is expected to continue.[6] Recreational sports and other group-oriented activities will be in demand, because they will offer the opportunity to meet other single people. Home food delivery services that now offer pizza may find a market for the delivery of gourmet meals to single people.

All of these social trends support the notion that the home will become a sanctuary for people in the future, and that sanctuary will be supported by a communication system bringing video and electronic messages from the global community into the living room.

Management Challenges

Complacency in the management of service industries, inattention to quality, disregard for customer concerns, and exclusive attention to short-term financial orientation all threaten to undermine the service sector of the economy. It is important to realize that under the pressures just mentioned, the service sector could become as vulnerable to foreign competition as the manufacturing sector has. The following discussion of the competitive challenges in services is based in part on a classic article by James Brian Quinn and Christopher E. Gagnon, in which they caution the reader that services could follow manufacturing into decline.[7]

Quinn and Gagnon point out that the economic trends in services are undeniable, and that they are similar to the recent experience in manufacturing. Since the early 1980s, the net positive trade balances in services have fallen steadily. For example, a serious loss of market share has been experienced in international airline travel as the once powerful carriers, Pan Am and TWA, de-

[5]Harold E. Johnson, "Older Workers Help Meet Employment Needs," *Personnel Journal,* May 1988, pp. 100–105.

[6]Edward Cornish, "The Coming of the Singles Society," *The Futurist,* July–August 1987, p. 2.

[7]J. B. Quinn and C. E. Gagnon, "Will Services Follow Manufacturing into Decline?" *Harvard Business Review,* November–December 1986, pp. 95–103.

clared bankruptcy in the face of foreign competitors that upgraded their fleets and emphasized quality of service.

Purely domestic services are not immune to foreign competition, either. Direct foreign investment in the U.S. service sector is substantial. Many famous names in services, such as 20th Century Fox, Stouffer's Hotels and Restaurants, Marshall Field, and Giant Foods, are now foreign-owned. In California, Japanese banks are changing the nature of competition and winning accounts by taking a much longer view in making business loans to new ventures at very competitive interest rates.

The nature of competition in services also is changing, because the forces of deregulation and new technologies have restructured service industries in recent years. Deregulation has caused significant restructuring in the domestic airline industry, with successful new regional carriers appearing (e.g., Southwest and Alaska) and old giants declaring bankruptcy (e.g., Eastern and Braniff). New route networks have formed around the hub-and-spoke concept to provide service in a more cost-effective manner. The use of computer reservation systems has allowed airlines to provide a variety of competitive fares based on preselling seats at a discount; thus, they can ensure high-load factors and profitable operations. Service managers need to understand these new competitive dimensions to take advantage of opportunities to improve service quality and performance, thereby creating barriers to the entry of foreign and domestic competitors. Competing on the traditional dimensions of quality, price, and availability will always be important, but consider the following additional dimensions based on the use of information technologies, which are the source of the value added by service firms.

Economies of Scale

Economies of scale are realized when fixed costs in new technology are allocated over increased volume; the result is reduced cost per transaction. For example, automation of the securities trading process changed the entire structure of the industry and made possible the handling of daily volumes in the millions of shares. The old system of transferring shares from seller to buyer manually has been replaced by an electronic clearinghouse. Without using a central electronic depository, Wall Street could not function as an efficient securities marketplace. New and expensive medical technologies, such as the CAT or MRI scanners, have resulted in regional treatment centers and the concentration of medical services at these large hospitals. Thus, we find that the introduction of capital-intensive technologies has resulted in the concentration of services and aggregation of demand.

Economies of Scope

Economies of scope, a new and somewhat controversial concept, describes the benefits that are realized when entirely new service products move through established distribution networks with little added cost. For example, once the communications and information-handling technologies are in place, a much wider set of services can be distributed to a more diffuse customer base at low marginal costs. In addition, this information technology base can offer strategic benefits through more rapid product introduction and faster response to competitors' moves. Insurance companies that automated their back-office operations in the 1960s to improve billing and collections found themselves with a competitive advantage during the interest rate explosion of the 1980s. Companies had to alter their products rapidly to attract interest-sensitive new customers and to avoid the losses from current customers borrowing against their policies at low interest rates. Only those companies with the flexibility of computer information systems could design and deploy their products quickly enough to obtain a competitive edge. Some companies added new computer-intensive financial services such as cash management accounts to attract funds. A very common example of economies of scope can be found at any local convenience store that has added self-service gasoline and microwave meal service to its original grocery stocks.

Complexity

Since deregulation, the domestic airline industry has witnessed an ever-changing fare structure so complex that fares can no longer be published in flight schedules. Computerized reservations systems allow airlines to analyze the status of flights and customer buying behavior in such detail that they can optimize margins on each type of demand and meet competitors' responses. The ability to monitor hundreds of flights and make seat allocation decisions on an hourly basis is accomplished with significant computer support and software algorithms. This special use of computer information to manage perishable capacity and to maximize revenues is called *yield management,* a topic that will be treated in detail in Chapter 13, Managing Capacity and Demand.

Sophisticated use of information systems to manage complexity also can be found in retail stores. Bar-code scanners give instant feedback on sales and inventory movements, which results in a better match of inventory to customers' needs. This information has enabled major chains to customize the stock featured at their stores so that they can accommodate regional preferences and compete better with small specialty shops.

Boundary Crossing

Competition among services once thought to be in different industries is now becoming commonplace. Some of the most striking examples are found in the financial services. Today, many consumers use their banks and brokers almost interchangeably, because neither is seriously restricted in its scope of operations. Banks, insurance companies, and brokerage houses offer a similar range of financial products and services and now compete in one market, without the traditional boundaries. As noted earlier, convenience stores now compete with fast-food restaurants as well as with service stations, and even manufacturing firms such as GM and Ford have entered the service arena by offering financing services to auto buyers. The ability of auto manufacturers to finance the sales of their cars has allowed them to offer loans at reduced interest rates as an incentive to buy their products. In fact, at present, General Motors Acceptance Corporation is the nation's largest single holder of consumer debt. Thus, we can readily see that competition in services can come from any quarter.

International Competitiveness

The worldwide service trade is growing with the help of cheaper and more flexible transportation and communication capabilities. During the 1960s, only 7 percent of the U.S. economy was exposed to foreign competition. Today, that figure is greater than 75 percent, and it is still climbing. With the world heading toward a single economy, or "global village," this trend toward greater international competition is expected to continue for both manufacturing and service firms.[8] For example, the purchase of Flying Tigers by Federal Express has enabled it to guarantee delivery anywhere in the world in two days; as a result, it joins DHL and others for a share in the growing business of global package delivery. Geographic distance is no longer a barrier between nations, and the challenges of ethnic diversity in the domestic market are multiplied by the difficulties of delivering a service in an international market with different cultural and language barriers.

SUMMARY

We have discovered that the modern industrial economies are dominated by employment in the service sector. Just as farming jobs migrated to manufacturing in the nineteenth century under the driving force of labor-saving technology, manufacturing jobs in due time migrated to services. Chapter 2 will conclude our discussion of the role of services in our new society and prepare us for developing new managerial skills by arguing that the distinctive characteristics of services require an approach to management significantly different from that found in manufacturing.

KEY TERMS AND DEFINITIONS

Clark-Fisher hypothesis a classification of economies according to the activity of the majority of the workforce.

Economies of scale allocation of the fixed costs of technology over an increased volume of sales (e.g., airline reservation system).

Economies of scope movement of new service products through established distribution networks (e.g., convenience stores adding self-serve gasoline pumps).

Industrial society a society dominated by factory work in mass-production industries.

Postindustrial society a service society in which people are engaged in information, intellectual, or creative-intensive activities.

Preindustrial society an agrarian society structured around farming and subsistence living.

Pull theory of innovation service innovations that are driven by customer needs.

Push theory of innovation product innovations that originate in scientific laboratories.

TOPICS FOR DISCUSSION

1. Illustrate how a person's lifestyle is influenced by the type of work that he or she does. For example, contrast a farmer, a factory worker, and a schoolteacher.
2. Is it possible for an economy to be based entirely on services?
3. Speculate on the nature of the society that may evolve after the postindustrial society.
4. What would be the impact on the service industry of the emerging social trend called *voluntary simplicity* (i.e., people choosing to spend less time working to enjoy life more)?
5. Comment on the role that marketing plays in the service innovation process.

[8]John Greenwald, "Down and Down the Dollar Goes," *Time*, Sept. 7, 1992, pp. 36–37.

Service Benchmark

In the 1990's the New Jobs Are in Services and Many Are High Paying!

More and more, Americans are serving each other. There has been a net increase of roughly 11 million jobs since the recession ended in early 1991, and almost all of the new ones are in industries that provide one kind of service or another. The fastest growth took place in business services, a catch-all category that includes everything from accountants and data processors to janitors and temporary workers; leisure services, from blackjack dealers to amusement park operators; and social services, like welfare workers. The industries that lost jobs at the greatest rate include clothing and textile manufacturing, oil and gas extraction and coal mining. Some fast-growing industries pay extraordinarily well: annual earnings at brokerage firms average more than $96,000. But some of the biggest gainers pay well below average: many providers of social welfare services work for nonprofit agencies and earn little more than those they try to help. All in all, the gap has widened between those at the top of the job ladder and those at the bottom. Researchers at the Bureau of Labor Statistics have found that the largest gains in job growth in recent years took place in the highest-paying job categories; relatively low-paying industries and occupations have also grown, but at a slower pace. Employment has actually shrunk among job categories in the middle range.

Source: "The New Jobs: A Growing Number Are Good Ones," Judith H. Dobrzynski, *The New York Times*, July 21, 1996, p. 10

Winners and Losers, Industry by Industry

(Industries ranked by how quickly they added or lost jobs from the first quarter of 1991 to the first quarter of 1996. Top 25 and bottom 25.)

	Total Jobs in First Quarter 1996 in 1000s	Avg. Annual Growth Rate, %	Avg. Annual Earnings in 1993, $
Business services	7,009	6.7	22,499
Leisure	1,505	6.2	21,018
Nonbanking financial institutions	496	5.7	NA
Social services	2,370	5.6	15,326
Brokerage	531	4.9	96,497
Local transit	439	4.7	20,496
Transportation services	430	4.4	31,617
Motion pictures	516	4.4	31,692
Agricultural services	599	4.2	NA
Museum and zoos	83	4.0	19,514
Auto repair and parking	1,059	3.6	20,430
Furniture stores	950	3.4	21,208
Building materials stores	883	3.3	22,914
Health services	9,463	3.3	34,200
Trucking and warehousing	1,879	3.2	27,289
Engineering and management	2,849	3.1	33,709
Special trade contractors	3,334	3.1	26,443
Education	1,982	3.0	20,088
Eating and drinking places	7,419	2.8	11,920
Misc. services	44	2.5	NA
Auto dealers and service stations	2,234	2.2	25,433
Rubber and plastics	962	2.2	33,103
Air transportation	828	2.2	43,093
Lumber products	754	2.1	27,713
State and local government	16,584	1.5	28,859
Legal services	926	0.3	61,224
Stone, clay, and glass	535	0.2	33,566
Food products	1,674	0.1	32,369
Paper products	682	0.1	42,178
Printing and publishing	1,532	–0.3	32,515
Primary metal industries	708	–0.7	47,020
Textile mills	642	–0.8	24,897
Chemicals	1,026	–0.9	56,289
Apparel and accessory stores	1,100	–1.1	13,971
Utility services	905	–1.2	55,722
Federal government	2,781	–1.2	NA
Transportation equipment	1,747	–1.2	NA
Banks and savings institutions	2,022	–1.7	35,252
Metal mining	51	–2.3	56,964
Petroleum and coal	140	–2.4	67,996
Railroads	234	–2.7	55,707
Apparel and textile	868	–2.8	19,225
Tobacco	41	–3.4	55,983
Instruments	831	–3.4	45,795
Leather	99	–4.8	22,664
Oil and gas extraction	312	–5.0	36,011
Pipelines	14	–5.9	54,011
Coal mining	101	–6.4	62,044

Sources: Regional Financial Associates, Bureau of Labor Statistics, as reprinted in *The New York Times,* July 21, 1996, p. 10.

SELECTED BIBLIOGRAPHY

BELL, DANIEL: *The Coming of Post-Industrial Society: A Venture in Social Forecasting,* Basic Books, Inc., New York, 1973.

COOK, JAMES: "You Mean We've Been Speaking Prose All These Years?" *Forbes,* April 11, 1983, pp. 143–149.

DAVIS, STANLEY M.: *Future Perfect,* Addison-Wesley, Reading, Mass., 1987.

FUCHS, VICTOR R.: *The Service Economy,* National Bureau of Economic Research, New York, 1968.

GERSHUNG, J. I.: *After Industrial Society,* The Macmillan Co., New York, 1978.

GERSUNY, C., and W. ROSENGREN: *The Service Society,* Schenkman Publishing Co., Cambridge, Mass., 1973.

GINZBERG, E., and G. VOJTA: "The Service Sector of the U.S. Economy," *Scientific American,* vol. 244, no. 3, March 1981, pp. 48–55.

GUILE, BRUCE E., and JAMES B. QUINN (ed.): *Managing Innovation: Cases from the Service Industries,* National Academy Press, Washington, D.C., 1988.

———: *Technology in Services: Policies for Growth, Trade, and Employment,* National Academy Press, Washington, D.C., 1988.

HESKETT, J. L.: "Lessons in the Service Sector," *Harvard Business Review,* March–April 1987, pp. 118–126.

———: *Managing in the Service Economy,* Harvard Business School Press, Boston, 1986.

———, W. E. SASSER, JR., AND C. W. L. HART: *Service Breakthroughs,* Free Press, New York, 1990.

HIRSCHHORN, L.: "The Post-Industrial Economy: Labour, Skills and the New Mode of Production," *The Service Industries Journal,* vol. 8, no. 1, 1988, pp. 19–38.

JOHNSTON, R.: "Service Industries: Improving Competitive Performance," *The Service Industries Journal,* vol. 8, no. 2, 1988, pp. 202–211.

KULONDA, D. J., and W. H. MOATES, Jr.: "Operations Supervisors in Manufacturing and Service Sectors in the United States: Are They Different?" *International Journal of Operations and Production Management,* vol. 6, no. 2, 1986, pp. 21–35.

LEWIS, R.: *The New Service Society,* Longman, New York, 1973.

LOVELOCK, C. H.: "Business Schools Owe Students Better Service," *Managing Services,* Prentice-Hall, Englewood Cliffs, N.J., 1988, pp. 22–24.

———, and R. K. SHELP: "The Service Economy Gets No Respect," *Managing Services,* Prentice-Hall, Englewood Cliffs, N.J., 1988, pp. 1–5.

QUINN, J. B., and C. E. GAGNON: "Will Services Follow Manufacturing into Decline?" *Harvard Business Review,* November–December 1986, pp. 95–103.

RIDDLE, D. I.: *Service-Led Growth,* Praeger, New York, 1986.

RIFKIN, JEREMY: *The End of Work: The Decline of the Global Labor Force and the Dawn of the Post-Market Era,* Tarcher/Putnam, New York, 1995.

TOFFLER, ALVIN: *The Third Wave,* William Morrow and Co., Inc., New York, 1980.

CHAPTER 2

The Nature of Services

LEARNING OBJECTIVES

After completing this chapter, you should be able to:

1. Classify a service into one of four categories using the service process matrix.
2. Describe a service using the four dimensions of the service package.
3. Discuss the managerial implications of the distinctive characteristics of a service operation.
4. Discuss the role of a service manager from an open-systems view of service operations.

In this chapter, we explore the distinctive features of services. The service environment is sufficiently unique to allow us to question the direct application of traditional manufacturing-based techniques to services without some modification, although many approaches are analogous. Ignoring the differences between manufacturing and service requirements will lead to failure, but more importantly, recognition of the special features of services will provide insights for enlightened and innovative management. Advances in service management cannot occur without an appreciation of the service system environment.

The distinction between a *product* and a *service* is difficult to make, because the purchase of a product is accompanied by some facilitating service (e.g., installation) and the purchase of a service often includes facilitating goods (e.g., food at a restaurant). Each purchase includes a bundle of goods and services in varying proportions, as shown in Table 2.1.

Services have a clear *front-office* (e.g., bank-teller interaction with a customer) and *back-office* (e.g., a bank's check-clearing operations) dichotomy in their operations, so we would be foolish to ignore the substantial opportunities for applying manufacturing techniques to the isolated back-office operations. These opportunities will be explored in Chapter 5, in which we consider the design of the service delivery system.

CHAPTER PREVIEW

The chapter begins with a classification of services based on the degree of customer interaction or customization and the degree of labor intensiveness. This classification allows us to focus on managerial issues that are found across similar service industries. An appreciation of the nature of services begins with the realization that a service is a package of explicit and implicit benefits performed within a supporting facility and using facilitating goods. These multiple dimensions of a service are central to the design and control of a service delivery system. The distinctive characteristics of service operations are discussed, and the implications for management are noted.

On the basis of these characteristics, the role of the service manager is viewed from an open-system perspective. That is, the service manager must deal with

TABLE 2.1. Proportion of Goods and Services in Typical Purchase Bundle

Goods					Services			
100%	75	50	25	0	25	50	75	100%

| .... Self-service gasoline......................... |
| .... Personal computer..................... |
| .... Office copier .... |
| .... Fast-food restaurant .... |
| .... Gourmet restaurant .... |
| .... Auto repair .... |
| .... Airline flight .... |
| .... Haircut .... |

Source: Adapted from W. E. Sasser, R. P. Olsen, and D. D. Wyckoff, *Management of Service Operations*, Allyn and Bacon, Boston, 1978, p. 11.

an environment in which the customers are present in the delivery system. This contrasts with manufacturing operations that are isolated or "buffered" from the customer by an inventory of finished goods. Thus, manufacturing traditionally has operated as a cost center, focusing on process efficiency. Service managers, who often operate as profit centers, must be concerned with both efficient and effective delivery of services.

SERVICE CLASSIFICATION

Concepts of service management should be applicable to all service organizations. For example, hospital administrators could learn something about their own business from the restaurant and hotel trade. Professional services such as consulting, law, and medicine have special problems, because the professional is trained to provide a specific clinical service (to use a medical example) but is not knowledgeable in business management. Thus, professional service firms offer attractive career opportunities for many college graduates.

A service classification scheme can help to organize our discussion of service management and break down the industry barriers to shared learning. As suggested, hospitals can learn about housekeeping from hotels. Less obviously, dry-cleaning establishments can learn from banks—cleaners can adapt the convenience of night deposits enjoyed by banking customers by providing laundry bags and after-hours drop-off boxes. For professional firms, scheduling a consulting engagement is similar to planning a legal defense or preparing a medical team for open heart surgery.

To demonstrate that management problems are common across service industries, Roger Schmenner proposed the *service process matrix* in Figure 2.1. In this matrix, services are classified across two dimensions that significantly affect the character of the service delivery process. The horizontal dimension measures

FIGURE 2.1. The service process matrix. *(From "How Can Service Businesses Survive and Prosper?" by Roger W. Schmenner,* Sloan Management Review, *vol. 27, no. 3, Spring 1986, p. 25, by permission of publisher. Copyright 1986 by the Sloan Management Review Association. All rights reserved.)*

Degree of Labor Intensity	**Degree of Interaction and Customization:** Low	High
Low	*Service factory:* • Airlines • Trucking • Hotels • Resorts and recreation	*Service shop:* • Hospitals • Auto repair • Other repair services
High	*Mass service:* • Retailing • Wholesaling • Schools • Retail aspects of commercial banking	*Professional service:* • Doctors • Lawyers • Accountants • Architects

the degree of labor intensity, which is defined as the ratio of labor cost to capital cost. Thus, capital-intensive services such as airlines and hospitals are found in the upper row because of their considerable investment in plant and equipment relative to labor costs. Labor-intensive services such as schools and legal assistance are found in the bottom row because their labor costs are high relative to their capital requirements.

The vertical dimension measures the degree of customer interaction and customization, which is a marketing variable that describes the ability of the customer to affect personally the nature of the service being delivered. Little interaction between customer and service provider is needed when the service is standardized rather than customized. For example, a meal at McDonald's, which is assembled from prepared items, is low in customization and served with little interaction occurring between the customer and the service providers. In contrast, a doctor and patient must interact fully in the diagnostic and treatment phases to achieve satisfactory results. Patients also expect to be treated as individuals and wish to receive medical care that is customized to their particular needs. It is important to note, however, that the interaction resulting from high customization creates potential problems for management of the service delivery process.

The four quadrants of the service process matrix have been given names, as defined by the two dimensions, to describe the nature of the services illustrated. *Service factories* provide a standardized service with high capital investment, much like a line-flow manufacturing plant.[1] *Service shops* permit more service customization, but they do so in a high-capital environment. Customers of a *mass service* will receive an undifferentiated service in a labor-intensive environment, but those seeking a *professional service* will be given individual attention by highly trained specialists.

Managers of services in any category, whether service factory, service shop, mass service, or professional service, share similar challenges, as noted in Figure 2.2. Services with high capital requirements (i.e., low labor intensity), such as airlines and hospitals, require close monitoring of technological advances to remain competitive. This high capital investment also requires managers to schedule demand to maintain utilization of the equipment. Alternatively, managers of highly labor-intensive services, such as medical or legal professionals, must concentrate on personnel matters. The degree of customization affects the ability to control the quality of the service being delivered and the perception of the service by the customer. Approaches to addressing each of these challenges are topics that will be discussed in later chapters.

THE SERVICE PACKAGE

Service managers have difficulty identifying their product. This problem is partly a result of the intangible nature of services, but it is the presence of the customer in the process that creates a concern for the total service experience. Consider the

[1]This concept of a service operated like a manufacturing factory is different from the more recent realization by manufacturing firms that operating a factory more like a service can achieve a competitive advantage. *See* R. B. Chase and D. A. Garvin, "The Service Factory," *Harvard Business Review*, vol. 67, no. 4, July/August 1989, pp. 61–69.

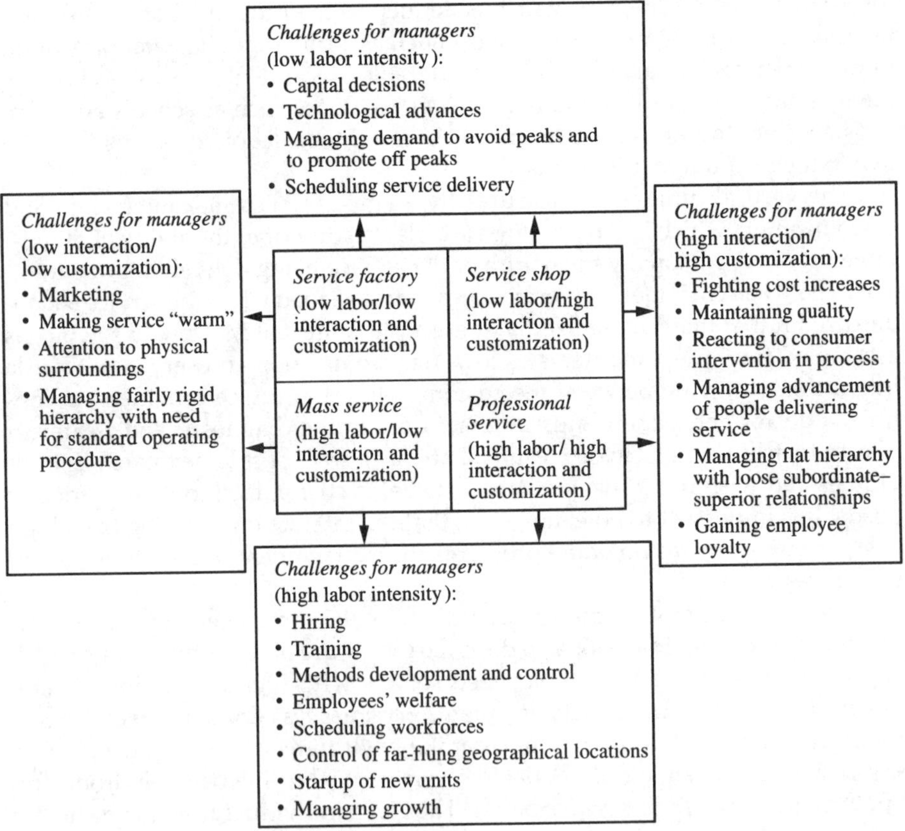

FIGURE 2.2. Challenges for service managers.
(From "How Can Service Businesses Survive and Prosper?" by Roger W. Schmenner, Sloan Management Review, *vol. 27, no. 3, Spring 1986, p. 27, by permission of publisher. Copyright 1986 by the Sloan Management Review Association. All rights reserved.)*

following examples. For a sit-down restaurant, atmosphere is just as important as the meal, because many diners regard the occasion as a way to get together with friends. A customer's opinion of a bank can be formed quickly on the basis of a teller's cheerfulness or length of the waiting line.

The *service package* is defined as a bundle of goods and services that is provided in some environment. This bundle consists of the following four features:

1. *Supporting facility.* The physical resources that must be in place before a service can be offered. Examples are a golf course, a ski lift, a hospital, and an airplane.
2. *Facilitating goods.* The material purchased or consumed by the buyer, or the items provided by the customer. Examples are golf clubs, skis, food items, replacement auto parts, legal documents, and medical supplies.
3. *Explicit services.* The benefits that are readily observable by the senses and that consist of the essential or intrinsic features of the service. Examples are the absence of pain after a tooth is repaired, a smooth-running automobile after a tune-up, and the response time of a fire department.
4. *Implicit services.* Psychological benefits that the customer may sense only

vaguely, or the extrinsic features of the service. Examples are the status of a degree from an Ivy League school, the privacy of a loan office, and worry-free auto repair.

All these features are experienced by the customer and form the basis of his or her perception of the service. It is important that the service manager offer a total experience for the customer that is consistent with the desired service package. Take, for example, a budget hotel. The supporting facility is a concrete-block building with austere furnishings. Facilitating goods are reduced to the minimum of soap and paper. The explicit service is a comfortable bed in a clean room, and implicit services might include a friendly desk clerk and the security of a well-lighted parking area. Deviations from this service package, such as adding bellhops, would destroy the bargain image. Table 2.2 lists criteria (with examples) for evaluating the service package.

The importance of facilitating goods in the service package can be used to classify services across a continuum from pure services to various degrees of mixed services. For example, psychiatric counseling with no facilitating goods would be considered a "pure" service. Automobile maintenance usually requires more facilitating goods than a haircut does.

Making general statements about service management is difficult when there are such variations in the nature of services. However, an appreciation of the unique features of the service environment is important for understanding the challenges facing service managers.

DISTINCTIVE CHARACTERISTICS OF SERVICE OPERATIONS

In services, a distinction must be made between *inputs* and *resources*. For services, inputs are the customers themselves, and resources are the facilitating goods, employee labor, and capital at the command of the service manager. Thus, to function, the service system must interact with the customers as participants in the service process. Because customers typically arrive at their own discretion and with unique demands on the service system, matching service capacity with demand is a challenge.

For some services, such as banking, however, the focus of activity is on processing information instead of people. In these situations, information technology, such as electronic funds transfer, can be substituted for physically depositing a payroll check; thus, the presence of the customer at the bank is unnecessary. Such exceptions will be noted as we discuss the distinctive characteristics of service operations. It should be noted here that many of the unique characteristics of services, such as customer participation and perishability, are interrelated.

The Customer as a Participant in the Service Process

The presence of the customer as a participant in the service process requires an attention to facility design that is not found in traditional manufacturing operations. That automobiles are made in a hot, dirty, noisy factory is of no concern to the eventual buyers, because they first see the product in the pleasant surroundings of a dealer's showroom. The presence of the customer on-site re-

TABLE 2.2. Criteria for Evaluating the Service Package

SUPPORTING FACILITY

1. *Location*
   Is it accessible by public transportation?
   Is it centrally located?
2. *Interior decorating*
   Is the proper mood established?
   Quality and coordination of furniture.
3. *Supporting equipment*
   Does the dentist use a mechanical or air drill?
   What type and age of aircraft does the charter airline use?
4. *Architectural appropriateness*
   Renaissance architecture for university campus.
   Unique recognizable feature of a blue tile roof.
   Massive granite facade of downtown bank.
5. *Facility layout*
   Is there a natural flow of traffic?
   Are adequate waiting areas provided?
   Is there unnecessary travel or backtracking?

FACILITATING GOODS

1. *Consistency*
   Crispness of french fries.
   Portion control.
2. *Quantity*
   Small, medium, or large drink.
3. *Selection*
   Variety of replacement mufflers.
   Number of menu items.
   Rental skis available.

EXPLICIT SERVICES

1. *Training of service personnel*
   Is the auto mechanic certified by the National Institute for Automotive Service Excellence (NIASE)?
   To what extent are paraprofessionals used?
   Are the physicians board certified?
2. *Comprehensiveness*
   Discount broker compared with full service.
   General hospital compared with clinic.
3. *Consistency*
   Airline's on-time record.
   Professional Standards Review Organization (PSRO) for doctors.
4. *Availability*
   24-hour ATM service.
   Is there a web site?
   Is there a toll-free number?

IMPLICIT SERVICES

1. *Attitude of service*
   Cheerful flight attendant.
   Police officer issuing traffic citation with tact.
   Surly service person in restaurant.
2. *Atmosphere*
   Restaurant decor.
   Music in a bar.
   Sense of confusion rather than order.
3. *Waiting*
   Joining a drive-in banking queue.
   Being placed on hold.
   Enjoying a martini in the restaurant bar.
4. *Status*
   College degree from Ivy League school.
   Box seats at sports event.
5. *Sense of well-being*
   Large commercial aircraft.
   Well-lighted parking lot.
6. *Privacy and security*
   Attorney advising client in private office.
   Magnetic key card for hotel room.
7. *Convenience*
   Use of appointments.
   Free parking.

quires attention to the physical surroundings of the service facility that is not necessary for the factory. For the customer, service is an experience occurring in the environment of the service facility, and the quality of service is enhanced if the service facility is designed from the customer's perspective. Attention to interior decorating, furnishings, layout, noise, and even color can influence the customer's perception of the service. Compare the feelings invoked by picturing yourself in a stereotypical bus station with those produced by imagining yourself in an airline terminal. Of course, passengers are not allowed in the terminal's back office (e.g., the luggage-handling area), which is operated in a factory-like environment. However, some innovative services have opened the back office to public scrutiny to promote confidence in the service (e.g., some restaurants provide a view into the kitchen, some auto repair bays can be observed through windows in the waiting area).

An important consideration in providing a service is the realization that the customer can play an active part in the process. A few examples will illustrate that the knowledge, experience, motivation, and even honesty of the customer all directly affect the performance of the service system:

1. The popularity of supermarkets and discount stores is predicated on the idea that customers are willing to assume an active role in the retailing process.
2. The accuracy of a patient's medical record can greatly influence the effectiveness of the attending physician.
3. The education of a student is determined largely by the student's own effort and contributions.

This strategy is best illustrated by the fast-food restaurants that have significantly reduced the typical number of serving and cleaning personnel. The customer not only places the order directly from a limited menu but also is expected to clear the table after the meal. Naturally, the customer expects faster service and less expensive meals to compensate for these inputs, but the service provider benefits in many subtle ways. First, there are fewer personnel who require supervision and such things as fringe benefits. Second, and more importantly, the customer provides the labor just at the moment it is required; thus, service capacity varies more directly with demand rather than being fixed by the size of the employed staff. The customer acts like a temporary employee, arriving just when needed to perform duties to augment the work of the service staff.

This strategy has received great acceptance in a society, such as the United States, where self-reliance is valued. Instead of being a passive buyer, the customer becomes a contributor to the gross national product.

Taking the customer out of the process, however, is becoming a common practice. Consider retail banking, in which customers are encouraged to use telephone or computer transactions, direct deposit, and automatic-debit bill paying instead of actually traveling to the bank. Moreover, the advent of Internet commerce gives new meaning to the phrase "window shopping." ☺

Simultaneous Production and Consumption of Services

The fact that services are created and consumed simultaneously and, thus, cannot be stored is a critical feature in the management of services. This inability to inventory services precludes using the traditional manufacturing strategy of relying on inventory as a buffer to absorb fluctuations in demand. An inventory of finished goods serves as a convenient system boundary for a manufacturer, separating the internal operations of planning and control from the external environment. Thus, the manufacturing facility can be operated at a constant level of output that is most efficient. The factory is operated as a *closed system*, with inventory decoupling the productive system from customer demand. Services, however, operate as *open systems*, with the full impact of demand variations being transmitted to the system.

Inventory also can be used to decouple the stages in a manufacturing process. For services, the decoupling is achieved through customer waiting. Inventory control is a major issue in manufacturing operations, whereas in services, the corresponding problem is customer waiting, or "queuing." The problems of selecting service capacity, facility utilization, and use of idle time all are balanced against customer waiting time.

The simultaneous production and consumption in services also eliminates many opportunities for quality-control intervention. A product can be inspected before delivery, but services must rely on other measures to ensure the quality of services delivered. We address this important topic in Chapter 10.

Time-Perishable Capacity

A service is a perishable commodity. Consider an empty airline seat, an unoccupied hospital or hotel room, or an hour without a patient in the day of a dentist. In each case, a lost opportunity has occurred. Because a service cannot be stored, it is lost forever when not used. The full utilization of service capacity becomes a management challenge, because customer demand exhibits considerable variation and building inventory to absorb these fluctuations is not an option.

Consumer demand for services typically exhibits very cyclic behavior over short periods of time, with considerable variation between the peaks and valleys. The custom of eating lunch between noon and 1 PM places a burden on restaurants to accommodate the noon rush. The practice of day-end mailing by businesses contributes to the fact that 60 percent of all letters are received at the post office between 4 and 8 PM.[2] The demand for emergency medical service in Los Angeles was found to vary from a low of 0.5 calls per hour at 6 AM to a peak of 3.5 calls per hour at 6 PM.[3] This peak-to-valley ratio of 7 to 1 also was true for fire alarms during an average day in New York City.[4]

For recreational and transportation services, seasonal variation in demand creates surges in activity. As many students know, flights home are often booked months in advance of spring break and the Christmas holiday.

[2]R. C. Cohen, R. McBridge, R. Thornton, and T. White, *Letter Mail System Performance Design: An Analytical Method for Evaluating Candidate Mechanization*, Report R-168, Institute for Defense Analysis, Washington, D.C., 1970.

[3]James A. Fitzsimmons, "The Use of Spectral Analysis to Validate Planning Models," *Socio-Economic Planning Sciences*, vol. 8, no. 3, June 1974, pp. 123–128.

[4]E. H. Blum, *Urban Fire Protection: Studies of the New York City Fire Department*, R-681, New York City Rand Institute, New York, January 1971.

Faced with variable demand and a perishable capacity to provide the service, the manager has three basic options:

1. Smooth demand by:
   a. Using reservations or appointments.
   b. Using price incentives (e.g., giving telephone discounts for evening and weekend calls).
   c. Demarketing peak times (e.g., advertising to shop early and avoid the Christmas rush).
2. Adjust service capacity by:
   a. Using part-time help during peak hours.
   b. Scheduling work shifts to vary workforce needs according to demand (e.g., telephone companies staff their operators to match call demand).
   c. Increasing the customer self-service content of the service.
3. Allow customers to wait.

The last option can be viewed as a passive contribution to the service process that carries the risk of losing a dissatisfied customer to a competitor. By waiting, the customer permits greater utilization of service capacity. The airlines explicitly recognize this by offering standby passengers a reduced price for their tickets.

Site Selection Dictated by Location of Customers

In manufacturing, products are shipped from the manufacturer to the wholesaler to the retailer, but in services, the customer and provider must physically meet for a service to be performed. Either the customer comes to the service facility (e.g., restaurant), or the service provider goes to the customer (e.g., ambulance service). Of course, there are exceptions, such as buying stock by phone or modem and taking university courses via teleconferencing. In fact, because of advances in information technology such as the Internet, opportunities for innovation in service systems abound (e.g., Federal Express allows its customers to track their packages using a web site).

Travel time and costs are reflected in the economics of site selection (e.g., in the case of Domino's Pizza). The result is that many small service centers are located close to prospective consumers. Of course, the tradeoff is between the fixed cost of the facility and the travel costs of the customers. The more expensive the facility, the larger or more densely populated the market area must be. For example, many a major-league baseball team has had trouble surviving in a medium-sized city.

The resulting small size of operation and the multisite locations of some services create several challenges.

Limited-Scale Economies

For services in which physical travel by the customer is necessary (e.g., restaurants), the immediate geographic market area limits the effective size of operations and removes the opportunity to gain economies of scale. However, some services such as franchised food firms have centralized many of their common functions (e.g., purchasing, advertising, and food preparation) to achieve these economies. Faced with a limited market area, some firms such as convenience stores have turned to an economy of scope strategy by offering a wide range of services from self-service gasoline to microwave meals.

Control of Decentralized Services

Unlike manufacturing, services are performed in the field, not in the controlled environment of a factory. For example, fast-food restaurants maintain service consistency across multiple locations through a standardized delivery process. In this case, the standardization may be achieved by designing special equipment (e.g., a french-fry scoop that measures the portion) or by offering a limited service (e.g., only burgers, fries, and shakes). More sophisticated services such as management consulting must rely on extensive training, licensing, and peer review.

For services that travel to the customer (e.g., telephone installations, delivery services, and maintenance and repair services), the problems of routing, dispatching, and scheduling become important. These aspects are examined in the supplement to Chapter 5, Vehicle Routing.

Labor Intensiveness

In most service organizations, labor is the key resource that determines the effectiveness of the organization. For these organizations, technological obsolescence is not fully accommodated by investments in new equipment; it is the skills of the labor force that age as new knowledge makes current skills obsolete. In an expanding organization, recruitment provides an avenue to acquiring this new knowledge. In a slow-growth or stable organization, however, the only successful strategy may be continuous retraining. The problem of aging labor skills is particularly acute in the professional service organization, in which extensive formal education is a prerequisite to employment.

The interaction between customer and employee in services creates the possibility of a more complete human work experience. In services, work activity generally is oriented toward people rather than toward things. There are exceptions, however, for services that process information (e.g., communications) or customers' property (e.g., brokerage services). In the limited customer-contact service industries, we now see a dramatic reduction in the level of labor intensiveness through the introduction of information technology.

Even the introduction of automation may strengthen personalization by eliminating the relatively routine impersonal tasks, thereby permitting increased personal attention to the remaining work. At the same time, personal attention creates opportunities for variability in the service that is provided. This is not inherently bad, however, unless customers perceive a significant variation in quality. A customer expects to be treated fairly and to be given the same service that others receive. The development of standards and of employee training in proper procedures is the key to ensuring consistency in the service provided. It is rather impractical to monitor the output of each employee, except via customer complaints.

The direct customer–employee contact has implications for service (industrial) relations as well. Auto workers with grievances against the firm have been known to sabotage the product on the assembly line. Presumably, the final inspection will ensure that any such cars are corrected before delivery. A disgruntled service employee, however, can do irreparable harm to the organization, because the employee is the firm's sole contact with customers. Therefore, the service manager must be concerned about the employees' attitudes as well as their performance. J. Willard Marriott, founder of the Marriott Hotel chain, has said, "In the service business you can't make happy guests with unhappy employees."[5] Through training and genuine concern for employee welfare, the organizational goals can be internalized.

Intangibility

Services are ideas and concepts; products are things. Therefore, it follows that service innovations are not patentable. To secure the benefits of a novel service concept, the firm must expand extremely rapidly and preempt any competitors. Franchising has been the vehicle to secure market areas and establish a brand name. Franchising allows the parent firm to sell its idea to a local entrepreneur, thus preserving capital while retaining control and reducing risk.

The intangible nature of services also presents a problem for customers. When buying a product, the customer is able to see it, feel it, and test its performance before purchase. For a service, however, the customer must rely on the reputation of the service firm. In many service areas, the government has intervened to guarantee acceptable service performances. Through the use of registration, licensing, and regulation, the government can assure consumers that the training and test performance of some service providers meet certain standards. Thus, we find that public construction plans must be approved by a registered professional engineer, a doctor must be licensed to practice medicine, and the telephone company is a regulated utility. In its efforts to "protect" the consumer, however, the government may be stifling innovation, raising barriers to entry, and generally reducing competition.

Difficulty in Measuring Output

Measuring the output of a service organization is a frustrating task for several reasons. Counting the number of customers served is seldom useful because it does not account for the uniqueness of the service that is performed. The problem of measurement is further complicated by the fact that not-for-profit service systems (e.g., universities, governments, and some hospitals) do not have a single criterion, such as maximizing profit, on which to base an evaluation of their performance. More importantly, can a system's performance be evaluated on the basis of output alone when this assumes a homogeneous input of service demands? A more definitive evaluation of service performance is a measure of the change in each customer from the input to the output state, a process known as *transactional analysis.* For example, consulting services and market research often involve providing clients with access to appropriate information and showing them how it relates to their situations, which is a very customized activity.

[5]G. M. Hostage, "Quality Control in a Service Business," *Harvard Business Review*, vol. 53, no. 4, July–August 1975, pp. 98–106.

AN OPEN-SYSTEMS VIEW OF SERVICES

Service organizations are sufficiently unique in their character to require special management approaches that go beyond the simple adaptation of the management techniques found in manufacturing a product. The distinctive characteristics suggest enlarging the system view to include the customer as a participant in the service process. As Figure 2.3 shows, the customer is viewed as an input that is transformed by the service process into an output with some degree of satisfaction.

The role of the service operations manager includes the functions of both production and marketing in an open system with the customer as a participant. The traditional manufacturing separation of the production and marketing functions, with finished-goods inventory as the interface, is neither possible nor appropriate in services. Marketing performs two important functions in daily-service operations: 1) educating the consumer to play a role as an active participant in the service process and 2) "smoothing" demand to match service capacity. This marketing activity must be coordinated with scheduling staff levels and with both controlling and evaluating the delivery process. By necessity, the operations and marketing functions are integrated for service organizations.

For services, *the process is the product*. The presence of the customer in the service process negates the closed-system perspective that is taken in manufacturing. Techniques to control operations in an isolated factory producing a tangible good are inadequate for services. No longer is the process machine-paced and the output easily measured for compliance with specifications. Instead, customers arrive with different demands on the service; thus, multiple measures of performance are necessary. Service employees interact directly with the cus-

FIGURE 2.3. Open-systems view of service operations.

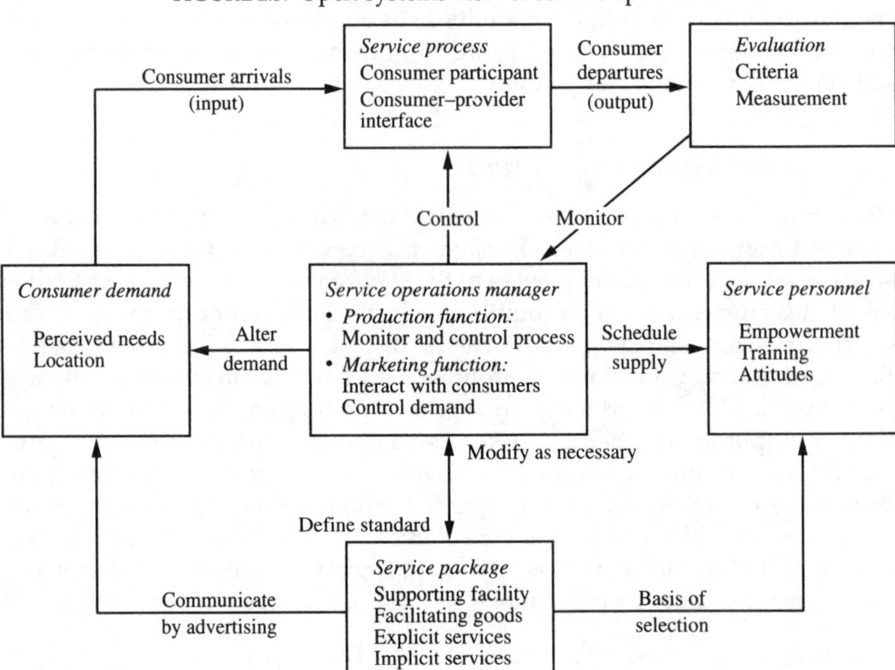

tomer, with little opportunity for management intervention. This requires extensive training and empowerment of employees to act appropriately in the absence of direct supervision.

Further, customer impressions of service quality are based on the total service experience, not just on the explicit service that is performed. A concern for employee attitudes and training becomes a necessity to ensure that the implicit service is also appreciated by the customer. When viewed from the customer's perspective, the entire service process raises concerns ranging from the aesthetic design of the facility to pleasant diversions in waiting areas.

An open-system concept of services also allows one to view the customer as a coproducer. Permitting the customer to participate actively in the service process (e.g., providing a salad bar at a restaurant) can increase productivity, which in turn can create a competitive edge.

SUMMARY

The management of an open system requires techniques and sensitivities different from those of a closed system. Service managers are faced with nonroutine operations in which only indirect control is possible. In services, it is the human element that is central to effective operations. For example, the unavoidable interaction between service provider and consumer is a source of great opportunity, as in direct selling. However, this interaction seldom can be fully controlled; thus, service quality may suffer. For this reason, the attitude and appearance of personnel in service organizations are important considerations. For services, the presence of the customer in the process materially alters what is viewed as the product. The unique characteristics of intangibility, perishability, and simultaneous provision and consumption introduce special challenges for service management. In many respects, the service manager adopts a style of management that incorporates the functions of marketing and operations.

In the next part of this book, we will examine strategic service issues, beginning in Chapter 3 with the formulation of a strategic service concept. We also will discover insights from a strategic classification system, discuss generic competitive service strategies, and conclude with a look at how customers are won in the marketplace.

KEY TERMS AND DEFINITIONS

Explicit services the essential or intrinsic features readily observable by the senses (e.g., on-time departure, quality of meal).

Facilitating goods material purchased or consumed by the buyer, or items provided by the customer (e.g., food, golf clubs).

Implicit services psychologic benefits or extrinsic features the customer may sense only vaguely (e.g., security of a well-lighted parking lot, privacy of a loan office).

Service process matrix a classification of services based on the degree of interaction and customization and the degree of labor intensity that results in four categories: service factory, service shop, mass service, and professional service.

Supporting facility the physical resources that must be in place before a service can be offered (e.g., golf course, hospital building, airplane).

The service package a description of a service based on four components: supporting facility, facilitating goods, explicit service, and implicit service.

Time-perishable capacity a service that is not used during some period of time and, therefore, is lost forever (e.g., an empty seat on an airplane).

TOPICS FOR DISCUSSION

1. What are some possible measures of performance for a fire department? For a fast-food restaurant?
2. Comment on why hospitals, given that they are so labor-intensive, are classified as a service shop in Figure 2.1.
3. Select a service with which you are familiar, and identify the seven "distinctive characteristics of service operations" that it has.
4. What factors are important for a manager to consider when attempting to enhance a service organization's image?
5. What contributions to the management of professional service firms can a business school graduate provide?

Service Benchmark

To Compete Better, Look Far Afield

How can companies best compete? One excellent and relatively underused way is to seek creative insights in industries far afield from their own.

Of course, in a time of fierce global competition businesses are hardly unaware of the need to improve performance. Many have relentlessly cut costs through downsizing and other strategies, for instance. Others have scrutinized similar companies in their quest for innovative processes, technologies and products.

But cost-cutting has its limits. And so does seeking inspiration only within one's own field. For example, many commercial real estate companies assumed during the last recession that once the economy picked up so would their business. Failing to look beyond their own realm, they could not see that more and more businesses were opting for portable and "at home" offices.

Enter the quest for creative ideas from beyond a company's own industry—from those normally unexplored regions that business strategists call "outside the box."

When Southwest Airlines wanted to improve the turnaround of its aircraft at airports, for instance, it could have examined the practices of other airlines' maintenance workers. Instead, the company went to the Indianapolis 500 to watch pit crews fuel and service race cars. The airline recognized that pit crews perform the same functions airplane maintenance crews do, just in a different industry and at much faster speed. The observations gave Southwest new ideas about equipment fittings, materials management, teamwork and speed that, in part, enabled the airline to cut its turnaround time by 50 percent.

Or consider Granite Rock. This company wanted to improve the way it loaded gravel into trucks in its yards. Before the gravel could be loaded, drivers had to leave their trucks and fill out paperwork to indicate how much gravel they needed. But, by observing automatic teller machines in banks, Granite Rock was able to revise this expensive and time-consuming procedure. Now, the truck drivers plug their "bank" cards into a machine so they do not have to leave the truck in order to make their requests for gravel.

Focusing on processes is the key to finding useful insights in apparently unrelated places. From a process standpoint, all companies do the same things—sell to customers, buy from suppliers, hire employees.

Understanding this broad connection, a major gas utility examined how Federal Express delivers packages overnight—and discovered ways to speed the delivery of its own product, fuel. Similarly, a major telecommunications company improved its billing system by visiting a package delivery concern. The telephone company recognized that the shipper's tracking of cargo was analogous to its tracking of invoices.

The lesson for businesses? Look for insights in apparently unrelated fields. An enterprise hoping to improve its production processes, for example, might do well to examine Domino's Pizza—a company that completes its order entry, manufacturing, distribution, billing and collection processes in 30 minutes. But the enterprise should perform this inquiry quickly. For, day by day, the global marketplace is growing more and more competitive.

Skeptical about "outside the box" thinking? Just recall Isaac Newton. The famous scientist gained his greatest insight into gravity not from learned, ancient treatises but from an apparently unlikely source: an apple.

Source: Robert Hiebeler, "To Compete Better, Look Far Afield," *The New York Times*, September 18, 1994, p. 11.

CASE: VILLAGE VOLVO

Village Volvo is the "new kid in town." It represents an effort by two former authorized Volvo dealer mechanics to provide quality repair service on out-of-warranty Volvos at a reasonable cost. On the basis of their 22 combined years of training and experience with the local Volvo dealer, they have earned a respected reputation and a following of satisfied customers, which make an independent service operation feasible. Village Volvo occupies a new Butler building (i.e., a prefabricated metal structure) that has four work bays in addition to an office, waiting area, and storage room.

The owners feel they have designed their operation to provide clients with a custom car care service that is unavailable at the local dealer. They have set aside specific times each week when clients may drive in for quick, routine services such as tune-ups and oil changes, but they encourage clients to schedule appointments for the diagnosis and repair of specific problems.

At the time of the appointment, the mechanic who will be working on the vehicle and the client discuss the problems the client has noticed. On occasion, the mechanic may take a short test drive with the client to be certain that both understand the area of concern.

Another source of information for the mechanic is the Custom Care Vehicle Dossier (CCVD). Village Volvo maintains a continuing file on each vehicle it services. This history can help the mechanic to diagnose problems and also provides a convenient record if a vehicle is returned for warranty service on an earlier repair. The owners are considering use of the CCVD as a way of "reminding" customers that routine maintenance procedures may be due.

After the mechanic has made a preliminary diagnosis, the service manager gives the vehicle owner an estimate of the cost and the approximate time when the repair will be completed if no unexpected problems arise. Company policy states that the owner will be consulted before any work other than the agreed-on job is done. Although the customer may speak with the mechanic during the repair process, the service manager is the main point of contact. It is the service manager's responsibility to be sure the customer understands the preliminary diagnosis, to advise the customer of any unexpected problems and costs, and to notify the customer when the vehicle is ready for pickup.

Village Volvo has no provisions for alternate transportation for customers at this time. A shuttle service two or three times a day is being considered, because the owners think their suburban location may deter some clients. The waiting room is equipped with a television set, comfortable chairs, coffee, a soft-drink vending machine, magazines, and the local newspaper. This facility is used almost exclusively by clients who come during the "drop-in" times (3 to 5 PM Wednesdays and 8 to 10 AM Thursdays) for quick, routine jobs such as tune-ups and buyer checks of used cars.

The owner-mechanics do no repairs between 7 and 8 AM and 5 and 6 PM, because these are heavy customer contact hours. They believe it is just as important to discuss with the client the repairs that have been done as it is to discuss what problems exist before that work is done. As repairs are made the owner-mechanic notes any other problems that might need attention in the future (e.g., fan and alternator belts show some wear and may need to be replaced in about 6000 miles). These notes are brought to the customer's attention at pickup time and also are recorded in the CCVD for future use, perhaps in the form of a reminder postcard to the owner.

All small worn-out parts that have been replaced are put in a clean box inside the car. More cumbersome replaced parts are identified and set aside for the client's inspection. Care is taken throughout the repair process to keep the car clean, and the inside is vacuumed as a courtesy before pickup. After the repairs are finished, the vehicle is taken for a short test drive. Then it is parked, ready for pickup.

The Village Volvo owners see their responsibility as extending beyond immediate service to their clients. The owners have developed a network of other service providers who assist in recycling used parts and waste products and to whom they can refer clients for work that is not part of Village Volvo's services (e.g., body work, alignments, and reupholstering). The owners also are considering the possibility of offering a mini-course one Saturday morning each month to teach clients what they can do to attain their 200,000-mile Volvo medals.

Questions

1. Describe Village Volvo's service package.

2. How are the distinctive characteristics of a service firm illustrated by Village Volvo?

3. How could Village Volvo manage its back office (i.e., repair operations) like a factory?

4. How can Village Volvo differentiate itself from Volvo dealers?

SELECTED BIBLIOGRAPHY

Collier, David A.: "Managing a Service Firm: A Different Management Game," *National Productivity Review,* Winter 1983–1984, pp. 36–45.

Killeya, J. C., and C. G. Armistead: "The Transfer of Concepts and Techniques between Manufacturing and Service Systems," *International Journal of Operations and Production Management,* vol. 3, no. 3, 1983, pp. 22–28.

Morris, B., and R. Johnston: "Dealing with Inherent Variability: The Difference between Manufacturing and Service?" *International Journal of Operations and Production Management,* vol. 7, no. 4, 1986, pp. 13–22.

Riddle, D. I.: *Service-Led Growth,* Praeger, New York, 1986.

Sasser, W. E., R. P. Olsen, and D. D. Wyckoff: *Management of Service Operations,* Allyn and Bacon, Inc., Boston, 1978.

Schmenner, Roger W.: "How Can Service Businesses Survive and Prosper?" *Sloan Management Review,* vol. 27, no. 3, Spring 1986, pp. 21–32.

PART TWO

The Service Concept and Competitive Strategy

The foundation for the theme of the book is presented in this section. An effective competitive strategy is particularly important for service firms, because they compete in an environment with relatively low barriers to entry. Consequently, service firms are always faced with new competition.

We begin in Chapter 3 with the elements of the strategic service concept. This is followed by a service classification focusing on the strategic opportunities that are available in the design of the service concept. The three generic competitive strategies—overall cost leadership, differentiation, and focus—are applied to services, and illustrations are provided.

Services and information technology are explored in Chapter 4. Information technology is the most important enabling technology in services, and a discussion of the innovation process in services focuses on the new technology process, which must include customers as well as employees and managers. Successful service firms have discovered the strategic value of information resulting from direct interaction with their customers. Use of this information is effective in creating barriers to entry, increasing revenues, and increasing productivity. Finally, the competitive importance of exploiting the virtual value chain is examined.

CHAPTER 3

Service Strategy

LEARNING OBJECTIVES

After completing this chapter, you should be able to:

1. Describe how a service has addressed each element in the strategic service concept.
2. Discuss the insights obtained from a strategic classification of services according to: nature of the service act, relationship with customers, degree of customization, nature of demand and supply, and method of service delivery.
3. Critically discuss the competitive environment of services.
4. Describe, with examples, how a service competes using the generic service strategies of overall cost leadership, differentiation, and focus.
5. Discuss the service purchase decision in the context of qualifiers, service winners, and service losers.

Most service firms compete in an economic environment that generally consists of a large number of small- and medium-sized firms, many of them privately owned. Of course, large service firms such as major airlines and hospitals also exist. In this type of economic environment, no firm has a significant market share; thus, no firm can dominate the industry (with the exception of government services, cable TV, and utilities). Since the deregulation of various industries in the 1980s, however, there has been some service industry consolidation, particularly with airlines and financial institutions. In any event, a thorough understanding of the competitive dimensions and limitations of the industry is necessary before a firm can begin to formulate its service strategy.

CHAPTER PREVIEW

The diversity of firms in the service sector makes generalizations concerning strategy difficult. Five schemes are presented, however, to classify services in ways that provide strategic insight and transcend narrow industry boundaries. These schemes can be used to think about the choices being made to position the service in relation to its competitors. *Positioning* is a marketing term that is used to describe the process of establishing and maintaining a distinctive place in the market.

Three generic strategies are successful in formulating methods that allow a firm to outperform competitors. The strategies of overall cost leadership, differentiation, and market focus are approaches that both manufacturing and service firms have adopted in various ways to gain a competitive advantage. With each of these strategies, however, management must not lose sight of the fact that only a focus on customers and satisfying their needs will result in a loyal customer base.

Winning customers in the marketplace means competing on several dimensions. Customers base their purchase decisions on many variables, including price, convenience, reputation, and safety. The importance of a particular variable to a firm's success depends on the competitive marketplace and the preferences of individual customers.

This chapter begins with a discussion of the strategic service concept, which contains all elements in the design of a competitive service. The service concept is divided into four structural elements: delivery system, facility design, location, and capacity planning. It also is divided into four managerial elements: service encounter, quality, managing capacity and demand, and information. These eight elements represent the competitive dimensions of a service firm, and each is treated separately in the chapters that follow.

THE STRATEGIC SERVICE CONCEPT

Chapter 2, The Nature of Services, introduced the idea of a *service package,* which contained four elements—supporting facility, facilitating goods, explicit service, and implicit service—as a way to describe an existing service or a vision of a new service. In this chapter, this service vision will be translated into a strategically focused *service concept* or *design* that contains eight dimensions.

Consider a building, which begins in the mind's eye of the architect and is translated onto paper in the form of engineering drawings for all the building's systems: foundation, structural, plumbing, and electrical. An analog to this design process is the strategic service concept with the system elements outlined here. These elements must be engineered to create a consistent service offering that achieves the strategic objectives. The service concept becomes a blueprint that communicates to customers and employees alike what service they should expect to give and to receive. These system elements are:

Structural:

Delivery system. Front and back office, automation, customer participation.

Facility design. Size, aesthetics, layout.

Location. Customer demographics, single or multiple sites, competition, site characteristics.

Capacity planning. Managing queues, number of servers, accommodating average or peak demand.

Managerial:

Service encounter. Service culture, motivation, selection and training, employment empowerment.

Quality. Measurement, monitoring, methods, expectations vs. perceptions, service guarantee.

Managing capacity and demand. Strategies for altering demand and controlling supply, queue management.

Information. Competitive resource, data collection.

A successful hospital located in Toronto, Canada, that performs only inguinal hernia operations will be used to illustrate how each element of the service concept contributes to the strategic mission. Shouldice Hospital is privately owned and uses a special operating procedure to correct inguinal hernias that has resulted in an excellent reputation. Its success is measured by the recurrence rate, which is twelve times lower than that of its competitors.[1]

The structural elements of Shouldice's service concept that support its strategy to target customers suffering from inguinal hernias are:

- *Delivery system.* A hallmark of the Shouldice approach is patient participation in all aspects of the process. For example, patients shave themselves before the operation, walk from the operating table to the recovery area, and are encouraged the evening after surgery to discuss the experience with new patients to alleviate their preoperative fears.
- *Facility design.* The facility is intentionally designed to encourage exercise and rapid recovery within four days, which is approximately one-half the time at traditional hospitals. Hospital rooms are devoid of amenities, and patients must walk to lounges, showers, and the cafeteria. The extensive hospital grounds are landscaped to encourage strolling, and the interior is carpeted and decorated to avoid any typical hospital "associations."

[1]Harvard Business School case, Shouldice Hospital Limited, ICCH no. 9-683-068, 1983, p. 3.

- *Location.* Being located in a large metropolitan community with excellent air service gives Shouldice access to a worldwide market. The large local population also provides a source of patients who can be scheduled on short notice to fill any canceled bookings.
- *Capacity planning.* Because hernia operations are elective procedures, patients can be scheduled in batches to fill the operating time available; thus, capacity is utilized to its maximum. This ease in scheduling operations allows Shouldice to operate like a fully occupied hotel; thus, the supporting activities, such as housekeeping and food service, also can be fully employed.

The managerial elements of the Shouldice service concept also support the strategy of delivering a quality medical procedure:

- *Service encounter.* All employees are trained to help counsel patients and encourage them to achieve a rapid recovery. A service culture fostering a family-type atmosphere is reinforced by communal dining for both workers and patients.
- *Quality.* The most important quality feature is the adherence of all physicians to the Shouldice method of hernia repair, which results in the low recurrence rate of inguinal hernias among these patients. In addition, patients with difficulties are referred back to the doctor who performed the procedure. Perceived quality is enhanced by the Shouldice experience, which is more like a short holiday than a typical hospital stay.
- *Managing capacity and demand.* Patients are screened by means of a mail-in questionnaire and are admitted by reservation only. Thus, the patient demand in terms of timing and appropriateness can be controlled effectively. As mentioned, walk-in patients or local residents on a waiting list are used to fill vacancies created by canceled reservations; thus, full use of hospital capacity is ensured.
- *Information.* A unique feature of the Shouldice service is the annual alumni reunion, which represents a continuing relationship of the hospital with its patients. Keeping information on patients allows Shouldice to build a loyal customer base, which is an effective word-of-mouth advertising medium. Providing free annual check-ups also allows Shouldice to build a unique data base on its procedure.

CLASSIFYING SERVICES FOR STRATEGIC INSIGHTS[2]

A general discussion of service strategy is complicated by the diversity of service firms in the economy and their differing customer relationships. However, strategic insights that transcend industry boundaries are needed to avoid the myopic view, which is prevalent among service managers, that concepts do not translate from one industry to another. For example, competitive strategies used by banking services could find an application in laundry services, because both

[2]Adapted from Christopher H. Lovelock, "Classifying Services to Gain Strategic Marketing Insights," *Journal of Marketing*, vol. 47, Summer 1983, p. 920.

deal with a customer's property. The new laundry drop-off and pick-up service available at commuter rail stations is similar in concept to bank automatic teller machines in supermarkets. The following classification schemes developed by Christopher Lovelock provide us with an appreciation of possible strategic dimensions that transcend industry boundaries.

Nature of the Service Act

As Figure 3.1 shows, the service act can be considered across two dimensions: who or what is the direct recipient of the service, and the tangible nature of the service. This creates four possible classifications: 1) tangible actions directed to the customer, such as passenger transportation and personal care; 2) tangible actions directed at the customer's possessions, such as laundry cleaning and janitorial services; 3) intangible actions directed at the customer's intellect such as entertainment; and 4) intangible actions performed on customer's assets, such as financial services.

This classification scheme raises questions about the traditional way in which services have been delivered. For example, does the customer need to be present physically throughout the service, only to initiate or terminate the transaction, or not at all? If customers must be present, then they must travel to the service facility and become part of the process, or the server must travel to the customer (e.g., ambulance service). This has significant implications for facility design and employee interaction, because the impressions that are made on the customer will influence his or her perceptions of the service. In addition, questions are raised concerning the impact of facility location and business hours on customer convenience. It is not surprising that retail banks have embraced ATMs and other electronic communication alternatives to personal interaction.

Thinking creatively about the nature of the service may identify more convenient forms of delivery or even a product that can substitute for the service.

FIGURE 3.1. Understanding the nature of the service act.
(Reprinted with permission of the American Marketing Association: Christopher H. Lovelock, "Classifying Services to Gain Strategic Marketing Insights," Journal of Marketing, *vol. 47, Summer 1983, p. 12.)*

Nature of the Service Act	**Direct Recipient of the Service** People	 Things
Tangible actions	*Services directed at people's bodies:* Health care Passenger transportation Beauty salons Exercise clinics Restaurants Haircutting	*Services directed at goods and other physical possessions:* Freight transportation Industrial equipment repair and maintenance Janitorial services Laundry and dry cleaning Landscaping/lawn care Veterinary care
Intangible actions	*Services directed at people's minds:* Education Broadcasting Information services Theaters Museums	*Services directed at intangible assets:* Banking Legal services Accounting Securities Insurance

For example, videotapes of lectures and CD recordings of concerts represent a convenient substitute for physical attendance, and they also serve as permanent library records of the events.

Relationship with Customers

Service firms have the opportunity to build long-term relationships, because customers conduct their transactions directly with the service provider, most often in person. In contrast, manufacturers traditionally have been isolated from the eventual end user by a distribution channel consisting of some combination of distributors, wholesalers, and/or retailers. Figure 3.2 contrasts the nature of the customer's "membership" with the nature of the service delivery. The value to the firm of customer membership is captured in this figure; however, a number of changes have occurred since it was first published in 1983. For example, car rental firms and major hotel chains have joined airlines in offering discounts through frequent flyer programs. In addition, some private toll highways offer annual passes, which can be attached to one's car. These passes electronically trigger a debit so that the driver need not stop to pay a toll.

Knowing your customers is a significant competitive advantage for a service organization. Having a data base of customers' names and addresses and their use of the service permits targeted marketing and individual treatment of customers. Customers benefit from membership because of the convenience of annual fixed fees and the knowledge that they are valued customers who will receive occasional perks (e.g., frequent flyer awards).

Customization and Judgment

Because services are created as they are consumed and the customer is often a participant in the process, an opportunity exists to tailor a service to the needs

FIGURE 3.2. Relationships with customers.
(Reprinted with permission of the American Marketing Association: Christopher H. Lovelock, "Classifying Services to Gain Strategic Marketing Insights," Journal of Marketing, *vol. 47, Summer 1983, p. 13.)*

	Type of Relationship between Service Organization and Its Customers	
Nature of Service Delivery	"Membership" relationship	No formal relationship
Continuous delivery of service	Insurance Telephone subscription College enrollment Banking American Automobile Association	Radio station Police protection Lighthouse Public highway
Discrete transactions	Long-distance phone calls Theater series subscription Commuter ticket or transit pass Sam's Wholesale Club Egghead computer software	Car rental Mail service Toll highway Pay phone Movie theater Public transportation Restaurant

Extent to Which Customer Contact Personnel Exercise Judgment in Meeting Individual Customer Needs	Extent to Which Service Characteristics Are Customized: High	Low
High	Professional services Surgery Taxi service Beautician Plumber Education (tutorials) Gourmet restaurant	Education (large classes) Preventive health programs College food service
Low	Telephone service Hotel services Retail banking (excl. major loans) Family restaurant	Public transportation Routine appliance repair Movie theater Spectator sports Fast-food restaurant

FIGURE 3.3. Customization and judgment in service delivery.
(Reprinted with permission of the American Marketing Association: Christopher H. Lovelock, "Classifying Services to Gain Strategic Marketing Insights," Journal of Marketing, *vol. 47, Summer 1983, p. 15.)*

of the customer. Figure 3.3 shows that customization proceeds along two dimensions: either the character of the service permits customization, or the service personnel have the discretion to modify the service.

Selecting the quadrant of Figure 3.3 in which to position a service is a strategic choice. For example, traditional movie theaters offer only one screen; thus, they are appropriately located in the low-low quadrant. Most new movie theaters, however, are built with multiple screens, allowing some degree of customization. Among fast-food restaurants, Burger King advertises "Have it your way," permitting some customization of its "Whopper." Within a particular industry, every quadrant could be occupied by different segments of that industry, as illustrated by the various types of food service operations in Figure 3.3. A strategic choice of offering more customization and allowing service personnel to exercise judgment, however, has implications for the service delivery system.

Nature of Demand and Supply

As noted in Chapter 2, the time perishability of service capacity creates a challenge for service managers, because these managers lack the option of producing and storing inventory for future sale. Even so, the extent of demand and supply imbalances varies across service industries, as shown in Figure 3.4.

To determine the most appropriate strategy in each case, it is necessary to consider the following questions:

1. What is the nature of the demand fluctuation? Does it have a predictable cycle (e.g., daily meal demand at a fast-food restaurant) that can be anticipated?
2. What are the underlying causes of these fluctuations in demand? If the causes are customer habits or preference, could marketing produce a change?
3. What opportunities exist to change the level of capacity or supply? Can part-time workers be hired during peak hours?

Extent to Which Supply Is Constrained	Extent of Demand Fluctuation over Time: Wide	Narrow
Peak demand can usually be met without a major delay	Electricity Natural gas Telephone Hospital maternity unit Police and fire emergencies	Insurance Legal services Banking Laundry and dry cleaning
Peak demand regularly exceeds capacity	Accounting and tax preparation Passenger transportation Hotels and motels Restaurants Theaters	Services similar to those above but with insufficient capacity for their base level of business

FIGURE 3.4. What is the nature of demand for the service relative to supply? *(Reprinted with permission of the American Marketing Association: Christopher H. Lovelock, "Classifying Services to Gain Strategic Marketing Insights,"* Journal of Marketing, *vol. 47, Summer 1983, p. 17.)*

Because managing capacity and demand is a central challenge to the success of a service firm, Chapter 13, Managing Capacity and Demand, is devoted entirely to this topic.

Method of Service Delivery

As Figure 3.5 shows, the method of service delivery has both a geographic component and a level-of-customer-interaction component.

Services with multiple sites have significant management implications for ensuring quality and consistency in the service offering. Detailed strategic implications of site location are discussed in Chapter 7. With advances in electronic communications, arm's-length transactions are becoming more common, because they offer customer convenience and efficient service delivery. For example, use of personal computers and modems allows businesses to customize their services and to decrease the amount of physical interaction between the cus-

FIGURE 3.5. Method of service delivery.
(Reprinted with permission of the American Marketing Association: Christopher H. Lovelock, "Classifying Services to Gain Strategic Marketing Insights," Journal of Marketing, *vol. 47, Summer 1983, p. 18.)*

Nature of Interaction between Customer and Service Organization	Availability of Service Outlets: Single site	Multiple site
Customer goes to service organization	Theater Barbershop	Bus service Fast-food chain
Service organization comes to customer	Lawn care service Pest control service Taxi	Mail delivery AAA emergency repairs
Customer and service organization transact at arm's length (mail or electronic communications)	Credit card company Local TV station	Broadcast network Telephone company

tomer and a human service provider. The strategic implications of the design of a service delivery system and its effect on the interaction between customer and service organization are discussed in Chapters 5 and 6.

The classification schemes described earlier are useful in suggesting strategic alternatives and avoiding industry myopia. Before a service strategy can be formulated, however, an understanding of the competitive nature of the industry is necessary.

UNDERSTANDING THE COMPETITIVE ENVIRONMENT OF SERVICES

In general, service firms compete in a difficult economic environment, and there are many reasons for this difficulty:

- *Relatively low overall entry barriers.* Service innovations are not patentable, and in most cases, services are not capital-intensive. Thus, innovations can easily be copied by competitors. However, other types of entry barriers exist, such as locating a resort hotel on the best beach of an island (e.g., the Club Med location on Moorea in French Polynesia).
- *Minimal opportunities for economies of scale.* Recall from Chapter 2 that because of the simultaneous production and consumption of services, the customer must travel to the service facility or the service must travel to the customer. The necessity of physical travel limits the market area and results in small-scale outlets. Franchised firms can realize some economies of scale by sharing purchasing or advertising costs; in other instances, electronic communications can be substituted for physical travel (e.g., ordering from L.L. Bean by telephone).
- *Erratic sales fluctuations.* Service demand varies as a function of the time of day and the day of the week (and sometimes seasonally), with random arrivals. Can you think of some exceptions?
- *No advantage of size in dealing with buyers or suppliers.* The small size of many service firms places them at a disadvantage in bargaining with powerful buyers or suppliers. Many exceptions should come to mind, however, such as McDonald's buying beef and Marriott buying mattresses.
- *Product substitution.* Product innovations can be a substitute for services (e.g., the home pregnancy test). Thus, service firms must not only watch other service competitors but also anticipate potential product innovations that might make their services obsolete.
- *Customer loyalty.* Established firms using personalized service create a loyal customer base, which becomes a barrier to entry by new services. For example, a hospital supply firm may place its own ordering computer terminals at customers' sites. These terminals then facilitate the placement of new orders to the extent that competitors are effectively excluded.
- *Exit barriers.* Marginal service firms may continue to operate despite low, or even nonexistent, profits. For example, a privately held firm may have employment of family members rather than maximizing profit as its goal. Other service firms, such as antique stores or scuba diving shops, have a hobby or romantic appeal that provides their owners with enough job satisfaction to offset low financial compensation. Thus, profit-motivated competitors would find it difficult to drive these privately held firms from the market.

For any particular service industry, there are firms that have overcome these competitive difficulties and prospered. For example, McDonald's has achieved a dominant position in the fast-food industry by overcoming many of the difficulties listed here. New entrants, however, must develop a service strategy that will address the important competitive features of their respective industries. Three generic strategies have been successful in providing a competitive advantage, and illustrations of how service firms have used these strategies will be our next topic.

COMPETITIVE SERVICE STRATEGIES[3]

Michael Porter has argued persuasively that three generic competitive strategies exist: overall cost leadership, differentiation, and focus.[4] Each strategy will be described in turn, with examples of how service firms use them to outperform their competition.

Overall Cost Leadership

An overall cost leadership strategy requires efficient-scale facilities, tight cost and overhead control, and often innovative technology as well. Having a low-cost position provides a defense against competition, because less efficient competitors will suffer first from competitive pressures. Implementing a low-cost strategy usually requires high capital investment in state-of-the-art equipment, aggressive pricing, and start-up losses to build market share. A cost leadership strategy sometimes can revolutionize an industry, as illustrated by the success of McDonald's, Wal-Mart, and Federal Express. Moreover, service firms have been able to achieve low-cost leadership using a variety of approaches.

Seeking Out Low-Cost Customers

Some customers cost less to serve than others, and they can be targeted by the service provider. For example, United Services Automobile Association (USAA) occupies a preeminent position among automobile insurers because it serves only military officers, a group that presents a lower-than-average risk of problems requiring compensation. This group also entails lower cost because its members, who are relatively nomadic, are willing to do business by telephone or mail and are accustomed to doing so. Consequently, USAA is able to conduct all of its business transactions by phone and mail, eliminating any need for the expensive sales force employed by traditional insurers. Another example of this strategy is provided by low-cost retailers such as Sam's Wholesale Club and Price Club, which target customers who are willing to buy in quantity, do without frills, and serve themselves.

Standardizing a Custom Service

Typically, income tax preparation is considered to be a customized service. H. & R. Block, however, has been successful in serving customers nationwide

[3]Adapted from James L. Heskett, "Positioning in Competitive Service Strategies," *Managing in the Service Economy,* Harvard Business School Press, Boston, 1986.
[4]Michael E. Porter, "Generic Competitive Strategies," *Competitive Strategy,* Free Press, New York, 1980.

when only routine tax preparation is required. Also, storefront legal services and family health care centers are attractive means of delivering routine professional services at low cost. The key word here is *routine.*

Reducing the Personal Element in Service Delivery

The potentially high-risk strategy of reducing the personal element in service delivery can be accepted by customers if increased convenience results. For example, convenient access to ATMs has weaned customers from personal interaction with live tellers and, consequently, has reduced transaction costs for banks.

Reducing Network Costs

Unusual start-up costs are encountered by service firms that require a network to knit together providers and customers. Electric utilities, which have substantial fixed costs in transmission lines, provide the most obvious example. Federal Express conceived a unique approach to reducing network costs by using a "hub-and-spoke" network. By locating a hub in Memphis with state-of-the-art sorting technology, the overnight air-package carrier was able to serve the United States with no direct routes between the cities that it served. Each time a new city is added to the network, Federal Express only needs to add one more route to and from the hub instead of adding routes between all the cities served. The efficiency of the hub-and-spoke network strategy has not been lost on passenger airline operators, either.

Taking Service Operations Off-Line

Many services, such as haircutting and passenger transportation, are inherently "on-line," because they can only be performed with the customer present. For services in which the customer need not be present, the service transaction can be "decoupled," with some content performed "off-line." For example, a shoe repair service could locate dispersed kiosks for customer drop-off/pick-up, thus consolidating orders for delivery to an off-site repair factory, which could even be located off-shore. Performing services off-line represents significant cost savings because of economies of scale from consolidation, low-cost facility location (e.g., American Airlines has one of its 800-number reservations centers located in the Caribbean), and absence of the customer in the system. In short, the decoupled service operation is run like a factory.

Differentiation

The essence of the *differentiation* strategy lies in creating a service that is perceived as being unique. Approaches to differentiation can take many forms: brand image (e.g., McDonald's golden arches), technology (e.g., Sprint's fiberoptics network), features (e.g., American Express's complete travel services), customer service (e.g., Nordstrom's reputation among department stores), dealer network (e.g., Century 21's nationwide real estate presence), and other dimensions. A differentiation strategy does not ignore costs, but its primary thrust lies in creating customer loyalty. As illustrated here, differentiation to enhance the service often is achieved at some cost that the targeted customer is willing to pay.

Making the Intangible Tangible

By their very nature, services often are intangible and leave the customer with no physical reminder of the purchase. Recognizing the need to remind customers of their stay, many hotels now provide complimentary toiletry items with the hotel name prominently affixed. The Hartford Steam Boiler Inspection and Insurance Company writes insurance on industrial power plants, but this company has enhanced its service to include regular inspections and recommendations to managers for avoiding potential problems.

Customizing the Standard Product

Providing a customized touch may endear a firm to its customers at very little cost. A hotel operator who is able to address a guest by name can make an impression that translates into repeat business. Hair salons have added many personalizing features (e.g., personal stylist, juice bar, relaxed surroundings, mood music) to differentiate themselves from barbershops. Burger King's efforts to promote a made-to-order policy is an attempt to differentiate itself from McDonald's classic make-to-stock approach to fast-food service.

Reducing Perceived Risk

Lack of information about the purchase of a service creates a sense of risk-taking for many customers. Lacking knowledge or self-confidence about services such as auto repair, customers will seek out providers who take the extra time to explain the work to be done, present a clean and organized facility, and guarantee their work (e.g., Village Volvo). Customers often see the "peace of mind" that is engendered when this trusting relationship develops as being worth the extra expense.

Giving Attention to Personnel Training

Investment in personnel development and training that results in enhanced service quality is a competitive advantage that is difficult to replicate. Firms that lead their industries are known among competitors for the quality of their training programs. In some cases, these firms have established college-like training centers (e.g., Arthur Andersen's facility in St. Charles, Illinois; McDonald's Hamburger University near Chicago).

Controlling Quality

Delivering a consistent level of service quality at multiple sites with a labor-intensive system is a significant challenge. Firms have approached this problem in a variety of ways, including personnel training, explicit procedures, technology, limits on the scope of the service, direct supervision, and peer pressure, among others. For example, to ensure consistency, the Magic Pan chain of restaurants designed a foolproof machine to produce its famous crêpes. The question of service quality is further complicated by the potential gap between customer expectations and experiences. Influencing customer quality expectations thus becomes an issue, and Chapter 10, Service Quality, provides a detailed look at this important topic of managing service quality.

Focus

The *focus* strategy is built around the idea of serving a particular target market very well by addressing the customers' specific needs. The market segment could be a particular buyer group (e.g., USAA and military officers), service (e.g., Shouldice Hospital and patients with inguinal hernias, Motel 6 and budget travelers, Federal Express and people who need guaranteed overnight package delivery), or geographic region (e.g., Wal-Mart and rural retail buyers, Southwest Airlines and other regional airlines). The focus strategy rests on the premise that the firm can serve its narrow target market more effectively and/or efficiently than other firms trying to serve a broad market. As a result, the firm achieves differentiation in its narrow target market by meeting customer needs better and/or by lowering costs.

Davidow and Uttal argue how important customer selection is to achieving a successful focus strategy.[5] They relate how one bank in Palo Alto, California, targets wealthy individuals and discourages others by policies such as closing an account after two checks have bounced. Davidow and Uttal's three-step approach to focus includes segmenting the market to design core services, classifying customers according to the value they place on service, and setting expectations slightly below perceived performance.

The focus strategy thus is the application of overall cost leadership and/or differentiation to a particular market segment, and the relationship of the three generic strategies to market position is shown in Figure 3.6. We conclude this chapter with discussions of winning customers in the marketplace.

WINNING CUSTOMERS IN THE MARKETPLACE

Depending on the competition and personal needs, customers select a service provider using criteria listed here. This list is not intended to be complete, because the very addition of a new dimension by a firm represents an attempt to engage in a strategy of differentiation. For example, initiation of the frequent flyer program "AAdvantage" by American Airlines was an attempt to add the dimension of customer loyalty to competition among airlines.

[5]W. H. Davidow and B. Uttal, "Service Companies: Focus or Falter," *Harvard Business Review*, July/August 1989, pp. 77–85.

FIGURE 3.6. Market position of generic strategies.
(Adapted with the permission of The Free Press, a Division of Macmillan, Inc., from Competitive Strategy: Techniques for Analyzing Industries and Competitors *by Michael E. Porter. Copyright © 1980 by The Free Press.)*

Target	**Strategic Advantage**	
	Low cost	Uniqueness
Entire market	Overall cost leadership	Differentiation
Market segment	Focus	

- *Availability.* How accessible is the service? The use of ATMs by banks has created 24-hour availability of some banking services (i.e., service beyond the traditional "banker's hours"). Use of 800-numbers by many service firms facilitates access after normal working hours.
- *Convenience.* The location of the service defines convenience for customers who must travel to that service. Gasoline stations, fast-food restaurants, and dry cleaners are examples of services that must select locations on busy streets if they are to succeed.
- *Dependability.* How reliable is the service? For example, once the exterminator is gone, how soon do the bugs return? A major complaint regarding automobile repair services is the failure to fix the problem on the first visit. For airlines, on-time performance is a statistic collected by the FAA.
- *Personalization.* Are you treated as an individual? For example, hotels have discovered that repeat customers respond to being greeted by their name. The degree of customization allowed in providing the service, no matter how slight, can be viewed as more personalized service.
- *Price.* Competing on price is not as effective in services as it is with products, because it often is difficult to compare the costs of services objectively. It may be easy to compare costs in the delivery of routine services such as an oil change, but in professional services, competition on price might be considered counterproductive because price often is viewed as being a surrogate for quality.
- *Quality.* Service quality is a function of the relationship between a customer's prior expectations of the service and his or her perception of the service experience both during and after the fact. Unlike product quality, service quality is judged by both the process of service delivery and the outcome of the service.
- *Reputation.* The uncertainty that is associated with the selection of a service provider often is resolved by talking with others about their experiences before a decision is made. Unlike a product, a poor service experience cannot be exchanged or returned for a different model. Positive word-of-mouth is the most effective form of advertising.
- *Safety.* Well-being and security are important considerations, because in many services, such as air travel and medicine, the customers are putting their lives in the hands of the service provider.
- *Speed.* How long must I wait for service? For emergency services such as fire and police protection, response time is the major criterion of performance. In other services, waiting sometimes may be considered a tradeoff for receiving more personalized services, such as reduced rates.

Writing about manufacturing strategy, Terry Hill used the term *order-winning criteria* to refer to competitive dimensions that sell products.[6] He further suggested that some criteria could be called *qualifiers,* because the presence of these dimensions is necessary for a product to enter the marketplace. Finally, Hill said that some qualifiers could be considered *order-losing sensitive.*

We will use a similar logic and the service criteria listed earlier to describe the service purchase decision. The purchase decision sequence begins with qual-

[6]Terry Hill, *Manufacturing Strategy,* Irwin, Homewood, Ill., 1989, pp. 36–46.

ifying potential service firms (e.g., must the doctor be on my PPO list?), followed by making a final selection from this subset of service firms using a service winner (e.g., which of the PPO doctors has the best reputation?). After the initial service experience, a return will be based on whether a "service loser" has occurred (e.g., the doctor was cold and impersonal).

Qualifiers

Before a service firm can be taken seriously as a competitor in the market, it must attain a certain level for each service-competitive dimension, as defined by the other market players. For example, in airline service, we would name safety, as defined by the air-worthiness of the aircraft and by the rating of the pilots, as an obvious qualifier. In a mature market such as fast foods, established competitors may define a level of quality, such as cleanliness, that new entrants must at least match to be viable contenders. For fast food, a dimension that once was a service winner, such as a drive-in window, over time could become a qualifier, because some customers will not stop otherwise.

Service Winners

Service winners are dimensions such as price, convenience, or reputation that are used by a customer to make a choice among competitors. Depending on the needs of the customer at the time of the purchase, the service winner may vary. For example, seeking a restaurant for lunch may be based on convenience, but a dinner date could be influenced by reputation. Note that a service winner can become an industry qualifier (e.g., ATM use by banks).

Service Losers

Failure to deliver at or above the expected level for a competitive dimension can result in a dissatisfied customer who is lost forever. For various reasons, the dimensions of dependability, personalization, and speed are particularly vulnerable to becoming *service losers*. Some examples might be failure of an auto dealer to repair a mechanical problem (i.e., dependability), rude treatment by a doctor (i.e., personalization), or failure of an overnight service to deliver a package on time (i.e., speed).

SUMMARY

The topic of service strategy began with a number of schemes to classify service industries to gain insights into possible strategic opportunities that transcend industry boundaries. We looked at the strategic service concept as a blueprint for implementing the service. Our discussion then turned to the economic nature of competition in the service sector. The fragmented nature of service industries populated with many small- to medium-sized firms suggests a rich environment for the budding entrepreneur.

The three generic competitive strategies of overall cost leadership, differentiation, and focus were used to outline examples of creative service strategies. Because of the transferability of concepts among service firms, strategies that are successful in one industry may find application in firms seeking a competitive advantage in another service industry.

Next, we looked at several dimensions of service competition and examined the concepts of service winners, qualifiers, and losers as competitive criteria. The application of the service concept to Shouldice Hospital illustrated how all eight elements support the service strategy. Chapter 4 will look at service process technology and, in particular, the contribution of information technology to service process design.

KEY TERMS AND DEFINITIONS

Differentiation a competitive strategy that creates a service that is perceived as being unique.

Focus a competitive strategy built around the concept of serving a particular target market very well by addressing the customers' specific needs.

Overall cost leadership a competitive strategy based on efficient operations, cost control, and innovative technology.

Qualifiers criteria used by a customer to create a subset of service firms meeting minimum performance requirements.

Service losers criteria representing failure to deliver a service at or above the expected level, resulting in a dissatisfied customer who is lost forever.

Service winners criteria used by a customer to make the final purchase decision among competitors that have been previously qualified.

Strategic service concept eight elements that define the service to be offered that are in turn grouped into structural and managerial categories.

TOPICS FOR DISCUSSION

1. What are the characteristics of services that will be affected most by the emerging electronic and communication technologies?
2. When does collecting information through service membership become an invasion of privacy?
3. What are some management problems that are associated with allowing service employees to exercise judgment in meeting customer needs?
4. What are the implications of the growing use of personal computers for the customization of services and elimination of human service interactions?
5. Give examples of service firms that use both the strategy of focus and differentiation and the strategy of focus and overall cost leadership.
6. Apply the strategic service concept to a service of your choice, and illustrate how all eight elements support the service strategy.

Service Benchmark

Central Market shuns conventional wisdom and big-name products

Central Market's opening in January prompted some friendly wagering among food-industry heavyweights who were left out in the cold.

The odds favored Frito-Lay's snacks appearing in the store, a specialty and fresh food supermarket, by the end of the summer. Other wagers bet that Coca-Cola and Budweiser trucks would pull up to the market's loading docks within six months. Now all bets are off.

Shunning big-name product lines is one reason why Central Market has caught the attention of the nation's $279.4 billion supermarket industry. The market—which within a year has become a flagship of the 225 Texas stores owned by parent-company H.E.B. Food Stores—has made it a practice to defy many of the standards that the country's 30,000 supermarkets embrace.

Although most supermarkets subscribe to the notion that customers want one-stop shopping. Central Market has proved that food alone sells well.

At Central Market, which carries virtually nothing except food, the average shopper spends $30 at the checkout counter, said Central Market general manager John Campbell. The national industry average, which also includes spending on general merchandise and health and beauty products, is $18.11, according to the Washington, D.C.-based Food Marketing Institute. The lower industry average results from shoppers who dash in for a few items, such as diapers or mascara, and then check out through the 10-items-or-fewer express lanes, Campbell said. "Here, they do serious shopping," he said.

Central Market also looks different from traditional stores. Its layout forces customers to walk through serpentine sections instead of straight aisles. It also houses a cooking school. There are 250 kinds of mustard, dozens of olive oils, and jams from all over the world on its shelves.

While at least half of the nation's 3.2 million supermarket workers are part-time employees, 90 percent of Central Market's 400 workers are full-time employees who receive health benefits, paid vacation time, tuition reimbursements and profit-sharing. It's an expensive staffing decision that Campbell says pays off by generating greater enthusiasm and product knowledge among workers, two factors that he says are vital to building customer satisfaction.

At Central Market at least 20 percent of the store's sales come from its roomy produce section which eats up almost a third of the store's 60,000 square feet of sales space. The section, kept at 65 degrees, stocks on any given day as many as 450 kinds of fruit and vegetables.

Seventy-five feet of refrigerator space displays fresh fish, while the 68-foot meat counter sells more than 100 types of meat, game and poultry. The cheese department offers 600 varieties.

In all, about two-thirds of the store's floor space is stocked with perishables. And each day, a truck from a local food bank comes by to take away the items that have failed Central Market's freshness guidelines.

Although the market risks losing money if too many of its meats and fruits aren't sold quickly, those items have higher profit margins than dry groceries. The margins for perishables are larger because those items are priced higher to make up for losses, refrigeration costs and the increased labor expenses that result from product displays.

"The more sales you can move to perishable, the better, because the amount you can charge for Coke, Pepsi or Tide is tight," said Kevin Coupe, executive editor of Progressive Grocer trade magazine in Stamford, Conn.

H.E.B. began discussing the Central Market concept in the mid 1980s when its market studies found that customers were increasingly interested in home cooking, nutrition and better-tasting foods.

"With Central Market, we were trying to get ahead of what we see as a definite trend and one that we feel like will only continue to grow," Ozmun said.

Source: Adapted from Diana Dworin, "Central Market proves it can thrive even as it shuns conventional wisdom and big-name products," ©*Austin American Statesman*, October 2, 1994, p. H1.

CASE: AMERICA WEST AIRLINES

America West Airlines was established in Phoenix as an employee-owned organization serving ten cities in the southwestern United States with a fleet of new Boeing 737 aircraft. Since then, it has grown to include 60 cities and extended its range westward to Hawaii and eastward to Boston.

This neophyte company showed remarkable daring by entering an arena where the majors, American Airlines and Delta Air Lines, already were firmly entrenched and where Southwest Airlines was digging in. Even more daring—some would say foolhardy—was the timing: deregulation was threatening to swallow up small airlines faster than they could refuel their planes.

America West, however, came into the game prepared with a skilled and creative management team, well-trained support personnel, and an effective inside pitch. Obviously, the fledgling company did not have the resources to provide the nationwide, much less the worldwide, coverage that American and Delta provided. Its smaller region, however, allowed it to do something the majors could not: America West established a major hub in Phoenix and offered more flights per day at lower cost between its cities than the two larger competitors could. In many cases, America West offered direct routing and, consequently, relatively short flight times between destinations. "Burdened" with serving everywhere from Tallahassee to Seattle, American and Delta were able to schedule flights between America West destinations, but with longer layovers and at premium prices because they were major carriers. For example, consider travel from Austin, Texas, to Los Angeles. America West has four flights scheduled each day, with each taking approximately 4.5 hours and requiring one layover of 30 minutes in Phoenix, and its least expensive fare is $238. American Airlines offers eight flights each day, with each lasting at least 5 hours, but the traveler has a 60-minute layover in Dallas and spends $298 for American's least expensive flight.

When America West passengers have a layover, it is almost always at the Phoenix hub. (America West has a "sub-hub" in Las Vegas, where layovers usually are overnight, an appeal not lost on many travelers.) Consequently, America West's "accommodations" at the Phoenix airport are as comfortable as one could hope for in a place that hosts such a large number of people each day. The waiting areas are spacious, with banks of well-padded seats placed farther apart than in most airports. Television monitors are mounted in several places throughout the facility, and because the concessions are run by nationally known fast-food franchises, the traveler has ample reason to "feel at home."

Southwest Airlines presented a competitive challenge somewhat different from that of American and Delta. Southwest was serving the same general region as America West and also was offering frequent, low-cost flights but with older Boeing 737 aircraft. Thus, it would seem that these two airlines were meeting head to head and might be destined to "flight"-to-the-finish of one of them.

Southwest established its hub at Love Field in Dallas, thereby offering its passengers easier access both to and from the city, which is especially attractive to commuters. (Landing at Love Field does, however, present a problem for those who must make connections in the Dallas–Fort Worth International Terminal.) Southwest began as the "fun airline," the one with attendants in hot pants and snappy commercials on television. Since then, however, it has met the competitive challenge by offering its frequent, low-cost, no-frills service. It generally has just two fares, peak and off-peak, and there is no need to call at 1 AM "to see if fares have changed in the past ten hours." Reservations for flights can be made by phone, but they must be paid for either through a travel agent or in person at the airport desk. There are no preassigned seats; seating is handled on a first-come, first-served basis according to a numbered boarding pass that is handed to the passenger at check-in time. On-board amenities usually are limited to free soft drinks, juice, and peanuts. Prepackaged cookies and crackers with cheese or peanut butter are available on long flights, and alcoholic beverages are available for a price. Except for short commuter flights, routing frequently involves several lengthy layovers, and it is not always possible to check baggage clear through to one's destination.

Thus far, America West has managed to meet Southwest's challenge in a variety of ways. With America West, the traveler can make reservations and pay for them with a credit card by telephone, a very real convenience for many people. Preassigned seating also can be done by telephone, and, in contrast to Southwest's ticketing policy, travel agents can ticket passengers using the SABRE reservation system. Onboard amenities include complimentary copies of *USA Today* and *The Wall Street Journal,* free beverages and peanuts, and on longer trips, an uncooked snack such as a sandwich, salad, cheese, fruit, and dessert. Baggage can be checked on all flights.

Clearly, America West's strategies have kept it in the game, although in recent times it has been struggling with some financial problems.

Questions

1. What generic competitive strategy has America West chosen to use in entering the air passenger market? What are the dangers of this strategy?

2. Identify the service winners, qualifiers, and service losers in America West's market.

3. How has America West addressed the eight elements in its strategic service concept?

4. Marketing analysts use market position maps to display visually the customers' perceptions of a firm in relation to its competitors regarding two attributes. Prepare a market position map for America West comparing it with American, Delta, and Southwest using the differentiation attributes of "cabin service" and "preflight service." You will need to define the endpoints on each scale to anchor the relative positioning of the airlines along the attribute (e.g., one extreme for cabin service is no amenities). The actual position is subjective, because no precise measurements are available.

SELECTED BIBLIOGRAPHY

DAVIDOW, W. H., and B. UTTAL: "Service Companies: Focus or Falter," *Harvard Business Review,* July–August 1989, pp. 77–85.

HESKETT, JAMES L.: *Managing in the Service Economy,* Harvard Business School Press, Boston, 1986.

HILL, TERRY: *Manufacturing Strategy,* 2nd ed., Irwin, Homewood, Ill., 1994.

LOVELOCK, CHRISTOPHER H.: "Classifying Services to Gain Strategic Marketing Insights," *Journal of Marketing,* Summer 1983, pp. 9–20.

———: *Services Marketing,* Prentice-Hall, Englewood Cliffs, N.J., 1984.

PORTER, MICHAEL E.: *Competitive Strategy,* Free Press, New York, 1980.

ROTH, A. V., and M. VAN DER VELDE: "Operations as Marketing: The Key to Effective Service Delivery Systems," Boston University Press, Boston, 1989.

SHOSTACK, LYNN G.: "Service Positioning through Structural Change," *Journal of Marketing,* January 1987, pp. 34–43.

THOMAS, DAN R. E.: "Strategy Is Different in Service Business," *Harvard Business Review,* July–August 1978, pp. 158–165.

ZEITHAML, VALARIE A.: "How Consumer Evaluation Processes Differ between Goods and Services," in James H. Donnelly and William R. George (eds.), *Marketing of Services,* American Marketing Association, Chicago, 1984.

———, A. PARASURAMAN, and L. L. BERRY: "Problems and Strategies in Services Marketing," *Journal of Marketing,* Spring 1985, pp. 33–46.

Services and Information Technology

LEARNING OBJECTIVES

After completing this chapter, you should be able to:

1. Discuss the role of the customer in service process innovation.
2. Place an example of service automation in its proper category.
3. Discuss the managerial issues associated with the adoption of new technology.
4. Discuss the competitive role of information in services.
5. Explain the concept of the virtual value chain and its role in service innovation.
6. Discuss the limits in the use of information.

As machine technology once changed an agricultural economy into an industrial economy, today's information technology is transforming our industrial economy into a service economy. The availability of computers and global communication technologies has created industries for collecting, processing, and communicating information. Today everyone on the globe can be in instant communication with everyone else, and this revolution is changing world society in many ways. Consider the impact of the emerging private satellite network industry, which provides uplinks and downlinks for personnel training, product introductions, credit checks, billing, financial exchanges, and overall telecommunications.

Kmart was among the first retail giants to establish a private satellite network using the new small-dish antenna VSAT (Very Small Aperture Terminal) placed on store roofs to receive and transmit masses of data. The VSAT at each Kmart is linked to the company's Troy, Michigan, data center via a satellite transponder leased from GTE Spacenet. The communication network has allowed Kmart to coordinate its multisite operations better and to realize substantial benefits, such as improved data transmission about the rate of sales, inventory status, product updates, and most important, credit authorizations for customers. The instant accessibility of credit histories can significantly lower the risk of nonpayment that credit card companies face, thus lowering the discount rate that reverts back to the retailer. This savings alone eventually will pay for the cost of the satellite network.[1]

CHAPTER PREVIEW

The chapter begins with a discussion of technological innovation in services. Because customers participate in the service delivery process, innovations such as the use of information technology (particularly in the front office) raise the issue of customer acceptance. In fact, information is viewed as the most important enabling technology in services.

A framework for viewing the contribution of information to the competitive strategy of the service firm also is presented. Using the dimensions of strategic focus (either external or internal) and competitive use of information (either on-line or off-line), four strategic roles for information are identified: creation of barriers to entry, revenue generation, data base asset, and productivity enhancement. For each role, examples are used to illustrate how firms have used information effectively.

Service product innovation is driven by an appreciation of the virtual value chain based on information gathered from customer transactions. This data base can be used to develop new services, creating value for the customer.

The chapter concludes with a discussion of limits in the use of information, dealing with questions of privacy, fairness, reliability, data accuracy, and anti-competitive behavior.

[1]From Bernie Ward, "Microspace, Maxiprofits," *Sky*, December 1990, pp. 22–31.

TECHNOLOGICAL INNOVATION IN SERVICES

The great gains in agricultural and manufacturing productivity came from the substitution of technology for human effort. Technology need not be confined to hardware and machines, however. It also includes innovative systems, such as electronic funds transfer or automated multiphasic health testing. In manufacturing, the introduction of technological innovations goes unnoticed by consumers, but such innovations become an integral part of the service that is provided. For example, many airlines have introduced automatic ticketing machines that accept credit cards and issue tickets according to a request entered by the passenger, who pushes the appropriate buttons. At many filling stations, a credit card reader located on the pump facilitates the purchase of gasoline.

Challenges of Adopting New Technology in Services

For services, "the process is the product," because customers participate directly in the service delivery. Therefore, the success of technological innovations, particularly for the front office, depends on customer acceptance. The impact on customers is not always limited to a loss of personal attention. Customers also may need to learn new skills (e.g., how to operate an automatic teller machine or pump gasoline), or they may have to forgo some benefit (e.g., loss of float through the use of electronic funds transfer). The contribution of customers as active participants or coproducers in the service process must be considered when making changes in the service delivery system.

As internal customers, employees also are affected by new technology and often need retraining. The example of scanning in retail stores was minor compared with the adoption of word processing by secretaries, who were used to typewriters.

Back-office innovation that does not directly affect the customer may raise complications of a different sort. For example, consider the use of magnetic-ink-character recognition equipment in banking. This technological innovation did not affect the customer at all; instead, it made the "hidden" check-clearing process more productive. The full benefits, however, could not be realized until all banks agreed to imprint their checks using a universal character code. Without such an agreement, the checks of uncooperative banks would need to be sorted by hand, which would limit severely the effectiveness of this technology. When all banks in the United States finally agreed on the use of the same magnetic-ink-character imprints on checks, the check-clearing process became much more efficient. The Bank of America took a leadership role in gaining acceptance for the concept, but the self-interest of banks was a principle motivation. The volume of check processing had exceeded their manual sorting capacity.

Other examples of this need to standardize occurred in retailing with the acceptance of the Universal Product Code (UPC) by manufacturers. Retailers who have adopted the UPC can use laser scanners to read a bar code (i.e., a series of vertical stripes of different widths) on products. Consequently, they can use a computer to register sales and update inventory levels simultaneously.

The incentive to innovate in services is hampered, however, because many ideas cannot be patented. One example is the idea of self-serve retailing. Much of the potential for technological and organizational progress is in this area. The prospective rewards for innovations are diminished, however, because the innovations may be freely imitated and quickly implemented by the competition.

Automation in Services

The back office has been the most logical place to introduce automation in services, because these operations often are repetitive and routine and thus amenable to labor-saving devices. Many applications have been in the hard automation category, such as replacing human manual activity with a machine (e.g., an automatic lawn sprinkler system at a hotel). More advanced programmable devices also have found application in services, sometimes interacting with the customer (e.g., automated answering systems that route callers by means of touch-tone phones).

Thus, a classification of automation applications in services must go beyond the traditional categories that are used in manufacturing because of the opportunities for interaction with the customer. In the following automation categories, first suggested by David Collier, we include the *expert system,* which is a form of mental automation (e.g., using a computer for reasoning and problem solving)[2]:

Fixed sequence (F). A machine that repetitively performs successive steps in a given operation according to a predetermined sequence, condition, and position, and whose set information cannot be changed easily. Service example: automatic parking lot gate.

Variable sequence (V). A machine that is the same as a fixed-sequence robot but whose set information can be changed easily. Service example: automated teller machine.

Playback (P). A machine that can produce operations from memory that were originally executed under human control. Service example: telephone answering machine.

Numerical controlled (N). A machine that can perform a given task according to a sequence, conditions, and a position as commanded by stored instructions that can be reprogrammed easily. Service example: animated characters at an amusement park.

Intelligent (I). A machine with sensory perception devices, such as visual or tactile receptors, that can detect changes in the work environment or task by itself and has its own decision-making abilities. Service example: autopilot for a commercial airplane.

Expert system (E). A computer program that uses an inference engine (i.e., decision rules) and a knowledge base (i.e., information on a particular subject) to diagnose problems. Service example: maintenance trouble-shooting for elevator repair.

Totally automated system (T). A system of machines and computers that performs all the physical and intellectual tasks that are required to produce a product or deliver a service. Service example: electronic funds transfer.

[2]David A. Collier, "The Service Sector Revolution: The Automation of Services," *Long Range Planning,* vol. 16, no. 6, December 1983, p. 11.

To illustrate the extent of automation in services, Table 4.1 provides examples of automation by service industry, with each example classified according to the preceding categories. The automation examples suggest that services are becoming more capital-intensive, and that the old notion of the service sector as being a low-skilled, labor-intensive operation must be reconsidered. Service workers will need more sophisticated skills to program, operate, and maintain the automated systems. More important, employee flexibility will be a valued attribute, because the nature of work is changed by new technology. For example, consider the many changes in the office that have occurred with the introduction of personal computers and word-processing capabilities.

Managing the New Technology Adoption Process

Innovation is a destroyer of tradition; thus, it requires careful planning to ensure success. By necessity, the productivity benefits of new technology will change the nature of work. Any introduction of new technology should include employee familiarization to prepare workers for new tasks and to provide input into the technology interface design (e.g., will typing skill be required, or will employees just point and click?). For services, the impact of new technology may not be limited to the back office. It could require a change in the role that customers play in the service delivery process. Customer reaction to the new technology, determined through focus groups or interviews, also could provide input into the design to avoid future problems of acceptance (e.g., consider the need for surveillance cameras at automated teller machines).

In writing about his experiences installing computer systems, Robert Radchuk has developed a ten-step planning guide to manage the implementation process. The following modified version of these steps includes the concerns for employees and customers[3]:

Step 1: Orientation and education. Become knowledgeable about the new technology and where it is headed. Visit trade shows and other users to gain hands-on familiarity. Secure the active involvement of a senior manager to champion the technology.

Step 2: Technology opportunity analysis. Undertake a feasibility study to define opportunities, estimate costs, and identify benefits. Benchmark the use of the technology in other industries.

Step 3: Application requirements analysis. Define the requirements for the new technology, and identify the hardware and software to be purchased. Refine cost and benefit estimates.

Step 4: Functional specification. Define the operating characteristics of the application, including the inputs, outputs, operator interface, and type of equipment to be used. This working document will be used in interactions with users of the system; thus, it should be an explicit definition in nontechnical terms of how the system will work.

Step 5: Design specification. Produce a specific engineering design with inputs from users, both employees and customers, to evaluate the effectiveness of the system interfaces. For example, as noted in Chapter 1, Burger King

[3]Adapted from Robert P. Radchuck, "Step-by-Step into High Tech," *CA Magazine*, vol. 115, no. 6, June 1982, pp. 72–73.

TABLE 4.1. Categories and Examples of Automation in Service Industries

	WHOLESALE AND RETAIL TRADE, 23.1%*		
F	Dry cleaner's conveyor	V	Point-of-sale electronic terminal
F	Newspaper dispenser	I	Self-serve grocery checkout
V	Automatic car wash	T	Automated distribution warehouse
V	Automatic window washers	T	Automated security systems
V	Optical supermarket	T	Telemarketing
	UTILITIES AND GOVERNMENT SERVICES, 17.9%*		
F	Automated one-person garbage trucks	I	Airborne warning and control systems
V	Mail-sorting machine	I	Doppler radar
V	Optical mail scanner	T	Electric power-generating plants
N	IRS Form 1040EZ reader	T	Electronic computer-originated mail
	HEALTH CARE SERVICES, 7.6%*		
F	Electronic beepers	I	Automated medication-delivery systems
F	Pacemakers	I	Electronic ambulance-dispatching systems
V	CAT and MRI scanners	I	Medical information systems
V	Dental chair system	E	Diagnostic expert systems
V	Fetal monitors		
	RESTAURANTS AND FOOD SERVICES, 6.0%*		
F	Assembly-line and rotating-service cafeterias	F	Vending machines
		V	Automatic french fryer
	FINANCIAL SERVICES, 4.9%*		
F	Pneumatic delivery systems	V	Master Card II—the electronic checkbook
V	Automated trust portfolio analysis	E	Stock trading
V	Automated teller machines	T	Electronic funds transfer systems
V	IBM 3890 encoded-check processor machine		
	TRANSPORTATION SERVICES, 4.9%*		
F	Automatic tollbooth	I	France's TGV trains
I	Air traffic control systems	I	Ship navigation systems
I	Autopilots	T	Space shuttle
I	Bay Area Rapid Transportation system		
	COMMUNICATION AND ELECTRONIC SERVICES, 2.2%		
V	Collating copying machines	T	Teleconference phone and Picturephone
V	Two-way cable television	T	Telephone switching systems
P	Telephone answering machines		
	EDUCATION SERVICES, 1.6%*		
F	Audiovisual machine	P	Language translation computers
V	Electronic calculators	P	Personal and home computers
V	Speak-and-Spell, Speak-and-Read	T	Library cataloging systems

TABLE 4.1 (*Continued*)

	HOTEL AND MOTEL SERVICES, 1.5%*		
F	Automatic sprinkler systems	V	Electronic key and lock systems
F	Elevator, escalator, and conveyor	T	Electronic reservation systems
	LEISURE SERVICES, 1.4%		
F	Movie projectors	I	Arcade and computer games
F	Wave machines	T	Disney World (e.g., Hall of Presidents)
P	Videodisk machines		

*Percentage of total workforce as reported in *Employment and Earnings,* U.S. Department of Labor, Bureau of Labor Statistics, December 1991, Table B-2, pp. 52–62.

Source: Adapted with permission from David A. Collier, "The Service Sector Revolution: The Automation of Services," *Long Range Planning,* vol. 16, no. 6, December 1983, pp. 12–13. Copyright © 1983 Pergamon Press Ltd.

has a mock-up of a typical store in a Miami warehouse where new technology ideas are tested in a simulated environment before their introduction into the marketplace.

Step 6: Implementation planning. Using project planning techniques, such as Microsoft® Project for Windows, develop a detailed implementation plan. This plan should account for all activities, such as personnel familiarization and training, facilities planning, prototype testing, and an initial operation in parallel with the current system until the new technology is debugged.

Step 7: Equipment selection and contract commitments. Contract for equipment purchases, and schedule the equipment for delivery as per the implementation plan.

Step 8: Implementation. Execute the implementation plan, and prepare progress reports for senior management.

Step 9: Testing of technology. Before committing to full-blown operations, test the technology. If a simulation is not possible, the new technology could be introduced at one or more trial sites before the entire service network is committed. Specific tests must be defined in advance to evaluate the system's response to anticipated demands.

Step 10: Review of results. Document information that has been learned from the implementation experience by comparing original expectations with actual results. This final step may be the most important, because expertise in managing the implementation of new technology can be a competitive advantage.

THE COMPETITIVE ROLE OF INFORMATION IN SERVICES[4]

For service management, information technology is helping to define the competitive strategy of successful firms. Figure 4.1 illustrates the different roles in

[4]Adapted from James A. Fitzsimmons, "Strategic Role of Information in Services," in Rakesh V. Sarin (ed.), *Perspectives in Operations Management: Essays in Honor of Elwood S. Buffa,* Kluwer Academic Publisher, Norwell, Mass., 1993.

Strategic Focus	Competitive Use of Information: On-line (Real time)	Off-line (Analysis)
External (Customer)	*Creation of barriers to entry:* Reservation system, Frequent user club, Switching costs	*Data base asset:* Selling information, Development of services, Micromarketing
Internal (Operations)	*Revenue generation:* Yield management, Point of sales, Expert systems	*Productivity enhancement:* Inventory status, Data envelopment analysis (DEA)

FIGURE 4.1. Strategic roles of information in services.
(Adapted from James A. Fitzsimmons, "Strategic Role of Information in Services," in Rakesh V. Sarin (ed.), Perspectives in Operations Management: Essays in Honor of Elwood S. Buffa, *Kluwer Academic Publishers, Norwell, Mass., 1993, p. 103.)*

which information technology can support a service firm's competitive strategy. We shall explore each of these roles in turn with illustrations from successful applications.

Creation of Barriers to Entry

As noted in Chapter 3, many services exist in markets that have low entry barriers. James L. Heskett, however, has argued that barriers to entry can be created by using economies of scale, building market share, creating switching costs, investing in communications networks, and using data bases and information technologies to strategic advantage.[5] We will discuss three uses of information for creating barriers to entry: reservation systems, frequent flyer or similar programs to gain customer loyalty, and development of customer relationships to increase switching costs.

Reservation Systems

A barrier to entry can be created by investing in on-line reservations systems that are provided to sales intermediaries such as travel agents. American Airline's SABRE System is an example of the kind of subtle barrier to entry that is created by a comprehensive information system. United and Delta have duplicated this reservations system at great cost, but most smaller carriers use these existing systems for a fee. The competitive importance of on-line reservations systems became evident in late 1982. At this time, the Civil Aeronautics Board (CAB) and the U.S. Department of Justice began a joint investigation of possible antitrust violations by airline reservations systems. In this investigation, Frontier Airlines filed charges accusing United of unfairly restricting competition in the use of its Apollo computerized reservations system.[6]

[5]James L. Heskett, "Operating Strategy Barriers to Entry," *Managing in the Service Economy,* Harvard Business School Press, Boston, 1986.

[6]For specific allegations, see "Frontier Airlines, Inc. (A)," Harvard Business School Case no. 9-184-041, HBS Case Services, 1983.

Frequent User Club

It was a small step for American Airlines, given its massive reservations system, to add up passenger accounts to accumulate travel credit for frequent flyer awards. These programs, which award free trips and several ancillary benefits, create strong brand loyalty among travelers, particularly business travelers who are not paying their own way. Thus, the discount fares of a new competitor have no appeal to these travelers, as People Express learned. A travel consultant has been quoted as saying, "It's one of the most anticompetitive programs ever erected."[7]

Alfred Kahn, the father of deregulation, headed the CAB in the late 1970s and did not foresee how airlines would create reservations systems and frequent flyer plans to stifle competition. He is quoted as saying, "Nobody recognized all the ways in which a carrier could insulate itself from competition."[8]

Switching Costs

Information technology in the form of on-line computer terminals has been used in the medical supplies industry to link hospitals directly to the suppliers' distribution networks. Both American Hospital Supply and McKesson, the drug distributor, have installed their on-line terminals in hospitals so that supplies and drugs can be purchased as the need arises. Significant switching costs are built into this arrangement, because the hospital is able to reduce inventory-carrying costs and has the convenience of on-line ordering for replenishments. The supplier benefits by a reduction in selling costs, because it is difficult for a competitor to entice away a customer who is already co-opted into its system.[9]

Revenue Generation

Real-time information technologies with a focus on internal operations can play a competitive role in increasing revenue opportunities. The concept of *yield management* is best understood as a revenue-maximizing strategy to make full use of service capacity. Advances in microcomputers have created opportunities for innovative point-of-sale devices, and the use of expert systems tied to 800-numbers allows increased customer service.

Yield Management

Through the use of its SABRE reservations system, American Airlines was the first to realize the potential of what is now called yield management. By constantly monitoring the status of both its upcoming flights and competitors' flights on the same route, American makes pricing and allocation decisions on unsold seats. Thus, the number of Supersaver fares allocated to a particular flight can be adjusted to ensure that remaining empty seats have a chance of being sold, but not at the expense of a full-fare seat. This real-time pricing strategy maximizes the revenue for each flight by ensuring that no seat goes empty for want of a

[7]R. L. Rose and J. Dahl, "Skies Are Deregulated, But Just Try Starting a Sizable New Airline," *The Wall Street Journal*, July 19, 1989, p. A1.
[8]Ibid., p. A8.
[9]From Harold S. Bott, "Information for Competitive Advantage," *Operations Management Review*, Fall 1985, p. 35.

bargain-seeking passenger while holding some seats in reserve for late arrivals who are willing to pay full fare.[10]

Thus, yield management is the application of information to improve the revenue that is generated by a time-perishable resource (e.g., airline seats, hotel rooms). The success of yield management for American has not gone unnoticed by other service industries; for example, Marriott Hotels has installed a nationwide yield management system to increase occupancy rates. In addition, American Airlines is capitalizing on its innovation by selling the yield management software to noncompetitive industries such as the French national railroad. The topic of yield management is covered in more detail in Chapter 13.

Point of Sale

Wal-Mart has discovered a new toy for the discount shopper: the VideOcart. As the shopper pushes the VideOcart through the store, information about the department at hand flashes onto the attached video screen. The cart also helps customers find items in the store by listing hundreds of products by department and then displaying a map of the store. The company supplying the cart claims that it has increased sales by $1 per visit in trials at supermarkets.[11] For another example, consider use of the palm-sized microcomputer transmitter. With this device, a server in a restaurant can transmit an order directly to the kitchen monitor and the bill to the cashier at the same time. This saves unnecessary steps and allows more time for suggestive selling.

Expert Systems

Otis Elevator Company puts an expert system together with laptop computers in the hands of its maintenance staff to speed repairs in the field. Collecting information on the behavior of its elevators over the years has led to a knowledge base that is incorporated into the expert system. Using a laptop computer, a repair person in the field can call up the system and receive diagnostic help in identifying the source of a problem. As a result, elevators are placed back in service quickly, and fewer repair people are needed. Some of the earlier applications of expert systems have been in the medical field, and conceivably, these systems could be accessed by physicians for a fee. As another example, an oil exploration expert system was able to identify promising drilling sites for a major oil company.

Data Base Asset

James L. Heskett observed that the data base a service firm possesses can be a hidden asset of strategic importance. The expense of assembling and maintaining a large data base is itself a barrier to entry by competitors. More important, however, the data base can be mined for profiles of customers' buying habits, and these present opportunities for developing new services.[12]

[10]Barry C. Smith, J. F. Leimkuhler, and R. M. Darrow, "Yield Management at American Airlines," *Interfaces*, vol. 22, no. 1, January–February 1992, pp. 8–31.

[11]From Kevin Helliker, "Wal-Mart's Store of the Future Blends Discount Prices, Department-Store Feel," *The Wall Street Journal*, May 17, 1991, p. B1.

[12]Heskett, op. cit., p. 44.

Selling Information

Dun & Bradstreet created a business by selling access to its data base of business credit information. American Home Shield, a provider of service contracts for individual home heating, plumbing, and electrical systems, also discovered that it had a valuable asset in its data base, accumulated over many years of repair experience; manufacturers now are invited to access this data base to evaluate the performance patterns of their products. American Express has detailed information about the spending habits of its cardholders and now offers breakdowns of customer spending patterns to its retail customers.

Developing Services

Club Med, an all-inclusive resort company with locations worldwide, has evolved to reflect the maturing of its membership. Studying the data base of member characteristics, Club Med realized that over time its once swinging singles members have become married with children. In order to continue capturing future vacation visits, Club Med modified some of their locations to accommodate families with young children. Now parents can enjoy the beach and water sports while their children are supervised by Club Med counselors at a children's park nearby. More recently, Club Med has added cruise ships to its vacation possibilities to attract the more senior members who are no longer interested in water sports. As this example illustrates, service firms that capture customer data at the time of the initial purchase have the opportunity to establish a lifetime relationship, with the potential for creating new or modified services for future purchase.

Micromarketing

Today, we can see a truly focused service strategy that can target customers at the micro level. Bar coding and checkout scanner technology creates a wealth of consumer buying information that can be used to target customers with precision. As Table 4.2 shows, analysis of this data base allows marketers to pinpoint their advertising and product distribution. To increase sales, Borden Inc. has used such information to select stores in which to feature its premium pasta sauce. Kraft USA saw its sales of cream cheese increase after targeting its flavors to the tastes of a particular store's shoppers.[13] American Express, by analyzing information about its customers and their changing spending patterns in meticulous detail, can even tell when they get married.

Productivity Enhancement

New developments in the collection and analysis of information have increased our ability to manage multisite service operations. Through use of notebook computers, retail inventory can be managed on a daily basis to make better use of shelf space by matching displayed products with sales. Information collected on the performance of multisite units can be used to identify the most efficient producers, and productivity is enhanced systemwide when the sources of these

[13]Michael J. McCarthy, "Marketers Zero in on Their Customers," *The Wall Street Journal*, March 18, 1991, p. B1.

successes are shared with other sites. The foundation for a learning organization is then established.

Inventory Status

Using a handheld computer, Frito-Lay sales representatives have eliminated paper forms. They download the data collected on their routes each day via telephone to the Plano, Texas, headquarters, and the company then uses this data to keep track of inventory levels, pricing, product promotions, and stale or returned merchandise. These daily updates on sales, manufacturing, and distribution keep fresh products moving through the system, matching consumer de-

TABLE 4.2. Example of Micromarketing Analysis

Hitting the Bull's-Eye Micromarketers can now target a product's best customers and the stores where they're most likely to shop. Here's one company's analysis of three products' best targets in the New York area.

Brand	Heavy User Profile	Lifestyle and Media Profile	Top 3 Stores
Peter Pan peanut butter	Households with kids headed by 18–54-year-olds, in suburban and rural areas	• Heavy video renters • Go to theme parks • Below average TV viewers • Above average radio listeners	**Foodtown Super Market** 3350 Hempstead Turnpike Levittown, NY **Pathmark Supermarket** 3635 Hempstead Turnpike Levittown, NY **King Kullen Market** 598 Stewart Ave. Bethpage, NY
Stouffer's Red Box frozen entrees	Households headed by people 55 and older, and upscale suburban households headed by 35–54-year-olds	• Go to gambling casinos • Give parties • Involved in public activities • Travel frequently • Heavy newspaper readers • Above average TV viewers	**Dan's Supreme Super Market** 69-62 188th St. Flushing, NY **Food Emporium** Madison Ave. & 74th St. New York, NY **Waldbaum Super Market** 196-35 Horace Harding Flushing, NY
Coors light beer	Head of household 21–34 years old, middle to upper income, suburban and urban	• Belong to a health club • Buy rock music • Travel by plane • Give parties, cookouts • Rent videos • Heavy TV sports viewers	**Food Emporium** 1498 York Ave. New York, NY **Food Emporium** First Ave. & 72nd St. New York, NY **Gristede's Supermarket** 350 E. 86th St. New York, NY

Source: Michael J. McCarthy, "Marketers Zero in on Their Customers," *The Wall Street Journal*, March 18, 1991, p. B1. Reprinted by permission of *The Wall Street Journal*,

mands. For a perishable product like potato chips, having the right product at the right place and in the proper amount is critical to Frito-Lay's success. One spokesperson said that the company saved more than $40 million in its first year because of reduced paperwork, reduced losses from stale products, and route consolidation.[14]

Data Envelopment Analysis

Data envelopment analysis (DEA) is a linear programming technique developed by A. Charnes, W. W. Cooper, and E. Rhodes to evaluate nonprofit and public sector organizations. Subsequently, it has found applications in for-profit service organizations. DEA compares each service delivery unit with all other service units for a multisite organization, and it computes an efficiency rating that is based on the ratio of resource inputs to outputs. Multiple inputs (e.g., labor-hours, materials) and multiple outputs (e.g., sales, referrals) are possible and desirable in measuring a unit's efficiency. Taking this information, the linear programming model determines the efficiency frontier on the basis of those few units producing at 100 percent efficiency. Areas for improvement can be identified by comparing the operating practices of efficient units with those of less efficient units. Sharing management practices of efficient units with less efficient units provides an opportunity for the latter's improvement and enhancement of total system productivity. Repeated use of DEA can establish a climate of organizational learning that fuels a competitive strategy of cost leadership.

Banker and Morey applied DEA to a 60-unit fast-food restaurant chain and found 33 units to be efficient.[15] In their analysis, three outputs (i.e., food sales for breakfast, lunch, and dinner) and six inputs (i.e., supplies and materials, labor, age of store, advertising expenditures, urban vs. rural location, and existence of a drive-in window) were used. It is interesting to note that the inputs included both discretionary and uncontrollable variables (e.g., the demographic variable of urban/rural locations, whether or not the unit had a drive-in window). The topic of data envelopment analysis is covered in more detail as a supplement to Chapter 14.

THE VIRTUAL VALUE CHAIN[16]

Today, businesses compete in two worlds: a physical world of things called a *marketplace*, and a virtual world of information called a *marketspace*. For example, when customers buy an answering machine to store phone messages, they are using products that are sold in the physical world. When customers contract with

[14]Peter H. Lewis, "Looking beyond Innovation, an Award for Results," *The New York Times*, June 23, 1991, p. 8.

[15]R. D. Banker and R. C. Morey, "Efficiency Analysis for Exogenously Fixed Inputs and Outputs," *Operations Research*, vol. 34, no. 4, July–August 1986, pp. 518–519.

[16]Adapted from Jeffrey F. Rayport and John J. Sviokla, "Exploiting the Virtual Value Chain," *Harvard Business Review*, November–December 1995, pp. 75–85.

their telephone company for electronic answering services, however, they are purchasing information services in the virtual world.

The process of creating value has long been described as stages linked together to form a *value chain.* The traditional physical value chain, as shown at the top of Figure 4.2, consists of a sequence of stages beginning with inbound logistics (i.e., raw materials) and ending with sales to a customer. The virtual value chain, as shown at the bottom of Figure 4.2, traditionally has been treated as information supporting physical value-adding elements, but not as a source of value itself. For example, managers use information on inventory levels to monitor the process, but they rarely use information itself to create new value for the customer. This is no longer the case for breakthrough service companies. For example, FedEx now exploits its information data base by allowing customers to track packages themselves using the company's web site on the Internet. Now customers can locate a package in transit by entering the airbill number, and they can even identify the name of the person who signed for it when delivered. The peace of mind of conveniently tracking a package has created added value for their customers and differentiates FedEx from its competitors.

To create value with information, managers must look to the marketspace. Although the value chain of the marketspace can mirror that of the marketplace, the value-adding process must first gather raw information that is processed and finally distributed. The value-adding steps are virtual in that they are performed through and with information. Creating value in any stage of a virtual value chain involves a sequence of five activities: gathering, organizing, selecting, synthesizing, and distributing information. This process is captured in Figure 4.2 for a firm that has some physical product to sell; however, for many services firms, only the virtual value chain would be shown.

The United Services Automobile Association (USAA), which provides financial services to military officers, has become a world-class competitor by exploiting the virtual value chain. As the name suggests, USAA began as an automobile insurance firm. Over time, it has used its information systems—installed to automate its core business of insurance sales and underwriting—to capture significant amounts of information about its customers. Unlike a typical insurance company, USAA had no sales force. All business was conducted by telephone or mail. Consequently, USAA had a ready data base and customers who were accustomed to doing business with relatively little human interaction, i.e., they were predisposed to using technological innovations. As data accumulated, USAA was able to prepare customer risk profiles and customize policies. Analyzing the flow of information harvested along the virtual value chain, USAA instituted business lines targeted to specific customers' needs, such as home owners insurance, mutual funds, and eventually became a full-fledged financial services firm.

LIMITS IN THE USE OF INFORMATION

So far only the benefits of using information as a competitive strategy have been addressed. Some of these strategies, however, raise questions of fairness, invasion of privacy, and anticompetitiveness. Also, if these strategies were abused, the result could harm consumers.

Anticompetitive

To create entry barriers, the use of reservation systems and frequent user programs has been identified as potentially anticompetitive. For example, how should a frequent flyer's free-trip award be considered, particularly when the passenger has been traveling on business at corporate expense? The IRS is considering taxing the free trip as income in kind, and corporations believe that the free tickets belong to the company. The long-run implication, however, is the removal of price competition in air travel.

Fairness

Perhaps the easiest way to start a riot is asking airline passengers on a flight how much their tickets cost. Under yield management, ticket prices can change every hour; therefore, price is a moving target and the ticketing process a lottery. At the extreme, is yield management fair and equitable to the public, or has every

FIGURE 4.2. Exploiting the Virtual Value Chain.
(Reprinted from Rayport, Jeffrey F., and J. J. Sviokla, "Exploiting the Virtual Value Chain," Harvard Business Review, *November–December 1995, pp. 78, 82.)*

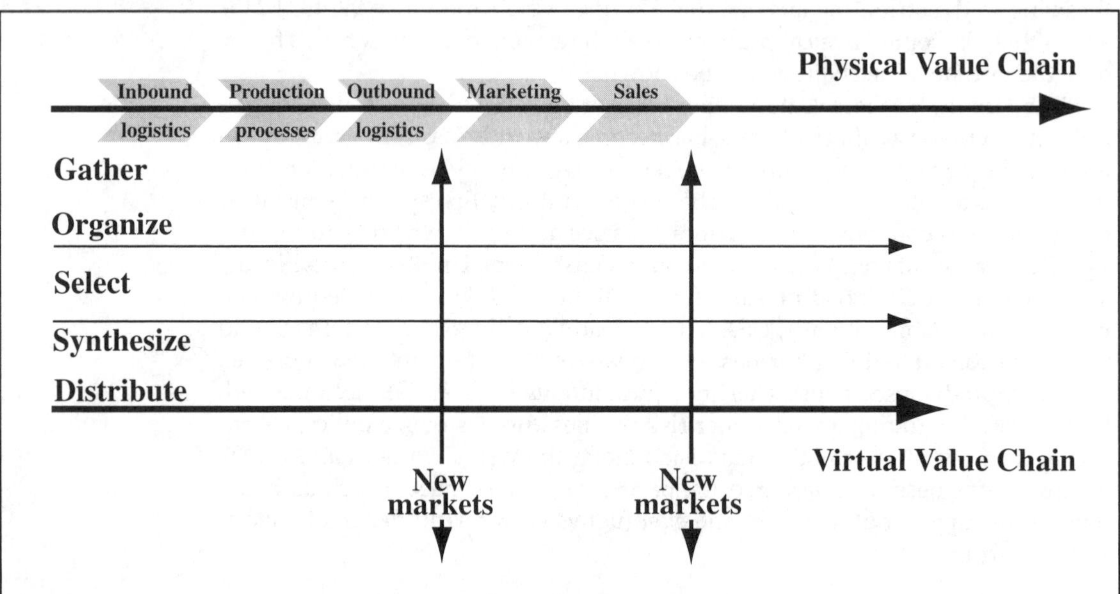

service price always been negotiable? Are customers only now becoming aware of their buying power?

Invasion of Privacy

The concept of micromarketing has the potential to create the most violent backlash from consumers because of the perceived invasion of privacy. When a record of your every purchase at the local supermarket is shared with eager manufacturers, very manipulative sales practices, such as targeting buyers of a competitor's soft drink with enticements to buy an alternative, could result. Lotus Development Corporation recently felt the sting of consumer displeasure after announcing the availability of its MarketPlace household data base to anyone with a PC and modem. Lotus received more than 30,000 requests from irate persons wanting to be removed from this data base. Lotus subsequently withdrew its offer of general availability, but it still sells access to the data base to large corporations.[17]

Data Security

Allowing information to get into hands of others for inappropriate use is a significant problem for government agencies such as the IRS; however, releasing personal medical records to insurance firms or potential employers without the consent of the patient is far more common—and damaging. Some businesses market lists of people who have filed worker compensation claims or medical malpractice suits, and such data bases can be used to blackball prospective employees or patients.

Reliability

Is the data accurate? Data kept on individuals can be corrupted and create havoc in people's lives. One U.S. law attempts to ameliorate such dilemmas by requiring credit-report agencies to allow individuals to review their credit records for accuracy.

SUMMARY

Information is the enabling technology for service process innovation. Because customers view the service process itself as the product, introduction of new technology requires attention to customer acceptance. Automation in services includes both hard technology and soft technology, with applications in both the front and back office.

The strategic role of information in service strategies is organized into four categories: creation of barriers to entry, revenue generation, data base asset, and

[17]"How Did They Get My Name?" *Newsweek,* June 3, 1991, p. 41.

productivity enhancement. Information-based competitive strategies were illustrated for each category.

Yield management, which was pioneered by American Airlines, is the most comprehensive use of information for strategic purposes and best illustrates the integrated nature of services. Using forecasting methods from operations management, pricing strategies from marketing, and consumer psychology from organizational behavior, American developed a computer-based method to sell airline seats at various prices to maximize the revenue for any given flight. This innovation directly attacks the classic service dilemma of matching supply and demand.

The concept of a virtual value chain provides a view of service innovation that creates value by using information gathered while serving customers. The discussion of the limits in the use of information suggests again that service managers always must be sensitive to the perceptions of their actions by the public they serve.

Thus far, we have discussed the role and nature of services in Part I, and service strategies and the enabling role of information in service process technology were explored in Part II. Part III, which begins with the next chapter, will examine ways of structuring services in a competitive market.

KEY TERMS AND DEFINITIONS

Data envelopment analysis a linear programming technique that measures the performance of service units to determine an efficiency frontier for internal benchmarking.

Expert system a computer program that can make inferences using a knowledge base and decision rules.

Marketspace the virtual world of information.

Value chain the stages and activities, from beginning to end, that are needed to produce a service, each of which has the potential to create value for the customer.

Yield management an information system that attempts to maximize revenue for services with time-perishable capacity (e.g., airlines, hotels).

TOPICS FOR DISCUSSION

1. What emerging technologies will have a significant effect on the delivery of services in the future?
2. As services are automated, what types of new demands are placed on marketing? Give an example to illustrate your answer.
3. Will the widespread use of yield management eventually erode the concept of fixed prices for any service?
4. What possible negative effects can yield management have on customer relations?
5. What ethical issues are associated with micromarketing?
6. Do you agree with the travel consultant's statement about frequent flyer awards that "It's one of the most anticompetitive programs ever erected"?
7. For each of the three generic strategies (i.e., cost leadership, differentiation, and focus), which of the four competitive uses of information is most powerful?

Service Benchmark

Frito-Lay Puts Handheld Computers in the Field

Frito-Lay Inc., the $4.9 billion snack-food division of Pepsico Inc. that is based in Plano, TX, took the prize in the category of business and related services for its work with handheld computers. The company's 10,000 sales representatives use them to sell more than 100 different brand-name products to more than 400,000 retail stores.

Using the bricklike Fujitsu computer, which replaced conventional paper forms, each route representative can send detailed sales and inventory information back to Frito-Lay headquarters each day. The computers keep track of prices, special promotions for each store, information on stale or returned products and other details. A printer in each delivery truck allows the sales representative to give the store manager a comprehensive receipt and invoice.

At the end of each day, instead of spreading paper receipts on the kitchen table and reaching for the calculator, pencil and aspirin, the sales representative simply hooks the Fujitsu to a telephone and sends the data to Frito-Lay's headquarters. The data are collected, compiled, and distilled. "We pick up every sale of every bag made to every customer every day," said Charles S. Feld, vice president of management information services for Frito-Lay. This information is then relayed to Frito-Lay's manufacturing and distribution centers as a "real-time" inventory system.

"The result is that we can keep fresh products moving through the system continuously," Mr. Feld said. "Having the right product in the right place at the right time is really critical to us." The daily sales data are also used to develop market strategies.

. . . The company spends about $2,500 to equip each of the 10,000 route salespeople with the Fujitsu computer and a printer for the delivery truck. And Mr. Feld and his team spent more than 18 months developing the software for the central system and for the system that returns the information to manufacturing and distribution centers.

Even so, Mr. Feld said, the system "paid for itself well within a year, and it has paid for itself more than once." A Frito-Lay spokesman said the company saved more than $40 million in its first year from reduced paperwork, reduced losses from stale products and route consolidation.

Mr. Feld said the company was now investigating systems that would hook directly into a customer's computer, handling accounts payable and receivables, and allowing store managers to assess which Frito-Lay products are most profitable.

Source: Reprinted with permission from Peter H. Lewis, "Looking Beyond Innovation, an Award for Results," *The New York Times*, Sunday, June 23, 1991, p. 8.

CASE: THE BEST LITTLE COOKIE HOUSE AROUND[18]

A chocolate chip cookie is a pretty straightforward thing—a bit of flour, a bit of sugar, a bit of shortening, a whole lot of chocolate chips, and not much more. Given those humble beginnings, one might not expect the stir created in 1992. We refer, of course, to the national controversy over who bakes the better cookie: Barbara Bush or Hillary Clinton?

Each of those stunning ladies undoubtedly makes superb creations that would grace any schoolkid's lunchbox. But, the truth be told, there has been a major revolution in the chocolate chip cookie industry that overshadows their efforts. This revolution was brought about by a young woman, Debbi Sivyer Fields, whose chocolate chip history goes back to her early years, when she baked just for family and friends.

Mrs. Fields (yes, *that* Mrs. Fields!) opened her first cookie shop in Palo Alto, California, in 1977. By 1980, she had established shops in other cities throughout northern California and Hawaii. During this expansion, she maintained control and personal involvement in all of them, and her success was as much a tribute to the personal relationship she felt with her customers and her natural business savvy as to the quality of her cookies.

As she began her expansion to other parts of the country, however, it became apparent that conventional methods of conducting a far-flung business would not allow her to maintain the personal control and involvement in day-to-day operations that she wanted. At that time, she felt that franchising, for example, would involve transferring a degree of authority to others and a concomitant loss of control over the quality of the cookies and the service, which was unacceptable to Mrs. Fields. So, initially, the challenge became one of cooking up an organizational and operational structure to meet Mrs. Fields's requirements.

Enter Mr. Fields. (Yes, folks, there is a Mr. Fields behind the cookie dough, too.) Randy Fields is an economist, and together, the Fields have developed a business that, according to a company spokesperson, in February 1993 included 348 domestic Mrs. Fields cookie stores, 23 Mrs. Fields bakeries, 94 La Petite Boulangerie bakeries, 36 international cookie stores, and bowing to the exigencies of the prevailing economic climate, 34 franchise operations.

The Fields solved the early problem of retaining direct control over their far-flung enterprises by developing a very flat organizational structure and an effective information system.

Organizational Structure

Each outlet has only one administrative person, a store manager. A district store manager (DSM) supervises several store managers and reports to a regional director of operations (RDO). The RDOs report to two directors of operations, who in turn report to Mrs. Fields. The regional and district managers make marketing decisions for the stores, and store controllers at the headquarters in Park City, Utah, manage the financial affairs.

Each day, the store controllers look at the computer reports of sales at each store. They also note the trends and any problems that have occurred during that time. Within 24 hours, the controllers relay their findings to Mrs. Fields via a vice president.

Operational Support

The MIS (Management Information Systems) people at Mrs. Fields implement and support the personal computer arrangement in each store, develop financial software, and manage telecommunications equipment and a voice-mail system. Each day, a single corporate data base tracks sales in all outlets and produces reports that allow corporate management personnel to spot and resolve problems quickly.

Before a proposed system is accepted, it is subjected to a cost/benefit analysis and then justified according to one of three criteria: 1) Does it offer an economic advantage? 2) Will it promote new sales? 3) Does it have any strategic importance? Mr. Fields sees information systems as a way for the company to grow without incurring the cost of expanding staff. We also note that the original MIS for Mrs. Fields has evolved

[18]Information for this case was gathered from several sources, including: Keri Ostrofsky, "Mrs. Fields Cookies," *Harvard Business School Case No. 9-189-056*, 1989; Tom Richman, "Mrs. Fields' Secret Ingredient," *Inc.*, October 1987, pp. 65–69; Jack Schember, "Mrs. Fields' Secret Weapon," *Personnel Journal*, September 1991, vol. 70, no. 9, pp. 56–58; and personal communication from Nina Macheel of Fields Software Group Inc.

into a "spin-off" business in its own right, Fields Software Group, headed by Mr. Fields, which markets its software product ROI (Retail Operations Intelligence) to other multi-unit retail and service organizations.

MIS in the Trenches

The computer system that is installed in each store has many applications. For example, it is used to monitor the financial records, schedule operations in the store, provide marketing support, make hourly sales projections, record employee work hours, track inventory, interview applicants, and support electronic mail.

At the beginning of each workday, the store manager enters the information for that day, such as day of the week, any special event in the area that might influence sales, and weather conditions, into the computer. The computer program responds with specific questions, then uses a mathematical model to outline the day's schedule. For example, it tells the manager how many sales per hour to expect and how many cookies per hour to bake. Next, the manager enters the types of cookies to be made that day, and the system prescribes the number of batches to mix, when the batches are to be mixed, and when any unused dough must be discarded.

Sales are entered into the computer throughout the day, and the system adjusts its projections and the mixing schedules accordingly. The system also makes suggestions, such as "offer samples" or "increase suggestive selling" when sales lag. Managers, however, are not obligated to follow these suggestions. Inventory also is tracked by the system, which then generates orders for supplies.

Mrs. Fields's information system plays an integral part in the hiring of employees. The information submitted by a job applicant is entered into a program that compares that applicant's qualifications with those of Mrs. Fields's employees. The program looks for a "fit" with the corporate culture, then advises the manager whether to call the applicant back for a follow-up interview, which is conducted interactively with the computer. The program once again recommends whether to hire the applicant, but the manager may appeal the recommendation directly to the personnel department.

In addition to the Day Planner and Interview applications, the capabilities of the information system most frequently used by store managers include: Form Mail, a menu-driven application used primarily for messages between the manager and staff; Labor Scheduler, an expert system that schedules the staff; Skills Test, a set of multiple-choice tests for employees being considered for raises and promotions; and Time Clock, a program that enables staff to punch in and out and that also facilitates the payroll process.

Questions

1. In what way has the management information system created a competitive advantage for Mrs. Fields?

2. How might the management information system contribute to a reported 100 percent turnover of store managers?

3. Will the management information system support or inhibit the expansion of Mrs. Fields's outlets? Why?

SELECTED BIBLIOGRAPHY

BANKER, RAJIV D., and R. C. MOREY, "Efficiency Analysis for Exogenously Fixed Inputs and Outputs," *Operations Research,* vol. 34, no. 4, July–August 1986, pp. 513–521.

BOTT, HAROLD S.: "Information for Competitive Advantage," *Operations Management Review,* Fall 1985, pp. 30–42.

HESKETT, JAMES L.: *Managing in the Service Economy,* Harvard Business School Press, Boston, Mass., 1986.

———, W. E. SASSER, and C. W. L. HART: *Service Breakthroughs,* The Free Press, New York, 1990.

MCFARLAN, WARREN F.: "Information Technology Changes the Way You Compete," *Harvard Business Review,* May–June 1984, pp. 98–103.

PORTER, E. MICHAEL: *Competitive Strategy,* The Free Press, New York, 1980.

———, and V. E. MILLAR: "How Information Gives You Competitive Advantage," *Harvard Business Review,* July–August 1985, pp. 149–160.

RAYPORT, JEFFREY F., and J. J. SVIOKLA; "Exploiting the Virtual Value Chain," *Harvard Business Review,* November–December 1995, pp. 75–85.

SHERMAN, DAVID H.: "Improving the Productivity of Service Businesses," *Sloan Management Review,* Spring 1984, pp. 41–43.

SMITH, BARRY C., J. F. LEIMKUHLER, and R. M. DARROW: "Yield Management at American Airlines," *Interfaces,* vol. 22, no. 1, January–February 1992, pp. 8–31.

PART THREE

Structuring the Service Enterprise

Now that the service concept and competitive strategy have been articulated, our attention moves to issues of service design. We begin by introducing a method of service process diagramming called *blueprinting* that can be used to evaluate existing or proposed service delivery designs much as an engineer uses drawings of a product to showcase a design. Several generic approaches to service design are discussed, and a walk-through audit of a restaurant illustrates how to validate a design from a customer perspective.

Questions of facility design such as aesthetics are important elements in creating an appropriate environment to support the service concept. Consideration also is given to the psychological need to avoid customer disorientation in an unfamiliar setting. The concepts of product layout and process layout as used in manufacturing are adapted for service layout applications. The issue of facility location is addressed, beginning with an estimation of spatial demand, use of appropriate location models, and final site selection considerations. Finally, several marketing innovations are discussed that question our assumptions concerning the role of location in service delivery.

CHAPTER 5

The Service Delivery System

LEARNING OBJECTIVES

After completing this chapter, you should be able to:

1. Prepare a blueprint for a service operation.
2. Describe a service process structure using the dimensions of divergence and complexity.
3. Use the taxonomy of service processes to classify a service operation.
4. Compare and contrast the generic approaches to service system design.
5. Contrast the use of information technology for employee empowerment and customer empowerment.

Designing a service delivery system is a creative process. It begins with a service concept and strategy to provide a service with features that differentiate it from the competition. The various alternatives for achieving these objectives must be identified and analyzed before any decisions can be made. Designing a service system involves issues such as location, facility design and layout for effective customer and work flow, procedures and job definitions for service providers, measures to ensure quality, extent of customer involvement, equipment selection, and adequate service capacity. The design process is never finished; once the service becomes operational, modifications in the delivery system are introduced as conditions warrant.

For an example of innovative service system design, consider Federal Express. The concept of guaranteed overnight air-freight delivery of packages and letters was the subject of a college term paper by the company's founder, Frederick W. Smith. As the story is told, the term paper received a C because the idea was so preposterous, but the business now is a model for the industry.

Traditionally, air freight has been slow and unreliable, an ancillary service provided by airlines that primarily are interested in passenger service. The genius of Smith, an electrical engineer, was in recognizing the analogy between freight transport and an electrical network connecting many outlets through a junction box. From this insight was born the "hub-and-spoke" network of Federal Express, with Memphis serving as the hub and sorting center for all packages. Arriving at night from cities throughout the United States, planes would unload their packages and wait approximately 2 hours before returning to their home cities with packages ready for delivery the next morning. Thus, a package from Los Angeles destined for San Diego would travel from Los Angeles to Memphis on one plane, then from Memphis to San Diego on another. With the exception of severe weather grounding an aircraft or a sorting error, the network design guaranteed that a package would reach its destination overnight. Thus, the design of the service delivery system itself contained the strategic advantage that differentiated Federal Express from the existing air-freight competitors. Today, Federal Express has expanded to several hubs (e.g., Newark and Los Angeles) and uses trucks to transport packages between nearby large urban centers (e.g., Boston and New York).

CHAPTER PREVIEW

Our discussion begins with the concept of *blueprinting,* which is an effective technique to describe the service delivery process in visual form. Using a *line of visibility,* we will differentiate between the front- and back-office portions of the service delivery system. The front office is where customer contact occurs, with concern for ambiance and effectiveness (e.g., a bank lobby) being necessary. The back office is hidden from the customer and often operated as a factory for efficiency (e.g., the check-sorting operations of a bank).

The analysis of structural alternatives in the system design will be considered in the context of the strategic objectives. Linking the concepts of production efficiency and sales opportunity will illustrate the necessity of integrating marketing and operations in service management.

Following a taxonomy for service process design, four generic approaches for viewing service system design—the production-line approach, customer as coproducer, customer contact, and information empowerment—are presented. Each approach advocates a particular philosophy, and the features of these approaches will be examined. A chapter supplement treats the problem of vehicle routing that occurs when a service makes deliveries to customer locations.

SERVICE BLUEPRINTING[1]

Developing a new service based on the subjective ideas contained in the service concept can lead to costly trial-and-error efforts to translate the concept into reality. When developing a building, the design is captured on architectural drawings called *blueprints,* because the reproduction is printed on special paper, creating blue lines. These blueprints show what the product should look like and all the specifications needed for its manufacture. G. Lynn Shostack has proposed that a service delivery system also can be captured in a visual diagram (i.e., a *service blueprint*) and used in a similar manner for the design of services.

As we explore the blueprint for a bank installment lending operation shown in Figure 5.1, many uses for this diagram will become apparent. First, the blueprint is a map or flowchart (called a *process chart* in manufacturing) of all transactions constituting the service delivery process. Some activities are processing information, others are interactions with customers, and still others are decision points. The decision points are shown as diamonds to highlight these important steps, such as providing protocols to avoid mistakes, for special consideration. Studying the blueprint could suggest opportunities for improvement and also the need for further definition of certain processes (e.g., the step "Print payment book" contains many activities, such as printing booklet, preparing check, and addressing and mailing envelope).

The *line of visibility* separates activities of the front office, where customers obtain tangible evidence of the service, from those of the back office, which is out of the customers' view. The high- and low-contact parts of the service delivery process are kept physically separate, but they remain linked by communications. This separation highlights the need to give special attention to operations above the line of visibility, where customer perceptions of the service's effectiveness are formed. A full treatment of this service encounter is the subject of Chapter 9. The physical setting, decor, employees' interpersonal skills, and even printed material all make a statement about the service, and the subject of facility design and layout is discussed in Chapter 6. Designing an efficient process is the goal of the back office, but the back-office operations have an indirect effect on the customer because of delays and errors.

The blueprinting exercise also gives managers the opportunity to identify potential *fail points* (F) and to design "foolproof" (*poka-yoke* is the term borrowed from Japan) procedures to avoid their occurrence, thus ensuring the delivery of high-quality service. In the installment lending example, several verification

[1]Adapted from G. Lynn Shostack, "Designing Services That Deliver," *Harvard Business Review,* January–February 1984, pp. 133–139.

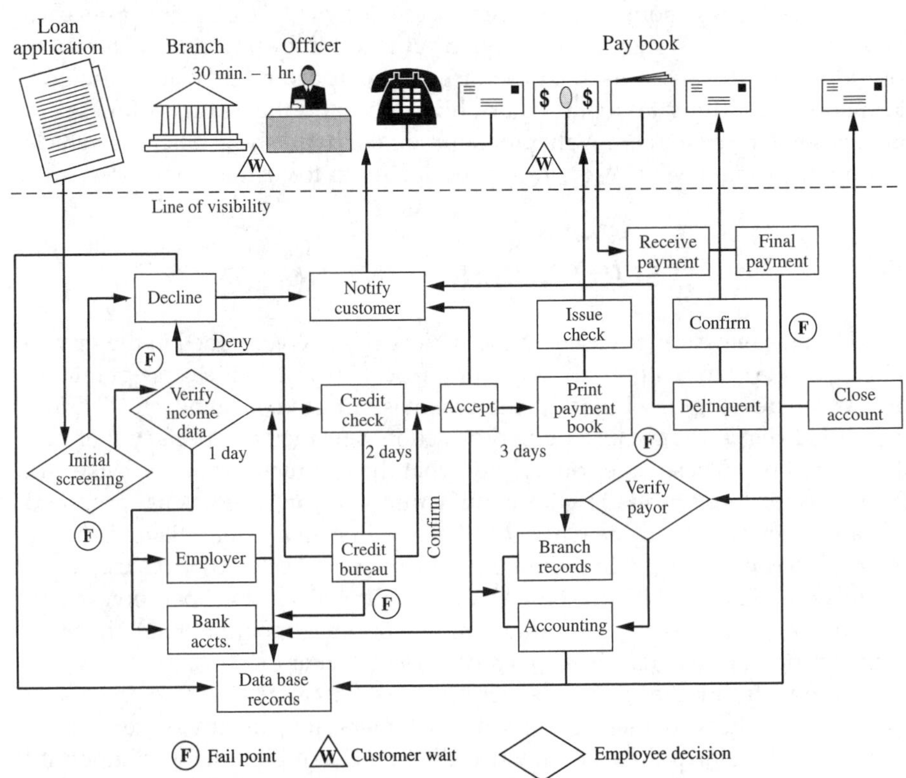

FIGURE 5.1. Blueprint for bank installment lending operation.
(Reprinted with permission of the American Marketing Association: G. Lynn Shostack, "Service Positioning through Structural Change," Journal of Marketing, *vol. 51, January 1987, p. 36.)*

points are included in the back-office activities. At these locations, *poka-yoke* devices such as check lists could be used to avoid errors. An automatic *poka-yoke* system could verify the mailing address by checking the compatibility of the city, state, and zip code as given by the customer with the U.S. Zip Code Registry.

For critical operations that are performance determinants of the service, we find that *standard execution times* are displayed. Some execution times will be represented as a range to account for the discretion necessary in some transactions (e.g., 30 minutes to 1 hour to apply for a loan). These standard times also will be useful in making capacity decisions and in setting expectations (e.g., loan check received 6 days after the application is approved).

Triangles are used to identify places in the process where customer waiting can be anticipated. Thus, customers who are waiting to see a loan officer will need a pleasant and adequate seating area with amenities such as coffee and reading material. The subject of managing queues is discussed in Chapter 11, Managing Queues. Separating the activity of preparing the payment book from issuing the loan check could significantly reduce the time a customer must wait for that check.

In summary, a blueprint is a precise definition of the service delivery system that allows management to test the service concept on paper before any final commitments are made. The blueprint also facilitates problem solving and creative thinking by identifying potential points of failure and highlighting opportunities to enhance customers' perceptions of the service.

STRATEGIC POSITIONING THROUGH PROCESS STRUCTURE

Preparing the service blueprint is the first step in developing a service process structure that will position a firm in the competitive market. Decisions still remain on the degree of complexity and divergence desired in the service. G. Lynn Shostack defined these concepts and used them to show how a service firm can position itself on the basis of process structure.[2]

The steps and sequences in the process captured by the service blueprint and measured by the number and intricacy of the steps represent the *degree of complexity* of the service delivery structure. For example, preparation of a take-out order at a fast-food restaurant is less complex than preparation of a gourmet dinner at a fine French restaurant. The amount of discretion or freedom permitted the server to customize the service is the *degree of divergence* that is allowed at each service process step. For example, the activities of an attorney, as contrasted with those of a paralegal, are highly divergent, because interaction with the client requires judgment, discretion, and situational adaptation.

The two dimensions of complexity and divergence, for example, allow us to create a market-positioning chart for the financial services industry, as shown in Figure 5.2. In all service industries, we can see movement in every direction of the process structure chart as firms position themselves in relation to their competitors.

Firms like H. & R. Block have sought high-volume, middle-class taxpayers by creating a *low-divergence* tax service for those seeking help in preparing standard tax returns. With low divergence, the service can be provided with narrowly skilled employees performing routine tasks, and the result is consistent quality at reduced cost.

A hair-styling salon for men represents a *high-divergence* strategy reshaping the

[2]G. Lynn Shostack, "Service Positioning through Structural Change," *Journal of Marketing*, vol. 51, January 1987, pp. 34–43.

FIGURE 5.2. Structural positioning of financial services.

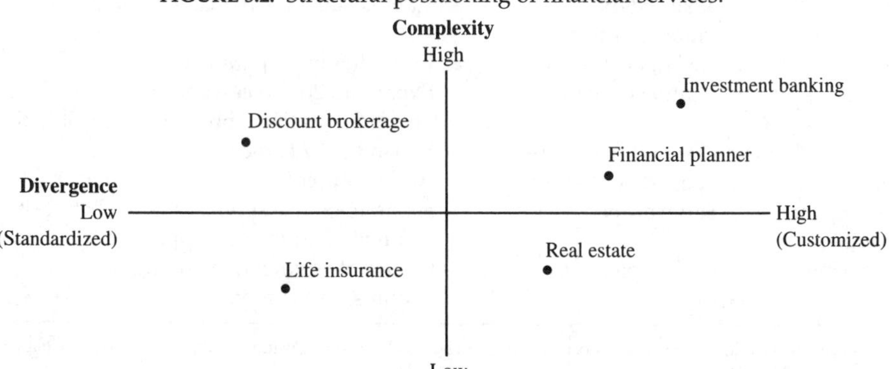

traditional barbering industry. High divergence is characterized as a niche strategy that seeks out customers who are willing to pay extra for the personalization.

Narrowing the scope of a service by specializing is a focused strategy that results in *low complexity.* Retailing recently has seen an explosion of specialty shops selling only one product, such as ice cream, cookies, or coffee. For such a strategy to succeed, the service or product must be perceived as being unique or of very high quality.

To gain greater market penetration or maximize the revenue from each customer, a strategy of adding more services can be initiated, thereby creating a structure with *high complexity.* For example, supermarkets have evolved into superstores through the addition of banking services, pharmacies, flower shops, books, video rentals, and food preparation.

Repositioning need not be limited to changes in only one dimension of the process structure (i.e., level of divergence or complexity). For a family restaurant seeking a strategy combining changes in levels of both complexity and divergence, consider Table 5.1

TAXONOMY FOR SERVICE PROCESS DESIGN

Service processes can be classified using the concept of divergence, the object toward which the service activity is directed, and the degree of customer contact. In Table 5.2, services are broadly divided into low divergence (i.e., standardized service) and high divergence (i.e., customized service). Within these two categories, the object of the service process is identified as goods, information, or people. The degree of customer contact ranges from no contact to indirect contact to direct contact (and is divided further into self-service and personal interaction with the service worker).

TABLE 5.1. Structural Alternatives for a Family Restaurant

Lower Complexity/Divergence	Current Process	Higher Complexity/Divergence
No reservations	Take reservation	Specific table selection
Self-seating, menu on blackboard	Seat guests, give menus	Recite menu, describe entrees and specials
Eliminate	Serve water and bread	Assortment of hot breads and hors d'oeuvres
Customer fills out form	Take orders	At table, taken personally by maitre d'
	Prepare orders:	
Pre-prepared, no choice	Salad (4 choices)	Individually prepared at table
Limit to 4 choices	Entree (15 choices)	Expand to 20 choices: add flaming dishes, bone fish at table, prepare sauces at table
Sundae bar, self-service	Dessert (6 choices)	Expand to 12 choices
Coffee, tea, milk only	Beverage (6 choices)	Add exotic coffees, wine list, liqueurs
Serve salad and entree together, bill and beverage together	Serve orders	Separate-course service, sherbet between courses, handgrind pepper
Cash only, pay when leaving	Collect payment	Choice of payment, including house accounts; serve mints

Source: Reprinted with permission of the American Marketing Association: G. Lynn Shostack, "Service Positioning through Structural Change," *Journal of Marketing,* vol. 51, January 1987, p. 41.

TABLE 5.2. Taxonomy of Service Processes

		Low Divergence (standardized service)			*High Divergence (customized service)*		
		Processing of goods	Processing of information or images	Processing of people	Processing of goods	Processing of information or images	Processing of people
No customer contact		Dry cleaning Restocking a vending machine	Check processing Billing for a credit card		Auto repair Tailoring a suit	Computer programming Designing a building	
Indirect customer contact			Ordering groceries from a home computer Phone-based account balance verification			Supervision of a landing by an air controller Bidding at a TV auction	
Direct customer contact	No customer-service worker interaction (self-service)	Operating a vending machine Assembling premade furniture	Withdrawing cash from an automatic bank teller Taking pictures in a photo booth	Operating an elevator Riding an escalator	Sampling food at a buffet dinner Bagging of groceries	Documenting medical history at a clinic Searching for information in a library	Driving a rental car Using a health club facility
	Customer-service worker interaction	Food serving in a restaurant Car washing	Giving a lecture Handling routine bank transactions	Providing public transportation Providing mass vaccination	Home carpet cleaning Landscaping service	Portrait painting Counseling	Haircutting Performing a surgical operation

Source: Reprinted with permission from Urban Wemmerlov, "A Taxonomy for Service Process and Its Implications for System Design," *International Journal of Service Industry Management*, vol. 1, no. 3, 1990, p. 29.

Degree of Divergence

A standardized service (i.e., low divergence) is designed for high volumes with a narrowly defined and focused service. The tasks are routine and require a workforce with relatively low levels of technical skills. Because of the repetitive nature of the service, opportunities to substitute automation for labor abound (e.g., use of vending machines, automatic car wash). Reducing the discretion of service workers is one approach to achieving consistent service quality, but one that also has possible negative consequences. These concepts will later be referred to as the *production-line approach* to service design.

For customized services (i.e., high divergence), more flexibility and judgment are required to perform the service tasks. In addition, more information is exchanged between the customer and the service worker. These characteristics of customized services require high levels of technical and analytic skills, because the service process is unprogrammed and not well defined (e.g., counseling, landscaping). To achieve customer satisfaction, decision making is delegated to service workers who can perform their tasks with some autonomy and discretion (i.e., the workers are empowered).

Object of the Service Process

When goods are processed, a distinction must be made between goods that belong to the customer and goods that are provided by the service firm (i.e., *facilitating goods*). For services such as dry cleaning or auto repair, the service is performed on the property of the customer; in this case, the property must be secured from damage or loss. Other services such as restaurants supply facilitating goods as a significant part of the service package. Therefore, appropriate stock levels and the quality of these facilitating goods become a concern, as illustrated by McDonald's attention to the purchase of food items.

Processing information (i.e., receiving, handling, and manipulating data) occurs in all service systems. In some cases, this is a back-office activity, such as check processing at a bank. For other services, the information is communicated indirectly by electronic means, as with telephone-based account balance verification. Service workers in these situations may spend hours before a video screen performing routine tasks, and motivation becomes a challenge. There are services such as counseling, however, in which information is processed through direct interactions between the customer and the service worker. For highly skilled employees in these services, the challenge of dealing with unstructured problems is important to job satisfaction.

Processing people involves physical changes (e.g., a haircut or a surgical operation) or geographic changes (e.g., a bus ride or a car rental). Because of the "high-touch" nature of these services, workers must possess interpersonal as well as technical skills. Attention also must be paid to service facility design and location, because the customer is physically present in the system. These topics are covered in Chapters 6 and 7.

Type of Customer Contact

Customer contact with the service delivery system can occur in three basic ways. First, the customer can be physically present and interact directly with the service providers in the creation of the service. In this instance, the customer has full sensory awareness of the service surroundings. Second, the contact may be indirect and occur via electronic media from the customer's home or office. Third, some service activities can be performed with no customer contact at all. Banking provides an example where all three options occur: making an application for an automobile loan requires an interview with a loan officer, payment on the loan can be accomplished by the electronic transfer of funds, and the financial record keeping for the loan is conducted in a back office of the bank.

Direct customer contact is subdivided into two categories: no interaction with service workers (i.e., self-service), and customer interaction with service workers. Self-service often is particularly attractive, because customers provide the necessary labor at the necessary time. Many cost-effective applications of technology in services, such as direct dialing and automatic teller machines, have relied on a market segment of customers who are willing to learn how to interact with machines. When customers desire direct interaction with service providers, all the issues addressed earlier concerning the processing of people (i.e., training in interpersonal skills and facility issues of location, layout, and design) become important to ensure a successful service experience. When customers are in the service process physically, additional management problems (e.g., managing queues to avoid creating a negative image) arise. The topic of customer waiting is discussed in Chapter 11, and the related issues of managing customer demand and scheduling service capacity are discussed in Chapter 13.

Service processes with indirect customer contact or with no customer contact need not be constrained by issues that arise from the physical presence of the customer in the system. Because the customer is decoupled from the service delivery system, a more manufacturing type of approach can be taken. Decisions regarding site location, facility design, work scheduling, and training of employees all can be driven by efficiency considerations. In fact, the no-customer-contact and goods-processing combination creates a category that normally is thought of in manufacturing. For example, dry cleaning is a batch process, and auto repair is a job shop.

This taxonomy of service processes presents a way to organize the various types of processes that are encountered in service systems and helps us to understand the design and management of services. This taxonomy also serves as a strategic positioning map for service processes and, thus, as an aid in the design or redesign of service systems.

GENERIC APPROACHES TO SERVICE SYSTEM DESIGN

In Chapter 2, we defined the service package as a bundle of attributes that a customer experiences. This bundle consists of four features: supporting facility, facilitating goods, explicit services, and implicit services. With a well-designed service system, these features are harmoniously coordinated in light of the desired service package. Consequently, the definition of the service package is key to designing the service system itself. This design can be approached in several ways.

At one extreme, we can deliver services through a *production-line approach.* With this approach, routine services are provided in a controlled environment to ensure consistent quality and efficiency of operation. Another approach is to encourage active customer participation in the process. Allowing the customer to take an active role in the service process can result in many benefits to both the consumer and provider. An intermediate approach divides the service into high- and low-customer-contact operations. This allows the low-contact operations to be designed as a technical core that is isolated from the customer.

It should be noted that combinations of these approaches also can be used. For example, banks isolate their check-processing operation, use self-serve automated tellers, and provide personalized loan service.

Production-Line Approach

We tend to see service as something personal: it is performed by individuals directly for other individuals. This humanistic perception can be overly constraining, however, and therefore can impede development of an innovative service system design. For example, we sometimes might benefit from a more technocratic service delivery system. Manufacturing systems are designed with control of the process in mind. The output often is machine-paced, and jobs are designed with explicit tasks to be performed. Special tools and machines are supplied to increase worker productivity. A service taking this production-line approach could gain a competitive advantage with a cost leadership strategy.

McDonald's provides the quintessential example of this manufacturing-in-the-field approach to service.[3] Raw materials (e.g., hamburger patties) are measured and prepackaged off-site, leaving the employees with no discretion as to size, quality, or consistency. In addition, storage facilities are designed expressly for the predetermined mix of products. No extra space is available for foods and beverages that are not called for in the service.

The production of french fries illustrates attention to design detail. The fries come precut, partially cooked, and frozen. The fryer is sized to cook a correct quantity of fries. This is an amount that will be not so large as to create an inventory of soggy fries or so small as to require making new batches very frequently. The fryer is emptied into a wide, flat tray near the service counter. This setup prevents fries from an overfilled bag from dropping to the floor, which would result in wasted food and an unclean environment. A special wide-mouthed scoop with a funnel in the handle is used to ensure a consistent measure of french fries. The thoughtful design ensures that employees never soil their hands or the fries, that the floor remains clean, and that the quantity is controlled. Further, a generous-looking portion of fries is delivered to the customer by a speedy, efficient, and cheerful employee.

This entire system is engineered from beginning to end, from prepackaged hamburgers to highly visible trash cans that encourage customers to clear their table. Every detail is accounted for through careful planning and design. The production-line approach to service system design attempts to translate a successful manufacturing concept into the service sector, and several features contribute to its success.

[3]Theodore Levitt, "Production-Line Approach to Service," *Harvard Business Review,* September–October 1972, pp. 41–52.

Limited Discretionary Action of Personnel

A worker on an automobile assembly line is given well-defined tasks to perform along with the tools to accomplish them. Employees with discretion and latitude might produce a more personalized car, but uniformity from one car to the next would be lost. Standardization and quality (defined as consistency in meeting specifications) are the hallmarks of a production line. For standardized routine services, consistency in service performance would be valued by customers. For example, specialized services like muffler replacement and pest control are advertised as having the same high-quality service at any franchised outlet. Thus, the customer can expect identical service at any location of a particular franchise operation (e.g., one Big Mac is as desirable as another), just as one product from a manufacturer is indistinguishable from another. If more personalized service is desired, however, the concept of employee empowerment becomes appropriate. The idea of giving employees more freedom to make decisions and to assume responsibility is discussed in Chapter 9, The Service Encounter.

Division of Labor

The production-line approach suggests that the total job be broken down into groups of simple tasks. Task grouping permits the specialization of labor skills (e.g., not everyone at McDonald's needs to be a cook). Further, the division of labor allows one to pay only for the skill that is required to perform the task. Of course, this raises the criticism of many service jobs as being minimum-wage, dead-end, and low-skill employment. Consider, for example, a new concept in health care called the *automated multiphasic testing laboratory.* Patients are processed through a fixed sequence of medical tests, which are part of the diagnostic work-up. Tests are performed by medical technicians using sophisticated equipment. Because the entire process is divided into routine tasks, the examination can be accomplished without an expensive physician.

Substitution of Technology for People

The systematic substitution of equipment for people has been the source of progress in manufacturing. This approach also can be used in services, as seen by the acceptance of automated teller machines in lieu of bank tellers. A great deal can be accomplished by means of the "soft" technology of systems, however. Consider, for example, the use of mirrors placed in an airplane galley. This benign device provides a reminder and an opportunity for flight attendants to maintain a pleasant appearance in an unobtrusive manner. Another example is the greeting card display that has a built-in inventory replenishment and reordering feature; when the stock gets low, a colored card appears to signal a reorder. Using a laptop computer, insurance agents can personalize their recommendations and illustrate the accumulation of cash values.

Service Standardization

The limited menu at McDonald's guarantees a fast hamburger. Limiting service options creates opportunities for predictability and preplanning; the service becomes a routine process with well-defined tasks and an orderly flow of customers. Standardization also helps to provide uniformity in service quality, because the process is easier to control. Franchise services take advantage of standardization to build national organizations and thus overcome the problem of demand being limited only to the immediate region around a service location.

Customer as Coproducer

For most service systems, the customer is present when the service is being performed. Instead of being a passive bystander, the customer represents productive labor just at the moment it is needed, and opportunities exist for increasing productivity by shifting some of the service activities onto the customer (i.e., making the customer a *coproducer*). Further, customer participation can increase the degree of customization. For example, Pizza Hut's lunch buffet permits customers to make their own salads and select pizza-by-the-slice while the cooks work continuously at restocking only the pizzas that are selling rather than at filling individual orders. Thus, involving the customer in the service process can support a competitive strategy of cost leadership with some customization if it is focused on customers who are interested in serving themselves.

Depending on the degree of customer involvement, a spectrum of service delivery systems, from self-service to complete dependence on a service provider, is possible. For example, consider the services of a real estate agent. A homeowner has the option of selling the home personally as well as of staying away from any involvement by engaging a real estate agent for a significant commission. An intermediate alternative is the "Gallery of Homes" approach. For a flat fee (e.g., $500), the homeowner lists the home with the Gallery. Home buyers visiting the Gallery are interviewed concerning their needs and are shown pictures and descriptions of homes that might be of interest. Appointments for visits with homeowners are made, and an itinerary is developed. The buyers provide their own transportation, the homeowners show their own homes, and the Gallery agent conducts the final closing and arranges financing, as usual. Productivity gains are achieved by a division of labor. The real estate agent concentrates on duties requiring special training and expertise, while the homeowner and buyer share the remaining activities.

The following features illustrate some of the contributions that customers can make in the delivery of services.

Substitution of Customer Labor for Provider Labor

The increasing minimum wage has hastened the substitution of customer labor for personalized services. Fewer hotel bellhops are seen today, and more salad bars are being used in restaurants. Airlines are encouraging passengers to use carry-on luggage. Technology also has helped to facilitate customer participation. Consider, for example, the use of automated teller machines at banks and of long-distance direct dialing. The modern customer has become a coproducer, receiving benefits for his or her labor in the form of lower-cost services. Interestingly, a segment of the customer population actually appreciates the control aspects of self-service. For example, the popularity of salad bars is a result of allowing the customer to individualize his or her salad in terms of quantity and items selected. Finally, coproduction addresses the problem of matching supply with demand in services, because the customer brings the extra service capacity at the time when it is needed.

Smoothing Service Demand

Service capacity is a time-perishable commodity. For example, in a medical setting, it is more appropriate to measure capacity in terms of physician-hours rather than in terms of the number of doctors on staff. This approach emphasizes the permanent loss to the service provider of capacity whenever the server is idle through lack of customer demand. The nature of demand for a service, however, is one of pronounced variation by the hour of the day (e.g., restaurants), the day of the week (e.g., theaters), or the season of the year (e.g., ski resorts). If variations in demand can be smoothed, the required service capacity will be reduced, and fuller, more uniform utilization of capacity can be realized. The result is improved service productivity.

To implement a demand-smoothing strategy, customers must participate, adjusting the timing of their demand to match the availability of the service. Typical means of accomplishing this are appointments and reservations; in compensation, customers expect to avoid waiting for the service. Customers also may be induced to acquire the service during off-peak hours by price incentives (e.g., reduced telephone rates after 5 PM, or midweek discounts on lift tickets at ski resorts).

If attempts to smooth demand fail, high utilization of capacity still may be accomplished by requiring customers to wait for service. Thus, customer waiting contributes to productivity by permitting greater utilization of capacity. Perhaps a sign such as the following should be posted in waiting areas: "Your waiting allows us to offer bargain prices!"

We would expect customers to be compensated for this input to the service process through lower prices, but what about "free" or prepaid government service? In this situation, waiting is a surrogate for the price that otherwise might be charged the user. The results are a rationing of the limited public service among users and high utilization of capacity. Using customers' waiting time as an input to the service process, however, may be criticized on the grounds that individual customers value their time differently.

The customer may need to be "trained" to assume a new, and perhaps more independent, role as an active participant in the service process. This educational role for the provider is a new concept in services. Traditionally, the service provider has kept the consumer ignorant and, thus, dependent on the server.

As services become more specialized, the customer also must assume a diagnostic role. For example, does the loud noise under my car need the attention of AAMCO (i.e., transmission) or Midas (i.e., muffler)? Further, an informed customer also may provide a quality-control check, which has been particularly lacking in the professional services. Thus, increased service productivity may depend on an informed and self-reliant customer. A more detailed discussion of demand smoothing is found in Chapter 13, Managing Capacity and Demand.

Customer Contact Approach

The manufacture of products is conducted in a controlled environment. The process design is totally focused on creating a continuous and efficient conversion of inputs into products without consumer involvement. Using inventory, the production process is decoupled from variations in customer demand and, thus, can be scheduled to operate at full capacity.

How can service managers design their operations to achieve the efficiencies of manufacturing when customers participate in the process? Richard B. Chase has argued persuasively that service delivery systems can be separated into high- and low-contact customer operations.[4] The low-contact, or back-office, operation is run as a plant, where all the production management concepts and automation technology are brought to bear. This separation of activities can result in a customer perception of personalized service while in fact achieving economies of scale through volume processing.

The success of this approach depends on the required amount of customer contact in the creation of the service, and on the ability to isolate a technical core of low-contact operations. In our taxonomy of service processes, this approach to service design would seem to be most appropriate for the processing-of-goods category (e.g., dry cleaning, where the service is performed on the customer's property).

Degree of Customer Contact

Customer contact refers to the physical presence of the customer in the system. The degree of customer contact can be measured by the percentage of time that the customer is in the system relative to the total service time. In high-contact services, the customer determines the timing of demand and the nature of the service by direct participation in the process. The perceived quality of service is determined to a large extent by the customer's experience. Consumers have no direct influence on the production process of low-contact systems, however, because they are not present. Even if a service falls into the high-contact category, it still may be possible to seal off some operations to be run as a factory. For example, the maintenance operations of a public transportation system and the laundry of a hospital are plants within a service system.

Separation of High- and Low-Contact Operations

When service systems are separated into high- and low-contact operations, each area can be designed separately to achieve improved performance. Different considerations in the design of the high- and low-contact operations are listed in Table 5.3. Note that high-contact operations require employees with excellent interpersonal skills. The service tasks and activity levels in these operations are uncertain, because customers dictate the timing of demand and, to some extent, the service itself. Note also that low-contact operations can be physically separated from customer contact operations; however, there is some need for communication across the line of visibility to track progress of customer orders or property (e.g., shoes dropped off at a kiosk for repair at a distant factory). The advantage of separation occurs because these back-office operations can be scheduled like a factory to obtain high utilization of capacity.

[4]Richard B. Chase, "Where Does the Customer Fit in a Service Operation?" *Harvard Business Review*, November–December 1978, pp. 137–142.

TABLE 5.3. Major Design Considerations for High- and Low-Contact Operations

Design Considerations	High-Contact Operation	Low-Contact Operation
Facility location	Operations must be near the customer.	Operations may be placed near supply, transportation, or labor.
Facility layout	Facility should accommodate the customer's physical and psychological needs and expectations.	Facility should enhance production.
Product design	Environment as well as the physical product define the nature of the service.	Customer is not in the service environment.
Process design	Stages of production process have a direct, immediate effect on the customer.	Customer is not involved in the majority of processing steps.
Scheduling	Customer is in the production schedule and must be accommodated.	Customer is concerned mainly with completion dates.
Production planning	Orders cannot be stored, so smoothing production flow will result in loss of business.	Both backlogging and production smoothing are possible.
Worker skills	Direct workforce makes up a major part of the service product and so must be able to interact well with the public.	Direct workforce need only have technical skills.
Quality control	Quality standards often are in the eye of the beholder and hence variable.	Quality standards generally are measurable and hence fixed.
Time standards	Service time depends on customer needs, and therefore time standards are inherently loose.	Work is performed on customer surrogates (e.g., forms), and time standards can be tight.
Wage payment	Variable output requires time-based wage systems.	"Fixable" output permits output-based wage systems.
Capacity planning	To avoid lost sales, capacity must be set to match peak demand.	Storable output permits setting capacity at some average demand level.
Forecasting	Forecasts are short-term and time-oriented.	Forecasts are long-term and output-oriented.

Source: Used by permission of the *Harvard Business Review.* Exhibit II from "Where Does the Customer Fit in a Service Operation," by Richard B. Chase (November–December 1978), p. 139.

Airlines have used this approach effectively in their operations. Airport reservation clerks and flight attendants wear uniforms designed in Paris and attend training sessions on the proper way to serve passengers. Baggage handlers seldom are seen, and aircraft maintenance is performed at a distant depot and run like a factory.

Sales Opportunity and Service Delivery Options

The commonly held view that organizations are information-processing systems is evident when considering information content requirements as a variable in designing service tasks. The service design matrix developed by Richard B. Chase, which is shown in Figure 5.3, illustrates the relationship between production efficiency and sales opportunity as a function of service delivery options.[5]

Service delivery options are ordered from left to right by increasing richness of information transfer. As discussed earlier, production efficiency is related to

[5]R. B. Chase and N. J. Aquilano, "A Matrix for Linking Marketing and Production Variables in Service System Design," *Production and Operations Management*, 6th ed., Irwin, Homewood, Ill., 1992.

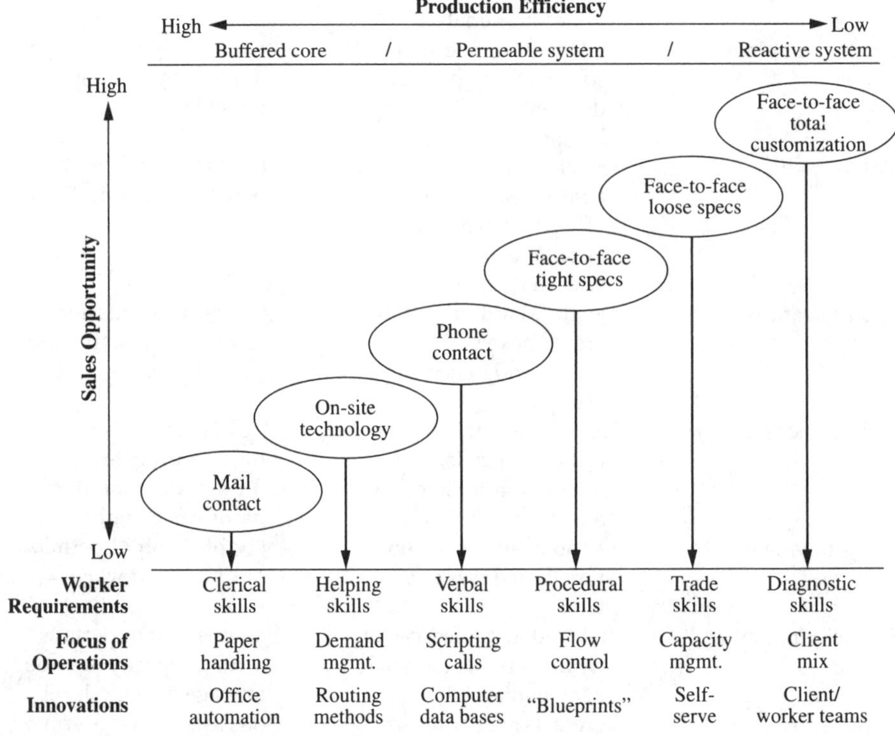

FIGURE 5.3. Sales opportunity and service system design.
(Reprinted with permission from R. B. Chase and N. J. Aquilano, "A Matrix for Linking Marketing and Production Variables in Service System Design," Production and Operations Management, *6th ed., Richard D. Irwin, Inc., Homewood, Ill., 1992, p. 123.)*

the degree of customer contact with the core service operations. Sales opportunity is a measure of the probability of making add-on sales and increasing the revenue that is generated from each customer. This matrix permits the explicit consideration of the tradeoffs made between marketing and production considerations when selecting the service delivery option.

We should not conclude that only one service delivery option must be selected. In order not to eliminate certain market segments, multiple channels of service should be considered. For example, gas stations have both full- and self-service pumps, and most banks still have live in addition to automated tellers.

Information Empowerment

Forget the "Age of Aquarius"—this is the age of information, and like it or not, we are all a part of it. Information technology (IT) is no longer just for computer "nerds." IT touches all of us everyday. The breakfast cereal on your table represents more than puffs, flakes, or shreds of grain. You can safely assume that three funny-looking little guys named Snap, Crackle, and Pop are not actually responsible for processing and packaging your rice, nor does a little sprite cavort around putting two scoops of raisins in each box of Raisin Bran. IT can be seen all the way from the rice paddy or wheat field, where it helps to manage the planting, propagating, harvesting, and transportation of the grain, to the processing and packaging facility to your market and even to your table (e.g., those traffic lights you passed between market and home are operated by an information-based technology). Essential services such as fire and police protection demand the use of IT, and the electricity and running water in our homes are brought to us by IT. In fact, IT is such a fundamental part of daily life throughout the entire world that the challenge is to find some aspect not touched by it.

Certainly, no service today could survive without use of IT, and successful managers will see that IT offers much more than simply a convenient way to maintain records. Indeed, one of its most important functions is to empower both employees and customers.

Employee Empowerment

The earliest use of IT was in record keeping. A business might have had a computerized data base of customer names and addresses, and perhaps another data base of the names and addresses for suppliers of essential goods and services. These various data bases made it a little easier to keep the shareholders—and the IRS—happy. They made record keeping a little faster and a little more accurate, but secretaries still just entered data, procurement clerks just ordered supplies or services, front-line service people smiled a lot, and production-floor workers still went about their routine duties. Top management held the task of juggling these diverse activities.

The development of *relational data bases,* however, changed everything. Relational, or integrated, data bases meant that information from all aspects of an operation could be used by anybody. A production manager could look at sales numbers and know immediately how much production to schedule in the next work period. A production-floor or front-line service worker could call for necessary supplies from inventory and even initiate an order for replacement inventory without having to go through the procurement office. The day of the empowered employee had arrived.

Of course, computers were the key to maintaining these data bases. The machines were powerful tools for keeping track of names and numbers, but when they began "talking to each other," another revolution was in store. Now employees of one organization could interact with each other across functional boundaries, and even with those in other organizations in "real time" and without the need to be together physically. This means, for example, that when a Delta flight is canceled, a Delta agent can book the stranded passengers not only on other Delta flights but also on those of other carriers from his or her computer terminal. It no longer is necessary for the agent or the passengers to scurry frantically from one airline counter to another in search of an available seat.

Customer Empowerment

In the previous discussion, we looked at how computers and IT empower employees, which translates into better service for customers. Customers, too, can be directly empowered by IT. The Internet, which links people together around the entire world, is one example of a very powerful tool. Customers no longer are dependent entirely on local service providers. A person with a medical question can search the world for answers, and we can shop around the world. Do you have a "sick" Mazda that defies the best of local mechanics? Just get on Internet and ask the folks at http://www.inslab.uky.edu/MailingLists/mazda-list.html to suggest solutions.

IT provides customers with other ways of taking an active part in the service process. For example, we can go to FedEx's home page, enter the airbill number of a package sent through FedEx, and find out exactly where the package is at that moment. If it has been delivered, we can find out who signed for it. We also can make our own travel reservations on-line and get information about our destination, which can enhance our trip immeasurably.

Our daily lives surely will be affected more and more by IT, and the impact will be measured in days and weeks rather than in years. Right now, customers in many supermarkets can speed up their checkout time by weighing and labeling their own produce. In some cases, the customer takes a sticky, bar-coded label from a dispenser over the cucumbers, and the integrated scale/checkout register automatically weighs the produce, reads the bar code, and prices the purchase. In other cases, the customer places lemons on a scale in the produce department. A sign over the lemons gives an item number, which the buyer enters on a number pad on the scale, and the scale spits out a sticky label with the total cost. Some scales are extremely user-friendly and have labeled buttons for different items so that the customer does not have to remember the code number from the item's bin to the scale. Very soon, many of us will be engaging in a "total" shopping experience: in addition to weighing and pricing our own produce, we will be scanning all our supermarket purchases ourselves, scanning our credit card, and bagging our groceries, too. (Some may think that's carrying customer empowerment too far!)

SUMMARY

We found that a service delivery system design can be captured in a visual diagram called a *service blueprint*. The line of visibility in this diagram introduced the concept of a front- and back-office partition of the service system. Competitive positioning of the service delivery system was accomplished using the dimensions of complexity and divergence to measure structural differentiation. We also looked at classifying services according to the concept of divergence, the object of the service, and the degree of customer contact. Four generic approaches to the design of service delivery systems were considered: production-line approach, customer participation, customer contact, and information empowerment. These approaches and their combinations provide many opportunities for innovative designs. Our look at the structuring of services will continue in Chapter 6 with a consideration of how design and layout of the supporting facility contribute to a competitive advantage.

KEY TERMS AND DEFINITIONS

Coproducer the productive role a customer can play in the service delivery process.

Complexity a dimension of service process structure that measures the number and intricacy of steps in the process.

Customer contact a measure of the physical presence of the customer in the system as a percentage of the total service time.

Divergence a dimension of service process structure that measures the degree of customization or decision making permitted of service employees.

Line of visibility a line drawn on the service blueprint showing separation of front-office from back-office activities.

Production-line approach a service design analogous to that in a manufacturing system with tight control, use of low-skilled labor, and the offering of a standard service.

Service blueprint a diagram of the service process showing activities, flows, fail points, customer waits, and a line of visibility.

TOPICS FOR DISCUSSION

1. Shostack's "line of visibility" on a service blueprint divides the service into front-office and back-office operations. How can this be useful to managers?
2. Select a service and prepare a "blueprint" identifying fail points, decision points, customer wait points, and the line of visibility.
3. What are the limits to the production-line approach to service?
4. Give an example of a service in which isolation of the technical core would be inappropriate.
5. What are some drawbacks of increased customer participation in the service process?
6. What ethical issues are involved in the promotion of sales opportunities in a service transaction?

Service Benchmark

PacBell's Experiment

The project, now called Infotel, was born in September 1991, when San Francisco-based PacBell sent a dozen managers to the Double Tree Inn in Santa Ana, Calif. Their familiar mission: think up ways to increase productivity.

Their leader, John Lewis, then general manager of PacBell's Los Angeles staff, wondered why the company was using traditional methods if it really wanted a quantum leap. Puzzling over the problem in the shower that first morning, he had an idea: He would "fire" his colleagues (and himself) and, unbeknownst to his bosses, change the agenda. He asked them to pretend that they had just inherited a phone company from "Uncle Herman" and found that the old man hadn't left enough money to buy a new computer system. Otherwise, they could invent a whole new phone company.

For the first few days, the participants got nowhere. They were simply too tangled in the PacBell culture, speaking in corporate acronyms and thinking old thoughts. So, Mr. Lewis imposed 25-cent fines for each peep of PacBell lingo. "We had lots of cocktails" with the proceeds, he says.

Then, changes came more easily. During "I wish" sessions, the managers offered ideas beginning with those words, as in: "I wish the first person who answered . . . the phone could solve my problem." That drill developed ideas for, among other things, changing office procedures so individual workers could perform many tasks quickly. Such an office could be set up, the managers thought, if they could invent software giving workers instant access to numerous databases.

A REALITY TEST

After some four weeks of brainstorming, Mr. Lewis told his boss, Marty A. Kaplan, PacBell's executive vice president for reengineering, that the group wanted to create and run a real Infotel within the phone company. Mr. Kaplan agreed, and Infotel spent the next year developing a business plan—despite the doubts of other senior managers. The group chose Santa Clarita as the site because it is small—its population is 30,000—but has a mix of business and residential accounts. For staffing, Infotel asked the Communications Workers of America for four union volunteers, who would bring along their old work but handle it with Infotel's new procedures, plus their own innovations.

Most of Infotel's cost savings come from small changes. Because of one software glitch, for instance, PacBell computers couldn't automatically process requests for voice mail from customers served by a certain kind of phone switch. Every day, the computers across the state kicked out hundreds of orders, and employees had to spend about 10 minutes processing each one.

Sandy Coash, an Infotel worker, identified the problem and told Mr. Lewis, to whom she wouldn't normally have had access. Within three months, PacBell software engineers fixed the problem for the whole state—and eliminated all that work. That and other software fixes allowed Infotel's four union workers to cut out 85% of the work they had brought with them from their old jobs, Mr. Lewis says.

There were many other changes. A new software program for repair workers' portable computers gives them all the information they need to fix a line; no longer do they have to call other PacBell employees for help. The computers also dispatch them to their next assignment; now they don't have to call in for those, either. Cellular telephones in their vans allow them to make phone calls on the road instead of pulling over at gas stations.

And that is just the beginning. Infotel has yet to implement its crowning achievement, a software program that should make customer-service computers as easy to use as a cash register at McDonald's. Once it's in place, workers will be able to point and click at a menu of orders when a customer calls, filling the order in minutes. The same workers will have remote access to switches and also will be able to perform tests on lines.

Currently, when a customer calls regular PacBell offices to start phone service, the worker who answers must type in the name, address, billing information and how the person wants to be listed in the directory. Then the worker fumbles through heavy manuals to look up corresponding computer codes for the whole order and type in the codes—sometimes making mistakes. The process takes an

Service Benchmark

PacBell's Experiment (cont.)

average of 22 minutes. A customer who also wants to report trouble on a line must transfer to a different department and talk to at least two more people.

PacBell's customers in Santa Clarita are already getting better service. They can now get new features such as call-waiting in seconds, instead of hours. And repair workers have developed a sixth sense. When Cindy Pascoe's daughter shorted out a phone line by knocking over a fish tank, a repairman arrived even before she knew the line was dead. "It was wonderful!" the department-store saleswoman exclaims.

Since the Infotel group didn't have enough money to buy a new, easy-to-use computer system, they jerry-rigged the one they had by writing a new software program. So far, the software has taken more than a year and more than $10 million to develop, but that is small change compared with the $4 billion Mr. Lewis estimates as the cost of replacing all of PacBell's current computers.

The bottom line: company-wide adoption of Infotel innovations, combined with other reengineering efforts, will allow PacBell to serve its existing customers with 10,000 fewer workers. Mr. Lewis is a bit sensitive about linking Infotel's success to the job cuts, which are to be completed by 1997. Infotel "is not laying them off. Competition is laying them off," he argues. Mr. Kaplan agrees: "We didn't say we're going to reengineer the business to cut 10,000 people. We said we've got to take a lot of costs out . . . and improve service."

A crucial question is how many well-paying jobs destroyed by technology will be offset by well-paying jobs created by technology. And many are being created. United Parcel Service of America Inc., for example, now has 3,000 information-technology employees, up from 90 in 1983. At many companies, more technicians will be needed to service computer networks, and more programmers to write software.

For at least a few years, however, technology-driven layoffs seem likely to dwarf new high-tech jobs. Many layoff victims will have to settle for the low-paying or part-time positions that are dominating recent job growth, because they generally aren't the ones who will get the new high-paying jobs. A telephone operator isn't qualified to install wireless communications equipment, for example. The danger is that America's work force could evolve into an elite minority of highly paid "knowledge workers" and frustrated masses of the underemployed or unemployed.

Already, many workers are aware that technology cuts two ways. Riding in an Infotel van, Steve Symach, a repairman, marvels at how technology has made his job easier. But he realizes it could cost him his job—before he plans to retire, in 12 years. "If the result of us being efficient is me being laid off," the silver-haired 18-year phone company veteran says, "I hate to say it, but I guess that's progress."

Source: Reprinted with permission from Joan E. Rigdon, "Retooling Lives: Technological Gains Are Cutting Costs, and Jobs, in Services," *The Wall Street Journal,* February 24, 1994, p. A5. Reprinted by permission of *The Wall Street Journal,* 1994, Dow Jones & Company, Inc. All Rights Reserved Worldwide.

CASE: 100 YEN SUSHI HOUSE[6]

Sang M. Lee tells of a meeting with two Japanese businessmen in Tokyo to plan a joint U.S.–Japanese conference to explore U.S. and Japanese management systems. As lunchtime drew near, his hosts told him with much delight that they wished to show him the "most productive operation in Japan."

Lee describes the occasion: "They took me to a sushi shop, the famous 100 Yen Sushi House, in the Shinzuku area of Tokyo. Sushi is the most popular snack in Japan. It is a simple dish, vinegared rice wrapped in different things, such as dried seaweed, raw tuna, raw salmon, raw red snapper, cooked shrimp, octopus, fried egg, etc. Sushi is usually prepared so that each piece will be about the right size to be put into the mouth with chopsticks. Arranging the sushi in an appetizing and aesthetic way with pickled ginger is almost an art in itself.

"The 100 Yen Sushi House is no ordinary sushi restaurant. It is the ultimate showcase of Japanese productivity. As we entered the shop, there was a chorus of 'Iratsai,' a welcome from everyone working in the shop—cooks, waitresses, the owner, and the owner's children. The house features an ellipsoid-shaped serving area in the middle of the room, where inside three or four cooks were busily preparing sushi. Perhaps 30 stools surrounded the serving area. We took seats at the counters and were promptly served with a cup of 'Misoshiru,' which is a bean paste soup, a pair of chopsticks, a cup of green tea, a tiny plate to make our own sauce, and a small china piece to hold the chopsticks. So far, the service was average for any sushi house. Then, I noticed something special. There was a conveyor belt going around the ellipsoid service area, like a toy train track. On it I saw a train of plates of sushi. You can find any kind of sushi that you can think of—from the cheapest seaweed or octopus kind to the expensive raw salmon or shrimp dishes. The price is uniform, however, 100 yen per plate. On closer examination, while my eyes were racing to keep up with the speed of the traveling plates, I found that a cheap seaweed plate had four pieces, while the more expensive raw salmon dish had only two pieces. I sat down and looked around at the other customers at the counters. They were all enjoying their sushi and slurping their soup while reading newspapers or magazines.

"I saw a man with eight plates all stacked up neatly. As he got up to leave, the cashier looked over and said, '800 yen, please.' The cashier had no cash register, since she can simply count the number of plates and then multiply by 100 yen. As the customer was leaving, once again we heard a chorus of 'Arigato Gosaimas' (thank you) from all the workers."

Lee continues his observations of the sushi house operations: "In the 100 Yen Sushi House, Professor Tamura [one of his hosts] explained to me how efficient this family-owned restaurant is. The owner usually has a superordinate organizational purpose such as customer service, a contribution to society, or the well-being of the community. Furthermore, the organizational purpose is achieved through a long-term effort by all the members of the organization, who are considered 'family.'

"The owner's daily operation is based on a careful analysis of information. The owner has a complete summary of demand information about different types of sushi plates, and thus he knows exactly how many of each type of sushi plates he should prepare and when. Furthermore, the whole operation is based on the repetitive manufacturing principle with appropriate 'just-in-time' and quality control systems. For example, the store has a very limited refrigerator capacity (we could see several whole fish or octopus in the glassed chambers right in front of our counter). Thus, the store uses the 'just-in-time' inventory control system. Instead of increasing the refrigeration capacity by purchasing new refrigeration systems, the company has an agreement with the fish vendor to deliver fresh fish several times a day so that materials arrive 'just-in-time' to be used for sushi making. Therefore, the inventory cost is minimum.

". . . In the 100 Yen Sushi House, workers and their equipment are positioned so close that sushi making is passed on hand to hand rather than as independent operations. The absence of walls of inventory allows the owner and workers to be involved in the total operation, from greeting the customer to serving what is ordered. Their tasks are tightly interrelated and everyone rushes to a problem spot to prevent the cascading effect of the problem throughout the work process.

"The 100 Yen Sushi House is a labor-intensive operation, which is based mostly on simplicity and common sense rather than high technology, contrary to American perceptions. I was very impressed. As I finished my fifth plate, I saw the same octopus sushi plate going around for about the 30th time. Perhaps I

[6]Reprinted with permission from Sang M. Lee, "Japanese Management and the 100 Yen Sushi House," *Operations Management Review,* Winter 1983, pp. 46–48.

had discovered the pitfall of the system. So I asked the owner how he takes care of the sanitary problems when a sushi plate goes around all day long, until an unfortunate customer eats it and perhaps gets food poisoning. He bowed with an apologetic smile and said, 'Well, sir, we never let our sushi plates go unsold longer than about 30 minutes.' Then he scratched his head and said, 'Whenever one of our employees takes a break, he or she can take off unsold plates of sushi and either eat them or throw them away. We are very serious about our sushi quality.' "

Questions

1. Prepare a service blueprint for the 100 Yen Sushi House operation.

2. What features of the 100 Yen Sushi House service delivery system differentiate it from the competition, and what competitive advantages do they offer?

3. How has the 100 Yen Sushi House incorporated the just-in-time system into its operation?

4. Suggest other services that could adopt the 100 Yen Sushi House service delivery concepts.

CASE: COMMUTER CLEANING—A NEW VENTURE PROPOSAL[7]

The service vision of Commuter Cleaning is to provide dry cleaning services for individuals with careers or other responsibilities that make it difficult for them to find the time to go to traditional dry cleaners. The company's goals are to provide a high-quality dry cleaning service that is both reliable and convenient.

The targeted market consists of office workers who live in the suburbs of large metropolitan areas. The service will be marketed primarily to single men and women as well as dual-career couples, because this segment of the population has the greatest need for a quality dry cleaning service but does not have the time to go to the traditional dry cleaners. The targeted cities are those surrounded by suburbs from which many people commute via mass transit.

The facilities where customers will drop-off and pick-up their dry cleaning will be located at sites where commuters meet their trains or buses into the downtown area (i.e., park-and-ride locations and commuter train stations). For each city, it will be necessary to determine who owns these transit stations and how land can be rented from the owner. In some locations, facilities where space could be rented already exist. In other locations, there may not be any existing facilities, and the pick-up and drop-off booths will need to be built.

The facilities for laundry pick-up and drop-off need not be large. The building or room at the station need only be large enough to accommodate racks for hanging the finished dry cleaning.

Initially, it may be necessary to restrict the service to laundering business-wear shirts, because these are the easiest of all clothing articles to clean and also will allow the operations to be simplified. Typically, a man or woman will need a clean shirt for each workday, so a large demand exists. One drawback would be the diminished customer convenience, because dry cleaning of garments would necessitate a separate trip to a traditional dry cleaner. If dry cleaning were outsourced, however, it would be possible to offer full-service cleaning very quickly, because a plant and equipment need not be purchased.

A decision also needs to be made about providing same-day or next-day service. One factor in this decision will be whether competitors in the area offer same-day service. These cleaners represent a serious threat only if they open early enough and close late enough to be convenient and accessible to customers. Most important, same-day service should be provided only where it is feasible to deliver on this promise consistently.

All advertisements will include a phone number that potential customers can call to inquire about the service. When a customer calls, he or she can request the service. That same day, the customer will be able to pick up a Commuter Cleaning laundry bag with the customer's name and account number on it and a membership card that is coded with the account number.

The delivery system will be a hub-and-spoke system, similar to the one that FedEx uses for package handling. Customers will have the convenience of dropping off their laundry at numerous neighborhood commuter stations. All dry cleaning will be picked up and delivered to one central plant, and once the shirts are clean, they will be returned to the customer's drop-off point. Same-day service is possible with pick-ups beginning at 8:00 AM and returns completed by 5:00 PM.

The customer will place the dirty shirts in the bag at home and simply leave the bag at the station on the

[7]Prepared by Mara Segal under the supervision of Professor James A. Fitzsimmons.

way to work. The station worker will attach a color-coded label on the bag to identify the location where the shirts were dropped off so that they can be returned to the same station. A laundry pick-up route will be established to bring bags from each location to the central cleaning plant. Once the bag reaches the central plant, the items will be counted and the number entered into the billing database. After the shirts have been cleaned, they will be put on hangers with the customer's laundry bag attached. The cleaned shirts will be segregated according to the location to which they need to be returned and then placed on a truck in reverse order of the delivery route. The customer will provide the station worker with his or her membership card, which will be used to identify and retrieve the customer's clothing and bag. Because all customers will be billed monthly, the time to pick up the laundry should be expedited and waiting lines avoided.

Initially, cleaning will be outsourced to a large dry cleaner with excess capacity. A favorable rate should be negotiated because of the predictable volume, convenience of aggregating the demand into one batch, and performing the pick-up and delivery service. Contracting for the cleaning will reduce the initial capital investment required to build a plant and buy equipment, and it also will provide time for the business to build a customer base that would support a dedicated cleaning plant. Further, contracting will limit the financial risk exposure if the concept fails. If the cleaning is outsourced, there will be no need to hire and manage a workforce to perform the cleaning; therefore, management can focus on building a customer base instead of supervising back-office activities. Also, with contract cleaning, it is more feasible to offer dry cleaning services in addition to laundering business shirts.

In the long run, however, contract cleaning may limit the potential profitability, expose the business to quality problems, and prevent the opportunity to focus cleaning plant operations around the pick-up-and-delivery concept. Ideally, once Commuter Cleaning has built a large client base and has access to significant capital, all cleaning will be done internally.

Most of the hiring will be targeted to area college students. Initially, two shifts of workers will be needed for the transit station facilities but just one van driver at any given time. As business expands, additional vans will be acquired and additional drivers hired. The first shift of drop-off station workers will begin at 6:00 AM and finish at 9:00 AM, at which time the van driver will transport the items from the drop-off sites to the cleaning site. The number of drivers needed and the hours they work will depend on how many pick-up and drop-off sites exist, their proximity to each other, the cleaning plant location, and the ability to develop efficient routing schedules. The second shift of drivers will deliver the cleaning from the plant to the transit stations from about 3:30 to 5:00 PM. The second shift of transit-site workers will begin at 5:00 PM and end when the last train or bus arrives, usually about 8:30 PM. Once cleaning is done internally, it will be possible to have plant employees also pick up the laundry and deliver it to the stations each day. This will allow Commuter Cleaning to hire some full-time workers, and it also will bring the back-office workers closer to the customers so that they can be more aware of problems and customer needs.

College students will be the best candidates for workers, because their schedules vary and classes usually are held in the middle of the day, from about 10 AM to 3 PM. Also, depending on course loads, some students may only have time to work 3 hours a day, while others may choose to work both the first and second shifts. The starting salary will be set slightly above the wage for typical part-time service jobs available to college students to discourage turnover.

When Commuter Cleaning is first introduced into a city, additional temporary workers will be needed to manage the customer inquiries for initiating the service. The week before introduction of the service, representatives will be at the station facilities to answer questions and perform the paperwork necessary to initiate service for interested customers. Because all advertisements will include the customer service number, it will be necessary to have additional representatives manning the phones to handle the inquiries. All employees will have the title "customer service representative" to stress the function of their jobs. These workers will be encouraged to get to know their customers and reach a first-name basis with them.

When customers initiate service, they will be encouraged to open an account for monthly billing rather than to pay each time that items are picked up. At this time, the customer service representative will collect all the necessary information, including name, address, phone number, location from where they commute, and credit card number. If a customer desires, the amount owed will be charged to the credit card each month. This is the most desirable form of payment, because it is efficient and involves no worry of delayed payments. This method also is becoming more common, and people generally now are comfortable having their credit card billed automatically. Each month, statements will be sent to all customers with transactions to verify the bill and request payment from those who do not use a credit card. If a customer is late in paying, a customer service representative will call and ask if he or she would like to begin paying with a credit card. Repeatedly delinquent customers will be required to pay at the time of pick-up, a stipulation that will be included in the customer's initial agreement for service. The customer service representatives will be responsible for answering all customer inquiries, including the initiation of new service, and one customer service representative will be responsible for customer billings. Each day, the laundry delivered to the plant will be entered into a data base that accumulates each customer's transactions for the month.

A smooth demand throughout the week is desirable to create a stable work load; however, actions likely will be needed to control fluctuations in demand and to avoid imbalances in the work load. One method of controlling demand is through price specials and promotions. Offering a discount on certain days of the week is common practice for dry cleaners, and one approach would be to offer special prices to different customer segments to entice them to bring in their laundry on a certain day. For example, Friday may be the busiest day of the week and Monday and Tuesday the slowest. In this case, the customer base could be divided (e.g., alphabetically) and each segment offered a discount price on a particular day. Other ideas include providing a complimentary cup of coffee to anyone bringing in laundry on Monday. These promotions can be implemented once demand fluctuations are observed. Attention also must be given to holidays, which may create temporary surges or lulls in business.

Questions

1. Prepare a service blueprint for Commuter Cleaning.

2. What generic approach to service system design is illustrated by Commuter Cleaning, and what competitive advantages does this design offer?

3. Using the data in Table 5.4, calculate a break-even price per shirt if monthly demand is expected to be 20,000 shirts and the contract with a cleaning plant stipulates a charge of $.50 per shirt.

4. Critique the business concept, and make suggestions for improvement.

TABLE 5.4. Commuter Cleaning Economic Analysis

Expense Item	Monthly Amount, $	Assumptions
Transit station rent	2,400	7 locations at $400 each
Delivery van	500	1 minivan (includes lease payment and insurance)
Station customer service representatives	5,544	7 locations, 2 shifts averaging 3 hours per shift at $6 per hour
Driver	528	1 driver, 2 shifts averaging 2 hours per shift at $6 per hour
Fuel	165	30 miles per shift at 12 mpg and $1.50 per gallon
Business insurance	100	
Office customer service representatives	4,000	2 office workers, each paid $24,000 a year
Laundry bags	167	Cost of 1,000 laundry bags at $2, each amortized over one year
Total Monthly Expenses	13,404	22-day month

SELECTED BIBLIOGRAPHY

BARTHOLDI, J. J. III, L. K. PLATZMAN, R. L. COLLINS, and W. H. WARDEN III: "A Minimal Technology Routing System for Meals on Wheels," *Interfaces*, vol. 13, no. 3, June 1983, pp. 1–8.

CHASE, RICHARD B.: "Where Does the Customer Fit in a Service Operation?" *Harvard Business Review,* November–December 1978, pp. 137–142.

———: "The Customer Contact Approach to Services: Theoretical Bases and Practical Extensions," *Operations Research,* vol. 29, no. 4, July–August 1981, pp. 698–706.

———, and N. J. AQUILANO: "A Matrix for Linking Marketing and Production Variables in Service System Design," *Production and Operations Management,* 6th ed., Irwin, Homewood, Ill., 1992.

———, G. B. NORTHCRAFT, and G. WOLF: "Designing High-Contact Service Systems: Application to Branches of a Savings and Loan," *Decision Sciences,* vol. 15, no. 4, 1984, pp. 542–556.

———, and D. A. TANSIK: "The Customer Contact Model for Organization Design," *Management Science,* vol. 29, no. 9, 1983, pp. 1037–1050.

COOK, T., and R. RUSSELL: "A Simulation and Statistical Analysis of Stochastic Vehicle Routing with Timing Constraints," *Decision Sciences,* vol. 9, no. 4, October 1978, pp. 673–687.

FITZSIMMONS, JAMES A.: "Consumer Participation and Productivity in Service Operations," *Interfaces,* vol. 15, no. 3, 1985, pp. 60–67.

HESKETT, J. L.: "Operating Strategy: Barriers to Entry," *Managing in the Service Economy,* Harvard Business School Press, Boston, 1986.

HILL, ARTHUR V.: "An Experimental Comparison of Dispatching Rules for Field Service Support," *Decision Sciences,* vol. 23, no. 1, January–February 1992, pp. 235–249.

———, V. A. MABERT, and D. W. MONTGOMERY: "A Decision Support System for the Courier Vehicle Scheduling Problem," *Omega,* vol. 16, no. 4, July 1988, pp. 333–345.

JOHNSTON, B., and B. MORRIS: "Monitoring Control in Service Operations," *International Journal of Operations and Production Management,* vol. 5, no. 1, 1985, pp. 32–38.

LEE, SANG M.: "Japanese Management and the 100 Yen Sushi House," *Operations Management Review,* Winter 1983, pp. 45–48.

LELE, M. M.: "How Service Needs Influence Product Strategy," *Sloan Management Review,* Fall 1986, pp. 63–70.

LEVITT, THEODORE: "Production-Line Approach to Service," *Harvard Business Review,* September–October 1972, pp. 41–52.

———: "The Industrialization of Service," *Harvard Business Review,* September–October 1976, pp. 63–74.

LOVELOCK, C. H., and R. F. YOUNG: "Look to Customers to Increase Productivity," *Harvard Business Review,* May–June 1979, pp. 168–178.

MILLS, P. K., R. B. CHASE, and N. MARGULIES: "Motivating the Client/Employee System as a Service Production Strategy," *Academy of Management Review,* vol. 8, no. 2, 1983, pp. 301–310.

ORLOFF, C. S.: "Routing a Fleet of M-Vehicles to/from a Central Facility," *Networks,* vol. 4, 1974, pp. 147–162.

RUSSELL, ROBERT: "An Effective Heuristic for the M-Tour Traveling Salesman Problem with Some Side Conditions," *Operations Research,* vol. 25, no. 3, May–June 1977, pp. 517–525.

SCHMENNER, ROGER: "How Can Service Business Survive and Prosper?" *Sloan Management Review,* Spring 1986, pp. 21–32.

SHOSTACK, G. L.: "Designing Services That Deliver," *Harvard Business Review,* January–February 1984, pp. 133–139.

———: "Service Positioning through Structural Change," *Journal of Marketing,* vol. 51, January 1987, pp. 34–43.

———: "How to Design a Service," *European Journal of Marketing,* vol. 16, no. 1, 1982, pp. 49–63.

CHAPTER 5 SUPPLEMENT: Vehicle Routing

Delivery of some services requires travel to the customer's location. In these cases, a method to develop vehicle routes quickly that minimize time and distance traveled becomes an important consideration in service design. An algorithm to perform this task will be developed and illustrated here.

On a typical Saturday, a college student may need to accomplish several tasks: work out at the gym, do some research in the library, go to the laundromat, and stop at a food market. Assuming no constraints on when these tasks may be done, the student faces no great obstacle in developing an itinerary that will require the least amount of time and distance traveled. The solution is straightforward and can be formulated in one's head.

Many services likewise must develop itineraries, but in these cases, the solutions may not be as obvious as the college student's. Examples range from Federal Express's ground transportation pick-up and delivery routes to bread deliveries at your local supermarket to a telephone repair person's route each day. Clearly, these cases require a useful tool to determine acceptable routing and scheduling without a great deal of hassle.

Enter G. Clarke and J. W. Wright, who in the 1960s developed the Clarke-Wright (C-W) algorithm to schedule vehicles operating from a central depot and serving several outlying points.[8] In practice, the C-W algorithm is applied to a problem through a series of iterations until an acceptable solution is obtained. Practical applications of the algorithm may not necessarily be optimal, but the short amount of time and the ease with which it can be applied to problems that are not elementary and straightforward make it an extremely useful tool. The logic of this algorithm, which involves a savings concept, serves as the basis for the more sophisticated techniques available in many commercial software programs.

The C-W savings concept considers the savings that can be realized by linking pairs of "delivery" points in a system that is composed of a central depot serving the outlying sites. As a very simple example, consider Bridgette's Bagel Bakery. Bridgette bakes her bagels during downtime at her brother Bernie's Beaucoup Bistro. Then she must transport her bagels to two sidewalk concession stands that are run by her sisters, Bernadette and Louise. Each stand is located 5 miles from the Bistro, but the stands themselves are 6 miles apart. The layout may be represented graphically as follows:

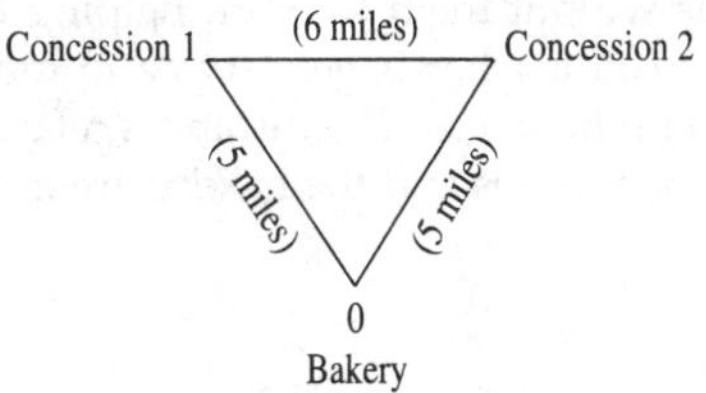

In this situation, the C-W algorithm first looks at the cost of driving from the bakery to one concession and back to the bakery, and then driving to the second concession and back to the bakery. Therefore, the total cost is equal to the sum of the costs (in miles) of driving from 0 to 1 and returning ($2C_{01}$) and driving from 0 to 2 and returning ($2C_{02}$), or

$$\text{Total cost} = 2C_{01} + 2C_{02}$$

Bridgette's total cost for following this route is 2×5 (miles) + 2×5 (miles), or 20 miles.

The C-W algorithm next considers the savings that can be realized by driving from the bakery to one concession, then to the second concession, and finally back to the bakery. This route saves Bridgette the cost of one trip from concession 1 back to the bakery and of one trip from the bakery to concession 2, but it adds the cost of the trip from concession 1 to concession 2. The net savings, S_{ij}, gained by linking any two locations i and j into the same route is expressed as

$$S_{ij} = C_{0i} + C_{0j} - C_{ij}$$

Bridgette would realize a net savings of 4 miles from linking the two concessions by creating one trip from the bakery to concession 1 and then traveling to concession 2 and returning to the bakery.

$$\begin{aligned} S_{12} &= C_{01} + C_{02} - C_{12} \\ &= 5 + 5 - 6 \\ &= 4 \end{aligned}$$

[8]G. Clarke and J. W. Wright, "Scheduling of Vehicles from a Central Depot to a Number of Delivery Points," *Operations Research*, vol. 12, no. 4, July–August 1964, pp. 568–581.

Admittedly, this example can be solved easily by inspection, and it does not require a sophisticated heuristic. Even so, it does serve as a convenient illustration of the savings concept that forms the basis of the C-W algorithm.

Using the C-W Algorithm Unconstrained

Application of the C-W algorithm to a less obvious situation proceeds through five steps, which will be described as we put them to work helping Bridgette, who is expanding her bagel service to four concessions in outlying areas. The distances related to each of these concessions and the bakery are given in Exhibit 5.1.

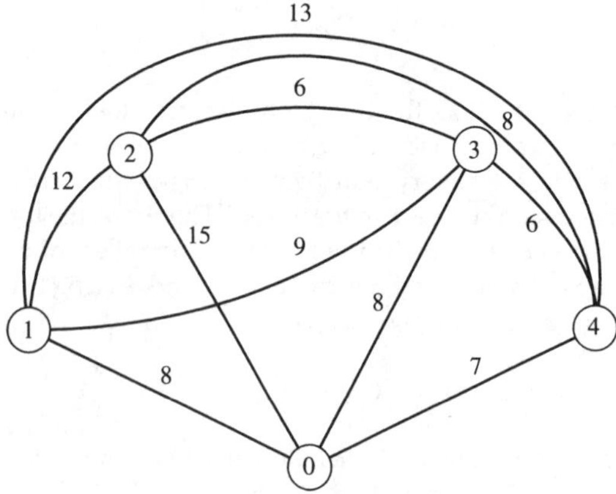

EXHIBIT 5.1. Network of bakery and four concessions with distances in miles.

1. *Construct a shortest-distance half-matrix (i.e., the matrix will contain the shortest distance between each pair of sites, including the starting location). A half-matrix is sufficient for this use, because travel distance or time is the same in both directions.* The shortest-distance half-matrix for Bridgette's bakery and the four outlying concessions is shown in Exhibit 5.2. (*Note:* For very large problems, the shortest distances may not be obvious. In these cases, computer software to make these calculations is available.)
2. *Develop an initial allocation of one round-trip to each destination.* Note in the diagram below that each concession is linked to the bakery by double lines with directional arrows. Four round-trips are represented.
3. *Calculate the net savings for each pair of outlying locations, and enter them in a net savings half-matrix.*

		Concessions			
		1	2	3	4
Bakery	0	8	15	8	7
		1	12	9	13
Concessions			2	6	8
				3	6

EXHIBIT 5.2. Shortest-distance half-matrix: miles between bakery and concessions.

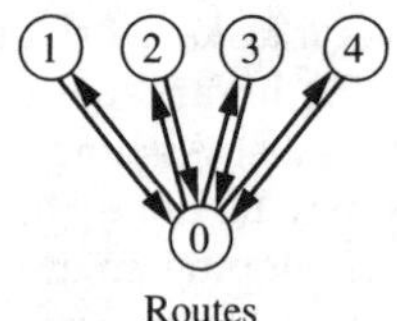

Routes

These net savings for each pair of outlying locations are calculated using the equation for S_{ij}, just as we did in Bridgette's initial problem. In this example, the net savings from linking concessions 1 and 2 is $8 + 15 - 12 = 11$. Similar calculations are made for each of the other possible pairs, and the values then are entered into a net savings half-matrix, as shown in Exhibit 5.3.

		Concessions			
		1	2	3	4
Bakery	0	...	...	...	...
		1	11	7	2
Concessions			2	17	14
				3	9

EXHIBIT 5.3. Net savings between all concession pairs.

4. *Enter values for a special trip indicator T into appropriate cells of the net savings half-matrix.* Our net savings calculation for linking each pair is based on how much is saved relative to the cost of the vehicle making a round-trip to each member of the pair. We will add to our net savings half-matrix the indicator T, which will show if two locations in question—for example, i and j or 0 (which represents the point of origin) and j—are directly linked. T may have one of three values, as given below:
   a. $T = 2$ when a vehicle travels from the point of origin (Bridgette's bakery in our example) to location j (concession 1, 2, 3, or 4 in our example) and then returns. This is designated as

$T_{0j} = 2$ and will appear only in the first row of the half-matrix. The appropriate value of T is entered into the net savings half-matrix and circled to distinguish it from the savings value. Remember, $T = 2$ indicates a *round-trip.*

b. $T = 1$ when a vehicle travels *one way directly* between two locations i and j. This is designated as $T_{ij} = 1$ and can appear anywhere in the half-matrix. Remember, $T = 1$ indicates a *one-way trip.*

c. $T = 0$ when a vehicle does *not* travel *directly* between two particular locations i and j. Accordingly, this is designated as $T_{ij} = 0$. Remember, $T = 0$ indicates that *no trip* is made between that pair of locations.

By convention, the $T = 0$ value is not entered; a cell without a T value of 1 or 2 noted in the matrix is understood to have a $T = 0$. It is important to recognize that for each location x, the sum of the T values in column x plus the sum of the T values in row x must equal 2 (i.e., a vehicle must arrive and depart for every location served).

Exhibit 5.4*a* shows Bridgette's net savings half-matrix for her four new concessions, with the appropriate T value of 2 listed in the cells representing round-trips between the bakery and each concession location. Note that the directional lines on the graphical depiction of this initial solution indicate a round-trip to each location.

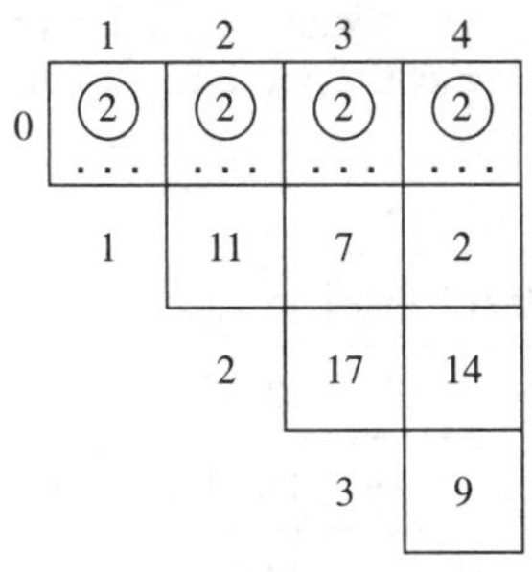

	1	2	3	4
0	(2)	(2)	(2)	(2)
1		11	7	2
2			17	14
3				9

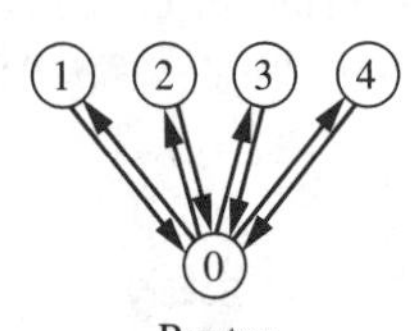

Routes

Routes: First trip: 0–1–0
Second trip: 0–2–0
Third trip: 0–3–0
Fourth trip: 0–4–0

EXHIBIT 5.4*a*. Initial solution.

5. *Identify the cell in the net savings half-matrix that contains the maximum net savings.* If the maximum net savings occurs in cell *(i, j)* in the half-matrix, then locations i and j can be linked if, and only if, the following conditions are met:

   a. T_{0i} and T_{0j} must be greater than zero.

   b. Locations i and j are not already on the same route or loop.

   c. Linking locations i and j does not violate any system constraints, which will be discussed later.

If all three conditions *are* met, set $T_{ij} = 1$. In Bridgette's case, cell (2, 3) has the highest net savings (i.e., 17). T_{02} and T_{03} are each greater than zero, locations 2 and 3 are not already on the same route, and at present, there are no constraints to linking locations 2 and 3. Thus, all conditions are met, and we may enter a T value of 1 in cell (2, 3), as shown in Exhibit 5.4*b*. This $T_{23} = 1$ in the cell indicates a *one-way trip* between concessions 2 and 3. At the same time that we have established the one-way trip between locations 2 and 3, we have eliminated a one-way trip from location 2 back to the bakery (0) and another one-way trip from the bakery to location 3. Therefore, it is necessary to reduce the $T = 2$ values in cells (0, 2) and (0, 3) to $T = 1$ in each. Exhibit 5.4*b* shows the appropriate T values for this new iteration, and the graphical depiction indicates the three new one-way routes.

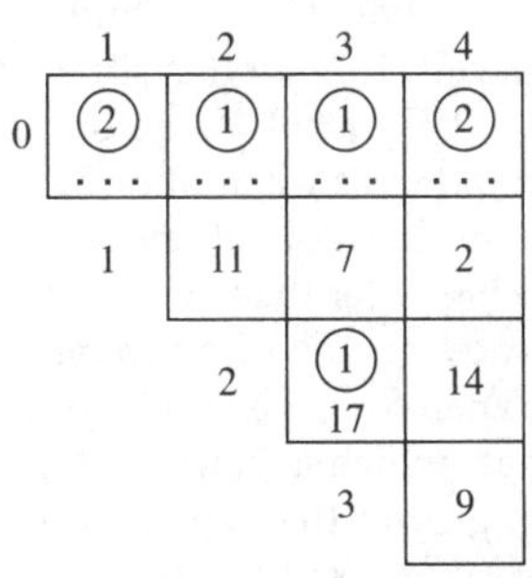

	1	2	3	4
0	(2)	(1)	(1)	(2)
1		11	7	2
2			(1) 17	14
3				9

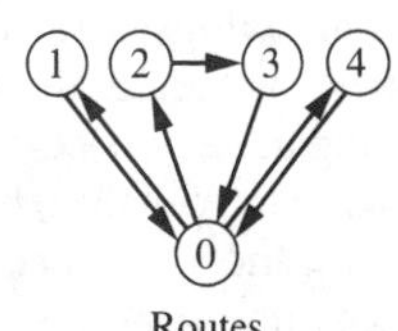

Routes

Routes: First trip: 0–1–0
Second trip: 0–2–3–0
Third trip: 0–4–0

EXHIBIT 5.4*b*. First iteration.

If any one of the conditions—5*a*, 5*b*, or 5*c*—is not met, then identify the cell with the next highest savings, and repeat step 5. If necessary, repeat this inspection until you have identified the cell with the highest savings that satisfies all three conditions, and set its T value equal to 1 (remember to reduce the appropriate $T = 2$ or $T = 1$ values in row 0). If no cell meets the conditions, then the algorithm ends. (The algorithm also ends when all locations are linked together on a single route, which we will discover as we proceed with Bridgette's problem.)

This first application of the C-W algorithm has saved Bridgette 17 miles, but still more savings can be realized by subjecting her data to another iteration of step 5. Looking again at Exhibit 5.4*b*, we can identify cell (2, 4) as having the next highest net savings value (i.e., 14). T_{02} and T_{04} are each greater than zero, locations 2 and 4 are not on the same route at present, and there are no constraints against having locations 2 and 4 on the same route. Therefore, we can link these two locations. Enter $T = 1$ in cell (2, 4), and reduce each of the T values in cells (0, 2) and (0, 4) by one trip, as shown in Exhibit 5.4*c*. Note in the graphical depiction that the trips from the bakery to concession 2 and from concession 4 back to the bakery have been eliminated, thus requiring an adjustment of the directional arrows.

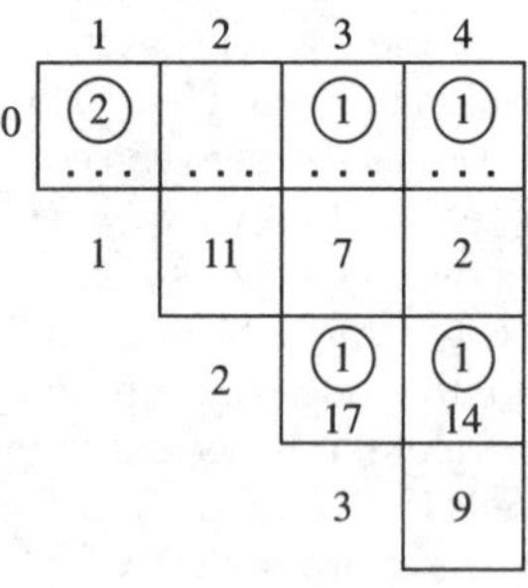

1 2 3 4
0 (2) (1) (1)
1 11 7 2
2 (1) (1) 17 14
3 9

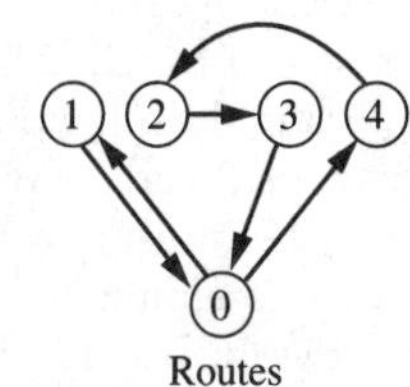

Routes: First trip: 0–1–0
Second trip:
0–4–2–3–0

EXHIBIT 5.4*c*. Second iteration.

Is further improvement possible? The next highest net savings is 11, found in cell (1, 2). In this situation, T_{01} is greater than zero, but T_{02} is not. Therefore, linking these two locations would violate condition 5*a*. Moving on, cell (3, 4) has the next highest net savings. The T_{03} and T_{04} values are each greater than zero, but concessions 3 and 4 are already on the same route, which violates condition 5*b*. Therefore, we must look at the next highest net savings, which is 7, in cell (1, 3). Here, T_{01} and T_{03} are each greater than zero, concessions 1 and 3 are not already on the same route, and no constraints exist. Therefore, we may link these two locations. We enter $T = 1$ in cell (1, 3) and reduce the T values in cells (0, 1) and (0, 3) by 1 each, as shown in Exhibit 5.4*d*. We have removed one trip between the bakery and concession 1 and one trip from concession 3 to the bakery. The directional arrows suggest that a counterclockwise route be used, but our assumption of equal time or distance traveling in either direction would permit the final route to be traversed in either direction.

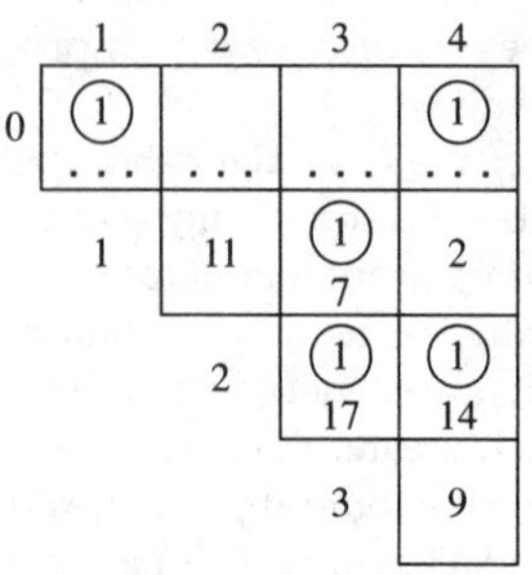

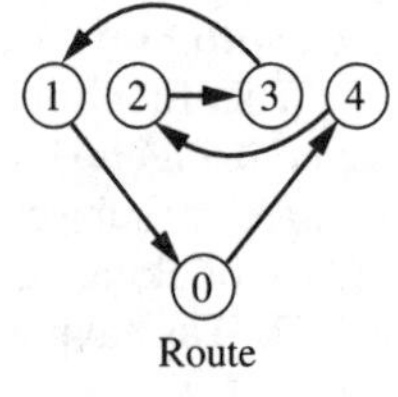

Route: Single trip:
0–4–2–3–1–0

EXHIBIT 5.4*d*. Final solution.

Using the C-W Algorithm with Constraints

Suppose that business booms and Bridgette decides to supply four new franchise operations, and that these franchises are located according to the schematic shown in Exhibit 5.5. Unfortunately, Bridgette cannot carry enough bagels in her Blue Bagel Beamer to supply all the new locations on a single route such as the one we constructed in the previous section. Each franchise requires 500 bagels per day, and she can transport a maximum of 1000 bagels per trip. How can we use the C-W algorithm to solve Bridget's problem? In general, the introduction of a constraint such as Bridgette's capacity limit or a delivery-time window does not alter the method of applying the algorithm. We need only account for the constraint so it does not violate step 5*c*.

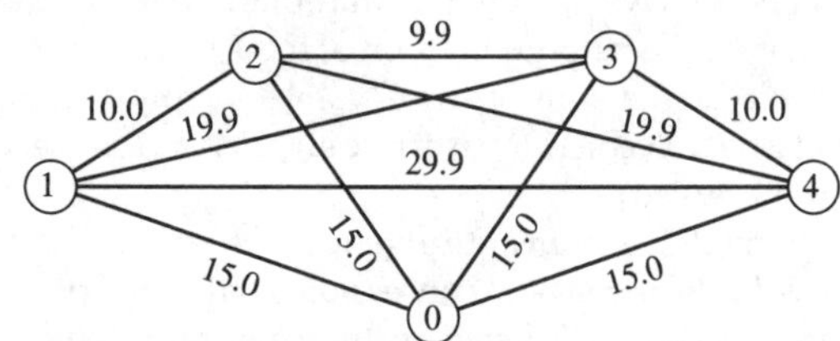

EXHIBIT 5.5. Network representation of a single bakery and four concessions.

In the present example, our first step again is to construct a shortest-distance half-matrix containing the distance between each pair of locations, as shown in Exhibit 5.6. Next, we construct the net savings half-

	1	2	3	4
Bakery 0	15.0	15.0	15.0	15.0
1		10.0	19.9	29.9
2			9.9	19.9
3				10.0

EXHIBIT 5.6. Shortest-distance half-matrix: miles between pairs of locations.

matrix and enter the appropriate $T = 2$ values for the initial solution, as shown in Exhibit 5.7*a*. (Note that we have not included graphical depictions of the individual trips and their directional arrows in this example, although some readers may find it helpful to add such sketches.)

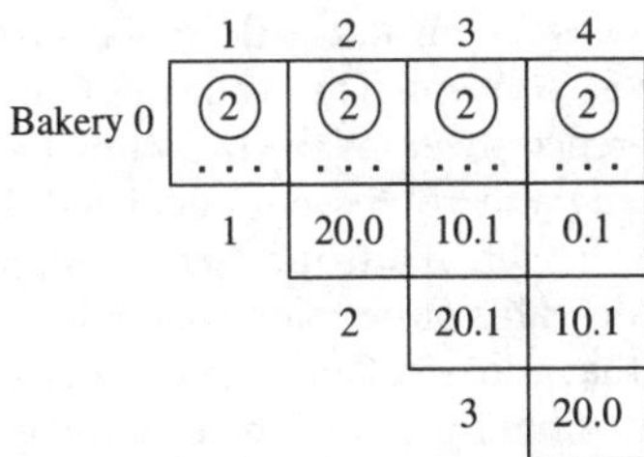

	1	2	3	4
Bakery 0	(2)	(2)	(2)	(2)
1		20.0	10.1	0.1
2			20.1	10.1
3				20.0

Routes: First trip: 0–1–0
Second trip: 0–2–0
Third trip: 0–3–0
Fourth trip: 0–4–0

EXHIBIT 5.7*a*. Initial solution.

Note that cell (2, 3) has the largest net savings and satisfies all the conditions under step 5 of the C-W algorithm. Therefore, we can link locations 2 and 3. Enter the $T = 1$ value in cell (2, 3), and reduce the T values in cells (0, 2) and (0, 3) to 1, as shown in Exhibit 5.7*b*.

	1	2	3	4
Bakery 0	(2)	(1)	(1)	(2)
1		20.0	10.1	0.1
2			(1) 20.1	10.1
3				20.0

Routes: First trip: 0–1–0
Second trip: 0–2–3–0
Third trip: 0–4–0

EXHIBIT 5.7*b*. First iteration.

The route just established from the bakery to franchise 2 to franchise 3 and back to the bakery (0–2–3–0) cannot have any more links added, because additional links would exceed Bridgette's capacity (a violation of condition 5*c*). Therefore, we must eliminate the following links: (1, 2), (1, 3), (2, 4), and (3, 4). The only link that remains possible is between locations 1 and 4. Adding the $T = 1$ value to cell (1, 4) and reducing the T values in cells (0, 1) and (0, 4) yields the final solution, as shown in Exhibit 5.7*c*.

Exhibit 5.8 shows the final routes that we constructed. The total mileage to be driven is 99.8; however, Exhibit 5.9 shows an alternate route devised from inspection that does the job in only 80 miles! As noted earlier, the C-W algorithm does not guarantee an optimal solution every time. In fact, in this simple case, the solution with the algorithm is approximately 25 percent poorer than the optimal solution. In general, however, the algorithm is highly effective, yielding very acceptable results, that, when combined with its simplicity of use, make it a very useful tool for developing vehicle routes.

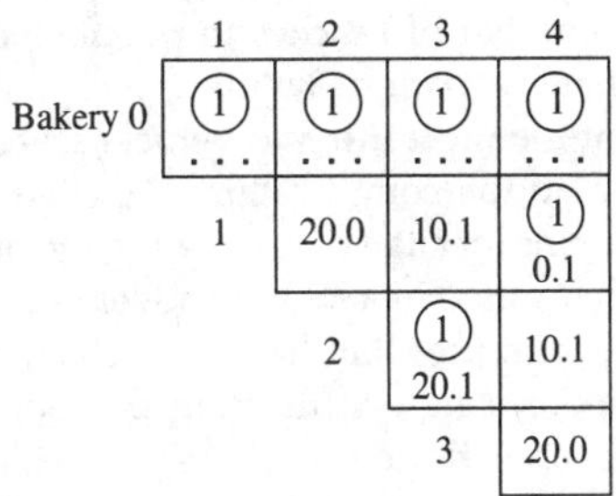

	1	2	3	4
Bakery 0	(1)	(1)	(1)	(1)
1		20.0	10.1	(1) 0.1
2			(1) 20.1	10.1
3				20.0

Routes: First trip: 0–2–3–0
Second trip: 0–1–4–0

EXHIBIT 5.7*c*. Final solution.

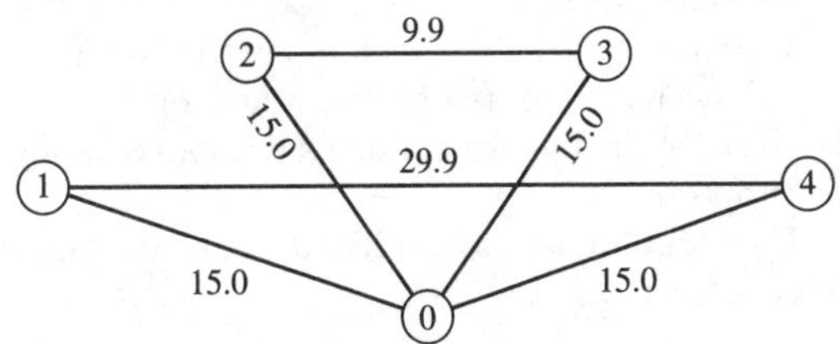

Total distance = 99.8 miles

EXHIBIT 5.8. Final routes developed.

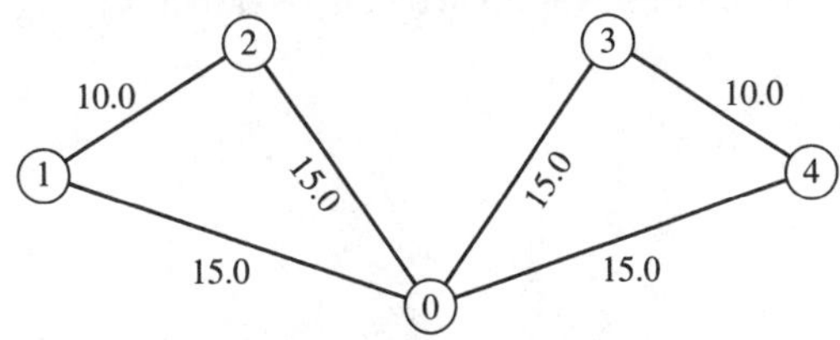

Total distance = 80 miles

EXHIBIT 5.9. Optimal solution.

Use of a "Minimal Technology Routing System"

Bartholdi et al. have reported using a very clever, manual method for routing vehicles that deliver Meals on Wheels (MOW) for Senior Citizens Services, Inc., in Atlanta, Georgia.[9] This program involved delivering a

[9]Adapted from J. J. Bartholdi III, L. K. Platzman, R. L. Collins, and W. H. Warden III, "A Minimal Technology Routing System for Meals on Wheels," *Interfaces*, vol. 13, no. 3, June 1983, pp. 1–8.

very large number of lunches to people located in a widely dispersed pattern within the city. This alone could daunt the most intrepid vehicle scheduler, but consider an added complication: the clientele being served were incapacitated, mostly by age and/or illness, which resulted in a high turnover of clients and, accordingly, in routes that had to be changed. Moreover, the sponsoring organization did not have the funding for sophisticated computers or skilled people to operate them. In fact, at the time of this study, one person was responsible for all administrative aspects of the program.

So, MOW needed a way of routing and scheduling that could accommodate the following constraints:

1. A large and frequently changing clientele made necessary the ability to add and remove both clients and locations easily.
2. It was necessary to allot the delivery work equally, because meals were delivered by four drivers who were paid by the hour and each was anxious to have his or her fair share of the work.
3. The program had to be utilized without computer support.
4. The program had to be utilized by an "unskilled" scheduler.

Very simply, the solution was first to assign each location on a grid of the Atlanta city map a Θ (theta) value. This part was done by the researchers using a traveling-salesperson heuristic based on a "space-filling curve" concept. The resulting Θ map would form a reference sheet for the MOW manager to use in scheduling the routes and vehicles. Next, two Rolodex cards were made for each client; the client's cards contained his or her name and address and the Θ value of that address. One card was inserted in one Rolodex alphabetically, and the other was filed in a second Rolodex according to increasing values of Θ. Using the system was an exercise in elegance and simplicity. First, the Θ file, which was organized according to Θ location, was manually divided into four relatively equal parts, and each part was assigned to one delivery person. Accommodating changes in clientele was equally easy. As a person was removed from the service, his or her card was pulled from the alphabetical file, the Θ value was noted, and the corresponding card was pulled from the Θ file. This automatically updated the route. Similarly, when a client was added to the service, his or her cards were added to the files, and again, the routing was automatically updated. In practice, this system proved to work exceedingly well.

Obviously, many methods exist to facilitate vehicle routing and scheduling, and it would not be possible to explore each and every one in this space. We have, however, looked at one of the most widely used methods, the Clarke-Wright algorithm, and at another method that is charming in its simplicity and usefulness.

SOLVED PROBLEMS

1. Unconstrained Route

Problem Statement

A cable TV installer has the new accounts shown on the map below to visit today for hook-up. Her office is located at node 0 with distances shown in miles between all places she must visit. What route will minimize her total distance traveled to visit each account and return to the office at the end of her workday?

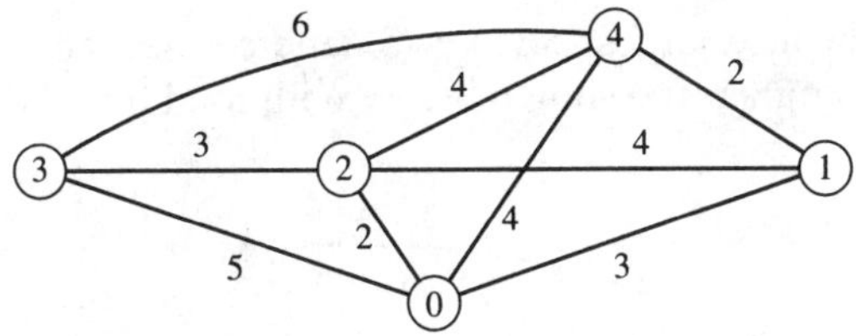

Solution

Step 1: Prepare shortest distance matrix

	1	2	3	4
0	3	2	5	4
	1	4	7	2
		2	3	4
			3	6

Step 2: Prepare savings matrix using the expression $S_{ij} = C_{0i} + C_{0j} - C_{ij}$

	1	2	3	4
0	...	...	...	...
	1	1	1	5
		2	4	2
			3	3

Step 3: Look for the largest savings (5), and connect accounts 1 and 4, creating the routes shown below:

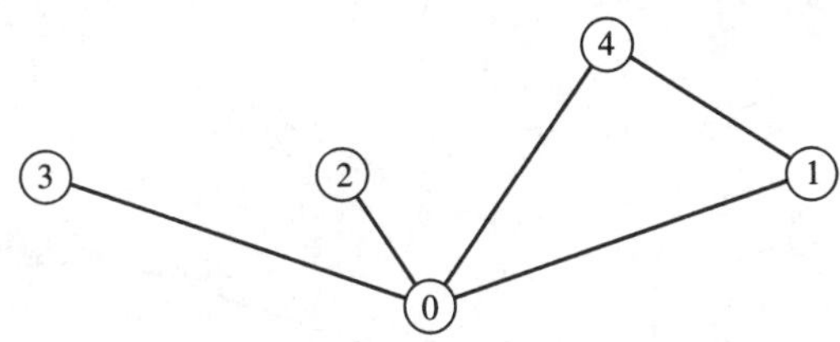

Step 4: Look for the next largest savings (4), and connect accounts 2 and 3, creating the routes shown below:

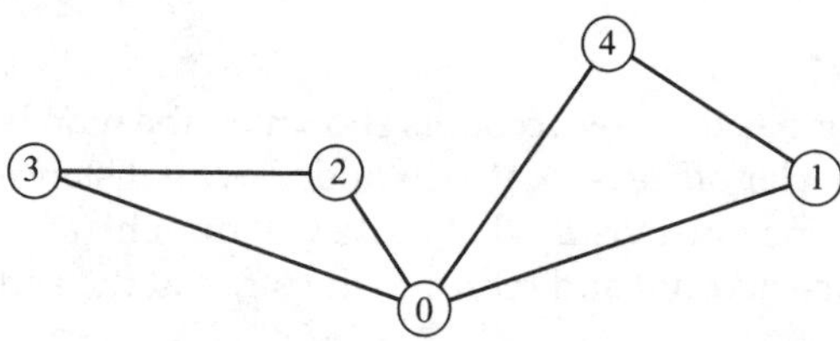

Step 5: Look for the next largest savings (3), and connect accounts 3 and 4, creating the final single route shown below with total travel distance of 16 miles:

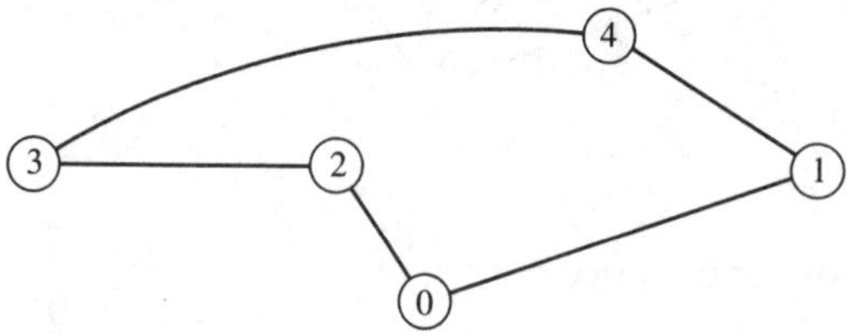

2. Route Constrained by Time Window

Problem Statement

For the cable TV installer, assume that the even-numbered accounts (2, 4) must be accomplished in the morning and the odd-numbered accounts (1, 3) in the afternoon.

Solution

Step 1: Using the savings matrix above, connect accounts 2 and 4, creating the route shown below. If more than two accounts had existed, we would find the largest savings and proceed to build a route with even-numbered accounts.

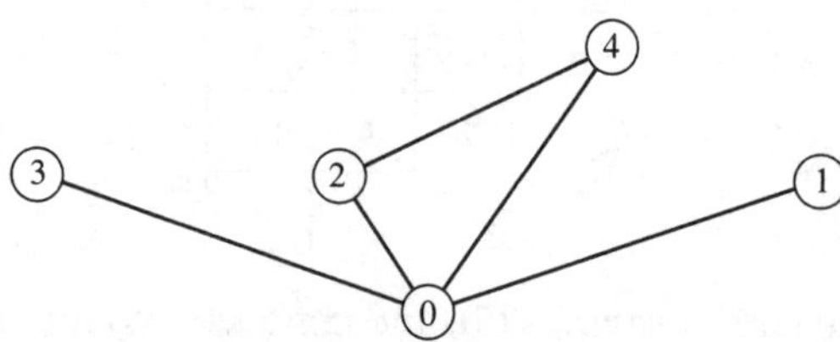

Step 2: Look for the largest savings (5), and connect accounts 1 and 4, creating the routes shown below:

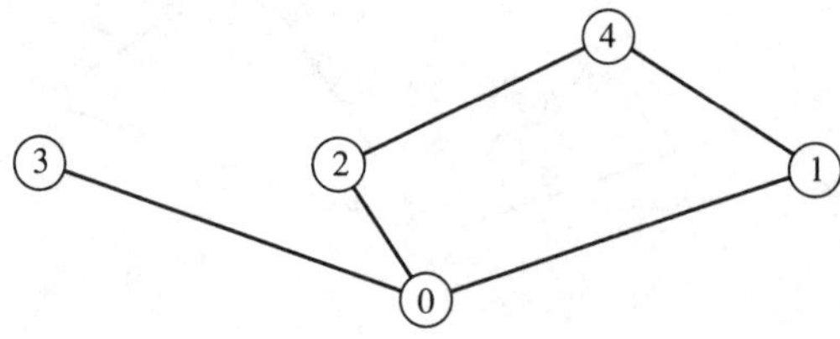

Step 3: Connect accounts 3 and 1, creating the final single route with total distance of 20 miles shown below. Note that accounts 3 and 2 could not be connected, because the resulting route would leave accounts 2 and 4 in the middle of a route violating the time window.

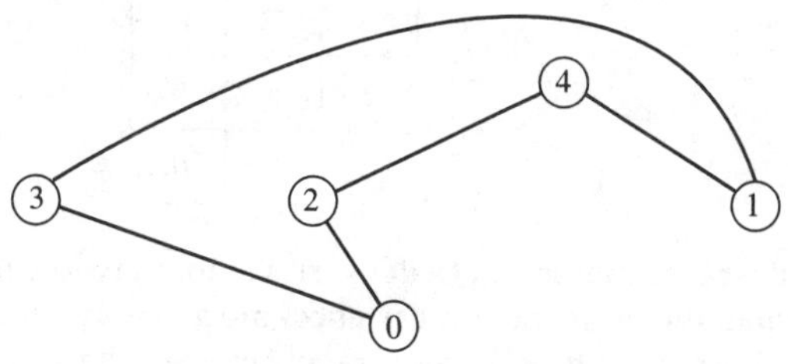

EXERCISES

5.1. For the following net savings matrix, find the recommended route.

	1	2	3	4
0	. . .	. . .	. . .	. . .
	1	3	2	5
		2	7	9
			3	8

5.2. For the following net savings matrix, find the recommended route.

	1	2	3	4
0	. . .	. . .	. . .	. . .
	1	2	4	3
		2	5	7
			3	2

5.3. The *New York Times* delivery service has customers at four apartments in the northwest part of town. Recommend an efficient route given the shortest-distance matrix in miles below for travel from the distribution center to and between the apartments.

	1	2	3	4
0	6	7	9	8
	1	12	13	12
		2	8	9
			3	14

5.4. A florist has received orders to deliver flowers to four office buildings. The matrix below contains the shortest distance in miles between the florist's shop and the offices. Construct a net savings matrix, and recommend a route to minimize the distance traveled.

	1	2	3	4
0	6	6	9	8
1		7	11	12
2			5	9
3				10

5.5. The Lone Star Beer distributor makes deliveries to four taverns from a central warehouse, as shown in the figure below. Distances are given in miles.
a Construct a shortest-route matrix for travel between all pairs of locations.
b. Construct a net savings matrix.
c. Recommend a delivery route to minimize the distance traveled.

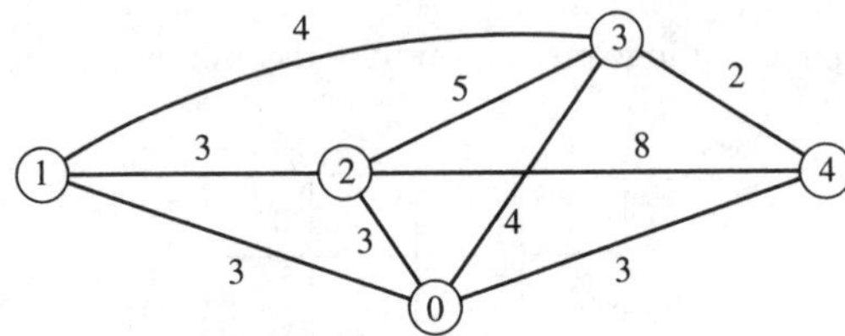

5.6. A university is planning to serve four off-campus apartments with a shuttle bus service. Given the net savings matrix below, recommend a bus route that minimizes the distance traveled.

	1	2	3	4
0	...	...	...	...
1		9	14	2
2			16	7
3				11

5.7. Wal-Mart has five distribution centers and one central warehouse. Below are the distances between all nodes (0 = warehouse). Construct the net savings matrix for this problem, and determine a route to minimize the distance traveled to serve all five distribution centers.

0-1	10 mi	1-2	7 mi	2-4	20 mi
0-2	10 mi	1-3	16 mi	2-5	19 mi
0-3	14 mi	1-4	13 mi	3-4	6 mi
0-4	12 mi	1-5	8 mi	3-5	18 mi
0-5	13 mi	2-3	5 mi	4-5	6 mi

5.8. The city refuse collection department uses a fleet of small trucks that collect trash around the city and make periodic deliveries to four staging sites. Currently, two dump trucks transport the trash from these staging sites to an incinerator. One truck is assigned to service sites 1 and 2 and the other to sites 3 and 4. The network in the figure below gives the miles between the staging sites and the incinerator, which is shown as node 0.

a. What is the cost per day to operate this two-truck system if gasoline is \$1.50 per gallon and the trucks average 5 miles per gallon and make 10 trips to each staging site per day? Truck drivers are paid \$80 per day.
b. A proposal has been made to purchase one large diesel truck with enough capacity to visit all four staging sites during one trip. What should be its route to minimize the distance traveled?
c. If diesel fuel costs \$1 per gallon and the truck averages 10 miles per gallon, determine the daily savings in operating costs.

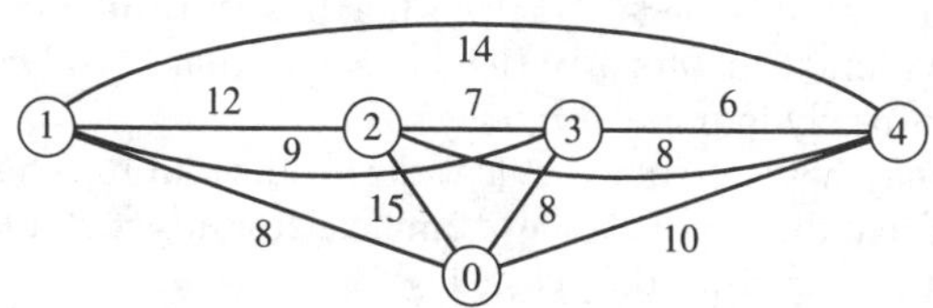

CASE: THE DALEY MONTHLY CAR POOL[10]

Alice Daley, owner and publisher of the local periodical *The Daley Monthly,* has a staff of six writers. Currently, employees drive in each morning from their homes, as shown in the figure below:

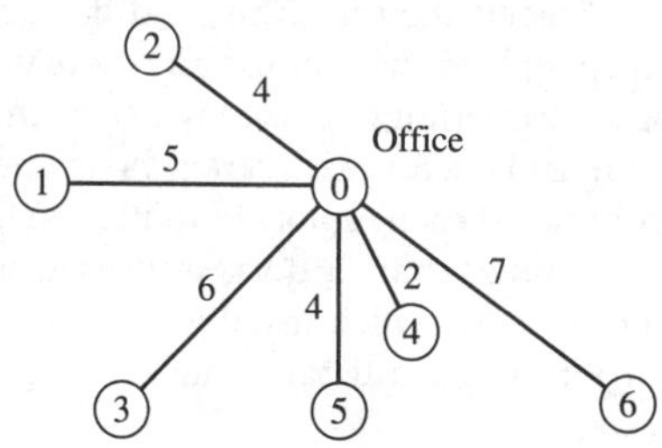

Because of increasing gasoline prices, however, the employees have approached Ms. Daley with a suggestion to use the company's nine-passenger van for a car pool. In considering this idea, Ms. Daley collected the additional data shown below on mileage between all pairs of employee locations.

1-2	2 mi	2-3	5 mi	3-5	5 mi
1-3	4 mi	2-4	6 mi	3-6	10 mi
1-4	6 mi	2-5	7 mi	4-5	3 mi
1-5	6 mi	2-6	11 mi	4-6	5 mi
1-6	12 mi	3-4	6 mi	5-6	5 mi

An alternative to using the company van is using an economy car. A compact car can hold only three passengers, however, so it would require two trips. Even so, the average of 26 miles per gallon for the compact compared with 12 miles per gallon for the van makes this option worth considering, particularly when gasoline is averaging 90 cents per gallon.

One final consideration is traffic congestion. The average possible speed is 30 miles per hour before 8 AM and 15 miles per hour between 8 and 9 AM.

Questions

1. What is the total cost of gasoline per day under the current arrangement of employees driving their own cars? Assume that fuel economy is 10 miles per gallon.

2. Find the least costly route for a car pool using the nine-passenger van. What would be the cost of gasoline per day for this arrangement?

3. What time would the van need to leave the office to return with all employees by 8 AM? By 9 AM?

4. If the employee living at location 6 offered to keep the van overnight, how is the route changed? To use the C-W algorithm, what must we now consider to be the origin?

5. If the compact car were used, what routes would you recommend to minimize the gasoline expense? What would the daily cost of gasoline be for this proposal?

6. At what time would the compact car need to leave the office to begin its pick-ups to be finished by 8 AM? By 9 AM?

7. Would your routes be modified if the employees living at locations 2 and 5 volunteered to use their compact cars and left from home to begin pick-ups?

8. What advantages and disadvantages are there to starting work at 8 AM?

[10]Prepared by Roland Bressler and Raymond Matthews under the supervision of James A. Fitzsimmons.

CASE: AIRPORT SERVICES, INC.[11]

Airport Services, Inc., is planning to implement a remote shuttle service among five terminals and the Port Welkin Airport. Mr. Kelly Mist has been given the task of developing the route and service schedules for the proposed operation to be used in the franchise application to the Port Welkin City Council. Mrs. Janet Rush, Mr. Mist's supervisor, asks him to create schedules with low operating costs for each round trip. Mrs. Rush states that with the locations currently in mind for terminal sites, Airport Services may have to run five buses, one between each terminal and the airport. She is hopeful, however, that fewer buses can be used.

Assignments

1. Mr. Mist is given the following information on which his analysis must be based:

Average operating cost: $0.455 per kilometer

Average operating speed: 60 kilometers per hour

Average layover time per stop: 9 minutes

From a city map, he develops a distance matrix for all proposed service locations, designating the airport as site 0. All distances are given in kilometers.

	1	2	3	4	5
0	10	4	5	5	7
	1	7	11	15	6
		2	8	9	8
			3	6	4
				4	9

Using the Clarke-Wright algorithm, recommend the best routing schedule under Mrs. Rush's least-cost objective.

[11]Prepared by James Vance under the supervision of James A. Fitzsimmons.

2. Mrs. Rush's initial reaction to Mr. Mist's work is very favorable; however, she has just been informed by the mayor that Port Welkin will require each bus to have a round-trip time (to and from the airport) of 40 minutes or less, excluding the loading and unloading time at the airport only. Although Mrs. Rush realizes that this will offer the shuttle users faster service, she is sure that it will cost the company more money.

Develop a new routing schedule that will meet this new time constraint yet still keep Airport Services's costs low.

3. The Port Welkin City Council awarded Airport Services a shuttle franchise on the basis of Mr. Mist's latest routing plan, and Mrs. Rush feels that initiation of the service has gone about as well as could be expected. Mr. Mist informs her that they are experiencing a recurring shortage of capacity at terminal 3; that is, there are more people boarding the bus than there are seats available. Mrs. Rush decides to seek a solution that meets the franchise conditions but does not require people to stand or use any more vehicles, even though the operating costs may rise slightly. Mr. Mist has analyzed the normal average boarding and alighting volumes at each remote terminal, as shown below. Also, he knows that Airport Services is using 48-passenger vehicles, which usually are full when leaving the airport on a multistop route.

Terminal	Avg. No. Boarding	Avg. No. Alighting
1	28	30
2	20	18
3	18	14
4	21	26
5	30	32

Develop a routing schedule that will incorporate the additional capacity constraint. How does this final solution compare with the previous two solutions regarding operating costs and round-trip time?

CHAPTER 6

The Supporting Facility

LEARNING OBJECTIVES

After completing this chapter, you should be able to:

1. Describe the critical design features of a service supporting facility.
2. Identify the bottleneck operation in a product layout, and regroup activities to create new jobs that will increase the overall service capacity.
3. Use operations sequence analysis to determine the relative locations of departments in a process layout that minimize total flow-distance.
4. Prepare a process flowchart for a service operation.
5. Recommend facility design features to remove the anxiety of disorientation.
6. Conduct a walk-through-audit.

Subtle differences in facility design are important. Consider customers' perceptions of the two leading discount giants, Kmart and Wal-Mart. In several independent surveys, shoppers have said they are more satisfied with Wal-Mart and generally view Wal-Mart with higher esteem than they do Kmart.[1] These companies offer similar merchandise at almost identical prices, and they operate stores that appear to be similar. What could explain this difference in customer perceptions?

On closer scrutiny, we find subtle differences in store decor and layout. At Wal-Mart, the main aisles are wider than those at Kmart. In addition, fluorescent lighting is recessed into the ceiling, creating a softer impression than the glare from the exposed fixtures at Kmart. The apparel departments are carpeted in a warm, autumnal orange, while Kmart's are tiled in off-white. Together, such features signal consumers that Wal-Mart is more upscale and that it carries merchandise of a little better quality than at Kmart. Wal-Mart's attention to the details of facility design has helped to shape shoppers' attitudes by striking that delicate balance needed to convince customers that its prices are low without making those customers feel cheap.

Wal-Mart has successfully used facility design to differentiate itself from its competitors. Using facility design as part of a differentiation strategy is very common. For example, the A-frame structure and blue roof of IHOP (International House of Pancakes) attract travelers to a pancake breakfast just as the "golden arches" of McDonald's signal a hamburger lunch.

Using a standard, or "formula," facility is an important feature in the overall cost leadership strategy. Major gasoline retailers have perfected the design of their service stations to facilitate construction (often completed within 2 weeks), lower costs, and create a consistent image awareness that will attract customers.

For theme restaurants and bars (e.g., a western bar, an Irish pub), facility design is central to the focus strategy of targeting a particular market and creating a unique ambiance. In retail banking, however, tradition still reigns, except for an innovative bank with headquarters in Columbus, Ohio, called Banc One. Banc One has designed branches that look more like mini-shopping malls than banks, with glass atriums, "boutiques" offering special services, signs of blue neon, comfortable seating areas, and fresh coffee. With its community focus, Banc One even has branches that are open on Saturdays and Sundays.[2]

CHAPTER PREVIEW

This chapter begins with a discussion of the issues to be considered in facility design. Layout is addressed with attention to traffic flow, space planning, and the need to avoid unnecessary travel. The concept of process flow analysis, which is used by industrial engineers, is modified for service operations and illustrated by a restaurant study in which a new credit card–processing procedure is evaluated.

The traditional product and process layouts from manufacturing are shown to have service counterparts, and they can be studied using the techniques of

[1]Francine Schwadel, "Little Touches Spur Wal-Mart's Rise," *The Wall Street Journal,* September 22, 1989, p. B1.

[2]Steve Lohr, "The Best Little Bank in America," *The New York Times,* July 7, 1991, sec. 3, p. 1.

assembly-line balancing and relative location analysis. The topic of disorientation caused by poor facility layout is treated from an environmental psychology viewpoint, and the importance of signage is stressed. Finally, a walk-through audit allows managers to assess the effectiveness of their service from the customer's viewpoint.

DESIGN

Service operations can be directly affected by the design of the facility. For example, a restaurant with inadequate ventilation for nonsmoking diners may discourage many customers. Alternatively, a physical fitness center with easy wheelchair access may be able to enlarge its services to include a new clientele.

Design and layout represent the supporting facility component of the *service package*. Together, they influence how a service facility is used and, sometimes, if it is even used at all. Consider again Toronto's Shouldice Hospital (discussed in Chapter 3). A good portion of its success in repairing inguinal hernias results from thoughtful facility design and layout. For example, operating rooms are grouped together so that surgeons may consult with each other easily during procedures. Because early ambulation promotes faster healing, the hospital is designed to provide ample pleasant places to walk—and even to climb a few steps. Meals are served only in community dining rooms rather than in patient rooms, which requires more walking and, as an added benefit, allows patients to get together and "compare notes." While functional and comfortable, patient rooms are not equipped with "extras" such as television sets, which might encourage patients to "lie around."

Other factors of design and layout can be "urgent." Consider the generally inadequate supply of rest-room facilities for women in most public buildings, especially during mass entertainment events. During intermission at your next concert or play, observe how long it takes individual females and males to use the rest rooms. Do you see any evidence of "potty parity" being designed into the building? In addition, count the number of rest rooms for men and the number for women in your classroom building. Chances are that equal numbers exist for each gender, but this does not necessarily ensure equality of access.

Clearly, good design and layout enhance the service, from attracting customers to making them feel more comfortable to ensuring their safety (e.g., adequate lighting, fire exits, proper location of dangerous equipment). Facility design also has an impact on the implicit service component of the service package—in particular, on criteria like privacy and security, atmosphere, and sense of well-being.

Several factors influence design: 1) the nature and objectives of the service organization, 2) land availability and space requirements, 3) flexibility, 4) aesthetic factors, and 5) the community and environment.

Nature and Objectives of Service Organizations

The nature of the core service should dictate the parameters of its design. For example, a fire station must have a structure that is large enough to house its vehicles, on-duty personnel, and maintenance equipment. A bank must be designed to accommodate some type of vault. Physicians' offices come in many shapes and sizes, but all must be designed to afford patients some degree of privacy.

Beyond such fundamental requirements, however, design can contribute much more to defining the service. It can engender immediate recognition, as in the case of McDonald's arches or IHOP's blue roof. External design also can provide a clue about the nature of the service inside. One would expect to see well-manicured grounds, freshly painted or marble columns, and perhaps a fountain in front of a funeral home. A school, however, might have colorful tiles on its facade and certainly a playground or athletic field nearby.

Appropriateness of design is important as well. A gasoline service station can be constructed of brightly colored, prefabricated sheet metal; however, would you deposit money in a bank that was using a trailer on wheels for a temporary branch?

Land Availability and Space Requirements

The land that is available for a service facility often comes with many constraints, such as costs, zoning requirements, and actual area. Good design must accommodate all these constraints. In an urban setting, where land is at a premium, buildings only can be expanded upward, and organizations often must exhibit great creativity and ingenuity in their designs to use a relatively small space efficiently. For example, in some urban areas (e.g., in Copenhagen), McDonald's has incorporated a second-floor loft to provide eating space.

Suburban and rural areas frequently offer larger, more affordable parcels of land that ameliorate the space constraints of urban facilities. Many sites, however, and especially urban ones, may have strict zoning laws on land usage and ordinances governing the exterior appearance of structures. Space for off-street parking also is a requirement. In any event, space for future expansion always should be considered.

Flexibility

Successful services are dynamic organizations that can adapt to changes in the quantity and nature of demand. How well a service can adapt depends greatly on the flexibility that has been designed into it. Flexibility also might be called "designing for the future." Questions to address during the design phase might be: how can this facility be designed to allow for later expansion of present services, and how can we design this facility to accommodate new and different services in the future? For example, many of the original fast-food restaurants built for walk-in traffic have had to modify their facilities to accommodate customer demands for drive-through window service.

Several airports face facility problems today because designers failed to anticipate either the tremendous growth in the numbers of people flying or the advent of the "hub-and-spoke" airline network following deregulation. Consequently, passengers often must tote carry-on luggage through a maze of stairways and long passageways to reach the departure gate of their connecting flights. In addition, consider the frustration facing passengers trying to retrieve checked luggage from a baggage-handling operation that was designed for circa 1960s air travelers!

Designing for the future often can translate into financial savings. For example, consider a church that locates in a developing community but does not have the resources to build the sanctuary it would like plus the necessary ancillary facilities it will need. Good design might lead the congregation to build a modest structure that can be used as a temporary sanctuary but later adapted easily and economically to serve as a fellowship hall, a Sunday school, and even a day care facility to meet the needs of a growing community.

In other instances, designing for the future may require additional expenses initially, but it will save financial resources in the long run. In fact, it may provide for growth that might not be possible otherwise. For example, cities often invest in oversized water and wastewater treatment plants in anticipation of future growth.

Aesthetic Factors

Compare two shopping trips to successful, upscale clothing stores. First, we go to an upscale department store such as Nordstrom's. As we enter the women's fine dresses department, we are aware of the carpeting beneath our feet, the ample space between clothing racks, the lack of crowding of dresses on the racks, the complimentary lighting, and most certainly, the very well-groomed salesperson who is ready to serve us immediately. Fitting rooms are located in an area separate from the display area, are roomy and carpeted, and have mirrors on three sides so that you can appreciate every aspect of your appearance. Everything in the department is designed to give a sense of elegance and attention to our needs.

Our second trip takes us to an Eddie Bauer Factory Outlet store. Within just a few steps of the entrance, we are confronted by tables piled high with a vast assortment of clothing. Along the walls and among the tables are racks packed as full as possible with more clothing. Only a maze of narrow pathways is visible around the floor. Salespersons are stationed at cash-register counters and are available to help when you seek them out. Fitting rooms are small "stalls" on the showroom floor and are equipped with only one mirror. (It helps to shop here with a companion, who can give you the advantage of "hindsight.") This is a large warehouse type of store rather than a modest-sized, serene, elegant place to shop; however, the outlet store offers great bargains in exchange for sacrificing plushness and lots of personal attention.

Both stores offer attractive, quality clothing. We feel very differently in each one, however, and their respective designs have played an important part in shaping our attitudes. Clearly, the aesthetic aspects of a design have a marked effect on the consumer's perceptions and behaviors, but they also affect the employees and the service they provide. Lack of attention to aesthetic factors during the design phase can lead to surly service rather than to "service with a smile."

The Community and Environment

The design of a service facility may be of greatest importance where it affects the community and its environment. Will the planned church allow enough space for parking, or will neighbors find it impossible to enter or exit their properties during church activities? Can Priscilla Price design a boarding kennel facility that will not "hound" neighboring businesses with undue noise and odor? How can a community design a detention facility that will provide adequately for the inmates' health and welfare yet still ensure the safety of the town's residents? Has the local dry cleaner designed his or her facility to keep hazardous chemicals out of the local environment?

These questions illustrate how crucial facility design can be in gaining community acceptance of a service. Zoning regulations and many public interest groups also can provide guidance in designing service facilities that are compatible with their communities and environment.

LAYOUT

In addition to facility design, the layout, or arrangement, of the service delivery system is important for the convenience of the customer as well as the service provider. No customer should be subjected to unnecessary aggravation from a poorly planned facility. Further, a poor layout can be costly in time that is wasted when service workers are engaged in unproductive activity. Consider the following experience of a citizen attempting to secure a building permit.

Suppose you want to build the home of your dreams. You have ordered plan #1006BHG from Columbia Design Group in Portland, Oregon, for its "Cozy Cottage." You have found just the right spot of land overlooking the lake and are eager to get that hammer in your hand. Are you all set to go now? Not quite. There is just one small detail: a building permit. You make a quick phone call to the county's building inspection department and are advised that obtaining a permit is very easy: "Just come downtown to our office and pay $200, and we'll take care of you." No problem, you think; you can handle that.

You arrive at the county services building with check in hand. (You did park in a legal spot, right?) A check of the black-felt signboard in the front lobby tells you that the building inspection department is in Office 3 1. (Is that supposed to be 31, or has a little white number fallen off?) Office 31 is on this floor, so you check there first. It turns out to be a rest room. You go to the third floor and find the office across from the elevator—the building inspector's office—a small, dark, dingy, windowless room with a high counter just inside the doorway. A surly old man levers himself out of a protesting chair behind a desk piled high with pink, turquoise, beige, and yellow papers. A coffee pot and a mountain of multihued papers are strewn on a table along one wall. The old man hobbles over to the counter to help you—at least there aren't 20 people in line ahead of you—and after hearing what you want, says that you are in the wrong office, that he just assigns inspectors to issue permits for occupancy at the end of construction. You have to go to "the other wing."

"The other wing" requires a return to the lobby, a check of the black-felt board, and a ride in another elevator—assuming the elevator is working. Just inside the door of Office 333 is a sign: "Take a number and sit." Your number is 21, and there are eight chairs facing a high counter. The room is well lit and has ten desks arranged in three rows behind the counter. There are two doors to back rooms on the east wall, and file cabinets line the west wall. Large maps are posted on the back wall. While waiting, you observe (many times) the typical interaction between an employee and a customer. They exchange pleasantries, then the employee goes to the first back room and returns with a packet of papers. The papers are shuffled back and forth between the employee and the customer, with each signing or making notations in turn. The packet is taken to the other back room and replaced by yet another packet, and the little waltz of fluttering papers and flying pens is repeated to the tune of subdued murmurs. This packet is reassembled and returned to the first office. The employee then retrieves a form from one of the file cabinets, fills it out (three pages in triplicate) on a typewriter at one of the desks, places two copies in other file cabinets, and, finally, hands the customer the treasured building permit.

After you witness 20 variations on this theme, it is your turn. You ask for your building permit. The employee goes to the first back room and returns empty-handed, saying "I can't seem to find your other permits."

"What other permits?" you ask.

"Why, electrical connection, water connection, and sewage connection permits, of course."

You explain that you are building by the lake and will not be on a community water or sewage system; you are going to have a well and a septic tank.

"Oh, then you need to file a geologist's report, a ground percolation test report, and permits to install a septic tank and a leach field before we can issue your building permit—and you'll still need to get the electrical permit. I can tell you where to go, if you like."

This episode illustrates the effect of design and layout on service providers and consumers. Providers' attitudes and responsiveness can be influenced profoundly by their surroundings and the work patterns imposed on them by the layout of their work space.

Sometimes, solutions are relatively easy. In our example, consider your first stop, the building inspection office. With adequate lighting and rearrangement of the furniture so that applicants could approach the employee's desk, the employee might be disposed to tell the customer how to find the building permit office—and also that preliminary permits and reports are necessary before a building permit can be issued. In addition, rearrangement of the work space in the building permit office might allow more efficient service by saving steps and time. These savings would translate into employees who provide service more quickly and, consequently, with more equanimity, because they would not have to deal with applicants who have grown surly during interminable waiting. Service could be improved even further by posting signs at the front desk detailing what preliminary permits and reports must be filed before the building permit can be issued, and this simple measure would benefit the provider and the customer alike.

A larger-scale improvement in layout could be considered as well. The building inspector's office, the building permit office, and other allied permit offices could be relocated in close proximity to each other within the building. Perhaps some offices could be combined physically, allowing easier communication between employees on related matters. Here again, customers would reap the benefits of more efficient service, reduced travel time between offices, and reduced waiting time.

Many improvements can be achieved with little cost either to the service provider or the consumer. In other situations, the layout of a service organization may involve significant expense, which would necessitate a critical analysis before implementation. Along these lines, we next consider two basic layout forms, product layout and process layout, each with its own associated challenge.

Product Layout and the Line-Balancing Problem

Some standard services can be divided into an inflexible sequence of steps or operations that all customers must experience. This is an example of a *product layout* most often associated with manufacturing assembly lines, where a product is assembled in a fixed sequence of steps. The most obvious analogy is to a cafeteria, where diners push their trays along as they assemble their meal. Staffing such a service requires allocating tasks among servers to create jobs that require nearly equal time. The job requiring the most time per customer creates a *bottleneck* and defines the capacity of the service line. Any change in the capacity of the service line requires that attention be given to the bottleneck activity. Several options are available: adding another worker to the job, providing some aid to reduce the activity time, or regrouping the tasks to create a new line balance with different activity assignments. A well-balanced line would have all jobs be of nearly equal duration to avoid unnecessary idleness and inequity in work assignments. A service line approach has the additional advantage of allowing for division of labor and use of dedicated special equipment, as illustrated by Example 6.1.

Example 6.1: Automobile Driver's License Office

The state automobile driver's license office is under pressure to increase its productivity to accommodate 120 applicants per hour with the addition of only one clerk to its present staff. The license renewal process currently is designed as a service line, with customers being processed in the fixed sequence listed in Table 6.1. Activity 1 (i.e., review application for correctness) must be performed first, and activity 6 (i.e., issue temporary license) must be the last step and, by state policy, be handled by a uniformed officer. Activity 5 (i.e., photograph applicant) requires an expensive instant camera.

The process flow diagram for the current arrangement, as shown in Figure 6.1*a*, identifies the bottleneck activity (i.e., the activity with the slowest flow rate per hour) as activity 3 (i.e., check for violations and restrictions), limits the current capacity to 60 applicants per hour. By focusing only on the bottleneck, one might think that assigning the additional clerk to perform activity 3 would double the flow through the bottleneck and achieve the goal

TABLE 6.1 License Renewal Process Times

Activity	Description	Time, *Sec*
1	Review application for correctness	15
2	Process and record payment	30
3	Check for violations and restrictions	60
4	Conduct eye test	40
5	Photograph applicant	20
6	Issue temporary license (state trooper)	30

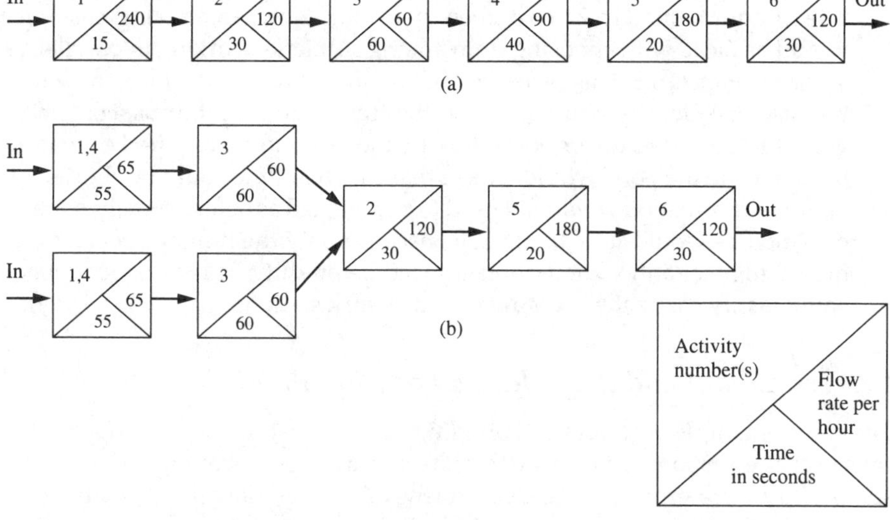

FIGURE 6.1. *(a)* Present and *(b)* proposed flow diagrams.

of 120 applicants per hour. However, the flow for this system would be limited to 90 applicants per hour, because the bottleneck would shift to activity 4.

The proposed process design, as shown in Figure 6.1*b* with seven clerks, can achieve the desired capacity of 120 applicants per hour, because activities 1 and 4 have been grouped together to create a new job (i.e., review applications for correctness and conduct eye test) that better balances the work load among the staff. How did we know to group these two activities together? First, remember that a flow rate of at least 120 applicants per hour must be achieved at each step in the process. Because activities 2 and 6 already are being performed at this rate, they need not be considered further. An additional clerk is required to perform activity 3, however, because only with two clerks working in parallel can we achieve a combined flow rate of 120 applicants per hour. Next, we must ask if it is possible to combine activities requiring small amounts of time to arrive at a job that can be performed in 60 seconds or less (i.e., achieve a flow rate of at least 60 applicants per hour)? By combining activity 1, which requires 15 seconds, with activity 4, which requires 40 seconds, we can achieve a combined job requiring 55 seconds per applicant (or a flow rate of 65 applicants per hour). Note that this solution requires the acquisition of one additional eye-testing machine. Another solution would be to combine activities 4 and 5 to create a job yielding a flow rate of 60 applicants per hour; however, an additional expensive camera would need to be purchased. Can you think of another process design that meets the capacity goal but could be viewed by customers and employees as offering more personalized service?

The example of the driver's license office lends itself to a radical rethinking of the product layout. If money were available to invest in computers, additional eye-testing equipment, and cameras, then the entire process could be reengineered. Consider training each clerk to perform all five activities with a combined time of 165 seconds, or an individual flow rate of approximately 22 customers per hour. Now, an arriving customer would be faced with choosing from among six clerks working in parallel, as shown in Figure 6.2. This system would be appealing to customers, however, because one clerk would handle all the transactions and, thus, customers would not be passed from one clerk to another and be required to wait in between. Further, one would expect that the total time could be shortened, because information would not need to be repeated as before. Finally, staffing of the office would now be flexible, because only the number of clerks required to meet anticipated demand need be on duty. This savings in labor could justify easily the investment in six work stations.

Process Layout and the Relative Location Problem

The earlier example of obtaining a building permit illustrates a *process layout*, because service personnel performing similar functions or having the same responsibility were grouped into departments. A process layout allows the customers to define the sequence of service activities to meet their needs and, thus, affords some degree of customization. The process layout also allows the service to be tailored to the customer's specifications, thereby delivering personalized

FIGURE 6.2. Reengineered Driver's License Office.

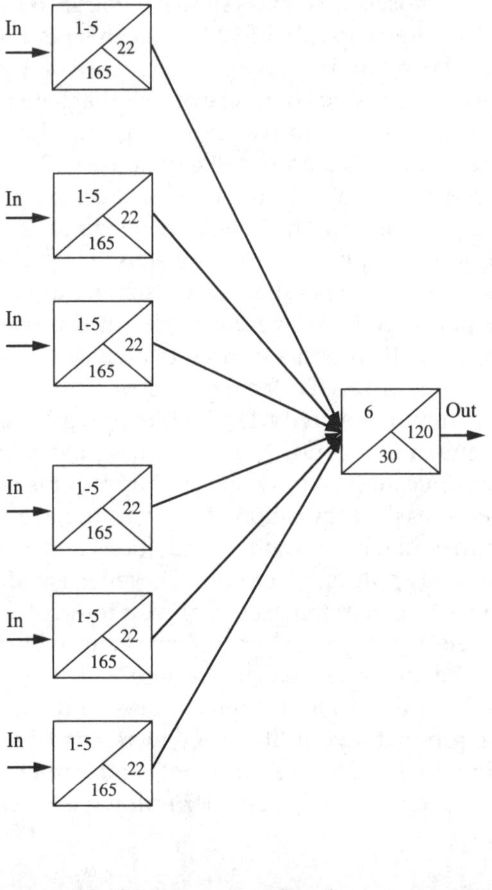

services. The ability to customize service requires more highly skilled service providers, who have discretion to personalize the service to customers' needs. Professional services such as law, medicine, and consulting, which are organized into specialties, provide examples.

From the service provider's perspective, the flow of customers appears to be intermittent, so there is a need for a waiting area in each department. The variability in demand at each department results when customers choose different sequences of services and place different demands on the service provided. On arriving at a particular department, customers often will find it busy and will need to join a queue, which usually operates on a first-come, first-served basis.

A dramatic and physical example of a service process layout is a university campus with buildings dedicated to various disciplines, giving students the flexibility of choosing classes from among them. The relative location problem can be seen in the layout of the campus. For both student and faculty convenience, we would expect selected departments such as engineering and physical sciences to be in close proximity to each other, while perhaps economics and business administration would be located together in another area. The library and administration offices would be located in a central part of the campus. One possible objective for selecting such a layout would be to minimize the total distance traveled by faculty, staff, and students between all pairs of departments. Many different layouts are possible, however. In fact, if we have identified n departments to be assigned to n locations, then n factorial layouts (i.e., 3,628,800 layouts for 10 departments) are possible. Because finding the best layout among these possibilities is beyond complete enumeration, we will use a heuristic approach to finding a good layout in Example 6.2.

Example 6.2: Ocean World Theme Park

The architect for Ocean World is beginning to formulate plans for the development of property outside Waco, Texas, to a second marine theme park after the success of its Neptune's Realm on the West Coast. Because of the hot and humid Texas weather during the summer months, ways to minimize the visitors' total travel distance between attractions are being considered. Data showing a typical day's flow of visitors between attractions at San Diego are given in Table 6.2 and will be used in the layout planning.

TABLE 6.2 Daily Flow of Visitors Between Attractions, Hundreds*

Flow matrix

	A	B	C	D	E	F
A	X	7	20	0	5	6
B	8	X	6	10	0	2
C	10	6	X	15	7	8
D	0	30	5	X	10	3
E	10	10	1	20	X	6
F	0	6	0	3	4	X

Net flow →

Triangularized matrix

	A	B	C	D	E	F
A	X	15	30	0	15	6
B	X	X	12	40	10	8
C	X	X	X	20	8	8
D	X	X	X	X	30	6
E	X	X	X	X	X	10
F	X	X	X	X	X	X

*Description of attractions: A = killer whale, B = sea lions, C = dolphins, D = water skiing, E = aquarium, F = water rides.

A heuristic called *operations sequence analysis* will be used to identify a good layout for this relative location problem.[3] This method uses as input the matrix of flows between departments and a grid showing the geographic center location for department assignments. In Table 6.2, we have created a triangularized form of the original flow matrix to sum the flows in either direction, because we are interested only in the total.

The heuristic begins with an initial layout, shown on the grid in Figure 6.3*a*. This initial layout is arbitrary but could be based on judgment or past experience. Table 6.2 suggests that attractions with high daily flow between them should be placed adjacent to each other. For example, we cannot see a need to place A adjacent to D, but it would be appropriate to place A close to C.

For nonadjacent attractions, the flow between them is multiplied by the number of grids that separate the attractions. Note we have assumed that diagonal separation is approximately equal to the distance of a grid side instead of using the Pythagorean theorem. These products are summed to arrive at a total flow distance of 124 for this initial layout. Considering the large contribution made to this sum by the separation of attractions A and C, we decide to move C adjacent to A to form the revised layout shown in Figure 6.3*b*, with a total flow distance of 96. The revised layout shown in Figure 6.3*c* is the result of exchanging attractions A and C. This exchange has placed attraction C adjacent to attractions D, E, and F, thereby reducing the total flow distance to 70. The final layout, in Figure 6.3*d*, is created by exchanging attractions B and E and by moving attraction F to form a rectangular space;

[3]Elwood S. Buffa, "Sequence Analysis for Functional Layouts," *Journal of Industrial Engineering*, vol. 6, no. 2, March–April 1955, pp. 12–13.

FIGURE 6.3. Ocean World site planning using operations sequence analysis.

(*a*) **Intial layout**

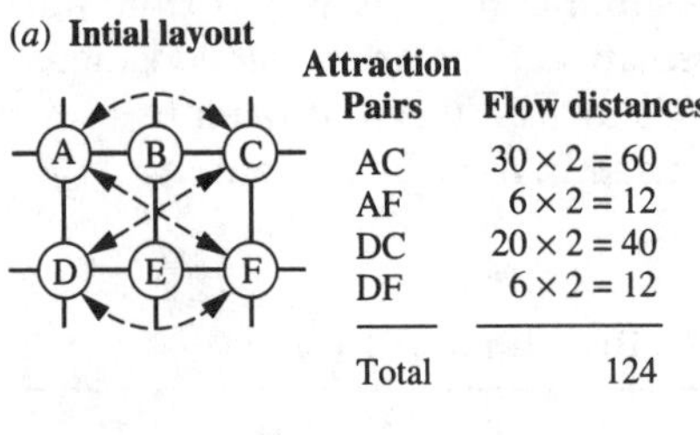

Attraction Pairs	Flow distances
AC	30 × 2 = 60
AF	6 × 2 = 12
DC	20 × 2 = 40
DF	6 × 2 = 12
Total	124

(*b*) **Move C close to A**

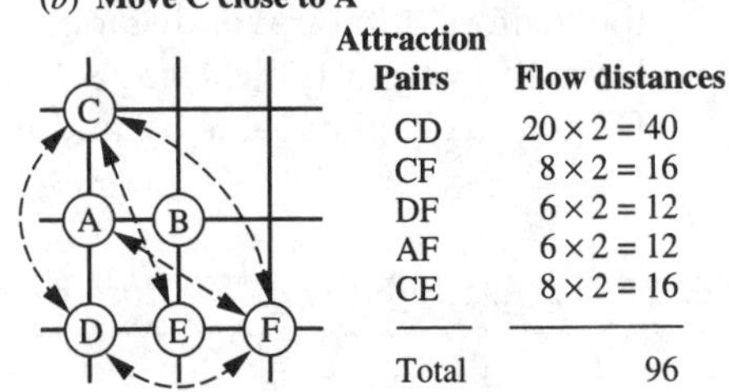

Attraction Pairs	Flow distances
CD	20 × 2 = 40
CF	8 × 2 = 16
DF	6 × 2 = 12
AF	6 × 2 = 12
CE	8 × 2 = 16
Total	96

(*c*) **Exchange A and C**

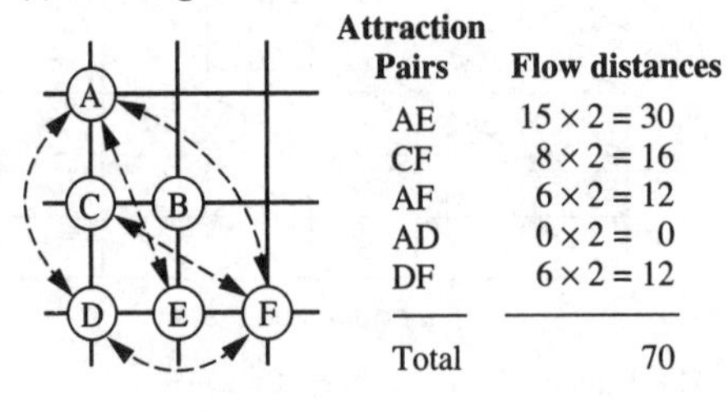

Attraction Pairs	Flow distances
AE	15 × 2 = 30
CF	8 × 2 = 16
AF	6 × 2 = 12
AD	0 × 2 = 0
DF	6 × 2 = 12
Total	70

(*d*) **Exchange B and E and move F**

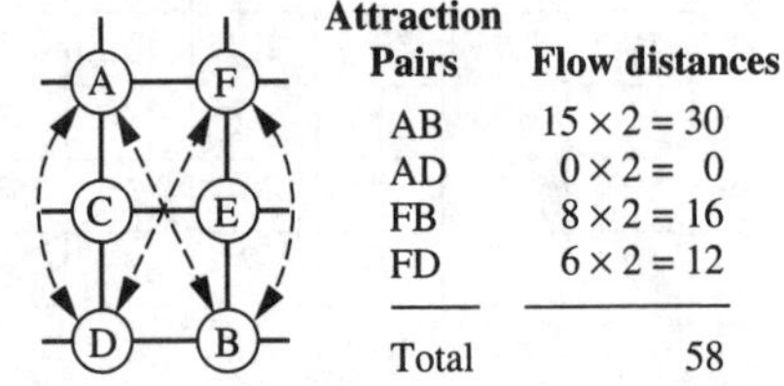

Attraction Pairs	Flow distances
AB	15 × 2 = 30
AD	0 × 2 = 0
FB	8 × 2 = 16
FD	6 × 2 = 12
Total	58

exchanging B and E keeps E and F adjacent as we move F to form a more compact space. By making high-flow attractions adjacent, we have reduced total nonadjacent flow distance to a value of 58 for our final site plan, which is shown in Figure 6.4.

The departmental exchange logic of operations sequence analysis was incorporated into a computer program known as *CRAFT* (Computerized Relative Allocation of Facilities Technique).[4] CRAFT requires the following inputs: an interdepartmental flow matrix, a cost matrix (i.e., cost/unit/unit distance moved), and an initial layout with exact departmental dimensions filling the space available. CRAFT can incorporate some constraints, such as fixing the location of a department. The program logic depicted in Figure 6.5 shows the incremental nature of the heuristic, which selects at each iteration the two departments that, if exchanged, will yield the most improvement in flow distance reduction. As can be seen in the Selected Bibliography at the end of this chapter, reports indicate the extensive use of CRAFT in service organization layout planning—for example, in insurance offices, hospitals, movie studios, and universities.

An objective other than minimization of travel distance also could be appropriate for designing the layout of a service. For example, if we had a core business with several ancillary businesses, we would want a layout that encouraged cus-

[4]E. S. Buffa, G. C. Armour, and T. E. Vollmann, "Allocating Facilities with CRAFT," *Harvard Business Review,* vol. 42, no. 2, March–April 1964, pp. 136–159.

FIGURE 6.4. Final site plan for Ocean World theme park.
(Map by Kate O'Brien, Desert Tale Graphics.)

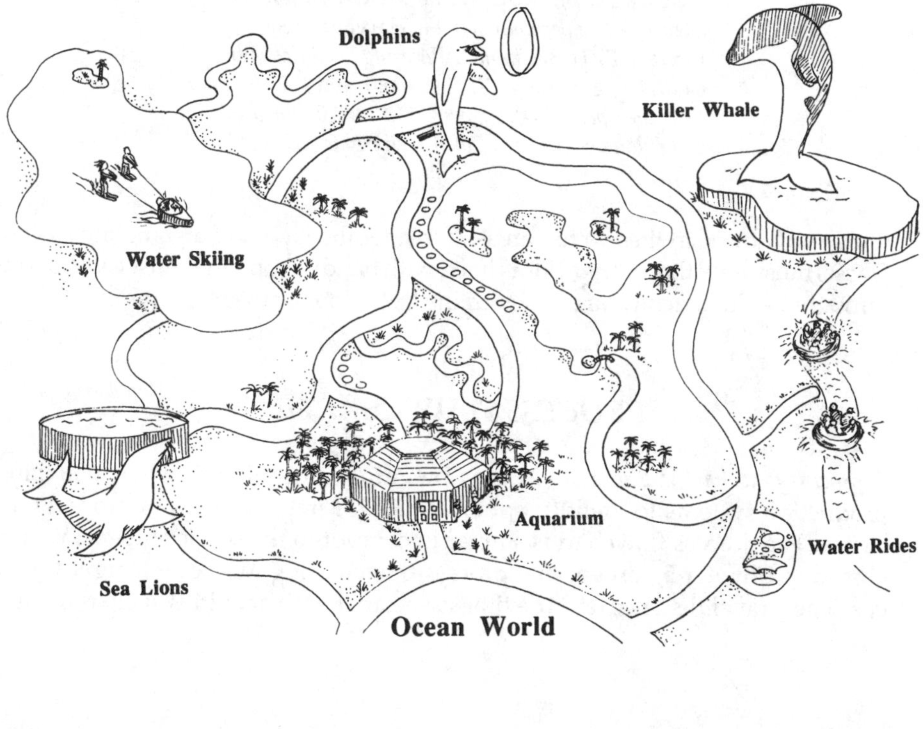

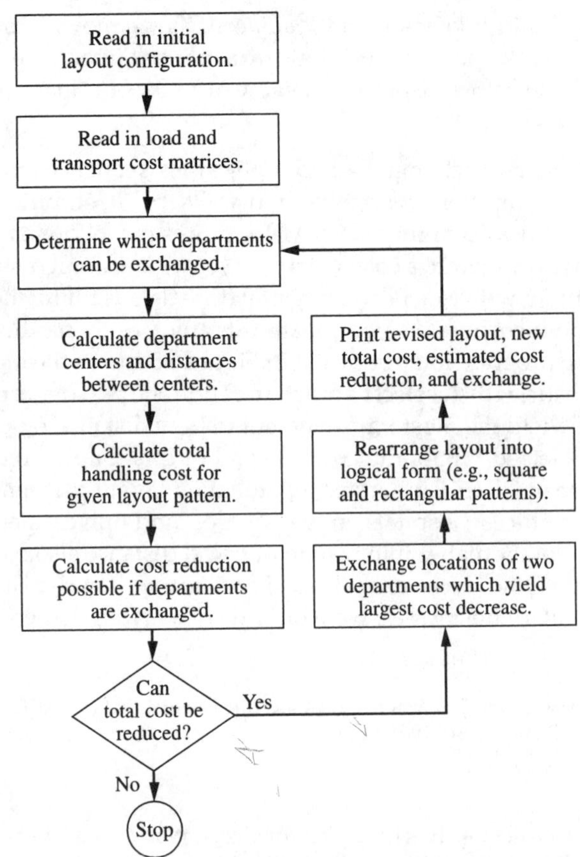

FIGURE 6.5. Flow diagram for CRAFT logic. *(Reprinted by permission of the* Harvard Business Review. *EXHIBIT from "Allocating Facilities with Craft," by E. S. Buffa, G. C. Armour, and T. E. Vollman (March–April 1964). Copyright © 1964 by the president and fellows of Harvard College; all rights reserved.)*

tomers to browse in these other areas. Consider the layout of a gambling casino. Guests must walk through corridors lined with trendy shops and must always pass through the slot machine area to reach the front door or the restaurant.

PROCESS FLOWCHARTING

A *process flowchart* is a visual aid used by industrial engineers when analyzing production systems to identify opportunities for improvement in process efficiency. The process flowchart is similar in concept to the service blueprint (discussed in Chapter 5), except that process flowcharting focuses on employee or customer travel distance and the time associated with activities such as delays, inspections, travel, and operations. Thus, the focus is on layout efficiency as measured in time and distance traveled.

For manufacturing layout analysis, the production process is broken down into the underlying sequence of operations, with the time required for each recorded and the distance measured when material is moved between operations. Delays, inspection activity, and storage of material also are noted. A description of the process in visual form helps to identify areas where efficiency can be improved by eliminating unnecessary activities (e.g., by reducing the distance that material is moved, by combining operations).

Because the customer is part of the process in services, the traditional industrial process chart is modified for use in studying service processes by redefining the customary symbols. This is shown in Table 6.3.

Service process flowcharting begins by observing the service to identify the sequence of steps involved. Each step is classified according to the five categories in Table 6.3 and listed in order. The process flow is drawn by connecting the symbols, and noting the time associated with each step and the distance traveled for movements.

Example 6.3: Credit Card Processing

For restaurants, credit card transactions are time-consuming for both guests and servers. A new procedure for processing such transactions has been suggested, however, and the benefits to servers and guests will be compared with the current procedure. The process flow analysis contained in Figures 6.6 and 6.7 comparing the two procedures was reported by Kimes and Mutkoski, only slightly modified here to use the service process categories as shown in Table 6.3.[5]

[5]S. E. Kimes and S. A. Mutkoski, "The Express Guest Check: Saving Steps with Process Design," *The Cornell HRA Quarterly*, vol. 30, no. 2, August 1989, p. 23.

TABLE 6.3. Service Process Chart Categories and Symbols

Category	Symbol	Description
Operation	○	An operation performed by the server off-line or by customer self-service. A possible service failure point.
Customer contact	∇	An occasion when server and customer interact. An opportunity to influence customer service perceptions.
Travel	→	The movement of customers, servers, or information between operations.
Delay	D	Delay resulting in a queue and a need for customer waiting space.
Inspection	□	An activity by customer or server to measure service quality.

Distance	Time	Activity
		Customer requests check
30 ft.	0.5 min.	Server walks
	0.5 min.	Server prepares check
30 ft.	0.5 min.	Server walks
	0.25 min.	Server presents check
30 ft.	0.5 min.	Server walks
	0.5 min.	Customer inspects, puts card out
30 ft.	0.5 min.	Server returns to table
	0.25 min.	Server picks up card
30 ft.	0.5 min.	Server walks to process
	0.5 min.	Server fills out slip
	0.5 min.	Server processes slip
	1.0 min.	Server obtains preauthorization
30 ft.	0.5 min.	Server walks
	0.25 min.	Server presents slip
30 ft.	0.5 min.	Server walks
	0.5 min.	Customer signs (leaves)
30 ft.	0.5 min.	Server walks
	0.25 min.	Server picks up slip
30 ft.	0.5 min.	(Customer leaves) Server walks
Total 270 ft.	9 min.	

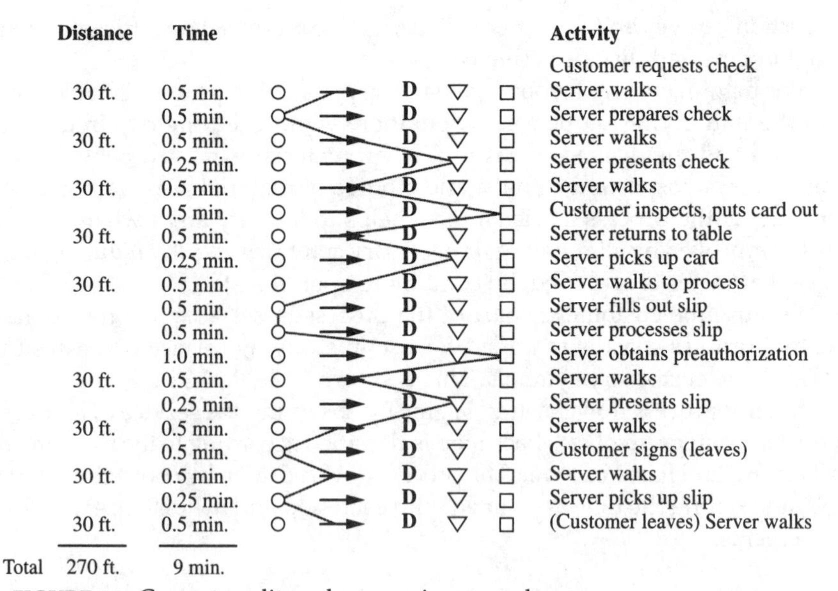

FIGURE 6.6. Current credit card–processing procedure.
(S. E. Kimes and S. A. Mutkoski, "The Express Guest Check: Saving Steps with Process Design," The Cornell HRA Quarterly, *August 1989, p. 23. © Cornell HRA Quarterly. Used by permission. All rights reserved.)*

A close examination of the process flowcharts reveals that the last three steps of the current credit processing procedure have been eliminated in the new procedure. Thus, the proposed card processing procedure has saved the server one round-trip to the table, or 60 feet of walking. Both the server and the guest benefit from a savings of 1.75 minutes in performing the transaction.

ENVIRONMENTAL PSYCHOLOGY AND ORIENTATION

Orientation is the first behavioral need of an individual on entering a place. It includes questions of place orientation (e.g., "Where am I?") as well as of function orientation (e.g., "How does this organization work, and what do I do next?"). On entering a physical setting, customers gain control when they can use spatial cues, along with previous experience, to identify where they are, where they should go, and what they need to do. Anxiety and a sense of helplessness can result if spatial cues are not present or previous experience cannot be used to avoid disorientation. Richard E. Wener argues that the causes of disorientation in service settings can be reduced by a facility design that incorporates the following: previous experience, design legibility, and orientation aids.[6]

[6]Richard E. Wener, "The Environmental Psychology of Service Encounters," in J. A. Czepiel, M. R. Solomon, and C. F. Surprenant (eds.), *The Service Encounter,* Lexington Books, Lexington, Mass., 1985, pp. 101–113.

Distance	Time	Activity
		Customer requests check
30 ft.	0.5 min.	Server walks
	0.5 min.	Server prepares check
	0.5 min.	Server fills out slip
30 ft.	0.5 min.	Server walks
	0.25 min.	Server presents check and slip
30 ft.	0.5 min.	Server walks
	0.5 min.	Customer inspects, puts card out, signs slip
30 ft.	0.5 min.	Server returns to table
	0.25 min.	Server picks up card and slip
30 ft.	0.5 min.	Server walks
	0.5 min.	Server processes slip and card
	1.0 min.	Server obtains authorization
30 ft.	0.5 min.	Server walks
	0.25 min.	Server presents card and receipt
30 ft.	0.5 min.	Server walks
		Customer leaves
Total 210 ft.	7.25 min.	

FIGURE 6.7. Proposed credit card–processing procedure.
(S. E. Kimes and S. A. Mutkoski, "The Express Guest Check: Saving Steps with Process Design," The Cornell HRA Quarterly, *August 1989, p. 23. © Cornell HRA Quarterly. Used by permission. All rights reserved.)*

Using formula facilities, franchised services have effectively removed the anxiety of disorientation so that customers know exactly what to do. Holiday Inn took this concept a step further by advertising that a guest will find no surprises at any of its locations, capitalizing on the need for familiarity to attract repeat customers.

Orientation also can be aided by facility designs that allow customers to see both into and through the space. Layouts for banks and hotels often use an entrance atrium that allows the entire space to be viewed and conceptualized at a glance. In addition, such a layout allows customers to observe the actions of others for behavioral cues.

Orientation aids and signage such as "You Are Here" maps, if properly aligned with the user's perspective (i.e., "up" on the sign equates to straight ahead for the user) and complete with environmental landmarks, can be effective as well. Strategically located plants and artwork can act as points of reference. Color-coded subway routes with corresponding color-coded connecting arrows represent an excellent use of signage to assist in self-service and to promote smooth flow of traffic.

WALK-THROUGH-AUDIT[7]

Delivery of a service should conform to the customer's expectations from the beginning to the end of the experience, because the customer is a participant in the service process and his or her impression of service quality is influenced by

[7]From J. A. Fitzsimmons and G. B. Maurer, "A Walk-Through-Audit to Improve Restaurant Performance," *The Cornell H.R.A. Quarterly,* February 1991, pp. 95–99.

many observations. An environmental audit can be a useful management tool for the systematic evaluation of a customer's view of the service being provided.

Such a walk-through-audit was developed by Fitzsimmons and Maurer for sit-down restaurants in which the customer is served. The audit consisted of 42 questions spanning the restaurant dining experience, beginning with approaching the restaurant from the parking area, then walking into the restaurant and being greeted, waiting for a table, being seated, ordering and receiving food and drinks, and finally, receiving the check and paying the bill. Sample questions from the walk-through-audit are shown in Figure 6.8. The questions span nine categories of variables: 1) maintenance items, 2) person-to-person service, 3) waiting, 4) table and place settings, 5) ambiance, 6) food presentation, 7) check presentation, 8) promotion and suggestive selling, and 9) tipping.

This audit was mailed to the owners or managers of 250 restaurants throughout Texas to study the relationship of tipping behavior to environmental vari-

Presented below are representative examples from among the 42 questions included in the audit used in our study.

Please answer all questions as they relate to your restaurant. There are no right or wrong answers. For each question, circle the number that best represents your restaurant for that item. Please check "Not Applicable" when the item does not apply to your restaurant's service.

1. How often is the parking area cleaned of trash items? (Not Applicable ____)	**Less than daily**				**At least hourly**
	1	2	3	4	5
			Time in minutes		
8. During busy periods, the wait before being seated is: (Not Applicable ____)	**Less than 15**	**15–29**	**30–44**	**45–59**	**60 or more**
a. Weekdays	1	2	3	4	5
b. Weekends	1	2	3	4	5
Are drinks served to customers who are waiting? Yes ____ No ____					
10. Once seated inside, the lighting level is: (Not Applicable ____)	**Like Candlelight**				**Brighter than a sunny day**
	1	2	3	4	5
22a. The average level of suggestive selling of appetizers is: (Not Applicable ____)	**Less than $2.00**	**$2–2.99**	**$3–3.99**	**$4–4.99**	**$5.00 or more**
	1	2	3	4	5
29. After the entree is served, what is the average number of visits to the table by the servers? (Not Applicable ____)	**1 or 2**	3	4	5	**6 or more**
	1	2	3	4	5
			Time in minutes		
40. Within how many minutes after the meal is finished is the final check presented? (Not Applicable ____) Before meal is finished = 0	**0 min.**	**1 min.**	**2 min.**	**3 min.**	**4 or more**
	1	2	3	4	5
			Percentage		
41. What is the average tip as a percentage of the bill? (Not Applicable ____)	**8 or less**	**9–11**	**12–14**	**15**	**Over 15**
	1	2	3	4	5

FIGURE 6.8. Sample questions from the walk-through-audit.
(J. A. Fitzsimmons and Gavin Maurer, "A Walk-Through-Audit to Improve Restaurant Performance," The Cornell HRA Quarterly, *vol. 31, no. 4, February 1991, p. 97. © Cornell HRA Quarterly. Used by permission. All rights reserved.)*

ables. Many of the comparisons within the study relate directly to the level of tipping as a percentage of the total bill. Tipping is a good measure of customer satisfaction. Clearly, however, some customers can be satisfied and still leave relatively low tips, and other customers will tip at a given level regardless of the quality of service they perceive. Within this study, tipping percentages ranged from less than 8 percent to more than 15 percent. Questions that relate to tipping behavior were grouped into the following categories: 1) person-to-person service, 2) service delays, 3) ambiance variables, 4) check presentation, and 5) promotion and suggestive selling.

Person-to-Person Service

It was anticipated that high levels of person-to-person service would relate to high customer satisfaction and, therefore, to large tips. This was confirmed by the study.

Several variables have a strong positive relationship to the size of the tip: 1) the time the server spends at the table doing extra food preparation, 2) the number of visits to the table by the server after the entree has been served, and 3) the average number of times the server refills coffee cups or drink glasses during the dessert portion of the meal. This indicates that extra attention at the table seems to generate higher tips, possibly because of greater customer satisfaction.

An important implication for management is that the initial training of servers should emphasize visits to the table as one strategy for achieving higher tips. Restaurants that promote high customer-server interaction may enjoy an additional competitive advantage because: 1) customers are more satisfied and more likely to return, and 2) the prospect of higher tips may attract and retain a better server staff.

Service Delays

The audit also indicates that tipping is high when customers are served drinks while they are waiting to be seated. This suggests that customers do not want to be ignored once they have arrived, and that they have more positive perceptions of the dining experience if they receive some level of service before they are seated. This may reveal an opportunity for restaurants to benefit by offering other activities or services to waiting customers. Chapter 11 discusses the effects of waiting during the service process.

Ambiance Variables

The ambiance, or aesthetic atmosphere, of a restaurant is one of the most important environmental variables for competitive differentiation. Four such variables—lighting level, music level, color scheme, and presence of cooking smells—were included in the study. Only lighting levels, however, proved to have a significant correlation with tipping behavior: a low lighting level was associated with large tips.

The level of light also is associated with other variables that have similar effects on tipping. For example, nearly two-thirds of the restaurants that used tablecloths and full place settings reported having "candlelight" or only slightly brighter lighting. Thus, tipping behavior may be associated with the complexity of the dining experience, a complex dining experience being defined as one in which overt sensory stimulation gives way to subtle appeals (e.g., those found in very "elegant" restaurants).

The extent to which cooking smells can be noticed supports this dining complexity dimension. Cooking smells are associated very closely with brighter light levels and "homey" or earth-tone color schemes. When comparing cooking smells with lighting, it appears that lower lighting levels are associated with low levels of cooking smells. Restaurants whose cooking smells are less noticeable also tend to have color schemes that utilize pastels, whereas restaurants with "very noticeable" cooking smells have schemes that utilize homey or earth-tone colors. This indicates that homey or earth-tone color schemes are associated with a less complex dining experience, whereas pastels appear to be the fashion in restaurants offering full table settings, tablecloths, and a more complex dining experience.

Creation and maintenance of the restaurant ambiance has management implications. Selection of lighting levels and color schemes as well as the control of cooking smells must present an ambiance that is consistent with the desired customer experience.

Check Presentation

There are two distinct ways of presenting the check, depending on whether management wants fast turnover of customers or diners to linger after the meal is finished. Both strategies may be positively perceived by customers and result in better tips.

One way to achieve fast turnover is to combine the clearing of each plate as the diner finishes and presentation of the check as closely as possible following the meal. This strategy did not necessarily mean lower tips in the audit, and it may lead to higher tips when customers want quick, efficient service without too many frills. In some cases, however, delayed presentation of the check also is associated with higher tipping. Unlike other service interactions that indicate long waiting times produce negative perceptions of service, a delay in presenting the check can carry a positive perception. In the audit, a group of restaurants reported that customers are given the bill no sooner than 3 minutes after the meal is finished. Most of these restaurants reported higher-than-average tips provided the wait did not exceed 4 minutes.

Again, the tip as a percentage of the bill was greater than for the sample as a whole, indicating there are some restaurants in which customers expect to be able to linger and will show their appreciation by tipping relatively higher than the sample. This may indicate that there is a point at which customers' perceptions change from pleasurable lingering to dissatisfied waiting.

Promotion and Suggestive Selling

Promotion variables include suggestive selling as well as promoting food and drink items at special prices. Promotional activity has a positive effect on the dining experience, as suggested by higher tips. Further, suggestive selling has a multiplier effect on tips, resulting from the added personal service and increased dollar amount of the bill. Thus, management can provide suggestive-selling vehicles as a way to increase both restaurant and server revenues.

Implications for Management

This study has demonstrated the importance of a walk-through-audit as an opportunity to evaluate the service experience from a customer's perspective, because the customer often becomes aware of cues that the owners and managers may have overlooked. There is no inherently superior service design. Instead, there are designs that are consistent and that provide a signal to customers about the service they can expect. Providing tangibility in a service involves giving the customer verbal, environmental, sensory, and service cues that define the service for the customer and encourage repeat visits.

THE WALK-THROUGH-AUDIT AS A DIAGNOSTIC TOOL

The walk-through-audit can be a useful diagnostic tool for management to evaluate the gaps in perception between customers and managers of the service delivery system. Customers visit a site less frequently than managers do and, thus, are more sensitive to subtle changes (e.g., peeling paint, worn rugs) than managers, who see the facility every day and likely overlook gradual deterioration of the supporting facility.

To test this use of a walk-through-audit, a movie theater audit was prepared and administered to movie-goers over several weekends. The same audit (i.e., questionnaire) also was given to the manager and assistant managers. The level of detail can be seen by reviewing the complete audit, which is shown in Figure 6.9. Note that the audit is divided into sections ordered in chronological sequence: general information, location, parking, ticketing, movies, lobby, concessions, restrooms, theater, and post-movie categories of questions. Thus, the entire customer experience is traced from beginning to end.

Responses for each item were averaged for the two groups and are displayed in Figure 6.10. This presentation highlights the gaps in service perception between management and customers. Some of these gaps are not surprising, such as "adequate parking" and "prices are clearly labeled" given that managers have assigned parking and set the prices. Other gaps suggest that some improvements are in order (e.g., "ticket staff are trained" and "concession staff are friendly"). It is telling that management scores were uniformly higher than the average customer scores for all audit questions.

Movie Theater Service Audit

Please take a few minutes and answer the following questions about your recent movie-going experience. There are no right or wrong answers. The purpose is to help analyze the quality of the service across several service dimensions. For each question, please circle the number that corresponds to your best answer. Please mark items "Not Applicable" when the item does not apply to your experience. Thank you for your help.

Name of Theater: _________ Movie: _________

Location: _________ Movie Rating: _________

Date: ________/________/________

Time: ________ AM or PM

General Information

Did the Movie Theater have a call-up information line?	No 1				Yes 5
If so, did it give adequate directions to the theater? (Not Applicable/Didn't use it ________)	No directions 1	2	3	4	Detailed directions 5
If so, did it give adequate details for the movies including times, brief abstract, sound system, etc.? (Not Applicable/Didn't use it ________)	Just movies & time 1	2	3	4	Novel on the movie and theater 5
If so, did the tape recorded message repeat, or must the customer call back? (Not Applicable/Didn't use it ________)	Must call back 1				Repeats forever 5

Location

Was the movie theater located in a safe part of town?	Heard gunshots 1	2	3	4	Extremely safe 5
Was the theater easily accessible from the major roads and streets?	Had to use an old dirt road 1	2	3	4	Right off the highway 5
Once in the vicinity of the theater, was the facility easily locatable?	Hidden behind shopping center 1	2	3	4	Easy to find 5
Was the theater located near where you live?	*Travel Time* More than 1 hour 1	2	15–45 min. 3	4	Fewer than 5 minutes 5
Was there a marquee in front of the theater?	No 1				Yes 5
If so, was the marquee easily viewed? (Not Applicable ________)	Not easily viewed 1	2	3	4	Needed sunglasses due to the bright lights 5
Is the theater stand-alone, or within a mall or other facility?	Stand-alone 1				In mall 5

Parking					
Was there adequate parking, even for the busiest nights?	Not a parking spot in sight				Every spot "on the front row" open
	1	2	3	4	5
Was the parking lot well lit?	Dark				Bright as a sunny day
	1	2	3	4	5
Was the majority of the parking close to the theater?	Short marathon				Car door hit front door of the theater
	1	2	3	4	5
Was the parking area monitored by security guards?	The owner can't spell security guard		Think I saw one		Guard camped out by my car
	1	2	3	4	5
Was there a passenger drop-off in front of the theater?	No drop-off area				Right beside my seat
	1	2	3	4	5
Ticketing					
Could you purchase your tickets ahead of time, via phone, etc.?	No				Yes
	1	2	3	4	5
Were there adequate ticket windows *available* to serve the largest of crowds?	1 window				Enough to service the largest crowds with no wait
	1	2	3	4	5
Were there adequate windows *open* to keep customer lines to a minimum?	Line stretches to the moon				No wait
	1	2	3	4	5
Were the ticketing staff friendly?	Permanent attitude				Part of the Walton family
	1	2	3	4	5
Were the ticketing staff trained on equipment, and did they have knowledge of the movies and times, etc.?	Dumber than a brick				Rocket scientists
	1	2	3	4	5
How reasonable were ticket prices?	Had to take out a loan				How do they stay in business?
	1	2	3	4	5
Regular prices?	More than $11.00		$5–$8		Less than $2.00
	1	2	3	4	5
Matinee?	More than $7.00		$3–$5		Less than $1.00
	1	2	3	4	5
Twilight?	More than $7.00		$3–$5		Less than $1.00
	1	2	3	4	5

Question	1	2	3	4	5
Did the theater accept credit cards? (Not Applicable, I'm a cash-kinda person ________)	No 1	2	3	4	Yes 5
Are ticket prices clearly labeled on the attraction board?	Needed a magnifying glass to read the prices 1	2	3	4	Can see the prices from the parking lot 5
Movies					
Did the movie theater offer a wide range of movies to cater to a broad audience, or does it focus on specialty movies?	Only "artsy" movies 1	2	3	4	I saw an "artsy," the kids saw Disney 5
Did the movie theater offer a large number of screens?	1 screen 1	2	3	4	Couldn't see all the screens due to the curvature of the earth 5
Lobby					
Was the lobby large enough to accommodate moviegoers before their movie?	"Sorry, you are going to have to wait outside!" 1	2	3	4	Enough to service the largest crowds 5
Were there entertainment and amenities such as payphones and video machines in the lobby to accommodate the moviegoers?	Boring 1	2	3	4	Was sad it was time to go into the movie 5
Did the lobby have a bar?	No 1	2	3	4	Yes 5
Was the lobby kept clean?	Was wondering if the janitor was on strike 1	2	3	4	Spotless 5
Was the lobby well lit?	Dark 1	2	3	4	Bright as a sunny day 5
How was the atmosphere of the theater?	Old and quaint 1	2	3	4	Bright and flashy 5
Was there adequate direction from the lobby to the proper movie theater?	Ended up in some B-movie by mistake 1	2	3	4	Runway lights led me right to my seat 5

Concessions

Question					
Were there adequate available concession stations to serve the largest of crowds?	1 station				Enough to service the largest crowds with no wait
	1	2	3	4	5
Were there adequate open concession stations to keep customer lines to a minimum?	Line stretched to the moon				No wait
	1	2	3	4	5
Were the concession staff friendly?	Permanent attitude				Part of the Walton family
	1	2	3	4	5
Were the concession staff trained on equipment, and did they have knowledge of concessions items and prices?	Dumber than a brick				Rocket scientists
	1	2	3	4	5
How were the prices of food?	What you'd expect at Sam's Club				Highway robbery
	1	2	3	4	5
Were you offered both healthy and regular popcorn?	No				Yes
	1	2	3	4	5
Was the quality of the concession food good?	Wouldn't feed it to my dog				Would have made the best restaurants list
	1	2	3	4	5
Was the selection at the concession broad, or was it limited to popcorn and sodas?	No selection		Std.		Broad as a candy store
	1	2	3	4	5

Restrooms

Question					
Were the restrooms within close proximity to the theater?	Wished I had a taxi to get there				Next to my seat
	1	2	3	4	5
Were there adequate restroom facilities to keep customer lines to a minimum?	Line stretched to the moon				No wait
	1	2	3	4	5
Are the restroom facilities kept clean?	Reminded me of the gas station down the street				Spotless
	1	2	3	4	5

Theater

Question	1	2	3	4	5
Was the size of the theater sufficient for providing good seating?	Was there 30 minutes early and had to sit on the first row				Came in 5 minutes late and had the best seat in the house
Were the seats spacious, and did the theater provide adequate leg room?	If I weighed 2 more pounds I couldn't have fit in the seat				Enough room in the seat for both me and my date
Was the theater clean?	Afraid to get up because I might slip on the popcorn and soda on the floor from last night				Spotless
Were the aisles well lit for movement during the movie?	Dark				Bright as a sunny day
How was the quality of the picture?	Bad as the old B/W TV at the camp house				Better than my new TV at home
How was the quality of the sound of the movie?	Like an AM station 300 miles away				Like my own personal CD player
How was the sound volume?	Needed earplugs or a stethoscope				Like I would set it if I had the remote control
How was the temperature of the theater?	Needed a parka or a personal air-conditioner				Felt good
Did the movie start on time?	10 minutes late		5 min.		On-time
Were technical difficulties handled properly? (Not Applicable __________)	I was sent home				No problem, didn't even know it happened

Post-Movie

Question	1	2	3	4	5
Was it easy to get out of the movie?	Like a slow moving cattle call				Could have sprinted if I wanted to

Was the lighting after the movie adequate?	Dark				Bright as a sunny day
	1	2	3	4	5
Were there ushers to assist you after the movie?	Didn't see an employee within 5 miles				Too many staff to count
	1	2	3	4	5
Was there access back to concessions, restroom after the movie?	Locked up tighter than Fort Knox				Had to walk right past it to get out of the place
	1	2	3	4	5

Name: ______________________________ Phone: ______________________

FIGURE 6.9 Movie theater walk-through-audit.
(Prepared by Angela Loftin and Deborah Yancey under the supervision of Professor James A. Fitzsimmons.)

SUMMARY

The strategic importance of facility design and layout was demonstrated by the reported perceptions of Wal-Mart and Kmart by their customers. Facility design using aesthetics and decor must be consistent with the objectives of the service package. Analytical approaches that have been developed for product and process production systems were applied to the analysis of service facility layouts. With modification for service operations, process flowcharting was shown to be useful in analyzing service layouts to identify unnecessary activities, highlight points of potential service failure and customer contact, and identify space needs for waiting customers. The psychological implications of poor service layout were addressed, along with the need for effective signage and thoughtful facility design to avoid customer disorientation. Finally, a walk-through-audit for restaurants and one for movie theaters were provided as examples of a management tool for ensuring that the service delivery system is meeting customer expectations.

Chapter 7 will consider several approaches to the facility location problem and its impact on creating a competitive advantage.

KEY TERMS AND DEFINITIONS

Bottleneck the activity in a product layout that takes the most time to perform and thus defines the maximum flow rate for the entire process.

CRAFT (Computerized Relative Allocation of Facilities Technique) a computer program that uses the departmental exchange logic of operations sequence analysis to solve the relative location problem of process layouts.

Operations sequence analysis a procedure to improve the flow distance in a process layout by arranging the relative location of departments.

Process flowchart a table listing the sequence of activities for a service operation noting the type of activity

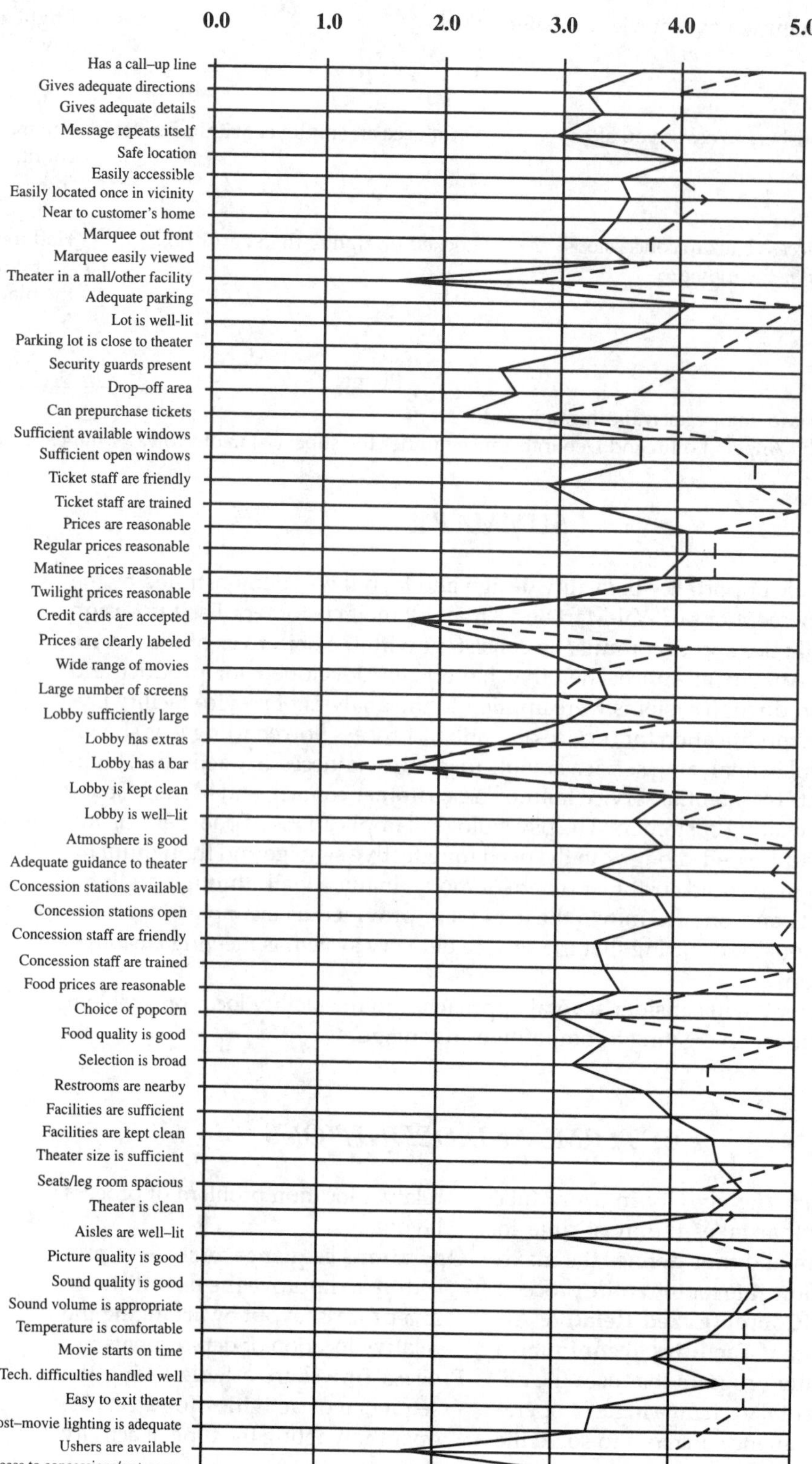

FIGURE 6.10. Movie theater walk-through-audit gap analysis.

with a symbol and the time and distance traveled.

Process layout a service permitting customization because customers determine their own sequence of activities (e.g., an amusement park).

Product layout a standardized service performed in a fixed sequence of steps (e.g., cafeteria).

Walk-through-audit a questionnaire administered to customers and managers to evaluate the perception of a service experience from beginning to end and across many detailed dimensions.

SOLVED PROBLEMS

1. Line-Balancing for Product Layout

Problem Statement

Arriving at JFK airport in New York from overseas requires a sequence of immigration and customs-clearing activities before a passenger can board a domestic flight for home. The table below lists the activities and their average times. Except for baggage claim, these activities must be performed in the sequence noted. What is the bottleneck activity and maximum number of passengers who can be processed per hour? What would you recommend to improve the balance of this process?

Activity	Average Time, *Sec*
1. Deplane	20
2. Immigration	16
3. Baggage claim	40
4. Customs	24
5. Check baggage	18
6. Board domestic flight	15

Solution

First, draw the product flow diagram, and identify the bottleneck activity. The slowest activity is "baggage claim," which results in a system capacity of 90 passengers per hour.

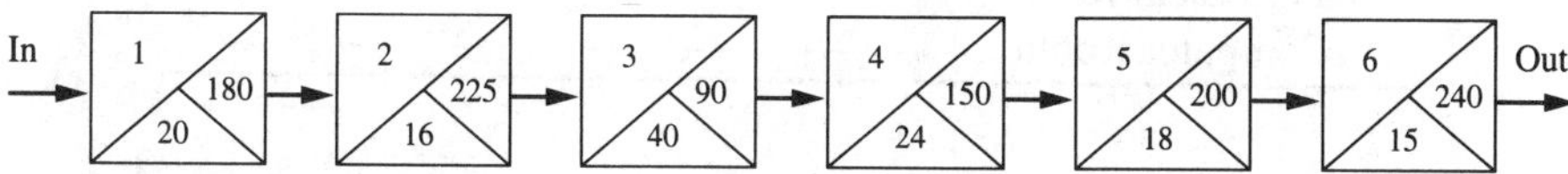

A recommendation for increasing system capacity could include doubling the capacity of the baggage claim area and combining the activities of the immigration and customs areas. This new product layout is shown in the flow diagram below, with the result of doubling the system capacity to 180 passengers per hour.

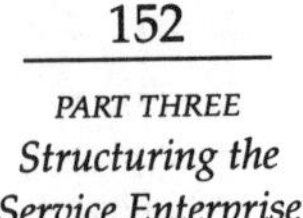

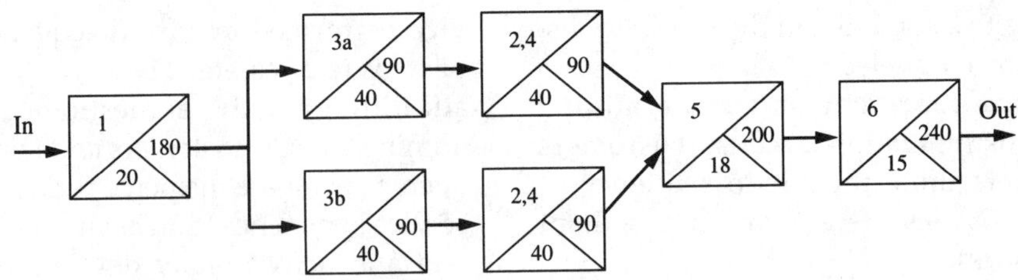

2. Relative Location for Process Layout

Problem Statement

The architect for the new undergraduate library is interested in a floor plan that would be viewed as convenient by users. Based on survey data from the old library, student movements between different areas in hundreds of trips per month are noted in the flow matrix below. Prepare a good initial rectangular layout that minimizes total flow distance between nonadjacent areas, then use operations sequence analysis to improve the layout.

Library Area	A	B	C	D	E	F
A Reserve Room	—	5	9	3	7	1
B Reference Room	3	—	8	2	6	2
C Copy Room	1	1	—	7	2	3
D Stacks	2	2	10	—	2	5
E Periodical Room	1	2	6	3	—	2
F Computer Room	1	1	1	4	2	—

Solution

First, create a triangularized total flow matrix by summing flows across the diagonal.

Library Area	A	B	C	D	E	F
A Reserve Room	—	8	10	5	8	2
B Reference Room	—	—	9	4	8	3
C Copy Room	—	—	—	17	8	4
D Stacks	—	—	—	—	5	9
E Periodical Room	—	—	—	—	—	4
F Computer Room	—	—	—	—	—	—

Second, locate library areas on the schematic rectangular layout shown below by placing high-flow areas adjacent to each other.

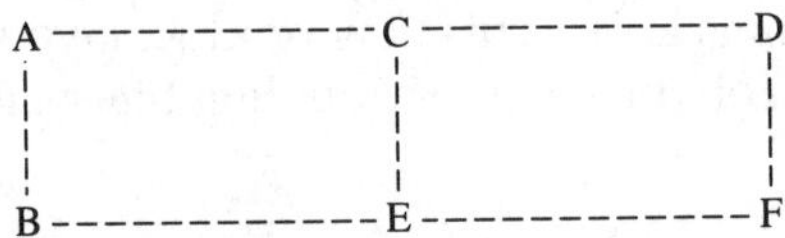

Next, calculate the total flow distance of nonadjacent pairs as shown below:

Nonadjacent Area Pairs	Flow	Distance		Total
AD	5	2	=	10
AF	2	2	=	4
BD	4	2	=	8
BF	3	2	=	6
				28

Finally, look for improvement by exchanging a pair of nonadjacent areas. Because no improvement is possible, accept the above layout.

TOPICS FOR DISCUSSION

1. Compare the attention given to aesthetics in different waiting rooms you have visited. How was your mood affected by the different environments?
2. For Example 6.2, the Ocean World theme park, make an argument for not locating popular attractions next to each other.
3. Select a service, and discuss how the design and layout of the facility meet the five factors: nature and objectives of the organization, land availability and space requirements, flexibility, aesthetics, and the community and environment.
4. Give examples of service designs and layouts that accentuate the service concept and examples that detract from the service concept. Explain the successes and failures.
5. The CRAFT program is an example of a heuristic programming approach to problem solving. Why may CRAFT not find the optimal solution to a layout problem?
6. Select a service, and prepare a list of questions and measures for a walk-through-audit.

EXERCISES

6.1. Revisit the Automobile Driver's License Office, and assume that some of our previous recommendations for investment have been implemented. For example, "checking for violations and restrictions" will be done on a computer terminal, with that activity now taking 30 instead of 60 seconds. However, no additional eye-test machines or cameras were purchased.

a. Assuming that one worker is assigned to each activity, what is the bottleneck activity and the maximum number of applicants who can be seen per hour?

b. Suggest a reallocation of activities among the six workers that would result in a service capacity of 120 applicants per hour. What investment would be required to implement your layout recommendation?

6.2. Getting a physical examination at a physician's office involves a series of steps. The table below lists these activities and their average times. The activities can occur in any order, but the doctor's consultation must be the last. Three nurses are assigned to perform activities 1, 2, and 4.

Activity	Average Time, *Min*
1. Blood pressure, wt., temp.	6
2. Medical history	20
3. Doctor's checkup	18
4. Lab work	10
5. Doctor's consultation	12

a. What is the bottleneck activity and the maximum number of patients who can be seen per hour?

b. Suggest a reallocation of nursing and/or doctor activities that would result in increased service capacity, and draw a product flow diagram. What is the capacity of your improved system?

6.3. A school cafeteria is operated by five persons performing the activities listed below in the average times shown.

Activity	Average Time, *Sec*
1. Serve salad and dessert	10
2. Pour drinks	30
3. Serve entree	60
4. Serve vegetables	20
5. Tally and collect payment	40

a. What is the bottleneck activity and the maximum service capacity per hour?

b. Suggest a reallocation of activities that would increase capacity and use only four employees, and draw a product flow diagram. What is the capacity of your improved system?

c. Recommend a way to maintain the serving capacity found in part b using only three employees.

6.4. Every fall, volunteers administer flu vaccine shots at a local supermarket. The process involves the following four steps:

Activity	Average Time, *Sec*
1. Reception	30
2. Drug allergy consultation	60
3. Fill out form and sign waiver	45
4. Administer vaccination	90

a. What is the bottleneck activity and maximum number of people who can be processed per hour?

b. If a fifth volunteer is assigned to help administer vaccinations, what activity now becomes the bottleneck? How has this arrangement influenced the capacity of the system?

c. Using five volunteers, suggest a reallocation of activities that would result in increased service capacity, and draw a product flow diagram. What is the capacity of your improved system?

6.5. Revisit the Ocean World Theme Park, and use the daily flow of visitors between attractions found in Example 6.2 for a different analysis.

a. Recommend a layout that would *maximize* the total travel distance between attractions.

b. What benefit would such a layout have for the owners of Ocean World Theme Park?

c. What reservations do you have about using the data from Table 6.2 for this new approach to the Ocean World Theme Park layout?

6.6. The Second Best Discount Store is considering rearranging its stockroom to improve customer service. Currently, stock pickers are given customer orders to fill from six warehouse areas. Movement between these areas is noted in the flow matrix below:

Using the initial layout below, perform an operations sequence analysis to determine a layout that minimizes total flow between nonadjacent departments. Calculate your flow improvement.

	A	B	C	D	E	F
A	—	1	4	2	0	3
B	0	—	2	0	2	1
C	2	2	—	4	5	2
D	3	0	2	—	0	2
E	1	4	3	1	—	4
F	4	3	1	2	0	—

6.7. A convenience store is considering changing its layout to encourage impulse buying. The triangular flow matrix below gives the measure of association between different product groups (e.g., beer, milk, magazines). A plus sign (+) indicates a high association, such as between beer and peanuts; a minus sign (–) indicates a repulsion, such as between beer and milk; and a zero (0) indicates no association.

	A	B	C	D	E	F
A		+	+	0	0	–
B			+	0	–	–
C				+	+	0
D					+	+
E						0
F						

Using the initial layout below, perform an operations sequence analysis to determine a layout that will encourage impulse buying by placing high-association product groups close to one another.

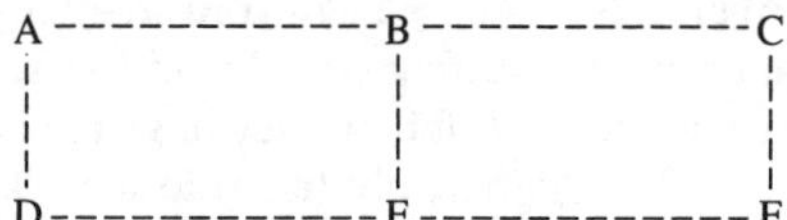

6.8. A community college that recently acquired a parcel of land is now preparing site plans. There is interest in locating academic departments in each of six buildings along a mall with three buildings on each side. Based on registration patterns, the daily flow of students between these six departments in hundreds is shown below.

	A	B	C	D	E	F
A. Psychology	—	6	4	8	7	1
B. English	6	—	2	3	9	5
C. Mathematics	6	1	—	12	2	4
D. Economics	3	2	10	—	3	5
E. History	7	11	2	1	—	6
F. Biology	6	2	8	10	3	—

Using the initial layout below, perform an operations sequence analysis to determine a site plan for the community college that will minimize the distance that students need to walk between classes.

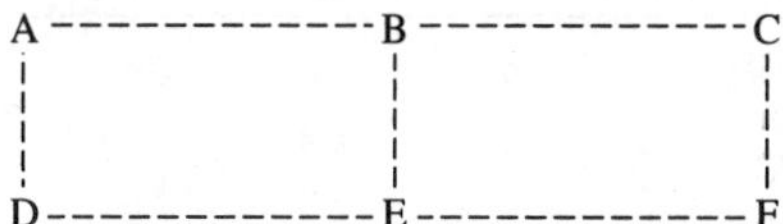

Service Benchmark

Software, Peripherals Take a Back Seat to Big Iron

The presentation of computer-related merchandise in consumer electronics superstores varies widely and reflects the different clientele and marketing strategies of the companies.

For Best Buy, computers are an important customer draw. As such , they are promoted heavily and assorted deeply, but are located in the back of the store. To get to the computers, customers must walk through the music CD, video-game or other departments.

For Circuit City Stores, computers are an important draw as well, but the customer needn't search for the systems. PCs are usually placed front and center, in front of a counter that resembles an island in the middle of the store. The rest of the computer-related merchandise is usually wrapped around this island.

At Incredible Universe, with the wide variety of merchandise on display in different departments, just finding the computer systems can be a challenge-let alone finding the software or computer accessories. The saving grace for the category, which takes a back seat to appliances and large-screen TVs in the chain's print ads, is that the consumer must walk through the computer department to get to the consumer electronics.

The different presentations are useful for these retailers in their efforts to differentiate themselves. But their strategies break down as soon as the customer looks beyond the heavy metal.

At Circuit City, the computers are all bunched together at the front of the store. The customer could not possibly fail to see that the chain is in the computer business with such an impressive assortment of hardware. But, software, peripherals and accessories are merchandised in different locations, depending on which Circuit City you visit. As a result, the company sells minimal quantities of these items, especially when compared with Best Buy.

Best Buy does a better job, but it can't hold a candle to the kind of presentation at CompUSA or Computer City SuperCenters. Best Buy offers several aisles of accessories, peripherals and software, and promotes the categories prominently in the stores and its advertising. The company also promotes system set-up-at home or in the store- as well as system upgrades and component installation.

Circuit City offers some of these same services, but for a much shorter assortment of products, offered in an inconsistent presentation. Incredible University is closer to Best Buy than to Circuit City in its assortment, presentation and available services. "Circuit City has fabulous merchandising, except for the computer department," said one supplier. "It's hit or miss."

Suppliers say Circuit City is promoting more software, but that the commissioned sales environment is a major hindrance. "In a commission environment like Circuit City, you don't want to sell a $30 mouse." one supplier said. "The same is true for Campo, Sun TV or The Good Guys!"

Best Buy, with a noncommissioned sales force, does better with software, but also offers a broader product assortment.

"All of the consumer electronics guys are trying to increase their sales in these categories," said Adam Levin, president of market research and consulting firm Levin Consulting, Beachwood, Ohio. "But first, they have to make a decision not to keep these products hidden. Circuit City has done a good job with its systems display, but has been inconsistent with peripherals and accessories. They need predictable, dedicated sections."

Levin said customers are looking for destination stores for accessories and peripherals. While electronics superstores are perceived as destination stores for systems and printers, only computer superstores and office-product superstores are seen as destinations for buying accessories, supplies and peripherals. "Our clients have found that the longer a store is in the market, the more software and peripherals it sells. It's a word-of-mouth and selection issue," he said.

Source: Adapted from Roger C. Lanctot, "Software, Peripherals Take a Back Seat To Big Iron," *Computer Retail Week,* © CMP Media, Inc., March 4, 1996, no. 628, p. 64

CASE: HEALTH MAINTENANCE ORGANIZATION (A)

In January 1996, Joan Taylor, the administrator of the Life-Time Insurance Company HMO in Buffalo, New York, was pleased with the Austin, Texas, location that was selected for a new ambulatory health center. (The process used to select this site is discussed in Chapter 7.) The center not only would serve as a clinic for the acutely ill but also as a center for preventive health services.

An important goal of the HMO was to offer programs that would encourage members to stay healthy. Various programs already had been planned, including those on smoking cessation, proper nutrition, diet, and exercise.

The clinic portion of the health center would be quite large; however, certain constraints in the layout would be necessary. Acutely ill patients would need to be separated from well patients. In addition, local safety regulations prohibited the radiography department from being adjacent to the main waiting room.

It was very important to Ms. Taylor to minimize the walking distance for both the patients and the HMO personnel. The matrix below provides the expected flow between departments based on 40 patients per day.

Questions

1. Beginning with a good initial layout, use operations sequence analysis to determine a better layout that would minimize the walking distance between different areas in the clinic.

2. Defend your final layout based on features other than minimizing walking distance.

		A	B	C	D	E	F
Reception	A	—	30	0	5	0	0
Waiting room	B	10	—	40	10	0	0
Examination	C	15	20	—	15	5	5
Laboratory	D	5	18	8	—	6	3
Radiography	E	0	4	1	2	—	4
Minor surgery	F	2	0	0	0	1	—

CASE: HEALTH MAINTENANCE ORGANIZATION (B)

The administrator of the Life-Time Insurance Company HMO, Ms. Taylor, was anxious to solve potential problems before their new clinic opened in Austin, Texas. In Buffalo, New York, where the original clinic is located, the pharmacy had been extremely busy from the beginning, and long waiting times for prescriptions to be filled presented a very real problem.

The Buffalo HMO pharmacy was modern, spacious, and well designed. The peak time for prescriptions was between 10 AM and 3 PM. During this period, prescriptions would back up, and the waiting time would increase. After 5 PM, the staff would be reduced to one pharmacist and one technician, but the two had no trouble providing very timely service throughout the evening.

Ms. Taylor became acutely aware of the long waiting times after several complaints had been lodged. Each stated that the waiting time had exceeded 1 hour. As shown in the table below, the pharmacy is staffed with five persons on duty until 5 PM.

Ms. Taylor personally studied the tasks of all the pharmacy personnel. She noted the time required to accomplish each task, and her results are listed below as well. Because the prescriptions were filled in an assembly-line fashion, each person performed only one task.

Activity	Time, *Sec*
Receive prescriptions	24
Type labels	120
Fill prescriptions	60
Check prescriptions	40
Dispense prescriptions	30

Note: The activities of filling, checking, and dispensing prescriptions must be performed by a registered pharmacist.

Questions

1. Identify the bottleneck activity, and show how capacity can be increased by using only two pharmacists and two clerks.

2. In addition to savings on personnel costs, what benefits does this arrangement have?

CASE: ESQUIRE DEPARTMENT STORE

Established by Arthur Babbitt, Sr., in 1971, Esquire Department Store has shown a recent decline in sales. The store manager, young Arthur Babbitt, Jr., has noticed a decrease in the movement of customers between departments. He believes that customers are not spending enough time in the store, and that this may result from the present layout, which is based on the concept of locating related departments close to each other. Babbitt, Sr., is not convinced. He argues that he has been in business for about 20 years, and that the loyal customers are not likely to quit shopping here simply because of the layout. He believes they are losing customers to the new factory outlet mall outside town, which seems to attract them away with discount prices.

Babbitt, Jr., explains that the greater the distance the customer travels between departments, the more products the customer will see. Customers usually have something specific in mind when they go shopping, but exposure to more products may stimulate additional purchases. Thus, to Babbitt, Jr., it seems that the best answer to this problem is to change the present layout so that customers are exposed to more products. He feels the environment today is different from the environment of 1971, and that the company must display products better and encourage impulse buying.

At this point, Babbitt, Sr., interrupts to say, "Son, you may have a point here about the store layout. But before I spend money on tearing this place up, I need to see some figures. Develop a new layout, and show me how much you can increase the time customers spend in the store."

Babbitt, Jr., returns to his office and pulls out some information that he has gathered about revising the store layout. He has estimated that on average, 57 customers enter the store per hour. The store operates 10 hours a day, 200 days a year. He has a drawing of the present layout, which is shown in Figure 6.11, and a chart depicting the flow of customers between departments, which is shown in Table 6.4.

Questions

1. Use CRAFT software to develop a layout that will maximize customer time in the store.

2. What percentage increase in customer time spent in the store is achieved by the proposed layout?

3. What other consumer behavior concepts should be considered in the relative location of departments?

FIGURE 6.11. Current layout of Esquire Department Store. (Figures in parentheses refer to rows and columns.)

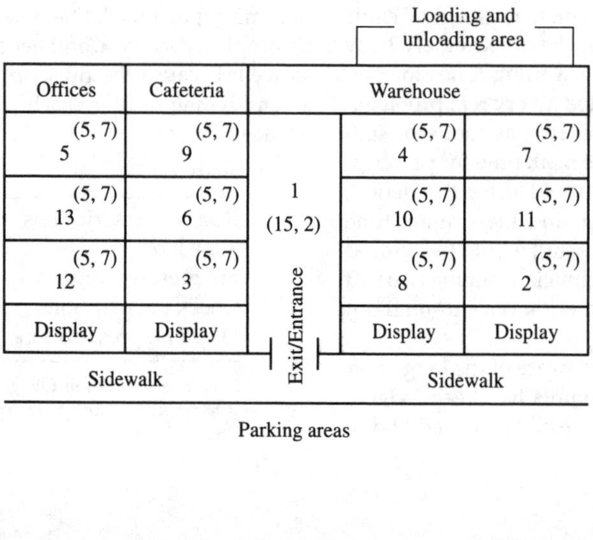

Loading and unloading area

Offices	Cafeteria		Warehouse	
(5, 7) 5	(5, 7) 9		(5, 7) 4	(5, 7) 7
(5, 7) 13	(5, 7) 6	1 (15, 2)	(5, 7) 10	(5, 7) 11
(5, 7) 12	(5, 7) 3		(5, 7) 8	(5, 7) 2
Display	Display	Exit/Entrance	Display	Display

Sidewalk | Sidewalk

Parking areas

TABLE 6.4. Flow of Customers Between Departments, in Thousands

	1	2	3	4	5	6	7	8	9	10	11	12	13
1	0	32	41	19	21	7	13	22	10	11	8	6	10
2	17	0	24	31	16	3	13	17	25	8	7	9	12
3	8	14	0	25	9	28	17	16	14	7	9	24	18
4	25	12	16	0	18	26	22	9	6	28	20	16	14
5	10	12	15	20	0	18	17	24	28	30	25	9	19
6	8	14	12	17	20	0	19	23	30	32	37	15	21
7	13	19	23	25	3	45	0	29	27	31	41	24	16
8	28	9	17	19	21	5	7	0	21	19	25	10	9
9	14	8	13	15	22	18	13	25	0	33	27	14	19
10	18	25	17	19	23	15	25	27	31	0	21	17	10
11	29	28	31	16	29	19	18	33	26	31	0	16	16
12	17	31	25	21	19	17	19	21	31	29	25	0	19
13	12	25	16	33	14	19	31	17	22	15	24	18	0

1. Exit-entrance
2. Appliances
3. Audio-stereo-TV
4. Jewelry
5. Housewares
6. Cosmetics
7. Ladies' ready-to-wear
8. Men's ready-to-wear
9. Boys' clothing
10. Sporting goods
11. Ladies' lingerie
12. Shoes
13. Furniture

SELECTED BIBLIOGRAPHY

ARMOUR, G. C.: "A Heuristic Algorithm and Simulation Approach to Relative Location of Facilities," *Management Science,* vol. 9, no. 1, September 1963, pp. 294–309.

ATKINSON, G. A., and R. J. PHILLIPS: "Hospital Design: Factors Influencing the Choice of Shape," *The Architects' Journal Information Library,* April 1964, pp. 851–855.

BITNER, MARY JO: "Evaluating Service Encounters: The Effects of Physical Surroundings and Employee Responses," *Journal of Marketing,* vol. 54, April 1990, pp. 69–82.

BUFFA, ELWOOD S.: "Sequence Analysis for Functional Layouts," *Journal of Industrial Engineering,* vol. 6, no. 2, March–April 1955, pp. 12–13.

———, G. C. ARMOUR, and T. E. VOLLMANN: "Allocating Facilities with CRAFT," *Harvard Business Review,* vol. 42, no. 2, March–April 1964, pp. 136–159.

FITZSIMMONS, J. A. and G. MAURER: "A Walk-Through Audit to Improve Restaurant Performance," *The Cornell HRA Quarterly,* vol. 31, no. 4, February 1991, pp. 94–99.

FRANCIS, R. L., and J. A. WHITE: *Facility Layout and Location: An Analytical Approach,* Prentice-Hall, Inc., Englewood Cliffs, N.J., 1974.

KIMES, S. E., and S. A. MUTKOSKI: "The Express Guest Check: Saving Steps with Process Design," *The Cornell HRA Quarterly,* vol. 30, no. 2, August 1989, pp. 21–25.

MARKIN, R. J., C. M. LILLIS, and C. L. NARAYANA: "Social-Psychological Significance of Store Space," *Journal of Retailing,* Spring 1976, pp. 43–54.

NORMAN, D. A.: *The Psychology of Everyday Things,* Basic Books, New York, 1988.

NUGENT, C. E., T. E. VOLLMANN, and J. RUML: "An Experimental Comparison of Techniques for the Assignment of Facilities to Locations," *Operations Research,* vol. 16, no. 1, January–February 1968, pp. 150–173.

SOMMERS, M. S., and J. B. KERNAN: "A Behavioral Approach to Planning, Layout and Display," *Journal of Retailing,* Winter 1965–1966, pp. 21–26, 62.

VOLLMANN, T. E., C. E. NUGENT, and R. L. ZARTLER: "A Computerized Model for Office Layout," *Journal of Industrial Engineering,* vol. 19, no. 7, July 1968, pp. 321–327.

———, and E. S. BUFFA: "The Facilities Layout Problem in Perspective," *Management Science*, vol. 12, no. 10, June 1966, pp. 450–468.

WENER, RICHARD A.: "The Environmental Psychology of Service Encounters," in J. A. Czepiel, M. R. Solomon, and C. F. Surprenant (eds.), *The Service Encounter*, Lexington Books, Lexington, Mass., 1985, pp. 101–113.

CHAPTER 7

Service Facility Location

LEARNING OBJECTIVES

After completing this chapter, you should be able to:

1. Discuss how a facility location is affected by selection of the criteria for judging customer service.
2. Locate a single facility using the cross-median approach.
3. Evaluate the business viability of a retail location by estimating expected revenues and market share using the Huff model.
4. Locate multiple facilities using the set covering model.
5. Discuss the nontraditional location strategies: competitive clustering, saturation marketing, marketing intermediaries, and substitution of communications for transportation.

In addition to the traditional role of creating entry barriers and generating demand, location also affects the strategic dimensions of flexibility, competitive positioning, demand management, and focus.

Flexibility of a location is a measure of the degree to which the service can react to changing economic situations. Because location decisions are long-term commitments with capital-intensive aspects, it is essential to select locations that can be responsive to future economic, demographic, cultural, and competitive changes. For example, locating sites in a number of states could reduce the overall risk of a financial crisis resulting from regional economic downturns. This portfolio approach to multisite location could be augmented by selecting individual sites near inelastic demand (e.g., locating a hotel near a convention center).

Competitive positioning refers to methods by which the firm can establish itself relative to its competitors. Multiple locations can serve as a barrier to competition through building a firm's competitive position and establishing a market awareness. Acquiring and holding prime locations before the market has developed can keep the competition from gaining access to these desirable locations and create an artificial barrier to entry (analogous to a product patent).

Demand management is the ability to control the quantity, quality, and timing of demand. For example, hotels cannot manipulate capacity effectively because of the fixed nature of the facility; however, a hotel can control demand by locating near a diverse set of market generators that supply a steady demand regardless of the economic condition, day of the week, or season.

Focus can be developed by offering the same narrowly defined service at many locations. Many multisite service firms develop a standard (or formula) facility that can be duplicated at many locations. While this "cookie-cutter" approach makes expansion easier, sites that are located in close proximity could siphon business from each other. This problem of demand cannibalization can be avoided if a firm establishes a pattern of desired growth for its multisite expansion.

Traditionally, location decisions have been based on intuition and had a considerable range of success. Although site selection often is based on opportunistic factors such as site availability and favorable leasing, a quantitative analysis can be useful to avoid a serious mistake. For example, regardless of how low the rent may be, being the only store in a deserted shopping mall offers no advantage.

CHAPTER PREVIEW

This chapter begins with an overview of the problem structure, including travel-time models, site selection, decision-making criteria, and estimation of geographic demand. Facility location models for both single- and multiple-facility systems also are explored. These models are illustrated with both public and private sector examples. The models are oriented toward selecting a site for a physical facility, but they could be used to deploy mobile units such as ambulances, police cars, and repair vehicles for field service.

Until now, we have assumed that the consumer and provider must be together physically for a service to be performed; however, alternatives exist if one is willing to substitute communication for transportation or to use marketing intermediaries. Such alternatives will be explored as possible methods of extending services beyond their immediate geographic area.

LOCATION CONSIDERATIONS

Many factors enter into the decision to locate a service facility. Figure 7.1 classifies location issues that will be used to guide our discussion throughout this chapter. The broad categories are geographic representation, number of facilities, and optimization criteria.

Geographic Representation

The traditional classification of location problems is based on how the geography is modeled. Location options and travel distance can be represented either on a plane or a network. Location on a plane (i.e., flat surface) is characterized by a solution space that has infinite possibilities. Facilities may be located anywhere on the plane and are identified by an *xy* cartesian coordinate (or, in a global context, by latitudes and longitudes), as shown in Figure 7.2. Distance between locations is measured at the extremes in one of two ways. One method is the *euclidian metric,* or vector, travel distance (remember the Pythagorean theorem), which is defined as:

$$d_{ij} = \left[(x_i - x_j)^2 + (y_i - y_j)^2 \right]^{1/2} \tag{1}$$

where d_{ij} = distance between points i and j,
x_i, y_i = coordinates of the ith point, and
x_j, y_j = coordinates of the jth point.

FIGURE 7.1. Classification of service facility location issues.

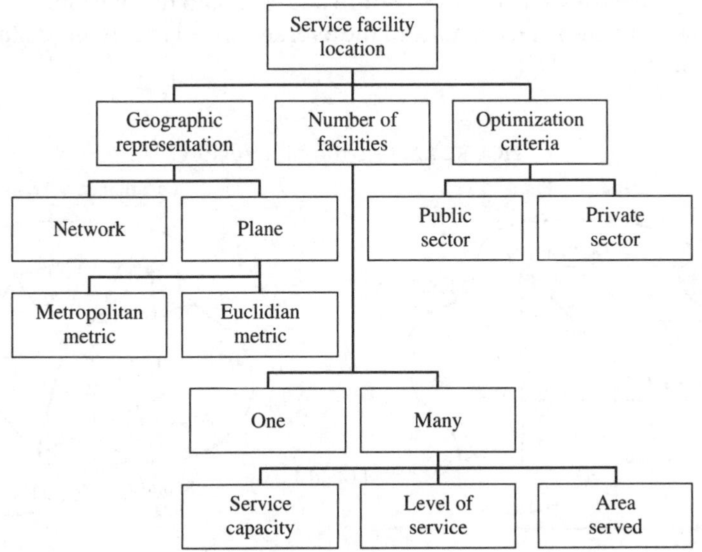

For example, if

the origin $x_i, y_i = 2, 2$ and the destination $x_j, y_j = 4, 4$

then

$$d_{ij} = \left[(2-4)^2 + (2-4)^2\right]^{1/2} = 2.83$$

The other method is the *metropolitan metric,* or rectangular displacement, travel distance (i.e., north-south and east-west travel in urban areas), which is defined as:

$$d_{ij} = |x_i - x_j| + |y_i - y_j| \tag{2}$$

Using the same example from above for the metropolitan metric:

$$d_{ij} = |2-4| + |2-4| = 4.0$$

Location on a network is characterized by a solution space that is restricted to the nodes of that network. For example, a highway system could be considered a network, with major highway intersections as nodes. The arcs of the network represent travel distance (or time) between pairs of nodes, calculated using the shortest route.

The selection of geographic representation and distance metric often is dictated by the economics of the data collection effort and the problem environment. Networks can represent more accurately the geographic uniqueness of an area (e.g., the travel restrictions caused by a river with few bridges or by mountainous terrain). Unfortunately, the cost of gathering the travel times between nodes can be prohibitive. When locating is done on a plane that represents an urban area, the metropolitan metric often is used, because streets for some cities are arranged in an east-west and north-south pattern. Both the metropolitan and euclidian metrics require an estimate of the average speed to convert distance traveled to time.

FIGURE 7.2. Geographic structure.

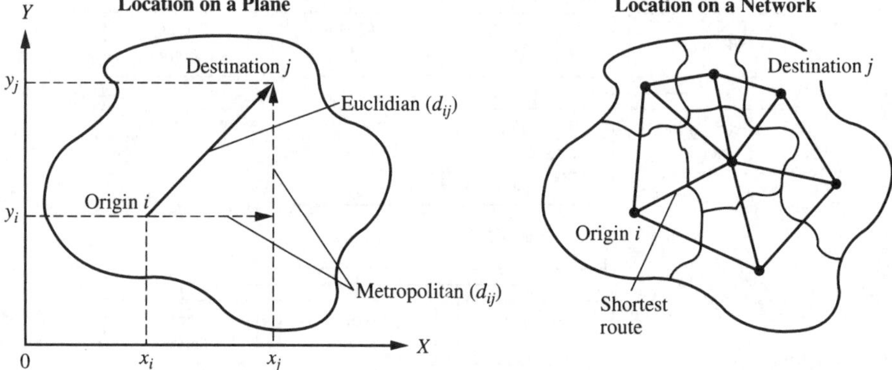

Number of Facilities

The location of a single facility generally can be treated mathematically with little difficulty. Unfortunately, the methods used to site a single facility do not guarantee optimal results when they are modified and applied to multisite location problems. Finding a unique set of sites is complicated by assigning demand nodes to sites (i.e., defining service areas for each site), and the problem is complicated further if the capacity at each site varies. In addition, for some services such as health care, a hierarchy of service exists. Private physicians and clinics offer primary care, general hospitals provide primary care plus hospitalization, and health centers add special treatment capabilities. Thus, the selection of services provided also may be a variable in multisite location studies.

Optimization Criteria

Private and public sector location problems are similar in that they share the objective of maximizing some measure of benefit. The location criteria that are chosen differ, however, because the "ownership" is different. Within the private sector, the location decision is governed by either minimization of cost (e.g., in the case of distribution centers) or maximization of profit (e.g., in the case of retail locations). In contrast, we like to think that public facility decisions are governed by the needs of society as a whole. The objective for public decision making is to maximize a societal benefit that may be difficult to quantify.

Private Sector Criteria

Traditional private sector location analysis focuses on a tradeoff between the cost of building and operating facilities and the cost of transportation. Much of the literature has addressed this problem, which is appropriate for the distribution of products (i.e., the warehouse location problem). These models may find some applications in services, however, when the services are delivered to the customers (e.g., consulting, auditing, janitorial, and lawn care services).

When the consumer travels to the facility, no direct cost is incurred by the provider. Instead, distance becomes a barrier restricting potential consumer demand and the corresponding revenue generated. Facilities such as retail shopping centers therefore are located to attract the maximum number of customers.

Public Sector Criteria

Location decisions in the public sector are complicated by the lack of agreement on goals and the difficulty of measuring benefits in dollars to make tradeoffs with facility investment. Because the benefits of a public service are difficult to define or quantify directly, surrogate (or substitute) measures of utility are used.

The average distance traveled by users to reach the facility is a popular surrogate. The smaller this quantity, the more accessible the system is to its users. Thus, the problem becomes one of minimizing the total average distance traveled, with a constraint on the number of facilities. The problem is additionally constrained by some maximum travel distance for the user. Another possibility is the creation of demand. Here the user population is not considered fixed but is determined by the location, size, and number of facilities. The greater the demand created or drawn, the more efficient the system is in filling the needs of the region.

These utility surrogates are optimized with constraints on investment. Analysis of cost-effectiveness usually is performed to examine tradeoffs between investment and utility. The tradeoffs for the surrogates are: 1) the decrease in average distance traveled per additional thousand-dollar investment, and 2) the increase in demand per additional thousand-dollar investment.

Effect of Criteria on Location

The selection of optimization criteria influences service facility location. For example, William J. Abernathy and John C. Hershey studied the location of health centers for a three-city region.[1] As part of that study, they noted the effect of health-center locations with respect to the following criteria:

1. *Maximize utilization.* Maximize the total number of visits to the centers.
2. *Minimize distance per capita.* Minimize the average distance per capita to the closest center.
3. *Minimize distance per visit.* Minimize the average per-visit travel distance to the nearest center.

The problem was structured so that each city had a population with a different mix of health care consumption characteristics. These characteristics were measured along two dimensions: 1) the effect of distance as a barrier to health care use, and 2) the utilization rate at immediate proximity to a health care center. Figure 7.3 shows a map of the three cities and the location of a single health care center under each of the three criteria. These criteria yield entirely different locations because of the different behavioral patterns of each city. For criterion 1 (maximize utilization), the center is located at city C, because this city contains a large number of elderly individuals for whom distance is a strong barrier. City B is selected under criterion 2 (minimize distance per capita), because this city is centrally located between the two larger cities. City A is the largest population center and has the most mobile and frequent users of health care; therefore, criterion 3 (minimize distance per visit) leads to this city being selected.

ESTIMATION OF GEOGRAPHIC DEMAND

The quality of service facility location analysis rests on an accurate assessment of geographic demand for the service (i.e., demand by geographic area). This requires the selection both of some geographic unit that partitions the area to be served and of some method for predicting demand from each of these partitions.

[1]W. J. Abernathy and J. C. Hershey, "A Spatial-Allocation Model for Regional Health-Services Planning," *Operations Research,* vol. 20, no. 3, May–June 1972, pp. 629–642.

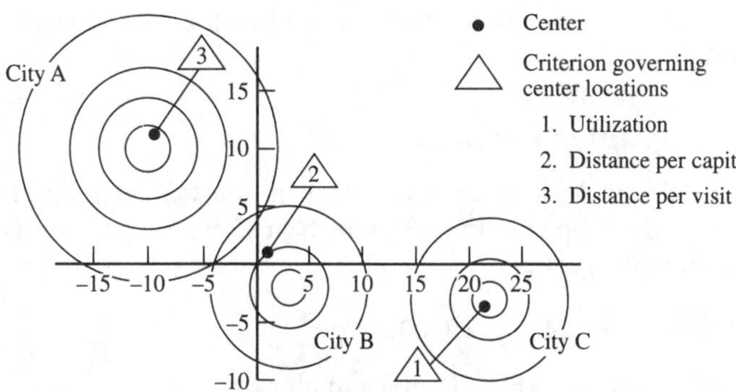

FIGURE 7.3. Location of one health center for three different criteria.
(W. J. Abernathy and J. C. Hershey, "A Spatial-Allocation Model for Regional Health-Services Planning." Reprinted with permission from Operations Research, *vol. 20, no. 3, 1972, p. 637. Operations Research Society of America. No further reproduction permitted without the consent of the copyright owner.)*

Census tracts or their smaller divisions, the block or block groups, are used. In many cases, the demand for service is collected empirically by searching past records for addresses of users and tallying these by district. The steps that define geographic demand will be illustrated by an example of a day care center.[2]

Define the Target Population

The characteristics that define the target population must be established. For example, if a system of day care centers for all families is being established, the target population might consist of families with children younger than 5 years and an employable adult. A private system also might include the ability to pay. In this example, the target population is defined as families that receive Aid to Families with Dependent Children (AFDC) support with children younger than 5 years and an employable parent.

Select a Unit of Area

For accuracy, geographic units should be as small as practicable. There are two limits: 1) the unit must be large enough to contain a sample size that is sufficient for estimating demand, and 2) the number of units must not exceed the computational capacity of the computers and facility location techniques. A census tract often is selected as the unit, because demographic data on the residents are readily available on computer tapes from the U.S. Census Bureau. In this study, block

[2]From L. A. Brown, F. B. Williams, C. Youngmann, J. Holmes, and K. Walby, "The Location of Urban Population Service Facilities: A Strategy and Its Application," *Social Science Quarterly,* vol. 54, no. 4, March 1974, pp. 784–799.

groups were selected as units, because census tracts were too large and single blocks too small.

Estimate Geographic Demand

Demographic data on block-group residents were analyzed statistically using linear regression to develop equation (3), which predicts the percentage of AFDC families in each block group:

$$Y_i = 0.0043X_{1i} + 0.0248X_{2i} + 0.0092X_{3i} \tag{3}$$

where Y_i = percentage of AFDC families in block group i,
X_{1i} = percentage of persons in block group i who are younger than 18 years and living in a housing unit with more than 1.5 persons per room,
X_{2i} = percentage of families in block group i with a single male head and children younger than 18 years, and
X_{3i} = percentage of families in block group i with a single female head and children younger than 18 years.

Once Y_i, a percentage, was estimated for each block group, it was multiplied by both the number of families in the block group and the average number of children younger than 5 years per family. This figure became the estimate for the number of children requiring day care service from each block group. For example, assume that 50 families live in block group 10 and they have an average of 2 children younger than 5 years per family. If Y_{10} is found to be 30 percent using equation (3), then the estimate of children from this block group who require day care would be equal to (.30)(50)(2) = 30.

Map Geographic Demand

The demand for each block group is plotted on a three-dimensional map to provide a visual representation of the geographic distribution of day care needs. The visual depiction of demand is useful for highlighting neighborhoods with concentrated demand that are possible candidates as sites for day care centers. Further, many facility location techniques require an initial set of locations that are improved on successively. Thus, the demand map is useful for selecting good starting locations.

FACILITY LOCATION TECHNIQUES

An understanding of the facility location problem can be gained from the results of locating a single facility on a line. For example, consider the problem of locating a beach mat concession along the beach front at Waikiki. Suppose you wish to find a location that would minimize the average walk to your concession from anywhere on the beach. Further, suppose you have data showing the density of bathers along the beachfront, which is related to the size and location of hotels. This problem is shown schematically in Figure 7.4.

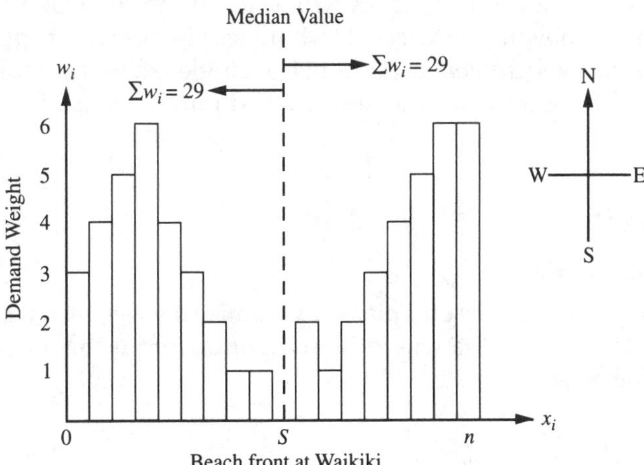

FIGURE 7.4. Locating a single facility along a line.

The objective is:

$$\text{Minimize} \quad Z = \sum_{i=0}^{s} w_i(s - x_i) + \sum_{i=s}^{n} w_i(x_i - s) \tag{4}$$

where w_i = relative weight of demand attached to the ith location on the beach,

x_i = location of the ith demand point on the beach in feet from the origin, in this case taken to be the west end of the beach, and

s = site of the beach mat concession.

The total-distance function Z is differentiated with respect to s and set equal to zero. This yields

$$\frac{dZ}{ds} = \sum_{i=0}^{s} w_i - \sum_{i=s}^{n} w_i = 0 \qquad \text{or}$$

$$\sum_{i=0}^{s} w_i = \sum_{i=s}^{n} w_i \tag{5}$$

This result suggests that the site should be located at the median with respect to the density distribution of bathers. That is, the site is located so that 50 percent of the potential demand is to each side (i.e., 29 in Figure 7.4). We probably should have expected this, because the median has the property of minimizing the sum of the absolute deviations from it.

The result for locating a site along a line can be generalized for locating a site on a plane if we use the metropolitan metric. Total travel distance will be minimized if the coordinates of the site correspond to the intersection of the x and y medians for their respective density distributions. We will refer to this as the *cross-median* approach.

The selection of a solution technique is determined by the characteristics of the problem, as outlined in Figure 7.1. Our discussion of location techniques is not exhaustive, but a few techniques will be discussed to illustrate various approaches to the problem. The selected techniques also represent approaches that deal with the various problem characteristics: single-facility vs. multiple-facility location, location on a plane or a network, and public vs. private optimization criteria.

Single Facility

Metropolitan Metric

Locating a single facility on a plane to minimize the weighted travel distances by means of the metropolitan metric is straightforward using the cross-median approach. The objective is:

$$Z = \sum_{i=1}^{n} w_i\{|x_i - x_s| + |y_i - y_s|\} \tag{6}$$

where w_i = weight attached to the ith point (e.g., population),
x_i, y_i = coordinates of the ith demand point,
x_s, y_s = coordinates of the service facility, and
n = number of demand points served.

Note that the objective function may be restated as two independent terms.

$$\text{Minimize } Z = \sum_{i=1}^{n} w_i|x_i - x_s| + \sum_{i=1}^{n} w_i|y_i - y_s| \tag{7}$$

Recall from our beach mat example that the median of a discrete set of values is such that the sum of absolute deviations from it is a minimum. Thus, our optimum site will have coordinates such that: 1) x_s is at the median value for w_i ordered in the x direction, and 2) y_s is at the median value for w_i ordered in the y direction. Because x_s, y_s, or both may be unique or lie within a range, the optimal location may be at a point, on a line, or within an area.

Example 7.1: Copying Service

A copying service has decided to open an office in the central business district of a city. The manager has identified four office buildings that will generate a major portion of its business, and Figure 7.5 shows the location of these demand points on an *xy* coordinate system. Weights are attached to each point and represent potential demand per month in hundreds of orders. The manager would like to determine a central location that will minimize the total distance per month that customers travel to the copying service.

Because of the urban location, a metropolitan metric is appropriate. A site located by the cross-median approach will be used to solve this problem. First, the median is calculated using equation (8):

$$\text{Median} = \sum_{i=1}^{n} \frac{w_i}{2} \tag{8}$$

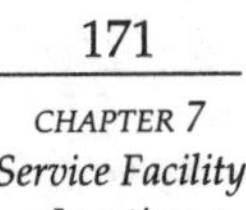

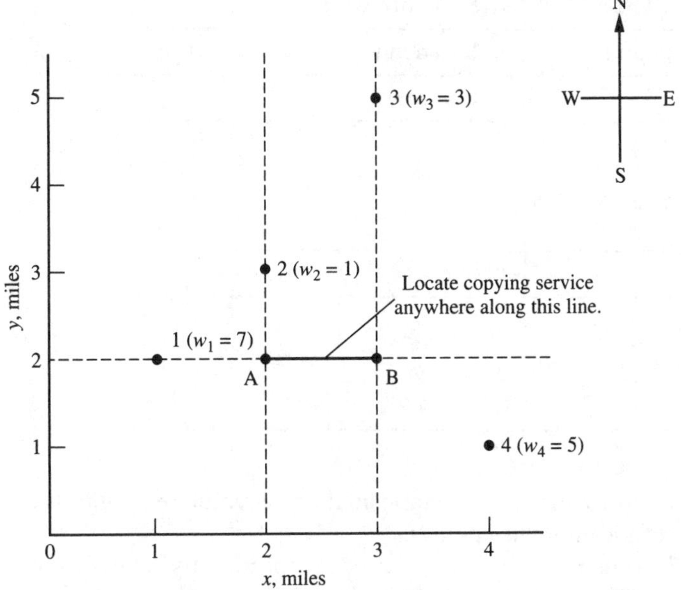

FIGURE 7.5. Locating a copying service.

TABLE 7.1. Median Value for x_s

Point i	Location x_i	$\Sigma\, w_i$
	ORDERING WEST TO EAST →	
1	1	7 = 7
2	②	7 + 1 = 8
3	3	
4	4	
	ORDERING EAST TO WEST ←	
4	4	5 = 5
3	③	5 + 3 = 8
2	2	
1	1	

From Figure 7.5, we find that the median has a value of $(7 + 1 + 3 + 5)/2 = 8$. To identify the x-coordinate median for x_s, we sum the values of w_i in the x direction both west to east and east to west. The top half of Table 7.1 lists in descending order the demand points from west to east as they appear in Figure 7.5 (i.e., 1, 2, 3, 4). The weights attached to each demand point are summed in descending order until the median value of 8 is reached or exceeded. The median value of 8 is reached when the weight of location 2 is added to the weight of location 1: thus, the first x-median is established at the value of 2 miles (i.e., the x-coordinate of location 2 is circled).

This procedure is repeated with demand points ordered from east to west, as shown in descending order in the bottom half of Table 7.1 (i.e., 4, 3,

TABLE 7.2. Median Value for y_s

Point i	Location y_i	Σw_i
	ORDERING SOUTH TO NORTH ↑	
4	1	5 = 5
1	②	5 + 7 = 12
2	3	
3	5	
	ORDERING NORTH TO SOUTH ↓	
3	5	3 = 3
2	3	3 + 1 = 4
1	②	3 + 1 + 7 = 11
4	1	

2, 1). The second x-median is established at the value of 3 miles (i.e., the x-coordinate of location 3 is circled).

Table 7.2 illustrates the same procedure for identifying the y-coordinate median for y_s. The top half of Table 7.2 lists in descending order the demand points from south to north as they appear in Figure 7.5 (i.e., 4, 1, 2, 3). In this case, the median value of 8 is first exceeded at location 1 when its weight is added to that of location 4 to yield a total of 12. The y-median is established at the value of 2 miles (i.e., the y-coordinate of location 1 is circled). At the bottom of Table 7.2, the demand points from north to south are listed in descending order as they appear in Figure 7.5 (i.e., 3, 2, 1, 4). Again, the median value is first exceeded at location 1 when its weight is added to those of locations 3 and 2 to yield a total of 11. Thus, we are left with only one y-median at 2 miles.

The cross-median approach of determining the median from all four points of the compass ensures that if a range of locations is appropriate, it will be readily identified. In this case, any location on the line segment AB minimizes total travel distance (e.g., coordinates $2 \leq x_s \leq 3$ and $y_s = 2$).

Note from Table 7.3 that the total weighted travel distance calculated for point A and point B are both equal to 35 miles; thus, any location either at point A or B or along the line between them will be acceptable. As this example illustrates, a location solution can be a line (i.e., a city street), a point

TABLE 7.3. Total Weighted Distance for Location A and B

Location A (2,2)							*Location B (3,2)*						
Office	Distance		Weight		Total		Office	Distance		Weight		Total	
1	1	×	7	=	7		1	2	×	7	=	14	
2	1	×	1	=	1		2	2	×	1	=	2	
3	4	×	3	=	12		3	3	×	3	=	9	
4	3	×	5	=	15		4	2	×	5	=	10	
					35							35	

(i.e., an intersection), or an area (i.e., a city block). Thus, the cross-median approach can result in some site selection flexibility.

Euclidian Metric

Changing the geographic structure to the straight-line distance between points complicates the location problem. The objective now becomes:

$$\text{Minimize } Z = \sum_{i=1}^{n} w_i \left[(x_i - x_s)^2 + (y_i - y_s)^2 \right]^{1/2} \tag{9}$$

Taking the partial derivatives with respect to x_s and y_s and setting them equal to zero results in two equations. Solving these equations for x_s and y_s yields the following pair of equations that identify the optimal location:

$$x_s = \frac{\sum_{i=1}^{n} \frac{w_i x_i}{d_{is}}}{\sum_{i=1}^{n} \frac{w_i}{d_{is}}} \tag{10}$$

$$y_s = \frac{\sum_{i=1}^{n} \frac{w_i y_i}{d_{is}}}{\sum_{i=1}^{n} \frac{w_i}{d_{is}}} \tag{11}$$

where

$$d_{is} = \left[(x_i - x_s)^2 + (y_i - y_s)^2 \right]^{1/2}$$

Unfortunately, these equations have no direct solution, because x_s and y_s appear on both sides of the equality (i.e., they are contained in the d_{is} term). The solution procedure begins with trial values of x_s and y_s. The formulas are used to calculate revised values of x_s and y_s, and the process is continued until the difference between successive values of x_s and y_s is negligible.[3]

Using the copying service example shown in Figure 7.5, the calculations shown in Table 7.4 were made to find an optimal location, assuming for now that a euclidian metric is appropriate. Beginning with a trial location of ($x_s = 2, y_s = 2$) and using equation (10), we find the revised value for $x_s = 20.78/11.19 = 1.857$. Using equation (11), we find the revised value for $y_s = 23.98/11.19 = 2.143$. Time—

[3]This form of the problem is referred to as the *generalized Weber problem* after Alfred Weber, who first formulated the problem in 1909.

TABLE 7.4. Euclidian Metric Calculations for Trial Location

Customer (i)	1	2	3	4
Location (x,y)	(1,2)	(2,3)	(3,5)	(4,1)
Weight (w_i)	7	1	3	5
Distance (d_{is})	1.0	1.0	3.16	2.24

and patience—permitting, we could continue until successive values of x_s and y_s were nearly identical and declare an optimal solution. The euclidian location always will result in a point, and only by accident will it agree with the metropolitan metric location.

In spite of the tedious mathematics, the euclidian location model is appropriate when vector travel is involved. The logic of the euclidian metric single-location model was not lost on Federal Express when it selected Memphis as the hub of its air package delivery network serving the entire United States. Memphis was considered to be close to the "center of gravity" for package movements in the United States.

Locating a Retail Outlet

When locating a retail outlet such as a supermarket, the objective is to maximize profit. In this case, a discrete number of alternative locations must be evaluated to find the most profitable site.

A gravity model is used to estimate consumer demand. This model is based on the physical analog that the gravitational attraction of two bodies is directly proportional to the product of their masses and inversely proportional to the square of the distance that separates them. For a service, the attractiveness of a facility may be expressed as:

$$A_{ij} = \frac{S_i}{T_{ij}^{\lambda}} \tag{12}$$

where A_{ij} = attraction to facility j for consumer i,
S_j = size of the facility j,
T_{ij} = travel time from consumer i's location to facility j, and
λ = parameter estimated empirically to reflect the effect of travel time on various kinds of shopping trips (e.g., where a shopping mall may have a $\lambda = 2$, convenience stores would have a $\lambda = 10$ or larger).

David L. Huff developed a retail location model using this gravity model to predict the benefit that a customer would have for a particular store size and location.[4] Knowing that customers also would be attracted to other competing stores, he proposed the ratio P_{ij}. For n stores, this ratio measures the probability of a customer from a given statistical area i traveling to a particular shopping facility j.

$$P_{ij} = \frac{A_{ij}}{\sum_{j=1}^{n} A_{ij}} \tag{13}$$

[4]David L. Huff, "A Programmed Solution for Approximating an Optimum Retail Location," *Land Economics*, August 1966, pp. 293–303.

An estimate of E_{jk}, the total annual consumer expenditures for a product class k at a prospective shopping facility j, then can be calculated as:

$$E_{jk} = \sum_{i=1}^{m} \left(P_{ij} C_i B_{ik} \right) \tag{14}$$

where P_{ij} = probability of a consumer from a given statistical area i traveling to a shopping facility j calculated by means of equation (13),
C_i = number of consumers at area i,
B_{ik} = average annual amount budgeted by consumer at area i for a product class k, and
m = number of statistical areas.

An estimate of M_{jk}, the market share captured by facility j of product class k sales, can be calculated as:

$$M_{jk} = \frac{E_{jk}}{\sum_{i=1}^{m} C_i B_{ik}} \tag{15}$$

An iterative procedure is used to calculate the expected annual profit of each potential site for various possible store sizes at the site. Net operating profit before taxes is calculated as a percentage of sales adjusted for the size of the store. The result is a list of potential sites with the store size at each that maximizes profit. All that remains is to negotiate a real estate deal for the site that comes closest to maximizing annual profit.

Example 7.2: Copying Service—Huff Analysis

Assume that the copying service in example 7.1 has been established at (x = 2, y = 2), as shown by location A in Figure 7.5 at the far left end of the optimal line. Further, assume that each customer order represents an expenditure of approximately \$10. Because convenience would be an important customer criterion, assume that $\lambda = 2$. If we wish to open a new store at location (x = 3, y = 2) (i.e., at location B on the far right end of the optimal line) but with *twice* the capacity of the existing copy center, how much market share would we expect to capture? Using the travel distances in Table 7.5 as input to the Huff model, the calculations shown in Tables 7.6 to 7.8 are obtained.

TABLE 7.5. Travel Distance in Miles (T_{ij}) [Using Metropolitan Metric]

	Customer Location (i)			
Site (j)	1	2	3	4
Proposed (3,2)	2	2	3	2
Existing (2,2)	1	1	4	3

TABLE 7.6. Attraction (A_{ij})

	Customer Location (i)			
Site (*j*)	1	2	3	4
Proposed ($S_1 = 2$)	0.5	0.5	0.2222	0.500
Existing ($S_2 = 1$)	1.0	1.0	0.0625	0.111
Total attraction	1.5	1.5	0.2847	0.611

TABLE 7.7. Probability (P_{ij})

	Customer Location (i)			
Site (*j*)	1	2	3	4
Proposed	.33	.33	.78	.82
Existing	.67	.67	.22	.18

TABLE 7.8. Monthly Expenditures (E_{jk}) and Market Share (M_{jk})

	Customer Expenditures ($)					
Site (*j*)	1	2	3	4	Monthly Total	Market Share (%)
Proposed	2,333	333	2,340	4,100	9,106	0.57
Existing	4,667	667	660	900	6,894	0.43
Totals	7,000	1,000	3,000	5,000	16,000	1.00

This example illustrates the result of an aggressive location strategy as used by well-financed national retail chains. For example, as the name might imply, Blockbuster Video has a reputation of moving into a community with supersized stores and driving out small, locally operated video-rental establishments.

Multiple Facilities

Location Set Covering Problem

The difficulty of evaluating decisions regarding public facility location has resulted in a search for surrogate, or substitute, measures of the benefit of the facility location. One such measure is the distance that the most distant customer would have to travel to reach the facility. This is known as the *maximal service distance.* We want to find the minimum number and location of facilities that will serve all demand points within some specified maximal service distance; this is known as the *location set covering* problem.

Example 7.3: Rural Medical Clinics

A state department of health is concerned about the lack of medical care in rural areas, and a group of nine communities has been selected for a pilot program in which medical clinics will be opened to serve primary health care needs. It is hoped that every community will be within 30 miles of at least one clinic. The planners would like to determine the number of clinics that are required and their locations. Any community can serve as a potential clinic site except for community 6, because facilities are unavailable there. Figure 7.6 shows a network identifying the cities as numbered circles; lines drawn between the sites show the travel distances in miles.

The problem is approached by first identifying for each community the other communities that can be reached from it within the 30-mile travel limit. Beginning with community 1, we see in Figure 7.6 that communities 2, 3, and 4 can be reached within the 30-mile distance limit. The results of similar inspections for each community are reported in the second column of Table 7.9 as the set of communities served from each site. An equivalent statement could be made that this set, less any communities that could not serve as a site, represents the set of sites that could cover the community in question for service within 30 miles. Thus, for community 5, a clinic located at site 3, 4, or 5 meets the maximal travel limit.

The third column of Table 7.9 represents the set of potential sites that could cover a given community. Several of these sets have been placed in

FIGURE 7.6. Travel network for a rural area.

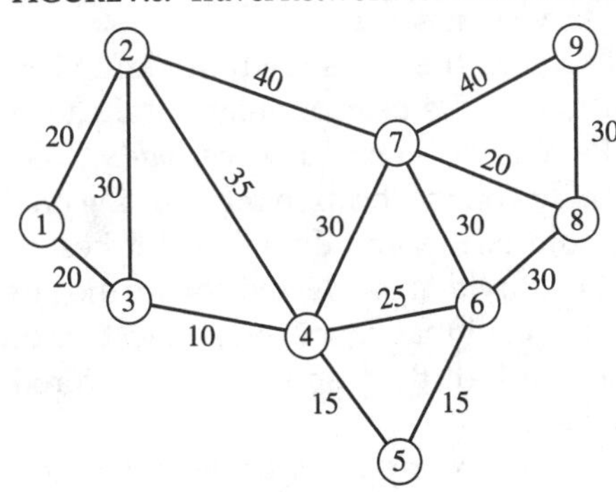

TABLE 7.9. Range of Service for Potential Sites

Community	Set of Communities Served from Site	Potential Sites that Could Serve the Community*
1	1,2,3,4	1,2,3,4
2	1,2,3	(1,2,3)†
3	1,2,3,4,5	1,2,3,4,5
4	1,3,4,5,6,7	1,3,4,5,7
5	3,4,5,6	(3,4,5)†
6	4,5,6,7,8	4,5,7,8
7	4,6,7,8	(4,7,8)†
8	6,7,8,9	7,8,9
9	8,9	(8,9)†

*Community 6 cannot serve as a clinic site.
†Subsets of potential sites.

parentheses, however, because they represent subsets of other potential locations. For example, because community 2 can only be served by sites 1, 2, and 3, one of these sites must be selected for a clinic location. Identifying these subsets reduces the problem size while ensuring that restrictions are satisfied.

Note that because of our desire to minimize the number of clinics to cover all the communities, any site common to two or more of these subsets is an excellent candidate for selection. In this case, sites 3, 4, and 8 are candidates. From inspection, we see that if sites 3 and 8 are selected, all subsets are accounted for; thus, all communities can be covered with just these two clinics. We also have identified the service region for each clinic; the clinic located at community 3 will serve communities 1 through 5, and the clinic located at community 8 will serve communities 6 through 9.

The location set covering problem often can yield more than one solution. In this example, if the maximal travel distance were set at 40 miles, the following five pairs of clinic site locations would provide coverage: (3, 8), (3, 9), (4, 7), (4, 8), and (4, 9).

Maximal Covering Location Problem

A variation of the location set covering problem is *maximal covering*. This problem is based on a very appealing objective: maximizing the population covered within a desired service distance.

A travel network such as the one shown in Figure 7.6 now would be augmented with information on the user population of each community. Richard Church and Charles ReVelle developed a *greedy adding (GA) algorithm* for solving this problem that builds on the location set covering analysis.[5] The algorithm begins with an empty solution set and then adds the best facility sites to this set one at a time. The first facility that is selected covers the largest population. Additional sites then are selected that cover the greatest amount of the remaining uncovered population until all the population is covered or the limit on the number of sites is reached.

For example, recall from Example 7.3 that sites 3, 4, and 8 were identified as candidates for the set covering problem. If we assume that each community has an equal population, then the GA algorithm would select site 4 as the first site to maximize population coverage. From Table 7.9, we see that site 4 covers communities 1, 3, 4, 5, 6, and 7. This exceeds the number of communities covered by either site 3 or site 8. Site 8 would be selected next, because it covers the uncovered communities 8 and 9 whereas site 3 only would cover the uncovered community 2.

SITE CONSIDERATIONS

Selection of the actual site requires other considerations beyond minimization of travel distance. Available real estate represents a major constraint on the final

[5]R. Church and C. ReVelle, "The Maximal Covering Location Problem," *Papers of the Regional Science Association*, vol. 32, Fall 1974, pp. 101–118.

TABLE 7.10. Site Selection Considerations

1. *Access:* Convenient to freeway exit and entrance ramps Served by public transportation	4. *Parking:* Adequate off-street parking
2. *Visibility:* Set back from street Sign placement	5. *Expansion:* Room for expansion
3. *Traffic:* Traffic volume on street that may indicate potential impulse buying Traffic congestion that could be a hindrance (e.g., fire stations)	6. *Environment:* Immediate surroundings should complement the service 7. *Competition:* Location of competitors 8. *Government:* Zoning restrictions Taxes

selection of a site. As indicated by Table 7.10, however, many considerations enter into the final decision.

BREAKING THE RULES

Before we leave the topic of service facility location, some caveats must be mentioned. Several creative exceptions to the assumed logic of the location models presented here need to be discussed. To this point, our location objective has been focused on customer convenience as measured in distance traveled to the planned facility. Consider, however, the success of the specialty mail-order business of L.L. Bean, located in Freeport, Maine, which calls into question the necessity of always finding a location that is convenient for customers' physical access.

In the following discussion, we will look at a marketing concept called *competitive clustering,* which is used for shopping goods, as well as a strategy called *saturation marketing* that defies the curse of cannibalization and has been successful for some urban retailers. A concept of *marketing intermediaries* is used to extend the service market well beyond the confines of geography, and, finally, the opportunity to substitute electronic communication for transportation is explored.

Competitive Clustering

Competitive clustering is a reaction to observed consumer behavior when they are choosing among competitors. When shopping for items such as new automobiles or used cars, customers like to make comparisons and, for convenience, seek out the area of town where many dealers are concentrated (i.e., the so-called motor mile).

Motel chains such as La Quinta have observed that inns located in areas with many nearby competitors experience higher occupancy rates than those located in isolation. It is surprising that locating near the competition is a strategy with profitable counterintuitive results for some services. Further, many motels are located by an interstate highway interchange, because their market is businesspeople and others traveling by car, not the local population.

Saturation Marketing

Au Bon Pain, a cafe known for its gourmet sandwiches, French bread, and croissants, has embraced the unconventional strategy of *saturation marketing* popularized in Europe. The idea is to group outlets of the same firm tightly in urban and other high-traffic areas. Au Bon Pain has clustered 16 cafes in downtown Boston alone, with many of them less than 100 yards apart—in fact, one group of five shops operates on different floors of Filene's department store. Although modest cannibalization of sales has been reported, the advantages of reduced advertising, easier supervision, and customer awareness, when taken together, overwhelm the competition and far outweigh the drawbacks. This strategy works best in high-density, downtown locations, where shops can intercept impulse customers with little time to shop or eat.[6]

The success of this approach became apparent to us during a summer visit to Helsinki, Finland, where we noticed ice cream vendors from the same firm with carts on nearly every corner of the downtown walking streets. The sight of a vendor seems to plant the idea of a treat in the mind of a passerby, who then takes advantage of the next, nearby opportunity.

Marketing Intermediaries

The idea that services are created and consumed simultaneously does not seem to allow for the "channel-of-distribution" concept as developed for goods. Because services are intangible and cannot be stored or transported, the geographic area for service would seem to be restricted. However, service channels of distribution have evolved that use separate organizational entities as intermediaries between the producer and the consumer.

James H. Donnelly provides a number of examples that illustrate how some services have created unlimited geographic service areas.[7] The retailer who extends a bank's credit to its customers is an intermediary in the distribution of credit. That Bank of America is a California bank does not limit use of the VISA card, which is honored worldwide. A health maintenance organization (HMO) performs an intermediary role between the practitioner and the patient by increasing the availability and convenience of "one-stop" shopping, and group insurance written through employers and labor unions is an example of how the insurance industry uses intermediaries to distribute its service.

Substitution of Communication for Transportation

An appealing alternative to moving people from one place to another is the use of telecommunications. One proposal that has met with some success is the use

[6]Suzanne Alexander, "Saturating Cities with Stores Can Pay," *The Wall Street Journal*, Sept. 11, 1989, p. B1.

[7]James H. Donnelly, "Marketing Intermediaries in Channels of Distribution for Services," *Journal of Marketing*, vol. 40, January 1976, pp. 55–70.

of telemetry to extend health care services into remote regions. Paramedics or nurse practitioners can use communication with a distant hospital to provide health care without transporting the patient. In addition, the banking industry has been promoting direct payroll deposit, which permits employees to have their pay deposited directly into their checking accounts. By authorizing employers to deposit salaries, the employees save trips to the bank; bankers also benefit through reduced check-processing paperwork and less congestion at their drive-in teller facilities.

A study by David A. Lopez and Paul Gray illustrates how an insurance company in Los Angeles decentralized its operations by using telecommunications and strategically locating its satellite offices.[8] An examination was made of the benefits and costs to the insurance firm when work was moved to the workers rather than when workers moved to their work. Insurance companies and other information-based industries are good candidates for employer decentralization, because members of their office staff perform routine clerical tasks using the firm's computer data bases. The proposed plan replaced the centralized operation in downtown Los Angeles with a network of regional satellite offices in the suburbs where the workers live.

The analysis also included a location study to determine the size, site, and number of satellites that would minimize the variable costs associated with employee travel and the fixed costs of establishing the satellite offices. The decentralization plan yielded several benefits to the company: 1) reduced staff requirements, 2) reduced employee turnover and training, 3) reduced salaries for clerical employees, 4) elimination of a lunch program, and 5) increased income from lease of the headquarters site. Employees whose travel to work was reduced by at least 5½ miles realized a net benefit over their reduced salary and loss of subsidized lunch. This employee benefit is important in light of increasing energy expenses for transportation.

It was found that underwriting life insurance and servicing insurance policies could be performed by means of a computer terminal. Phone communications usually were sufficient for personal contacts, and few face-to-face meetings were needed. These findings substantiate those of other studies in Britain and Sweden indicating that individuals require face-to-face contacts only for initial meetings and periodic refreshing; they do not require continual face-to-face contact to reach decisions and conduct routine business.

With the introduction of the Internet in the mid 1990s, the potential for electronic commerce has become a reality—customers shop from a desk at home and surf the World Wide Web for interesting home pages to visit.

[8]D. A. Lopez and P. Gray, "The Substitution of Communication for Transportation: A Case Study," *Management Science*, vol. 23, no. 11, July 1977, pp. 1149–1160.

Service Benchmark

Saturating Cities with Stores Can Pay

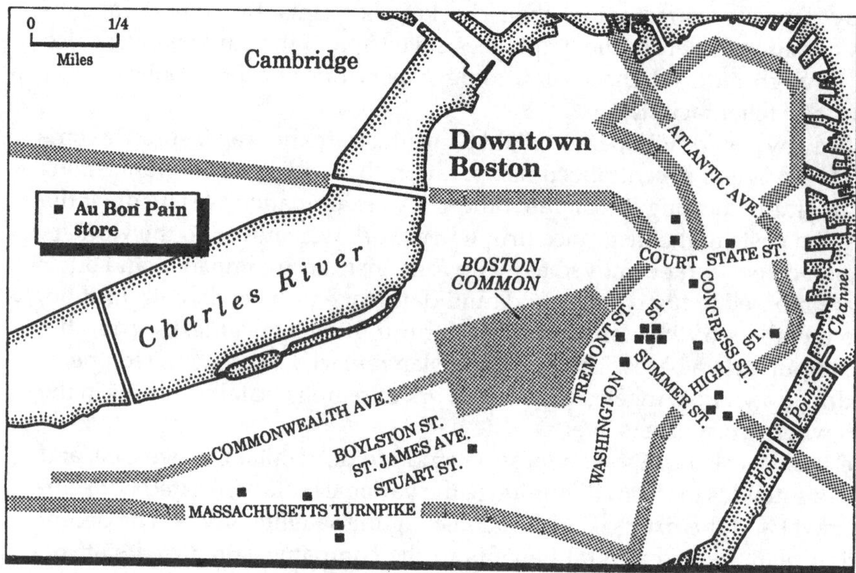

Locations of Au Bon Pain cafes in downtown Boston.

Boston commuters hurrying to work from South Station can't avoid walking past an Au Bon Pain cafe no matter how hard they try.

There's one inside the station, and one across the street at 1 Financial Center. There's another two blocks away, at 176 Federal St., another two blocks away from that at 75-101 Federal St., and still another two more blocks away, at 14 Milk St.

"We like to say you can toss a football from unit to unit," says Louis Kane, cochairman of the fast-growing chain best known for its gourmet sandwiches, freshly squeezed orange juice and freshly baked French bread, croissants and muffins.

Au Bon Pain Co. is among the latest to embrace the unconventional strategy of saturation marketing. The idea, relatively new to the U.S., is to group outlets tightly in urban and other high-traffic areas. Au Bon Pain has clustered 16 cafes in downtown Boston alone—with many less than 100 yards apart, and one group of five shops operating on different floors of Filene's department store.

The chain is so confident of the success of saturation marketing that it now plans to export the strategy to other cities, where it has only a handful of units so far. It will open more than 15 stores a year in cities 500 miles or less from here, including New York, Philadelphia and Washington, D.C. In New York, it's focusing on downtown and midtown, where there are already three Rockefeller Center outlets.

While putting too many sites too close together can cannibalize sales—as it has done modestly at some Au Bon Pain locations—proponents say the advantages outweigh the drawbacks. Clustering shops can reduce advertising expenses, make for easier supervision and attract customers from the competition.

DEVELOPING BRAND IDENTITY

"The concept of saturation marketing makes perfect sense," says Richard Winger, a vice presidential at Boston Consulting Group, a management consulting firm. "It's the developing of brand identity, that gives [companies] that extra push. When you think of croissants [in Boston], you think Au Bon Pain."

It's too soon to tell whether saturation marketing will catch on as the latest marketing trend. Apparently only a few other companies have tried it seriously. BayBanks Inc., a second-tier regional bank here, has nonetheless managed to become a leader in retail banking by saturating the city and suburbs with automated teller machines. In downtown alone, it has 75 machines—almost three times as many as its major competitors. "We're every place," says Donald Issachs, a spokesman for the bank. "And the public loves it."

Benetton S.p.A., the Italian clothing company, was among the first in the U.S. to adopt the strategy, using saturation marketing to become a major player in the mid 1980s. Some New York neighborhoods sprouted three or four stores carrying only Benetton clothes and promoting slightly different themes or fashions.

While good for Benetton, the strategy alienated some store owners, who operate the shops independently. Some Benetton dealers, in fact, have sued the company, charging that their sales dropped after another Benetton-only shop opened nearby.

Indeed, some merchants question the merits of saturation marketing. McDonald's Corp, for example, won't put its restaurants too close together because it doesn't want them to compete with each other. "We're not coming in, looking at 20 square blocks and saying, 'Where are we going to put the next one?' We're interested in building sales at existing restaurants. That's one of our strategies for growth," says Chuck Ebeling, a McDonald's spokesman.

LIMITATIONS OF STRATEGY

Au Bon Pain concedes that its strategy has limitations. Saturation wouldn't work for Au Bon Pain in suburban or residential areas because it's not a "destination restaurant" that people will drive to. Instead, the strategy works best in high-density, downtown locations, where shops can intercept the hordes of impulse customers with little time to shop or eat lunch. In addition, the company acknowledges that there can be too much of a good thing. While it will open some more shops here, it expects most of its growth in other cities.

Au Bon Pain was formed about a decade ago when Mr. Kane, owner of the original Au Bon Pain, merged his two stores with a cookie company owned by Ronald Shaich, now cochairman. The new closely held Au Bon Pain didn't immediately embrace saturation marketing. Like many new fast-food businesses seeking to expand rapidly, Au Bon Pain turned to franchising after opening a handful of shops here. It franchised several units along the East Coast and in the Midwest, and more in airports around the U.S.

But it found that some franchisees were a headache to deal with. At the same time, it discovered that the more company-owned shops it opened in downtown Boston, the better it did. As a result, it bought out some of the franchisees and for several years has concentrated instead on saturation marketing here. The company now has 70 stores—51 company-owned and 19 franchised—with average sales of more than $1.25 million a year and about 10,000 customers a week.

"Why do we do this craziness? We do it because we continue to make money at it," says Mr. Shaich. "In the morning, people probably don't walk more than 50 feet for breakfast and they won't walk more than a block for lunch. So if the walls of the market are a block, then we have to be in each of those mini-markets."

Cannibalization has been limited so far, the company says. The Au Bon Pain at 75-101 Federal St., for example, recently saw sales drop 5% in the two weeks after a new Au Bon Pain opened a couple of blocks away. But, even though the new store had sales of about $60,000 in its first four weeks, sales at the older shop quickly recovered to the normal $100,000 a month. Customers of that store—mostly workers at two nearby banks—apparently tried the new Au Bon Pain, but then came back to the first store because it was closer and more convenient for them, says Marianne Graziadei, general manager of the store.

Even when sales don't fully recover, the gains at new stores more than offset any marginal loss at existing stores, the company maintains. Sales at the Au Bon Pain at Summer and Hawley streets have fallen 5% since a new store opened a block away four months ago. Still, the new store's projected yearly sales of $850,000 more than offsets the $75,000 drop at the older store.

Moreover, if the new store hadn't been opened, another restaurant likely would have taken the location—and a competitor would be getting the additional sales, says Mr. Kane.

ZERO AD BUDGET

The danger of cannibalization is further offset by other benefits of saturation marketing. "We've never spent a penny on advertising," boasts Mr.

Shaich. Yet the awareness level of the chain in Boston is "phenomenal," he says.

This awareness, of course, stems from the proximity of the stores, says Marc Particem, senior vice president at Booz, Allen & Hamilton Inc., a management consulting firm in New York. "It's like having outdoor billboards on every block; the stores are a substitute for advertising."

The company also benefits from close supervision. Regional managers can walk from store to store, visiting as many in one day as managers of scattered chains might visit in a week. "Our guys live in our stores," says Mr. Kane.

Source: Reprinted with permission from Suzanne Alexander, "Saturating Cities with Stores Can Pay," *The Wall Street Journal,* Monday, September 11, 1989, p. B1. Reprinted by permission of *The Wall Street Journal,* 1989, Dow Jones & Company, Inc. All Rights Reserved Worldwide.

SUMMARY

Facility location plays an important role in the strategy of a service firm through its influence on the competitive dimensions of flexibility, competitive positioning, demand management, and focus. Our approach to service facility location began with a discussion of issues that must be considered, such as geographic representation, number of facilities, and optimization criteria and their effect on the location selected. The first step in the facility location analysis is estimating geographic demand. This requires a definition of the target population, selection of the unit of area, and, often, the use of regression analysis.

The discussion of facility location techniques began with the single-facility problem. Two simple models were presented that identified an optimal location for minimizing the total distance traveled by customers using the two most common travel patterns (i.e., metropolitan and euclidian). The location of a single retail outlet to maximize profit is an important decision that has been studied by David Huff using a gravity model to predict customer attractiveness to a store based on its size and location. For the multiple-facility location problem, the concept of location set covering is central to understanding the many approaches to identifying multiple-site locations.

A section on "breaking the rules" presents several location strategies that appear to be counterintuitive compared with the analytical models presented earlier. Strategies such as competitive clustering are common for shopping goods, and saturation marketing has been successful for some small retail outlets. In addition, use of marketing intermediaries can decouple the provider from the consumer. Finally, if the requirement for face-to-face interaction between server and consumer is relaxed, then the advantages of substituting communication for transportation become possible.

The next chapter concludes our discussion of structuring services for competitive advantage by considering the management of service projects that are encountered during the design of new services.

KEY TERMS AND DEFINITIONS

Competitive clustering the grouping of competitors (e.g., automobile dealerships) in close proximity for convenience in comparative shopping by customers.

Cross-median an approach to the location of a single facility using the metropolitan metric to minimize the total weighted distance traveled.

Euclidian metric a measure of distance traveled assuming vector travel from one point to another (e.g., the flight of an airplane between two cities).

Location set covering an approach to finding the minimum number and location of facilities that will serve all demand points within a specified maximum travel distance.

Marketing intermediaries a business entity in the channel of distribution between the final customer and the service provider (e.g., a bank extending credit to a retailer through a credit card).

Metropolitan metric a measure of distance traveled assuming rectangular displacement (e.g., north-south and east-west travel in urban areas).

Saturation marketing the location of a firm's individual outlets (e.g., ice cream vendors) in close proximity to create a significant presence that attracts customer attention.

SOLVED PROBLEMS

1. Cross-Median Location Problem

Problem Statement

A health clinic is being planned to serve a rural area in west Texas. The service area consists of four communities at the following *xy* coordinate locations in miles: A(6, 2), B(8, 6), C(5, 9), D(3, 4), with populations of 2000, 1000, 3000, and 2000, respectively. Recommend a "cross-median" location for the health clinic minimizing the total weighted metropolitan distance traveled.

Solution

First, calculate the median value in thousands:

$$\text{Median} = (2 + 1 + 3 + 2)/2 = 4$$

Second, plot the four communities on the grid below with population in thousands as subscripts:

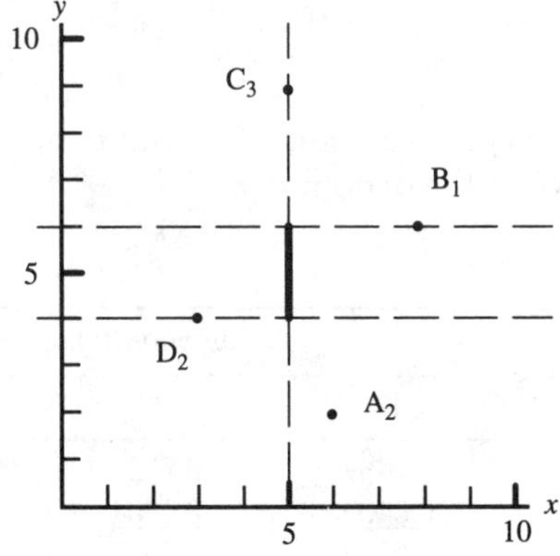

Third, draw the x-median dotted line (i.e., vertical line) on the plot by moving from left-to-right, adding the weights until the sum is equal to or exceeds the median (i.e., $D_2 + C_3 = 5$). The result is one vertical line at $x = 5$. Moving from right-to-left, add the weights until the sum is equal to or exceeds the median (i.e., $B_1 + A_2 + C_3 = 6$). The result is the same vertical line at $x = 5$.

Fourth, draw the y-median dotted line (i.e., horizontal line) on the plot by moving from top-to-bottom, adding the weights until the sum is equal to or exceeds the median (i.e., $C_3 + B_1 = 4$). The result is a horizontal line at $y = 6$. Moving from bottom to top, add the weights until the sum is equal to or exceeds the median (i.e., $A_2 + D_2 = 4$). The result is another horizontal line at $y = 4$. The recommended location results in a line segment shown as a dark line in the plot with xy coordinates of (5,4 to 5,6).

2. Retail Location Using the Huff Model

Problem Statement

The west Texas area in the plot above is served by a grocery store in community D. A proposed store with three times the floor space is being considered for location in community C. Assume that monthly expenditures per customer average about $100. Then, using the metropolitan metric for travel and $\lambda = 2$, use the Huff model to estimate the impact on monthly expenditures and market share for the existing store in community D if the proposed store in community C is constructed.

First, determine the travel distances using the metropolitan metric:

Travel Distance in Miles (T_{ij}) [Using Metropolitan Metric]

	Community (i)			
Site (*j*)	A (6,2)	B (8,6)	C (5,9)	D (3,4)
Proposed C (5,9)	8	6	0	7
Existing D (3,4)	5	7	7	0

Second, using equation (12), calculate the attraction matrix with $\lambda = 2$. For example, the attraction of community A to the proposed location at C (with $S = 3$ to account for the larger floor space) would be calculated as:

$$A_{ij} = \frac{S_j}{T_{ij}^{\lambda}} = \frac{S_1}{T_{11}^2} = \frac{3}{8^2} = \frac{3}{64} = 0.0469$$

Note that the attraction is given a value of ∞ where the store is located in the same community ($T_{ij} = 0$ in the denominator).

Attraction (A_{ij})

	Community Location (i)			
Site (*j*)	A	B	C	D
Proposed $S_1 = 3$	0.0469	0.8333	∞	—
Existing $S_2 = 1$	0.0400	0.0204	—	∞
Total attraction	0.0869	0.8537		

Third, using equation (13), calculate the probability using the total attraction as the denominator. For example, the probability of residents in community A traveling to the proposed grocery store location at C would be calculated as:

$$P_{ij} = \frac{A_{ij}}{\sum_{j=1}^{n} A_{ij}} = \frac{A_{11}}{A_{11} + A_{12}} = \frac{0.0469}{0.0469 + 0.04} = 0.54$$

Probability (P_{ij})

	Community Location (*i*)			
Site (*j*)	A	B	C	D
Proposed	.54	.98	1.0	0
Existing	.46	.02	0	1.0

Fourth, using equation (14), the monthly expenditures are calculated, and using equation (15), the market shares are determined. For example, expenditures from residents of community A at the proposed grocery store location at C would be calculated as:

$$E_{jk} = \sum_{i=1}^{m} \left(P_{ij}C_iB_{ik}\right) = P_{11}C_1B_1 = (.54)(2000)(100) = \$108{,}000$$

Monthly Expenditures (E_{jk}) and Market Share (M_{jk})

	Community Expenditures ($)					
Site (*j*)	A	B	C	D	Monthly Total	Market Share (%)
Proposed	108,000	98,000	300,000	0	506,000	0.63
Existing	92,000	2,000	0	200,000	294,000	0.37
Totals	200,000	100,000	300,000	200,000	800,000	1.00

TOPICS FOR DISCUSSION

1. Pick a particular service, and identify shortcomings in its site selection.
2. How would you proceed to estimate empirically the parameter λ in the Huff retail location model for a branch bank?
3. Why do you think set covering is an attractive approach to public sector facility location?
4. What are the characteristics of a service that would make communication a good substitute for transportation?
5. What are the benefits of using intermediaries in the service distribution channel?

EXERCISES

7.1. Revisit the copying service in Example 7.1, and assume that over the years, the monthly demand from the four customers has increased to the following weights: $w_1 = 7$, $w_2 = 9$, $w_3 = 5$, and $w_4 = 7$. If we previously located the copying service at point A in Figure 7.5, should we now consider a relocation?

7.2. A temporary-help agency wants to open an office in a suburban section of a large city. It has identified five large corporate offices as potential customers. The locations of these offices in miles on an xy coordinate grid for the area are: $c_1 = (4, 4)$, $c_2 = (4, 11)$, $c_3 = (7, 2)$, $c_4 = (11, 11)$, and $c_5 = (14, 7)$. The expected demand for temporary help from these customers is weighted as: $w_1 = 3$, $w_2 = 2$, $w_3 = 2$, $w_4 = 4$, and $w_5 = 1$. The agency reimburses employees for travel expenses incurred by their assignments; therefore, recommend a location (i.e., xy coordinates) for the agency that will minimize the total weighted metropolitan distance for job-related travel.

7.3. Four hospitals located in one county are cooperating to establish a centralized blood-bank facility to serve them all. On an xy coordinate grid of the county, the hospitals are found at the following locations: $H_1 = (5, 10)$, $H_2 = (7, 6)$, $H_3 = (4, 2)$, and $H_4 = (16, 3)$. The expected number of deliveries per month from the blood bank to each hospital is estimated at 450, 1200, 300, and 1500, respectively. Using the metropolitan metric, recommend a location for the blood bank that will minimize the total distance traveled.

7.4. A pizza delivery service has decided to open a branch near off-campus student housing. The project manager has identified five student apartment complexes in the northwest area of the city, the locations of which on an xy coordinate grid in miles are: $C_1 = (1, 2)$, $C_2 = (2, 6)$, $C_3 = (3, 3)$, $C_4 = (4, 1)$, and $C_5 = (5, 4)$. The expected demand is weighted as: $w_1 = 5$, $w_2 = 4$, $w_3 = 3$, $w_4 = 1$, and $w_5 = 5$. Using the metropolitan metric, recommend a location for the pizza branch that will minimize the total distance traveled.

7.5. A small city airport is served by four airlines. The terminal is rather spread out, with boarding areas located on an xy coordinate grid at: $A = (1, 4)$, $B = (5, 5)$, $C = (8, 3)$, and $D = (8, 1)$. The number of flights per day, of approximately equal capacity, is: $A = 28$, $B = 22$, $C = 36$, and $D = 18$. A new central baggage claim area is under construction.

a. Using the metropolitan metric, recommend a location for the new baggage claim area that will minimize the total weighted distance from the boarding areas.

b. Using the euclidian metric and the result found in part **a** as an initial solution, find the optimum location assuming vector travel.

7.6. You have been asked to help locate a catering service in the central business district of a city. The locations of potential customers on an xy coordinate grid are: $P_1 = (4, 4)$, $P_2 = (12, 4)$, $P_3 = (2, 7)$, $P_4 = (11, 11)$, and $P_5 = (7, 14)$. The expected demand is weighted as: $w_1 = 4$, $w_2 = 3$, $w_3 = 2$, $w_4 = 4$, and $w_5 = 1$.

a. Using the metropolitan metric, recommend a location for the catering service that will minimize the total weighted distance traveled to serve the customers.

b. Using the euclidian metric and the result found in part **a** as an initial solution, find the optimum location assuming vector travel.

7.7. Revisit the copying service Huff analysis in Example 7.2. Recalculate the monthly customer expenditures and market share for the proposed copying center at location B if the new store will be *three* times the capacity of the existing store at location A and the new demand weights from Exercise 7.1 above are used.

7.8. A locally owned department store samples two customers in each of five geographic areas to estimate consumer spending in its home appliances department. It is estimated that these customers are a good sample of the 10,000 customers the store serves. The number of customers in each area is: $C_1 = 1500$, $C_2 = 2500$, $C_3 = 1000$, $C_4 = 3000$, and $C_5 = 2000$. It is found that the two consumers have the following budgets in dollars for home appliances per year: $B_{11} = 100$, $B_{12} = 150$, $B_{21} = 75$, $B_{22} = 100$, $B_{31} = 125$, $B_{32} = 125$, $B_{41} = 100$, $B_{42} = 120$, $B_{51} = 120$, and $B_{52} = 125$. Using the Huff retail location model, estimate annual home appliance sales for the store.

7.9. Bull's-Eye, a chain department store, opens a branch in a shopping complex near the store mentioned in Exercise 7.8. The Bull's-Eye branch is three times larger than the locally owned store. The travel times in minutes from the five areas to the two stores ($j = 1$ for the locally owned store, $j = 2$ for Bull's-Eye) are: $T_{11} = 20$, $T_{12} = 15$, $T_{21} = 35$,

$T_{22} = 20$, $T_{31} = 30$, $T_{32} = 25$, $T_{41} = 20$, $T_{42} = 25$, $T_{51} = 25$, and $T_{52} = 25$. Use the Huff retail location model to estimate the annual consumer expenditures in the home appliance section of each store assuming that $\lambda = 1$.

7.10. A community is currently being served by a single self-serve gas station with six pumps. A competitor is opening a new facility with twelve pumps across town. Table 7.11 shows the travel times in minutes from the four different areas in the community to the sites and the number of customers in each area.

a. Using the Huff retail location model and assuming that $\lambda = 2$, calculate the probability of a customer traveling from each area to each site.

b. Estimate the proportion of the existing market lost to the new competitor.

7.11. Recall the rural medical clinics in Example 7.3, and suppose that each community were required to be 25 miles at most from the nearest clinic. How many clinics would be needed, and what would their locations be? Give all possible location solutions.

7.12. A bank is planning to serve the rural communities shown in Figure 7.7 with automated teller machines (ATMs). The travel time in minutes between communities in the service area is shown on the network in Figure 7.7. The bank is interested in determining the number and location of ATMs necessary to serve the communities so that a machine will be within 20 minutes travel time of any community.

7.13. The volunteer fire department serving the communities in Figure 7.7 has just purchased two used fire engines auctioned off by a nearby city.

a. Select all possible pairs of communities in which the fire engines could be located to ensure that all communities can be reached in 30 minutes or less.

b. What additional consideration could be used to make the final site selection from the community pairs found in part **a**?

TABLE 7.11. Travel Times to Gas Stations

Area	1	2	3	4
Old station	5	10	9	15
New competitor	20	8	12	6
Customers (c_i)	100	150	80	50

FIGURE 7.7. Service area network.

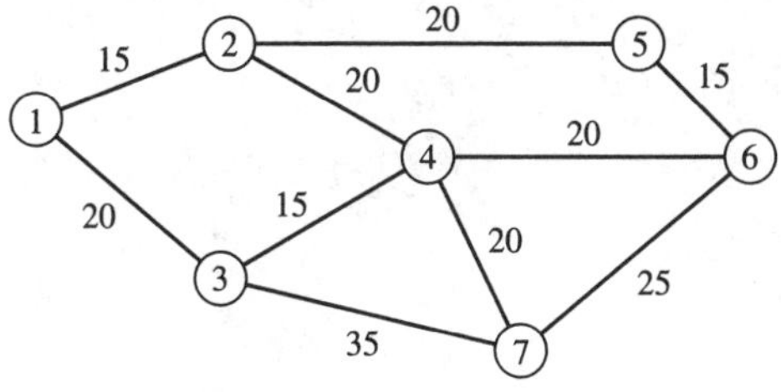

CASE: HEALTH MAINTENANCE ORGANIZATION (C)

Joan Taylor, the administrator of Life-Time Insurance Company, which is based in Buffalo, New York, was charged with establishing a health maintenance organization (HMO) satellite clinic in Austin, Texas. The HMO concept would offer Austin residents an alternative to the traditional fee-for-service medical care. Individuals could enroll in the HMO voluntarily and, for a fixed fee, be eligible for health services. The fee would be paid in advance.

Ms. Taylor carefully planned the preliminary work that would be required to establish the new clinic in Austin, and when she arrived, most of the arrangements had been completed. The location of the ambulatory health center (clinic), however, had not been selected. Preliminary data on the estimated number of potential enrollees in the HMO had been determined by census tract, and these data are presented in Table 7.12. Using the cross-median approach and the census-tract map in Figure 7.8, recommend a location for the clinic.

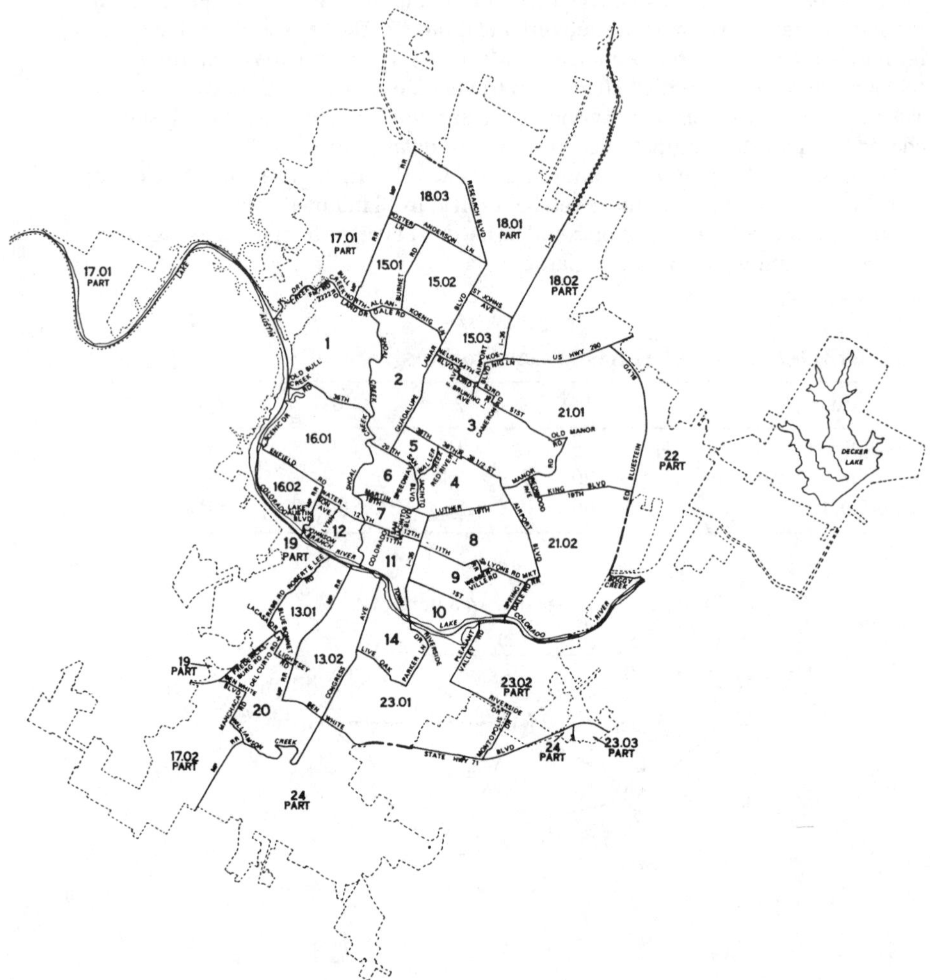

FIGURE 7.8. Census-tract map of Austin, Texas.

TABLE 7.16. Minimum Travel Time Between Potential and Existing Sites and Block Groups in Minutes

	Census Block Group											
Site	1	2	3	4	5	6	7	8	9	10	11	12
A	7	5	5	9	1	3	4	5	7	10	14	17
B	10	8	8	10	7	3	3	2	1	2	2	5
X	16	14	14	16	13	8	7	6	4	4	2	2
Y	12	10	10	12	9	5	4	3	2	4	2	5
Z	7	5	5	7	4	2	1	4	3	10	10	13

TABLE 7.17. Relationship of Size of Store to Margin on Sales, Expenses, and Net Operating Profit as a % of Sales

	Operating Data		
Sales Area (sq ft)	Margin on Sales	Expenses	Net Operating Profit before Taxes
10,000	16.2	12.3	3.9
15,000	15.6	12.0	3.6
20,000	14.7	11.8	2.9

increments) up to the maximum allowable sales area for each potential site.

2. What is the expected annual net operating profit before taxes and expected market share for the outlet you have recommended? Defend your recommendation.

3. Try two other values of λ (e.g., 0.5 and 5.0) to measure the sensitivity of customer travel propensity on your recommended location.

4. Briefly state any shortcomings you may perceive in this model.

SELECTED BIBLIOGRAPHY

ABERNATHY, W. J., and J. C. HERSHEY: "A Spatial-Allocation Model for Regional Health-Services Planning," *Operations Research,* vol. 20, no. 3, May–June 1972, pp. 629–642.

BROWN, L. A., F. B. WILLIAMS, C. YOUNGMANN, J. HOLMES, and K. WALBY; "The Location of Urban Population Service Facilities: A Strategy and Its Application," *Social Science Quarterly,* vol. 54, no. 4, March 1974, pp. 784–799.

CHHAJED, D., R. L. FRANCIS, and T. J. LOWE: "Contributions of Operations Research to Location Analysis," *Location Science,* vol. 1, no. 4, 1993, pp. 263–287.

CHURCH, R., and C. REVELLE: "The Maximal Covering Location Problem," *Papers of the Regional Science Association,* vol. 32, Fall 1974, pp. 101–118.

CRAIG, C. S., A. GHOSH, and S. MCLAFFERTY: "Models of the Retail Location Process: A Review," *Journal of Retailing,* vol. 60, no. 1, Spring 1984, pp. 5–36.

DANIELS, P. W.: "Technology and Metropolitan Office Location," *The Service Industries Journal,* vol. 7, no. 3, 1982, pp. 276–291.

DONNELLY, JAMES H.: "Marketing Intermediaries in Channels of Distribution for Services," *Journal of Marketing,* vol. 40, January 1976, pp. 55–70.

FITZSIMMONS, JAMES A.: "A Methodology for Emergency Ambulance Deployment," *Management Science,* vol. 19, no. 6, February 1973, pp. 627–636.

———, and L. A. ALLEN: "A Warehouse Location Model Helps Texas Comptroller Select Out-of-State Audit Offices," *Interfaces*, vol. 13, no. 5, September–October 1983, pp. 40–46.

———, and B. N. SRIKAR: "Emergency Ambulance Location Using the Contiguous Zone Search Routine," *Journal of Operations Management*, vol. 2, no. 4, August 1982, pp. 225–237.

GELB, B. D., and B. M. KHUMAWALA: "Reconfiguration of an Insurance Company's Sales Regions," *Interfaces*, vol. 14, no. 6, 1984, pp. 87–94.

HUFF, DAVID L.: "A Programmed Solution for Approximating an Optimum Retail Location," *Land Economics*, August 1966, pp. 293–303.

KHUMAWALA, B. M.: "An Efficient Algorithm for the *p*-Median Problem with Maximum Distance Constraint," *Geographical Analysis*, vol. 5, no. 4, October 1973, pp. 309–321.

KIMES, S. E., and J. A. FITZSIMMONS: "Selecting Profitable Hotel Sites at La Quinta Motor Inns," *Interfaces*, vol. 20, no. 2, March 1990, pp. 12–20.

LOPEZ, D. A., and P. GRAY: "The Substitution of Communication for Transportation: A Case Study," *Management Science*, vol. 23, no. 11, July 1977, pp. 1149–1160.

MAHAJAN, V., S. SHARMA, and D. SRINIVAS: "An Application of Portfolio Analysis for Identifying Attractive Retail Locations," *Journal of Retailing*, vol. 61, no. 4, Winter 1985, pp. 19–34.

MANDELL, MARVIN B.: "Modeling Effectiveness-Equity Trade-offs in Public Service Delivery Systems," *Management Science*, vol. 37, no. 4, April 1991, pp. 467–482.

MIN, H.: "Location Planning of Airport Facilities Using the Analytic Hierarchy Process," *Logistics and Transportation Review*, vol. 30, no. 1, March 1995, pp. 79–94.

PRICE, W. L., and M. TURCOTTE: "Locating a Blood Bank," *Interfaces*, vol. 16, no. 5, 1986, pp. 17–26.

ROSENBERG, L. J., and E. C. HIRSCHMAN: "Retailing without Stores," *Harvard Business Review*, July–August 1980, pp. 103–112.

SAVAS, E. S.: "On Equity in Providing Public Services," *Management Science*, vol. 24, no. 8, April 1978, pp. 800–808.

SWERSEY, ARTHUR J., and LAKSHMAN S. THAKUR: "An Integer Programming Model for Locating Vehicle Emissions Testing Stations," *Management Science*, vol. 41, no. 3, March 1995, pp. 496–512.

CHAPTER 8

Managing Service Projects

LEARNING OBJECTIVES

After completing this chapter, you should be able to:

1. Describe the characteristics of a project and its management challenges.
2. Illustrate the use of a Gantt chart, and discuss its limitations.
3. Construct a project network.
4. Perform critical path analysis on a project network.
5. Allocate limited resources to a project.
6. Crash activities to reduce the project completion time.
7. Analyze a project with uncertain activity times to determine the project completion distribution.

Projects can vary widely in their complexity, resource requirements, time needed for completion, and risk. Consider, for example, projects that might be undertaken by a passenger airline: opening a new route, overhauling an aircraft, implementing a new marketing strategy, installing a new data processing system, purchasing a new fleet of aircraft, changing in-flight service, and installing a new inventory control system. In this age of time-based competition, successful project management can bring new products to the marketplace sooner, thereby preempting rivals and capturing market share. For example, in the construction industry, Lehrer McGovern Bovis became famous for its construction management services by achieving significant time savings when it used an overlapping phased design-construction process in which the foundation was poured before the final drawings were completed.

The risks that are inherent in a project can threaten the survival of a company. For example, failure to complete a project on time can bankrupt a small construction firm when the contract includes a penalty cost for delay. The potential risks and rewards associated with a project are factors that enter into building a project team, selecting a project leader, and developing a strategy for successful completion of the project.

CHAPTER PREVIEW

Project management is concerned with planning, scheduling, and controlling activities to achieve timely project completion within budget and quality expectations. Relevant questions that need to be addressed include:

1. What activities are required for completing a project?
2. In what sequence should these activities be performed?
3. When should each activity be scheduled to begin and end?
4. Which activities are critical to completing the project on time?
5. How should resources be allocated to the activities?
6. What is the probability of meeting the scheduled project completion date?
7. Is the project on schedule?
8. How should a delayed project be managed to get back on schedule?

This chapter begins with an overview of the functions that characterize a project management system, then traditional bar-chart methods for project management are presented and discussed. As an alternative to such traditional methods, several network-based methods are described in detail. Microsoft Project for Windows is used to illustrate the ease and power of project management software.

Characteristics of Projects

Projects have certain characteristics in common that should be noted. First, they are relatively large-scale and can be massively complex, as illustrated by Boeing's development of the 777 aircraft, which had many partners who required extensive coordination. Projects also involve a substantial commitment of resources and management attention.

Another characteristic is that the projects are complex in terms of the number and interdependence of the activities, and they involve many activities that should be performed in a specified sequence. The sequence generally is dictated by technological or strategic considerations. Also, the time and resources that the activities will require must be estimated. This is particularly difficult for activities that have never been performed previously, which often is the case in research and development projects.

A final characteristic is that the projects are relatively nonroutine. This means that organizations do not engage in a particular project in an on-going and repetitive fashion. (One exception, however, would include the periodic maintenance that airlines perform on their aircraft.) Generally, each project has novel features that require customized managerial attention.

Activities of Project Managers

Organizations initiate projects for a variety of reasons, such as constructing a new facility, introducing a new service, or beginning a consulting engagement. All these reasons are catalysts that lead to the inception of a project. The management functions of planning, scheduling, and controlling are actively pursued from project conception to project completion.

Planning

A project usually begins with a statement of work. This statement is a written description of the objectives and contains a tentative schedule that specifies starting and completion dates as well as a proposed budget. An aid to planning is development of a *work breakdown structure* (WBS), which is a family tree subdivision of the efforts that are required to achieve the objective. A WBS is developed by starting with the end objective and successively subdividing work into manageable components, such as tasks, subtasks, and work elements. As an example, consider the project of moving a hospital across town to a new location. The project (or "program" if it is a multiyear project) is defined as "move the hospital." One task is "move patients." A subtask is "arrange for ambulance transportation." A work element is "prepare patients for the move." The detailed project definition as provided by the WBS helps to identify the skills that are necessary to achieve the project goals, and it provides a framework for budgeting.

Scheduling

After the initial plans are developed and accepted, a more detailed schedule is prepared. Scheduling begins with decomposing the project into individual activities. The sequencing of the activities is specified, and time and resource requirements are estimated. Computer software then is used to determine the start and finish dates for each activity in the project. Allocation of resources to specific activities are planned at this time, and this process can influence the project duration and cost. Development of project schedules will be addressed extensively later in the chapter.

Controlling

The final project schedule becomes the basis on which the project is implemented and monitored for progress against intermediate completion steps (called *milestones*). Expenditures against the budget also can be tracked using the project schedule. Controlling is concerned with making sure that all aspects of project implementation are performed according to both time and budget. If they are not, then the schedule and plan are revised as necessary to ensure that the project objectives are achieved.

The importance of projects has attracted much attention recently and yielded a number of techniques to help managers. Our discussion begins with Gantt charts and concludes with personal computer software that analyzes projects that are modeled as networks.

TECHNIQUES FOR PROJECT MANAGEMENT

Gantt Project Charts

Developed by Henry Gantt in 1916, a *Gantt chart* is used to determine the timing of individual activities in a project. This chart plots a time line for each activity against a *calendar.* Gantt charts are a useful tool for portraying visually the schedule of activities and monitoring the progress of a project against its plan.

The first step in using a Gantt chart is to break down the project into discrete activities. "Discrete" means that each activity has a distinct beginning and end. After the project has been decomposed into its activities, the sequence of those activities is determined. This task is easier said than done, however. Usually, there are several possible strategies for carrying out a project, and it may not be obvious which one is best. The skill of the project manager, along with the input of other people interested in the project, ultimately determines the sequence that is adopted. A Gantt chart also requires time estimates for each activity. The durations of the activities are assumed to be deterministic and known, which means that we presume to know exactly how long each activity will take. Of course, this is not realistic, but it does provide estimates that are helpful for managing a project.

Example 8.1: Servicing a Boeing 747

A Gantt chart can be used to schedule a periodic or repetitive project, because the sequence of activities is well understood and past experience has determined how long each activity takes. Consider the required activities in a routine, 50-minute layover of a Boeing 747 passenger aircraft. Figure 8.1 is a Gantt chart that displays each activity with a horizontal bar indicating its du-

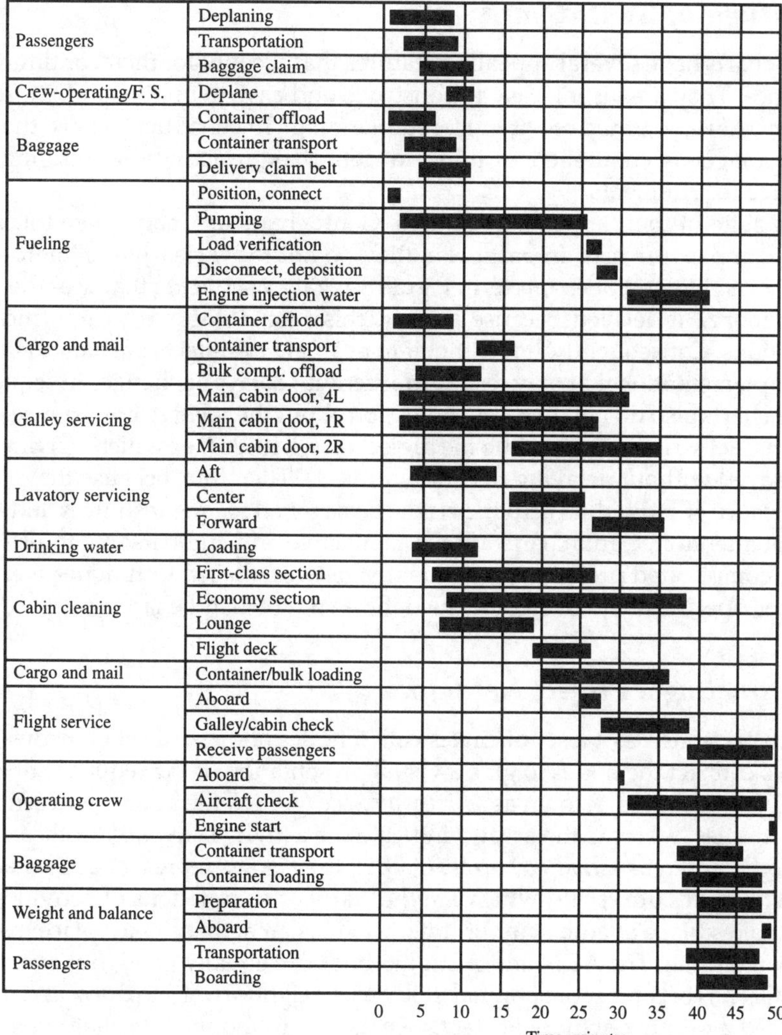

FIGURE 8.1. Gantt Chart Schedule of service activities for a Boeing 747.

ration in minutes and the scheduled beginning and ending times. Many activities, such as galley servicing, can be accomplished concurrently with others, because the corresponding horizontal bars overlap each other and, thus, are scheduled to be performed during the same time period. For lavatory servicing, however, the aft, center, and forward sections are serviced in sequence, not concurrently. This chart can be used to determine the labor and equipment resources that are required to complete the project on time. Once under way, activities that fall behind schedule can be noted by drawing a vertical line representing the current time and noting which activities have not finished as scheduled and, consequently, need attention to get back on schedule and finish the project in 50 minutes.

A Critique of Gantt Charts

Gantt charts have several appealing features that account for their continued acceptance. They are visual, easy to construct, and easy to understand. More important, however, they result in forced planning. To construct a chart, the project manager is compelled to think in detail about activity scheduling and resource requirements.

In spite of their appealing features, Gantt charts are inadequate for large-scale, complex projects. In particular, they do not show clearly the interdependence of activities. For example, in Figure 8.1, galley servicing that uses the main cabin door 2R is delayed, because access to this door is blocked by cargo and mail operations. Consequently, it is difficult to evaluate the effects of changes in project implementation that may result from activity delays or changes in sequence. These charts also do not give any indication about the relative importance of individual activities in completing the project on schedule (i.e., which activities can be delayed without delaying the entire project). Therefore, because the relative importance of individual activities is the basis for allocating resources and managerial attention, Gantt charts are too ineffective and cumbersome to use with large, complicated projects. Consequently, network-based techniques were developed specifically to overcome the deficiencies of Gantt charts.

Constructing a Project Network

A network consists of a set of circles called nodes and also a set of arrows. The arrows connect the nodes to give a visual presentation of the sequence of activities. In one method, known as *activity on node* (AON), the nodes represent project activities, whereas the arrows indicate the activity sequence. In the second method, known as *activity on arrow* (AOA), the arrows represent project activities. The nodes are *events,* which are the starts or completions of activities. An event takes place at an instant of time, whereas an activity takes place over an interval of time. The AON and AOA methods are equally good, but over time, the AON has become more popular. It is very straightforward to draw, and it does not need a dummy activity artifact such as that found in AOA diagrams. Both diagrams will be illustrated here, but all critical path analyses will use the AON convention, which we will call a *PERT chart* (the accepted name given to project management diagrams).

A key assumption underlying critical path analysis is that an activity cannot begin until *all* immediate predecessor activities are completed. Also, a PERT chart generally has a single node that indicates the project beginning and a single node that indicates the project end. PERT charts are *connected* and *acyclic.* "Connected" means that it is possible to get to any network node by following arrows leaving the start node. "Acyclic" means that the sequence of activities progresses without interruption from the start node to the end node without looping around in circles.

Example 8.2: Tennis Tournament—Project Network

Planning a tennis tournament is an opportunity to use project management. The goal is to hold a successful weekend tournament at a future date, and

TABLE 8.1. Tennis Tournament Activities

Activity Description	Code	Immediate Predecessor	Estimated Duration (days)
Negotiate for location	A	—	2
Contact seeded players	B	—	8
Plan promotion	C	A	3
Locate officials	D	C	2
Send RSVP invitations	E	C	10
Sign player contracts	F	B,C	4
Purchase balls and trophies	G	D	4
Negotiate catering	H	E,F	1
Prepare location	I	E,G	3
Tournament	J	H,I	2

preparations for the tournament require that all activities be identified. We also need to estimate the durations of these activities and note any constraints in sequence or precedence. Table 8.1 lists the activities that are required for the tournament along with their precedence requirements and durations.

Figure 8.2 shows an AOA project network for the tennis tournament. Note the use of three dummy activities (i.e., the broken arrows) to ensure that activity precedence is not violated. For example, the dummy activity joining nodes 3 and 7 ensures that activity F follows the completion both of activity C and activity B. Dummy activities do not consume time but are included only to maintain the proper activity sequence. The length of an activity arrow has no meaning, although each activity is subscripted to note its duration. Nodes are numbered according to a convention: the node at the arrow head must have a larger number than the node at the tail to indicate the direction of the activity. For example, if the arrow representing the dummy activity that joins nodes 3 and 7 were reversed (i.e., pointing to node 3 instead of node 7), then the precedence interpretation would change (i.e., activity D would follow activity B, which is not correct). Preparing an AOA network requires much care and is prone to errors.

Figure 8.3 is a PERT chart (AON network) of the same tennis tournament project. In this case, arrows represent the sequence of activities, and nodes represent the activities themselves. Preparing a PERT chart is a simple mat-

FIGURE 8.2. AOA network for tennis tournament.

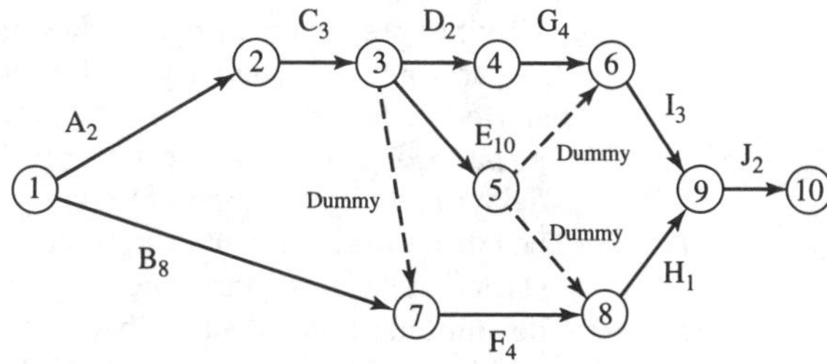

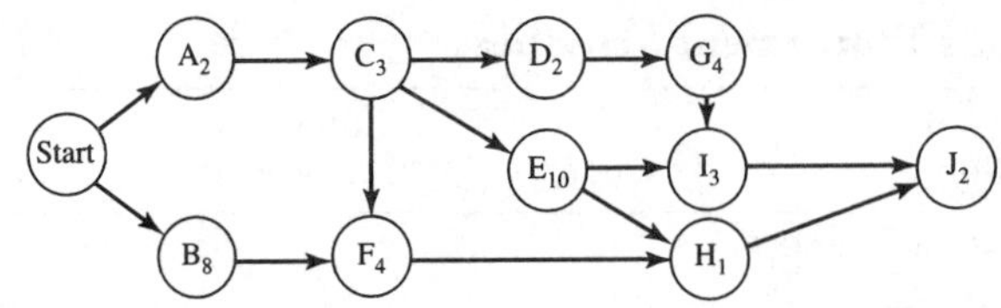

FIGURE 8.3. PERT Chart (AON network) for tennis tournament.

ter of drawing nodes in approximate sequence from beginning to end and joining the nodes with arrows in the appropriate direction. Sometimes a start or finish node is added, as in the tennis tournament example. It should be clear that the AOA and AON networks describe the same sequence of activities.

Critical Path Method

The *critical path method (CPM)* is an approach to determine the start and finish dates for individual activities in a project. A result of this method is the identification of a *critical path,* or unbroken chain of activities from the start to the end of the project. A delay in the starting time of any critical path activity results in a delay in the project completion time. Because of their importance for completing the project, *critical activities* receive top priority in the allocation of resources and managerial effort. In the spirit of *management by exception,* the critical activities are the exceptions that need close scrutiny.

CPM involves some simple calculations, and Table 8.2 lists the notations that are used in this analysis. Note that we have not indicated how the expected activity duration t is determined. In many cases, these values are assumed to be deterministic (i.e., constants) and are based on expert judgment and past experience. In other cases, the expected durations are assumed to be the arithmetic means of known probability distributions. We shall discuss the deterministic case first and treat probability distributions later.

TABLE 8.2. Notation for Critical Path Method

Item	Symbol	Definition
Expected activity duration	t	The expected duration of an activity
Early start	*ES*	The earliest time an activity can begin if all previous activities are begun at their earliest times
Early finish	*EF*	The earliest time an activity can be completed if it is started at its early start time
Late start	*LS*	The latest time an activity can begin without delaying the completion of the project
Late finish	*LF*	The latest time an activity can be completed if it is started at its latest start time
Total slack	*TS*	The amount of time an activity can be delayed without delaying the completion of the project

CPM involves calculating early times (*ES* and *EF*), late times (*LS* and *LF*), and a slack time (*TS*). Early times are calculated for each activity beginning with the first activity and moving successively forward through the network to the final activity. Thus, the early times (*ES* and *EF*) are calculated by a *forward pass* through the project. The early start for the first activity is set equal to zero, and the early times for a particular activity are calculated as:

$$ES = EF_{predecessor} \tag{1}$$

$$EF = ES + t \tag{2}$$

Note that $EF_{predecessor}$ is the early finish of an immediately preceding activity and that t is the duration of the activity under consideration. When there are several immediate predecessors, the one with the *largest* early finish time is used. The early finish for the last activity is the early finish for the project as a whole.

Late times (*LS* and *LF*) are calculated for each activity, beginning with the last activity in the network and moving successively backward through the network to the first activity. The late times thus are calculated by a *backward pass* through the project. By convention, the late finish for the last activity is set equal to the early finish (i.e., $LF = EF$). If a project completion date is known, then this date can be used as the late finish for the last activity. For any particular activity, the late times are calculated as follows:

$$LF = LS_{successor} \tag{3}$$

$$LS = LF - t \tag{4}$$

Note that $LS_{successor}$ is the late start of an immediately succeeding activity. When there are several immediate successors, the one with the *smallest* late start is used.

Slack times are determined from the early and late times. Total slack (*TS*) for an activity can be calculated in either of two equivalent ways:

$$TS = LF - EF \quad \text{or} \tag{5}$$

$$TS = LS - ES \tag{6}$$

Slack is one of the most important aspects of critical path analysis. Activities that have zero slack are critical, meaning that they cannot be delayed without also delaying the project completion time. When displayed on a Gantt chart, the set of critical activities always forms a complete and unbroken path from the initial node to the completion node of the network. Such a path is referred to as the *critical path;* in terms of duration time, this is the longest path in the network. A project network has *at least* one critical path, and it could have two or more.

Example 8.3: Tennis Tournament—Critical Path Analysis

The PERT chart of the tennis tournament is shown in Figure 8.4. Each node is labeled with the activity code, and the duration is a subscript. Next to each

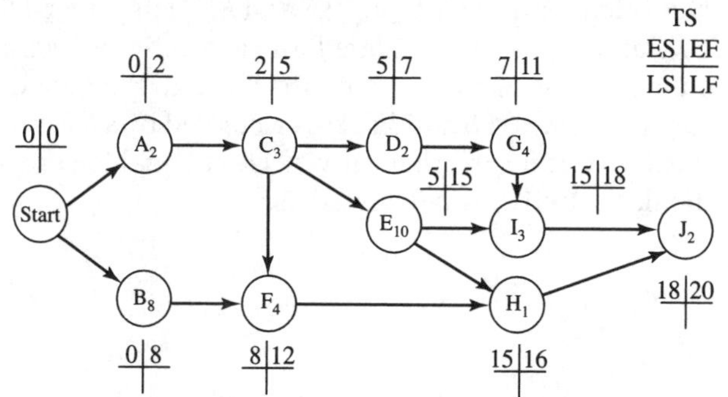

FIGURE 8.4. PERT chart for tennis tournament with early time calculations.

node is a cross to be filled in with the activity schedule times, which are calculated as shown below (note that t represents the activity time):

$$TS = LS - ES$$

$ES = EF_{predecessor}$	$EF = ES + t$
$LS = LF - t$	$LF = LS_{successor}$

Early times are calculated beginning with the "start" node (i.e., forward pass) and are recorded in the top row of the cross for each activity, after which we see that the project will take 20 days to complete (i.e., *EF* for the last activity). Note that we need to be especially careful to select the predecessor with the *largest EF* as the time for the *ES* of the activity in question, which occurs when more than one arrow comes into a node (i.e., activities E and F converge on node H). Because no single activity begins the project, an artificial activity or "start" node is created with a duration of zero. Using this convention, we have a single "start" and a single "finish" node for the project. (Artificial "finish" nodes are used when a project does not have a single concluding activity.)

Figure 8.5 on page 205 shows the completed critical path analysis. Note that per convention, the late finish for the last activity is set equal to 20 days. This value is the starting point for calculating late times (i.e., backward pass), which are entered into the bottom row of the cross for each activity. Again, we must use caution to select the successor with the *smallest LS* as the time for the *LF* of the activity in question, which occurs when more than one arrow departs from a node (i.e., activities D, E, and F following node C).

The critical activities have zero slack, which is easily seen as the difference between *ES* and *LS* or between *EF* and *LF*; thus, these activities have no scheduling flexibility. The critical path is defined by the critical activities A-C-E-I-J. As shown in Figure 8.6, the critical path represents the unbroken line of activities from beginning to end of the project. Any delay in activities on this path will delay the completion of the project beyond the 20 days.

Figure 8.6 on page 206 is a modified activity-on-arrow PERT chart (recall Figure 8.2), without dummy arrows, on which each activity is plotted

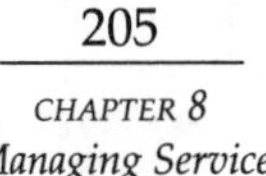

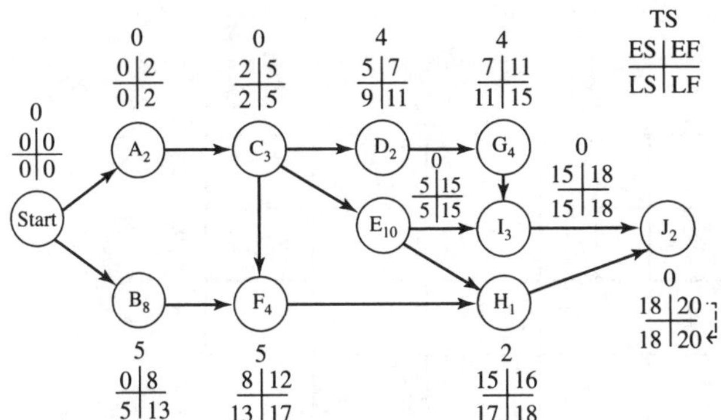

FIGURE 8.5. Completed critical path analysis for tennis tournament.

with an arrow equal to its duration in days and scheduled to begin at its early start date. The dotted lines following activities G, F, and H represent slack on noncritical paths. This figure provides a visual picture of a project schedule. For example, activity G has 4 days of total slack. The start of this activity can be delayed, or its duration may take longer than expected, up to a total of 4 days without affecting the project completion time. Note that the 5 days of total slack for activities B and F include the 2 days of total slack of activity H. Thus, if used to its maximum limit, total slack for an activity can drive a following activity to become critical. For example, if the start of activity F were delayed 5 days until the beginning of day 14, then activity H must be accomplished on day 18 with no slack available. Activity F could be delayed 3 days, however, without affecting the *ES* of the following activity (i.e., H). The length of the dotted lines immediately following activities F, G, and H represent what is called *free slack,* because these delays have no effect on the early start of following activities.

Microsoft Project for Windows Analysis

The tennis tournament also can be analyzed using the software program Microsoft Project for Windows. Data are entered using the Gantt chart format shown in Figure 8.7, and a calendar is included noting the dates and days in the week. Each activity's duration and precedence relationship are entered, creating an early start schedule after the last activity has been entered. The critical path is identified by the cross-hatched bars of the critical activities on the Gantt chart. Note these critical activities are bars that begin immediately after each other and, together, add up to the 20-day project duration, excluding weekend days (i.e., Saturday and Sunday), because in this example, no work is accomplished on the weekend. The program does not break the bar of an activity for the weekend, however, and continues uninterrupted from Friday to the following Monday (see activities 2 and 5).

A Microsoft Project for Windows PERT chart is shown in Figure 8.8. The critical path is shown with darkened boxes and heavy arrows. Corresponding to the Gantt chart, the scheduled start (i.e., beginning of day) and scheduled finish (i.e., end of day) dates are noted for each activity under the activity ID number. The

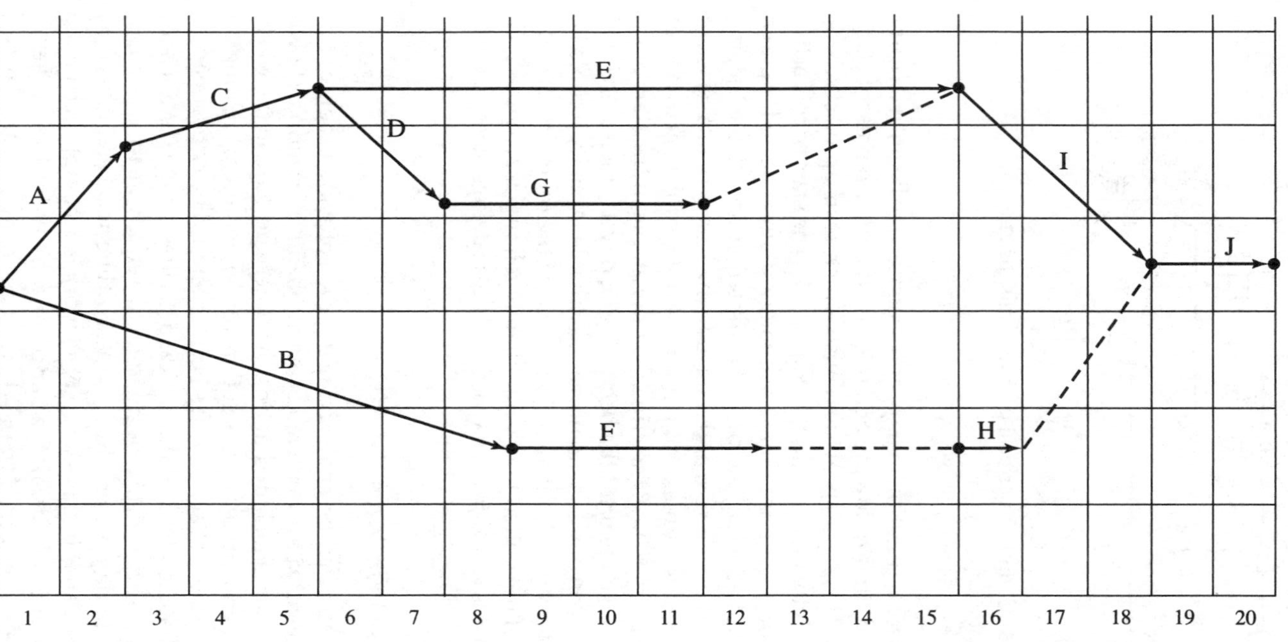

FIGURE 8.6. PERT early start schedule for tennis tournament.

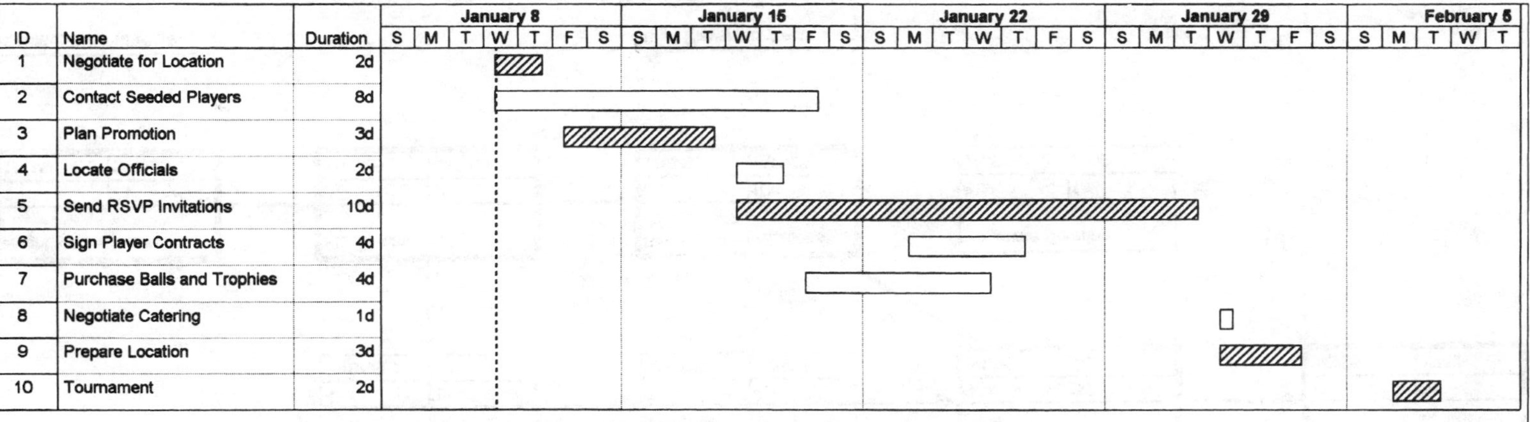

FIGURE 8.7. Microsoft Project for Windows Gantt chart.

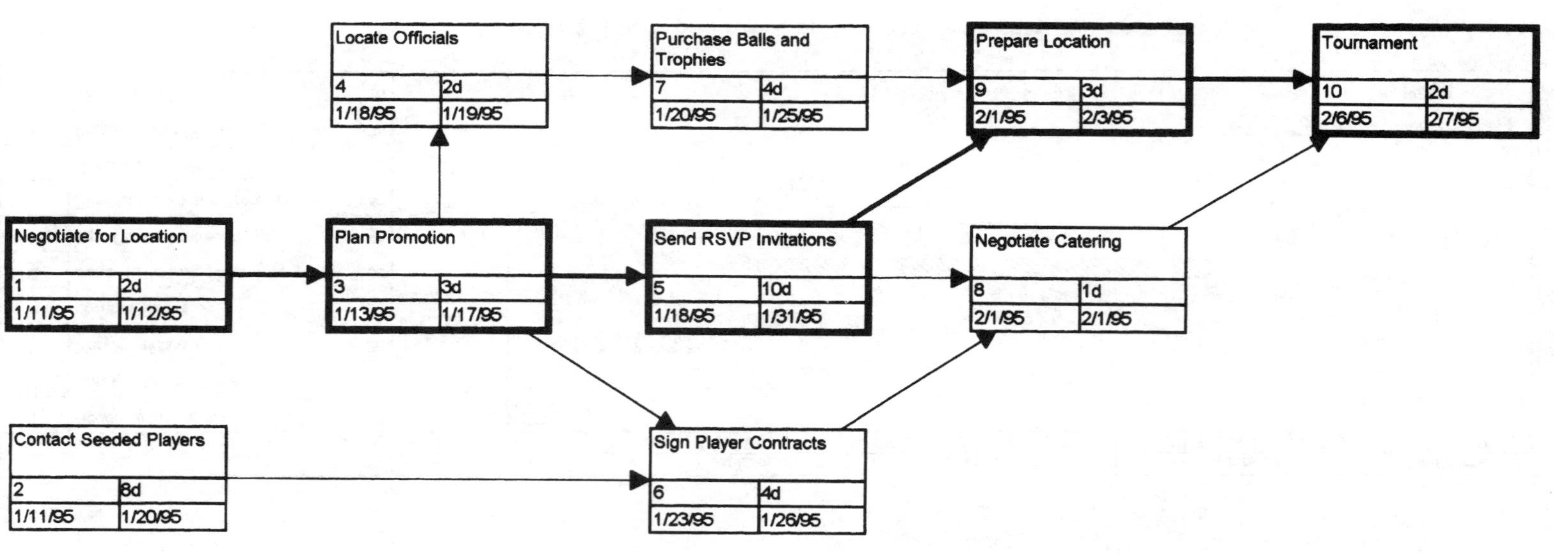

FIGURE 8.8. Microsoft Project for Windows PERT chart.

days of duration for each activity also are noted. For example, the first activity, "Negotiate for Location," which requires 2 days to accomplish, begins at the start of day 1/11/95 and finishes at the end of day 1/12/95.

Of what value is the information provided by critical path analysis? First, we know which activities likely will determine the project completion time if everything goes according to plan. We have identified the activities that cannot be delayed and, consequently, require more intense managerial attention. We also have identified noncritical activities that have some scheduling flexibility and can be used to advantage (e.g., the 4 slack days needed to purchase balls and trophies can be used to shop for bargains). Related to this, of course, is the allocation of resources. For example, workers might be shifted from activities with slack time to critical activities to reduce the risk of a project overrun or to make up for delays.

RESOURCE CONSTRAINTS

To this point in our analysis of project networks, we have assumed (although not explicitly) that resources are available to perform many activities concurrently. As shown in Figure 8.8, our PERT chart reveals three paths in parallel, with only the longest being critical and, thus, determining the project completion time. For example, while RSVP invitations are being extended (i.e., the critical path activity), balls and trophies are being purchased and player contracts are being signed. During this time period, if one person were required to perform each task, then at least three people would be required to support our project schedule. In addition to workers, resource constraints also could include equipment availability (e.g., construction crane), shared facility (e.g., laboratory), and specialists (e.g., computer programmers). Ignoring the effect of resource constraints can result in a project schedule being infeasible; thus, the expected project completion date would be unattainable.

Returning to the tennis tournament example, an early start Gantt chart is shown in Figure 8.9. An early start schedule is created simply by starting each activity at its early start time (i.e., every line is drawn as far left as possible). In Figure 8.9, the critical path activities are drawn with a heavy line, indicating that the scheduling of these activities cannot be changed if we wish to complete the project in 20 days. The noncritical path activities (i.e., those with slack) are drawn with a light line, indicating that flexibility exists in their schedules. Assuming that one person is required to perform each activity, we have added a "Personnel Required" row at the bottom to indicate the staffing levels for each day in the project. As shown, the scheduled use of resources varies greatly, from one person during the last 4 days to 3 people during the sixth through eleventh days.

Using the scheduling flexibility of the noncritical activities, the resource leveled schedule shown in Figure 8.10 can be created. Note that all the noncritical activities except B have delayed start dates, with activities F and H starting on their late start dates. If only two persons are available to arrange this tournament, however, then the project duration must be extended by 1 day, because our leveled schedule shows that three persons are required on day 14. As might be expected, resource constraints result in stretching out the completion time of a project.

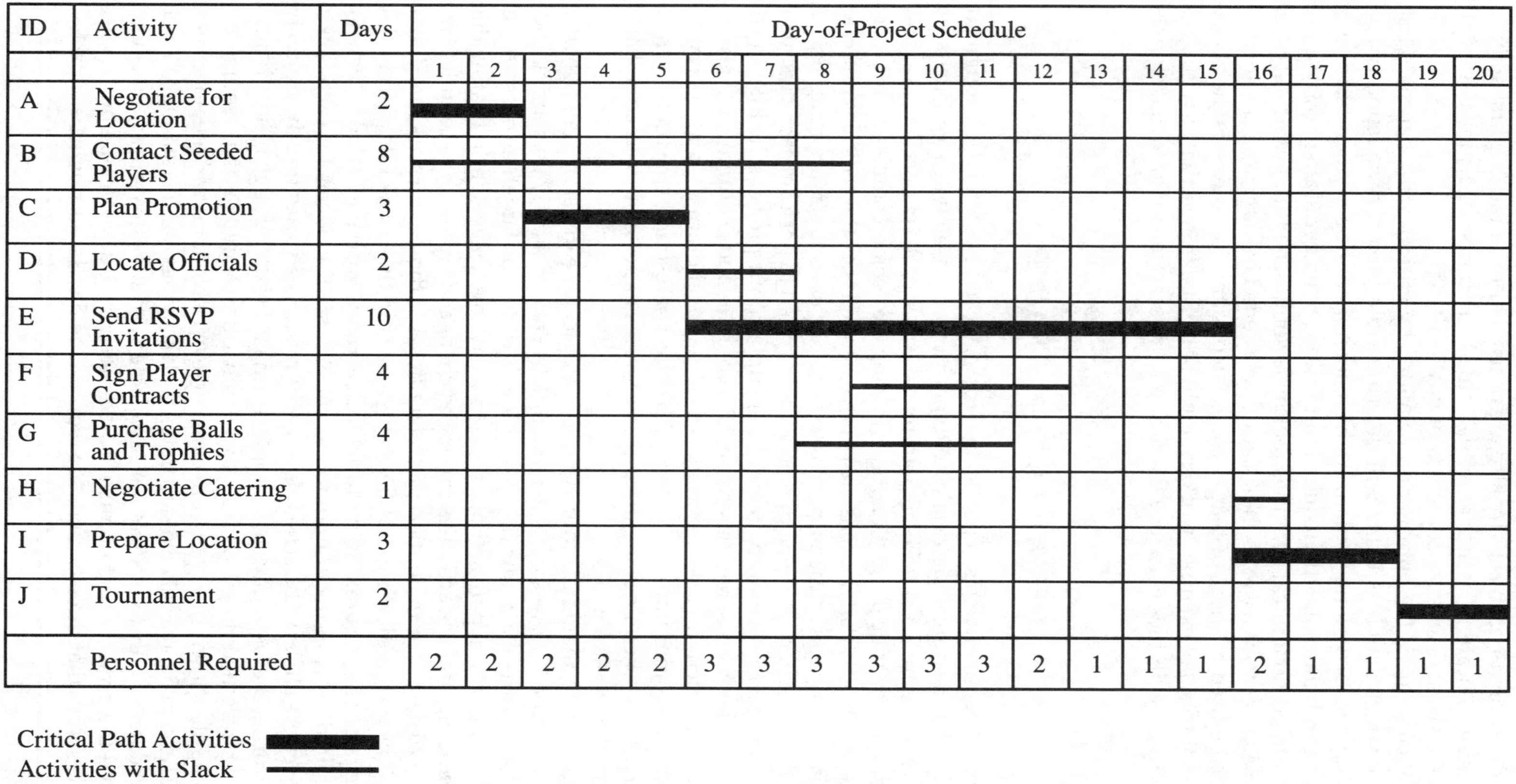

ID	Activity	Days	Day-of-Project Schedule																			
			1	2	3	4	5	6	7	8	9	10	11	12	13	14	15	16	17	18	19	20
A	Negotiate for Location	2																				
B	Contact Seeded Players	8																				
C	Plan Promotion	3																				
D	Locate Officials	2																				
E	Send RSVP Invitations	10																				
F	Sign Player Contracts	4																				
G	Purchase Balls and Trophies	4																				
H	Negotiate Catering	1																				
I	Prepare Location	3																				
J	Tournament	2																				
	Personnel Required		2	2	2	2	2	3	3	3	3	3	3	2	1	1	1	2	1	1	1	1

Critical Path Activities
Activities with Slack

FIGURE 8.9. Early start Gantt chart.

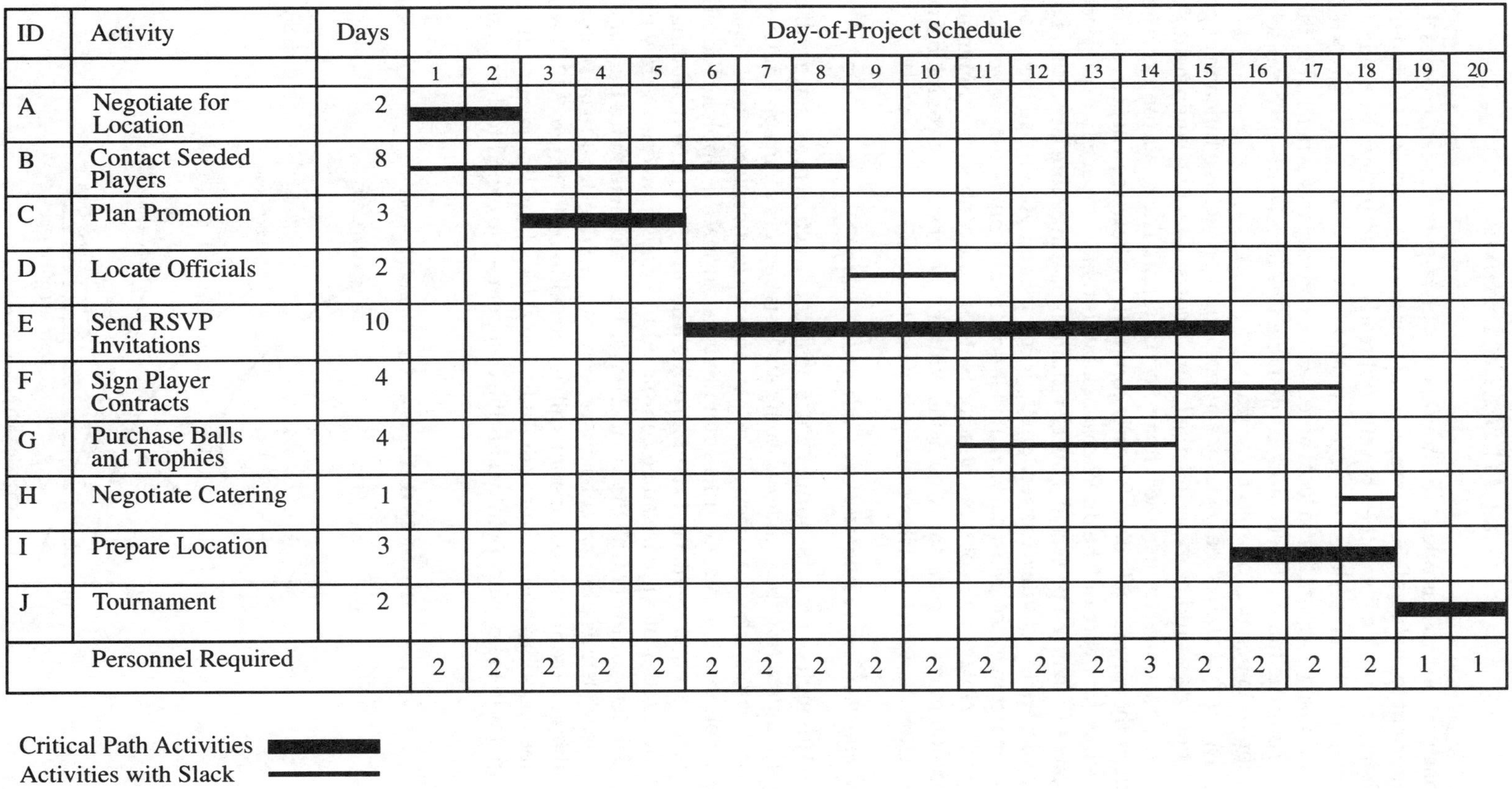

ID	Activity	Days	Day-of-Project Schedule																			
			1	2	3	4	5	6	7	8	9	10	11	12	13	14	15	16	17	18	19	20
A	Negotiate for Location	2																				
B	Contact Seeded Players	8																				
C	Plan Promotion	3																				
D	Locate Officials	2																				
E	Send RSVP Invitations	10																				
F	Sign Player Contracts	4																				
G	Purchase Balls and Trophies	4																				
H	Negotiate Catering	1																				
I	Prepare Location	3																				
J	Tournament	2																				
	Personnel Required		2	2	2	2	2	2	2	2	2	2	2	2	2	3	2	2	2	2	1	1

Critical Path Activities

Activities with Slack

FIGURE 8.10. Resource-leveled schedule.

ACTIVITY CRASHING

Construction projects often are undertaken with target completion dates that are important to the client. For example, consider the construction of a student dormitory at a university. If the project is not ready for occupancy by the last week of August, then a serious disruption would occur. At one university, students were housed temporarily in local hotels at the contractor's expense. For this reason, construction contracts often contain clauses to reward early project completion or to penalize a project overrun.

Figure 8.11 shows the costs for a hypothetical project as a function of project duration. As would be expected, the indirect costs of renting equipment, supervision, and insurance increase with project duration. The opportunity cost curve reflects the contractual bonus for early completion (shown as a negative cost) and penalties for overrun. The direct cost of labor is related inversely to project time, because finishing a project in a hurry requires applying more labor than normal to critical path activities to speed up their completion. Adding all these costs results in a convex total cost curve that identifies a minimum-cost project duration from the vantage point of the contractor. Note that the contractor's minimum cost duration may not necessarily coincide with the client's target completion date. Therefore, how could such a discrepancy be resolved?

Example 8.4: Tennis Tournament—Activity Crashing

Although our tennis tournament is not a construction project, we will use it for illustrating the activity crashing analysis because all the preliminary critical path analysis has been done. An activity is considered to be "crashed" when it is completed in less time than is normal by applying additional labor or equipment. For example, using a normal two-person painting crew, the interior of a home can be completed in 4 days; however, a crew of four painters could "crash" the job in 2 days. This information for time and cost of each tennis tournament activity is shown in Table 8.3. The last column of this table contains a calculation called "expedite-cost." Figure 8.12 illustrates the cost-time tradeoff for activity E. The slope of the line joining the crash point to the normal point yields the cost per day to expedite the activity as-

FIGURE 8.11. Costs for hypothetical project.

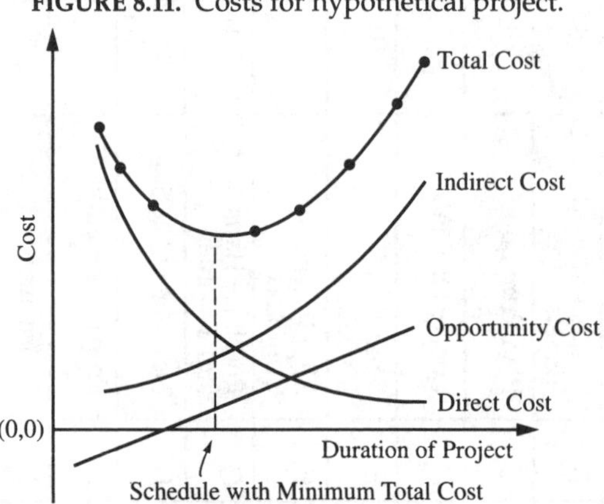

TABLE 8.3. Cost-Time Estimates for Tennis Tournament

Activity	*Time Estimate (days)*		*Direct Cost ($)*		Expedite Cost ($/day)
	Normal	Crash	Normal	Crash	
A	2	1	5	15	10
B	8	6	22	30	4
C	3	2	10	13	3
D	2	1	11	17	6
E	10	6	20	40	5
F	4	3	8	15	7
G	4	3	9	10	1
H	1	1	10	10	—
I	3	2	8	10	2
J	2	1	12	20	8
			115		

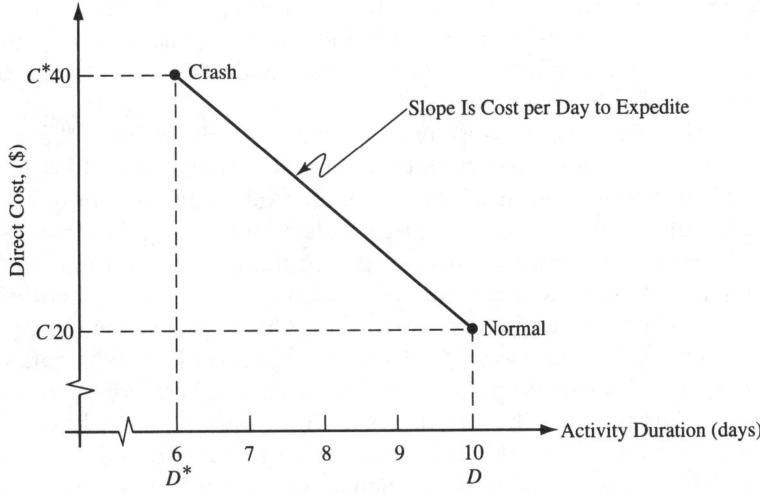

FIGURE 8.12. Activity cost-time tradeoff.

suming a constant rate of cost increase. The values for the expedite-cost slope are calculated using equation (7), which is a ratio of the difference in cost (crash – normal) divided by the difference in duration (normal – crash), yielding an expedite-cost per day.

$$S = \frac{C^* - C}{D - D^*} \tag{7}$$

where C = activity cost (* for crash cost) and
D = activity duration (* for crash duration).

In performing the complete analysis that results in a total cost determination for various project durations, schedules for indirect costs and opportunity costs are required. Table 8.4 shows the indirect cost schedule, ranging from 45 to 13, and the opportunity costs, ranging from 8 to –8. The

TABLE 8.4. Total Cost Calculations

Project Duration	Activity Crashed	Direct Cost	Indirect Cost	Opportunity Cost	Total Cost
20	Normal	115	45	8	168
19	I*	117	41	6	164
18	C*	120	37	4	161
17	E	125	33	2	160
16	E	130	29	0	159
15	E	135	25	−2	158
14	J*	143	21	−4	160
13	E*, B	152	17	−6	163
12	A*, B*	166	13	−8	171

analysis begins with the first row showing the normal project duration and costs (the direct cost of 115 came from Table 8.3). The project duration is incrementally reduced 1 day at a time by crashing an activity on the critical path. Using the expedite-cost as a guide, the critical activity with the least expedite-cost is selected (e.g., for the critical path A-C-E-I-J, we find that activity I costs only 2 to crash 1 day).

Table 8.5 is used to keep track of changes in *all* project paths as we reduce the time of activities on the critical path(s). Note that we have given activity I an asterisk, because it cannot be crashed further (i.e., only 1 day was available) and, thus, is no longer a candidate for crashing. In Table 8.5 under the I* column, we have the revised path durations for the project and find that path A-C-E-I-J, with a duration of 19 days, remains the only critical path. We next turn to activity C to crash for 1 day, followed by crashing activity E for 3 straight days until we create two critical paths of 15 days' duration. With both path A-C-E-I-J and path B-F-H-J being critical, any reduction in project duration must reduce the duration of each path simultaneously. Candidates include selecting activity E on one path and B on the other, at a combined cost of 9, or selecting activity J, which is common to both paths, at a cost of 8. As seen in Table 8.5, further crashing involves multiple critical paths. Once the project duration reaches 12 days, it cannot be reduced further in duration, because critical path A-C-E-I-J now contains all activities with an asterisk (i.e., no candidates remain to be crashed). From Table 8.4, however, we see that a project duration of 15 days reaches a minimum total cost. This du-

TABLE 8.5. Project Path Durations Following Crashing

Project Paths	Normal Duration	*Duration After Crashing Activity*							
		I*	C*	E	E	E	J*	E*, B	A*, B*
A-C-D-G-I-J	16	15	14	14	14	14	13	13	12
A-C-E-I-J	20	19	18	17	16	15	14	13	12
A-C-E-H-J	18	18	17	16	15	14	13	12	11
A-C-F-H-J	12	12	11	11	11	11	10	10	9
B-F-H-J	15	15	15	15	15	15	14	13	12

ration would be acceptable to the client, because a bonus of 2 is received if the project is completed in 15 days.

The crashing procedure can be summarized as:

1. Calculate the expedite-cost for each activity using equation (7).
2. List all the paths in the project network and their normal duration.
3. Crash by 1 day the least costly (i.e., minimum expedite-cost) activity on the critical path or the least costly combination of activities on common critical paths. Record the cost of the crashed schedule.
4. Update the duration for each path in the project network.
5. If an activity has reached its crash time, note with an asterisk and do not consider it as a further candidate.
6. If a critical path contains activities all noted with an asterisk, STOP; otherwise, GO to 3.

INCORPORATING UNCERTAINTY IN ACTIVITY TIMES

In the Example 8.4, we assumed that activity duration t was a constant. For many situations, however, this assumption is not practical because of the uncertainties involved in carrying out the activities. These durations generally are random variables that have associated probability distributions. Therefore, we do not know in advance the exact durations of all activities; consequently, we cannot determine the exact completion time of the project.

Estimating Activity Duration Distributions

To this point in our analysis, we have assumed that activity durations are known with certainty. However, for projects requiring creativity and experimentation (e.g., staging a Broadway play) or construction projects in adverse locations (e.g., the Alaska crude-oil pipeline), activity durations are random variables. Figure 8.13 shows a typical Beta distribution that is commonly used to describe the duration of uncertain activities. This distribution captures the "skewness" in the

FIGURE 8.13. Beta distribution of activity duration.

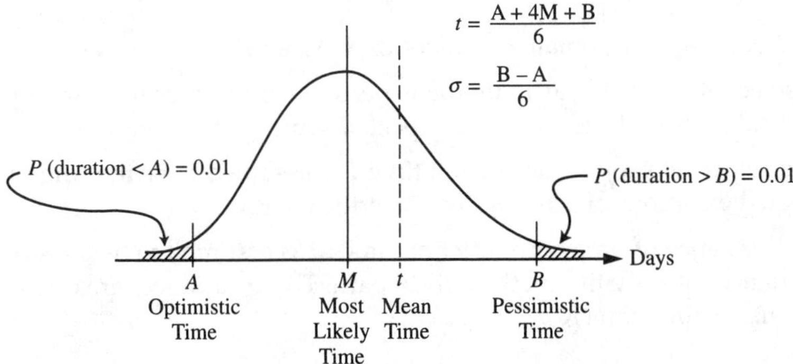

distribution of activity duration that is likely to have a mean that is greater than the mode. Further, the Beta distribution can be approximated by simple formulas that require only three critical time estimates:

1. *Optimistic time (A).* This is the duration of an activity if no complications or problems occur. As a rule of thumb, there should be about a one percent chance of the actual duration being less than *A*.
2. *Most likely time (M).* This is the duration that is most likely to occur. In statistical terms, *M* is the modal value.
3. *Pessimistic time (B).* This is the duration of an activity if extraordinary problems arise. As a rule of thumb, there should be about a one percent chance of the actual duration ever exceeding *B*.

Using these three time estimates, the following formulas can be used to calculate the mean and the variance of each activity distribution. The formula for the mean is a weighted average, with the modal value being given a weight of four:

$$t = (A + 4M + B)/6 \tag{8}$$

Recall that our definitions of optimistic and pessimistic times stipulate that 98 percent of the distribution should be contained within the range *A-B*. Thus, the standard deviation formula assumes that the optimistic time *A* and the pessimistic time *B* are six standard deviations apart.

$$\sigma = (B - A)/6 \tag{9}$$

The activity variance, which we will use in calculating the project completion time distribution, becomes:

$$\sigma^2 = (B - A)^2/36 \tag{10}$$

Project Completion Time Distribution

Because each activity has a distribution, the project itself will have a completion time distribution that is based on the path of longest duration. The steps involved in the analysis are:

1. For every activity, obtain estimates of *A*, *M*, and *B*.
2. Use equation (8) to calculate the expected activity durations, and perform critical path analysis using the expected activity durations *t*.
3. The expected project completion time *T* is assumed to be the sum of the expected durations of activities on the critical path.
4. The variance of project completion time σ_T^2 is assumed to be the sum of the variances of activities on the critical path. These variances are calculated by means of equation (10).

5. The project completion time is assumed to be distributed normally.[1]
6. Probabilities regarding project completion time can be determined from standard normal tables. (*See* Appendix A, Areas of a Standard Normal Distribution)

Example 8.5: Tennis Tournament—Project Completion Time Distribution

We revisit the tennis tournament project once again, but now we assume that the activity durations are uncertain and obtain the three time estimates as recorded in Table 8.6 below. Because the tennis facility is booked for other matches, you are asked to find the probability of finishing the tournament within 24 days of initiating negotiations (i.e., of completing the entire project).

The variances and expected activity durations are calculated by means of equations (8) and (10) and are given in Table 8.6. Note that the expected activity durations are identical to the values that were used in the critical path analysis performed in Example 8.3. Thus, the critical path A-C-E-I-J, which was identified earlier in Figure 8.5, will be the focus of our determination of the project completion time distribution.

We would expect the sum of activity durations on this path to take 20 days and, thus, to determine the expected project completion time T. The variance of project completion time is calculated by summing the variances that are associated with the critical activities. This yields:

$$\sigma_T^{\,2} = 4/36 + 4/36 + 144/36 + 36/36 + 0 = 188/36 = 5.2$$

[1]This assumption is based on the central limit theorem from statistics, which states that the sum of many independent random variables is a random variable that tends to be distributed normally. In this case, the project completion time is the sum of the individual durations of activities on the critical path.

TABLE 8.6. Variances and Expected Activity Durations

	Time Estimates				
Activity	*A*	*M*	*B*	Variance (σ^2)	Expected Duration (t)
A	1	2	3	4/36	2
B	5	8	11	36/36	8
C	2	3	4	4/36	3
D	1	2	3	4/36	2
E	6	9	18	144/36	10
F	2	4	6	16/36	4
G	1	3	11	100/36	4
H	1	1	1	0	1
I	2	2	8	36/36	3
J	2	2	2	0	2

We can now use T and σ_T^2 to determine the probability of finishing the project within 24 days. The Z value for the standard normal deviate is calculated using equation (11):

$$Z = \frac{X - \mu}{\sigma} \tag{11}$$

Thus, for the tennis tournament:

$$Z = \frac{X - \mu}{\sigma} = \frac{24 - T}{\sigma_T} = \frac{24 - 20}{\sqrt{5.2}} = 1.75$$

From the standard normal table with $Z = 1.75$, we find the probability of completing the project within 24 days to be approximately 0.96. Figure 8.14 shows the normal distribution of the project completion time with a 0.04 probability of exceeding 24 days' duration.

A Critique of the Project Completion Time Analysis

The key assumption underlying our analysis leading to a project completion time distribution is that the critical path as calculated from expected activity durations will actually be the true critical path. This is a critical assumption, because it suggests that we know the critical path before all the uncertain activities have been completed. In reality, the critical path itself is a random variable that is not known for certain until the project is completed. We know that the duration of the critical path is uncertain and has a probability distribution associated with it; likewise, the durations of other paths are uncertain. Consequently, it is possible for a path with an expected duration of less than the critical path to become the realized critical path because activities on this path have taken much longer than expected. The net effect is that a path not identified as being critical could determine project completion. Thus, estimates of expected completion time and variance of completion time for the project are biased when they are based only on the single critical path. For the variance, the bias can be either on the high or the low side, but the expected project completion time is always biased optimistically. That is, the true expected completion time is always greater than or equal to the estimate.

FIGURE 8.14. Project completion time distribution.

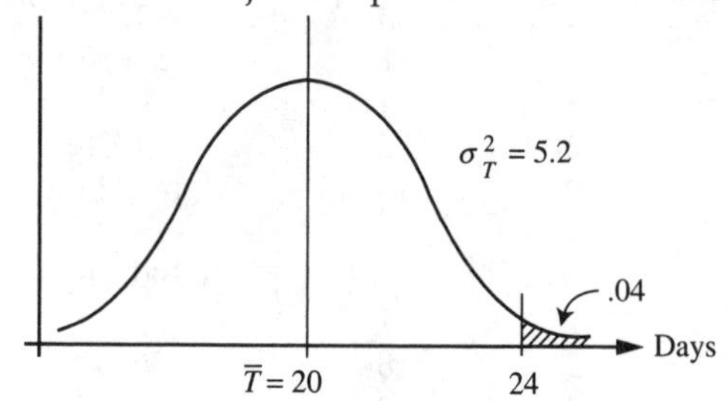

A simple guideline can assist in giving a feel for the accuracy of these estimates: if the expected duration of the critical path is much longer than that of any other path, then the estimates likely will be good. In this case, the critical path very likely will actually determine the project completion time. If the project network contains noncritical paths with very little total slack time, however, these paths may well affect project completion time. This situation is called *merge node bias.* That is, the project completion node has several paths coming into it, any one of which could be the critical path that determines the project completion time. In our analysis, only the most likely path is assumed to be critical; thus, our project completion time distribution is biased optimistically because other near critical paths are ignored. Example 8.6 illustrates the effect on the probability of completing a project when a near-critical path contains an activity with a large variance.

Example 8.6: Tennis Tournament—Merge Node Bias

A few days into the project, we discover that the purchase of balls and a trophy (i.e., activity G) may take longer than expected, with revised estimates of $A = 2$, $M = 3$, and $B = 28$. What effect does this have on the probability of completing the project in 24 days?

First, we recalculate the expected duration and variance of activity G using equations (8) and (10) and find that $t = 7$ and $\sigma^2 = 676/36$. Recall from Figure 8.6 that activity G initially had a 4-day expected duration and total slack of 4 days. Thus, with a revised duration of 7 days, activity G still is noncritical, with a $TS = 1$. The large variance of activity G, however, will have an impact on the likelihood of this path A-C-D-G-I-J becoming critical. A completion time distribution can be determined for this near-critical path in the following manner:

Near-Critical Path	t	σ^2
A	2	4/36
C	3	4/36
D	2	4/36
G	7	676/36
I	3	36/36
J	2	0
	$T = 19$	$\sigma_T^2 = 724/36 = 20$

We now can use T and σ_T^2 of the near-critical path to determine the probability of finishing the project within 24 days. The Z value for the standard normal deviate is calculated using equation (11):

$$Z = \frac{X - \mu}{\sigma} = \frac{24 - T}{\sigma_T} = \frac{24 - 19}{\sqrt{20}} = 1.12$$

Referring to the standard normal table with $Z = 1.12$, we find that the probability of completing the project within 24 days is approximately 0.87. The completion time distribution for this near-critical path is shown in Figure 8.15.

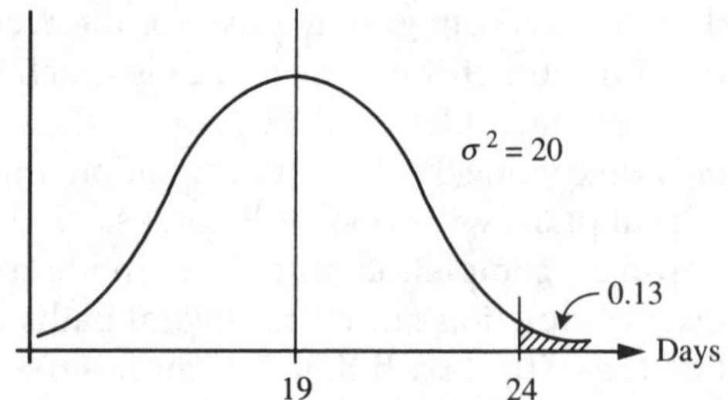

FIGURE 8.15. Near-critical path completion time distribution.

Thus, a near-critical path with a high variance activity should not be ignored, because in fact, such a path may become critical and delay the project completion time. Monte Carlo simulation has been suggested as an approach to determine the project completion time distribution more accurately.[2]

PROBLEMS WITH IMPLEMENTING CRITICAL PATH ANALYSIS

The mechanics of critical path analysis make the use of network models appear to be deceptively simple. After all, the calculations are straightforward. Network analysis does not resolve all the problems inherent in project management, however. Two major concerns are developing the project network and eliciting time estimates for activities.

The project network indicates the sequence in which activities are to be performed. For most projects, several different strategies may be adopted. The technological factors along with the influences of people who are concerned with the project generally determine which strategy is selected. As the project is implemented, the project network is subject to review and possible revision, which may be needed because some activities get off schedule or resources may not be available when needed.

Reviewing and revising the project network can be very time-consuming. The individuals involved with the project must be consulted about anticipated changes. The process of reviewing and revising the project network is an ongoing process that is made easier with the use of computer software.

The second concern in using network models is eliciting time estimates for activities. Obviously, poor estimates would impact the accuracy of project planning. Resident experts often are sought out for their experience in past projects. It is difficult to get good time estimates, however, because people disagree and consensus may be difficult to achieve.

Another problem is that of bias introduced into estimates of activity durations. For example, an individual actually may expect to carry out an activity in

[2]R. M. Van Slyke, "Monte Carlo Methods and the PERT Problem," *Operations Research,* vol. 11, no. 5, September–October 1963, pp. 839–860.

8 days but gives an estimate of 10 days. Thus, the individual provides a few days leeway by padding the estimate. To avoid these problems, a data base of actual times on past projects could be developed to provide time estimates for common activities. For example, painting the walls of a room could be estimated based on the time per square foot from past experience.

Service Benchmark

Project Management Software in Use

The project manager's job has been made easier with the use of computer software that goes beyond the planning and scheduling of activities as illustrated by Microsoft Project for Windows to the motivation and management of people. In the effort of getting a project finished on time, many managers are so consumed in daily tasks that they may forget to manage the project employees. A new software program called Managepro for Windows does just that. It reminds the executive that there are important management issues that go beyond deadlines.

"In today's corporation you see a rapidly expanding scope of management, or span of control, and the result is that you wind up with a manager being responsible for more and more people," said Kerry N. Diehl, a general manager at a large Eastern electric utility that he asked not be named. "Unless you can come up with a good tool or mechanism for controlling and delegating projects and activities, you end up spending more time trying to figure out what you gave to whom than you do actually managing."

For Mr. Diehl, that tool is Managepro for Windows, which pairs people management with project management. A dash of philosophy and psychology, in the form of an expert system that offers online advice, is tossed in for good measure. The combination is powerful and effective. Managepro for Windows should not be confused with simpler project management software, which helps executives set goals and timetables for a given work activity. And indeed it can be quite helpful at planning most common business tasks.

But Managepro for Windows prefers to call itself a new type of software: goal and people management. That reflects how it works: separate but integrated sets of operations, one for goals and one for people. As a manager, you set the goal and assign tasks toward reaching that goal to various people. You want to know how the project is going, and that means keeping track of how the people are doing.

"I use it to track projects, due dates and the people who are responsible," said Stacey Richardson, manager of management information systems at the Ridge Tahoe, a timesharing condominium resort in South Lake Tahoe, Nev. "And then you can get your reports out either on project information, showing progress on all the steps, or a completely different view, showing all the steps that have to be taken by a given individual."

The goals part of the software helps managers define, as specifically as possible, the broad company goals. Examples might be to reduce shipping errors to less than 1 percent by June 15, or to double sales in Minnesota by the end of the year. The goals are listed on a scoreboard similar to a spreadsheet showing for each one a description of the deadline, the person or teams responsible for achieving the goal, and an indicator for how the project is going—whether it is on track, behind schedule or critical.

The goals are listed in what is commonly known as a collapsed outline form. If the manager wants more information—Why is our shipping project behind schedule?—she clicks on that item to reveal greater levels of detail: Aha! Linda in the shipping department was going to report by April 1 on alternative shipping services. She's behind schedule.

Now the manager can shift to the people dimension—finding out, for example, whether Linda has a pattern of missing deadlines and might benefit from more oversight of interim progress. A series of buttons on screen can be clicked to summon information for each employee: goals, progress, feedback, review, recognition, development, commitment, calendar, details and notes. The information is kept confidential with a simple password protection scheme.

"It's a manager's dream come true," said Randy Dugger, who manages work station local area network support for Tandem Computers Inc. of Cupertino, CA. "Before Managepro, you typically had to write down all this information in some word processing file, and you'd print it out and put the paper in the employee's file," he said. "It was all paper tracking, searching through files to find the right piece of information. With Managepro, everything concerning your project is two or three clicks away. "I keep track of everything concerning my employees, the good messages as well as the bad, as well as counseling sessions. Everything is fully documented. I can print out a report and use it during the employee review process."

Another button on screen, the supervisor, offers experts' wisdom on human relations management. How does a manager help nurture and develop the skills of workers? How does she become a more effective manager? How do managers deal with workers who are not doing their assigned jobs, or those who do the jobs but wreak havoc along the way?

The Managepro adviser notes that some employees are like war canoes, getting from point A to point B swiftly and without a ripple. Others are like garbage scows: They get there eventually, but they are noisy, smelly and leave an oil slick. "The people in Department X tell me they don't ever want to work with you again because of your aggressive behavior," the adviser says as an example of how to pilot a garbage scow. "Fix that relationship in the 60 days left in this project so that they tell me they look forward to working with you again."

Managepro may also remind the manager that it's time to reward a promising employee with a pair of tickets to a ballgame or dinner for two.

"It does come with what is basically a human resources philosophy behind it," said Mr. Diehl, the utility manager. "By taking the broader look, not just being a task manager but addressing the ideas of employee evaluation and the issues of compensation and recognition, it provides a much-needed dimension to project management. It's not that people don't think of it, but the software helps as a reminder."

Mr. Dugger of Tandem said: "I wouldn't say that it has changed my management style. It's just made my job a lot easier. The nice thing is that you can use as much or as little of it as you want. It doesn't force you to use the whole thing all at once. You can grow into it."

Source: Adapted from Peter H. Lewis, "Pairing People Management with Project Management," *The New York Times*, April 11, 1993, p. 12.

SUMMARY

Managers of organizations typically are immersed in the detailed operations of ongoing projects. They also are responsible for generating new projects. The vitality of an organization can be seen in the way that projects are conceived and carried out. For dynamic organizations, project management has important dimensions; it involves planning, scheduling, and controlling the activities that are necessary to carry out a project successfully.

For small, uncomplicated projects, Gantt charts are a good tool for assisting project managers. For large projects that involve many interdependent activities, however, Gantt charts are cumbersome. Network techniques using critical path analysis were developed as tools for aiding managers of complex projects.

Network techniques are very important tools for project management. They indicate the activities that likely will affect project completion, and they also facilitate the evaluation of changes in project implementation. Further, advances are being made with regard to the accuracy and efficiency of network approaches. In conjunction with the availability of faster and cheaper computer resources, this will make network techniques even more valuable to service operations managers.

KEY TERMS AND DEFINITIONS

Calendars specifications of the days and hours that resources such as people and equipment are available for work.

Critical path the sequence of activities in a project that has the longest duration, thus defining the project completion time.

Critical path method (CPM) the process for determining the start and finish dates for individual activities, thus creating the *critical path* for the project.

Critical activities activities on the critical path that, if delayed, would result in the delay of the project as a whole.

Gantt chart a graphical representation of the project schedule containing horizontal bars for each activity with the length of the bars corresponding to the duration of the activity.

Milestone the completion of a major achievement, phase, or measurable goal.

PERT chart a graphical representation of the relationship between activities using arrows to show precedence and nodes for activity descriptions.

Predecessor an activity that must precede another activity.

Project a collection of related activities or steps that are performed in a specified sequence for the purpose of meeting a defined, nonroutine goal.

Successor an activity that follows another activity.

Work breakdown schedule a family tree subdivision of the effort that is required to achieve the project objective.

SOLVED PROBLEMS

1. Critical Path Analysis

Problem Statement

You have been asked to head a special project team at McDonald's to bring out a new breakfast item called the McWaffle. You have prepared the network diagram below showing the necessary activities with their expected times in days. Calculate the scheduling times *ES, LS, EF, LF,* and slack time *TS* for each activity. What are the critical path and project duration?

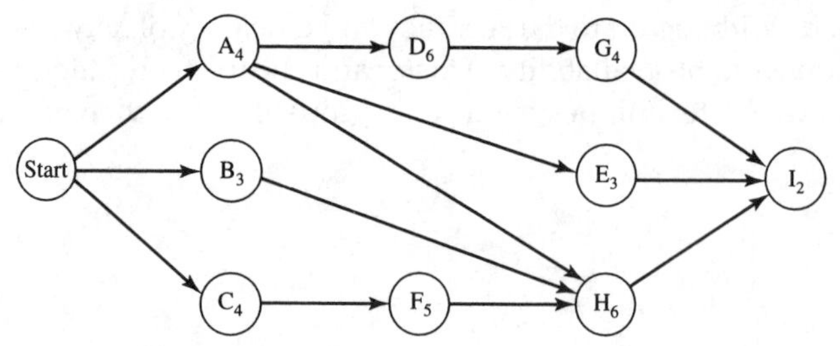

Solution

Activity	Time	*Forward Pass* ES	EF	*Backward Pass* LF	LS	TS = LS – ES
A	4	0	4	5	1	1
B	3	0	3	9	6	6
C	4	0	4	4	0	0
D	6	4	10	11	5	1
E	3	4	7	15	12	8
F	5	4	9	9	4	0
G	4	10	14	15	11	1
H	6	9	15	15	9	0
I	2	15	17	17	15	0

The critical path activities are C, F, H, and I, because $TS = 0$ in each case. The project duration is 17 days, the sum of the critical path activity times.

2. Activity Crashing

Problem Statement

For the network above, assume that an activity's daily expedite-cost in dollars per day is equal to the activity's time (e.g., the cost to reduce the activity time of H by one day is $6.) Further, assume that each activity may be crashed only 1 day. What activities should be crashed to reduce the project duration by 3 days at least cost?

Solution

In the table below, the circled numbers represent the project duration, starting with 17 days. After activity C is crashed, two paths become critical; thus, two activities must be crashed (one on each path) to achieve a 14-day project duration.

Project Path	Normal Time	*Activities Crashed* I	C	F&A or F&G
A-D-G-I	16	15	(15)	(14)
A-E-I	9	8	8	8 or 7
A-H-I	12	11	11	11 or 10
B-H-I	11	10	10	10
C-F-H-I	(17)	(16)	(15)	(14)

3. Incorporating Uncertainty in Activity Times

Problem Statement

Assume the McWaffle project above contained some uncertain activity times as shown below. Calculate the mean and variance of all activities, and determine the probability of completing the project within 20 days without crashing any activities.

Solution

First, calculate the mean and variance for each activity using equations (8) and (10):

Activity	*A*	*M*	*B*	Mean	Variance
A	3	4	5	4	4/36
B	3	3	3	3	0
C	3	4	5	4	4/36
D	4	6	8	6	16/36
E	2	3	4	3	4/36
F	2	4	12	5	100/36
G	3	4	5	4	4/36
H	4	5	12	6	64/36
I	2	2	2	2	0

Second, determine the critical path. This calculation yields activity means that are identical to those of the original problem statement. Thus, the critical path is C-F-H-I, with an expected time of $T = 17$ days. The variance of the project completion time is the sum of the critical activity variances. This yields $\sigma_T^2 = 4/36 + 100/36 + 64/36 + 0 = 168/36 = 4.67$. Using equation (11), we calculate the Z value for a project completion within 20 days:

$$Z = \frac{X - \mu}{\sigma} = \frac{20 - T}{\sigma_T} = \frac{20 - 17}{\sqrt{4.67}} = 1.39$$

Using Appendix A, Areas of a Standard Normal Distribution, we find a probability of $0.5 + 0.4177 = 0.9177$, or approximately a 92 percent chance of competing the project within 20 days.

TOPICS FOR DISCUSSION

1. Give examples of large, complex projects undertaken by a major urban bank that might benefit from project management techniques.
2. Project management is concerned with planning, scheduling, and controlling activities. Explain what each of these means in terms of project management.
3. Are Gantt charts still viable project management tools? Explain.
4. Determining the activity sequence and estimating activity durations often are the most difficult aspects of project analysis. Explain.
5. Give a critique of project analysis with uncertain activity times.
6. Explain why the PERT estimate of expected project duration is always optimistic. Can we get any feel for the magnitude of this bias?

7. What are some typical problems with implementing critical path analysis?
8. Costs and resource utilization are major concerns in project management. Can you suggest methods for integrating these into critical path analysis?

EXERCISES

8.1. An electric utility is planning its annual project of shutting down one of its steam boilers for maintenance and repair. An analysis of this project has identified the following principal activities and their expected times and relationships.

Activity	Time (days)	Immediate Predecessor
A	4	—
B	3	—
C	4	—
D	6	A
E	3	A
F	5	C
G	4	D
H	6	A,B,F
I	2	E,G,H

a. Prepare a project network diagram.
b. Calculate the scheduling times and total slack for each activity.
c. List the critical path activities and project duration.
d. Assuming that one worker is required for each activity, prepare a resource-leveled schedule. What is the maximum number of workers required to finish the project on time?

8.2. A consulting firm is planning a reengineering project for a client. The following activities and time estimates have been identified:

Activity	Time (days)	Immediate Predecessor
A	1	—
B	2	—
C	2	—
D	2	A,B
E	4	A,C
F	1	C
G	4	D
H	8	G,E,F

a. Draw a project network diagram.
b. Calculate the scheduling times and total slack for each activity.
c. List the critical path activities and project duration.
d. Assuming that one worker is required for each activity, prepare a resource-leveled schedule. What is the maximum number of workers required to finish the project on time?

8.3. Slippery Rock College is planning a basketball tournament. The following information has been collected on each activity in the project:

Activity	Time (days)	Immediate Predecessor	Description
A	3	—	Select teams
B	5	A	Mail out invitations
C	10	—	Arrange accommodations
D	3	B,C	Plan promotion
E	5	B,C	Print tickets
F	10	E	Sell tickets
G	8	C	Complete arrangements
H	3	G	Develop schedules
I	2	D,H	Practice
J	3	F,I	Conduct tournament

a. Draw a network diagram of this project, and label the activities and events.
b. Calculate the total slack and scheduling times for all activities. What is the critical path?
c. When should team selection begin if the tournament is scheduled to start on the morning of December 27? (Include Saturday and Sunday as working days.)

8.4. A simple network consisting of four activities has the following network diagram:

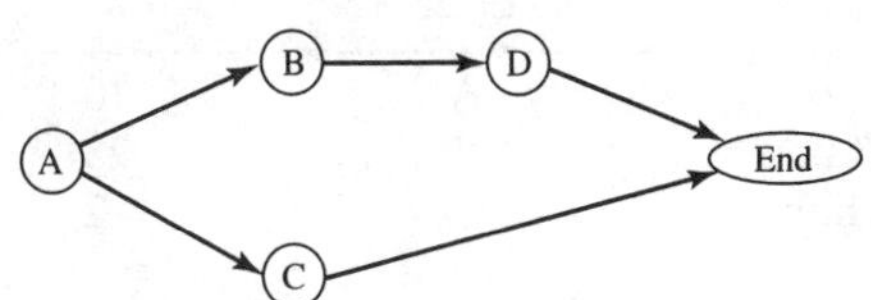

The cost/time relationships for the activities are:

Activity	Minimum Time (weeks)	Maximum Time (weeks)	Cost/Time Relationship ($1000)
A	5	10	100 – (3 × activity time)
B	5	10	100 – (2 × activity time)
C	10	30	100 – (2 × activity time)
D	10	15	100 – (5 × activity time)

For example, if completed in 5 weeks, activity A would require $85,000, and if completed in 10 weeks, it would require $70,000.
a. What would be the minimum cost of completing this project in 20 weeks?
b. If the desired completion date is 33 weeks and the profit markup is 20 percent above cost, what should be the bid price for this project?

8.5. The following project network and table provide the normal times and costs as well as the crash times and costs for the activities required to complete a project. Crash the completion time to the minimum level.

Activity	Normal Time (weeks)	Cost ($)	Crash Time (weeks)	Cost ($)
A	4	2500	2	6000
B	5	4000	4	5000
C	2	3000	1	5000
D	2	2000	1	3000
E	6	3000	4	4000
F	3	2000	1	5000
G	1	2000	1	2000

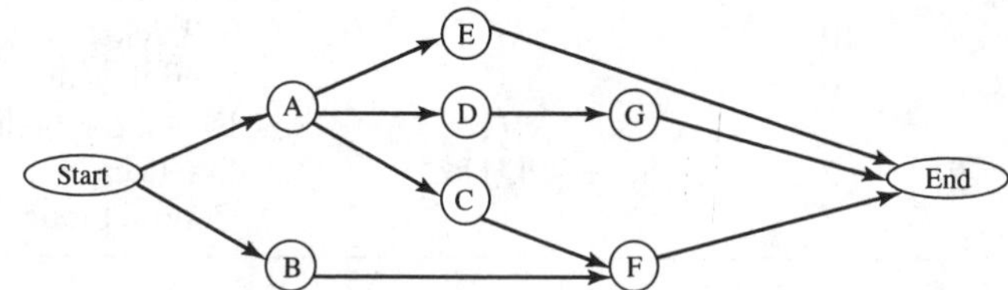

8.6. A construction firm has been commissioned to renew a portion of the Alaska crude-oil pipeline that has fallen into a state of disrepair. The project activities with the estimated times and their relationships are:

Activity	Code	Time (days)	Immediate Predecessor
Assemble crew for job	A	10	—
Build inventory with old line	B	28	—
Measure and sketch old line	C	2	A
Develop materials list	D	1	C
Erect scaffolding	E	2	D
Procure pipe	F	30	D
Procure valves	G	45	D
Deactivate old line	H	1	B,D
Remove old line	I	6	E,H
Prefabricate new line	J	5	F
Place valves	K	1	E,G,H
Place new pipe	L	6	I,J
Weld pipe	M	2	L
Connect valves	N	1	K,M
Insulate	O	4	K,M
Pressure test	P	1	N
Remove scaffolding	Q	1	N,O
Clean up	R	1	P,Q

a. Prepare a project network.
b. List the critical path activities and the expected project duration.
c. Determine the scheduling times and total slack for all activities.
d. In the contract, a bonus of $100,000 per day will be paid for each day the project is completed earlier than its expected duration. Evaluate the following alternatives to shorten the project duration and then make a recommendation:
   1. Crash activity B by 4 days at a cost of $100,000.

2. Crash activity G by 1 day at a cost of $50,000.
3. Crash activity O by 2 days at a cost of $150,000.
4. Crash activity O by 2 days by drawing resources from activity N, thereby extending the time of N by 2 days.

8.7. The following activities have been identified by a consulting firm that is developing an information system for an insurance firm to make a transition to a "paperless" organization:

Activity	Immediate Predecessor	*Activity Duration (months)* Optimistic	Most Likely	Pessimistic
A	—	4	6	8
B	—	1	2	3
C	A	4	4	4
D	A	4	5	6
E	B	7	10	16
F	B	8	9	10
G	C	2	2	2
H	D,E,G	2	3	7
I	F	1	3	11

a. Draw the project network showing the activities with their expected times.
b. What is the critical path and the expected duration of the project?
c. What is the probability of completing the project within 2 years?

8.8. The following activities are required for completing a project:

Activity	Immediate Predecessor	*Activity Duration (days)* Optimistic	Most Likely	Pessimistic
A	—	3	6	15
B	—	2	5	14
C	A	6	12	30
D	A	2	5	8
E	C	5	11	17
F	D	3	6	15
G	B	3	9	27
H	E,F	1	4	7
I	G	4	19	28
J	H,I	1	1	1

a. Draw a network diagram of this project showing the activities and their expected duration times.
b. What is the critical path and the expected completion time of the project?
c. What is the probability of completing the project in 41 days or less?

8.9. The project network and table below show the expected number of weeks to complete a series of activities and the corresponding variances:

Activity	Expected Duration (weeks)	Variance (weeks)
A	5	1
B	10	2
C	4	1
D	7	1
E	6	2
F	8	1
G	4	2
H	3	1
I	5	1
J	7	2
K	8	3

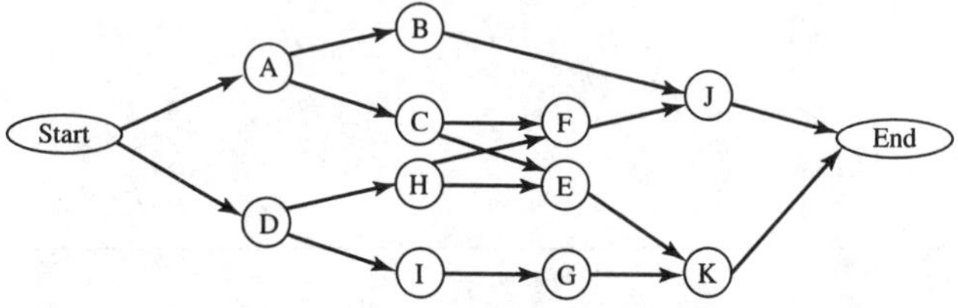

a. Determine the critical path and the earliest expected completion time.
b. What is the probability of completing the project in 24 weeks or less?

8.10. You have been asked to plan the following covert operation for the AIC:

		Activity Duration (days)		
Activity	Immediate Predecessor	Optimistic	Most Likely	Pessimistic
A	—	1	2	3
B	A	3	3	3
C	B	4	6	8
D	A	2	8	8
E	A	6	9	12
F	D,C	4	7	10
G	D	10	10	16
H	D,E	4	5	6
I	F,G,H	2	2	2

a. Draw a network diagram for this project.
b. Calculate the expected time and variance for each activity.
c. Determine the critical path and the expected project completion time.
d. What is the probability of the project taking more than 25 days to complete?

CASE: INFO-SYSTEMS, INC.

Info-Systems is a rapidly growing firm that specializes in information systems consulting. In the past, its projects have been relatively short term and not required extensive project scheduling or close management surveillance. Recently, however, Info-Systems was awarded a contract to develop and implement a large inventory system for a manufacturing firm.

During the initial proposal study, Info-Systems determined that the manufacturing firm's current hardware configuration was inadequate to meet its long-term needs, and new general hardware specifications were developed. Therefore, as part of its assignment, Info-Systems is to perform a vendor evaluation and selection for this new hardware. The initial study also proposed that the system would comprise a combination of batch and on-line processing and estimated a minimum of 1 year for completion.

Info-Systems plans to divide the project into four major areas involving the activities to support: 1) hardware selection and installation, 2) batch processing development, 3) on-line processing development, and 4) conversion from the old system to the new one. Further, it feels the use of a project management system would be very beneficial in providing a more definitive estimate of the probable project completion, in controlling the project once it is under way, and in assigning personnel to the project at the appropriate times. Therefore, Info-Systems has assigned several of its senior staff to develop a detailed task list, which is presented below:

Tasks	Work Duration (days)	Immediate Predecessor
A. Evaluate and select hardware.	30	—
B. Develop batch processing system requirements (e.g., data definition, transaction volume).	60	—
C. Develop on-line processing requirements (e.g., volume response times).	40	—
D. Define specific hardware requirements; order and receive equipment.	100	A,B,C
E. Design report layouts for batch system.	30	B
F. Design input forms for batch system.	20	E
G. Design screen layouts for on-line system.	25	C
H. Design file layouts.	20	F,G
I. Prepare program specifications for *daily* batch cycle.	30	H
J. Prepare program specifications for *weekly* batch cycle.	20	H
K. Prepare program specifications for *monthly* batch cycle.	15	H
L. Prepare program specifications for on-line processing.	20	H
M. Install and test new hardware.	15	D
N. Code programs for *daily* batch cycle.	20	I
O. Code programs for *weekly* batch cycle.	15	J
P. Code programs for *monthly* batch cycle.	10	K
Q. Code programs for on-line cycle.	18	L
R. Document batch system.	35	I,J,K
S. Document on-line system.	25	L
T. Test *daily* cycle.	20	M,N
U. Test *weekly* cycle.	15	M,O
V. Test *monthly* cycle.	12	M,P

W.	Test on-line processing.	15	M,Q
X.	Test total system.	20	T,U,V,W
Y.	Design conversion requirements, programs, and files.	30	H
Z.	Prepare conversion programs.	20	Y
AA.	Test conversion programs.	15	Z
BB.	Run actual conversion.	3	X,AA
CC.	Operate system in parallel and train users.	60	R,S,BB
DD.	Gain user acceptance.	5	CC
EE.	Implement production system.	5	DD

Questions

1. Using Microsoft Project for Windows, prepare a network and identify the critical path activities, the expected project duration, and scheduling times for all activities.

2. The elapsed time for delivery of the hardware is estimated at 90 days. Would the project completion time be affected if delivery of the hardware were delayed by 30 days? Would the critical path change?

3. Using the original network and critical path, what strategies could management consider to complete the project on time if activity B were delayed by several weeks?

CASE: WHITTIER COUNTY HOSPITAL

After some 50 years at its present location, Whittier County Hospital is preparing to move into a new building sometime in the near future, when construction and outfitting are completed. The hospital's board of directors has appointed a special management committee to control the entire procedure, including coordination with outside agencies as well as internal departments. As a first step in its mission, the committee wishes to develop a base of information that will be used to: 1) establish an initial sketch plan for proceeding through the detailed planning and moving phases, and 2) provide a fundamental management and scheduling tool for day-to-day operations during the transition period.

The management staff believes that a PERT analysis of a sketch plan would be very helpful to the committee's understanding of the moving process, so it begins to develop a network of activities and duration estimates for the task. After consultation with the general contractor at the building site, it is estimated that completion of construction and checking the newly installed equipment likely will take 50 more days, with 40 and 60 days being the optimistic and pessimistic estimates, respectively. At this point the structure will be vacated by the contractor and turned over to the board.

Before this occurs, however, a detailed plan of action for each hospital department must be drawn up for approval by the Move Committee (as it is formally known). The staff estimates this will take at least 10 days, perhaps as many as 20 days, and most likely 15 days to develop and secure approval.

Once the detailed plan has received an initial go-ahead, the staff will have a number of activities to perform before a trial run and subsequent evaluation of the plan are made:

1. Develop and distribute an information newsletter to all hospital employees outlining the general procedures, with specific procedures attached for each department; it is estimated that this will take at least 3, probably 4, and at most, 7 days.
2. Develop information and generate media coverage for the upcoming events; this is estimated to take at least (and probably) 2 days, and 3 days at most.
3. Negotiate with local EMS and private ambulance services for transferring the patients; this is estimated to take at least 10, probably 14, and at most, 20 days.
4. Negotiate with professional moving companies for transferring equipment, records, and supplies; this is estimated to take at least 4, probably 5, and at most, 8 days.
5. Coordinate the procedures with, and determine the responsibilities of, the local police and fire de-

partments; this is estimated to take at least 3, probably 5, and at most, 10 days.

6. Coordinate the admissions and exchange procedures during the transition period with other hospitals in the surrounding area; this is estimated to take at least 2, probably 3, and at most, 5 days.

Once the construction and equipment checkout is completed, the new facility must be cleaned thoroughly by hospital staff before the actual move so that it will conform to the required levels for such institutions. Also, after the contractor vacates the premises, the employees can be oriented to the layout and workings of the new building. Because this orientation process is very important, the management staff wants to ensure that it begins after the newsletter is distributed and that it is completed before the trial run of the move. The staff estimates that cleaning and orientation can occur at the same time without problems. Cleaning will take at least 2, probably 3, and at most, 5 days; the employee orientation will take at least 4, probably 5, and at most, 7 days.

Although the actual trial run will take only 1 day, the entire activity, including evaluation, is estimated to need at least (and most likely) 3 days, with 5 days at most if serious problems are encountered. Once this step is finished, coordination of final plans and schedules with the patient and equipment carriers, local agencies, and area hospitals should take 2 days (3 at most). Finally, the completed schedules and procedures will be discussed in each department throughout the hospital on the day before moving day, and this discussion is expected to run the entire day because of the normal work schedules and tasks that all employees will be maintaining.

For the moving day, the staff has broken the entire process into seven different activities for the sketch plan:

	Activity Duration (days)		
	Optimistic	Most Likely	Pessimistic
Administration, accounting, and business office	0.25	0.5	1.0
Library and medical/personnel records	0.25	0.5	0.75
Laboratory and purchasing/stores	0.3	0.8	1.0
Housekeeping and food services	0.5	0.75	1.3
Other equipment and supplies that must move the same day as patients	0.8	1.0	1.2
Patients	0.4	1.0	1.0
Other equipment and supplies (noncritical) that will be moved after patients	1.0	2.0	2.5

The staff feels confident that basic operations will be fully under way at the new location once the first six activities are complete, and this is the critical goal established by the hospital's board of directors. The new location will not, of course, be fully operational until the remaining, noncritical equipment and supplies are moved.

Questions

1. Assume that you are part of the management staff whose task is to develop this sketch plan. Using Microsoft Project for Windows, develop the PERT network as outlined above, identify the critical path, and determine the expected time to reach basic operational status at the new facility.

2. The board of directors has said that it would like to try to move on a Sunday to minimize interference with weekday traffic. If there are Sundays which fall 46, 53, 60, 67, and 74 days from now, determine the probability (using a normal distribution) of reaching basic operational status at the new location on the two Sundays that are closest to the expected time you calculated previously.

3. Briefly assess the potential problems you see in applying critical path analysis to the sketch plan for moving Whittier County Hospital.

SELECTED BIBLIOGRAPHY

BRANCH, M. A.: "Where Do Wal-Marts Come From?" *Progressive Architecture,* vol. 9, 1993, pp. 66–69.

BRASSARD, MICHAEL, and DIANE RITTER: *The Memory Jogger II,* GOAL/QPC, Methuen, MA, 1994.

CLELAND, DAVID I.: "The Age of Project Management," *Project Management Journal,* vol. 22, no. 1, March 1991, pp. 19–24.

———, and W. R. KING: *Project Management Handbook,* Van Nostrand Reinhold, New York, 1983.

FERSKO-WEISS, HENRY: "Project Management Software Gets a Grip on Usability," *PC Magazine,* July 1992, pp. 323–369.

KATZENBACH, JON R., and DOUGLAS K. SMITH: *The Wisdom of Teams,* HarperBusiness, New York, 1994.

LEVY, F. K., G. L. THOMPSON, and J. D. WIEST: "The ABC's of the Critical Path Method," *Harvard Business Review,* vol. 41, no. 5, October 1963, pp. 413–423.

MACCRIMMON, K. R., and C. C. RYAVEC: "An Analytical Study of PERT Assumptions," *Operations Research,* vol. 12, no. 1, January–February 1964, pp. 16–37.

RANDOLPH, W. A., and BARRY Z. POSNER: "What Every Manager Needs to Know About Project Management," *Sloan Management Review,* Summer 1988, pp. 65–73.

STALK, GEORGE, JR.: "Time—The Next Source of Competitive Advantage," *Harvard Business Review,* July–August 1988, pp. 41–51.

WIEST, J. D., and F. K., LEVY; *A Management Guide to PERT/CPM,* 2d ed., Prentice-Hall, Inc., Englewood Cliffs, NJ, 1977.

PART FOUR

Managing Service Operations

The day-to-day operation of a service is a constant challenge, because the objectives of the organization, needs of the customer, and attention to service employees all must be managed simultaneously in an ever-changing environment. We begin by exploring how to manage the encounter between customer and service provider within the context of meeting organizational objectives. This discussion leads naturally to the issue of service quality, which is measured by the gap between customer expectations and customer perceptions of the service. The important topic of service quality is addressed by illustrating a number of approaches to managing service quality, including measurement issues, quality service by design, service process control, and personnel programs for quality improvement.

The inability of services to inventory output (as is done in manufacturing) creates a management challenge to match customer demand with service capacity. This challenge illustrates the inseparability of marketing and operations in service management. Therefore, marketing approaches that can influence customer demand are explored, including a continuation of our earlier discussion regarding the concept of yield management as pioneered by American Airlines. Adjusting service capacity to match demand is accomplished by workshift scheduling methods and use of part-time employees. A perfect match is seldom possible, however, and this results in waiting customers. Thus, managing queues becomes an important skill to avoid customer perceptions of a poor service experience.

Finally, we conclude with a discussion of inventory systems to manage the facilitating goods found in all service organizations.

CHAPTER 9

The Service Encounter

LEARNING OBJECTIVES

After completing this chapter, you should be able to:

1. Use the service encounter triad to describe a service firm's delivery process.
2. Identify organizational features that describe the culture of a service firm.
3. Discuss the role of information technology in employee empowerment.
4. Prepare abstract questions and write situational vignettes to screen service recruits.
5. Discuss the role of the customer as coproducer.
6. Describe how elements of the service profit chain lead to revenue growth and profitability.

Most services are characterized by an encounter between a service provider and a customer. Recall from Chapter 5, the Service Delivery System, that this encounter occurs above the "line of visibility" on the service blueprint. This interaction, which defines the quality of the service in the mind of the customer, has been called a "moment of truth" by Richard Normann.[1] The often brief encounter is a moment in time when the customer is evaluating the service and forming an opinion of its quality. A customer experiences many encounters with a variety of service providers, and each moment of truth is an opportunity to influence the customer's perceptions of the service quality. For example, an airline passenger experiences a series of encounters, beginning with purchasing the ticket from a telephone reservation clerk and continuing with baggage check-in at the airport, in-flight service, baggage claim on arrival, and finally, the award of frequent flyer credit.

Realizing that such moments of truth are critical in achieving a reputation for superior quality, Jan Carlzon, the CEO of Scandinavian Airlines System (SAS), focused on these encounters in the reorganization of SAS to create a distinctive and competitive position in terms of quality of service. According to Jan Carlzon's philosophy, the organization exists to serve the front-line workers who have direct customer contact. His revolutionary thinking stood the old organization chart on its head, placing the customer-encounter personnel (formerly at the bottom) now at the top of the chart. It then became everyone else's responsibility to serve those front-line personnel who in turn served the customer. Changing the organization chart signaled a move to refocus on satisfying the customer and managing moments of truth. It is interesting that this implementation required dividing the company into various profit centers down to the route level and allowing managers (now close to the customers) the authority to make decisions on their own.[2]

CHAPTER PREVIEW

In this chapter, the service encounter is depicted as a triangle formed by the interacting interests of the customer, service organization, and contact personnel. Each participant in the service encounter attempts to exert control over the transaction, leading to the need for flexibility and the empowerment of contact personnel. A discussion of service organization culture follows, with examples of how the founders of successful service firms established a set of values and expectations encouraging their employees to focus on delivering exceptional service.

The activities of selecting and training contact personnel are addressed next. Then, the many expectations and attitudes of customers are explored, as well as the concept of the customer as coproducer. The high correlation of service quality perceptions that are shared by contact personnel and customers leads to a discussion of management's contribution to creating a customer service orientation among its employees. A chapter supplement addresses the topic of work measurement.

[1]Richard Normann, *Service Management,* John Wiley & Sons, New York, 1984, p. 89.
[2]Jan Carlzon, *Moments of Truth,* Ballinger, Cambridge, Mass., 1987.

One of the unique characteristics of services is the active participation of the customer in the service production process. Every moment of truth involves an interaction between a customer and a service provider; each has a role to play in an environment staged by the service organization. The *service encounter triad* shown in Figure 9.1 captures the relationships between the three parties in the service encounter and suggests possible sources of conflict.

The managers of a for-profit service organization have an interest in delivering service as efficiently as possible to protect their margins and remain competitive. Nonprofit service organizations might substitute effectiveness for efficiency, but they still must operate under the limits imposed by a budget. To control service delivery, managers tend to impose rules and procedures on the contact personnel to limit their autonomy and discretion when serving the customer. These same rules and procedures also are intended to limit the extent of service provided for the customer and the resulting lack of customization that might result in a dissatisfied customer. Finally, the interaction between contact personnel and the customer has the element of perceived control by both parties. The contact people want to control the behavior of the customer to make their own work more manageable and less stressful; at the same time, the customer is attempting to gain control of the service encounter to derive the most benefit from it.

Ideally, the three parties gain much by working together to create a beneficial service encounter. The moment of truth can be dysfunctional, however, when one party dominates the interaction by focusing solely on his or her own control of the encounter. The following examples illustrate the conflict that arises when each party in turn dominates control of the encounter.

Encounter Dominated by the Service Organization

To be efficient and, perhaps, to follow a cost leadership strategy, an organization may standardize service delivery by imposing strict operating procedures and,

FIGURE 9.1. The service encounter triad.
(Adapted from John E. G. Bateson, "Perceived Control and the Service Encounter," in J. A. Czepiel, M. R. Solomon, and C. F. Surprenant (eds.), The Service Encounter, *Lexington Books, Lexington, Mass., 1985, p. 76.)*

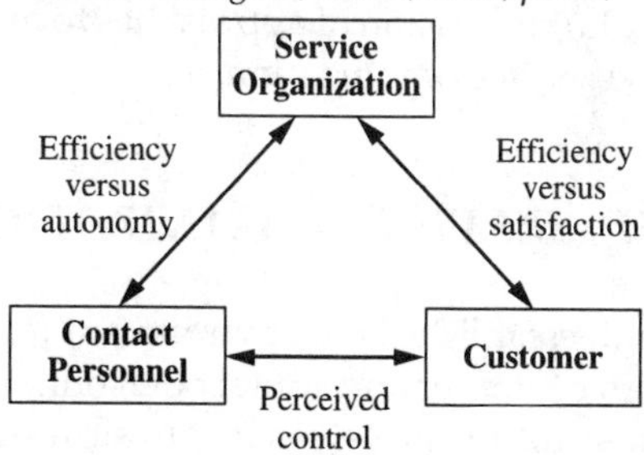

thus, severely limiting the discretion of the contact personnel. Customers are presented with a few standard service options from which to choose, and personalized service is not available. Many franchise services such as McDonald's, Jiffy Lube, and H. & R. Block have been successful with a structural organization and environment that dominates the service encounter. Much of their success has resulted from teaching customers what *not* to expect from their service; however, much of the frustration that customers experience with other institutions, labeled pejoratively as "bureaucracies," is the result of contact personnel having no autonomy to deal with individual customer's needs. Contact personnel in such organizations may sympathize with the customer but are forced to go "by the book," and their job satisfaction is diminished in the process.

Contact Personnel–Dominated Encounter

In general, service personnel attempt to limit the scope of the service encounter to reduce their own stress in meeting demanding customers. When contact personnel are placed in an autonomous position, they may perceive themselves as having a significant degree of control over customers. The customer is expected to place considerable trust in the contact person's judgment because of the service provider's perceived expertise. The relationship between physician and patient best illustrates the shortcomings of the contact personnel–dominated encounter. The patient, who is not even referred to as a "customer," is placed in a subordinate position with no control over the encounter. Further, an allied organization, such as a hospital in this case, is subjected to tremendous demands placed on it by individual staff physicians with no regard for matters of efficiency.

Customer-Dominated Encounter

The extremes of standardized and customized services represent opportunities for customers to control the encounter. For standardized services, self-service is an option that gives customers complete control over the limited service that is provided. For example, at a self-service gasoline station that is equipped with a credit card reader, the customer need not interact with anyone. The result can be very efficient and satisfying to the customer who needs or desires very little service. For a customized service such as legal defense in a criminal case, however, all the organization's resources may be needed, at great cost in efficiency.

A satisfactory and effective service encounter should balance the need for control by all three participants. The organization's need for efficiency to remain economically viable can be satisfied when contact personnel are trained properly and the customer's expectations and role in the delivery process are communicated effectively. Our discussion of approaches to managing the service encounter begins with the service organization.

THE SERVICE ORGANIZATION

The service organization establishes the environment for the service encounter. The interaction between customer and contact personnel occurs within the context of an organization's culture as well as its physical surroundings.

Culture

Why do you choose one service over another—supermarket A over supermarket B, copying service X over copying service Y, or family practitioner M over family practitioner D? Cost, you may answer . . . or ambiance or any of several other good reasons. The bottom line, however, may be corporate *culture,* because the underlying culture helps to determine the value that customers place on the service. Several definitions of organizational culture have been proposed:

- Culture is a pattern of beliefs and expectations that is shared by the organization's members and produces norms that powerfully shape the behavior of individuals or groups in organizations.[3]
- Culture is the traditions and beliefs of an organization that distinguish it from other organizations and infuse a certain life into the skeleton of structure.[4]
- Organizational culture is a system of shared orientations that hold the unit together and give a distinctive identity.[5]

The founders and/or senior managers of a service organization establish, whether purposely or unintentionally, a climate or culture that prescribes a norm of behavior or set of values to guide employee decision making in the firm. Take, for example, ServiceMaster, a very profitable company that provides hospitals and other organizations with housekeeping services. Writing about ServiceMaster, Carol Loomis discovered that the company's name embodied its value of "Service to the Master."

> Founded by a devout Baptist, the late Marion E. Wade, the company has always described itself as driven by religious principle. The first of its corporate objectives is "to honor God in all we do." The cafeteria wall at ServiceMaster's suburban headquarters proclaims that "Joy cometh in the morning," and although there are no "Cleanliness is next to Godliness" signs around, the neatness and shine of the office project the thought.[6]

Choice of language is another approach to communicate values, as illustrated by the Walt Disney Corporation. At Disney theme parks, show business terms are used because they are in the entertainment business. Instead of Personnel there is Casting. Employees are referred to as "cast members" to instill the appropriate frame of mind. Cast members work either "onstage" or "backstage," but both kinds of employees are required to "put on the show."

The examples above illustrate how an organization's values, when consistently communicated by management, permit contact personnel to act with considerable autonomy, because their judgment is founded on a shared set of values. These values often are communicated by stories and legends about individual risk-taking on behalf of the organization and its customers. Federal Express, with a motto of "absolutely positively overnight," has many stories of extraordinary employee feats to safeguard that service guarantee. Consider, for

[3]H. M. Schwartz and S. M. Davis, "Matching Corporate Culture and Business Strategy," *Organizational Dynamics,* vol. 59, 1981, p. 33.

[4]Henry Mintzberg, *Mintzberg on Management: Inside Our Strange World of Organizations,* The Free Press, New York, 1989, p. 98.

[5]Wayne K. Hoy, C. John Tarter, and Robert B. Kottkamp, *Open Schools/Healthy Schools,* Sage Publications, London, 1991, p. 5.

[6]Carol J. Loomis, "How the Service Stars Managed to Sparkle," *Fortune,* June 11, 1984, p. 117.

example, the pick-up driver who was faced with a collection box he was unable to open—instead of leaving it standing on the street corner until someone could come out to repair it, he wrestled the entire box into his vehicle so that the packages it contained could be liberated and delivered the next day.

The organization benefits from a shared set of values, because contact personnel are empowered to make decisions without the need for the traditional level of supervision, which assumes that only management is vested with authority to act on behalf of the organization.

Empowerment

For years, McDonald's has served as the model of efficient service delivery. Incorporating the traditional mass-production philosophy of industry, McDonald's has been successful in delivering a consistent meal to billions of customers through an organization that could be described as "manufacturing in the field." The discretion of contact personnel is limited by procedures and design (e.g., the french fry scoop that guarantees portion control). Most employees are minimum-wage teenagers, and high turnover is the norm. The organization's structure is pyramid-shaped, with layers of supervision from the assistant store manager, store manager, and regional manager to corporate "consultants," to ensure consistency of service delivery across all locations.

A new model of service organization now is emerging that has a structure best described as an inverted T. In this organization, the layers of supervision are drastically reduced, because contact personnel are trained, motivated, and supplied with timely, computer-based information that enables them to manage the service encounter at the point of delivery.

Jan Carlzon, the innovative president of SAS, is quoted as saying:

> Instructions only succeed in providing employees with knowledge of their own limitations. Information, on the other hand, provides them with a knowledge of their opportunities and possibilities . . . To free someone from rigorous control by instructions, policies and orders, and to give that person freedom to take responsibility for his ideas, decisions and actions, is to release hidden resources which would otherwise remain inaccessible to both the individual and the company . . . A person who has information cannot avoid taking responsibility.[7]

Perhaps it is surprising that Taco Bell has become the new service model of employee *empowerment*. Other firms adopting this new model include ServiceMaster, Marriott, and Dayton Hudson. Senior managers of these firms all share a belief that people want to do good work—and will do so if given the opportunity. Consequently, they have made the following commitments: 1) to invest in people as much as, or more than, in machines; 2) to use technology to support contact personnel rather than to monitor or replace them; 3) to consider the recruitment and training of contact personnel as critical to the firm's success; and 4) to link compensation to performance for employees at all levels. In this type of organization, a much-reduced middle management no longer has the traditional supervisory role; instead, middle managers become facilitators for the front-line or contact personnel. More important, investment in computer infor-

[7]W. E. Sasser, Jr., C. W. L. Hart, and J. L. Heskett, *The Service Management Course*, The Free Press, New York, 1991, p. 97.

mation systems is necessary to supply the front-line personnel with the ability to resolve problems as they arise and to ensure a quality service encounter.[8]

Empowered contact personnel must be motivated, informed, competent, committed, and well-trained. Front-line personnel should exhibit the ability to take responsibility, manage themselves, and respond to pressure from customers.

CONTACT PERSONNEL

Ideally, customer contact personnel should have personality attributes that include flexibility, tolerance for ambiguity, an ability to monitor and change behavior on the basis of situational cues, and empathy for customers. The last attribute (i.e., empathy for customers) has been found to be more important than age, education, sales-related knowledge, sales training, and intelligence.

Some individuals may find front-line service to be boring and repetitive, whereas others see the job as providing an opportunity to meet and interact with a variety of people. Those with the necessary interpersonal skills may gravitate toward high-contact service jobs, but a selection process still is required to ensure high-quality moments of truth.

Selection

No reliable tests exist to measure a person's service orientation; however, a variety of interviewing techniques have proven to be useful. Abstract questioning, the situational vignette, and role playing all have been used in evaluating potential front-line employees.

Abstract Questioning

The questions asked in the abstract interview are open-ended. They provide insights regarding an applicant's ability to relate the immediate service situation to information collected from past experience. An example of a question that assesses an applicant's attention to the environment would be "From your past work experience, what type of customer was most difficult for you to deal with and why?" To determine if an applicant actively collects information, a questioner might ask, "What was the customer's primary complaint or negative characteristic?" Some final questions to evaluate the applicant's interpersonal style could be "How did you handle the customer?" and "What would be the ideal way to deal with that type of customer?"

Abstract questioning also can be used to reveal a person's willingness to adapt. An effective employee will take notice of details in his or her personal life as well as on the job. People who consider the events around them and can describe their significance usually are able to learn more as well as faster.

Because of their nature and preparation for the interview, some applicants will be better able than others to talk extensively about their past experiences. Careful listening and probing by the interviewer for the substance of an answer to an abstract question will lessen the possibility of being deceived with

[8]L. A. Schlesinger and J. L. Heskett, "The Service-Driven Service Company," *Harvard Business Review*, September–October 1991, p. 72.

"puffery." Finally, there is no assurance that the ability to reflect on past events necessarily will guarantee that such perceptiveness and flexibility will transfer to the job.

Situational Vignette

A *situational vignette* interview requires the applicant to answer questions regarding a specific situation. For example, consider the following situational vignette:

> The day after a catering service has catered a large party, a customer returns some small cakes, claiming they were stale. Although the man is demanding a refund, he is so soft-spoken and timid that you can hardly hear him across the counter. You know that your business did not make those cakes, because they don't look like your chef's work. What would you do?

Presenting a situation like this may reveal information regarding an applicant's instincts, interpersonal capabilities, common sense, and judgment. To gain more information about a candidate's adaptability, further questions about the situation can be asked: "How would you handle the man if, suddenly, he were to become irate and insistent? What steps would you take to remedy the situation?"

Situational vignettes provide an opportunity to determine whether applicants are able to "think on their feet." An applicant with good communication skills, however, still may not indicate clearly a genuine desire to serve customers or an empathic nature. Again, the interviewer must pay close attention to the substance of an applicant's response in addition to the way it is delivered.

Role Playing

Role playing is an interviewing technique that requires applicants to participate in a simulated situation and to react as if this service environment were real. Role playing often is used in the final phase of recruitment, and others in the organization are asked to cooperate by posing as "actors" for the situation.

Role playing provides a way for an interviewer to observe an applicant under stress. Interviewers using this technique may probe and change the situation as the session progresses. This method allows for more realistic responses than either the abstract questioning or situational vignette interviews; applicants are required to use their own words and react to the immediate situation instead of describing them.

Although role playing provides an excellent opportunity to observe a candidate's strengths and weaknesses in a realistic customer encounter, direct comparison of applicants is difficult. Role playing does require careful scripting, and the "actors" need to rehearse their roles before the interview.

Training

Most training manuals and employee handbooks for customer-contact personnel are devoted to explaining the technical skills that are needed to perform the jobs. For example, they often detail explicitly how to fill out guest reports, use cash registers, dress properly, and enforce safety requirements, but customer interaction skills are dismissed with a simple comment to be pleasant and smile.

TABLE 9.1. Difficulties with Interactions Between Customers and Contact Personnel

Unrealistic Customer Expectations	Unexpected Service Failure
1. Unreasonable demands	1. Unavailable service
2. Demands against policies	2. Slow performance
3. Unacceptable treatment of employees	3. Unacceptable service
4. Drunkenness	
5. Breaking of societal norms	
6. Special-needs customers	

Source: Adapted from J. D. Nyquist, M. J. Bitner, and B. H. Booms, "Identifying Communication Difficulties in the Service Encounter: A Critical Incident Approach," in J. A. Czepiel, M. R. Solomon, and C. F. Surprenant (eds.), *The Service Encounter*, Lexington Books, Lexington, Mass., 1985, pp. 195–212.

Difficulties with interactions between customers and contact personnel fall into two major groups and nine categories. These are shown in Table 9.1.

Unrealistic Customer Expectations

Approximately 75 percent of the reported communication difficulties arise from causes other than a breakdown in the technical service delivery. These difficult encounters involve customers with unrealistic expectations that cannot be met by the service delivery system. Examples include passengers who bring oversize luggage aboard an airplane or diners who snap fingers and yell at servers. Unrealistic customer expectations can be broken down into six categories:

1. *Unreasonable demands.* Services that the firm cannot offer, or customer demands that require inappropriate time and attention (e.g., "I want to carry all my luggage on board," or "Please sit with me; I'm afraid of flying").
2. *Demands against policies.* Requests that are impossible to fulfill because of safety regulations, laws, or company policies (e.g., "We've been waiting an hour for takeoff, and I must have my smoke," or "Our party of ten wants separate checks for the meal").
3. *Unacceptable treatment of employees.* Mistreatment of employees with verbal or physical abuse (e.g., "You idiot! Where is my drink?" or a diner pinching a waitress).
4. *Drunkenness.* Intoxicated customer requiring special attention (e.g., "Bring me another drink!" or an intoxicated passenger who requires assistance to get off the plane).
5. *Breaking of societal norms.* Customers breaking societal norms in general (e.g., "We can't sleep because of the loud TV in the next apartment," or guests swimming nude in the pool).
6. *Special-needs customers.* Special attention to customers with psychological, medical, or language difficulties (e.g., "My wife is hemorrhaging," or "Wieviel kostet das?").

Unexpected Service Failure

A failure in the service delivery system places a communication burden on the contact personnel. Service failures, however, provide a unique opportunity for contact personnel to demonstrate innovation and flexibility in their recovery. Three categories of service failures can be identified:

1. *Unavailable service.* Services that normally are available or expected are lacking (e.g., "I reserved a table by the window," or "Why is the ATM out of order?").
2. *Slow performance.* Service is unusually slow, creating excessive customer waiting (e.g., "Why hasn't our plane arrived?" or "We've been here for an hour, and no one has taken our order").
3. *Unacceptable service.* Service does not meet acceptable standards (e.g., "My seat doesn't recline," or "Eeegads, there's a hair in my soup!").

Unavoidable communication difficulties with customers require contact personnel whose training and interpersonal skills can prevent a bad situation from becoming worse. Programs can be developed to train contact personnel to use prescribed responses in given situations. For example, when faced with unreasonable demands—as illustrated above for category 1 difficulties—the server can appeal to the customer's sense of fairness by pointing out that the needs of other customers would be jeopardized. Actual scripts also can be developed and rehearsed for each anticipated situation. For example, in response to "I want to carry all my luggage on board," the employee need only say, "I'm very sorry, but federal safety regulations permit a passenger only two carry-on pieces small enough to be stored under the seat or overhead. May I check your larger pieces all the way to your final destination?"

Another approach involves general training in communication skills. This approach should help contact personnel to anticipate the types of exchanges they might encounter, expand their repertoire of possible responses, and develop decision rules for choosing appropriate responses to a given situation. Role playing can provide an ideal setting for gaining this communication experience. Contact personnel who are well trained will be able to control the service encounter in a professional manner, and the results will be increased satisfaction for the customer and decreased stress and frustration for the provider.

THE CUSTOMER

Every purchase is an event of some importance for the customer, whereas the same transaction usually is routine for the service provider. The emotional involvement that is associated with the routine purchase of gasoline at a self-serve station or an overnight stay at a budget hotel is minor, but consider the very personal and dramatic roles played by a customer taking an exotic vacation or seeking medical treatment. Unfortunately, it is very difficult for the bored contact personnel, who see hundreds of customers a week, to maintain a corresponding level of emotional commitment.

Expectations and Attitudes

Service customers are motivated to look for a service much as they would for a product; similarly, their expectations govern their shopping attitudes. Gregory Stone developed a now-famous topology in which shopping-goods customers were classified into four groups.[9] The definitions that follow have been modified for the service customer:

1. *The economizing customer.* This customer wants to maximize the value obtained for his or her expenditures of time, effort, and money. He or she is a demanding and sometimes fickle customer who looks for value that will test the competitive strength of the service firm in the market. Loss of these customers serves as an early warning of potential competitive threats.
2. *The ethical customer.* This customer feels a moral obligation to patronize socially responsible firms. Service firms that have developed a reputation for community service can create such a loyal customer base; for example, the Ronald McDonald House program for the families of hospitalized children has helped the image of McDonald's in just this way.
3. *The personalizing customer.* This customer wants interpersonal gratification, such as recognition and conversation, from the service experience. Greeting customers on a first-name basis always has been a staple of the neighborhood family restaurant, but computerized customer files can generate a similar personalized experience when used skillfully by front-line personnel in many other businesses.
4. *The convenience customer.* This customer has no interest in shopping for the service; convenience is the secret to attracting him or her. Convenience customers often are willing to pay extra for personalized or hassle-free service; for example, supermarkets that provide home delivery may appeal to these customers.

The attitude of customers regarding their need to control the service encounter was the subject of a study investigating customers' decision-making processes when they were confronted with the choice between a self-service option and the traditional full-service approach.[10] Customers who were interviewed appeared to be using the following dimensions in their selection: 1) amount of time involved, 2) customer's control of the situation, 3) efficiency of the process, 4) amount of human contact involved, 5) risk involved, 6) amount of effort involved, and 7) customer's need to depend on others.

It is not surprising that customers who were interested in the self-service option found the second dimension (i.e., customer's control of the situation) to be the most important factor in choosing that option. The study was conducted over a variety of services, ranging from banks and gas stations to hotels and airlines.

[9]Gregory P. Stone, "City Shoppers and Urban Identification: Observations on the Social Psychology of City Life," *American Journal of Sociology,* July 1954, pp. 36–43.
[10]John E. G. Bateson, "The Self-Service Consumer: Empirical Findings," in L. Berry, L. Shostack, and G. Upah (eds.), *Marketing of Services,* American Marketing Association, Chicago, 1983, pp. 76–83.

Services competing on a cost leadership strategy can make use of this finding by engaging the customer as a *coproducer* to reduce costs.

The Customer as Coproducer[11]

In the service encounter, both the provider and the customer have roles to play in transacting the service. Society has defined specific tasks for service customers to perform, such as the procedure required for cashing checks at a bank. Diners in some restaurants may assume a variety of productive roles, such as assembling their meals and carrying them to the table in a cafeteria, serving themselves at a salad bar, or busing their own tables. In each case, the customer has learned a set of behaviors that is appropriate for the situation. The customer is participating in the service delivery as a partial employee with a role to play and is following a script that is defined by societal norms or implied by the particular design of the service offered.

Customers possess a variety of scripts that are learned for use in different service encounters. Following the appropriate script allows both the customer and service provider to predict the behavior of each other as they play out their respective roles. Thus, each participant expects some element of perceived control in the service encounter. Difficulties can arise, however, when new technology requiring a new or redefined script is introduced into the service encounter.

Customer resistance to new forms of service transactions—such as the introduction of Universal Product Codes in supermarkets, which removed the need for item pricing, and automated teller machines (ATMs) in banking, which eliminated the need for human interaction—may be explained by the need to learn a radically new script. What once was a "mindless" routine service encounter now requires some effort to learn a new role. For example, when ATMs were first introduced, a sample machine was placed in the bank lobby so that customers could practice their new role.

Teaching customers a new role can be facilitated if the transition becomes a logical modification of past behavior. Public acceptance of the Windows operating system for PCs can be attributed to the fact that all applications share the same interface; thus, only one script must be learned.

CREATING A CUSTOMER SERVICE ORIENTATION[12]

A study of 23 branch banks revealed a high correlation between customers' and employees' perceptions of service quality. Each dot in Figure 9.2 represents data from a different branch bank. Employees were asked: "How do you think the customers of your bank view the general quality of the service they receive in your branch?" Customers were asked: "Describe the general quality of the ser-

[11]Adapted from M. R. Solomon, C. F. Surprenant, J. A. Czepiel, and E. G. Gutman, "A Role Theory Perspective on Dyadic Interactions: The Service Encounter," *Journal of Marketing*, vol. 49, Winter 1985, pp. 99–111.

[12]Adapted from Benjamin Schneider, "The Service Organization: Climate Is Crucial," *Organizational Dynamics*, Autumn 1980, pp. 52–65.

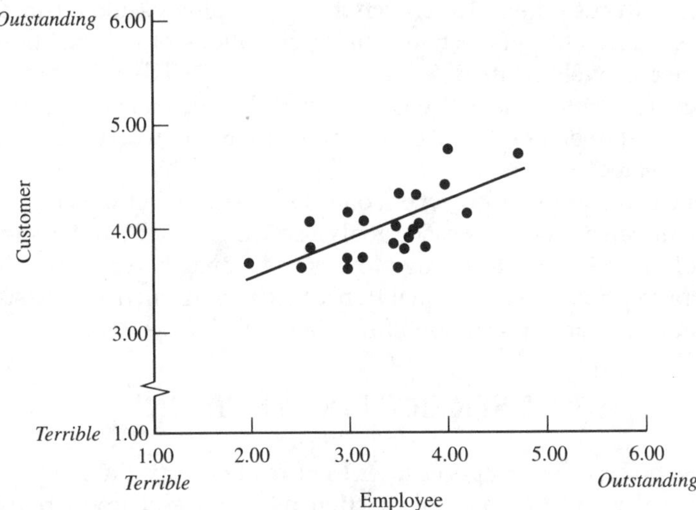

FIGURE 9.2. Relationship between customer and employee perceptions of customer service.
(After Benjamin Schneider, "The Service Organization: Climate Is Crucial," Organizational Dynamics, *Autumn 1980, p. 62. Copyright by Benjamin Schneider. All rights reserved.)*

vice received in your branch." Both groups graded service on the same six-point scale.

Further analysis showed that customers perceived better service in branches where employees reported the following:

1. There is a more enthusiastic service emphasis.
2. The branch manager emphasizes service as personnel perform their roles.
3. There is an active effort to retain all customer accounts, not just large-account holders.
4. The branch is staffed with sufficient, well-trained tellers.
5. Equipment is well maintained, and supplies are plentiful.

In addition, when employees described their branch as one in which the manager emphasized customer service, customers not only reported that service was superior but, more specifically, that:

1. Tellers were courteous and competent.
2. Staffing levels were adequate.
3. The branch appeared to be well administered.
4. Teller turnover was low.
5. The staff had positive work attitudes.

From this study, it appears that when employees perceive a strong service orientation, customers report superior service. Creating a customer service orientation results in superior service practices and procedures that are observable by customers and, further, seem to fit employee views of the appropriate style for dealing with customers. Thus, even though employees and customers view service from different perspectives, their perceptions of organizational effectiveness are positively related.

A lesson for management also is suggested. The way management relates to the contact personnel (or internal customers) is reflected in how the external customers are treated.

As shown in Figure 9.3, however, some discrepancies between employee and management perceptions of service goals also were evident in this same study. This lack of congruence between employees and management eventually affects customer perceptions of service quality, because management emphasis in a service organization cannot be hidden from those who are served.

THE SERVICE PROFIT CHAIN[13]

The service profit chain proposes a series of relationships linking profitability, customer loyalty, and employee satisfaction, retention, and productivity. As Figure 9.4 shows, profitability and revenue growth are derived from loyal customers, and loyal customers result from satisfaction, which is influenced by the perceived value of the service. Service value is created by satisfied, committed, and productive employees, and employee satisfaction is generated by investing in information technology, training, and a policy of employee empowerment.

1. *Internal quality drives employee satisfaction.* Internal quality describes the environment in which employees work, and it includes employee selection and development, rewards and recognition, access to information to serve the customer, workplace technology, and job design. For example, at USAA, a financial services company serving military officers, telephone service representatives are supported by a sophisticated information system that puts complete customer information files on their monitor when a customer gives them a membership number. The facility is located in suburban San Antonio on acres of property and resembles a small college campus. Using 75 classrooms, state-of-the-art job-related training is an expected part of everyone's work experience.
2. *Employee satisfaction drives retention and productivity.* In most service jobs, the real cost of employee turnover is loss of productivity and decreased customer satisfaction. In personalized service firms, low employee turnover is linked closely to high customer satisfaction. For example, the cost of losing a valued broker at a securities firm is measured by the loss of commissions during the time his or her replacement is building relationships with customers. Employee satisfaction also can contribute to productivity. Southwest Airlines has consistently been the most profitable airline in part because of its high rate of employee retention, with turnover of less than 5 percent per year—the lowest in the industry.
3. *Employee retention and productivity drives service value.* At Southwest Airlines, customer perceptions of value are very high even though the airline does not assign seats, offer meals, or integrate its reservation system with other car-

[13]Adapted from J. L. Heskett, T. O. Jones, G. W. Loveman, W. E. Sasser, Jr., and L. A. Schlesinger, "Putting the Service-Profit Chain to Work," *Harvard Business Review,* March–April 1994, pp. 164–174.

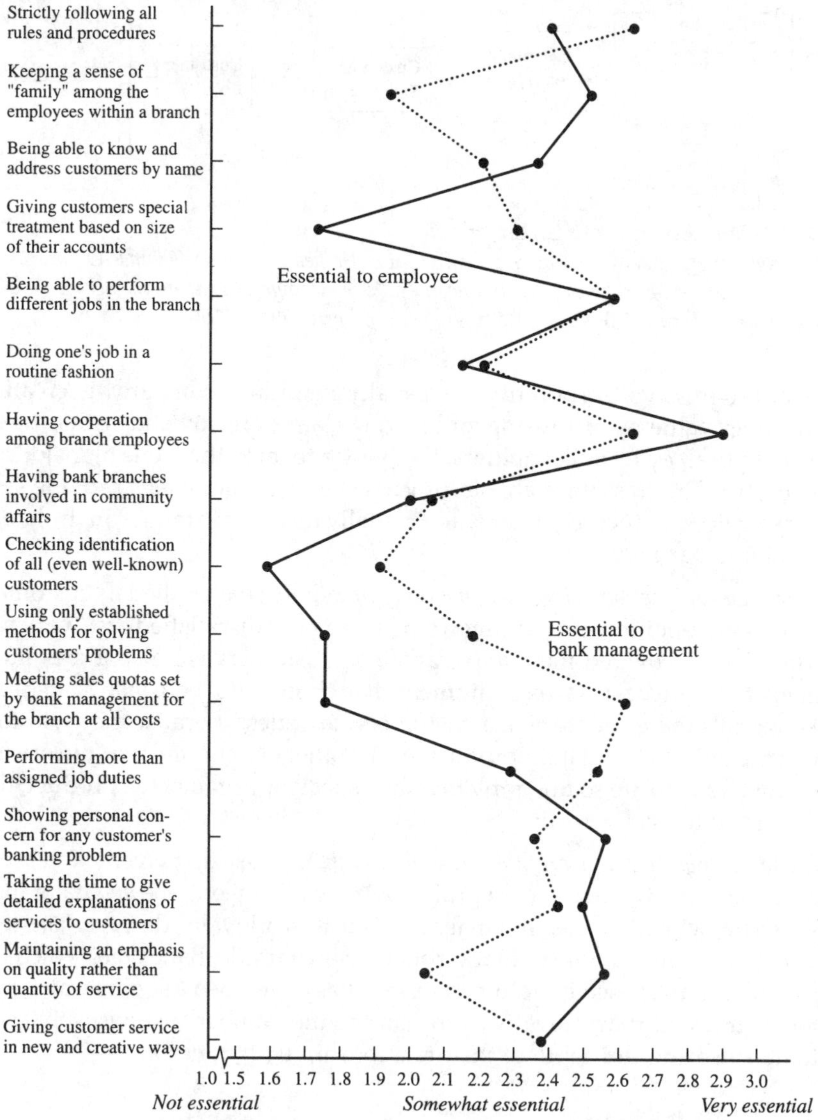

Strictly following all rules and procedures
Keeping a sense of "family" among the employees within a branch
Being able to know and address customers by name
Giving customers special treatment based on size of their accounts
Being able to perform different jobs in the branch
Doing one's job in a routine fashion
Having cooperation among branch employees
Having bank branches involved in community affairs
Checking identification of all (even well-known) customers
Using only established methods for solving customers' problems
Meeting sales quotas set by bank management for the branch at all costs
Performing more than assigned job duties
Showing personal concern for any customer's banking problem
Taking the time to give detailed explanations of services to customers
Maintaining an emphasis on quality rather than quantity of service
Giving customer service in new and creative ways

Essential to employee
Essential to bank management

1.0 1.5 1.6 1.7 1.8 1.9 2.0 2.1 2.2 2.3 2.4 2.5 2.6 2.7 2.8 2.9 3.0
Not essential *Somewhat essential* *Very essential*

FIGURE 9.3. Discrepancies between employee and management perceptions of service delivery goals.
(After Benjamin Schneider, "The Service Organization: Climate Is Crucial," Organizational Dynamics, *Autumn 1980, p. 64. Copyright by Benjamin Schneider. All rights reserved.)*

riers. Customers place high value on frequent departures, on-time service, friendly employees, and very low fares (60 to 70 percent lower than existing fares in the markets it enters). These low fares are possible in part because highly trained, flexible employees can perform several jobs and turn around an aircraft at the gate in 15 minutes or less.

4. *Service value drives customer satisfaction.* Customer value is measured by comparing the results received to the total costs incurred in obtaining the ser-

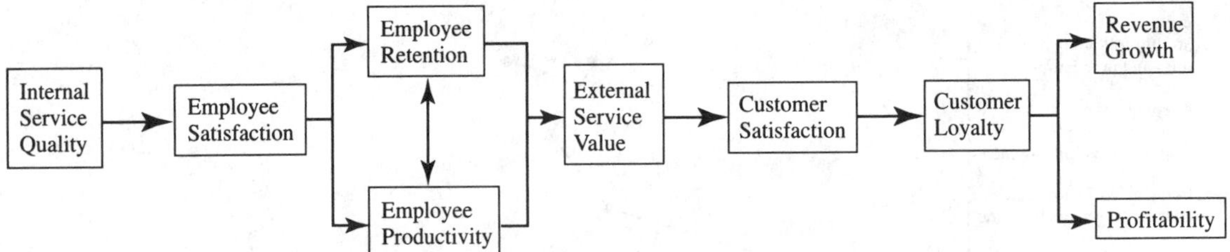

FIGURE 9.4 The Service Profit Chain
Adapted from The Links in the Service Profit Chain *[James L. Heskett, Thomas O. Jones, Gary W. Loveman, W. Earl Sasser, Jr., and Leonard A. Schlesinger: "Putting the Service-Profit Chain to Work,"* Harvard Business Review, *March–April 1994, p. 166.]*

vice. Progressive Corporation, a casualty insurance company, is creating customer value by processing and paying claims quickly and with little effort required by its policyholders. By flying a team to the scene of major catastrophes, Progressive is able to process claims immediately, provide support services, reduce legal costs, and actually place more money in the hands of injured parties.

5. *Customer satisfaction drives customer loyalty.* When Xerox polled its customers using a five-point scale ranging from "extremely dissatisfied" to "very satisfied," it discovered that "very satisfied" customers were six times more likely to repurchase Xerox equipment than those who were just "satisfied." Xerox calls these very satisfied customers "apostles," because they will convert the uninitiated to their product. At the other extreme are the "terrorists," customers who are so unhappy that they speak out against the product; this is a group to avoid creating.
6. *Customer loyalty drives profitability and growth.* Because a 5 percent increase in customer loyalty can increase profits by 25 to 85 percent, the *quality* of market share, which is measured in terms of customer loyalty, deserves as much attention as the *quantity* of market share. For example, Banc One, which is a profitable bank based in Columbus, Ohio, has developed a sophisticated system to track customer loyalty by measuring the number of services that customers use and the depth of their relationship with Banc One.

SUMMARY

The service encounter is viewed as a triad, with the customer and contact personnel both exercising control over the service process in an environment that is defined by the service organization. The importance of flexibility in meeting customer needs has resulted in many service organizations empowering their contact personnel to exercise more autonomy.

Giving employees more discretion requires a selection process that identifies applicants with the potential for adaptability in their interpersonal behaviors. Communication difficulties with customers will arise even in the best of circumstances, however. Unrealistic customer expectations and unexpected service failures must be dealt with by the contact personnel as they arise. Training to anticipate possible situations and developing "scripts" to respond to problems are two important measures that contribute to the professionalism of service providers.

Customers can be classified by their service expectations. Those with a need for control are candidates for self-service options. Viewing customers as coproducers returns us to the concept of "scripts." In this case, customers follow scripts to facilitate the service, and the scripts provide some behavioral predictability in the encounter.

Finally, the concept of creating a customer service orientation was discussed with reference to a study of branch banks. In this study, it was discovered that customers and contact personnel share similar views of the quality of service delivered.

Another aspect of the service encounter is service quality, which will be explored in Chapter 10.

KEY TERMS AND DEFINITIONS

Abstract questioning an open-ended question used to screen potential employees by revealing a candidate's ability to adapt and use interpersonal skills.

Culture the shared beliefs and values of an organization that guide employee decision making and behavior in the firm.

Coproducer viewing the customer as a productive resource in the service delivery process, which requires roles to play (e.g., busing his or her lunch table) and scripts to follow (e.g., using an ATM).

Empowerment providing contact personnel with the training and information to make decisions for the firm without close supervision.

Service encounter triad a triangle depicting the balance of goals among the service organization, contact personnel, and customer.

Situational vignette a service encounter situation that can test a candidate's ability to "think on her or his feet" and to use good judgment.

TOPICS FOR DISCUSSION

1. How does the historical image of service as servitude affect today's customer expectations and service employee behavior?
2. What are the organizational and marketing implications of considering a customer as a "partial employee"?
3. Comment on the different dynamics of one-on-one service and group service in regard to perceived control of the service encounter.
4. How does use of a "service script" relate to service quality?
5. If the roles played by customers are determined by cultural norms, how can services be exported?

Service Benchmark

Miss Manners on Complaint Handling

In the standard exchange involving a person making a complaint and one who is receiving the complaint, usually on behalf of a commercial establishment, there are, Miss Manners has observed, two obligatory roles.

One person must say something along the lines of: "This is the most outrageous thing that ever happened. I can't imagine how anyone could be so stupid. I'm going to find out exactly how this came about, and believe me, I'm going to do something about it right away."

And the other must say: "Look, mistakes happen. This is just not all that important. There's no use getting upset, because these things happen all the time. It's not really anybody's fault."

Now here comes the peculiar part: The person at whom the complaint is directed gets to choose which role he or she wants to play, and the complainer has to take the other.

Miss Manners realizes that this is a difficult concept. It must be, because those who are obliged to receive complaints, either occasionally or as a wearisome way to earn a living, don't seem to have caught on to the possibilities of the *switcheroo.*

Here is the way the standard exchange goes:

Complainer (in more or less normal voice, with just a small edge to it): "This is an outrage."

Complainee (in bored tone): "Oh, calm down. It's nobody's fault; it just happens occasionally. It's really too late to do anything about it."

Complainer (shrieking): "You mean it's happened before? Is everyone here an idiot? I've never seen such bungling in all my life. There is no excuse for this, none whatsoever." And so on and on and on.

But here is the same situation, except that the complainee has decided not to take abuse, and so has preempted that function.

Complainee (with note of abject desperation): "It certainly is. I can't imagine how this could have happened, but you may be sure I'm going to do something about it. I can't apologize to you enough. We pride ourselves on getting things right, and this is intolerable. Please give us another chance—let me see what I can do to make it up to you."

Complainer (grudgingly at first, but warming up to the subject to counter threat of Complainee continuing in the same vein): "Oh, that's OK. We all make mistakes. It's not all that important."

The essential ingredients to pull off the switch are the apology and the promise to do something, but what makes it work is the tone. Two people can't keep up an argument in which both are carrying on like that.

Miss Manners is astonished that so few people avail themselves of this simple technique to neutralize what is otherwise a nasty exchange.

Source: Judith Martin, "Complaint-Handling Requires a Deft 'Switcheroo'," Associated Press as printed in *Austin American Statesman*, November 1, 1992, p. E14.

CASE: AMY'S ICE CREAM[14]

Amy's Ice Cream is a business that was founded in Austin, Texas, and has expanded to several other Texas cities. When asked about the driving force behind it, Phil Clay, the production manager, explained that "while the product is of excellent quality and does come in some unique flavors, ultimately ice cream is ice cream. One can just as easily go to Swensen's or the Marble Slab to get great ice cream. Service is what differentiates Amy's from other ice cream stores and keeps customers coming back again and again." And indeed, the service at Amy's is unique.

Amy Miller, the owner and founder, got her start in the ice cream business when she worked for Steve's Ice Cream in Boston, a store whose gimmick was mashing toppings into ice cream. She recalls how Harvard and M.I.T. graduates would work at the store—obviously for reasons other than the great salary and fringe benefits. She quickly realized that this was a business that instantly made its customers happy. Working in an ice cream store was a "feel-good" occupation, which lured such bright workers who could easily make much more money working almost anywhere else.

When she opened the first Amy's Ice Cream in October 1984, she had two philosophies: one that an employee should enjoy what he or she does, and another that the service as well as the ice cream should make the customer smile. These philosophies have provided the foundation for a business that more than one decade later is firmly established and thriving.

In the beginning, theater majors and artists often were hired as servers, because the idea of enjoying what they were doing was just as appealing to them as making money. These outgoing and creative employees were very skilled at projecting their colorful personalities across the counter. They joked and interacted with customers while filling their orders. Customers were drawn to the fun and variety of the service, which might be described as "ice cream theater," and once drawn, the customers returned again and again for repeat performances.

How does Amy's recruit employees who are up to "performing"? Originally, the employment application form was rather casual, simply handwritten and mimeographed. Mr. Clay recalls, however, that one day he was out of forms when a very large man asked for a copy. The man became somewhat belligerent at being told none was available, so Mr. Clay whipped out a white paper bag—the only writing surface under the counter—and offered it as an "alternate" form. The applicant was satisfied and carried away his form to complete! When Mr. Clay relayed this story to Amy, she said the white paper bag would work just fine, and it became the new "official" application form. In fact, it has proven to be a very good indicator of whether an applicant is willing and able to express herself or himself both easily and creatively. A person who uses the bag just to write down the usual biographical information (i.e., name, address, Social Security number, and so on) probably will not be as entertaining a scooper as one who makes it into a puppet or hot air balloon. Getting "the sack" at Amy's takes on a whole new meaning. Applicants who pass the sack test are then interviewed.

New employees go through an on-the-job training process. One part of this training concerns ice cream procedures so that servers can deliver a consistent product. The other part teaches them to express themselves from behind the counter, which includes recognizing which customers enjoy the revelry and which just want to be left alone, as well as how far the kidding can be taken with different customers. In general, employees are free to interact theatrically with those customers who want to do so.

Amy's operates on an approximate three-percent profit margin. Consequently, the servers are minimum-wage, and about 80 percent of them are part-time workers who receive no additional benefits. In fact, most managers make less than $15,000 per year, and there is a $30,000 cap for all employees—including Amy. In view of the low remuneration, how is Amy's Ice Cream always able to recruit the high-quality help that translates into satisfied customers?

Well, they do get Amy's Ice Cream T-shirts at cost and all the ice cream they can eat! Perhaps the major reason, however, is that Amy's is freedom-oriented rather than rules-oriented. The only "uniform" an employee must wear is an apron, whose primary function is to project a sense of continuity behind the counter. A hat also is de rigueur, but the employee is free to choose any hat as long as it effectively restrains the hair. In addition, the employee may wear any clothing that suits his or her mood that day as long as it is not soiled, political, or excessively revealing.

Employees can bring their own music, keeping in mind their type of clientele, to play in their stores. For example, an Amy's located in a downtown nightspot district draws a young, exuberant crowd that would appreciate lively music, whereas an Amy's located in

[14]Prepared by Bridgett Gagne, Sandhya Shardanand, and Laura Urquidi under the supervision of Professor James A. Fitzsimmons.

an upscale shopping mall attracts a clientele whose musical tastes might be a bit more quiet.

The design of each store and the artwork displayed there tend to be colorful and eclectic, but again, the employees are free to make contributions. Amy's employs a local artist to decorate all stores; still, the individual managers have considerable say in what they feel is desirable for their own location. Often, the artwork is an exhibition of local artists' efforts.

Everyone does everything that needs to be done in the store. If the floor needs to be cleaned, the manager is just as likely to do it as a scooper. There is a very strong sense of teamwork and camaraderie. Employee meetings are usually held at 1 AM, after the last Amy's Ice Cream has closed for the night. Door prizes are offered to encourage attendance.

Apparently, it is a lifestyle choice to work for Amy's. These employees are people who do not want a "real job" in which they would have to wear certain clothes, work certain hours, and not have nearly as much fun. Obviously, money is not the major motivation, and it may be that the lack of big money is one of the unifying forces among employees.

Amy's Ice Cream has created what is definitely a "nonmainstream environment," which many feel is responsible for the legions of happy customers who keep the business merrily dipping along.

Questions

1. Describe the service organization culture at Amy's Ice Cream.

2. What are the personality attributes of the employees who are sought by Amy's Ice Cream?

3. Design a personnel selection procedure for Amy's Ice Cream using abstract questioning, a situational vignette, and/or role playing.

SELECTED BIBLIOGRAPHY

ALBRECHT, KARL: "Achieving Excellence in Service," *Training and Development Journal,* vol. 39, no. 12, December 1985, pp. 64–67.

BATESON, J.: "Perceived Control and the Service Encounter," in J. A. Czepiel, M. R. Solomon, and C. F. Surprenant (eds.), *The Service Encounter,* Lexington Books, Lexington, Mass., 1985, pp. 76–83.

BERRY, L. L.: "The Employee as Customer," *Journal of Retailing Banking,* vol. 3, no. 1, March 1981, pp. 33–40.

BITNER, MARY JO: "Evaluating Service Encounters: The Effects of Physical Surroundings and Employee Responses," *Journal of Marketing,* vol. 54, no. 2, April 1990, pp. 69–82.

———, B. H. BOOMS, AND L. A. MOHR: "Critical Service Encounters: The Employee's Viewpoint," *Journal of Marketing,* vol. 58, October 1994, pp. 95–106.

BITRAN, GABRIEL R., and JOHANNES HOECH: "The Humanization of Service: Respect at the Moment of Truth," *Sloan Management Review,* vol. 31, no. 2, Winter 1990, pp. 89–96.

BOWEN, D. E., and E. L. LAWLER: "Empowering Service Employees," *Sloan Management Review,* Summer 1995, pp. 73–84.

CARLZON, JAN: *Moments of Truth,* Ballinger, Cambridge, Mass., 1987.

CHASE, R. B.: "The 10 Commandments of Service System Management," *Interfaces,* vol. 15, no. 3, May–June 1985, pp. 68–72.

GRONROOS, CHRISTIAN: *Service Management and Marketing,* Lexington Books, Lexington, Mass., 1990.

HESKETT, J. L.: "People and the Service Culture," *Managing in the Service Economy,* Harvard Business School Press, Boston, 1986, pp. 117–134.

———, T. O. JONES, G. W. LOVEMAN, W. E. SASSER, JR., and L. A. SCHLESINGER: "Putting the Service-Profit Chain to Work," *Harvard Business Review,* March–April 1994, pp. 164–174.

HOLLANDER, S. C.: "A Historical Perspective on the Service Encounter," in J. A. Czepiel, M. R. Solomon, and C. F. Surprenant (eds.), *The Service Encounter,* Lexington Books, Lexington, Mass., 1985, pp. 49–65.

KELLY, J., J. DONNELLY, and S. SKINNER: "Customer Participation in Service Production and Delivery," *Journal of Retailing,* vol. 66, no. 3, 1990, pp. 315–335.

JONES, T. O., and W. E. SASSER, JR.: "Why Satisfied Customers Defect," *Harvard Business Review,* November–December 1995, pp. 88–99.

MILL, R. C.: "Managing the Service Encounter," *The Cornell H.R.A. Quarterly,* February 1986, pp. 39–46.

MILLS, P. K., R. B. CHASE, and N. MARGULIES: "Motivating the Client/Employee System as a Service Production Strategy," *Academy of Management Review,* vol. 8, no. 2, 1983, pp. 301–310.

NYQUIST, J. D., M. J. BITNER, and B. H. BOOMS: "Identifying Communication Difficulties in the Service Encounter: A Critical Incident Approach," in J. A. Czepiel, M. R. Solomon, and C. F. Surprenant (eds.), *The Service Encounter,* Lexington Books, Lexington, Mass., 1985, pp. 195–212.

SCHLESINGER, LEONARD A.: "Enfranchisement of Service Workers," *California Management Review,* Summer 1991, pp. 83–101.

———: "Breaking the Cycle of Failure in Services," *Sloan Management Review,* Spring 1991, pp. 17–28.

———, and J. L. HESKETT: "The Service-Driven Service Company," *Harvard Business Review,* September–October 1991, pp. 71–81.

SCHNEIDER, BENJAMIN, and DANIEL SCHECHTER: "Development of a Personnel Selection System for Service Jobs," in S. W. Brown, E. Gummesson, B. Edvardsson, and B. Gustavsson (eds.), *Service Quality: Multidisciplinary and Multinational Perspectives,* Lexington Books, Lexington, Mass., 1991, pp. 217–235.

———, and D. E. BOWEN: *Winning the Service Game,* Harvard Business School Press, Boston, 1995.

SHIFFLER, R. E., and R. W. COYE: "Monitoring Employee Performance in Service Operations," *International Journal of Operations and Production Management,* vol. 8, no. 2, 1988, pp. 5–13.

SOLOMON, M. R.: "Packaging the Service Provider," *The Service Industries Journal,* vol. 5, no. 1, 1985, pp. 65–72.

———, C. F. SURPRENANT, J. A. CZEPIEL, and E. G. GUTMAN: "A Role Theory Perspective on Dyadic Interactions: The Service Encounter," *Journal of Marketing,* vol. 49, Winter 1985, pp. 99–111.

WALKER, J. A.: "Service Encounter Satisfaction: Conceptualized," *Journal of Services Marketing,* vol. 9, no. 1, 1995, pp. 5–14.

WEHRENBERG, STEPHEN B.: "Front-line Interpersonal Skills a Must in Today's Service Economy," *Personnel Journal,* vol. 66, no. 1, January 1987, pp. 115–118.

Chapter 9 Supplement: Work Measurement

Time Study

This technique of work measurement known as *time study* is used to develop standards of performance. Management can use these standard times for many purposes, such as to determine staffing needs, allocate tasks to jobs, develop standard costs, evaluate employee performance, and establish wage payment plans. (Recall the standard times attached to critical operations on the service blueprint.)

Time study involves identifying and measuring the individual work *elements* of repetitive jobs. These repetitive jobs also are called work *cycles.* For example, consider the responsibilities of the person who serves salads at your local cafeteria. A particular work cycle for this server might include the elements of retrieving a dish, filling the dish, adding a dressing, and handing the dish to the diner.

Measurements are made with a stopwatch, and the time when each element is completed is recorded on an observation sheet such as that shown in Table 9.2. The variability of the element times and the level of confidence or accuracy that is desired provide a statistical basis for determining the number of cycles to observe.

Our example worksheet contains a record of the observations of a server who wraps silverware into napkins and repeats the sequence, or cycle, ten times. Each column represents one finished place setting. The stopwatch is started as the server begins positioning the napkin. The first reading (*R*), in hundredths of a minute on the watch, is noted when the server reaches for the silverware. The second reading is made after the last piece of silverware is placed on the napkin, and the third reading is noted after the napkin is rolled around the silverware. The final reading for cycle 1 is made after the rolled napkin is placed in a box. In our example, the actual readings for elements 1 through 4 in cycle 1 are noted at 3, 8, 15, and 23 one-hundredths of a minute, respectively, after the stopwatch is started. After the server is timed through nine more repetitions of the work cycle, each elapsed time (*T*) is calculated. For example, the time the server took between the end of the first element and the end of the second element in cycle 1 is 8 − 3 = 5 one-hundredths of a minute, which is written in the chart as 0.05.

The next step in using the time study sheet is to find the sum of the elapsed times for each element across all the cycles and then calculate the average time for each element. These average times provide information for this particular server, but if he or she is significantly faster or slower than an average server, management would not want to base decisions on such times. Therefore, the values are adjusted by means of a *performance rating* to reflect what reasonably may be expected of an "average" worker.

A performance rating represents a subjective judgment by the person who is conducting the time study. Expert analysts are trained to estimate efficiency rates by viewing films of people working at different rates. For example, a poor worker might work at what the analyst would consider to be 90 percent of normal, and the average time would be adjusted downward by a factor of 0.9. A very fast worker might be rated at 110 percent of normal, and the average time would be adjusted upward by a factor of 1.10. The adjusted times are called *normal element times* and are derived according to the following formula:

$$NT_i = R_i(OT_i) \tag{1}$$

where NT_i = normal time of the *i*th work element,

OT_i = average observed time of the *i*th work element, and

R_i = proficiency rating of the employee in performing the *i*th work element expressed as a decimal percentage (e.g., 0.90 for 90 percent of normal).

In our example, the server's normal time for the first element, position napkin, therefore is

$$\begin{aligned} NT_1 &= (1.10)(0.050) \\ &= 0.055 \end{aligned}$$

Similar calculations are made to obtain normal times for the remaining elements. It should be noted, however, that because of their subjective nature, performance ratings as used in the example above can be a source of contention.

The sympathetic reader already may recognize the need to qualify the normal element times just calculated. The server cannot be expected to fold silverware into napkins in a robot-like manner for 8 solid hours during a working day. Allowances must be made for breaks, personal needs, and perhaps other interruptions such as obtaining more napkins and sil-

TABLE 9.2 Time Study Observation Sheet

Activity: *Folding silverware into napkins* Date: *1/10/97*

Began timing: *2:32*
Ended timing: *2:35*

Study no. *13*

Observer *C.C.*

Std time *0.326 min/item*

Element description		Cycles										Sum	Avg. time	Rating	Normal time
		1	2	3	4	5	6	7	8	9	10				
1 *Position napkin*	T	0.03	0.05	0.05	0.06	0.06	0.06	0.05	0.05	0.05	0.04	0.50	0.050	1.10	0.055
	R	3	28	65	95	25	57	85	13	42	67				
2 *Group knife, fork, and spoon*	T	0.05	0.08	0.09	0.08	0.08	0.07	0.08	0.09	0.06	0.08	0.76	0.076	1.00	0.076
	R	8	36	74	103	33	64	93	22	48	75				
3 *Roll silverware*	T	0.07	0.15	0.06	0.06	0.07	0.06	0.06	0.06	0.07	0.07	0.73	0.073	0.90	0.065
	R	15	51	80	9	40	70	99	28	55	82				
4 *Place in box*	T	0.08	0.09	0.09	0.10	0.11	0.10	0.09	0.09	0.08	0.09	0.92	0.092	1.05	0.097
	R	23	60	89	19	51	80	208	37	63	91				
5	T														
	R														
6	T														
	R														
7	T														
	R														
8	T														
	R														
9	T														
	R														

Note: T = time
R = reading

Foreign elements:

Normal cycle time *0.294*
÷
[1–Allowance (10%)] *0.9*
=
Standard time *0.327*

verware. These allowances are figured as a percentage of the job time (i.e., a 10-percent allowance would translate into 6 minutes every working hour). The resulting adjusted times, known as the *standard element times,* and their sum, known as the *standard cycle time,* are calculated according to the following formulas:

$$ST_i = \frac{NT_i}{1 - A} \tag{2}$$

$$CT = \sum_{i=1}^{n} ST_i \tag{3}$$

where ST_i = standard time for the ith work element,
A = allowance expressed as a decimal percentage (e.g., 0.10 for 10 percent),
CT = standard cycle time, and
n = number of work elements in the work cycle.

We complete our example time study sheet by adding the normal element times to obtain a normal cycle time of 0.294. This result is adjusted by an allowance of 10 percent, or 0.10, to yield a standard cycle time of 0.327. Note that the sample time study sheet has a space to record any foreign elements observed (e.g., setting aside a dirty fork). These random occurrences are not included explicitly in the work cycle, but they are accounted for in selecting the allowance when deriving standard times. The standard cycle time now can be used by management to assign a server sufficient time to prepare enough folded silverware and napkins for the next mealtime.

Work Sampling

Time studies are used to determine how long it takes to complete a task; *work sampling* is used to determine how people allocate their time among various types of activities. Suppose we are interested in the proportion of time an employee spends at various activities that occur randomly during the workday. Tallying observations of worker activity that are noted at random times during the day would lead to our desired proportions.

Consider, for example, a server at a Red Lobster restaurant. This server must take drink and food orders, serve drinks, dish up and serve salads, grind fresh pepper on the salads, serve biscuits, serve entrees, take dessert orders, serve desserts, and present the check as well as clear away dirty dishes and refill drinks as required throughout. Obviously, there is much variation in the server's duties: one diner may require information on how particular foods are prepared before the order can be taken, another may drink his or her water as fast as the glass is filled, some may eat quickly and require little attention beyond the basic service, and still others may request much extra service.

To study worker activity that is as complex and seemingly random as we have just described, we can use the work sampling method, which is concerned with the proportion of time that a worker is engaged in different activities rather than with the actual time that is spent performing an activity. This technique is most useful in the design and redesign of contact personnel jobs because of the nonprogrammed nature of direct customer contact activities.

As described by Sheryl E. Kimes and Stephen A. Mutkoski, work sampling involves seven steps.[15]

1. *Define the activities.* Divide the work into as few categories as possible that do not overlap.
2. *Design the observation form.* The form should be designed with ease of use and ease of future analysis in mind.
3. *Determine the length of the study.* The study must be long enough to provide a random sample of activities.
4. *Test the form.* Try the form in actual practice to see if the categories are well defined and if it is easy to use and accurate. Does the test application suggest any changes that should be made in the definition of the categories or the design of the form?
5. *Determine the sample size and observation pattern.* Common statistical methods can be used to select the size of the sample to study and an observation schedule. In general, the larger the sample size, the more accurate and representative the sample will be. A formula can be used to determine how many observations must be made to achieve the desired level of confidence or accuracy, and a schedule for making those observations must be devised. Details of the statistical methods involved are described later in this supplement in the section called "Sample Size."

[15]S. E. Kimes and S. A. Mutkoski, "Customer Contact in Restaurants: An Application of Work Sampling," *The Cornell HRA Quarterly,* May 1991, pp. 82–88.

6. *Conduct the study.* Observers must be trained to use the form properly. Kimes and Mutkoski also point out the importance of considering the effect the study can have on the behavior of those who are being observed, and they suggest two approaches to mediate any adverse effect on the subjects: to inform and assure them that they are not being evaluated, and to make very discreet, unobtrusive observations without informing them. In addition, data for the first day or two could be discarded to allow the workers to feel more at ease with the data collection process.
7. *Analyze the data.* Again, common statistical methods can be used to calculate the information required by management. In simplest terms, it is necessary only to total the number of observations in each category and calculate the percentage of time spent on that activity.

Kimes and Mutkoski describe an application of work sampling in a study of servers working in two different types of restaurants: family and "mid-scale." The major difference between these two restaurant types for the purposes of their study is in the nature and amount of customer-server interaction: they hypothesized that the emphasis in the family restaurants "would be on efficiency with an eye toward increasing table turnover, while in a mid-scale restaurant, the emphasis would be more on guest service with the idea of increasing 'add-on' sales and guest satisfaction."

Above all, their sampling plan needed to provide "a good random representative sample" of servers' activities. Therefore, they selected six different family restaurants and six different mid-scale restaurants and conducted their studies during the peak lunch and dinner times. They observed two servers at each restaurant for at least 1 1/2 hours.

For this study, the servers' activities were divided into the following eight categories:

1. *Guest contact.* Any interaction with the customer.
2. *Walk—empty.* Walking without carrying anything.
3. *Walk—full.* Walking while carrying food, beverages, or dirty dishes.
4. *Bus.* Clearing a vacated table.
5. *Prepare.* Preparing food and beverages before service.
6. *Can't see.* Server is out of sight.
7. *Check.* Delivering or processing the check.
8. *Rest.* Server's break time.

These categories were listed on the form shown in Table 9.3, which was to be used by the student observers who visited each restaurant anonymously to minimize any effect they might have on the subjects. Observations were recorded at 1-minute intervals: one server was checked on the minute, and the other server was checked on the half minute. Because observations made at such regular intervals are not random, the researchers compensated by drawing a random sample of the student observations at each restaurant for their final analysis.

Kimes and Mutkoski suggest ways that management can use the information from their study. If servers are spending more or less time with customers than desired, perhaps the jobs can be redesigned to increase or decrease the customer contact time. If servers are spending too much time on busing tables, perhaps more bus help could be employed. If servers are off the floor too much, perhaps a type of "front-waiter, back-waiter" system would be helpful.

Sample Size

Consider the following situation: The nursing supervisor at a major hospital must make up a new work schedule for her staff and needs information on which to base her decisions. Therefore, she is interested in determining the actual proportion of time that nurses (RNs) spend in direct patient care. She believes the RNs spend approximately 20 percent of their time in direct patient care but wants to conduct a work sampling study to validate her estimate. For this study, she wants to be 95 percent confident that the resulting estimate will be within 5 percent of the true proportion.

Given the desired confidence level defined above, we can calculate the size of the sample that would be required for the study. The size of the sample (or the number of observations) depends on both an estimate of the proportion of time spent in a particular activity and the accuracy that is desired. The formula for calculating the sample size is:

$$N = \frac{Z^2 P(1 - P)}{E^2} \tag{4}$$

where N = sample size,
Z = standard normal deviate for desired level of confidence,
P = assumed proportion expressed as a decimal percentage, and
E = maximum error allowed expressed as a decimal percentage.

TABLE 9.3 Work Sampling Form for Retaurant Study

Restaurant ______________ Lunch ____ Dinner____
Date ____ Time ____

Key OB#	Guest Contact	Walk— Empty	Walk— Full	Bus	Prepare	Can't See	Check	Rest	Key OB#
1		√							1
2	√								2
3	√								3
4		√							4
5						√			5
6						√			6
34						√			34
35						√			35
36						√			36
37			√						37
38	√								38
39		√							39
40							√		40
Sum									Sum

By noting what the server is doing once each minute, an observer can obtain a sampling of which tasks occupy the server's time. The 40 observation points indicated in the above form would not constitute a sufficient sample by themselves, but would be part of a lengthier study.

Source: S. E. Kimes and S. A. Mutkoski, "Customer Contact in Restaurants: An Application of Work Sampling," *The Cornell HRA Quarterly*, May 1991, p. 86. © Cornell HRA Quarterly. Used by permission. All rights reserved.

In actual practice, an estimate of the proportion of time spent on a particular activity (P) can be made by conducting small initial studies or by assigning a conservative value of 50 percent, or 0.5 (which will guarantee that the sample size is large enough to achieve the desired level of confidence). A third way of estimating P is to make a reasonable assumption based on experience, as the supervisor did in our hospital example above when she set P equal to 0.2 (i.e., 20 percent). For this example, $E = 0.05$, and $Z = 1.96$ (for a two-tailed 0.95 confidence level as found in the end-of-book Appendix table "Areas of a Standard Normal Distribution"). Substituting these values in equation (4) yields:

$$N = \frac{(1.96)^2(0.2)(1-0.2)}{(0.05)^2} = 246 \text{ observations}$$

The supervisor now needs to construct a schedule of random observations made over a period of time that is long enough to ensure adequate representation of all activities. For this example, assume that the study will be conducted for 20 weekdays. This means that 13 observations per day ($246/20 = 12.3$) are required. These observations should be made at random times during each workday, and the hour and minute for each observation can be determined using a random-number table.

Work Methods Charts

The flow of work activities and the interactions between customers and workers can be represented graphically. The most commonly used graphical tools are *worker-customer charts* and *activity charts.*

Worker-Customer Charts

When the server's work cycle time is shorter than that required by the supply of customers, the interaction can be shown on a time scale. The resulting worker-customer chart can be used to schedule work activities so that one employee can serve more than one customer at a time.

Figure 9.5 shows a worker-customer chart for a bank in which one drive-in teller serves two lanes. We simplify this example by using average times and ignoring randomness. On the average, a customer takes 15 seconds to approach the service area, 48 seconds to be served, and 9 seconds to depart. Note that the customer's average cycle time is 72 seconds, but the teller's average cycle time is 48 seconds. You also can see that while the teller is occupied with the first customer, a second customer has entered the system and is waiting for service in the second lane.

Activity Charts

The worker-customer chart described above is a useful tool in simple situations, but a situation involving multiple servers and many customers may benefit from use of a more complex graphical depiction called an activity chart. An activity chart also uses a time scale, as shown in Figure 9.6. In this example, two tellers at a drive-in bank are located in a single station. The bank has three lanes, one served directly from the teller station window and the other two from pneumatic tubes that transfer materials to and from the teller station. The average service time at each position is 48 seconds per customer. Each customer requires an average of 15 seconds to enter the service area and an average of 9 seconds to depart. We can see from this chart that the system is operating efficiently; that is, the system quickly adapts to avoid waiting by customers and idle time for tellers. Also, note that we have created a two-server queuing system with a single waiting line in spite of the physical need for multiple lanes. (For a discussion of queuing systems, *see* Chapter 11.)

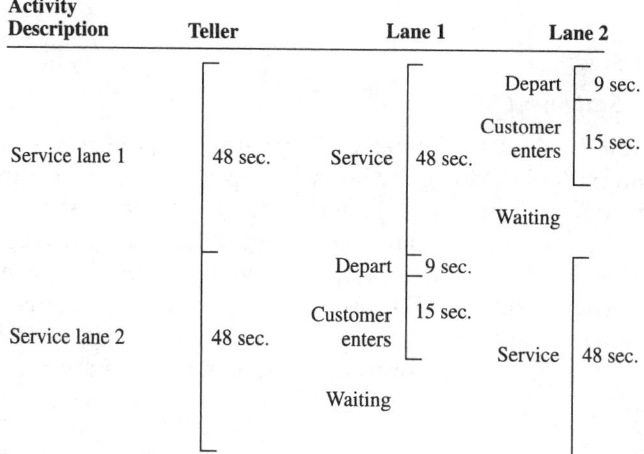

Total cycle time: 96 seconds
Idle-teller time per cycle: 0
Working-teller time per cycle: 96 seconds
Idle-lane time per cycle: 48 seconds
Working-lane time per cycle: 144 seconds

FIGURE 9.5. Worker-customer chart: teller serving two lanes of a drive-in bank.

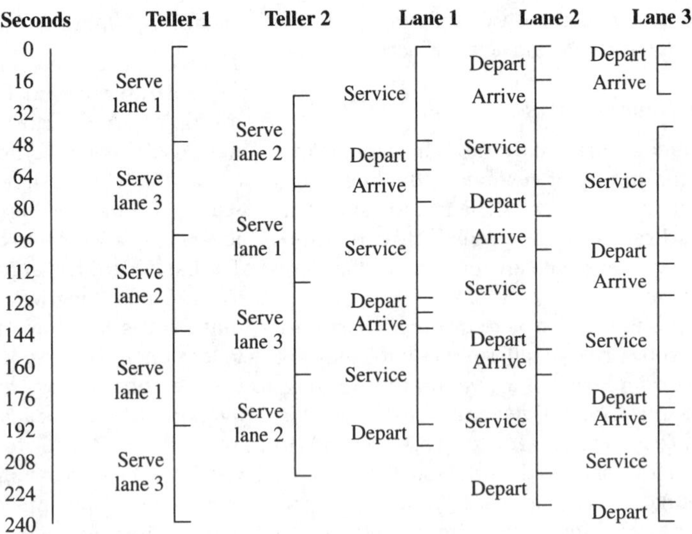

FIGURE 9.6. Activity chart: two tellers serving three lanes of a drive-in bank.

SOLVED PROBLEMS

1. Time Study

Problem Statement

A discount tire dealer is interested in determining the optimal staffing level for his mechanics during busy hours to avoid excessive customer waiting. Using a stopwatch during one afternoon, he observed a mechanic taking an average of 18 minutes to spin balance and mount four tires on a car. He judged that this experienced mechanic had a proficiency rating of about 110 percent. What is the normal time for this activity? If the allowance for fatigue and personal time is 15 percent, what should the standard time for this activity be? For planning purposes, how many cars can one mechanic service per hour?

Solution

Using equation (1), we calculate the normal time as:

$$NT_i = R_i(OT_i) = (1.10)(18) = 19.8 \text{ minutes}$$

Using equation (2), we calculate the standard time as:

$$ST_i = \frac{NT_i}{1-A} = 19.8/(1-.15) = 23.3 \text{ minutes}$$

Therefore, the number of cars a mechanic can service in one hour = 60/23.3 ≅ 2.5 cars per hour.

2. Work Sampling

Problem Statement

The discount tire owner is concerned about the excessive waiting of customers and wants to determine the percentage of time that his mechanics are idle. He wants an estimate within a ± 5 percent degree of accuracy at a 95-percent confidence level.

Solution

A work sampling study over a 10-day period is suggested. Because no estimate of the percentage idle time is given, we will use 0.5 to guarantee a conservative sample size, which is calculated using equation (4):

$$N = \frac{Z^2P(1-P)}{E^2} = \frac{(1.96)^2(0.5)(1-0.5)}{(0.05)^2} = 384$$

Thus, 38 random observations of the work area should be made during each day, or approximately one every 12 minutes assuming an 8-hour workday.

EXERCISES

9.1. We want to estimate the proportion of time when a car wash facility is unused. It is known that the facility is busy for at least 80 percent of the day, and a study is conducted for 1 week. If we need an estimate within ± 5 percent at a 90-percent confidence level, how many observations are required each day?

9.2. If a team of workers takes 14 minutes on average to wash and handwipe a typical car, how many cars per hour can be serviced if an allowance of 10 percent is allowed for fatigue and personal needs?

9.3. One of the cleaning staff at the Last Resort Motel was observed making beds at an average rate of 8 minutes per bed. The proficiency rating of the staff person is estimated to be 90 percent.

a. What is the normal time for this task?

b. If the allowance for fatigue and personal needs is 10 percent, what is the standard time for this task?

9.4. A restaurant manager has noticed that tables are not cleared fast enough and diners are kept waiting during the busy lunch period. To justify hiring a part-time person to clear tables, she has decided to conduct a time study to determine how many tables one person can clear per hour. After observing tables being cleared for 1 week, an average of 3 minutes per table has been observed.

a. What is the normal time for clearing a table if the proficiency rating of the person observed was 85 percent?

b. If the allowance for fatigue and personal needs is 10 percent, what is the expected number of tables that can be cleared per hour?

9.5. A check-out line at a supermarket consists of two activities in sequence, one performed by a cashier and the other by a grocery packer. The cashier was observed taking 4 minutes on average to process a shopper, whereas the packer was able to finish bagging the groceries in 3 minutes. The proficiency ratings of the cashier and packer are estimated to be 80 percent and 90 percent, respectively.

a. What is the normal time for the check-out process?

b. If the allowance for fatigue and personal needs is 15 percent, how many shoppers can be processed per hour?

9.6. The cleaning staff at the Last Resort Motel has complained of being overworked. Management has decided to conduct a work sampling study to verify its contention that the staff is busy only about 60 percent of the time. The study should yield an estimate of idle time with a ± 5 percent degree of accuracy at a 95-percent confidence level.
   a. How many random observations should be made?
   b. Explain how you would select each observation time during a typical 8-hour day (the study will be conducted for 10 days).

9.7. The telephone company is considering taking public telephones out of service if their utilization rate is less than 20 percent. A 10-day work sampling study is conducted. The estimate of utilization should be within a ± 5 percent degree of accuracy at a 95-percent confidence level.
   a. How many random observations should be made per day?
   b. If the telephone is located in a restaurant, explain how you could enlist a waitperson to conduct the study using a fixed observation interval of 15 minutes.

9.8. One station attendant serves a full-service gas station that has a total of three pumps. On the average, a car takes 10 seconds to pull up to a pump; the attendant takes 15 seconds to find out customer needs and to begin pumping gas. It takes 40 seconds for the gas to be pumped (the attendant is free during this time), and cleaning the windshield takes 15 seconds. Finally, it takes 30 seconds to replace the nozzle on the pump and for payment to be made. Customers enter the station every 60 seconds (deterministic). Assume a customer goes to an empty pump if available or to any pump otherwise. Draw a worker-customer chart for a five-minute observation of this scenario.

CASE: COUNTY GENERAL HOSPITAL[16]

County General is a large public hospital serving a major metropolitan area in the growing Sunbelt region of the United States. A significant portion of the hospital's budget is consumed by labor costs, and the total number of employees can be broken down as follows:

Administrative and management	18
Professional	
MDs	67
RNs	145
LVNs	196
Support	368
Total	794

The hospital's top management has been concerned for some time that the labor costs for professional staff, particularly the registered nurses, have not been kept under control as closely as the annual operating plan envisioned at its inception. In attempting to see how the nursing staff could be utilized better, management has decided to undertake a work sampling study of the registered nurses to see what proportions of their time actually are spent on various tasks.

In designing the study, management established eight general categories of activities for defining the registered nurse's typical workday: 1) direct patient care, 2) indirect patient care (i.e., preparation of medicine, equipment, and so on), 3) paperwork, 4) communication and teaching, 5) escorting and errands, 6) housekeeping, 7) travel, and 8) nonproductive (i.e., idle time, mealtime, and so on).

Observers who perform the actual sampling will be given lists of specific duties that would define each category and also would ensure that the study has a high degree of consistency in the allocation of a nurse's daily duties to the correct categories. On the basis of a pilot study, County General's management estimates that the proportions of time spent in each of the above

[16]Prepared by James Vance under the supervision of Professor James A. Fitzsimmons.

categories are 15, 12, 10, 40, 5, 3, 5, and 10 percent, respectively. The study will be conducted during a 14-day period from each of three workshifts, and management wants to ensure that the estimates come within ±2 percent of the true proportions with a 98-percent confidence level.

Questions

1. How many observations will be required to ensure that all categories have enough data collected to meet the established parameters for accuracy? Assume there is a normal distribution.

2. The study was accomplished as designed, and the hospital management team was given the following summary data:

Category	% of Time	Category	% of Time
1	13.8	5	3.1
2	12.3	6	4.5
3	11.9	7	3.1
4	39.7	8	11.6

On the basis of your knowledge of hospital functions and the general goal of providing a high level of service to patients, suggest at least one or two strategies management might apply to utilize better the time of the registered nursing staff. Describe the effects that your strategies might have on the time requirements for other staff groups and on the general level of health care in County General.

Service Quality

LEARNING OBJECTIVES

After completing this chapter, you should be able to:

1. Describe and illustrate the five dimensions of service quality.
2. Use the service quality gap model to diagnose quality problems for a service firm.
3. Describe how the SERVQUAL survey instrument is used to measure gaps in a service firm's quality.
4. Illustrate how Taguchi methods and poka-yoke methods are applied to quality design in services.
5. Construct a "house of quality" as part of a quality function deployment project.
6. Construct a statistical process control chart for service operation.
7. Use a fishbone chart in a cause-and-effect analysis.
8. Compare and contrast the quality program features espoused by Philip Crosby and W. Edward Deming.
9. Describe the features of an unconditional service guarantee and its managerial benefits.
10. Discuss the concept of a service recovery.

Service "with a smile" used to be enough to satisfy most customers. Today, however, some service firms differentiate themselves in the marketplace by offering a "service guarantee." Unlike a product warranty, which promises to repair or replace the faulty item, service guarantees typically offer the dissatisfied customer a refund, discount, or free service. Take, for example, the First Interstate Bank of California. After interviewing its customers, the bank management discovered that they were annoyed by a number of recurring problems, such as inaccurate statements and broken automatic teller machines (ATMs). Account retention improved after the bank began to pay customers $5 for reporting each such service failure. What is surprising, however, is that the service guarantee also had a motivating effect on the employees. When an ATM failed at a branch, the employees, out of pride, decided to keep the branch open until the machine was repaired at 8:30 PM.

Another hidden benefit of a guarantee is customer feedback. Now customers have a reason and motivation to talk to the company instead of just to their friends.

In addition to advertising the firm's commitment to quality, a service guarantee focuses employees by defining performance standards explicitly and, more important, builds a loyal customer base. The experience of Hampton Inns, an early adopter of a "100 percent satisfaction guarantee," illustrates that superior quality is a competitive advantage. In a survey of 300 guests who invoked the guarantee, more than 100 already had stayed again at a Hampton Inn. The hotel chain figures that it has received $8 in revenue for every $1 paid to a disgruntled guest.[1]

CHAPTER PREVIEW

Service quality is a complex topic, as shown by the need for a definition containing five dimensions: reliability, responsiveness, assurance, empathy, and tangibles. Using these dimensions, the concept of a service quality gap is introduced; it is based on the difference between a customer's expectations of a service and the perceptions of that service as it is delivered. A survey instrument that measures service quality, called SERVQUAL, is based on implementing the service quality gap concept. The discussion of measurement also includes the concept of benchmarking, which is a process of comparing one's service delivery system with those of other firms with a reputation of being best in class.

Quality begins, however, with the design of the service delivery system. Thus, concepts borrowed from manufacturing (e.g., Taguchi methods, poka-yoke, and quality function deployment) are applied to the design of service delivery systems. In addition, applications of statistical process control to services are illustrated by the construction of quality-control charts. Achieving service quality through the use of quality tools is illustrated by the example of Midway Airlines.

Finally, programs to improve quality and create an organization that is focused on providing excellence in quality are discussed. The teachings of Dem-

[1]Daniel Pearl, "More Firms Pledge Guaranteed Service," *The Wall Street Journal,* July 17, 1991, p. B1.

ing and Crosby, the concept of an unconditional service guarantee, and the Malcolm Baldrige National Quality Award all are explored.

DEFINING SERVICE QUALITY

For services, the assessment of quality is made during the service delivery process, which usually occurs with an encounter between a customer and a service contact person as discussed in Chapter 9. Customer satisfaction with service quality can be defined by comparing perceptions of the service received with expectations of the service desired. When expectations are exceeded, service is perceived to be of exceptional quality—and also to be a pleasant surprise. When expectations are not met, however, service quality is deemed unacceptable. When expectations are confirmed by perceived service, quality is satisfactory. As Figure 10.1 shows, these expectations are based on several sources, including word of mouth, personal needs, and past experience.

Dimensions of Service Quality

The dimensions of service quality as shown in Figure 10.1 were identified by marketing researchers studying several different service categories: appliance repair, retail banking, long-distance telephone service, securities brokerage, and credit card companies. They identified five principal dimensions that customers use to judge service quality—reliability, responsiveness, assurance, empathy, and tangibles, which are listed in order of declining relative importance to customers.[2]

Reliability. The ability to perform the promised service both dependably and accurately. Reliable service performance is a customer expectation and means that the service is accomplished on time, in the same manner, and without errors every time. For example, receiving mail at approximately

[2]A. Parasuraman, V. A. Zeithaml, and L. L. Berry, "SERVQUAL: A Multiple-Item Scale for Measuring Consumer Perceptions of Service Quality," *Journal of Retailing*, vol. 64, no. 1, Spring 1988, pp. 12–40.

FIGURE 10.1. Perceived service quality.
(Reprinted with permission of the American Marketing Association: adapted from A. Parasuraman, V. A. Zeithaml, and L. L. Berry, "A Conceptual Model of Service Quality and Its Implications for Future Research," Journal of Marketing, *vol. 49, Fall 1985, p. 48.)*

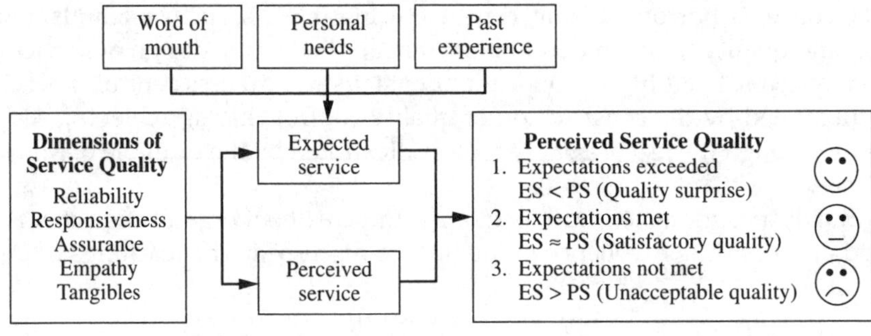

the same time each day is important to most people. Reliability also extends into the back office, where accuracy in billing and record keeping is expected.

Responsiveness. The willingness to help customers and to provide prompt service. Keeping customers waiting, particularly for no apparent reason, creates unnecessary negative perceptions of quality. If a service failure occurs, the ability to recover quickly and with professionalism can create very positive perceptions of quality. For example, serving complimentary drinks on a delayed flight can turn a potentially poor customer experience into one that is remembered favorably.

Assurance. The knowledge and courtesy of employees as well as their ability to convey trust and confidence. The assurance dimension includes the following features: competence to perform the service, politeness and respect for the customer, effective communication with the customer, and the general attitude that the server has the customer's best interests at heart.

Empathy. The provision of caring, individualized attention to customers. Empathy includes the following features: approachability, sensitivity, and effort to understand the customer's needs. One example of empathy is the ability of an airline gate attendant to make a customer's missed connection the attendant's own problem and find a solution.

Tangibles. The appearance of physical facilities, equipment, personnel, and communication materials. The condition of the physical surroundings (e.g., cleanliness) is tangible evidence of the care and attention to detail that are exhibited by the service provider. This assessment dimension also can extend to the conduct of other customers in the service (e.g., a noisy guest in the next room at a hotel).

Customers use these five dimensions to form their judgments of service quality, which are based on a comparison between expected and perceived service. The gap between expected and perceived service is a measure of service quality; satisfaction is either negative or positive.

Gaps in Service Quality

Measuring the gap between expected service and perceived service is a routine customer feedback process that is practiced by leading service companies. For example, Club Med, an international hotel chain operating resort villages worldwide, uses the questionnaire shown in Figure 10.2. This questionnaire is mailed to all guests immediately after their departure from a Club Med vacation to assess the quality of their experience. Note that the first question explicitly asks the guest to evaluate the gap between his or her expectations and the actual Club Med experience.

In Figure 10.3, the gap between customer expectations and perceptions is defined as GAP 5. It is shown to depend on the size and direction of the four gaps that are associated with delivery of the service.

The first gap is the discrepancy between customer expectations and management perceptions of these expectations. GAP 1 arises from management's lack of full understanding about how customers formulate their expectations on the

G.M. Questionnaire

Club Med Village: ______________________

Dates of your stay: From: ______________ to: ______________
Month/Day/Year Month/Day/Year

Name: ______________________ Member # ______________

Address: ______________________

City: ______________ State: ______________ Zip: ______________

	•OVERALL IMPRESSION	•ORGANIZATION	•TEAM OF G.O.s	•FOOD	•BAR	•SPORTS	•DAYTIME AMBIANCE	•EVENING ENTERTAINMENT	•MUSIC AND DANCE	•MINI CLUB	•EXCURSIONS	•ACCOMMODATIONS	•CLUB FLIGHTS AND TRANSFERS	•CLEANLINESS
EXCELLENT	6	6	6	6	6	6	6	6	6	6	6	6	6	6
VERY GOOD	5	5	5	5	5	5	5	5	5	5	5	5	5	5
GOOD	4	4	4	4	4	4	4	4	4	4	4	4	4	4
FAIR	3	3	3	3	3	3	3	3	3	3	3	3	3	3
POOR	2	2	2	2	2	2	2	2	2	2	2	2	2	2
VERY POOR	1	1	1	1	1	1	1	1	1	1	1	1	1	1

Your Comments: ______________________

1. Did Club Med meet your expectations?
   ☐ Far below expectations ☐ Surpassed expectations
   ☐ Fell short of expectations ☐ Far surpassed expectations
   ☐ Met expectations
2. If this was not your first Club Med, how many other times have you been to a Club Med village? ______________
3. How did you make your Club Med reservations?
   ☐ Through a travel agent ☐ Through Club Med Reservations
4. Quality of your reservations handling (pre-travel information):
   ☐ Very poor ☐ Poor ☐ Fair ☐ Good ☐ Excellent
5. Which one factor was most important in your choosing Club Med for your vacation?
   ☐ Previous stay with us ☐ Advertisement ☐ Editorial Article
   ☐ Travel Agent Recommendation ☐ Friend/Relative Recommendation
6. Kindly indicate your age bracket:
   ☐ Under 25 ☐ 25-34 ☐ 35-44 ☐ 45-54 ☐ 55 or over
7. Kindly indicate your marital status: ☐ Married ☐ Single
8. Would you vacation with Club Med again? ☐ Yes ☐ No
9. If you answered yes to question 8, where would you like to go on your next Club Med vacation?
   ☐ U.S.A. ☐ Mexico ☐ French West Indies ☐ Caribbean ☐ Europe
   ☐ Other: ______________

FIGURE 10.2. Customer satisfaction questionnaire.
(After Club Med, 40 West 57 Street, New York, NY 10019.)

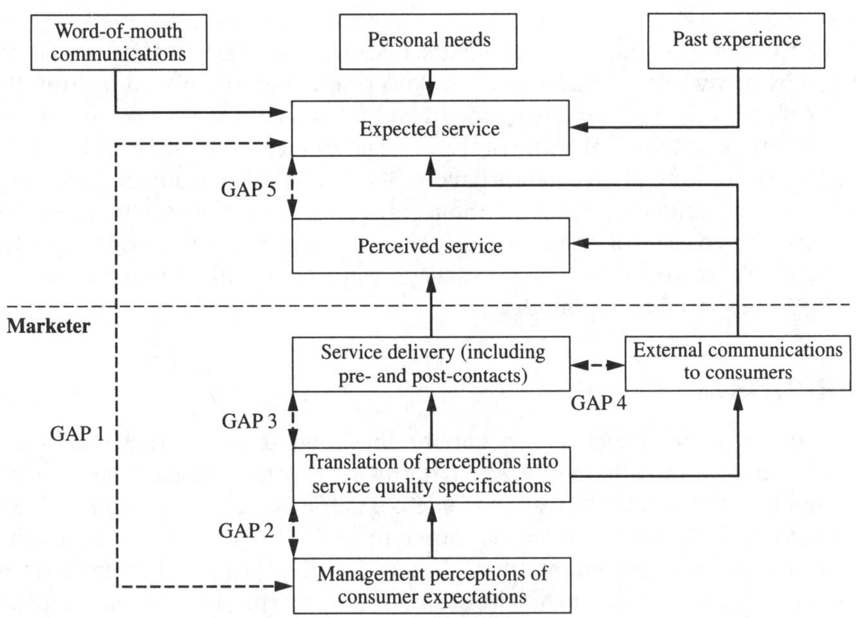

FIGURE 10.3. Service quality gap model.
(Reprinted with permission of the American Marketing Association: V. A. Zeithaml, L. L. Berry, and A. Parasuraman, "Communication and Control Processes in the Delivery of Service Quality," Journal of Marketing, *vol. 52, April 1988, p. 36.)*

basis of a number of sources: advertising, past experience with the firm and its competitors, personal needs, and communications with friends. Strategies for closing this gap include improving market research, fostering better communication between management and its contact employees, and reducing the number of levels of management that distance the customer.

The second gap results from management's inability to formulate target levels of service quality to meet perceptions of customer expectations and translate these into workable specifications. GAP 2 may result from a lack of management commitment to service quality or a perception of the unfeasibility of meeting customers' expectations; however, setting goals and standardizing service delivery tasks can close this gap.

The third gap is referred to as the service performance gap, because actual delivery of the service does not meet the specifications set by management. GAP 3 can arise for a number of reasons, including lack of teamwork, poor employee selection, inadequate training, and inappropriate job design.

Customer expectations of the service are formed by media advertising and other communications from the firm. GAP 4 is the discrepancy between service delivery and external communications in the form of exaggerated promises and lack of information provided to contact personnel.

The remainder of this chapter will address ways of closing these gaps in service quality. We begin by considering approaches to measuring service quality.

MEASURING SERVICE QUALITY

Measuring service quality is a challenge, because customer satisfaction is determined by many intangible factors. Unlike a product with physical features that can be objectively measured (e.g., the fit and finish of a car), service quality contains many psychological features (e.g., the ambiance of a restaurant). In addition, service quality often extends beyond the immediate encounter, because, as in the case of health care, it has an impact on a person's future quality of life. The multiple dimensions of service quality are captured in the SERVQUAL instrument, which is an effective tool for surveying customer satisfaction that is based on the service quality gap model.

SERVQUAL[3]

The authors of the service quality gap model shown in Figure 10.3 developed a multiple-item scale called *SERVQUAL* for measuring the five dimensions of service quality (i.e., reliability, responsiveness, assurance, empathy, and tangibles). This two-part instrument, which is shown in Table 10.1, has an initial section to record customer expectations for a class of services (e.g., budget hotels), followed by a second section to record a customer's perceptions for a particular service firm. The 22 statements in the survey describe aspects of the five dimensions of service quality.

A score for the quality of service is calculated by computing the differences between the ratings that customers assign to paired expectation and perception statements. This score is referred to as GAP 5, as was shown in Figure 10.3. Scores for the other four gaps also can be calculated in a similar manner.

This instrument has been designed and validated for use in a variety of service encounters. The authors have suggested many applications for SERVQUAL, but its most important function is tracking service quality trends through periodic customer surveys. For multisite services, SERVQUAL could be used by management to determine if any unit has poor service quality (indicated by a low score); if so, management can direct attention to correcting the source of customers' poor perceptions. SERVQUAL could be used in marketing studies to compare a service with a competitor's and again identify the dimensions of superior or inadequate service quality.

Benchmarking

The measure of the quality of a firm's performance can be made by comparison with the performance of other companies known for being "best in class," which is a process known as *benchmarking*. For example, Singapore Airlines has a reputation for outstanding cabin service, Federal Express for consistent overnight delivery, Hampton Inns for clean rooms, and Nordstrom's department store for attentive salespersons. For every quality dimension, some firm has earned the

[3]From A. Parasuraman, V. A. Zeithaml, and L. L. Berry, "SERVQUAL: A Multiple-Item Scale for Measuring Consumer Perceptions of Service Quality," *Journal of Retailing*, vol. 64, no. 1, Spring 1988, pp. 12–40.

TABLE 10.1. The SERVQUAL Instrument*

DIRECTIONS: This survey deals with your opinions of ______ services. Please show the extent to which you think firms offering ______ services should possess the features described by each statement. Do this by picking one of the seven numbers next to each statement. If you strongly agree that these firms should possess a feature, circle the number 7. If you strongly disagree that these firms should possess a feature, circle 1. If your feelings are not strong, circle one of the numbers in the middle. There are no right or wrong answers—all we are interested in is a number that best shows your expectations about firms offering ______ services.

E1 They should have up-to-date equipment.
E2 Their physical facilities should be visually appealing.
E3 Their employees should be well dressed and appear neat.
E4 The appearance of the physical facilities of these firms should be in keeping with the type of services provided.
E5 When these firms promise to do something by a certain time, they should do so.
E6 When customers have problems, these firms should be sympathetic and reassuring.
E7 These firms should be dependable.
E8 They should provide their services at the time they promise to do so.
E9 They should keep their records accurately.
E10 They shouldn't be expected to tell customers exactly when services will be performed.(–)[†]
E11 It is not realistic for customers to expect prompt service from employees of these firms.(–)
E12 Their employees don't always have to be willing to help customers.(–)
E13 It is OK if they are too busy to respond to customer requests promptly.(–)
E14 Customers should be able to trust employees of these firms.
E15 Customers should be able to feel safe in their transactions with these firms' employees.
E16 Their employees should be polite.
E17 Their employees should get adequate support from these firms to do their jobs well.
E18 These firms should not be expected to give customers individual attention.(–)
E19 Employees of these firms cannot be expected to give customers personal attention.(–)
E20 It is unrealistic to expect employees to know what the needs of their customers are.(–)
E21 It is unrealistic to expect these firms to have their customers' best interests at heart.(–)
E22 They shouldn't be expected to have operating hours convenient to all their customers.(–)

DIRECTIONS: The following set of statements relate to your feelings about XYZ. For each statement, please show the extent to which you believe XYZ has the feature described by the statement. Once again, circling a 7 means that you strongly agree that XYZ has that feature, and circling a 1 means that you strongly disagree. You may circle any of the numbers in the middle that show how strong your feelings are. There are no right or wrong answers—all we are interested in is a number that best shows your perceptions about XYZ.

P1 XYZ has up-to-date equipment.
P2 XYZ's physical facilities are visually appealing.

TABLE 10.1 The SERVQUAL Instrument* (*Continued*)

P3	XYZ's employees are well dressed and appear neat.
P4	The appearance of the physical facilities of XYZ is in keeping with the type of services provided.
P5	When XYZ promises to do something by a certain time, it does so.
P6	When you have problems, XYZ is sympathetic and reassuring.
P7	XYZ is dependable.
P8	XYZ provides its services at the time it promises to do so.
P9	XYZ keeps its records accurately.
P10	XYZ does not tell customers exactly when services will be performed.(–)
P11	You do not receive prompt service from XYZ's employees.(–)
P12	Employees of XYZ are not always willing to help customers.(–)
P13	Employees of XYZ are too busy to respond to customer requests promptly.(–)
P14	You can trust employees of XYZ.
P15	You feel safe in your transactions with XYZ's employees.
P16	Employees of XYZ are polite.
P17	Employees get adequate support from XYZ to do their jobs well.
P18	XYZ does not give you individual attention.(–)
P19	Employees of XYZ do not give you personal attention.(–)
P20	Employees of XYZ do not know what your needs are.(–)
P21	XYZ does not have your best interests at heart.(–)
P22	XYZ does not have operating hours convenient to all their customers.(–)

*A seven-point scale ranging from "Strongly Agree" (7) to "Strongly Disagree" (1), with no verbal labels for the intermediate scale points (i.e., 2 through 6), accompanied each statement. Also, the statements were in random order in the questionnaire. A complete listing of the 34-item instrument used in the second stage of data collection can be obtained from the first author.

†Ratings on these statements were reverse-scored prior to data analysis.

Source: Reprinted with permission of the *Journal of Retailing* from A. Parasuraman, V. A. Zeithaml, and L. L. Berry, "SERVQUAL: A Multiple-Item Scale for Measuring Consumer Perceptions of Service Quality," *Journal of Retailing*, vol. 64, no. 1, Spring 1988, pp. 38–40.

reputation for being "best in class" and, thus, is a benchmark for comparison. Benchmarking, however, involves more than comparing statistics. It also includes visiting the leading firm to learn firsthand how management has achieved such outstanding performance. For obvious proprietary reasons, this often requires going outside one's own field. Some manufacturers, for example, have visited the pit stops at automobile races to learn methods of reducing the time for production-line changeovers. Others have visited Domino's Pizza to understand how it delivers customized products within 30 minutes.

For a typical example, consider an electronics company seeking to improve its purchasing function. This company formed a study team that visited Ford to learn how it reduced the number of its suppliers, talked with Toyota about vendor relationships, and observed the buying process at Reliance Electric. The team returned with quantifiable measures that benchmarked the superior performance of these leading firms and with knowledge of how these gains were accomplished.[4]

[4]A. Steven Walleck, "A Backstage View of World-Class Performers," *The Wall Street Journal*, Aug. 26, 1991, p. A10.

Scope of Service Quality

A comprehensive view of the service system is necessary to identify the possible measures of service quality. We will use health care delivery as our example service, and we will view quality from five perspectives: content, process, structure, outcome, and impact. For health care, the scope of service quality obviously extends beyond the quality of care that is provided for the patient; it also includes the impact on the family and community. This comprehensive view of service quality need not be limited to health care, however, as demonstrated by the negative economic impact of failed savings-and-loan institutions on their customers as well as on the community as a whole.

Content

Are standard procedures being followed? For example, is the dentist following accepted dental practices when extracting a tooth? For routine services, standard operating procedures generally are developed, and service personnel are expected to follow these established procedures. In health care, a formal peer-review system, called Professional Standards Review Organization (PSRO), has been developed as a method of self-regulation. Under this system, physicians in a community or specialty establish standards for their practices and meet regularly to review peer performance so that compliance is assured.

Process

Is the sequence of events in the service process appropriate? The primary concern here is maintaining a logical sequence of activities and a well-coordinated use of service resources. Interactions between the customer and the service personnel are monitored. Also of interest are the interactions and communications among the service workers. Check sheets such as the one shown in Table 10.2 are common measurement devices. For emergency services such as fire and ambulance, disaster drills in a realistic setting are used to test a unit's performance; problems with coordination and activity sequencing can be identified and corrected through these practice sessions.

Structure

Are the physical facilities and organizational design adequate for the service? The physical facilities and support equipment are only part of the structural dimension, however. Qualifications of the personnel and the organizational design also are important quality dimensions. For example, the quality of medical care in a group practice can be enhanced by an on-site laboratory and x-ray facilities. More important, the organization may facilitate consultations among the participating physicians. A group medical practice also provides the opportunity for peer pressure to control the quality of care that its members provide.

Adequacy of the physical facilities and equipment can be determined by comparison with set standards for quality conformance. One well-known fast-food restaurant is recognized for its attention to cleanliness. Store managers are subjected to surprise inspections in which they are held responsible for the appearance of the parking lot, sidewalk, and restaurant interior. Personnel quali-

TABLE 10.2. Quality-Control Check Sheet for an Emergency Room

Head Injuries

Date of visit: ______ MRN: ______
Nurse: ______ Physician: ______
Nurse reviewer initials: ______ Physician reviewer initials: ______

Nursing criteria	Yes	No	N/A
1. Are the patient's vital signs assessed on arrival?	☐	☐	☐
2. Does the triage note include time and mechanism of injury?	☐	☐	☐
3. Does the triage note include history of loss of consciousness and presence/absence of associated symptoms (nausea/vomiting/focal neurologic complaints)?	☐	☐	☐
4. Does the triage note include a brief neurologic assessment (Glasgow scale)?	☐	☐	☐
5. Does the triage list patient's current medications, including time of last dose recorded?	☐	☐	☐
6. Does triage note include past medical history?	☐	☐	☐
7. Is the patient's cervical spine immobilized?	☐	☐	☐
8. If history of LOC > 5 minutes or neurologic findings are present, is supplemental O_2 applied, cardiac monitor applied, i.v. line established, and physician notified immediately?	☐	☐	☐
9. Is the patient's mental status reassessed every 30 minutes?	☐	☐	☐
10. Are the discharge instructions reviewed with the patient and other responsible adult?	☐	☐	☐
Physician assessment criteria			
1. Is the chief complaint including time, mechanism of injury, and loss of consciousness recorded?	☐	☐	☐
2. Does the note include presence/absence of other injuries?	☐	☐	☐
3. Is a HEENT exam noting: scalp lacerations or contusions, pupil size and reactivity, tympanic membranes, and neck exam recorded?	☐	☐	☐
4. Is Chest, Lung, Heart, and Abdominal exam recorded?	☐	☐	☐
5. Is a Neurologic exam including: Glasgow scale, motor and sensory examination, and gait recorded?	☐	☐	☐
Physician action criteria			
1. Is a CAT scan obtained if there is a history of LOC or neurologic findings?	☐	☐	☐
2. Is a CAT scan obtained if there is a history of blood clotting disorder, thrombocytopenia, lethargy, or patient taking coumadin?	☐	☐	☐
3. Are x-rays of the c-spine obtained?	☐	☐	☐
4. If the patient is discharged, is the mental status at the time of discharge recorded?	☐	☐	☐
5. Are discharge instructions including indications for return to the ED, aftercare plan, and referral for follow-up care given to patient and other responsible adult?	☐	☐	☐
Patient outcome criteria			
1. Does the patient and responsible adult verbalize understanding of signs and symptoms indicating need to return?	☐	☐	☐
2. If the CAT scan reveals emergent intracranial hematoma, is surgical intervention initiated within 2 hours?	☐	☐	☐
3. Did the patient require second visit due to missed diagnosis?	☐	☐	☐

fications for hiring, promotion, and merit increases also are matters of meeting standards. University professors seldom are granted tenure unless they have published, because the ability to publish in a refereed journal is considered to be independent evidence of research quality. A measure of organizational effectiveness in controlling quality would be the presence of active self-evaluation procedures and members' knowledge of their peers' performances.

Outcome

What change in status has the service effected? The ultimate measure of service quality is a study of the end result. Is the consumer satisfied? We are all familiar with the cards on restaurant tables that request our comments on the quality of service. Complaints by consumers are one of the most effective measures of the quality outcome dimension. For public services, the assumption often is made that the status quo is acceptable unless the level of complaints begins to rise. The concept of monitoring output quality by tracking some measure (e.g., the number of complaints) is widely used. For example, the performance of a hospital is monitored by comparing certain measures against industry norms. The infection rate per 1000 surgeries might be used to identify hospitals that may be using substandard operating room procedures.

Clever approaches to measuring outcome quality often are employed. For example, the quality of trash pick-up in a city can be documented by taking pictures of the city streets after the trash vehicles have made their rounds. One often-forgotten measure of outcome quality is the satisfaction of empowered service personnel with their own performance.

Impact

What is the long-range effect of the service on the consumer? Are the citizens of a community able to walk the streets at night with a sense of security? The result of a poll asking that question would be a measure of the impact of police performance. The overall impact of health care often is measured by life expectancy or the infant mortality rate, and the impact of education often is measured by literacy rates and performance on nationally standardized tests.

It should be noted, however, that the impact also must include a measure of service and accessibility, which usually is quoted as the population served per unit area. Health care in the United States is criticized for the financial barriers to patient accessibility in general but especially in rural and large inner-city areas. As a result, this country's impact measures of life expectancy and infant mortality are far worse than those in all other industrial countries and even several Third World countries. In a similar fashion, the literacy rate is a measure of the impact of the education system, and again, the United States lags behind many other nations. Health care and education are perhaps the two most essential services in the United States today. Clearly, they are in great need of managers who can devise and implement excellent and innovative service operations strategies.

A commercial example of an impact measurement is the number of hamburgers sold, which once was displayed in neon lights by McDonald's. In addition, a bank's lending rate for minorities could be a measure of that institution's economic impact on a community.

TABLE 10.3. Measuring Service Quality for a Health Clinic

Quality Perspective	Description	Possible Measures
Content	Evaluation of medical practice	Review medical records for conformance with national standards of medical care.
Process	The sequence of events in the delivery of care and the interactions between patients and medical staff	Use checklists to monitor conformance with procedures. Conduct exit interviews with patients.
Structure	The physical facilities, equipment, staffing patterns, and qualifications of health personnel	Record times patients wait to see a doctor. Note ratio of doctors to registered nurses on duty. Record utilization of equipment.
Outcome	The change in the patient's health status as a result of care	Record deaths as a measure of failures. Note the level of patient dissatisfaction by recording the number of complaints. Record the number of diseased organs removed in surgery.
Impact	Appropriateness, availability, accessibility, and overall effect on the community of the health clinic	Note number of patients turned away because of lack of insurance or financial resources. Record the mode of travel and distance patients travel to reach the clinic.

Table 10.3 illustrates how this service quality perspective can be applied to measuring the quality of service delivered by a health clinic.

QUALITY SERVICE BY DESIGN

Quality can neither be inspected into a product nor somehow added on, and this same observation applies to services. A concern for quality begins with the design of the service delivery system. How can quality be designed into a service? One approach is to focus on the four dimensions of the service package that we explored in Chapter 2, The Nature of Services.

Incorporation of Quality in the Service Package

Consider the example of a budget hotel competing on overall cost leadership:

1. *Supporting facility.* Architecturally, the building is designed to be constructed of materials that are maintenance-free, such as concrete blocks. The grounds are watered by an automated underground sprinkler system. The air-conditioning and heating system is decentralized by using individual room units to confine any failure to just one room.

2. *Facilitating goods.* Room furnishings are durable and easy to clean (e.g., bedside tables are supported from the wall to facilitate carpet cleaning). Disposable plastic cups are used instead of glass, which is more expensive, requires cleaning, and, thus, would detract from the budget image.
3. *Explicit services.* Maids are trained to clean and make up rooms in a standard manner. Every room has the same appearance, including such "trivial" matters as the opening of the drapes.
4. *Implicit services.* Individuals with a pleasant appearance and good interpersonal skills are recruited as desk clerks. Training in standard operating procedures (SOPs) ensures uniform and predictable treatment for all guests. An on-line computer tracks guest billing, reservations, and registration processing. This system allows guests to check out quickly and automatically notifies the cleaning staff when a room is free to be made up.

Table 10.4 illustrates how the budget hotel has taken these design features and implemented a quality system to maintain conformance to the design requirements. The approach is based on Philip Crosby's definition of quality as

TABLE 10.4. Quality Requirements for Budget Hotel

Service Package Feature	Attribute or Requirement	Measurement	Nonconformance Corrective Action
Supporting facility	Appearance of building	No flaking paint	Repaint
	Grounds	Green grass	Water grass
	Air-conditioning and heating	Temperature maintained at 68° ± 2°	Repair or replace
Facilitating goods	TV operation	Reception clear in daylight	Repair or replace
	Soap supply	Two bars per bed	Restock
	Ice	One full bucket per room	Restock from ice machine
Explicit services	Room cleanliness	Stain-free carpet	Shampoo
	Swimming-pool water purity	Marker at bottom of deep end visible	Change filter and check chemicals
	Room appearance	Drapes drawn to width of 3 ft	Instruct maid
Implicit services	Security	All perimeter lights working	Replace defective bulbs
	Pleasant atmosphere	Telling departing guests "Have a nice day"	Instruct desk clerk
	Waiting room	No customer having to wait for a room	Review room cleaning schedule

"conformance to requirements."[5] This example illustrates the need to define explicitly, in measurable terms, what constitutes conformance to requirements. Quality is seen as an action-oriented activity requiring corrective measures when nonconformance occurs.

Taguchi Methods

The example above illustrates the application of *Taguchi methods,* which are named after Genichi Taguchi, who advocated "robust design" of products to ensure their proper functioning under adverse conditions.[6] The idea is that for a customer, proof of a product's quality is in its performance when abused. For example, a telephone is designed to be far more durable than necessary, because more than once it will be pulled off a desk and dropped on the floor. In our budget hotel example, the building is constructed of concrete blocks and furnished with durable furniture.

Taguchi also applied the concept of robustness to the manufacturing process. For example, the recipe for caramel candy was reformulated to make plasticity, or chewiness, less sensitive to the cooking temperature. Similarly, our budget hotel uses an on-line computer to notify the cleaning staff automatically when a room has been vacated. Keeping the maids posted on which rooms are available for cleaning allows this task to be spread throughout the day, thus avoiding a rush in the late afternoon that could result in quality degradation.

Taguchi believed that product quality was achieved by consistently meeting design specifications. He measured the cost of poor quality by the square of the deviation from the target, as shown in Figure 10.4. Once again, note the attention to standard operating procedures (SOPs) used by the budget hotel to promote uniform treatment of guests and consistent preparation of the rooms.

[5]Philip B. Crosby, *Quality Is Free: The Art of Making Quality Certain,* McGraw-Hill Book Company, New York, 1979.
[6]G. Taguchi and D. Clausing, "Robust Quality," *Harvard Business Review,* January–February 1990, pp. 65–75.

FIGURE 10.4. Taguchi quality loss function.

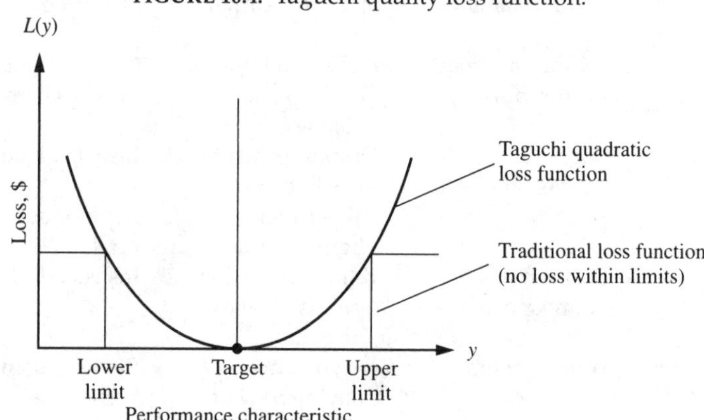

Poka-yoke

Shigeo Shingo believed that low-cost, in-process quality-control mechanisms and routines used by employees in their work could achieve high quality without costly inspection. He observed that errors occurred not because employees were incompetent, but because of lapses in attention or the worker being interrupted. He advocated the adoption of *poka-yoke* methods, which can be translated roughly as "foolproof" devices. The poka-yoke methods use checklists or manual devices that do not let the employee make a mistake.[7]

For example, recall McDonald's use of the french fry scoop, which measures out a consistent serving of potatoes. This poka-yoke device also enhances cleanliness and, hence, the aesthetic quality of the service as well. The emergency room checksheet in Table 10.2 is another poka-yoke device that reminds workers of steps often forgotten in hurrying to satisfy patients in a timely manner. Limiting employee discretion by physical design or the institution of SOPs is an important strategy in service quality control. Because it is difficult for management to intervene in the service process and impose a quality-appraisal system (i.e., inspection and testing), limiting discretion and incorporating poka-yoke methods facilitate mistake-free service. It is interesting to note how these unobtrusive design features channel service behavior without the slightest hint of coercion—as many of us experience when we hear a "beep" from Microsoft Word for Windows to warn us that an invalid keystroke has been made.

Quality Function Deployment

To provide customer input at the product design stage, a process called *quality function deployment* (QFD) was developed in Japan and used extensively by Toyota and its suppliers. The process results in a matrix, referred to as a "house of quality," for a particular product that relates customer attributes to engineering characteristics. The central idea of QFD is the belief that products should be designed to reflect the customers' desires and tastes; thus, the functions of marketing, design engineering, and manufacturing must be coordinated. The "house of quality" provides a framework for translating customer satisfaction into identifiable and measurable conformance specifications for product or service design.[8]

Although QFD was developed for use in product planning, its application to the design of service delivery systems is very appropriate, as shown by the following example.

Example 10.1: Quality Function Deployment for Village Volvo

Recall the Village Volvo case from Chapter 2. Village Volvo is an independent auto service garage that specializes in Volvo auto maintenance and competes with Volvo dealers for customers. Village Volvo has decided to assess its service delivery system in comparison with that of the Volvo dealer

[7]Shigeo Shingo, *Zero Quality Control: Source Inspection and the Poka-Yoke System,* Productivity Press, Stamford, Conn., 1986.

[8]J. R. Hauser and D. Clausing, "The House of Quality," *Harvard Business Review,* May–June 1988, pp. 63–73.

to determine areas for improving its competitive position. The steps in conducting the QFD project and constructing a "house of quality" follow:

1. *Establish the aim of the project.* In this case, the objective of the project is to assess Village Volvo's competitive position. QFD also could be used when a new service delivery system is being considered for the first time.
2. *Determine customer expectations.* Based on the aim of this project, identify the customer group to be satisfied and determine their expectations. For Village Volvo, the target customer group are Volvo owners with nonroutine repairs (i.e., exclude routine maintenance for this study). Customer expectations could be solicited by interviews, focus groups, or questionnaires. In this example, we will use the five dimensions of service quality to describe customer expectations. As shown in Figure 10.5, these are the *rows* of the house of quality. In a more sophisticated QFD project, customer expectations are broken down into primary, secondary, and tertiary levels of detail; for example, the primary expectation of "reliability" could be further specified with "accuracy" at the secondary level and "correct problem diagnosed" as the tertiary level of detail.
3. *Describe the elements of the service.* The *columns* of the house of quality matrix contain the service elements that management can manipulate to satisfy customer expectations. For Village Volvo, we have selected training, attitudes, capacity, information, and equipment.
4. *Note the strength of relationship between the service elements.* The *roof* of the house of quality provides an opportunity to note the strength of correlation between pairs of service elements. We have noted three levels of strength of

FIGURE 10.5. "House of quality" for Village Volvo.

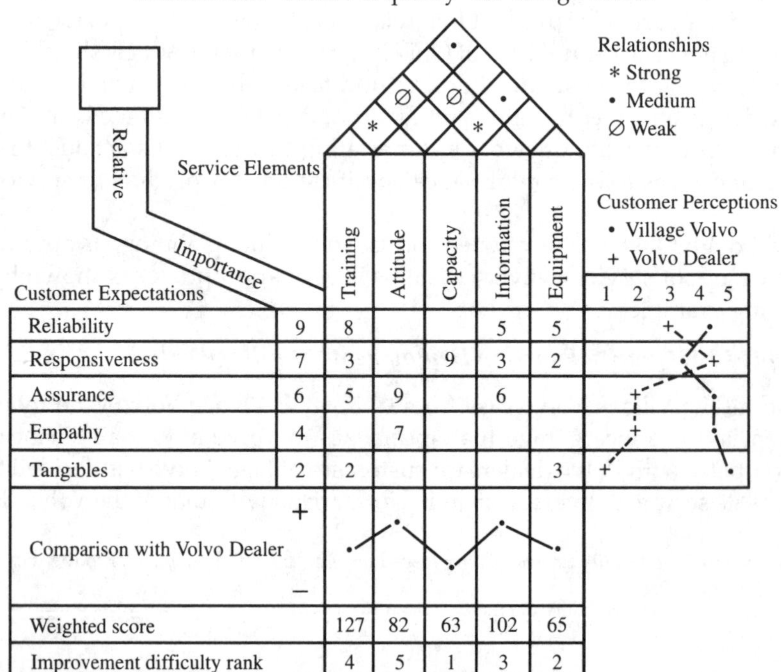

Customer Expectations	Relative Importance	Training	Attitude	Capacity	Information	Equipment
Reliability	9	8			5	5
Responsiveness	7	3		9	3	2
Assurance	6	5	9		6	
Empathy	4		7			
Tangibles	2	2				3
Weighted score		127	82	63	102	65
Improvement difficulty rank		4	5	1	3	2

relationship: ∗ = strong, • = medium, and ∅ = weak. As you might expect, we note a strong relationship between training and attitudes. Noting these relationships between elements may provide useful points of leverage to improve service quality.

5. *Note the association between customer expectations and service elements.* The *body* of the matrix contains numbers between 0 and 9 (9 indicating a very strong link) to indicate the strength of the link between a service element and a corresponding customer expectation. These numbers would follow a discussion by the project team about how various service elements affect the firm's capacity to satisfy the different customer expectations.

6. *Weighting the service elements.* This step is taken to measure the importance of a customer's assessment of the service element. The *chimney* of the house of quality contains a listing of the relative importance of each customer expectation. These weights on a scale of 1 to 9 indicate the importance that customers place on each of their expectations and could be determined by a customer survey. The relative importance will be multiplied by the strength of the link number in the body of the matrix under each service element to arrive at a weighted score for that element. For example, the training element would have a weighted score, which is calculated as:

$$(9)(8) + (7)(3) + (6)(5) + (4)(0) + (2)(2) = 127$$

The weighted scores are entered in the *basement* of the house of quality and represent a measure of each service element's importance to satisfying customer needs. These weighted results should be treated with caution and common sense, however, because they depend on uncertain estimates of relative importance and relationship scores.

7. *Service element improvement difficulty rank.* In the basement of the house is a ranking for the difficulty of improving each service element, with a rank of 1 being the most difficult. Capacity and equipment have a high rank because of their capital requirements. This exercise demonstrates that even though customers may give a service element a high rank, the firm may be unable to deliver it.

8. *Assessment of competition.* A study of the Volvo dealer is made to assess customers' perceptions of service at the dealer compared with that at Village Volvo. The result of a customer survey (using customers who have experienced both providers) using a five-point scale is plotted to the *right* of the matrix. Based on knowledge of the dealer (perhaps from mechanics), a relative comparison of the level (plus or minus) of each service element is plotted at the *bottom* of the matrix. This information will be used to assess the competitive strengths and weaknesses of Village Volvo.

9. *Strategic assessment and goal setting.* Looking at the completed house of quality, Village Volvo can see some strengths and weaknesses in its strategic position relative to the Volvo dealer. Except for responsiveness, it is viewed favorably by its customers. This result must be viewed with caution, however, because these data were obtained from a survey of Village Volvo customers and, thus, were not unexpected. The comparison of service elements with the Volvo dealer and weighted scores yields some possible directions for im-

provement in service. In the area of attitudes and information, Village Volvo is in a superior position, but there appears to be a problem with capacity, training, and equipment. The high-weighted score given to training suggests that a first-priority goal of an investment in training might be in order. In addition, leverage would be achieved, because training has relationships, from strong to weak, with attitudes, capacity, and equipment. Finally, the improvement difficulty rank for training is fourth out of five.

ACHIEVING SERVICE QUALITY

Services are difficult for customers to evaluate before the fact. As we have already noted, they are intangible and consumed simultaneously with production. This presents a challenge to the service manager, because quality-inspection intervention between the customer and the contact employee is not an option as in manufacturing (e.g., no slip of paper can be placed in the box by Inspector Number 12).

Cost of Quality

Caveat emptor—"let the buyer beware"—has become obsolete. As American businesses discovered in the late 1980s and early 1990s, impersonal service, faulty products, and broken promises all carry a price. A very visible example of this reality today is the prominent part that liability concerns and insurance play in almost every service imaginable. Poor quality can lead to bankruptcy. A gourmet soup company, for example, was forced out of business when its vichyssoise was found to contain poison-producing botulism organisms. Announcements of automobile recalls for correcting defects are commonplace as well.

Products can be returned, exchanged, or fixed, but what recourse does the customer of a faulty service have? Legal recourse! Medical malpractice lawsuits have been notorious for their large settlements, and although some cases of abuse by the legal system surely have occurred, the possibility of malpractice litigation does promote a physician's sense of responsibility to the patient. The threat of a negligence suit might induce a responsible doctor to take more time in an examination, seek more training, or avoid performing a procedure for which he or she is not competent. Unfortunately, as evidenced by the frequent claims of physicians that extra testing is necessary to defend against potential malpractice claims, the cost of care may increase without any improvement in quality.

No service has immunity from prosecution. For example, a Las Vegas hotel was sued for failing to provide proper security when a guest was assaulted in her room. An income tax preparer can be fined up to $500 per return if a taxpayer's liability is understated because of the preparer's negligence or disregard of Internal Revenue Service rules and regulations.

A noted quality expert, Joseph M. Juran, has advocated a cost-of-quality accounting system to convince top management of the need to address quality issues.[9] He identified four categories of costs: internal failure costs (from defects

[9]J. M. Juran and F. M. Gryna, Jr., *Quality Planning and Analysis,* McGraw-Hill Book Company, New York, 1980.

discovered before shipment), external failure costs (from defects discovered after shipment), detection costs (for inspection of purchased materials and during manufacture), and prevention costs (for keeping defects from occurring in the first place). Juran found that in most manufacturing companies, external and internal failure costs together accounted for 50 to 80 percent of the total cost of quality. Thus, to minimize this total cost, he advocated that more attention be paid to prevention. Suggestions have been made that $1 invested in prevention is worth $100 in detection costs and $10,000 in failure costs.

In Table 10.5, we have adapted Juran's cost-of-quality system for use by service firms with a banking example. In the prevention row, recruitment and selection of service personnel are viewed as ways to avoid poor quality. Identifying people with appropriate attitudes and interpersonal skills can result in hiring contact persons with the natural instincts that are needed to serve customers well.

Inspection is included in the detection row, but it generally is impractical except in the back-office operations of a service.

Because service is an experience for the customer, any failure becomes a story for that customer to tell others. Service managers must recognize that dissatisfied customers not only will take their future business elsewhere but also tell others about the unhappy experience, thus resulting in a significant loss of future business.

TABLE 10.5. Costs of Quality for Services

Cost Category	Definition	Bank Example
Prevention	Costs associated with operations or activities that keep failure from happening and minimize detection costs	Quality planning Recruitment and selection Training programs Quality improvement projects
Detection	Costs incurred to ascertain the condition of a service to determine whether it conforms to quality standards	Periodic inspection Process control Checking, balancing, verifying Collecting quality data
Internal failure	Costs incurred to correct nonconforming work before delivery to the customer	Scrapped forms and reports Rework Machine downtime
External failure	Costs incurred to correct nonconforming work after delivery to the customer or to correct work that did not satisfy a customer's specified needs.	Payment of interest penalties Investigation time Legal judgments Negative word-of-mouth Loss of future business

Source: Adapted from C. A. Aubry and D. A. Zimbler, "The Banking Industry: Quality Costs and Improvement," *Quality Progress*, December 1983, pp. 16–20.

Tools for Achieving Service Quality

Service Process Control

The control of service quality can be viewed as a feedback control system. In a feedback system, output is compared with a standard. The deviation from that standard is communicated back to the input, and adjustments then are made to keep the output within a tolerable range. A thermostat in a home provides a common example of feedback control. Room temperature is monitored continually; when the temperature drops below some preset value, the furnace is activated and will continue to operate until the correct temperature is restored.

Figure 10.6 shows the basic control cycle as applied to service process control. The service concept establishes a basis for setting goals and defining measures of system performance. Output measures are taken and monitored for conformance to requirements. Nonconformance to requirements is studied to identify its causes and determine corrective action.

Unfortunately, it is difficult to implement an effective control cycle for service systems. Problems begin with the definition of service performance measures. The intangible nature of services makes direct measurement difficult, but it is not impossible. Many surrogate measures of service quality exist. For example, the waiting time of customers might be used. In some public services, the number of complaints that are received is used.

Monitoring service performance is frustrated by the simultaneous nature of production and consumption. This close interface between customer and provider prevents any direct intervention in the service process to observe conformance to requirements. Consequently, consumers may be asked to express their impression of service quality "after the fact" by filling out questionnaires. Monitoring only the final customer impressions of service quality, however, may be too late to avoid the loss of future sales. These difficulties in controlling service quality may be addressed by focusing on the delivery process itself and by employing a technique borrowed from manufacturing called *statistical process control.*

FIGURE 10.6. Service process control.

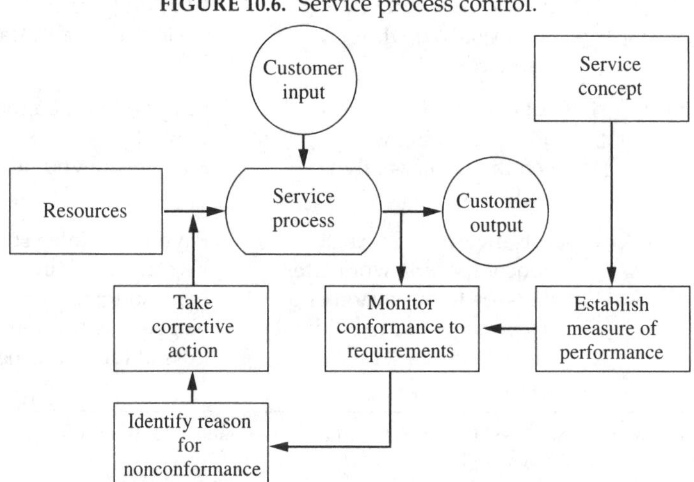

The performance of a service often is judged by key indicators. For example, the educational performance of a high school is measured by the Scholastic Aptitude Test (SAT) scores of its students. The effectiveness of a police department's crime-prevention program is judged by the crime rate, and a bank teller's performance is judged by the accuracy of his or her end-of-day balances.

What happens if the service process is not performing as expected? Generally, an investigation is conducted to identify the cause of the problem and to suggest corrective action; however, performance variations may result from random occurrences and not have a specific cause. The decision maker wants to detect true degradation in service performance and avoid the failure costs that are associated with poor service. On the other hand, making an unnecessary change in a system that is performing correctly should be avoided. Thus, two types of risks are involved in controlling quality, as shown in Table 10.6. These risks have been given names to identify the injured party. If a process is deemed to be out of control when it in fact is performing correctly, a Type I error has occurred, which is the producer's risk. If a process is deemed to be functioning properly when it in fact is out of control, a Type II error has occurred, which is the consumer's risk.

A visual display called a *control chart* is used to plot values of a measure of process performance (e.g., the time a directory assistance operator spends with a caller) to determine if the process is in control (e.g., the time is less than 30 seconds in the operator example). For example, Figure 10.7 shows a control chart that is used to monitor emergency ambulance response time. This chart is a daily plot of mean response time that permits monitoring performance for unusual deviations from the norm. When a measurement falls outside the control limits—

TABLE 10.6. Risks in Quality-Control Decisions

	Quality-Control Decision	
True State of Service	Take Corrective Action	Do Nothing
Process in control	Type I error (producer's risk)	Correct decision
Process out of control	Correct decision	Type II error (consumer's risk)

FIGURE 10.7. $\bar{X}$-chart for ambulance response.

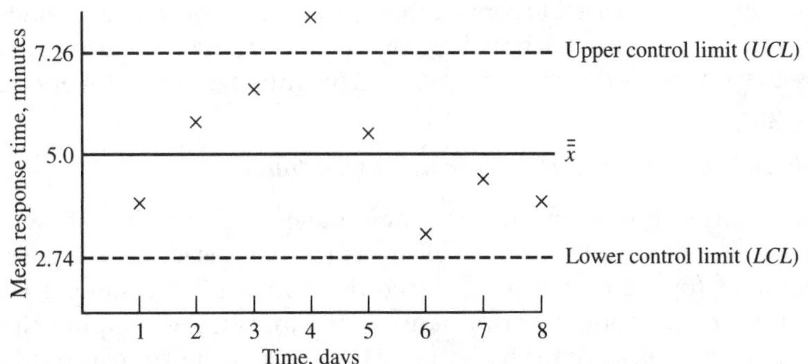

that is, above the upper control limit (UCL) or below the lower control limit (LCL)—the process is considered to be out of control; consequently, the system is in need of attention. For our ambulance example, day 4 signaled a need for investigation by the supervisor. An excessive mean response time for that day occurred because a nearby ambulance was out of commission and our vehicle needed to travel longer distances. Since day 4, ambulance performance has remained within the control limits, so no action is required.

Constructing a control chart is similar to determining a confidence interval for the mean of a sample. Recall from statistics that sample means tend to be distributed normally according to the central-limit theorem (i.e., although the underlying statistic may be distributed in any manner, mean values drawn from this statistic have a normal distribution). We know from standard normal tables that 99.7 percent of the normal distribution falls within 3 standard deviations of the mean. Using representative historical data, both the mean and standard deviation for some system performance measure are determined. These parameters then are used to construct a 99.7-percent confidence interval for the mean of the performance measure. We expect future sample means that are collected at random to fall within this confidence interval; if they do not, then we conclude that the process has changed and the true mean has shifted.

The steps in constructing and using a quality-control chart can be summarized as:

I. Decide on some measure of service system performance.
II. Collect representative historical data from which estimates of the population mean and variance for the system performance measure can be made.
III. Decide on a sample size, and using the estimates of population mean and variance, calculate (by convention) ± 3 standard deviation control limits.
IV. Graph the control chart as a function of sample mean values versus time.
V. Plot sample means collected at random on the chart, and interpret the results as follows:
    A. Process in control (i.e., sample mean falls within control limits).
    B. Process out of control (i.e., sample mean falls outside control limits, or a run of seven means falling either above or below the average). In this case:
        1. Evaluate the situation.
        2. Take corrective action.
        3. Check results of action.
VI. Update the control chart on a periodic basis, and incorporate recent data.

Control charts for means fall into two categories based on the type of performance measure. A variable control chart ($\bar{X}$-chart) records measurements that permit fractional values, such as length, weight, or time. An attribute control chart (*p*-chart) records discrete data, such as the number of defects or errors as a percentage.

Example 10.2: Control Chart for Variables ($\bar{X}$-Chart)

The quality-control chart for mean ambulance response time shown in Figure 10.7 is an example of a variable measure. It is based on taking a random sample of four ambulance calls each day to calculate a sample mean response time to monitor performance. The range of the sample values (i.e., the difference between the highest and the lowest value) will be used instead of the standard deviation to calculate the control limits. Assume that past records of ambulance system performance yield an estimated population mean response time of 5.0 minutes, with an estimated average range of 3.1 minutes. Appropriate formulas for calculating the control limits for an $\bar{X}$-chart using the range $\bar{R}$ as a substitute for the standard error of the mean are:

$$UCL = \bar{\bar{X}} + A_2\bar{R} \qquad (1)$$

$$LCL = \bar{\bar{X}} - A_2\bar{R} \qquad (2)$$

where $\bar{\bar{X}}$ = estimate of population mean,
$\bar{R}$ = estimate of population range, and
A_2 = value from Table 10.7 for sample size n.

For the ambulance response time control chart shown in Figure 10.7, the control limits for a sample size of four are calculated as follows:

$$UCL = \bar{\bar{X}} + A_2\bar{R} = 5.0 + (.729)(3.1) = 7.26$$

$$LCL = \bar{\bar{X}} - A_2\bar{R} = 5.0 - (.729)(3.1) = 2.74$$

We also could monitor the variance of the ambulance response times using the range (i.e., largest value minus the smallest value in the sample) as a measure of variance. A range or $\bar{R}$-chart can be constructed in a manner similar to the $\bar{X}$-chart by using the following formulas:

TABLE 10.7. Variable Control Chart Constants

		R-chart	
Sample Size (n)	$\bar{X}$-chart A_2	D_3	D_4
2	1.880	0	3.267
3	1.023	0	2.574
4	.729	0	2.282
5	.577	0	2.114
6	.483	0	2.004
7	.419	.076	1.924
8	.373	.136	1.864
9	.337	.184	1.816
10	.308	932	1.777
12	.266	.283	1.717
14	.235	.328	1.672
16	.212	.363	1.637
18	.194	.391	1.608
20	.180	.415	1.585
22	.167	.434	1.566
24	.157	.451	1.548

Source: Adapted from Table 27 of *ASTM Manual on Presentation of Data and Control Chart Analysis*, copyright 1976 American Society for Testing and Materials, Philadelphia.

$$UCL = D_4\overline{R} \tag{3}$$

$$LCL = D_3\overline{R} \tag{4}$$

where $\overline{R}$ = estimate of population range,
D_4 = UCL value from Table 10.7 for sample size n, and
D_3 = LCL value from Table 10.7 for sample size n.

For our ambulance case, the range control limits are calculated using the constants in Table 10.7 for a sample size of four:

$$UCL = D_4\overline{R} = (2.282)(3.1) = 7.1$$

$$LCL = D_3\overline{R} = (0)(3.1) = 0$$

Example 10.3: Control Chart for Attributes (p-Chart)

In some cases, system performance is classified as either "good" or "bad." Of primary concern is the percentage of bad performance. For example, consider the operator of a mechanized sorting machine in a post office. The operator must read the ZIP code on a parcel and, knowing its location in the city, divert the package by conveyor to the proper route truck. From past records, the error rate for skilled operators is about 5 percent, or a fraction defective of 0.05. Management wants to develop a control chart to monitor new operators to ensure that personnel who are unsuited for the job can be identified. Equations (5) and (6) below are used to construct a percentage or p-chart. These formulas should be familiar, because they represent the ± 3 standard deviation confidence interval for a percentage.

$$UCL = \overline{p} + 3\sqrt{\frac{\overline{p}(1-\overline{p})}{n}} \tag{5}$$

$$LCL = \overline{p} - 3\sqrt{\frac{\overline{p}(1-\overline{p})}{n}} \tag{6}$$

where $\sqrt{\frac{\overline{p}(1-\overline{p})}{n}}$ = standard error of percentage,
$\overline{p}$ = estimate of population percentage, and
n = sample size.

The p-chart control limits for the sorting operation are calculated using equations (5) and (6) and random samples of 100 parcels drawn from the route trucks. Note that if the calculation of an LCL results in a negative number, then LCL is set equal to zero.

$$UCL = 0.05 + 3\sqrt{\frac{(0.05)(0.95)}{100}} = 0.05 + 3(0.0218) = 0.1154 \approx 0.11$$

$$LCL = 0.05 - 3\sqrt{\frac{(0.05)(0.95)}{100}} = 0.05 - 3(0.0218) = -0.0154\ [\text{set} = 0.0]$$

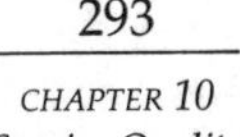

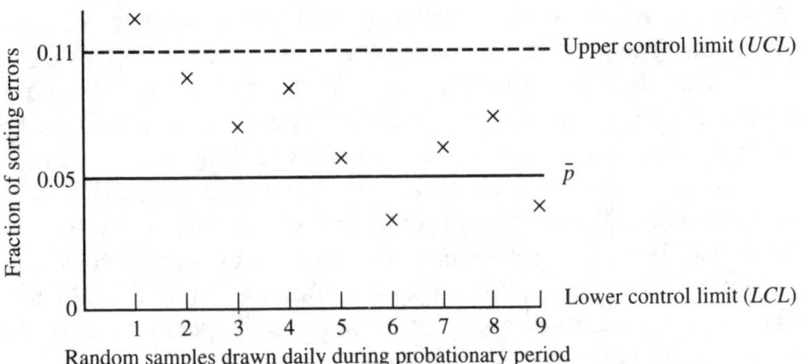

FIGURE 10.8. *p*-Chart for ZIP code sorting operator.

The *p*-chart for this operation is shown in Figure 10.8. Given this 9-day probationary experience for the new employee, would you conclude that the person is suitable for the sorting position?

Statistical Process Control at Midway Airlines[10]

Midway Airlines was once a successful regional carrier, with a major hub at the Midway Airport in Chicago and service to other midwestern and northeastern cities. Midway was unable to compete with the major carriers and eventually filed for bankruptcy, but this was not for lack of attention to quality. It used the hub-and-spoke network that requires on-time departures to avoid delays, which would compromise the efficient transfer of passengers during their multileg journeys. Figure 10.9 shows a *p*-chart used by Midway's employees to monitor this important measure of schedule performance. It is interesting to note that just the effort of tracking the percentage of on-time departures resulted in marked

[10]Adapted from D. Daryl Wyckoff, "New Tools for Achieving Service Quality," *The Cornell HRA Quarterly,* November 1984, pp. 78–91.

FIGURE 10.9. Control chart of Midway Airlines departure delays.
(D. Daryl Wyckoff, "New Tools for Achieving Service Quality," The Cornell HRA Quarterly, *November 1984, p. 87. © Cornell HRA Quarterly. Used by permission. All rights reserved.)*

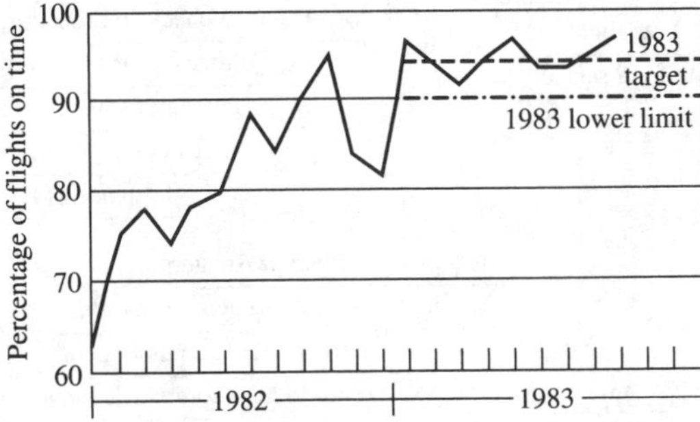

improvement during the early months of 1982. In November and December, however, the on-time performance was severely eroded.

Additional study was deemed necessary to determine the underlying causes of late departures. Midway turned to a cause-and-effect tool called *fishbone analysis,* or an Ishikawa chart, which was so-named after its originator. Figure 10.10 shows a fishbone analysis that identifies possible causes of flight departure delays. The analysis begins with the problem at the head and traces the major categories of causes back along the spine. The usual causes are labeled under the broad categories of Personnel, Procedure, Equipment, Material, and Other. From personal experience, Midway's employees suggested specific causes of late departures, which are noted below each broad category.

The fishbone chart now can be used to eliminate the causes of delayed departure through a process of discussion and consensus; the remaining possibilities are targeted for additional data gathering. Data were collected on possible causes of departure delay as noted in Table 10.8, and Midway used a technique

FIGURE 10.10 Portion of Midway Airlines fishbone analysis: causes of flight departure delays.
(D. Daryl Wyckoff, "New Tools for Achieving Service Quality," The Cornell HRA Quarterly, *November 1984, p. 89. © Cornell HRA Quarterly. Used by permission. All rights reserved.)*

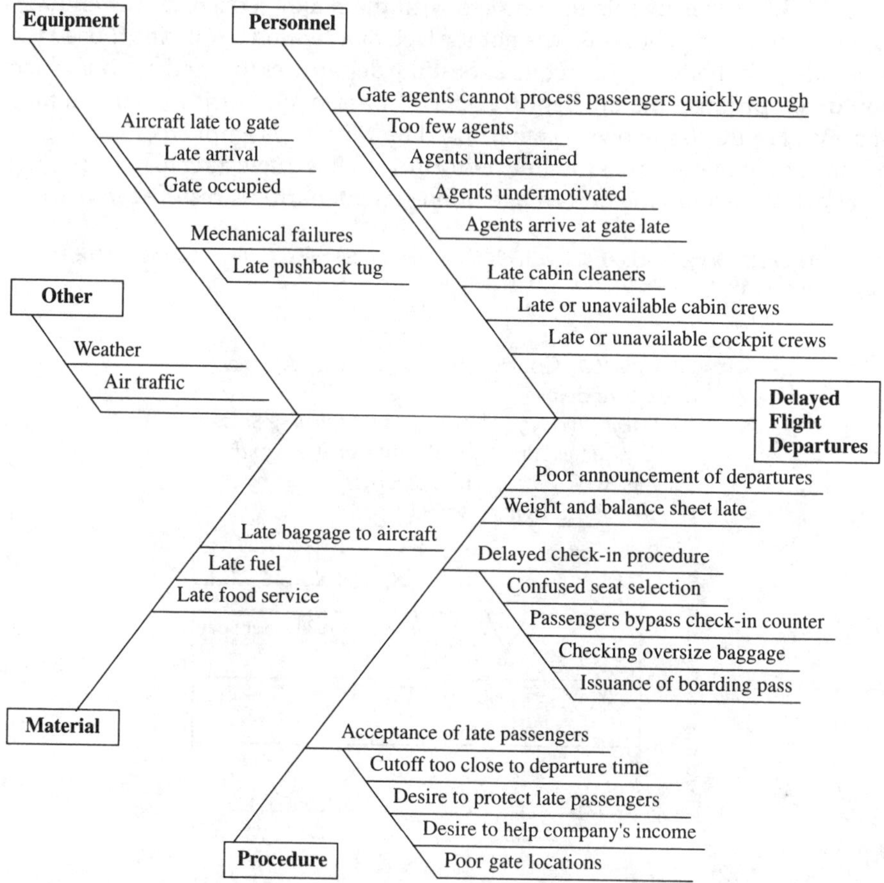

TABLE 10.8 Pareto Analysis of Flight Departure Delays

All Stations, Except Hub			*Newark*			*Washington (National)*		
	Percentage of Incidences	Cumulative Percentage		Percentage of Incidences	Cumulative Percentage		Percentage of Incidences	Cumulative Percentage
Late passengers	53.3	53.3	Late passengers	23.1	23.1	Late passengers	33.3	33.3
Waiting for pushback	15.0	68.3	Waiting for fueling	23.1	46.2	Waiting for pushback	33.3	66.6
Waiting for fueling	11.3	79.6	Waiting for pushback	23.1	69.3	Late weight and balance sheet	19.0	85.6
Late weight and balance sheet	8.7	88.3	Cabin cleaning and supplies	15.4	84.7	Waiting for fueling	9.5	95.1

Source: D. Daryl Wyckoff, "New Tools for Achieving Service Quality," *The Cornell HRA Quarterly*, November 1984, p. 89.

called *Pareto analysis* that arranges data so that causes of a problem are ordered in descending frequency of occurrence. Pareto, a nineteenth-century Italian economist, observed that 80 percent of the country's wealth resided with 20 percent of its citizens. This principle, known as the *80/20 rule,* has been observed in many situations. For example, 80 percent of a retailer's sales are generated by 20 percent of the customers. Applying this rule to Midway, 80 percent of the departure delays should be accounted for by 20 percent of the causes. As seen in Table 10.8, approximately 90 percent of departure delays were explained by four causes.

Acceptance of late passengers proved to be the number-one cause of departure delays. Because gate agents were anxious to avoid losing the fares of latecomers, they delayed flight departures and, thus, inconvenienced punctual passengers. Midway established a policy of on-time departure, and soon thereafter, the number of late arrivals declined. Other causes of delays (e.g., waiting for "pushback" and a cabin-cleaning problem at Newark) then were addressed.

In January 1983, once the flight departure process was under control, the company set an on-time departure target of 95 percent and a lower control limit of 90 percent. The experience of Midway illustrates the reason why statistical process control is successful in improving service quality. The collection, recording, and analysis of data are accomplished by employees, who view the activity as an opportunity for self-improvement and learning.

PROGRAMS FOR SERVICE QUALITY IMPROVEMENT

Service quality begins with people. All our measurements to detect nonconformance by means of statistically based control charts do not produce a quality service; instead, quality begins with the development of positive attitudes among all people in the organization. How is this accomplished? Positive attitudes can be fostered through a coordinated program that begins with employee selection and progresses through training, initial job assignments, and other aspects of career advancements. To avoid complacency, an ongoing quality-improvement program is required. These programs emphasize preventing poor quality, taking personal responsibility for quality, and building an attitude that quality can be made certain.

Personnel Programs for Quality Assurance

Multisite service firms face special problems of maintaining consistent service across all units. For example, customers expect the same service from a hotel unit in Chicago that they found previously in a New Orleans unit of the same chain. In fact, the idea of "finding no surprises" is used as a marketing feature.

G. M. Hostage[11] believes the success of Marriott Corporation results in part from personnel programs that stress training, standards of performance, career

[11]G. M. Hostage, "Quality Control in a Service Business," *Harvard Business Review,* vol. 53, no. 4, July–August 1975, pp. 98–106.

development, and rewards. He finds that service quality is enhanced by the attitude a company takes toward its employees. The following eight programs have been the most effective:

1. *Individual development.* Using programmed instruction manuals, new management trainees acquire the skills and technical knowledge that are needed for the entry-level position of assistant manager. For a geographically dispersed organization, these manuals ensure that job skills are taught in a consistent manner.
2. *Management training.* Management personnel through the middle levels attend one management development session each year. A variety of professional management topics are addressed in 2- and 3-day seminars that are attended by lower-level managers from various operating divisions.
3. *Human resources planning.* The kinds of people who will be needed to fill key company positions in the coming years are identified, and an inventory of good prospects is created for future promotion. A key element of the plan is periodic performance review of all management personnel.
4. *Standards of performance.* A set of booklets was developed to instruct employees in how to conduct themselves when dealing with guests and, in some cases, even in how to speak. The *Marriott Bellman* stresses how to make a guest feel welcome and special. The *Switchboard Operator* tells in detail how to speak with a guest and handle a variety of specific situations. The *Housekeeper* tells precisely how a room is to be made up, right down to the detail of placing the wrapped soap bar on the proper corner of the washbasin with the label upright. In many cases, booklets are accompanied by an audiovisual film or a videotape to demonstrate proper procedures. Adherence to these standards is checked by random visits from a flying squad of inspectors.
5. *Career progression.* A job-advancement program with a ladder of positions of increasing skill and responsibility gives employees the opportunity to grow with the company.
6. *Opinion surveys.* An annual rank-and-file opinion survey is conducted by trained personnel at each unit. Subsequently, the results are discussed at a meeting. This survey has acted as an early warning system to head off the build-up of unfavorable attitudes.
7. *Fair treatment.* Employees are provided with a handbook of company expectations and obligations to its personnel. The formal grievance procedure includes access to an ombudsperson to help resolve difficulties.
8. *Profit sharing.* A profit-sharing plan recognizes that employees are responsible for much of the company's success and that they deserve more than just a paycheck for their efforts.

Quality-Improvement Program to Achieve Zero Defects

Philip Crosby, a former vice president for quality at ITT and now a sought-after quality-management consultant, advocates a 14-step zero-defects quality-improvement program.[12] His program has been implemented at a number of service firms, such as the Paul Revere Insurance Company, and has the following 14 sequential steps:

1. *Management commitment.* The need for quality improvement first is discussed with members of management to gain their commitment. This raises the level of visibility and concern for quality at the highest levels, and it ensures everyone's cooperation.
2. *Quality-improvement team.* Representatives from each department are selected to form a team that runs the quality-improvement program, which ensures each department's participation.
3. *Quality measurement.* The status of quality throughout the organization is audited. This requires that quality measurements be reviewed and established where they do not exist. Once quality becomes measurable, an objective evaluation is made to identify nonconformance and to monitor corrective action. Developing quality measures for services is a difficult task, but it represents an opportunity for worker participation. Service personnel most often respond with enthusiasm and pride when asked to identify quality measures for their work.
4. *Cost-of-quality evaluation.* To avoid any bias in the calculations, the comptroller's office identifies the cost of quality, which is composed of items such as litigation, rework, engineering changes, and inspection labor. Measuring the cost of quality provides an indication of where corrective action will be profitable for an organization.
5. *Quality awareness.* The cost of poor quality is communicated to supervisors and employees through the use of booklets, films, and posters. This helps to change attitudes about quality by providing visible evidence of the concern for quality improvement.
6. *Corrective action.* A systematic process of facing problems, talking about them, and resolving them on a regular basis is needed. The habit of identifying quality problems and correcting them at the local level is encouraged.
7. *Establishment of a zero-defects program.* Three or four members of the team are selected to investigate the zero-defects concept and to implement the program. The committee should understand the literal meaning of the phrase *zero defects.* The idea that everyone should do his or her work right the first time must be communicated to all employees.
8. *Supervisor training.* A formal orientation is conducted for all levels of management to enable them to explain the program to their people.
9. *Zero-defects day.* An event is created that employees can recognize as a turning point in the organization's attitude toward quality. From this day on, zero defects will be the performance standard for the organization.
10. *Goal setting.* Employees are encouraged to think in terms of establishing improvement goals for themselves and their groups. Supervisors should help their employees to set specific and measurable goals.

[12]Philip B. Crosby, *Quality Is Free: The Art of Making Quality Certain,* McGraw-Hill Book Company, New York, 1979.

11. *Error-cause removal.* People are asked to describe on a simple, 1-page form any problem that keeps them from performing error-free work. The appropriate department is asked to respond to the problem expeditiously.
12. *Recognition.* Award programs are established to recognize those employees who meet their goals. With genuine recognition of performance, continued support for the program will result.
13. *Quality councils.* The quality professionals are brought together on a regular basis to discuss actions that are necessary to improve the program.
14. *Do it over again.* A typical program takes more than 1 year, and by then, employee turnover necessitates a new educational effort. Such repetition makes the program a permanent part of the organization.

Deming's 14-Point Program

W. Edwards Deming generally is credited with initiating the highly successful Japanese quality revolution. In Deming's view, management was responsible for 85 percent of all quality problems and, therefore, had to provide the leadership in changing the systems and processes that created them. Management needed to refocus attention on meeting customer needs and on continuous improvement to stay ahead of the competition. His philosophy is captured in a 14-point program[13]:

1. *Create constancy of purpose for improvements of product and service.* Management must stop its preoccupation solely with the next quarter and build for the future. Innovation in all areas of business should be expected.
2. *Adopt the new philosophy.* Refuse to allow commonly accepted poor levels of work, delays, and lax service.
3. *Cease dependence on mass inspection.* Inspection comes too late and is costly. Instead, focus on improving the process itself.
4. *End the practice of awarding business on price tag alone.* The purchasing department should buy on the basis of statistical evidence of quality, not on the basis of price. Reduce the number of vendors, and reward high-quality suppliers with long-term contracts.
5. *Constantly and forever improve the system of production and service.* Search continually for problems in the system, and seek ways of improvement. Waste must be reduced and quality improved in every business activity, both front-office and back-office.
6. *Institute modern methods of training on the job.* Restructure training to define acceptable levels of work. Use statistical methods to evaluate training.
7. *Institute modern methods of supervising.* Focus supervision on helping workers to do a better job. Provide the tools and techniques to promote pride in one's work.

[13]W. Edwards Deming, *Quality, Productivity, and Competitive Position,* MIT Center for Advanced Engineering Study, Cambridge, Mass., 1982.

8. *Drive out fear.* Eliminate fear by encouraging the communication of problems and expression of ideas.
9. *Break down barriers between departments.* Encourage problem solving through teamwork and use of quality-control circles.
10. *Eliminate numerical goals for the workforce.* Goals, slogans, and posters cajoling workers to increase productivity should be eliminated. Such exhortations cause worker resentment, because most of the necessary changes are outside their control.
11. *Eliminate work standards and numerical quotas.* Production quotas focus on quantity, and they guarantee poor quality in their attainment. Quality goals such as an acceptable percentage of defective items do not motivate workers toward improvement. Use statistical methods for continuing improvement of quality and productivity.
12. *Remove barriers that hinder hourly workers.* Workers need feedback on the quality of their work. All barriers to pride in one's work must be removed.
13. *Institute a vigorous program of education and training.* Because of changes in technology and turnover of personnel, all employees need continual training and retraining. All training must include basic statistical techniques.
14. *Create a structure in top management that will push every day on the above 13 points.* Clearly define management's permanent commitment to continuous improvement in both quality and productivity.

Unconditional Service Guarantee[14]

Whenever you buy a product, a warranty to guarantee its performance is expected—but to guarantee a service? Impossible! Not so, according to Christopher Hart, who writes that service guarantees exist and have five important features:

1. *Unconditional.* Customer satisfaction is unconditional, without exceptions. For example, L. L. Bean, a Maine mail-order house, accepts all returns without question and provides a replacement, refund, or credit.
2. *Easy to understand and communicate.* Customers should know precisely what to expect from a guarantee in measurable terms. For example, Bennigan's promises that if a lunch is not served within 15 minutes, the diner receives a free meal.
3. *Meaningful.* The guarantee should be important to the customer in financial as well as in service terms. Domino's Pizza guarantees that if an order is not delivered within 30 minutes, the customer gets $3 off rather than a free pizza, because its customers consider a rebate to be more desirable.
4. *Easy to invoke.* A dissatisfied customer should not be hassled with filling out forms or writing letters to invoke a guarantee. Cititravel, a service of Citibank, guarantees the lowest airfares or a refund of the difference; a toll-free call to an agent is all that is necessary to confirm a lower fare and get a refund.

[14]From Christopher W. L. Hart, "The Power of Unconditional Service Guarantees," *Harvard Business Review,* July–August 1988, pp. 54–62.

5. *Easy to collect.* The best guarantees are resolved on the spot, as illustrated by Domino's Pizza and Bennigan's.

A service guarantee has obvious marketing appeal. More important, however, the service guarantee can redefine the meaning of service for an industry by setting quality standards. For example, Federal Express defined small-parcel delivery with its overnight delivery guarantee. A service guarantee promotes organizational effectiveness in several ways:

1. *Focuses on customers.* A guarantee forces a company to identify its customers' expectations. In a survey of its passengers, British Airways found that they judged its service on four dimensions: care and concern, initiative, problem solving, and—to the airline's surprise—recovery when things go wrong.
2. *Sets clear standards.* A specific, unambiguous guarantee for the customer also sets clear standards for the organization. The Federal Express guarantee of delivery "absolutely positively by 10:30 AM" defines the responsibilities of all its employees.
3. *Guarantees feedback.* Customers invoking a guarantee provide valuable information for quality assessment. Dissatisfied customers now have an incentive to complain and to get management's attention. Manpower Inc., a temporary-worker agency, takes a proactive approach by calling the client after the first day to get feedback on customer satisfaction.
4. *Promotes an understanding of the service delivery system.* Before a guarantee is made, managers must identify the possible failure points in their system and the limits to which these can be controlled. Burger Bug Killers, Inc., a Florida exterminator, will not guarantee or accept a job unless the client adheres to recommended facility improvements such as sealing doors and windows from insect penetration. Federal Express adopted a hub-and-spoke network to ensure that all packages would be brought to Memphis in the evening for sorting and flown out that very night for delivery by 10:30 the next morning.
5. *Builds customer loyalty.* A guarantee reduces the customer's risk, makes expectations explicit, and builds market share by retaining dissatisfied customers who otherwise would leave for the competition.

Malcolm Baldrige National Quality Award

The Malcolm Baldrige National Quality Award was created by Congress on August 20, 1987. The award is named for Malcolm Baldrige, who served as Secretary of Commerce from 1981 until his death in a rodeo accident in 1987. The award is given annually to recognize U.S. companies that excel in quality achievement and management. There are three eligibility categories for the award: manufacturing companies, service companies, and small businesses.

Each company participating in the award process submits an application, which includes an Award Examination; sample examination items and point values are listed in Figure 10.11. Note the heavy emphasis on "business results" and

1996 Categories/Items		Point Values
1.0 Leadership		**90**
1.1 Senior Executive Leadership	45	
1.2 Leadership System and Organization	25	
1.3 Public Responsibility and Corporate Citizenship	20	
2.0 Information and Analysis		**75**
2.1 Management of Information and Data	20	
2.2 Competitive Comparisons and Benchmarking	15	
2.3 Analysis and Use of Company-Level Data	40	
3.0 Strategic Planning		**55**
3.1 Strategy Development	35	
3.2 Strategy Deployment	20	
4.0 Human Resources Development and Management		**140**
4.1 Human Resource Planning and Evaluation	20	
4.2 High Performance Work Systems	45	
4.3 Employee Education, Training, and Development	50	
4.4 Employee Well-Being and Satisfaction	25	
5.0 Process Management		**140**
5.1 Design and Introduction of Products and Services	40	
5.2 Process Management: Product and Service Production and Delivery	40	
5.3 Process Management: Support Services	30	
5.4 Management of Supplier Performance	30	
6.0 Business Results		**250**
6.1 Product and Service Quality Results	75	
6.2 Company Operational and Financial Results	110	
6.3 Human Resource Results	35	
6.4 Supplier Performance Results	30	
7.0 Customer Focus and Satisfaction		**250**
7.1 Customer and Market Knowledge	30	
7.2 Customer Relationship Management	30	
7.3 Customer Satisfaction Determination	30	
7.4 Customer Satisfaction Results	160	
TOTAL POINTS		1000

FIGURE 10.11. Malcolm Baldrige National Quality Award criteria.

"customer focus and satisfaction." The Award Examination is designed not only to serve as a reliable basis for making awards but also to permit a diagnosis of the applicant's overall quality management. All applicants receive feedback prepared by teams of U.S. quality experts. Because of this quality-audit aspect of the award, Motorola requires all its vendors to apply for the award.

ISO 9000

ISO 9000 is a series of quality standards defined by the International Standards Organization (ISO), which is a consortium of virtually all the world's industrialized nations. The most difficult standard to attain is ISO 9001, which provides quality standards for organizations that design, produce, service, and install products. ISO 9002 is similar but applies to organizations that do not perform design and service activities. Service firms fall under ISO 9003. Information about the quality standard program series is contained in ISO 9004.

Documentation of processes and consistent performance are the key features of ISO standards. ISO 9000 seeks to achieve this by requiring that businesses implement a three-component cycle:

1. *Planning.* Activities affecting quality must be planned to ensure that goals, authority, and responsibility are both defined and understood.
2. *Control.* Activities affecting quality must be controlled to ensure that specified requirements at all levels are met, problems are anticipated and averted, and corrective actions are planned and carried out.
3. *Documentation.* Activities affecting quality must be documented to ensure an understanding of quality objectives and methods, smooth interaction within the organization, feedback for the planning cycle, and to serve as objective evidence of quality system performance.

The motivation for considering ISO 9000 arises from the fact that the European Economic Community has adopted this certification as a requirement for doing business in their countries. Many companies follow and implement the ISO 9000 quality standards for reasons other than compulsory requirements, however. Companies have found that the very process of implementing the standard and the benefits from quality improvement are significant enough to justify this effort.

SERVICE RECOVERY

A service failure can be turned into a service delight by empowering front-line employees with the discretion to "make things right." For example, when an airplane full of anxious passengers is delayed for some minor mechanical problem, break out complementary drinks. More heroic efforts become legends, such as the story of a Federal Express employee who hired a helicopter to repair a downed telephone line during a snowstorm. Expenses that are incurred to accomplish a recovery are "pennies on the dollar" compared with the possible adverse "word-of-mouth" stories that now are turned into good stories of how an employee went the extra mile to accommodate a customer.

TABLE 10.9. Customer Feedback and Word-of-Mouth

- The average business only hears from 4 percent of its customers who are dissatisfied with the products or service. Of the 96 percent who do not bother to complain, 25 percent of them have serious problems.
- The 4 percent who complain are more likely to stay with the supplier than the 96 percent who do not complain.
- About 60 percent of the complainers would stay as customers if their problem were resolved, and 95 percent would stay if the problem were resolved quickly.
- A dissatisfied customer will tell from 10 to 20 other people about his or her problem.
- A customer who has had a problem resolved by a company will tell approximately 5 people about her or his situation.

Table 10.9 contains some statistics on the behavior of dissatisfied customers suggesting that a quick resolution to service failure is an important way to create loyal customers.

STAGES IN QUALITY DEVELOPMENT

In this chapter, we have looked at the most important issues of incorporating quality into the delivery of services. Some aspects of quality assurance in a service organization may occur simultaneously, but it is useful to look at such development in a systematic way.

The service quality ladder shown in Figure 10.12 summarizes the progressive steps in quality development. Inspection is shown as the first rung, because organizations usually begin here with their first attempts to address quality problems (e.g., checking hotel rooms after cleaning). Quality function deployment is shown as the top rung, because quality finally must be recognized as a basic customer requirement that should be incorporated in the design of the service delivery process.

SUMMARY

We began our study of quality issues in services by noting that customers are the ultimate judges of a service's value. Market researchers have identified five principal dimensions that customers use to judge service quality. Customers use these dimensions to make their assessments, which are based primarily on a comparison of their expectations for the service that is desired with their perceptions of the service that is delivered. We then looked at the different types of gaps that can occur when customers' expectations do not meet their perceptions.

Next, we turned to the problem of measuring service quality and discussed five aspects concerning the scope of services—their content, process, structure, outcome, and impact. Benchmarking and SERVQUAL are two useful approaches that can be used to measure quality in a variety of services.

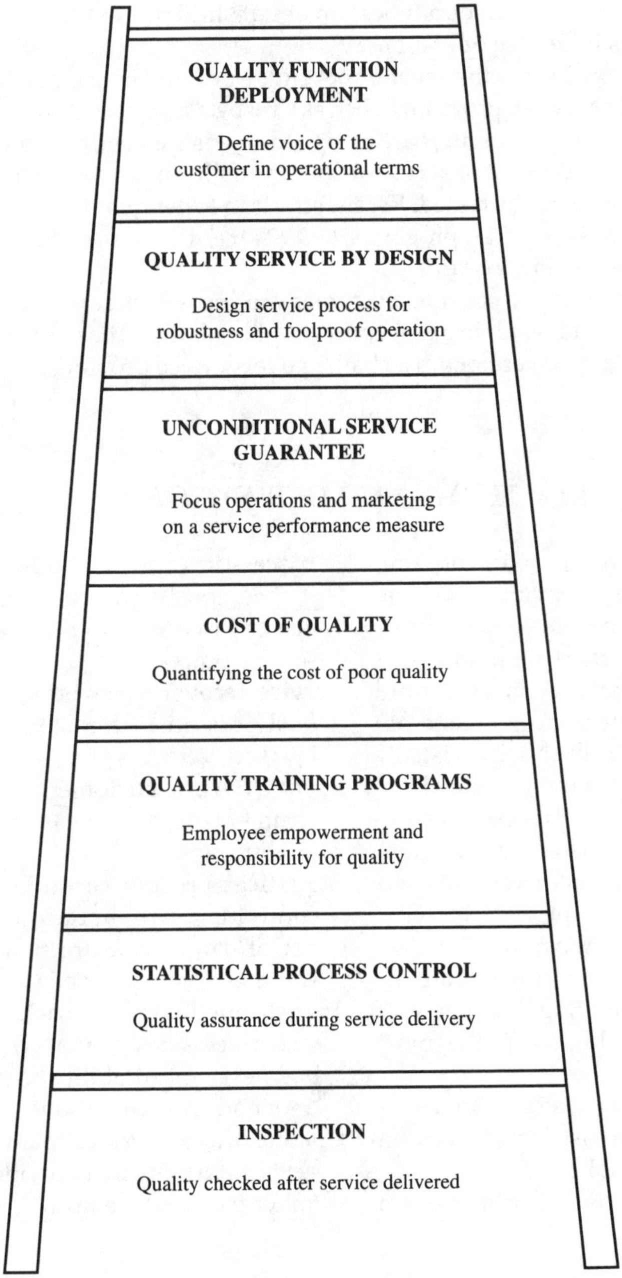

QUALITY FUNCTION DEPLOYMENT
Define voice of the customer in operational terms

QUALITY SERVICE BY DESIGN
Design service process for robustness and foolproof operation

UNCONDITIONAL SERVICE GUARANTEE
Focus operations and marketing on a service performance measure

COST OF QUALITY
Quantifying the cost of poor quality

QUALITY TRAINING PROGRAMS
Employee empowerment and responsibility for quality

STATISTICAL PROCESS CONTROL
Quality assurance during service delivery

INSPECTION
Quality checked after service delivered

FIGURE 10.12. The service quality ladder.

We noted the necessity of "designing in" quality. We also examined the Taguchi concept of robustness, poka-yoke fail-safe strategies, and quality function deployment methods of incorporating customer requirements in design for quality.

The costs of quality are categorized as failure costs, detection costs, and prevention costs. We illustrated the application of statistical process control to avoid high failure costs in service operations.

Finally, we considered the most important aspect of service quality—people—and looked at several programs, such as Crosby's zero-defects program and Deming's 14-point program, that are designed to ensure continuous improvement in quality. The concept of service recovery and the importance of word-of-mouth stories also were discussed. Recent efforts to foster quality in services include unconditional guarantee programs, ISO 9000 certification, and the Malcolm Baldrige National Quality Award.

In the next chapter, we consider customer waiting, which sometimes can exceed expectations and result in a perception of poor quality. The management of queues and waiting perceptions is a challenge for service providers.

KEY TERMS AND DEFINITIONS

Benchmarking the practice of comparing one's performance with that of other firms that are "best in class."

Control chart a chart with an upper control limit and a lower control limit on which sample means are plotted periodically to show visually when a process is out of control.

Fishbone analysis a process of cause-and-effect analysis using a diagram to trace back possible causes of a service quality problem.

Pareto analysis arrangement of data so that causes of a problem are ordered in descending frequency of occurrence to highlight the most likely one.

Poka-yoke a "foolproof" device or checklist to assist employees in avoiding a mistake.

Quality function deployment a process in which a "house of quality" is constructed to incorporate customer needs into the design of a service process.

Service recovery converting a previously dissatisfied customer into a loyal customer.

SERVQUAL a customer survey instrument used to measure service quality gaps.

Statistical process control use of a control chart to monitor a process performance measure that signals when intervention is needed.

Taguchi methods approaches to service process design that ensure "robustness" or an ability to function under adverse conditions.

Unconditional service guarantee a service warranty that provides a customer focus for the firm.

TOPICS FOR DISCUSSION

1. How do the five dimensions of service quality differ from those of product quality?
2. Why is measuring service quality so difficult?
3. Illustrate the four components in the cost of quality for a service of your choice.
4. Why do service firms hesitate to offer a service guarantee?
5. How can recovery from a service failure be a blessing in disguise?

Service Benchmark

Service Winners of the Malcolm Baldrige National Quality Award

1990
Federal Express Corporation
Memphis, TN

1992
AT&T Universal Card Services
Jacksonville, FL

The Ritz-Carlton Hotel Company
Atlanta, GA

1994
AT&T Consumer Communications Services
Basking Ridge, NJ

GTE Directories Corporation
Dallas/Ft. Worth Airport, TX

SOLVED PROBLEMS

1. Control Chart for Variables

Problem Statement

To become productive, Resort International is interested in setting standards for the time that telephone reservation clerks spend with vacationers making tour arrangements. Collecting data on the amount of time the reservation clerks spend with customers has been proposed to determine the mean time and average range as well as to establish a process control chart for this operation. The table below records the time in minutes that reservation clerks spent answering calls as found by observing one call each day during a typical week. The fifth row contains the $\overline{X}$ values for each day. The last row contains the range (i.e., high-low) values for each day (e.g., the high for Monday was 14 and the low was 5, yielding a range of 9).

Clerk	Mon.	Tue.	Wed.	Thur.	Fri.
Alice	5	11	12	13	10
Bill	6	5	12	10	13
Janice	14	13	10	9	9
Mike	8	6	9	12	14
$\overline{X}$	8.25	8.75	10.75	11.0	11.5
Range	9	8	3	4	5

Solution

First, we establish the population mean and range using the sample results from the 5 days shown above:

$$\overline{X} = \frac{8.25 + 8.75 + 10.75 + 11.0 + 11.5}{5} = 10.05$$

$$\overline{R} = \frac{9 + 8 + 3 + 4 + 5}{5} = 5.8$$

Second, we establish the control limits for an $\overline{X}$ -chart using equations (1) and (2) when sampling four random calls each day for each clerk. The sample size of 4 was selected for convenience.

$$UCL = \overline{\overline{X}} + A_2\overline{R} = 10.05 + (.729)(5.8) = 14.28$$

$$LCL = \overline{\overline{X}} - A_2\overline{R} = 10.05 - (.729)(5.8) = 5.82$$

Third, we also establish limits for the range of call times for these samples of four calls by constructing an *R*-chart using equations (3) and (4).

$$UCL = D_4\overline{R} = (2.282)(5.8) = 13.2$$

$$LCL = D_3\overline{R} = (0)(5.8) = 0$$

Plotting the average call time, which is based on a random sample of four calls for each clerk for each day, provides a record of performance for each clerk. If the average call time for any clerk falls outside the control limits, then an explanation is in order. If the average is above the *UCL*, too much time is being spent taking reservations, which results in lost productivity. If the average falls below the *LCL*, the clerk may be too curt, which results in a customer perception of unresponsiveness.

2. Control Chart for Attributes

Problem Statement

A regional airline is concerned about its record of on-time performance. The Memphis hub experiences 20 flight operations each day of the week, with the following record of on-time departures for the previous 10 days: 17, 16, 18, 19, 16, 15, 20, 17, 18, and 16. Prepare a *p*-chart with a sample size consisting of 1 week's average on-time departure percentage.

Solution

First, we calculate the expected population fraction of on-time departures, which is the sum of the 10-day experience divided by a total of 200 flights:

$$\overline{p} = \frac{17 + 16 + 18 + 19 + 16 + 15 + 20 + 17 + 18 + 16}{(10)(20)} = 0.86$$

Then, the control limits are determined using equations (5) and (6) with a sample size of 7:

$$UCL = \bar{p} + 3\sqrt{\frac{\bar{p}(1-\bar{p})}{n}} = 0.86 + 3\sqrt{\frac{.86(1-.86)}{7}} = 0.86 + 3(0.13)$$
$$= 1.25\ [\text{set} = 1.00]$$

$$LCL = \bar{p} - 3\sqrt{\frac{\bar{p}(1-\bar{p})}{n}} = 0.86 - 3(0.13) = 0.47$$

As often is the case for p-charts, one limit is set equal to the extreme value (i.e., $UCL = 1.00$ or $LCL = 0.0$). In this case, an average percentage of on-time departures for the week would be calculated, and only if this is found to be less than 47 percent (or 9 out of 20 departures late) would action be taken to investigate the abnormal occurrence for cause.

EXERCISES

10.1. In **Example 10.1,** Village Volvo wants to test the results of the QFD exercise for sensitivity to changes in the relative importance of customer expectations. Recalculate the weighted scores for the QFD exercise when customer expectations are given equal relative importance (e.g., five). Has this changed the previous recommendation to focus on training?

10.2. In **Example 10.2,** the ambulance supervisor now has decided to double the response time sample size to eight calls per day. Calculate the new UCL and LCL for a revised $\bar{X}$-chart. For the next week, you record the following sample of daily mean response times: 5.2, 6.4, 6.2, 5.8, 5.7, 6.3, and 5.6. Would you be concerned?

10.3. The time to make beds at a motel should fall into an agreed on range of times. A sample of four maids was selected, and the time needed to make a bed was observed on three different occasions as noted below:

	Service Time (sec)		
Maid	Sample 1	Sample 2	Sample 3
Ann	120	90	150
Linda	130	110	140
Mary	200	180	175
Michael	165	155	140

a. Determine the upper and lower control limits for an $\bar{X}$-chart and an R-chart with a sample size of four.

b. After the control chart was established, a sample of four observations had the following times in seconds: 185, 150, 192, and 178. Is corrective action needed?

10.4. The management of the Diners Delight franchised restaurant chain is in the process of establishing quality-control charts for the time that its service people give to each customer. Management thinks the length of time that each customer is given should remain within certain limits to enhance service quality. A sample of six service people was selected, and the customer service they provided was observed four times. The activities that the service people were performing were identified, and the time to service one customer was recorded as noted below:

Service Person	Service Time (sec)			
	Sample 1	Sample 2	Sample 3	Sample 4
1	200	150	175	90
2	120	85	105	75
3	83	93	130	150
4	68	150	145	175
5	110	90	75	105
6	115	65	115	125

a. Determine the upper and lower control limits for an $\bar{X}$-chart and an R-chart with a sample size of 6.

b. After the control chart was established, a sample of six service people was observed, and the following customer service times in seconds were recorded: 180, 125, 110, 98, 156, and 190. Is corrective action called for?

10.5. After becoming familiar with their jobs, the sorting machine operators of **Example 10.3** now average only two address errors per 100 parcels sorted. Prepare a p-chart for experienced sorting operators.

10.6. Several complaints recently have been sent to the Gotham City police department regarding the increasing incidence of congestion on the city's streets. The complaints attribute the cause of these traffic tie-ups to a lack of synchronization of the traffic lights. The lights are controlled by a main computer system, and adjusting this program is costly. Therefore, the controllers are reluctant to change the situation unless a clear need is shown.

During the past year, the police department has collected data at 1000 intersections The data were compiled on a monthly basis as shown below:

Month	Congestion Incidence
January	14
February	18
March	14
April	12
May	16
June	8
July	19
August	12
September	14
October	7
November	10
December	18

a. Construct a p-chart based on the above data.

b. Should the system be modified if, during the next 3 months, reports of congestion at these 1000 intersections indicate the following:

Month	Congestion Incidence
January	15
February	9
March	11

10.7. The Speedway Clinical Laboratory is a scientific blood-testing facility that receives samples from local hospitals and clinics. The blood samples are passed through several automated tests, and the results are printed through a central computer that reads and stores the information about each sample that is tested.

Management is concerned about the quality of the service it provides and wants to establish quality-control limits as a measure for the quality of its tests. Such managerial practice is viewed as significant, because incorrect analysis of a sample can lead to a wrong diagnosis by the physician, which in turn may cost the life of a patient. For this reason, 100 blood samples were collected at random each day after they had gone through testing. After retesting was performed manually on this sample, the results were:

Day	Incorrect Analysis	Day	Incorrect Analysis
1	8	11	4
2	3	12	6
3	1	13	5
4	0	14	10
5	4	15	2
6	2	16	1
7	9	17	0
8	6	18	6
9	3	19	3
10	1	20	2

a. Construct a *p*-chart to be used in assessing the quality of the service described above.

b. On average, what is the expected number of incorrect tests per 100 samples?

c. Later, another sample of 100 was taken. After the accuracy of the tests was established, 10 samples were found to have been analyzed incorrectly. What is your conclusion about the quality of this service?

10.8. The Long Life Insurance Company receives applications to buy insurance from its salespeople, who are specially trained in selling insurance to new customers. After the applications are received, they are processed through a computer. The computer is programmed so that it prints messages whenever it runs through an item that is not consistent with company policies. The company is concerned with the accuracy of the training that its salespeople receive, and it contemplates recalling them for more training if the quality of their performance is below certain limits. Five samples of 20 applications received from specific market areas were collected and inspected with the following results:

Sample	Applications with Errors
1	2
2	2
3	1
4	3
5	2

a. Determine the upper and lower control limits for a *p*-chart using a sample size of 20.

b. After the control limits were established, a sample was taken and four applications were found to have mistakes. What can we conclude from this?

CASE: CLEAN SWEEP, INC.

Clean Sweep, Inc. (CSI), is a custodial-janitorial services company specializing in contract maintenance of office space. Although not a large company compared with its primary competitors, CSI does have several major contracts to service some of the state government's offices. To enter and stay in the custodial service business, CSI adopted the strategy of having a small workforce that performs high-quality work at a reasonably rapid pace. At present, management feels that CSI has a staff that is more productive on an individual basis than those of its competition. Management recognizes that this single factor is the key to the company's success, so maintaining a high worker productivity level is critical.

Within the staff, the organizational structure is divided into four crews, each of which is composed of a crew leader and six to nine other crew members. All crews are under the direction of a single crew supervisor. Within the state building complex, there are nine buildings included in CSI's contracts, and the custodial assignments have been distributed as shown in Table 10.10 to balance the work-load distribution among the crews (on the basis of gross square feet of floor space per member).

The responsibilities of each crew involve the following general tasks, which are listed in no order of importance: 1) vacuum carpeted floors, 2) empty trash cans and place trash in industrial waste hoppers, 3) dry-mop and buff marble floors, 4) clean rest rooms, 5) clean snack bar area(s), and 6) dust desk tops.

Each crew works an 8½-hour shift, during which it gets two 15-minute paid rest breaks and one 30-minute lunch break, which is unpaid. There is some variation among the crews in choosing break and lunch times, however, primarily because of the personalities of the crew leaders. The leaders of crews 2 and 3 are the strictest in their supervision, whereas the leaders of crews 1 and 4 are the least strict, according to the crew supervisor.

CSI's management is aware that the department of the state government overseeing the custodial service contracts makes periodic random inspections and rates the cleaning jobs that CSI does. This department also receives any complaints about the custodial service from office workers. Table 10.11 contains the monthly ratings and number of complaints received (by building) during CSI's current contracts. Because the renegotiation of CSI's contracts is several months away, company management would like to maintain a high level of quality during the remaining months to improve its competitive stance.

As with other custodial service operations, employee turnover in CSI's staff has been fairly high but is still lower than the turnover experienced by many competitors. Management attributes this to the higher pay scale that CSI offers relative to that of the competition. Even though individual staff costs are higher, the greater productivity levels of a smaller-than-average workforce have resulted in greater-than-average profits for the company. Nevertheless, problems are reported by the crew supervisor, and complaints are voiced by the crew members. These complaints fall into two general categories: 1) inequity in crew leaders' attitudes and performance expectations, and 2) lack of opportunities for personal advancement. Table 10.12 shows a historical distribution of monthly complaints from each crew according to these two categories for the same period as that covered by the ratings reported in Table 10.11.

Questions

1. Prepare an $\bar{X}$-chart for complaints, and plot the average complaints per building for each crew during

TABLE 10.10. Custodial Assignments

Crew	No. of Members*	Buildings Assigned and Gross Ft^2	Total Ft^2 Assigned
1	6	Bldg. A, 30,000; Bldg. C, 45,000; Bldg. F, 35,000	110,000
2	8	Bldg. B East, 95,000; Bldg. H, 55,000	150,000
3	9	Bldg. B West, 95,000; Bldg. G, 85,000	180,000
4	8	Bldg. D, 40,000; Bldg. E, 75,000; Bldg. I, 42,000	157,000

*Excludes crew leader

TABLE 10.11 Complaints about and Ratings of Cleaning Crews*

Month	A	Be	Bw	C	D	E	F	G	H	I
	Building									
1	2	5	7	3	2	3	2	4	3	4
	7	5	3	6	7	5	6	5	4	5
2	1	6	8	2	1	1	2	3	2	5
	7	5	3	6	6	5	6	5	5	4
3	0	6	8	1	0	2	2	4	0	1
	8	5	4	6	8	5	6	6	6	7
4	1	5	4	1	0	1	1	4	1	3
	7	5	5	8	8	6	7	5	6	6
5	1	3	2	2	0	1	1	3	1	2
	6	6	6	7	8	6	7	5	6	6
6	2	5	3	0	1	0	0	2	1	0
	7	6	6	7	7	8	6	5	5	7
7	0	4	2	1	0	0	0	0	0	1
	8	7	7	6	6	8	8	6	7	7
8	1	2	4	2	1	0	1	2	1	1
	6	6	5	7	7	8	7	5	6	7
9	1	2	4	1	1	0	1	1	3	0
	7	7	5	6	7	8	6	5	5	8

*First-row numbers for each month represent total number of complaints. Second-row numbers for each month represent ratings on a 1-to-10 scale; any rating under 5 is felt to be poor, and 8 or above is good.

TABLE 10.12 Job-Related Complaints from Crew Members

	Crew 1		*Crew 2*		*Crew 3*		*Crew 4*	
Month	Inequity	No Advance-ment	Inequity	No Advance-ment	Inequity	No Advance-ment	Inequity	No Advance-ment
1	0	1	3	3	4	3	0	2
2	0	0	2	1	1	1	0	1
3	1	0	2	1	2	2	1	2
4	0	0	1	2	3	1	0	2
5	1	1	3	1	2	1	0	2
6	1	0	1	2	2	1	0	1
7	0	1	1	1	1	3	0	1
8	0	0	2	2	1	2	1	1
9	0	0	2	1	2	2	0	2

the 9-month period. Do the same for the performance ratings. What does this analysis reveal about the service quality of CSI's crews?

2. Discuss possible ways to improve service quality.
3. Describe some potential strategies for reducing CSI's staffing problems.

CASE: THE COMPLAINT LETTER

Most service problems are solved by direct communication between the server and the customer during the moment of service. Occasionally, however, a customer may be motivated to communicate some thoughtful and detailed feedback to a service provider after the encounter, as illustrated in the following letter:

THE COMPLAINT LETTER

October 13, 1986
123 Main Street
Boston, Massachusetts

Gail and Harvey Pearson
The Retreat House on Foliage Pond
Vacationland, New Hampshire

Dear Mr. and Mrs. Pearson:

This is the first time that I have ever written a letter like this, but my wife and I are so upset by the treatment afforded by your staff that we felt compelled to let you know what happened to us. We had dinner reservations at the Retreat House for a party of four under my wife's name, Dr. Elaine Loflin, for Saturday evening, October 11. We were hosting my wife's brother and his wife, visiting from Atlanta, Georgia.

We were seated at 7:00 PM in the dining room to the left of the front desk. There were at least four empty tables in the room when we were seated. We were immediately given menus, a wine list, ice water, dinner rolls, and butter. Then we sat for 15 minutes until the cocktail waitress asked us for our drink orders. My sister-in-law said, after being asked what she would like, "I'll have a vodka martini straight-up with an olive." The cocktail waitress responded immediately, "I'm not a stenographer." My sister-in-law repeated her drink order.

Soon after, our waiter arrived, informing us of the specials of the evening. I don't remember his name, but he had dark hair, wore glasses, was a little stocky, and had his sleeves rolled up. He returned about ten minutes later, our drinks still not having arrived. We had not decided upon our entrees, but requested appetizers, upon which he informed us that we could not order appetizers without ordering our entrees at the same time. We decided not to order appetizers.

Our drinks arrived and the waiter returned. We ordered our entrees at 7:30. When the waiter asked my wife for her order, he addressed her as "young lady." When he served her the meal, he called her "dear."

At ten minutes of eight we requested that our salads be brought to us as soon as possible. I then asked the waiter's assistant to bring us more rolls (each of us had been served one when we were seated). Her response was, "Who wants a roll?," upon which, caught off guard, we went around the table saying yes or no so she would know exactly how many "extra" rolls to bring to our table.

Our salads were served at five minutes of eight. At 25 minutes past the hour we requested our entrees. They were served at 8:30, one and one-half hours after we were seated in a restaurant which was one-third empty. Let me also add that we had to make constant requests for water refills, butter replacement, and the like.

In fairness to the chef, the food was excellent, and as you already realize, the atmosphere was delightful. Despite this, the dinner was a disaster. We were extremely upset and very insulted by the experience. Your staff is not well trained. They were overtly rude, and displayed little etiquette or social grace. This was compounded by the atmosphere you are trying to present and the prices you charge in your dining room.

Perhaps we should have made our feelings known at the time, but our foremost desire was to leave as soon as possible. We had been looking forward to dining at the Retreat House for quite some time as part of our vacation weekend in New Hampshire.

We will be hard-pressed to return to your establishment. Please be sure to know that we will share our experience at the Retreat House with our family, friends, and business associates.

Sincerely,
Dr. William E. Loflin

Source: Martin R. Moser, "Answering the Customer's Complaint: A Case Study," *The Cornell HRA Quarterly,* May 1987, p. 10.

Experience has shown that complaint letters receive "mixed reviews." Some letters bring immediate positive responses from the providers, whereas other letters bring no response or resolution. The restaurateur's response to the complaint letter in this case was:

THE RESTAURATEUR'S REPLY

The Retreat House on Foliage Pond
Vacationland, New Hampshire
November 15, 1986

Dr. William E. Loflin
123 Main Street
Boston, Massachusetts

Dear Dr. Loflin:

My husband and I are naturally distressed by such a negative reaction to our restaurant, but very much appreciate your taking the time and trouble to apprise us of your recent dinner here. I perfectly understand and sympathize with your feelings, and would like to tell you a little about the circumstances involved.

The Lakes Region for the past four or five years has been notorious for its extremely low unemployment rate and resulting deplorable labor pool. This year local businesses found that the situation had deteriorated to a really alarming nadir. It has been virtually impossible to get adequate help, competent or otherwise! We tried to overhire at the beginning of the season, anticipating the problems we knew would arise, but were unsuccessful. Employees in the area know the situation very well and use it to their advantage, knowing that they can get a job anywhere at any time without references, and knowing they won't be fired for incompetency because there is no one to replace them. You can imagine the prevailing attitude among workers and the frustration it causes employers, particularly those of us who try hard to maintain high standards. Unhappily, we cannot be as selective about employees as we would wish, and the turnover is high. Proper training is not only a luxury, but an impossibility at such times.

Unfortunately, the night you dined at the Retreat House, October 11, is traditionally one of the busiest nights of the year, and though there may have been empty tables at the time you sat down, I can assure you that we served 150 people that night, despite the fact that no fewer than four members of the restaurant staff did not show up for work at the last minute, and did not notify us. Had they had the courtesy to call, we could have limited reservations, thereby mitigating the damage at least to a degree, but as it was, we, our guests, and the employees who were trying to make up the slack all had to suffer delays in service far beyond the norm!

As to the treatment you received from the waitress and waiter who attended you, neither of them is any longer in our employ, and never would have been had the labor situation not been so desperate! It would have indeed been helpful to us had you spoken up at the time—it makes a more lasting impression on the employees involved than does our discussing it with them after the fact. Now that we are in a relatively quiet period we have the time to properly train a new and, we hope, better waitstaff.

Please know that we feel as strongly as you do that the service you received that night was unacceptable, and certainly not up to our normal standards.

We hope to be able to prevent such problems from arising in the future, but realistically must acknowledge that bad nights do happen, even in the finest restaurants. Believe me, it is not because we do not care or are not paying attention!

You mentioned our prices. Let me just say that were you to make a comparative survey, you would find that our prices are about one half of what you would expect to pay in most cities and resort areas for commensurate cuisine and ambience. We set our prices in order to be competitive with other restaurants in this particular local area, in spite of the fact that most of them do not offer the same quality of food and atmosphere and certainly do not have our overhead!

I hope that this explanation (which should not be misconstrued as an excuse) has shed some light, and that you will accept our deep regrets and apologies for any unpleasantness you and your party suffered. We should be very glad if someday you would pay us a return visit so that we may provide you with the happy and enjoyable dining experience that many others have come to appreciate at the Retreat House.

Sincerely,
Gail Pearson

Source: Martin R. Moser, "Answering the Customer's Complaint: A Case Study," *The Cornell HRA Quarterly*, May 1987, p. 11.

Questions

1. Briefly summarize the complaints and compliments in Dr. Loflin's letter.

2. Critique the letter of Gail Pearson in reply to Dr. Loflin. What are the strengths and weaknesses of the letter?

3. Prepare an "improved" response letter from Gail Pearson.

4. What further action should Gail Pearson take in view of this incident?

SELECTED BIBLIOGRAPHY

BEHARA, R. S., and R. B. CHASE: "Service Quality Deployment: Quality Service by Design," in Rakesh V. Sarin (ed.), *Perspectives in Operations Management: Essays in Honor of Elwood S. Buffa*, Kluwer Academic Publisher, Norwell, Mass., 1993.

BERRY, L. L., and A. PARASURAMAN: "Prescriptions for a Service Quality Revolution in America," *Organizational Dynamics*, vol. 20, no. 4, 1992, pp. 5–15.

———, V. A. ZEITHAML, and A. PARASURAMAN: "Five Imperatives for Improving Service Quality," *Sloan Management Review Association*, vol. 31, no. 4, Summer 1990, pp. 29–38.

BROWN, T. J., G. A. CHURCHILL, and J. P. PETER: "Improving the Measurement of Service Quality," *Journal of Retailing*, vol. 69, no. 1, Spring 1993, pp. 127–139.

CARR, L. P.: "Applying Cost of Quality to a Service Business," *Sloan Management Review*, Summer 1992, p. 72–77.

CHASE, R. B., and D. M. STEWART: "Make Your Service Fail-Safe," *Sloan Management Review*, Spring 1994, pp. 35–44.

COLLIER, DAVID A.: "The Customer Service and Quality Challenge," *The Service Industries Journal*, vol. 7, no. 1, 1987, pp. 77–90.

CRONIN, J. J., and S. A. TAYLOR: "SERVPERF Versus SERVQUAL: Reconciling Performance-Based and Perceptions-Minus-Expectations Measurement of Service Quality," *Journal of Marketing*, vol. 58, January 1994, pp. 125–131.

CROSBY, PHILIP B.: *Quality Is Free: The Art of Making Quality Certain*, McGraw-Hill Book Company, New York, 1979.

DEMING, W. EDWARDS: *Quality, Productivity, and Competitive Position*, M.I.T. Center for Advanced Engineering Study, Cambridge, Mass., 1982.

GARVIN, DAVID A.: "Competing on the Eight Dimensions of Quality," *Harvard Business Review*, November–December 1987, pp. 101–109.

GRANT, ROBERT M., R. SHANI, and R. KRISHNAN: "TQM's Challenge to Management Theory and Practice," *Sloan Management Review*, Winter 1994, pp. 25–35.

HALSTEAD, D.: "Five Common Myths About Customer Satisfaction," *Journal of Services Marketing*, vol. 7, no. 3, 1993, pp. 4–12.

HART, CHRISTOPHER W. L.: "The Power of Unconditional Service Guarantees," *Harvard Business Review*, July–August 1988, pp. 54–62.

———, J. L. HESKETT, and W. E. SASSER, JR.: "The Profitable Art of Service Recovery," *Harvard Business Review,* July–August 1990, pp. 148–156.

HAUSER, J. R.: "How Puritan-Bennet Used the House of Quality," *Sloan Management Review,* Spring 1993, pp. 61–70.

———, and D. CLAUSING: "The House of Quality," *Harvard Business Review,* May–June 1988, pp. 63–73.

HAYWOOD-FARMER, JOHN: "Towards a Conceptual Model of Service Quality," *International Journal of Operations and Production Management,* vol. 8, no. 6, 1988, pp. 19–29.

HOSTAGE, G. M.: "Quality Control in a Service Business," *Harvard Business Review,* vol. 53, no. 4, July–August 1975, pp. 98–106.

JOHNSON, PERRY L.: *ISO 9000: Meeting the New International Standards,* McGraw-Hill, New York, 1993.

KLAUS, PETER G.: "Quality Epiphenomenon: The Conceptual Understanding of Quality in Face-to-Face Service Encounters," in J. A. Czepiel, M. R. Solomon, and C. F. Surprenant (eds.), *The Service Encounter,* Lexington Books, Lexington, Mass., 1985, pp. 17–35.

LEES, J., and B. G. DALE: "Quality Circles in Service Industries: A Study of Their Use," *The Service Industry Journal,* vol. 8, no. 2, 1988, pp. 143–154.

PARASURAMAN, A., V. A. ZEITHAML, and L. L. BERRY: "A Conceptual Model of Service Quality and Its Implications for Future Research," *Journal of Marketing,* vol. 49, Fall 1985, pp. 41–50.

———: "SERVQUAL: A Multiple-Item Scale for Measuring Consumer Perceptions of Service Quality," *Journal of Retailing,* vol. 64, no. 1, Spring 1988, pp. 12–40.

———: "More on Improving Service Quality Measurement," *Journal of Retailing,* vol. 69, no. 1, Spring 1993, pp. 140–147.

REICHHELD, F. F., and W. E. SASSER: "Zero Defections: Quality Comes to Services," *Harvard Business Review,* September–October 1990, pp. 105–111.

TAGUCHI, G., and D. CLAUSING: "Robust Quality," *Harvard Business Review,* January–February 1990, pp. 65–75.

TAKEUCHI, H., and J. A. QUELCH: "Quality Is More than Making a Good Product," *Harvard Business Review,* vol. 61, no. 4, July–August 1983, pp. 139–145.

WYCKOFF, D. D.: "New Tools for Achieving Service Quality," *The Cornell HRA Quarterly,* vol. 25, no. 3, November 1984, pp. 78–91.

ZEITHAML, V. A., L. L. BERRY, and A. PARASURAMAN: "Communication and Control Processes in the Delivery of Service Quality," *Journal of Marketing,* vol. 52, April 1988, pp. 35–48.

CHAPTER 11

Managing Queues

LEARNING OBJECTIVES

After completing this chapter, you should be able to:

1. Describe how queues form.
2. Apply Maister's two "laws of service."
3. Describe the psychology of waiting components, and suggest management strategies to deal with each.
4. Describe the essential features of a queuing system.
5. Explain why the negative exponential distribution of time between arrivals is equivalent to the Poisson distribution of arrival rates.

The management of queues at Burger King represents an evolving process of refinement. When these stores first opened, a "conventional" lineup was used that required customers to arrange themselves in single file behind a single cash register, where orders were taken. Assemblers prepared the orders and presented them to customers at the far end of the counter. This conventional style of line-up often is called the "snake," as mentioned in the following *Wall Street Journal* article.[1]

Louis Kane hates snakes.

The restaurant executive means the single lines that feed customers one at a time to a group of cashiers. He thinks snakes are much too "institutional." Besides, he says, he would rather try to guess which line will move the fastest. But surveys show that customers prefer snakes to multiple lines because they hate "getting stuck behind some guy ordering nine cappuccinos, each with something different on top," says Mr. Kane, co-chairman of the Boston-based Au Bon Pain soup-and-sandwich chain.

The customers have won. Over the past couple of years, Au Bon Pain has instituted snakes at every restaurant that has enough room. But the debate lives on. "We talk about this a great deal," Mr. Kane says.

The issue is queues. Experts suggest that no aspect of customer service is more important than the wait in line to be served. The act of waiting—either in person or on the phone—"has a disproportionately high impact" on customers, says David Maister, a Boston consultant who has studied the psychology of waiting. "The wait can destroy an otherwise perfect service experience."

A customer waiting in line is potentially a lost customer. According to one study, up to 27% of customers who can't get through on the telephone will either buy elsewhere or skip the transaction altogether, says Rudy Oetting, a senior partner at Oetting & Co., a New York company that consults on telephone use. Adds Russell James, an official at Avis Rent a Car Inc.: "You can't be outlined by a competitor or you will lose business."

Today's customers are also more demanding than ever. "The dramatic difference between 1980 and 1990 can be described in one word: speed," says N. Powell Taylor, manager of GE Answer Center, a General Electric Co. operation that fields three million calls a year. "People expect quicker answers. No one has the time any more."

In the past few years particularly, many companies have stepped up efforts to shorten waits—or at least make them more tolerable. Here are some of the methods they are trying:

Animate

Some contend that a wait isn't a wait if it's fun. At Macy's in New York now, the line to see Santa Claus wends its way through displays of dancing teddy bears, elves and electric trains. "It's part of the adventure of going to see Santa Claus," says Jean McFaddin, a vice president at the big department store, where 300,000 people see Santa in 30 days.

At Disneyland and Walt Disney World, the waits—which can be up to 90 minutes long—are planned along with the attractions themselves. Visitors waiting for rides that board continuously pass animated displays that are designed to be viewed as people walk along. Waits for theater shows include such attractions as singers and handicraft displays aimed at audiences that will be waiting in one place as long as 30 minutes. Indeed, the waits themselves are called

[1]Reprinted with permission. Amanda Bennett, "Their Business Is on the Line," *The Wall Street Journal*, Dec. 7, 1990, p. B1. Reprinted by permission of *The Wall Street Journal*, 1989, Dow Jones & Company, Inc. All Rights Reserved Worldwide.

"preshows." Says Norman Doerges, executive vice president of Disneyland, "that's what makes the time pass, is the entertainment."

At the Omni Park Central Hotel in New York, when a line exceeds six people, assistant managers are dispatched to the hotel restaurant to bring out orange and grapefruit juice to serve to the people in line. "We are trying to tell the guest 'we know you are here,' " says Philip Georgas, general manager and regional vice president.

Still, not all diversions are suitable. Many callers don't like listening to recordings while they're on hold. GE plays its corporate theme for customers while they wait, but it draws the line at playing recorded advertising. "We tend to stay away from commercials," says Mr. Taylor, because of the fear that customers will think company employees "are probably sitting there doing nothing," making customers wait so they will have to listen to the commercials.

Discriminate

"The key thing is not just moving people out of the line," says Mr. James at Avis. "The key is who you move out of the line." For the past two years, high-volume renters at Avis have been able to sign a permanent rental agreement in advance and be driven directly to their cars when they arrive at many Avis locations. Somewhat less-frequent renters check in at a kiosk near the car park. Other car rental concerns are offering similar preferential services.

Such service is increasingly common in the travel, banking and credit-card industries. But "one needs a great deal of creativity in this area" lest less-favored customers be offended, says Mr. Maister. "Those businesses that want to serve priority customers faster are best advised to do it out of sight of the regular customers." He cites some airlines that locate first-class check-in counters away from the economy counters. "You don't want to rub the noses of the economy passengers in it."

Automate

While assembly-line techniques can accelerate manufacturing operations, they often slow the delivery of services. When callers must speak to several different people to get a complete answer, "crew interference" sets in, says Warren Blanding, editor of Customer Service Newsletter in Silver Spring, Md. "The most efficient way to do a job is to have one person do it."

So Employers Health Insurance, Green Bay, Wis., has assembled a complex computer data base of scripts that employees can read to customers on the telephone. The employee keys in the caller's name, location and type of health insurance question. The computer then pops up a question-and-answer format that can be read verbatim.

"We know that 75% of the calls we get in are standard questions," says Sterling L. Phaklides, an assistant vice president in the claims division. "Because people are sticking to the scripts, they are giving up-to-date information" without consulting technicians, he says. But callers who ask questions that aren't covered in the scripts can be referred to specialists at any point. "It does save telephone time," the official says. The claims area handles 3,700 calls a day; only about 1% of callers hang up before they are connected—which is better than average, he says.

Obfuscate

Mr. Maister says the perceived wait is often more important than the actual wait. In a paper on the psychology of waiting, he notes that some restaurants deliberately announce longer waiting times, thus pleasing customers when the wait is actually shorter. At Disneyland in Anaheim, Calif., lines snake around corners, Mr. Maister says. Thus people focus more on how fast the line is moving than on how long the line is.

Disneyland says its aim isn't to deceive. It posts waiting times at the start of each line. "A big danger in disguising a line is that people don't know what

> they are getting into," says Mr. Doerges. "If you do it without proper preparation, people get frustrated."
>
> Still, some think that even that information will be too depressing. Technology is available that will announce a caller's place in line, but Penny Rhode, vice president, customer service, at First Gibralter Bank in Dallas, chose not to use it. "I felt like . . . focusing on the positive, rather than perhaps saying that there are 14 callers ahead of you."
>
> Under First Gibralter's system, after 1½ minutes a phone voice offers the caller the option of continuing to wait or leaving a message. Since it started the system in October, the bank has averaged about 100 messages a day out of between 3,000 and 3,200 calls.

Dissatisfaction with the slowness of a single-line arrangement led Burger King to try the "hospitality" line-up, in which cash registers are evenly spaced along the counter and customers select a line (in effect betting on which of several will move the fastest). In this arrangement, the cashier who takes an order also assembles the order. Although the hospitality line-up proves to be very flexible in meeting peak-period demand, it does tend to be more labor-intensive than the conventional line-up. Consequently, Burger King made yet another change, this time to what is called a "multiconventional" lineup, which is a hybrid of both earlier systems. The restaurant returned to a single line, but a new cash register now allows up to six orders to be recorded at the same time. Assemblers prepare the orders and distribute them at the end of the counter. Returning to a single line has guaranteed fairness, because customers are served in the order of their arrival. In addition, customers have enough time to make their meal selection without slowing the entire order-taking process.

Burger King's concern with reducing customer waiting time represents a trend toward providing faster service. In many cases, speed of delivery is viewed as a competitive advantage in the marketplace. For example, many hotels today will total your bill and slide it under your room door during the last night of your stay, thereby achieving "zero waiting time" at the check-out counter.

Fluctuations in demand for service are difficult to cope with, because the consumption and production of services occur simultaneously. Customers typically arrive at random and place immediate demands on the available service. If service capacity is fully utilized at the time of his or her arrival, then the customer is expected to wait patiently in line. Varying arrival rates and service time requirements result in the formation of queues (i.e., lines of customers waiting their turn for service). The management of queues is a continuing challenge for service managers.

CHAPTER PREVIEW

Our understanding of waiting lines begins with a definition of queuing systems and the inevitability of waiting, and then the implications of asking people to wait are studied further from a psychological perspective. We shall discover that the perception of waiting often is more important to the consumer than the actual time spent waiting, suggesting that innovative ways should be found to reduce the negative aspects of waiting. The economic value of waiting as a cost for the provider and currency for the consumer also is considered. Finally, the essential features of a service system are discussed in terms of a schematic queuing model, and queuing terminology is defined.

QUEUING SYSTEMS

A *queue* is a line of waiting customers who require service from one or more servers. The queue need not be a physical line of individuals in front of a server, however. It might be students sitting at computer terminals that are scattered around a college campus, or a person being placed on "hold" by a telephone operator. Servers typically are considered to be individual stations where customers receive service. The stereotypical queue—people waiting in a formal line for service—is seen at the check-out counters of a supermarket and the teller windows in a bank, yet queuing systems occur in a variety of forms. Consider the following variations:

1. Servers need not be limited to serving one customer at a time. Transportation systems such as buses, airplanes, and elevators are bulk services.
2. The consumer need not always travel to the service facility; in some systems, the server actually comes to the consumer. This approach is illustrated by urban services such as fire and police protection as well as by ambulance service.
3. The service may consist of stages of queues in a series or of a more complex network of queues. For example, consider the haunted-house attraction at amusement parks like Disneyland, where queues are staged in sequence so that visitors can be processed in batches and entertained during the waiting periods (e.g., first outside on the walk, then in the vestibule, and finally on the ride itself).

In any service system, a queue forms whenever current demand exceeds the existing capacity to serve. This occurs when servers are so busy that arriving consumers cannot receive immediate service. Such a situation is bound to occur in any system for which arrivals occur at varying times and service times also vary.

THE INEVITABILITY OF WAITING

As Figure 11.1 shows, waiting is part of everyone's life, and it can involve an incredible amount of time. For example, a typical day might include waiting at several stoplights, waiting for someone to answer the telephone, waiting for your meal to be served, waiting for the elevator, waiting to be checked out at the supermarket—the list goes on and on.

In the old Soviet Union and even the newly independent countries that have formed since its recent break-up, we find dramatic examples of the role that queuing can play in people's daily lives. A noted Russian scholar, Hedrick Smith, observed that the queue in that country is a national pastime:

> Personally, I have known of people who stood in line 90 minutes to buy four pineapples, three hours for a two-minute roller coaster ride, three and a half hours to buy three large heads of cabbage only to find the cabbages were gone

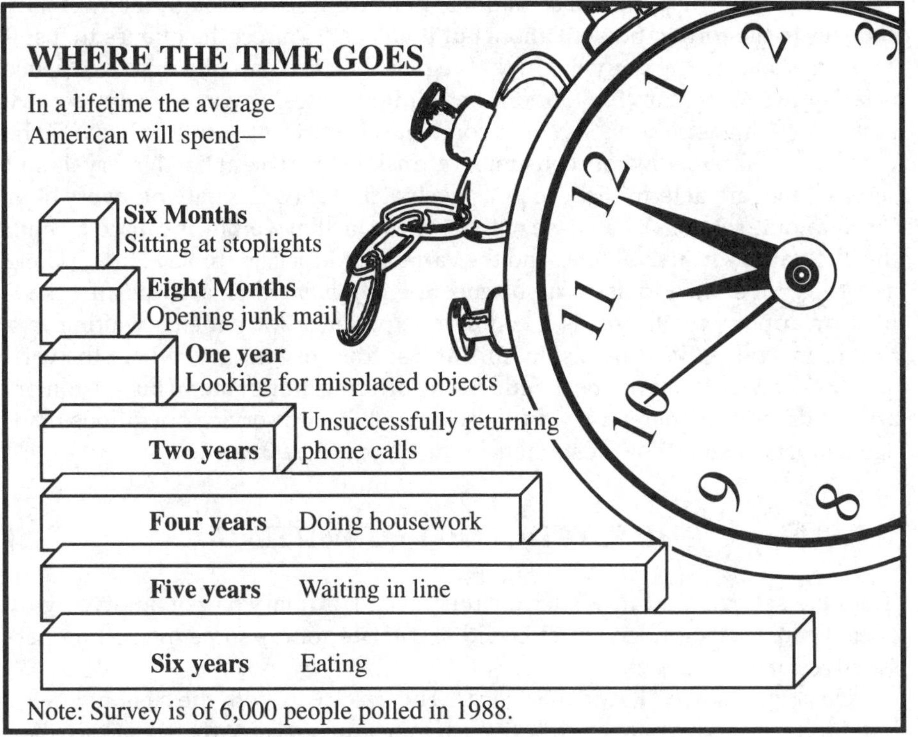

FIGURE 11.1. Where the time goes.
Source: Copyright, 1989, U.S. News & World Report, *January 30, 1989, p. 81.*

> as they approached the front of the line, 18 hours to sign up to purchase a rug at some later date, all through a freezing December night to register on a list for buying a car, and then waiting 18 more months for actual delivery, and terribly lucky at that. Lines can run from a few yards long to half a block to nearly a mile, and usually they move at an excruciating creep.[2]

He also found that there was a matter of line etiquette. Line jumping by serious shoppers was accepted for ordinary items but not for scarce ones. Smith observed:

> "People know from experience that things actually run out while they are standing in line," advised one young [woman]. "So if the line is for something really good and you leave it for very long, people get very upset. They fly off the handle and curse you and try to keep you from getting back in when you return. It's up to the person behind you to defend your place in line. So it's serious business asking someone to hold your place. They take on a moral obligation not only to let you in front of them later on but to defend you. You have to be stubborn yourself and stand your ground in spite of the insults and the stares. And when you get to the front of the line, if the sales clerks are not limiting the amount, you can hear people, maybe six or eight places back, shouting at you not to take so much, that you are a person with no scruples or that you have no consideration for other people. It can be rather unpleasant."[3]

[2]Hedrick Smith, *The Russians,* Quadrangle Press, New York, 1975, pp. 64–65.
[3]Ibid., p. 67.

Since Smith made his observations, perestroika has brought about many changes in the former Soviet Union, but it has yet to affect the queues that still are so much a part of daily life in that region. The Russian queuing experience is far more severe than that found in the United States; however, in any service system, waiting is bound to occur. A complete absence of waiting only would be possible in a situation where consumers are asked to arrive at fixed intervals and service times are deterministic (e.g., a psychiatrist schedules patients every hour for 50-minute sessions). Later, we will demonstrate that waiting is caused by both the fluctuations in arrival rates and the variability in service times. Thus, as long as service times vary, delays can be encountered even when arrivals are scheduled by appointment. This is a common experience for patients waiting in a physician's office. Waiting also occurs at fast-food restaurants, where the variability of service times has been reduced by offering a short menu but customers arrive at random. Therefore, waiting is inevitable, and service operations managers must consider how customers in queue are to be treated.

THE PSYCHOLOGY OF WAITING[4]

If, as noted above, waiting is such an integral and ordinary part of our lives, why does it cause us so much grief? David H. Maister offers some interesting perspectives on this subject.

He suggests two "Laws of Service." The first deals with the customer's expectations versus his or her perceptions. If a customer receives better service than he or she expects, then the customer departs a happy, satisfied person, and the service may benefit from a trickle-down effect (i.e., the happy customer will tell friends about the good service). Note, however, that the trickle-down effect can work both ways: a service can earn a bad reputation in the same manner (and create more interesting stories for the customer to pass along).

Maister's second law states that it is hard to play "catch-up ball." By this, he means that first impressions can influence the rest of the service experience; thus, a service that requires its customers to wait would be advised to make that period a pleasant experience. To do the "impossible"—to make waiting at least tolerable and, at best, pleasant and productive—a creative and competitive service management must consider the following aspects of the psychology of waiting.

That Old Empty Feeling

Just as "nature abhors a vacuum," people dislike "empty time." Empty, or unoccupied, time feels awful. It keeps us from other productive activities; frequently is physically uncomfortable; makes us feel powerless and at the mercy of servers, whom we may perceive as uncaring about us; and, perhaps worst of all, seems to last forever. The challenge to the service organization is obvious: fill this time in a positive way. It may require no more than comfortable chairs and a fresh coat of paint to cheer up the environment. Furnishings in a waiting area can affect indirectly the perception of waiting. The fixed, bench-like seating in

[4]Adapted from David H. Maister, "The Psychology of Waiting Lines," in J. A. Czepiel, M. R. Solomon, and C. F. Surprenant (eds.), *The Service Encounter*, Lexington Press, Lexington, Mass., 1985, pp. 113–123.

bus and rail terminals discourages conversation. The light, movable table-and-chair arrangement of a European sidewalk cafe brings people together and provides opportunities for socializing. In another situation, a music recording may be enough to occupy a telephone caller who is on hold and, at the same time, reassure the caller that he or she has not been disconnected.

Perhaps the strategy most widely noted in the literature is that of installing mirrors near elevators. Hotels, for example, record fewer complaints about excessive waits for elevators that are surrounded by mirrors. The mirrors allow people to occupy their time by checking their grooming and surreptitiously observing others who are waiting.

Services often can make waiting times productive as well as pleasurable. Instead of treating the telephone caller mentioned above to the strains of Mozart or Madonna, the service can air some commercials. Such a practice involves risk, however, because some people resent being subjected to this tactic when they are being held captive. At The Olive Garden restaurants, diners who are waiting for tables can spend their time in the bar, which benefits the restaurant with added sales, or can wait in the lobby and watch a chef prepare fresh pastas, which certainly stimulates appetites. No need to play "catch-up ball" here. Each diner reaches the table happily anticipating an agreeable experience rather than sourly grumbling, "It's about time!"

Services that consist of several stages, such as one might find at a diagnostic clinic, can conceal waiting by asking people to walk between successive stages. There are innumerable other ways to fill time: reading matter, television monitors, live entertainment, posters, artwork, toys to occupy children, and cookies and pots of coffee. The diversions are limited only by management's imagination and desire to serve the customer effectively.

A Foot in the Door

As noted above, some diversions merely fill time so that waiting doesn't seem so long, and others also can provide the service organization with some ancillary benefits. Happy customers are more likely than unhappy customers to be profitable customers. Another aspect of diversions is important, however.

Maister points out that "service-related" diversions themselves, such as handing out menus to waiting diners or medical history forms (and paper cups) to waiting patients, "convey a sense that service has started." One's level of anxiety subsides considerably once service has started. In fact, people generally can tolerate longer waits, within reason, if they feel service has begun better than they can tolerate such waits if service has not even started. Another view is that customers become dissatisfied more quickly with an initial wait than with subsequent waits after the service has begun.

The Light at the End of the Tunnel

There are many anxieties at work before service begins. Have I been forgotten? Did you get my order? This line doesn't seem to be moving; will I ever get served? If I run to the rest room, will I lose my turn? When will the plumber get here? Will the plumber get here at all? Whether rational or not, anxieties may be the single biggest factor influencing the waiting customer.

Managers must recognize these anxieties and develop strategies to alleviate them. In some cases, this may be a simple matter of having an employee acknowledge the customer's presence. At other times, telling the customer how long he or she will have to wait is sufficient reassurance that the wait at some point will end. Signs can serve this purpose as well. As you approach the Port Aransas, Texas, ferry landing, for example, you see signs posted along the road noting the number of minutes you have left to wait if you are stopped in line at that point.

When appropriate, scheduling appointments is one strategy to reduce waiting time, but it is not foolproof. Unforeseen events might interfere, or prior appointments may require more time than expected. If the appointed time comes and goes, the anxiety of not knowing how long the wait will be sets in—along with some measure of irritation at the "insult" of being stood up. A simple explanation and apology for the delays, however, usually will go a long way in reestablishing goodwill.

Excuse Me, but I Was Next

Uncertain and unexplained waits create anxieties and, as noted above, occasionally some resentment in customers. The moment a customer sees a later arrival being served first, however, anxiety about how long the wait will be is transformed into anger about the unfairness of it all. This can lead to a testy—if not explosive—situation, and the service provider is just as likely as the usurper to be the target of the anger.

A simple strategy for avoiding violations of the first-come, first-served (FCFS) queuing policy is the take-a-number arrangement. For example, customers entering a meat market take a number from a dispenser and wait for it to be called. The number currently being served may be displayed so that the new customer can see how long the wait will be. With this simple measure, management has relieved the customer's anxiety over the length of the wait—and the possibility of being treated unfairly. As an ancillary benefit, it also encourages "impulse buying" through allowing the customer to wander about the shop instead of needing to protect a place in line. As equitable as it is, however, this system is not totally free from producing anxiety; it does require the customer to stay alert for the numbers being called or risk losing his or her place in line.

Another simple strategy for fostering FCFS service when there are multiple servers is use of a single queue. Banks, post offices, and airline check-in counters commonly employ this technique. A customer who enters one of these facilities joins the back of the line; the first person in line is served by the next available server. Anxiety is relieved, because there is no fear that later arrivals will "slip" ahead of their rightful place.[5] Often, customers who have been "guaranteed" their place in this way will relax and enjoy a few pleasantries with others in the line. Note that such camaraderie also occupies the customer's empty time and makes the waiting time seem shorter. Queue configurations are examined in more detail later in this chapter.

Not all services lend themselves to such a straightforward prioritization, however. Police service is one example; for obvious reasons, an officer on the way

[5]For a discussion of slips and skips, see Richard C. Larson, "Perspectives on Queues: Social Justice and the Psychology of Queuing," *Operations Research*, vol. 35, no. 6, November–December 1987, pp. 895–905.

to a call about a "noisy dog next door" will change priorities when told to respond to a "robbery-in-progress." In this case, the dispatcher can ameliorate the "noisy-dog" caller's wait anxiety by explaining the department's response policy and providing the caller with a reasonable expectation of when an officer will arrive.

Other services may wish to give preferential treatment to special customers. Consider the express check-in for "high rollers" at Las Vegas hotels, or for first-class passengers at airline check-in counters. Keep in mind, however, that such special "perks" also can engender irritation among the unfavored who are standing in long lines nearby. A management sensitive to the concerns of all its customers will take measures to avoid an image of obvious discrimination. In the example just mentioned, one solution might be to "conceal" the preferential treatment by locating it in an area that is separate from the regular service line.

They Also Serve, Who Sit and Wait

Management must remember that one of the most important parts of its service package is attention to the needs of its customers during the waiting process. The customer who is subjected to unnecessary anxiety or aggravation during this period likely will be a demanding and difficult customer—or, worse, a former customer.

THE ECONOMICS OF WAITING

The economic cost of waiting can be viewed from two perspectives. For a firm, the cost of keeping an employee (i.e., an internal customer) waiting may be measured by unproductive wages. For external customers, the cost of waiting is the forgone alternative use of that time. Added to this are the costs of boredom, anxiety, and other psychological distresses.

In a competitive market, excessive waiting—or even the expectation of long waits—can lead to lost sales. How often have you driven by a filling station, observed many cars lined up at the pumps, and then decided not to stop? One strategy to avoid lost sales is to conceal the queue from arriving customers. In the case of restaurants, this often is achieved by diverting people into the bar, a tactic that frequently results in increased sales. Amusement parks such as Disneyland require people to pay for their tickets outside the park, where they are unable to observe the waiting lines inside. Casinos "snake" the waiting line for nightclub acts through the slot-machine area both to hide its true length and to foster impulsive gambling.

The consumer can be considered a resource with the potential to participate in the service process. For example, a patient who is waiting for a doctor can be asked to complete a medical history record and thereby save valuable physician time (i.e., service capacity). The waiting period also can be used to educate the person about good health habits, which can be achieved by making health publications or filmstrips available. As another example, restaurants are quite innovative in their approaches to engaging the customer directly in providing the service. After giving your order to a waiter in many restaurants, you are asked to go to the salad bar and prepare your own salad, which you eat while the cook prepares your meal.

Consumer waiting may be viewed as a contribution to productivity by permitting greater utilization of limited capacity. The situation of customers waiting in line for a service is analogous to the work-in-process inventory for a manufacturing firm. The service firm actually is inventorying customers to increase the overall efficiency of the process. In service systems, higher utilization of facilities is purchased at the price of customer waiting. Prominent examples can be found in public services such as post offices, medical clinics, and welfare offices, where high utilization is achieved with long queues.

Yoram Barzel reports the following event to illustrate the economic value of waiting[6]:

> On June 14, 1972, the United States of America Bank (of Chicago) launched an anniversary sale. The commodity on sale was money, and each of the first 35 persons could "buy" a $100 bill for $80 in cash. Those farther down the queue could each obtain similar but declining bonuses: the next 50 could gain $10 each; 75, $4 each; 100, $2 each; and the following 100, $1 each. Each of the next 100 persons could get a $2 bill for $1.60 and, finally, 800 (subsequently, it seems, expanded to 1800) persons could gain $0.50 each. The expected waiting time in such an unusual event was unpredictable; on the other hand, it was easy to assess the money value of the commodity being distributed.
>
> First in line were four brothers aged 16, 17, 19, and 24. Because the smallest was 6′2″, their priority was assured. "I figured," said Carl, the youngest brother, "that we spent 17 hours to make a $20 profit. That's about $1.29 an hour."
>
> "You can make better than that washing dishes," added another of the brothers. Had they been better informed they could have waited less time. The 35th person to join the line arrived around midnight, had to wait just 9 hours, and was the last to earn $20—$2.22 per hour. To confirm her right, she made a list of all those ahead of her in the line.
>
> "Why am I here?" she asked. "Well, that $20 is the same as a day's pay to me. And I don't even have to declare it on my income tax. It's a gift, isn't it?"

The experience described above demonstrates that those in line considered their waiting time as the cost of securing a "free" good. While waiting can have a number of economic interpretations, its true cost is always difficult to determine. For this reason, the tradeoff between the cost of waiting and the cost of providing service seldom is made explicit, yet service providers must consider the physical, behavioral, and economic aspects of the consumer waiting experience in their decision making.

ESSENTIAL FEATURES OF QUEUING SYSTEMS

Figure 11.2 depicts the essential features of queuing systems. These are: 1) calling population, 2) arrival process, 3) queue configuration, 4) queue discipline, and 5) service process.

Services obtain customers from a *calling population.* The rate at which they arrive is determined by the *arrival process.* If servers are idle, then the customer is immediately attended; otherwise, the customer is diverted to a queue, which can have various configurations. At this point, some customers may *balk* when confronted with a long or slow-moving waiting line and seek service elsewhere. Other customers, after joining the queue, may consider the delay to be intolera-

[6]Yoram Barzel, "A Theory of Rationing by Waiting," *The Journal of Law and Economics,* vol. 17, no. 1, April 1974, p. 74.

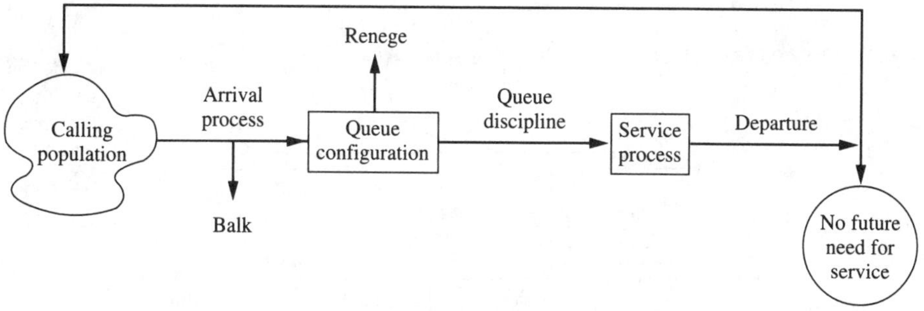

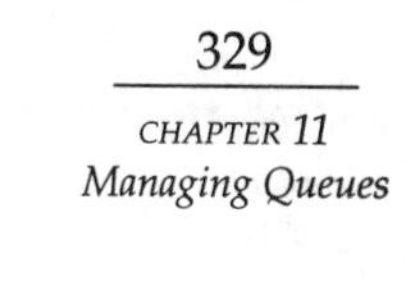

FIGURE 11.2. Queuing system schematic.

ble, and so they *renege,* which means that they leave the line before service is rendered. When a server does become available, a customer then is selected from the queue, and service begins. The policy governing the selection is known as the *queue discipline.* The service facility may consist of no servers (i.e., self-service), one or more servers, or complex arrangements of servers in series or in parallel. After the service has been rendered, the customer departs the facility. At that time, the customer may either rejoin the calling population for future return or exit with no intention of returning.

We shall now discuss in more detail each of these five essential features of queuing systems.

Calling Population

The calling population need not be homogeneous; it may consist of several subpopulations. For example, arrivals at an outpatient clinic can be divided into walk-in patients, patients with appointments, and emergency patients. Each class of patient will place different demands on services, but more important, the waiting expectations of each will differ significantly.

In some queuing systems, the source of calls may be limited to a finite number of people. For example, consider the demands on an office copier by a staff of three secretaries. In this case, the probability of future arrivals depends on the number of persons who currently are in the system seeking service. For instance, the probability of a future arrival becomes zero once the third secretary joins the copier queue. Unless the population is quite small, however, an assumption of independent arrivals or infinite population usually suffices. Figure 11.3 shows a classification of the calling population.

Arrival Process

Any analysis of a service system must begin with a complete understanding of the temporal and spatial distribution of the demand for that service. Typically, data are collected by recording the actual times of arrivals. These data then are used to calculate interarrival times. Many empirical studies indicate that the distribution of interarrival times will be exponential, and the shape of the curve in Figure 11.4 is typical of the exponential distribution. Note the high frequency at the origin and the long tail that tapers off to the right. The exponential distribution also can be recognized by noting that both the mean and the standard deviation are theoretically equal ($\mu = 2.4$ and $\sigma = 2.6$ for Figure 11.4).

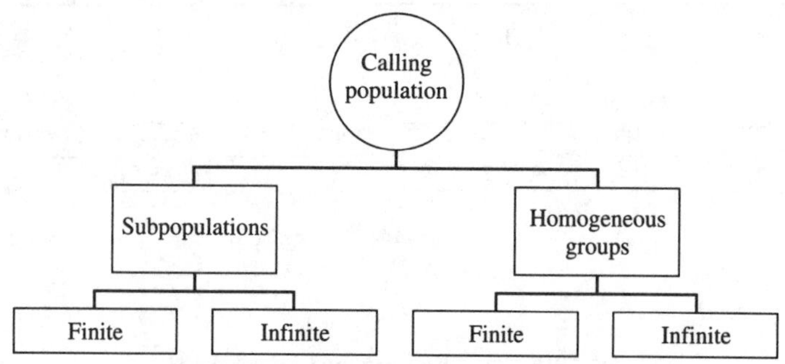

FIGURE 11.3. Classification of calling population.

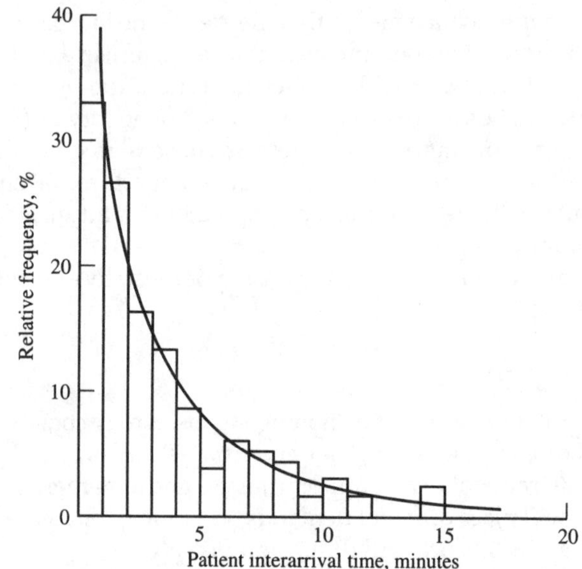

FIGURE 11.4. Distribution of patient interarrival times for a university health clinic.
(E. J. Rising, R. Baron, and B. Averill, "A Systems Analysis of a University Health-Service Outpatient Clinic." Reprinted with permission from Operations Research, *vol. 21, no. 5, Sept.–Oct. 1973, p. 1038, Operations Research Society of America. No further reproduction permitted without the consent of the copyright owner.)*

The exponential distribution has a continuous probability density function of the form

$$f(t) = \lambda e^{-\lambda t} \qquad t \geq 0 \tag{1}$$

where λ = average arrival rate within a given interval of time (e.g., minutes, hours, days),
t = time between arrivals,
e = base of natural logarithms (2.718 . . .),
mean = $1/\lambda$, and
variance = $1/\lambda^2$.

The cumulative distribution function is:

$$F(t) = 1 - e^{-\lambda t} \qquad t \geq 0 \qquad (2)$$

Equation (2) gives the probability that the time between arrivals will be t or less. Note that λ is the inverse of the mean time between arrivals. Thus, for Figure 11.4, the mean time between arrivals is 2.4 minutes, which implies that λ is $1/2.4 = 0.4167$ arrival per minute (i.e., an average rate of 25 patients per hour). Substituting 0.4167 for λ, the exponential distribution for the data displayed in Figure 11.4 is:

$$f(t) = 0.4167e^{-0.4167t} \qquad t \geq 0 \qquad (3)$$

$$F(t) = 1 - e^{-0.4167t} \qquad t \geq 0 \qquad (4)$$

Equation (4) now can be used to find the probability that if a patient has already arrived, another will arrive in the next 5 minutes. We simply substitute 5 for t, and so

$$\begin{aligned} F(5) &= 1 - e^{-0.4167(5)} \\ &= 1 - 0.124 \\ &= 0.876 \end{aligned}$$

Thus, there is an 87.6 percent chance that another patient will arrive in the next 5-minute interval. Test this phenomenon the next time you are waiting in a physician's office

Another distribution, known as the *Poisson distribution,* has a unique relationship to the exponential distribution. The Poisson distribution is a discrete probability function of the form

$$f(n) = \frac{(\lambda t)^n e^{-\lambda t}}{n!} \qquad n = 0, 1, 2, 3, \ldots \qquad (5)$$

where λ = average arrival rate within a given interval of time (e.g., minutes, hours, days),
t = number of time periods of interest (usually $t = 1$),
n = number of arrivals $(0, 1, 2, \ldots)$,
e = base of natural logarithms $(2.718\ldots)$,
mean = λt, and
variance = λt.

The Poisson distribution gives the probability of n arrivals during the time interval t. For the data of Figure 11.4, substituting for $\lambda = 25$, an equivalent description of the arrival process is

$$f(n) = \frac{(25)^n e^{-25}}{n!} \qquad n = 0, 1, 2, 3, \ldots \qquad (6)$$

This gives the probability of 0, 1, 2, . . . patients arriving during any 1-hour interval. Note that we have taken the option of converting $\lambda = 0.4167$ arrival per minute to $\lambda = 25$ arrivals per hour. Equation (6) can be used to calculate the interesting probability that no patients will arrive during a 1-hour interval by substituting 0 for n as shown below:

$$
\begin{aligned}
f(0) &= \frac{(25)^0 e^{-25}}{0!} \\
&= e^{-25} \\
&= 1.4 \times 10^{-11} \text{ which is a very small probability.}
\end{aligned}
$$

Figure 11.5 shows the relationship between the Poisson distribution (i.e., arrivals per hour) and the exponential distribution (i.e., minutes between arrivals). As can be seen, they represent alternative views of the same process. Thus, an exponential distribution of interarrival times with a mean of 2.4 minutes is equivalent to a Poisson distribution of number of arrivals per hour with a mean of 25 (i.e., 60/2.4).

Service demand data often are collected automatically (e.g., by trip wires on highways), and the number of arrivals over a period of time is divided by the number of time intervals to arrive at an average rate per unit of time. The demand rate during the unit of time should be stationary with respect to time (i.e., lambda [λ] is a constant); otherwise, the underlying fluctuations in demand rate as a function of time will not be accounted for. This dynamic feature of demand is illustrated in Figure 11.6 for hours in a day, in Figure 11.7 for days of the week, and in Figure 11.8 for months of the year.

Variation in demand intensity directly affects the requirements for service capacity. When possible, service capacity is adjusted to match changes in demand, perhaps by varying the staffing levels. Another strategy is to smooth demand by asking customers to make appointments or reservations. Differential pricing is used by the telephone company to encourage callers to use off-peak hours, and movie theaters provide ticket discounts for patrons arriving before 6 PM. Smoothing demand and adjusting supply are important topics, which are covered in depth in Chapter 13 "Managing Capacity and Demand." Figure 11.9 presents a classification of arrival processes.

Our discussion has focused on the frequency of demand as a function of time, but the spatial distribution of demand also may vary. This is particularly true of emergency ambulance demand in an urban area, which has a spatial shift in demand resulting from the temporary movements of population from residential areas to commercial and industrial areas during working hours.

FIGURE 11.5. Poisson and exponential equivalence.

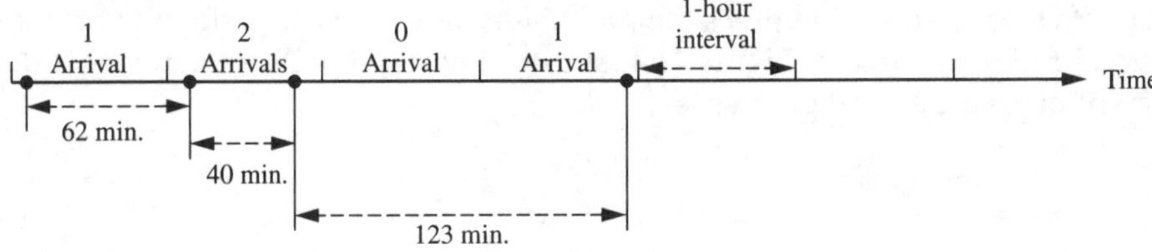

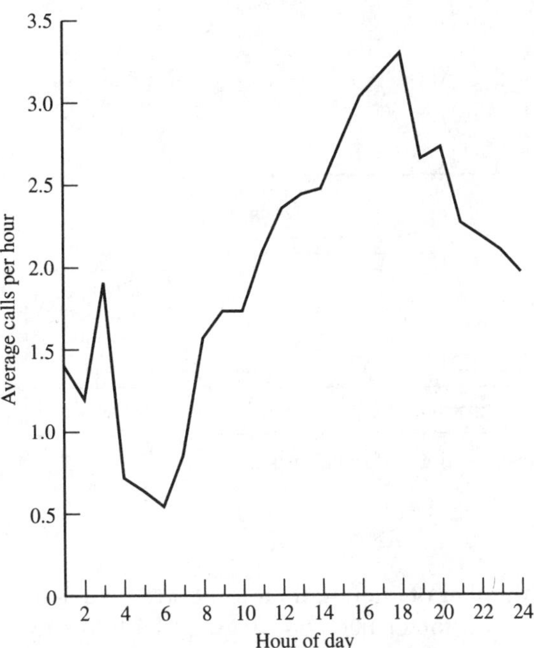

FIGURE 11.6. Ambulance calls by hour of day. *(Reprinted with permission from James A. Fitzsimmons, "The Use of Spectral Analysis to Validate Planning Models,"* Socio-Economic Planning, *vol. 8, no. 3, June 1974, p. 127. Copyright © 1974, Pergamon Press Ltd.)*

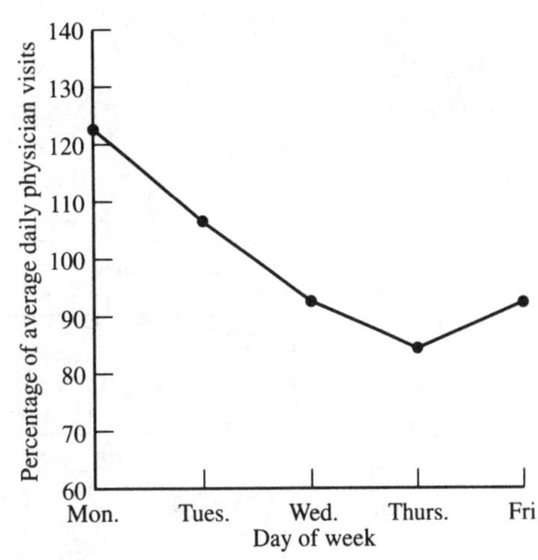

FIGURE 11.7. Patient arrivals at health clinic by day of week. *(E. J. Rising, R. Baron, and B. Averill, "A Systems Analysis of a University Health-Service Outpatient Clinic." Reprinted with permission from* Operations Research, *vol. 21, no. 5, Sept.–Oct. 1973, p. 1035, Operations Research Society of America. No further reproduction permitted without the consent of the copyright owner.)*

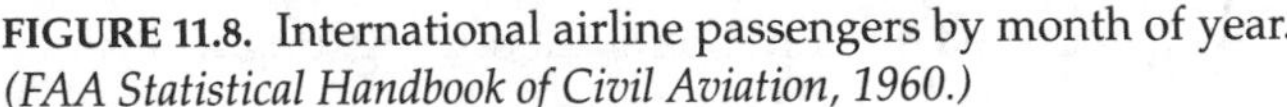
FIGURE 11.8. International airline passengers by month of year. *(FAA Statistical Handbook of Civil Aviation, 1960.)*

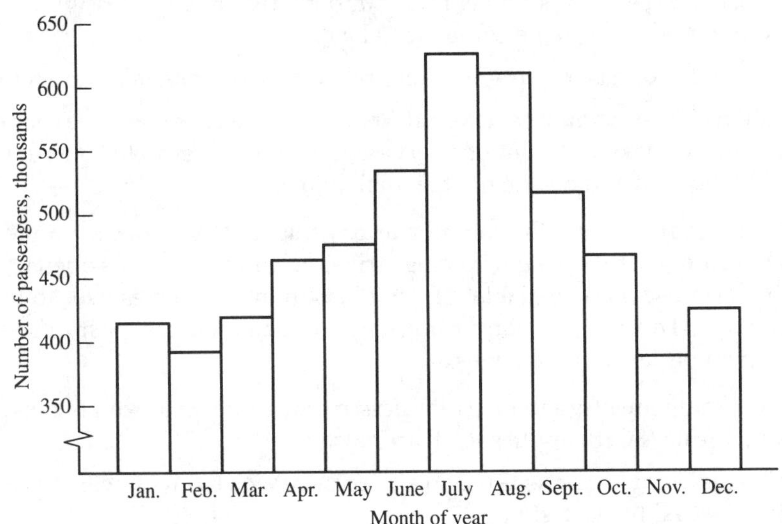

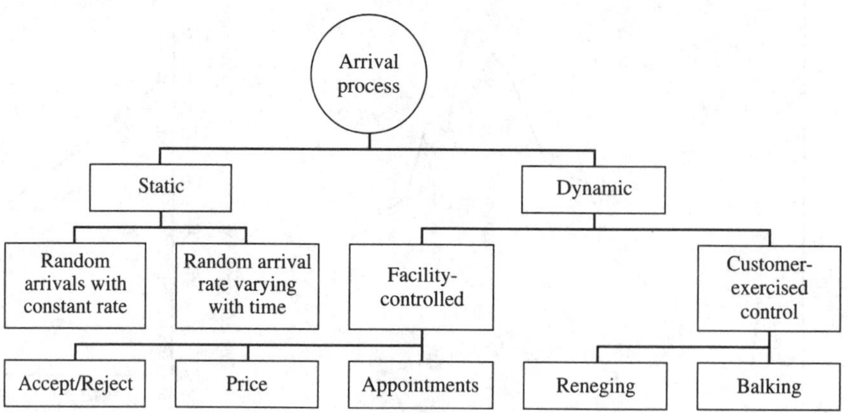

FIGURE 11.9. Classification of arrival processes.

Queue Configuration

Queue configuration refers to the number of queues, their locations, their spatial requirements, and their effects on customer behavior. Figure 11.10 illustrates three alternative waiting configurations for a service, such as a bank, a post office, or an airline counter, where multiple servers are available.

For the multiple-queue alternative shown in Figure 11.10*a*, the arriving customer must decide which queue to join. The decision need not be irrevocable, however, because one may switch to the end of another line. This line-switching activity is called *jockeying*. In any event, watching the line next to you moving faster than your own is a source of aggravation, but the multiple-queue configuration does have the following advantages:

1. The service provided can be differentiated. The use of express lanes in supermarkets is an example. Shoppers with small demands on service can be isolated and processed quickly, thereby avoiding long waits for little service.
2. Division of labor is possible. For example, drive-in banks assign the more experienced teller to the commercial lane.
3. The customer has the option of selecting a particular server of preference.
4. Balking behavior may be deterred. When arriving customers see a long, single queue snaked in front of a service, they often interpret this as evidence of a long wait and decide not to join that line.

Figure 11.10*b* depicts the common arrangement of brass posts with red velvet ropes strung between them, forcing arrivals to join one sinuous queue. Whenever a server becomes available, the first person in line moves over to the service counter. This is a popular arrangement in bank lobbies, post offices, and amusement parks. Its advantages are:

1. The arrangement guarantees fairness by ensuring that a first-come, first-served rule (FCFS) applies to all arrivals.
2. There is a single queue; thus, no anxiety is associated with waiting to see if one selected the fastest line.

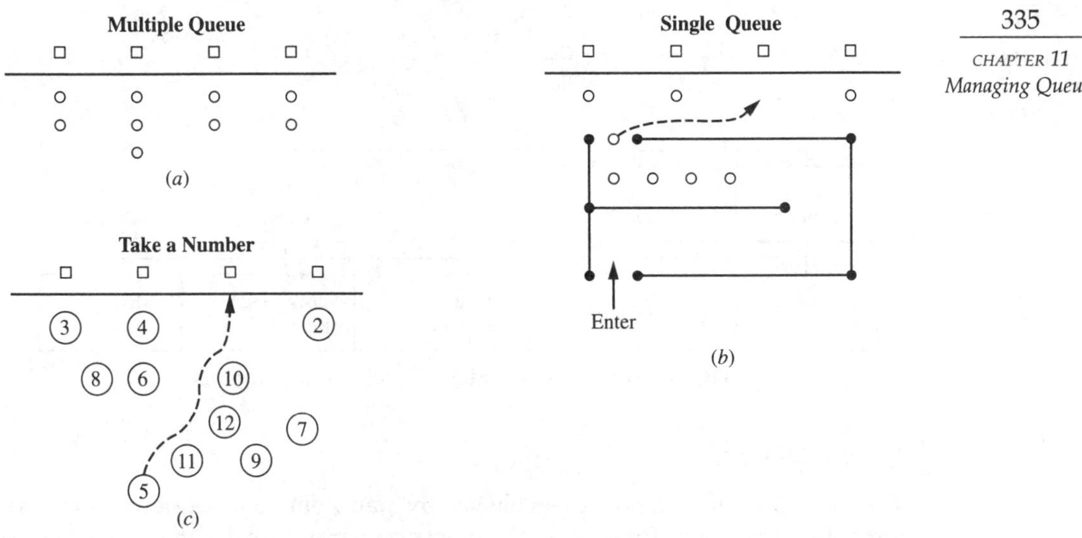

FIGURE 11.10. Alternative waiting-area configurations.

3. With only one entrance at the rear of the queue, the problem of cutting-in is resolved and reneging made difficult.
4. Privacy is enhanced, because the transaction is conducted with no one standing immediately behind the person being served.
5. This arrangement is more efficient in terms of reducing the average time that customers spend waiting in line.

Figure 11.10*c* illustrates a variation on the single queue in which the arriving customer takes a number to indicate his or her place in line. When using such numbers to indicate positions in a queue, there is no need for a formal line. Customers are free to wander about, strike up a conversation, relax in a chair, or pursue some other diversion. Unfortunately, as noted earlier, customers must remain alert to hear their numbers being called or risk missing their turns for service. Bakeries make subtle use of the "take-a-number" system to increase impulse sales. Customers who are given the chance to browse among the tantalizing pastries often find that they purchase more than just the loaf of fresh bread for which they came.

If the waiting area is inadequate to accommodate all customers desiring service, then they are turned away. This condition is referred to as a *finite queue.* Restaurants with limited parking may experience this problem to a certain extent. A public parking garage is a classic example, because once the last stall is taken future arrivals are rejected with the word *FULL* until a car is retrieved.

Finally, concealment of the waiting line itself may deter customers from balking. Amusement parks often process waiting customers by stages. The first stage is a line outside the concession entrance, the second is the wait in an inside vestibule area, and the final stage is the wait for an empty vehicle to convey a party through the attraction. Figure 11.11 shows a classification of queue configurations.

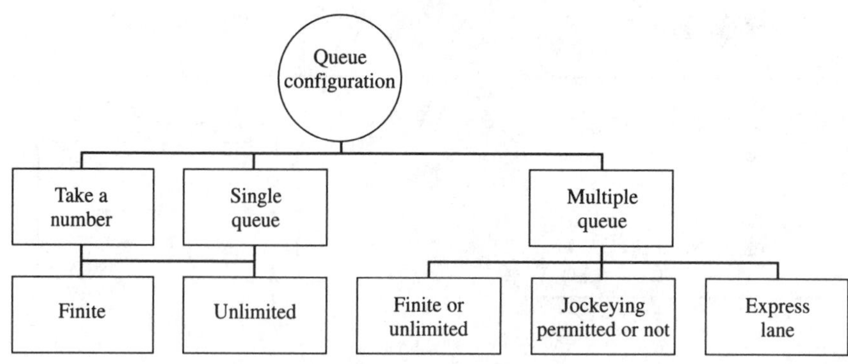

FIGURE 11.11. Classification of queue configurations.

Queue Discipline

The *queue discipline* is a policy established by management to select the next customer from the queue for service. The most popular service discipline is the first-come, first-served (FCFS) rule. This represents an egalitarian approach to serving waiting customers, because all customers are treated alike. The rule is considered to be static, because no information other than position in line is used to identify the next customer for service.

Dynamic queue disciplines are based on some attribute of the customer or status of the waiting line. For example, computer installations typically give first priority to waiting jobs with very short processing times. This shortest-processing-time (SPT) rule has the important feature of minimizing the average time that a customer spends in the system.[7] This rule is seldom used in its pure form, however, because jobs with long operation times would continually be set aside for more recent arrivals with shorter times. By selecting next the job with the shortest service time, excessive delays result for jobs with long service times. Typically, arrivals are placed in priority classes on the basis of some attribute, and the FCFS rule is used within each class. An example is the express checkout counter at supermarkets, where orders of ten or fewer items are processed. This allows large stores to segment their customers and, thereby, compete with the neighborhood convenience stores that provide prompt service. In a medical setting, the procedure known as *triage* is used to give priority to those who would benefit most from immediate treatment.

The most responsive queue discipline is the preemptive priority rule. Under this rule, the service currently in process for a person is interrupted to serve a newly arrived customer with higher priority. This rule usually is reserved for emergency services, such as fire or ambulance service. An ambulance that is on the way to a hospital to pick up a patient for routine transfer will interrupt this mission to respond to a suspected-cardiac-arrest call.

The queue discipline can have an important effect on the likelihood that a waiting customer will renege. For this reason, information on the expected waiting time

[7]R. W. Conway, W. L. Maxwell, and L. W. Miller, *Theory of Scheduling*, Addison-Wesley Publishing Company, Reading, Mass., 1967, p. 27.

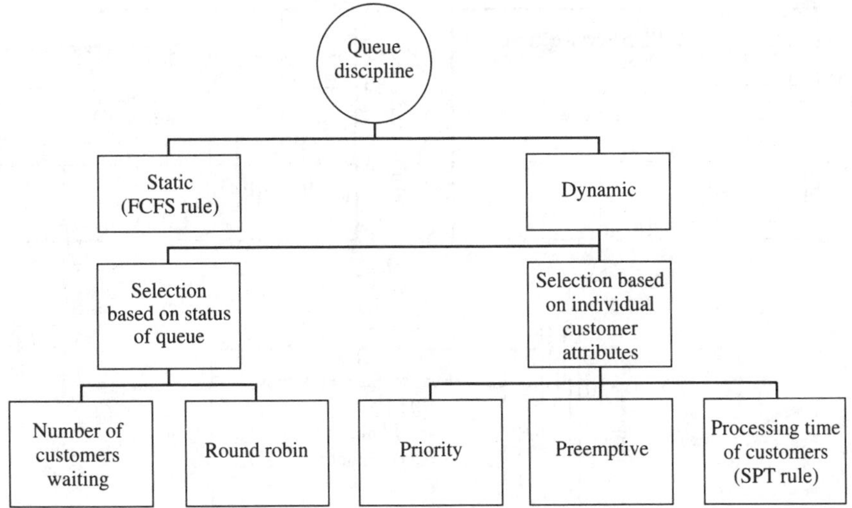

FIGURE 11.12. Classification of queue disciplines.

might be made available to the arriving customer, and updated periodically for each waiting customer. This information usually is available to computer-center users who are interested in the status of their jobs waiting in queue to be processed.

Some fast-food chains (e.g., Wendy's) take a more direct approach to avoid customer reneging. When long lines begin to form, a service person begins to take orders while customers are waiting in line. Taking this idea further is the concept of round-robin service as used by time-shared computer systems. In these systems, a customer is given partial service, and then the server moves on to the next waiting customer. Thus, customers alternate between waiting and being served. Figure 11.12 shows a classification of queue disciplines.

Service Process

The distribution of service times, arrangement of servers, management policies, and server behavior all contribute to service performance. Figure 11.13 contains histograms of several service time distributions in an outpatient clinic, and as the figure shows, the distribution of service times may be of any form. Conceivably, the service time could be a constant, such as the time to process a car through an automated car wash; however, when the service is brief and simple to perform (e.g., preparing orders at a fast-food restaurant, collecting tolls at a bridge, or checking out items at a supermarket), the distribution of service times frequently is exponential (*see* Figure 11.4). The histogram for second-service times, Figure 11.13*c*, most closely approximates an exponential distribution. The second-service times represent those brief encounters in which, for example, the physician prescribes a medication or goes over your test results with you. The distribution of service times is a reflection of the variations in customer needs and server performances.

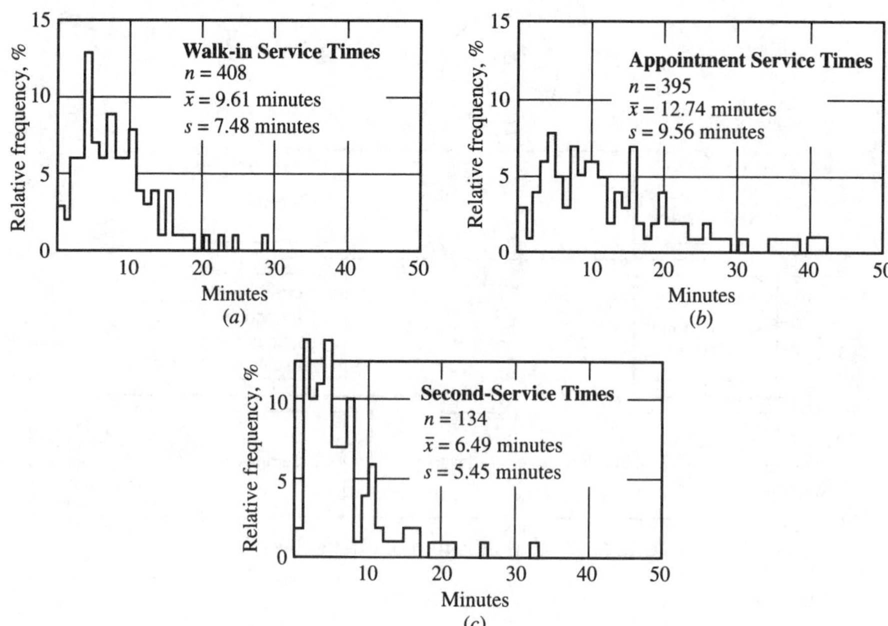

FIGURE 11.13. Histograms of outpatient-clinic service times.
(E. J. Rising, R. Baron, and B. Averill, "A Systems Analysis of a University Health-Service Outpatient Clinic." Reprinted with permission from Operations Research, *vol. 21, no. 5, Sept.–Oct. 1973, p. 1039, Operations Research Society of America. No further reproduction permitted without the consent of the copyright owner.)*

Table 11.1 illustrates the variety of service facility arrangements that are possible. With servers in parallel, management gains flexibility in meeting the variations in demand for service. Management can vary the service capacity effectively by opening and closing service lines to meet changes in demand. At a bank, additional teller windows are opened when the length of queues becomes excessive. Cross-training employees also adds to this flexibility. For example, at supermarkets, stockers often are used as cashiers when lines become long at the check-out counters. A final advantage of parallel servers is that they provide redundancy in case of equipment failures.

The behavior of service personnel toward customers is critical to the success of the organization. Under the pressure of long waiting lines, a server may speed

TABLE 11.1. Service Facility Arrangements

Service Facility	Server Arrangement
Parking lot	Self-service
Cafeteria	Servers in series
Toll booths	Servers in parallel
Supermarket	Self-serve, first stage; parallel servers, second stage
Hospital	Many service centers in parallel and series, not all used by each patient

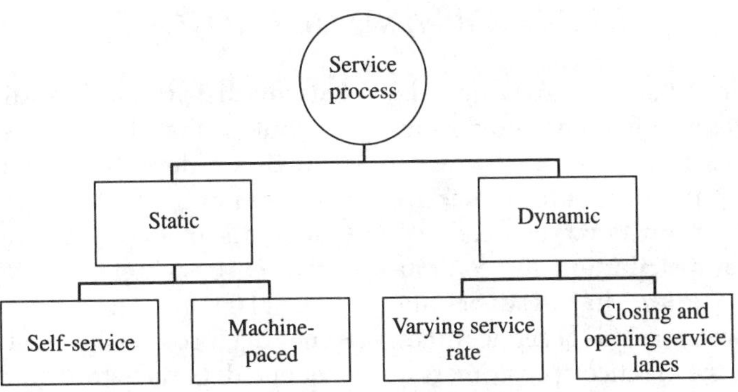

FIGURE 11.14. Classification of service processes.

up and spend less time with each customer; unfortunately, a gracious and leisurely manner then becomes curt and impersonal. Sustained pressure to hurry may increase the rate of customer processing, but it also sacrifices quality. This behavior on the part of a pressured server also can have a detrimental effect on other servers in the system. For example, a busy emergency telephone operator may dispatch yet another patrol car before properly screening the call for its critical nature; in this situation, the operator should have spent more time than usual to ensure that the limited resources of patrol cars were being dispatched to the most critical cases. Figure 11.14 suggests a classification of service processes.

SUMMARY

An understanding of the queuing phenomenon is necessary before creative approaches to the management of service systems can be considered. An appreciation of the behavioral implications of keeping customers waiting reveals that the perception of waiting often is more important than the actual delay. Waiting also has economic implications for both the service firm and its customers.

A schematic queuing model identified the essential features of queuing systems: calling population, arrival process, queue configuration, queue discipline, and service process. An understanding of each feature provides insights and identifies management options for improving customer service.

In Chapter 17, "Queuing Models and Capacity Planning," we will explore applications of several analytical queuing models that are useful for predicting customer waiting times. These models will suggest further insights that will be helpful in capacity planning and scheduling decisions.

KEY TERMS AND DEFINITIONS

Balk occurs when an arriving customer sees a long queue and decides not to seek service.

Calling population source of service customers from a market area.

Exponential distribution the continuous distribution that describes the time between arrivals or service times.

Jockeying the practice of customers in a multiple queue system leaving one queue to join another.

Poisson distribution the discrete distribution that describes random arrivals or departures from a busy server per time interval (e.g., hour).

Queue discipline a rule for selecting the next customer in line to be served (e.g., FCFS).

Reneging occurs when a customer in queue departs before obtaining service.

TOPICS FOR DISCUSSION

1. Suggest some strategies for controlling the variability in service times.
2. Suggest diversions that could make waiting less painful.
3. Select a bad and good waiting experience, and contrast the situations with respect to the aesthetics of the surroundings, diversions, people waiting, and attitude of servers.
4. Suggest ways that service management can influence the arrival times of customers.
5. When the line becomes long at some fast-food restaurants, an employee will walk along the line taking orders. What are the benefits of this policy?

Service Benchmark

Conquering Those Killer Queues

Five o'clock at a Grand Union market in Greenwich Village. One line swelled to five people, then fell back to three. Another hit four, whereupon the woman at the end maneuvered her cart to the next lane just in time to beat out a less dexterous man. Two express lanes stayed steady at two or three deep. It was pretty much what the computer said should happen. Supermarkets have found from research that customers will put up with a line of seven people before getting fed up enough to leave, so many use computers to schedule cashiers.

Grand Union tries to keep lines at no more than three. At its 300-store chain, it has determined three peak periods: 8:30 to 10 AM, 11:30 to 1 PM, and 4:30 to 7 PM. To deal with these bursts, Grand Union, like some others in the business, relies heavily on part-timers. As many as 65 percent of its cashiers are elderly, housewives or high school students who work four hours a day.

Additional help has come from electronic scanners, which Grand Union has installed in about half its stores. All large stores also have at least one express checkout. In May, Grand Union opened a 65,000-square-foot expanse in Kingston, N.Y. It boasts 20 checkouts, six of them express lanes. Two of them are a new concept being tested: the super-express lane, which takes six items or less and only cash. "Our goal is to get people through the cash registers in about five to seven minutes," the Grand Union spokesman said. "That's what we assume is tolerable."

One way to take some of the sting out of waiting is to entertain customers. Since 1959, the Manhattan Savings Bank has offered live entertainment during the frenzied noontime hours. In 13 branches, a pianist performs and one branch has an organ player (Willard Denton, the former Chemical chairman who dreamed up the idea, liked organs, though present management thinks they are a trifle loud for a bank). Occasionally, to make line-waiting even more wonderful, Manhattan Savings has scheduled events such as a fancy-cat exhibit, a pure-bred dog show and a boat show.

Because of all this, Manhattan Savings believes customers endure long waits better than those who go to banks where the only music is the person in front of you grinding his teeth. "At very hectic times, we get very few complaints," said Jean Madsen, a senior vice president.

At hotels and office buildings, mirrors affixed to elevator doors make people less maniacal during waits. Instead of deciding whom to kill, they can comb their hair. A study done by Russel Ackoff showed that hotels that had mirrors received far less grumbling about elevator delays than ones without mirrors.

Just telling people how long they have to wait often cheers them up. Disneyland is sensitive to waiting, since the line for a hot attraction like Star Tours can run to 1,800 people. Like many amusement parks, Disney employs entertainment for waiters, but it is also big on feedback. At various spots along lines, signs give estimated delays from those points. Queuing experts say nothing is worse than the blind waiting familiar to people at bus stops, who don't know if the next bus is one minute or 15 minutes away. Disney's feedback permits parents to weigh odd options: Is it wiser to wait 25 minutes for Mr. Toad's Wild Ride or 30 minutes for Dumbo?

There are lots more tricks to be tried. The Port Authority of New York and New Jersey once figured out that the best way to move cars through the Holland Tunnel was to have stoplights space the cars into clusters of 14. Last year, when PATH train fares rose to $1 from 75 cents, the Port Authority found that lines moved quickest when quarters-only machines collected fares.

Peter Kolesar, a professor of operations research at the Columbia University Business School, thinks there ought to be more efforts to shift demand by altering pricing. Some rail lines, for example, charge less for off-peak trains and restaurants offer early-bird discounts.

During a whimsical moment, Dick Larson speculated that if the average American waited half an hour a day in one line or another, then the population expended 37 billion hours a year in lines. It strikes him, he said, that businesses ought to consider merchandising products to idle waiters to take their minds off pulling out their hair. "Like those flower peddlers outside tunnels and bridges," he said. "They're very shrewd."

Source: N. R. Kleinfield, "Conquering Those Killer Queues," *The New York Times*, September 25, 1988, p. 1.

CASE: THRIFTY CAR RENTAL

Thrifty Car Rental has become one of the U.S. southwest's major rental agencies, even though it competes with several national firms. It definitely is the largest regional company, with offices and outlets in 19 cities and five states, and it primarily operates off-site from the airport terminals of those major cities. Thrifty's rental fleet consists almost entirely of fuel-efficient compact and subcompact automobiles. Its clientele utilizes these vehicles for tourism and business purposes, obtaining service at any location with or without prior arrangements. Thrifty does lose customers on occasion when the desired vehicles are unavailable at a given location, but this "stockout" situation occurs less than 10 percent of the time.

The service counter where customers are processed by Thrifty's personnel has a simple design. In the "old days," it varied only in the number of cubbyholes that keep various forms within easy reach of the servers. Today, the cubbies and forms have given way to computer terminals for more streamlined service. The number of servers varies with the size of the local market and the level of demand at specific times. In smaller markets, Thrifty may need three people at one time behind the counter, but in the largest markets, this number could be as high as eight when demand is heaviest. Usually, these peak-demand times reflect the airport's inbound-outbound flight schedule; as they occur, one or more attendants may deal exclusively with clients who have made prior arrangements to pick up a vehicle or with those who are returning vehicles. When this situation exists, these attendants hang appropriate messages above their chosen stations to indicate their special service functions to clientele. Because the speed of customer service is an important factor in maintaining Thrifty's competitive edge, management and service personnel have worked very hard to ensure that each client is processed without unnecessary delay.

Another important factor in Thrifty's competitive stance is the ability to turn incoming vehicles around and quickly prepare them for new clients. The following steps are necessary to process a vehicle from incoming delivery to outgoing delivery: 1) confirmation of odometer reading, 2) refueling and confirmation of fuel charge, 3) visual damage inspection, 4) priority assessment, 5) interior cleaning, 6) maintenance assessment, 7) maintenance and check-out, 8) exterior cleaning and polishing, 9) refueling and lot storage, and 10) delivery to customer.

When a client returns a vehicle to any location, one of Thrifty's crew will confirm the odometer reading, drive about 200 meters to the service lot, and confirm any fuel charge necessary to refill the car's tank. In some cases, the crew member may be able to process all this information on a hand-held computer, and the customer can be on her or his way without having to queue up in the office. In less streamlined locations, the crew member will relay the information to all attendants immediately so that the client may complete payment inside and be released as soon as possible. (If the crew member notices any interior or exterior damage to the vehicle, the attendant will notify the manager on duty; the client must clarify his or her responsibility in the circumstances and may be delayed while this is occurring.) After the damage-inspection step, the fleet supervisor assigns a priority status to incoming cars on the basis of the company's known (i.e., certain) demand and reserve policy (for walk-up clients): high-priority treatment for cars that are needed within the next 6-hour period, and normal treatment for everything else. High-priority vehicles get preferential treatment for servicing.

After the vehicle's interior is cleaned thoroughly and sprayed with a mild air freshener, a mechanic examines the vehicle's maintenance record, gives the vehicle a test drive, and notes on a form any maintenance actions he or she deems necessary. Thrifty has certain policies covering periodic normal maintenance, such as oil and filter changes, tire rotation and balancing, lubrication, coolant replacement, and engine tune-ups. Major special maintenance actions, such as brake repair, transmission repair or adjustment, or air-conditioning and heating repair, are performed as needed.

Typically, a garage in Thrifty's system has a standard side-by-side, three-bay design: two bays always are used for normal maintenance, and the third is used for either normal or special maintenance. About 20 percent of the time is spent on special maintenance in this third bay. In general, Thrifty uses a team of five mechanics for its garages: one master mechanic (who is the garage manager), two journeymen mechanics, and two apprentices. The apprentices who are responsible for all normal maintenance tasks except the engine tune-up are stationed to service every vehicle in each outside bay, and alternate on vehicles in the middle bay. The journeyman mechanics are responsible for all other maintenance, and they also alternate on servicing vehicles in the middle bay.

After servicing, the vehicle is moved outside to the car wash area, and a team of two people washes, rinses, and buffs the exterior to ensure a good appearance. Because part of the rinse cycle contains a wax-type liquid compound, the vehicle usually does not require a time-consuming wax job. From this point, the vehicle's fuel tank again is topped off, and the vehicle is placed in the lot for storage. When the vehicle is called for by an attendant, a driver will take it to the rental area for the client.

Assignment

On the basis of your experience and the description of Thrifty's operations, describe the five essential features of the queuing systems at the customer counter, the garage, and the car wash.

CASE: EYE'LL BE SEEING YOU[8]

Mrs. F arrives 15 minutes early for a 1:30 PM appointment with her Austin, Texas, ophthalmologist, Dr. X. The waiting room is empty, and all the prior names on the sign-in sheet are crossed out. The receptionist looks up but does not acknowledge her presence. Mrs. F, unaware of the drama about to unfold, happily anticipates that she may not have to wait long beyond her scheduled time and settles into a chair to read the book she has brought with her. Large windows completely surround three sides of the waiting room. The receptionist sits behind a large opening in the remaining wall. Attractive artwork decorates the available wall space, and trailing plants rest on a shelf above the receptionist's opening. It is an appealing, comfortable waiting room.

At 1:25 PM, another patient, Jack, arrives. Mrs. F knows his name must be Jack, because the receptionist addresses him by first name and the two share some light-hearted pleasantries. Jack takes a seat and starts looking through a magazine.

At 1:40 PM, a very agitated woman enters and approaches the receptionist. She explains that she is very sorry she missed her 1 o'clock appointment and asks if it would be possible for Dr. X to see her anyway. The receptionist replies very coldly, "You're wrong. Your appointment was for 11."

"But I have 1 o'clock written down!" responds the patient, whose agitation now has changed to distress.

"Well, you're wrong."

"Oh dear, is there any way I can be worked in?" pleads the patient.

"We'll see. Sit down."

Mrs. F and her two "companions" wait until 1:50 PM, when staff person number 2 (SP2) opens the door between the waiting room and the hallway leading to the various treatment areas. She summons Jack, and they laugh together as she leads him to the back. Mrs. F thinks to herself, "I was here first, but maybe he just arrived late for an earlier appointment," then goes back to her book. Five minutes later, Ms. SP2 appears at the door and summons the distressed patient. At this point, Mrs. F walks to the back area (she's a long-time patient and knows the territory), seeks out Ms. SP2, and says, "I wonder if I've been forgotten. I was here before those two people who have just been taken in ahead of me."

Ms. SP2 replies very brusquely, "Your file's been pulled. Go sit down."

Once again occupying an empty waiting room, Mrs. F returns to her reading. At 2:15 PM (no patient has yet emerged from a treatment area), Ms. SP2 finally summons Mrs. F and takes her to room 1, where she uses two instruments to make some preliminary measurements of Mrs. F's eyes. This is standard procedure in Dr. X's practice. Also standard is measuring the patient's present eyeglass prescription on a third instrument in room 1. Mrs. F extends her eyeglasses to Ms. SP2, but Ms. SP2 brushes past her and says curtly, "This way." Mrs. F then is led to a seat in the "dilating area," although no drops have been put in her eyes to start dilation.

The light in the dilating area is dimmed to protect dilating eyes, but Mrs. F is able to continue reading her book. No one else is seated in the dilating area. At 2:45 PM, Ms. SP2 reappears, says "this way" (a woman of very few words, our Ms. SP2), and marches off to examining room 3. "Wait here," she commands, leaving Mrs. F to seat herself in the darkened room.

Mrs. F can hear Dr. X and Jack laughing in the next examining room. At 2:55 PM, she hears the two men say good-bye and leave the room. Mrs. F expects Dr.

[8]This case, sad to say, is true in its entirety. The names of the physician and his staff have been omitted, not to protect them but because such treatment of patients is so pervasive in the U.S. health care system that it serves no purpose to identify them. We offer the case for two reasons: first, because it is so wonderfully instructive regarding important material in this chapter; and second, because we wish to point out that customers and providers must work together in our emerging service society. Service providers must be sensitive to the needs of customers, and customers must demand and reward good service.

X to enter her room shortly. At 3:15 PM, however, when he still has not appeared, she walks forward and interrupts Ms. SP2, the receptionist, the bookkeeper, and Ms. SP3, who are socializing. "Excuse me, but have I been forgotten?" she asks.

Ms. SP2 turns her head from her companions and replies, "No, he's in the line. Go sit down."

Mrs. F wonders what that means but returns to her assigned place. She is here, after all, for a particular visual problem, not just for a routine check-up.

All good things, however, including Mrs. F's patience and endurance of abusive treatment, eventually end. At 4:00 PM, Mrs. F does some marching of her own—to the front desk, where she announces to the assembled Mss. SP1 through SP4 that she has been waiting since 1:30 PM, that she has been sitting in the back for 2½ hours, and that not once during that time has one member of the staff come to let her know what the problem is, how much longer she can expect to wait, or, indeed, that she has not been forgotten. She adds that she will wait no longer, and she feels forced to seek the services of a physician who chooses to deliver health care. There are several patients seated in the waiting room at the time.

There is an epilogue to this case. Mrs. F went directly home and wrote the following letter to Dr. X informing him of the treatment she had (not) received at his office and stating that she and her family would seek care elsewhere:

____

____

January 5, 1989

________, M.D.
Austin, Texas

Dear Dr. ______:

It is with very real regret that I am transferring our eye care to another physician, and I want you to know the reason for my decision.

It is 4:22 PM, and I have just returned home from a 1:30 PM appointment with(out) you. The appointment was made because I had received an adverse report from Seton Hospital's recent home vision test. I was kept waiting in the dilation area and in examining room 3 for more than two-and-one-half hours, during which time not one single member of your staff gave me any explanation for the delay or assured me I had not been forgotten. When I finally asked if I were forgotten, I was treated with a very bad attitude ("how dare I even ask!") and still was given no reason for the delay or any estimate of how much longer I would have to wait. Consequently, I left without seeing you.

As I stated above, I make this change with very real regret, because I value your expertise and the treatment you personally have given the four of us during these past many years. But I will not tolerate the callous treatment of your staff.

Sincerely yours,

Mrs. __________

Questions

1. In this chapter, we referred to Maister's First and Second Laws of Service. How do they relate to this case?

2. What features of a good waiting process are evident in Dr. X's practice? List the shortcomings that you see.

3. Do you think that Mrs. F is typical of most people waiting for a service? How so? How not?

4. If Dr. X were concerned with keeping the F family as patients, how could he have responded to Mrs. F's letter? Write a letter on Dr. X's behalf to Mrs. F.

5. How could Dr. X prevent such incidents in the future?

6. List constructive ways in which customers can respond when services fall seriously short of their requirements or expectations.

SELECTED BIBLIOGRAPHY

BARZEL, YORAM: "A Theory of Rationing by Waiting," *The Journal of Law and Economics,* vol. 17, no. 1, April 1974, pp. 73–94.

DAVIS, MARK M., and M. J. MAGGARD: "An Analysis of Customer Satisfaction with Waiting Times in a Two-Stage Service Process," *Journal of Operations Management,* vol. 9, no. 3, August 1990, pp. 324–334.

KATZ, K. L., B. M. LARSON, and R. C. LARSON: "Prescription for the Waiting-in-Line Blues: Entertain, Enlighten, and Engage," *Sloan Management Review,* vol. 32, no. 2, Winter 1991, pp. 44–53.

LARSON, RICHARD C.: "Perspectives on Queues: Social Justice and the Psychology of Queuing," *Operations Research*, vol. 35, no. 6, November–December 1987, pp. 895–905.

———: "There's More to a Line Than Its Wait," *Technology Review*, July 1988, pp. 61–67.

MAISTER, D. H.: "The Psychology of Waiting Lines," in J. A. Czepiel, M. R. Solomon, and C. F. Surprenant (eds.), *The Service Encounter*, Lexington Press, Lexington, Mass., 1985, pp. 113–123.

RISING, E. J., R. BARON, and B. AVERILL: "A Systems Analysis of a University Health-Service Outpatient Clinic," *Operations Research*, September 1973, pp. 1030–1047.

SCHWARTZ, BARRY: *Queuing and Waiting*, University of Chicago Press, Chicago, 1975.

SMITH, HEDRICK: *The Russians*, Quadrangle Press, New York, 1975.

TAYLOR, SHIRLEY: "Waiting for Service: The Relationship Between Delays and Evaluations of Services," *Journal of Marketing*, vol. 58, April 1994, pp. 56–69.

CHAPTER 12

Managing Facilitating Goods

LEARNING OBJECTIVES

After completing this chapter, you should be able to:

1. Discuss the role of information technology in the management of inventory.
2. Describe the function, characteristics, and costs of an inventory system.
3. Determine the order quantity for various inventory applications.
4. Determine the reorder point and safety stock for inventory systems with uncertain demand.
5. Design a continuous or periodic review inventory-control system.
6. Conduct an ABC analysis of inventory items.
7. Use either expected value or incremental analysis to determine the order quantity for the single-period inventory model.
8. Describe the rationale behind the retail discounting model.

All agree that well-stocked shelves make happy customers, but do well-stocked shelves make providers happy as well? Consider a pharmacy with a shelf-full of a particular prescription medicine. If all of that medicine does not sell quickly, the pharmacy may have a shelf-full of medication that has passed its expiration date and no longer can be sold. The obvious dilemma is to match "stores-on-hand" to demand. The pharmacy certainly does not want to turn away sick customers because it is out of the requested medicine; on the other hand, it also does not want to incur the losses that result from an inventory of out-of-date medicine.

In the "old" days, inventory management required workers to monitor sales and stock-on-hand, then to mail or phone orders for new supplies when it "seemed" to be advisable. This system frequently resulted in excess inventories or stockouts (i.e., the empty-shelf syndrome). Information management, however, has transformed inventory management into a process allowing the service to meet customer demands without incurring the expense of excess inventory. Use of computer-based information systems in inventory management represents one of the earliest and most successful applications of information technology. All of us are familiar with the bar codes, as shown in Figure 12.1, that are found on nearly every inventory item purchased in retail stores. The bar code supplies information that allows management to track where inventory is located and how fast it is moving. For example, most supermarkets use computerized inventory systems to maintain automatically records of inventory balances based on point-of-sale (POS) scanning of the bar codes on items. When stock levels are depleted (or reach a predetermined reorder point), a purchase order to a preapproved vendor is initiated automatically using electronic data interchange (EDI). When the order is received, the inventory balance is adjusted accordingly. Such use of information technology saves costs by avoiding paperwork, facilitating cash management, and creating a system that responds quickly to inventory needs among suppliers, service providers, and customers.

Clearly, few service enterprises can eliminate inventories of goods and supplies entirely. Auto parts stores must have a reserve of motor oil and commonly used parts to meet daily demand. A Pizza Hut restaurant must have a reserve of cheese and other food items. A document-copying business must have stores of

FIGURE 12.1. Bar code applications.

Bar code printed on a 20 ounce can of Hunt's Big John's Beans 'n Fixin's

Bar code stapled to an eight foot length of 1" × 2"

paper, printer ink, and toner, and your community's fire department must have a ready supply of fuel for its trucks. Because such inventories of goods often represent large capital investments, we must have effective ways of managing them. Keeping track of a wide variety of items (i.e., stock-keeping units [SKUs]), both those on hand and those that should be ordered, as well as when they should be ordered is a significant challenge for management, and it requires a knowledge of inventory theory.

CHAPTER PREVIEW

Managing the facilitating goods component of a service package involves cost tradeoffs, customer service, and information systems. This chapter begins with a discussion of the role of inventory in services, its characteristics, and costs. A fundamental inventory management question concerns what quantity to order, and order quantity models are developed for various inventory applications.

When to place an order (called a *reorder point*) is another inventory management question. This decision is complicated when services are faced with uncertain demand and, thus, the need for safety stocks to protect against stockouts. The continuous review system and the periodic review system are computer information systems for implementing these decisions. Design parameters for each of these systems are developed with illustrations. The ABC classification of inventory items is used to identify which computer inventory system to install.

The chapter concludes with a discussion of two special inventory situations. For perishable goods, a model is developed to identify the optimal order quantity to balance the opportunity cost of underestimating demand with the lost investment in inventory resulting from overestimating demand. Finally, a retail discounting model is proposed to determine the discount price for items that are not selling to generate cash to buy more popular goods.

INVENTORY THEORY

Inventory theory covers several aspects of the inventory of goods and supplies, including the role that inventory plays in the operation of a service, the characteristics of various inventory systems, and the costs that are involved in maintaining inventories.

Role of Inventory in Services

Inventories serve a variety of functions in service organizations, such as decoupling the stages in the distribution cycle, accommodating a heavy seasonal demand, and maintaining a supply of materials as a hedge against anticipated increases in their cost. We will look at these and other functions in more detail later; first, we will examine the inventory distribution system.

- *Decoupling inventories.* Consider the system depicted in Figure 12.2. Two types of flow exist within the system. One is the flow of information beginning with the customer and proceeding back to the original source(s) of the goods or service, and the other is the actual movement of goods—in this case, from the producer to the customer—by way of inventory reserves at each stage of the system.

Following the diagram, we see that the customer makes a demand, and for the purposes of our analysis, we will consider this demand to be a random variable with an associated probability distribution. When, for example, demand for a box of cereal occurs at a grocery retailer, the item is withdrawn from the available stock (either on the shelf or in the retailer's inventory). As the demand continues, the stock must be replenished, and an order is placed with the distributor. From the time the order is made until it is received, however, the available stock continues to decline. This interval is called the *replenishment lead time,* and it may vary from a day to a week or even more. It also may vary from one order period to another. This flow of information originating with the customer's demand is directed in turn along the distribution channel to the producer.

If we follow the movement of the item itself, we see that it makes its way through the distribution channel with stops at the various inventory sites where it is held in readiness for the next leg of its journey to the customer. Each of these inventory stages serves as a buffer, allowing each organization in the interdependent system to operate somewhat independently and without interruption. Here, we can see the *decoupling function* of inventory systems. The retailer, distributor, wholesaler, and factory are stages in the system, and a stockout at any stage would have immediate and drastic consequences for the others. Inventories, however, decouple these stages and help to avoid expensive interruptions of service.

- *Seasonal inventories.* Some services involve significant seasonal demands. Consider toy stores and the year-end holidays, camping-gear retailers and summer vacation time, or garden-supply stores and spring planting time.

FIGURE 12.2. Inventory distribution system.

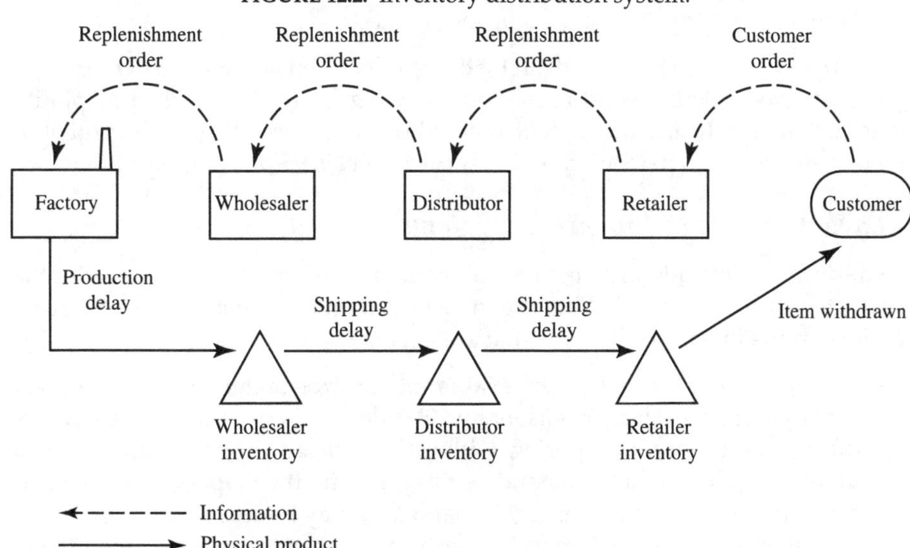

Services that experience such cyclical high-demand times may accumulate large inventories in advance of the high-demand season to accommodate their customers.

- *Speculative inventories.* A service that anticipates a significant increase in the cost of a good in which it deals may find it more economical to accumulate and maintain a large inventory at present prices rather than to replenish its supplies after the increase. The strategy of maintaining a speculative inventory is known as *forward buying*. The reverse of this strategy occurred in the spring of 1996, when U.S. oil companies anticipated the reentry of Iraq into the international petroleum market, which would decrease the market value of the resource. These companies did not want to have huge reserves of "pre-Iraq" expensive oil when the world price dropped; therefore, they allowed their reserves (i.e., their inventory) to decline drastically—*forward hedging!*
- *Cyclical inventories.* The term *cyclical inventory* refers to normal variations in the level of inventories. In other words, the level of stock in inventory is at its highest just after an order is received, and it declines to its lowest point just before a new order is received.
- *In-transit inventories.* The term *in-transit inventories* is used for stock that has been ordered but has not yet arrived.
- *Safety stocks.* An effective service maintains an inventory of stock that will meet expected demand. Services operate in a dynamic environment, however, which means that uncertainties in replenishment lead time and demand always exist. To deal with such unexpected fluctuations, many services maintain inventory in excess of the inventory that is kept to meet the expected demand. This excess inventory is referred to as *safety stock.*

Inventory management is concerned with three basic questions:

1. What should be the *order quantity?*
2. When should an order be placed (called a *reorder point*)?
3. How much *safety stock* should be maintained?

Later, we will see that determining the reorder point is related to determining the safety stock. Both are influenced by the *service level,* which is the probability that all demand during the replenishment lead time is met (e.g., if the probability of a stockout is 5 percent, then the service level is 95 percent).

Characteristics of Inventory Systems

To design, implement, and manage an inventory system, we must consider the characteristics of the stocks that are to be stored and understand the attributes of the various inventory systems that are available.

- *Type of customer demand.* When evaluating the type of demand, we first look for any trends, cycles, or seasonality. Has demand been increasing steadily during the observation period without significant drops, or do we see a monthly cycle in which demand begins high and then tapers off by the end of the month? As noted earlier, demand also may be seasonal.

  Other attributes of demand also are important to consider. Demand may occur in discrete units, such as the number of scuba-diving masks sold per day. It also may be continuous, such as gallons of water consumed, or bulk, such as passengers on an airline flight. If final customer demand can be described as a probability distribution, it is referred to as *independent demand,* and we then can forecast future demand. In other cases, the demand for one type of inventory item may be related to the demand for another; for example, the demand for catsup at McDonald's restaurant is dependent on the number of hamburgers and french fries that are sold. This type of demand is called *dependent demand.*

- *Long-term planning.* Management must consider whether it will stock an inventory of a particular item indefinitely or if the need for the item is temporary. For example, a hospital will always need tanks of oxygen, but a sports clothing retailer will not need an endless supply of Atlanta Olympics sweatshirts.
- *Replenishment lead time.* The replenishment lead time has an obvious impact on inventory needs. If we expect a relatively long time between placing an order and receiving it, we must carry a larger inventory than if we anticipate a short lead time, especially when critical items are involved. If lead time is stochastic with an associated probability distribution, we may be able to use this information to determine our inventory needs during the lead time.
- *Constraints and relevant inventory costs.* Some constraints are straightforward. For example, available storage space determines the maximum amount of goods that can be stored, and the "shelf life" of a good likewise may limit the number of perishable items that can be held in inventory. Other constraints are more complex, such as the costs of maintaining an inventory, and there are obvious costs such as the capital expenditures for the storage facility, be it a warehouse or a walk-in refrigerator. Items held in inventory also represent a capital expenditure (i.e., they represent an opportunity cost of capital). Other costs include those of personnel and the maintenance required to manage the inventory as well as "incidentals" such as insurance and taxes on the inventoried assets. Yet another cost to consider is that of overcoming existing constraints (e.g., what would it cost to expand the size of the warehouse or refrigerator?).

Relevant Costs of an Inventory System

The performance of an inventory system usually is gauged by its average annual cost. Relevant costs to be considered include holding costs, ordering costs, stockout costs, and the purchase cost of the items; Table 12.1 provides a detailed listing of the sources of these costs. The inventory holding cost is the cost that varies directly with the number of items held in stock. The opportunity cost associated with capital tied up in inventory is a major component of the holding cost. Other components are insurance cost, obsolescence cost, deterioration cost, and direct handling cost. The ordering cost is the cost that varies directly with the number of orders that are placed. Order preparation, transportation, receiving, and inspection on arrival are major contributors to the ordering cost of purchases from suppliers. The stockout cost varies directly with the number of units out of stock, and this cost includes the margin on a lost sale and the potential loss of future sales. The purchase cost of the item can be a function of the order size when quantity discounts are offered by the supplier.

TABLE 12.1 Inventory Management Costs

Ordering costs
- Preparing specifications for items to be purchased
- Locating or identifying potential suppliers and soliciting bids
- Evaluating bids and selecting suppliers
- Negotiating prices
- Preparing purchase orders
- Issuing or transmitting purchase orders to outside suppliers
- Following up to ensure purchase orders are received by suppliers

Receiving and inspection costs
- Transportation, shipping, and pick-up
- Preparing and handling records of receipts and other paperwork
- Examining packages for visible damage
- Unpacking items
- Counting or weighing items to ensure the correct amount has been delivered
- Withdrawing samples and transmitting them to inspection and testing organizations
- Inspecting or testing items to ensure they conform to purchase specifications
- Transferring items into storage areas

Holding or carrying costs
- Interest charges on money invested in inventories
- Opportunity cost of capital tied up in inventory items, warehouses, and other parts of the inventory system
- Taxes and insurance
- Moving items into and out of inventory stores, and keeping records of the movements
- Theft or pilferage
- Providing security systems for protecting inventories
- Breakage, damage, and spoilage
- Obsolescence of parts and disposal of out-of-date materials
- Depreciation
- Storage space and facilities (size usually is based on maximum rather than average inventories)
- Providing controlled environments of temperature, humidity, dust, etc.
- Managing (tasks such as supervising stores personnel, taking physical inventory periodically, verifying and correcting records, etc.)

Shortage costs
- Lost sales and profits
- Customer dissatisfaction and ill-will; lost customers
- Penalties for late delivery or nondelivery
- Expediting orders to replenish exhausted stock

In the following section, we will develop models that determine the appropriate size of the order quantity based on minimizing the total annual cost of the inventory system.

ORDER QUANTITY MODELS

Many different models have been developed to answer the question: How much do we order? All these models use relevant inventory costs as the criteria for

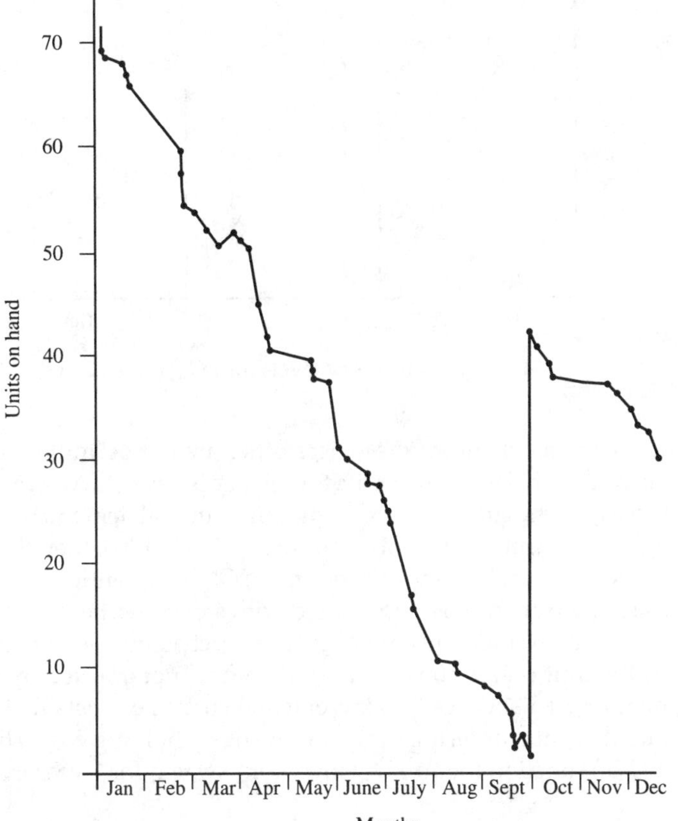

FIGURE 12.3. Actual stock record for an auto part.

gauging performance; however, each is based on a particular inventory situation that is best described by a plot of inventory level versus time. Figure 12.3 shows the actual stock record (i.e., inventory behavior) during a year for an item at an auto parts store. As shown, the demand rate can be considered to be approximately constant; thus, replenishment orders (40 units in this case) can be placed to arrive when units on hand approach zero but still are sufficient to avoid a stockout.

The inventory stock behavior over time is modeled to account for the costs both of holding and of ordering inventory over a typical year. Using calculus, the functional form of the inventory costs is differentiated to arrive at an optimal value for the order quantity, which is referred to as Q^*. The best-known inventory model is a simple formula to determine an economic order quantity for purchased lots.

Economic Order Quantity

The simple *economic order quantity (EOQ)* model, which assumes a constant rate of demand and no stockouts, is a surprisingly accurate model for retail grocery items such as sugar, flour, and other staples. In this situation, demand appears to be constant, because a large number of customers make periodic purchases in

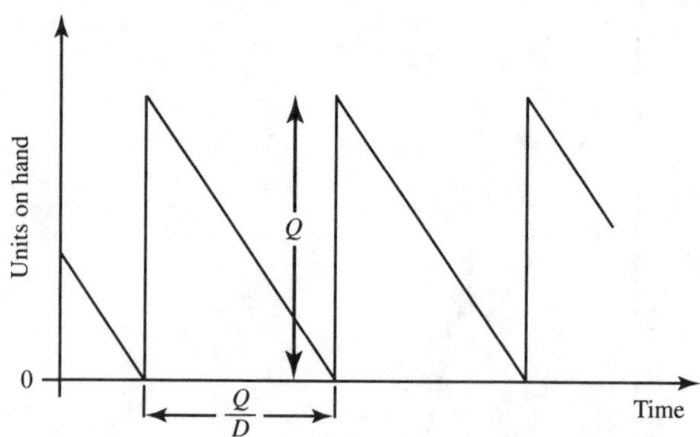

FIGURE 12.4. Inventory levels for *EOQ* model.

small amounts and stockouts of these necessities are not permitted. Figure 12.4 depicts the inventory balances over time for this simple system, with a cycle being repeated every Q/D fraction (i.e., order quantity/annual demand) of a year. For example, if Q is 100 units and the annual demand D is 1200, then the cycle will be repeated each month. We want to determine Q^*, the quantity that minimizes relevant costs. There are no costs associated with stockouts, because they do not occur. Also, we will exclude the annual cost of purchasing the item, because we assume that the unit cost is constant and, therefore, not affected by the size of the order quantity. This leaves two incremental costs (i.e., costs that vary with the order quantity): the ordering cost and inventory holding cost. The *total cost purchase lot* (TC_p) function for an *EOQ* inventory system for 1 year is:

$$TC_p = \text{ordering cost } \textit{plus} \text{ average holding cost} \tag{1}$$

We can express equation (1) in a more usable form. First, we define some notation:

D = demand in units per year,
H = holding cost in dollars per unit per year,
S = cost of placing an order in dollars per order, and
Q = order quantity in units.

Note that D and H must be in same time units (e.g., months, years).

The annual ordering cost is easy to derive. Because all demand D must be satisfied with orders of size Q, then D/Q orders are placed annually. Each time an order is placed, it costs S dollars, and this results in an annual ordering cost of $S(D/Q)$. The annual cost to hold inventory also is straightforward. If one unit is kept in inventory for 1 year, the holding cost is H dollars. From Figure 12.4, the maximum inventory balance is Q, whereas the minimum balance is zero. This gives an average inventory level of $Q/2$ units. Thus, the annual inventory holding cost becomes $H(Q/2)$.

We now can rewrite the relevant annual cost of the inventory system with purchase lots as

$$TC_p = S(D/Q) + H(Q/2) \tag{2}$$

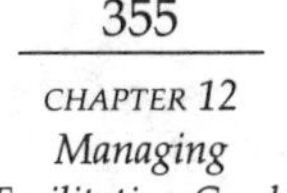

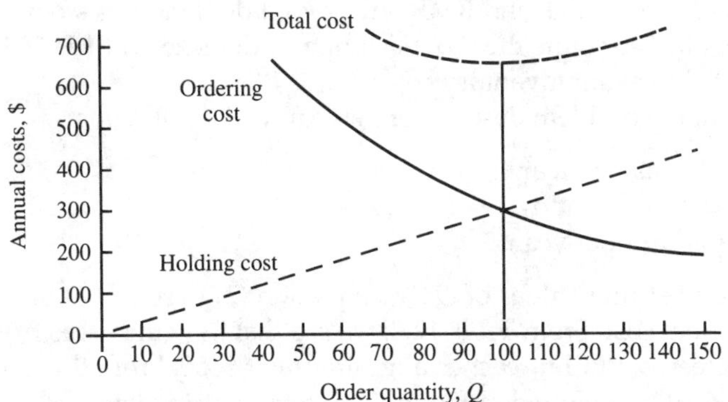

FIGURE 12.5. Relevant annual costs for *EOQ* model.

As Figure 12.5 shows, both the holding cost and the ordering cost change with different values of Q, and the total cost curve is shaped as a shallow bowl. Thus, there is a unique value of Q that gives a minimum total annual cost for the inventory system. This value, of course, is the *EOQ*; however, other nearby values of Q are only slightly more costly.

There are several ways to determine *EOQ*. For example, we can take the derivative of equation (2) with respect to Q, set the derivative equal to zero, and solve for *EOQ*.[1] There is another, easier way to solve for *EOQ*, however. Observe that the minimum of TC_p occurs where the ordering cost equals the inventory holding cost. Therefore, we can equate the two costs and solve for *EOQ*.

$$S(D/Q) = H(Q/2)$$

$$Q^2 = 2DS/H$$

$$EOQ = \sqrt{\frac{2DS}{H}} \qquad (3)$$

Example 12.1: Rocky Mountain Power—EOQ

Rocky Mountain Power (RMP) maintains an inventory of spare parts that is valued at nearly $8 million. This inventory is composed of thousands of different stock-keeping units (SKUs) used for power generation and utility line maintenance, and the inventory balances are updated on a computerized information system.

Glass insulators (i.e., SKU 1341) have a relatively stable usage rate, averaging 1000 items per year. RMP purchases these insulators from the manufacturer at a cost of $20 per unit delivered to the Denver warehouse. An order for replenishment is placed whenever the inventory balance reaches a predetermined reorder point. The cost that is associated with placing an order is estimated to be $30. This includes the cost of order processing, receiving, and distribution to outlying substations.

An estimate of the annual inventory holding cost for SKU 1341 is $6 per unit. This holding cost represents a 30 percent opportunity cost of capital.

[1] $dTC_p/dQ = -DS/Q^2 + H/2 = 0$; thus $Q^2 = 2DS/H$, and $Q^* = \sqrt{2DS/H}$.

SKU 1341 is essential, and RMP must avoid depleting its stock of this item. We want to determine the replenishment order size for SKU 1341 that minimizes the relevant inventory costs.

From the problem description, we know the following:

$D = 1000$ units per year,
$S = \$30$ per order, and
$H = \$6$ per unit per year.

We can substitute values of Q into equation (2) to see what happens to the total annual cost. From Table 12.2, we see that as Q increases from 70 units, TC_p decreases, until it reaches a minimum at \$600. From this point on, TC_p increases. When plotted in Figure 12.5, these values demonstrate the bowl-shaped total annual cost curve. Of course, we can calculate the EOQ directly by using equation (3), which gives:

$$EOQ = \sqrt{\frac{2DS}{H}}$$

$$EOQ = \sqrt{\frac{2(1000)(30)}{6}}$$

$$= 100 \text{ units}$$

The annual relevant cost when $Q^* = 100$ units, as shown in Table 12.2, is \$600 equally divided between ordering cost and holding cost. Nearby values of Q could be considered as being more appropriate, however. For example, an order of 120 units (10 boxes of a dozen each) has a TC_p exceeding the EOQ by only \$10 per year.

Inventory Model with Quantity Discounts

Suppliers have their own interest in the size of the order quantity. Production runs cost money to set up and often result in an economical batch size. For example, the time and effort that are necessary to make a batch of four dozen

TABLE 12.2. Tabulation of Inventory Costs

Order Quantity (Q)	Order Cost, \$30	Inventory Holding Cost, \$6	Total Cost (TC_p)
70	428.57	210.00	638.57
80	375.00	240.00	615.00
90	333.33	270.00	603.33
100	300.00	300.00	600.00
110	272.73	330.00	602.73
120	250.00	360.00	610.00
130	230.77	390.00	620.77

chocolate chip cookies is not much more than for baking a batch of one dozen. Similarly, manufacturing firms have an interest in encouraging customers to buy in full batch sizes. Further, savings in transportation costs are available to shippers who require a full truckload instead of a less-than-full truckload. Offering a per-unit price discount to customers who order in large quantities permits the savings in manufacture and transportation to be shared between both parties. Very often, the price break occurs at an order quantity much larger than the customer's EOQ. Thus, a tradeoff occurs between a savings on the cost of purchasing the inventory and the expense of holding a larger-than-desired quantity. To study this tradeoff, we must recognize that the price of the item now is a variable and must be included in the total annual cost function. Thus, our TC_p equation (2) is modified by adding the purchase cost, and this new equation is called *total cost with quantity discounts* (TC_{qd}).

$$\text{Total Cost} = \text{Purchase Cost} + \text{Ordering Cost} + \text{Holding Cost}$$

$$TC_{qd} = CD + S(D/Q) + I(CQ/2) \tag{4}$$

where C = unit cost of item in dollars and I = annual inventory holding cost expressed as a percentage of the cost of the item (note that $IC = H$).

To demonstrate the trade-off analysis in the evaluation of a quantity discount offer, we return to the Rocky Mountain Power example.

Example 12.2: Rocky Mountain Power—Quantity Discount Problem

The supplier of the glass insulators, SKU 1341, is negotiating with RMP to place replenishment order quantities in lots greater than the current 100-unit size. The following quantity discount schedule has been proposed:

Order Quantity	Unit Price ($)
1–239	20.00
240–599	19.50
≥600	18.75

How should RMP respond? Because the price of the item now varies with the order quantity, the appropriate inventory cost model now becomes equation (4), using $I = 30$ percent. How does one proceed, however, to use equation (4) to determine the order quantity that minimizes the total annual inventory cost, which now includes the purchase cost as well as the ordering and holding costs? Figure 12.6 illustrates one option, which is plotting the total cost as a function of order quantity and noting the lowest point of the resulting *discontinuous* curve (in this case, at the price break of 240 units).

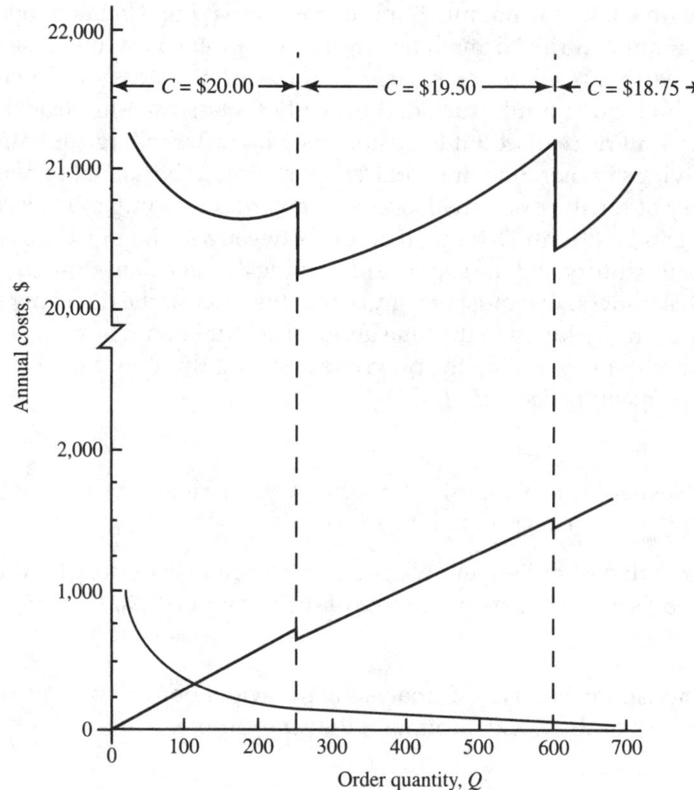

FIGURE 12.6. Annual costs for the quantity discount model.

We can arrive at this same conclusion, however, using the following analytical steps:

1. Compute *EOQ* for the *lowest* price per unit, substituting $IC = H$ in equation (3):

$$EOQ = \sqrt{\frac{2DS}{IC}}$$

$$= \sqrt{\frac{2(1000)(30)}{(.30)(18.75)}}$$

$= 103$, but the price of \$18.75 is appropriate only for $EOQ \geq 600$.

2. If the *EOQ* falls outside the appropriate price range (as occurred in the last paragraph), then we recalculate *EOQ* for the next lowest price and proceed until the *EOQ* is found in the appropriate price range. Therefore, we recalculate the *EOQ* for a price of \$19.50 (i.e., substitute 19.50 for C) and obtain a revised *EOQ* of 101. This result is not useful, however, because the *EOQ* of 101 is outside the appropriate range of 240 to 599 for a unit price of \$19.50. Next, we calculate the *EOQ* with C = \$20 and obtain a value of 100, which is appropriate because it falls within the range of 1 to 239 for a unit price of \$20.

The table below summarizes the series of calculations we make to arrive at an appropriate *EOQ*:

Order Quantity	Unit Price ($)	*EOQ*
≥600	18.75	103
240–599	19.50	101
1–239	20.00	100 (appropriate *EOQ*)

3. Calculate TC_{qd} using equation (4) for the *EOQ* found in step 2, and compare with TC_{qd} when substituting for the *Q*'s that just obtain all higher price discounts (the discontinuity points in the TC_{qd} function as shown in Figure 12.6). Select the *Q* that minimizes TC_{qd}.

$$\begin{aligned} TC_{qd}(EOQ = 100) &= 20(1000) + 30(1000)/100 + .30(20)(100)/2 \\ (C = 20) & \\ &= 20{,}000 + 300 + 300 \\ &= 20{,}600 \end{aligned}$$

$$\begin{aligned} TC_{qd} \quad (Q = 240) &= 19.50(1000) + 30(1000)/240 + .30(19.50)(240)/2 \\ (C = 19.50) & \\ &= 19{,}500 + 125 + 702 \\ &= 20{,}327 \end{aligned}$$

$$\begin{aligned} TC_{qd} \quad (Q = 600) &= 18.75(1000) + 30(1000)/600 + .30(18.75)(600)/2 \\ (C = 18.75) & \\ &= 18{,}750 + 50 + 1687.5 \\ &= 20{,}487.5 \end{aligned}$$

Total annual costs are minimized with an order quantity of 240 units.

Inventory Model with Planned Shortages

When customers are willing to tolerate stockouts, an inventory system with planned shortages is possible. For example, a tire store may not stock all sizes of high-performance tires, knowing that a customer is willing to wait a day or two if the particular tire is out-of-stock. For this strategy to be acceptable to customers, however, the promised delivery date must be adhered to, and it must be within a reasonable length of time. Otherwise, customers would fault the retailer for being unreliable.

Using *electronic data interchange (EDI)* and predictable delivery from suppliers, a strategy of minimal inventory stocking can be implemented. The benefits of such a system are captured by the tradeoff between the cost of holding inventory and the cost that is associated with a stockout that can be *backordered.* An item is considered to be backordered when a customer is willing to wait for delivery; thus, the sale is not lost. Some subjective cost should be associated with customer inconvenience, however. Software manufacturers have taken this tolerance of stockouts to the extreme by creating "vaporware," which is software that is planned but not yet available. Such a company would advertise this software to gauge the level of demand; however, excessive use of this strategy risks the credibility of the firm in the mind of customers. For retailers, this strategy can attract customers when the inventory cost savings are passed along as everyday low prices.

Figure 12.7 illustrates the idealized behavior of a planned shortage inventory system assuming a constant rate of demand and customers who will wait until the next order quantity Q is received to satisfy backorders that have accumulated to a maximum of K units. A new total inventory cost equation, which is called *total costs with backorders* (TC_b), now is required:

$$(TC_b) = \text{ordering cost } \textit{plus} \text{ holding cost } \textit{plus} \text{ backorder cost}$$

$$= S\frac{D}{Q} + H\frac{(Q-K)^2}{2Q} + B\frac{K^2}{2Q} \qquad (5)$$

where K = number of stockouts backordered when order quantity arrives and
B = backorder cost in dollars per unit per year.

Using the similar-triangles argument from geometry (i.e., the sides and heights of right triangles are proportional) and noting that inventory is held physically only for a fraction of the inventory cycle, the expression for average inventory can be derived as follows:

Average inventory held during the inventory cycle $= \left(\frac{Q-K}{2}\right)\left(\frac{T_1}{T}\right)$, but by similar triangles, $T_1/T = (Q-K)/Q$ and, by substitution we obtain $(Q-K)^2/2Q$.

In a similar manner, we can derive the expression for average backorders as follows:

Average number of backorders held during the inventory cycle $= \left(\frac{K}{2}\right)\left(\frac{T_2}{2}\right)$, but by similar triangles, $T_2/T = K/Q$ and, by substitution, we obtain $K^2/2Q$.

FIGURE 12.7. Inventory levels for the planned shortages model.

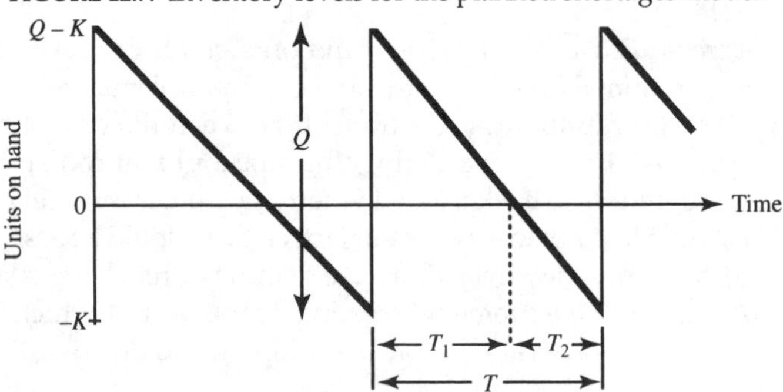

Because the total inventory cost expression shown in equation (5) contains two decision variables, Q and K, we must take partial derivatives and solve for each variable to obtain the following values for order quantity and size of backorders[2]:

$$Q^* = \sqrt{\frac{2DS}{H}\left(\frac{H+B}{B}\right)} \tag{6}$$

$$K^* = Q^*\left(\frac{H}{H+B}\right) \tag{7}$$

The planned shortages model and the resulting equations (6) and (7) provide considerable insight into inventory systems when the backorder cost B is permitted to take on values from 0 to ∞ as shown in Table 12.3. Substituting ∞ for B in equation (6) reduces the equation to the classic *EOQ* equation (3). Thus, when a business uses the classic *EOQ*, the implication is that backorder cost is infinitely large and no stockout should occur. Because the cost of a backorder has a finite value, however, using the *EOQ* equation results in an inventory system that is more costly than necessary.

Letting the backorder cost decrease to zero results in an undefined value for *EOQ* because we have division by zero. However, inventory models that fit this situation do exist. For example, consider patients waiting for heart transplants. Because the donors cannot be inventoried, we have a queue or inventory of recipients in backorder status who are waiting for an available donor.

[2] Taking the partial derivative of equation (5) with respect to K yields $-2H(Q-K)/2Q+2BK/2Q$, which is set $=0$ and solved for $K^*=Q[H/(H+B)]$. Note that $Q-K=Q[B/(H+B)]$ and substituting for K in equation (5) yields $TC_b = DS/Q + H[BQ/(H+B)]^2/2Q + B[HQ/(H+B)]^2/2Q$. Taking the partial derivative with respect to Q yields $-DS/Q^2 + HB^2/2(H+B)^2 + BH^2/2(H+B)^2$, which is set $=0$ and solved for $Q^* = \sqrt{2DS(H+B)/HB}$.

TABLE 12.3. Values for Q^* and K^* as a Function of Backorder Costs

B	Q^*	K^*	Inventory levels
$B \to \infty$	$\sqrt{\frac{2DS}{H}}$	0	
$0 < B < \infty$	$\sqrt{\frac{2DS}{H}\left(\frac{H+B}{B}\right)}$	$Q^*\left[\frac{H}{H+B}\right]$	
$B \to 0$	Undefined	Q^*	

Example 12.3: Rocky Mountain Power—Planned Shortages Problem

Assume that the cost of a backorder for the glass insulator is the price of a \$50 overnight FedEx package. Using equations (6) and (7), calculate a new order quantity and maximum backorder accumulation. Has a savings in total annual costs been realized compared with the classic *EOQ* approach?

$$Q^* = \sqrt{\frac{2DS}{H}\left(\frac{H+B}{B}\right)} = \sqrt{\frac{2(1000)(30)}{6}\left(\frac{6+50}{50}\right)} = 106$$

$$K^* = Q^*\left(\frac{H}{H+B}\right) = 106\left(\frac{6}{6+50}\right) = 11$$

$$TC_b = S\frac{D}{Q} + H\frac{(Q-K)^2}{2Q} + B\frac{K^2}{2Q}$$

$$= 30\frac{1000}{106} + 6\frac{(106-11)^2}{2(106)} + 50\frac{11^2}{2(106)}$$

$$= 283 + 255 + 29 = 567$$

Recall that the TC_p for the *EOQ* of 100 was \$600, a value \$33 in excess of the TC_b calculated above. Thus, using the simple *EOQ* model can be costly because of the implied assumption that stockouts cannot occur. Note that on an annual basis, both ordering and holding costs have been reduced significantly below the \$300 value for the *EOQ* model at the small cost of \$29 for backordering.

INVENTORY MANAGEMENT UNDER UNCERTAINTY

The simple *EOQ* formula does not consider uncertainties in demand rate or in replenishment lead time. Each time an order is placed, these uncertainties pose a risk of stockouts occurring before the replenishment order arrives. To reduce the risk of stockouts during this time, extra inventory can be held in excess of expected demand during the lead time. A tradeoff exists between the cost of investing in and holding excess inventory and the cost of stockouts, however. In any event, except by good luck, either some stock remains in inventory or stockouts have occurred and the shelves are bare when the replenishment order arrives.

The key to inventory management under uncertainty is the concept of a *service level.* This is a customer-oriented term and is defined as the percentage of demand occurring during the lead time that can be satisfied from inventory. Some analytical approaches for determining the optimal service level have been suggested, but in practice, selecting a service level is a policy decision. Consider, for example, a convenience store. Depending on competition and the patience of customers, cold beer might require a 99-percent service level, but a 95-percent service level might be appropriate for fresh bread.

The service level is used to determine a *reorder point (ROP)*, which is the level of inventory on hand when a replenishment order is initiated. The reorder point is set to achieve a prespecified service level. This, of course, requires information on the frequency distribution of demand during the replenishment lead time. When we set the reorder point, we also are determining the *safety stock* level (SS) which is the excess inventory that is held during the reorder lead time to achieve the desired service level. The reorder point equals the safety stock level plus the *average demand during the lead time* (d_L). That is,

$$ROP = SS + d_L \tag{8}$$

The demand during lead time distribution now can be described in the following general manner, where the daily demand has a mean μ and standard deviation σ:

$$d_L = \mu(LT) \tag{9}$$

$$\sigma_L = \sigma\sqrt{LT} \tag{10}$$

The Central Limit Theorem allows us to assume that the demand during lead time distribution has a normal distribution no matter what the daily demand distribution is. The safety stock now can be calculated using the following equation, where z_r is the standard normal deviate for r-percent service level:

$$SS = z_r\sigma\sqrt{LT} \tag{11}$$

Figure 12.8 illustrates the concept of establishing a demand during lead time distribution for the case in which daily demand has a mean of 3 and standard deviation of 1.5 and the lead time is 4 days. Note that the ROP is the stock level that is on-hand when an order is placed and, thus, should be sufficient to satisfy r percent of demand during the lead time. We assume that daily demand is an independent variable. The independence assumption permits the summation of individual daily demand means and variances to arrive at a total demand during the lead time, which has a normal distribution based on the Central Limit Theorem.

FIGURE 12.8. Demand during lead time.

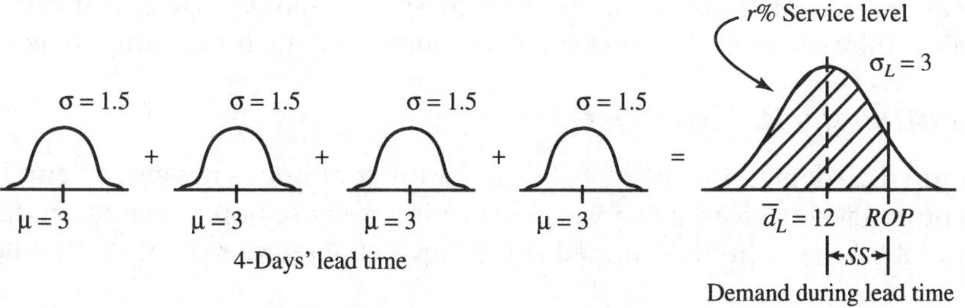

Example 12.4: Rocky Mountain Power—Reorder Point

Recall inventory item SKU 1341, the glass insulator. RMP's computerized information system has tracked the daily demand rate for this item. Daily demand appears to be distributed normally with a mean, $\mu = 3$ and standard deviation, $\sigma = 1.5$. The replenishment lead time has been a constant 4 days. Because SKU 1341 is an important item for utility line maintenance, it is company policy to achieve a 95-percent service level for such items. What reorder point and safety stock should be recommended?

Using equations (9) and (10), the demand during lead time for RMP becomes:

$$d_L = \mu(LT) = 3(4) = 12$$

$$\sigma_L = \sigma\sqrt{LT} = 1.5\sqrt{4} = 3$$

Then, we turn to the Standard Normal Distribution in Appendix A to find that a $z = 1.645$ leaves 5 percent in one tail to guarantee a 95-percent service level. The safety stock that is required to ensure the desired service level is calculated using equation (11):

$$\begin{aligned} SS &= z_r\sigma\sqrt{LT} \\ &= (1.645)(1.5)\sqrt{4} \\ &= 5 \end{aligned}$$

Using equation (8), we find the reorder point for RMP to be:

$$\begin{aligned} ROP &= SS + d_L \\ &= 5 + 12 \\ &= 17 \end{aligned}$$

INVENTORY CONTROL SYSTEMS

Many different inventory control systems are used in actual practice. They differ in the methods for determining the order quantity and when a replenishment order should be made. We shall restrict our discussion here to two of the most common inventory control systems: the continuous review system (Q,r), and the periodic review system (i.e., order-up-to). In all inventory control systems, two questions must be answered: 1) When should an order be placed? and 2) What size is the order quantity? Because inventory control systems face uncertainty in demand, we will find that when one of these questions is answered using a fixed value, the answer to the other must accommodate the uncertainty in demand.

Continuous Review System

Figure 12.9 depicts inventory balances for the continuous review system. The inventory level decreases in a variable fashion because of uncertainty in demand until it reaches a predetermined trigger level, the reorder point *ROP*. When the inventory balance reaches the *ROP*, an order for replenishment is placed with the vendor. For this inventory system, the order quantity *EOQ* is fixed (i.e., *EOQ* units always are ordered each time an order is placed). An example of this "two bin" system is the Hallmark greeting card stand that has a reorder card, containing the stock number, placed near the back of the card display to remind the retailer to reorder the item before the remaining cards are sold.

From the time the reorder point is reached until the replenishment is received, the inventory level continues to decline. Generally, there will be some inventory remaining just before the replenishment is received. The average inventory balance just when the replenishment arrives is the safety stock level *SS*. This inventory is maintained to protect against stockouts that might result from unusually high levels of demand and/or longer-than-expected replenishment lead time. On occasion, however, a stockout does occur. For this system, unsatisfied demand during the lead time period is backordered until the replenishment order is received, in which case the backordered items are set aside and the remaining part of the *EOQ* placed in stock.

Note that for the continuous review system, the order quantity is fixed, but the cycle time between orders varies. A computerized information system using bar codes for each SKU can track inventory balances continuously to indicate when the reorder point is reached. Retailers like Wal-Mart use *point-of-sale (POS)* cash registers to record up-to-the-minute status of stock levels, with an end-of-day report on all items that have reached their reorder points. In many cases, the purchase order is generated automatically by the computer and sent to the vendor or, in the case of Wal-Mart, to its distribution center for the next shipment.

FIGURE 12.9. Continuous review system (Q, r).

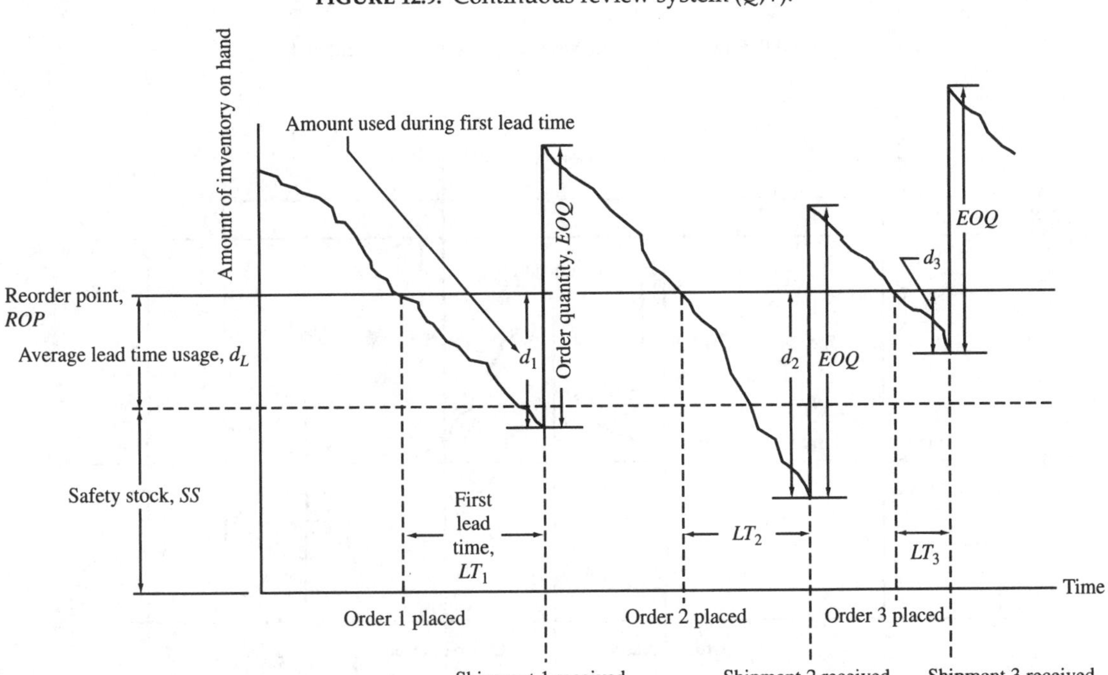

Again, the parameter equations for the continuous review system are:

$$EOQ = \sqrt{\frac{2DS}{H}}$$

$$ROP = SS + \mu LT$$

$$SS = z_r \sigma \sqrt{LT}$$

Periodic Review System

Figure 12.10 depicts inventory balances for the periodic review system. Orders for replenishment are placed after a fixed review period *RP* has elapsed. The order quantity varies and is calculated to be that needed to bring the total inventory (i.e., on-hand plus on-order) up to some predetermined target inventory level *TIL*. Note that occasional backorders can occur with this system, just as with the continuous review system. With the periodic review system, the order quantity varies in response to the demand rate, whereas the cycle time between orders is fixed.

To determine the fixed-review period, first calculate an *EOQ*, then divide the resulting value by the average daily demand to arrive at an expected cycle time. The resulting review period thus balances the holding and ordering costs to achieve a minimum total incremental cost for the system.

The periodic review system generally is used when orders for many different SKUs are consolidated for replenishment from a distributor or regional warehouse that resupplies on a periodic basis (e.g., restocking a convenience store once a week).

FIGURE 12.10. Periodic review system (order-up-to).

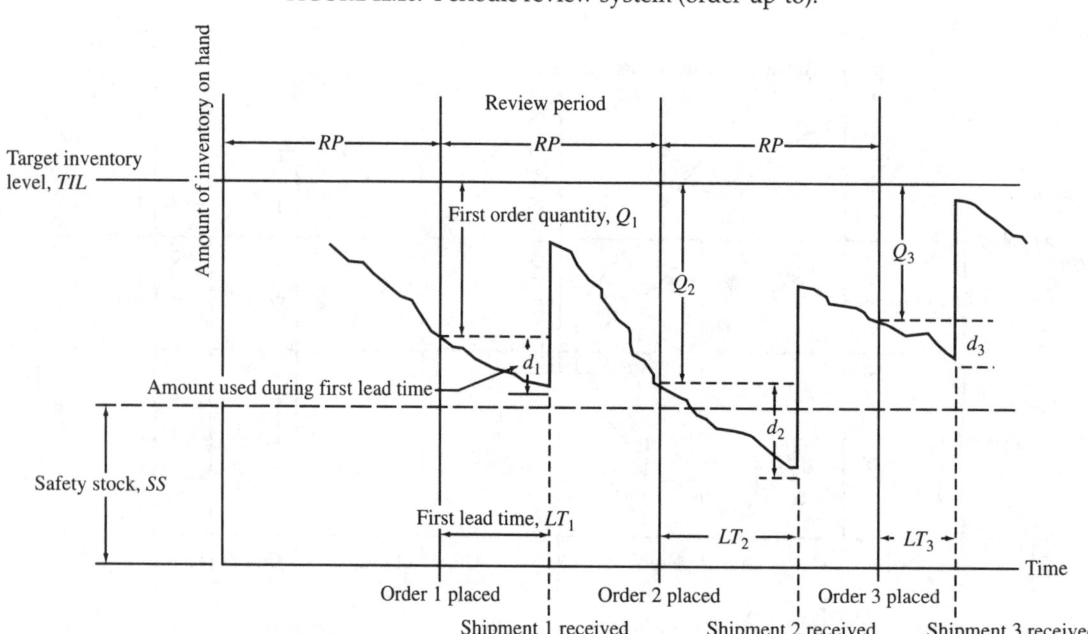

The parameter equations for the periodic review system are noted below, where the daily demand has a mean of μ and standard deviation of σ. Note that exposure to a stockout for the periodic review system is the review period plus the lead time (i.e., $RP + LT$) instead of just the lead time (LT) as in the continuous review system. Thus, carrying extra inventory is the cost that is paid for lack of continuous information on the inventory status.

$$RP = EOQ/\mu \tag{12}$$

$$TIL = SS + \mu(RP + LT) \tag{13}$$

$$SS = z_r\sigma\sqrt{RP + LT} \tag{14}$$

Example 12.5: Rocky Mountain Power—Periodic Review System

Recall from Example 12.4 that for inventory item SKU 1341, the glass insulator, daily demand is distributed normally, with a mean, $\mu = 3$ and standard deviation $\sigma = 1.5$. In Example 12.1, the EOQ was calculated to be 100 units. The replenishment lead time has been a constant 4 days. Again, because SKU 1341 is an important item for utility line maintenance, it is company policy to achieve a 95-percent service level for such items. If a periodic review system is selected to control glass insulator inventory, what are the recommended review period, target inventory level, and safety stock?

Using equation (12), the review period $RP = 100/3 = 33$ days, or approximately once each month. The safety stock is calculated using equation (14):

$$\begin{aligned} SS &= z_r\sigma\sqrt{RP + LT} \\ &= (1.645)(1.5)\sqrt{33 + 4} \\ &= 15 \end{aligned}$$

The target inventory level is determined using equation (13):

$$\begin{aligned} TIL &= SS + \mu(RP + LT) \\ &= 15 + 3(33 + 4) \\ &= 126 \end{aligned}$$

Thus, once every month the inventory of SKU 1341 on hand is noted with an order placed for an amount that is equal to the difference between that inventory and the target level of 126 units.

The ABCs of Inventory Control

Usually, a few inventory items or SKUs account for most of the inventory value as measured by dollar volume (i.e., demand multiplied by item cost). Thus, we must pay close attention to these few items that control most of the inventory value. The 80-20 rule, or Pareto analysis, introduced in Chapter 10, Service Quality, is useful for inventory classification. The ABC classification system, shown graphically in Figure 12.11, often is used to organize SKUs into three groups depending on their value. The A class typically contains about 20 percent of inventory items but accounts for 80 percent of dollar volume. These significant items need close attention. At the other extreme are the insignificant class C items, which usually represent 50 percent of inventory items but account for only about 5 percent of the dollar volume. In the middle is class B, which represents 30 percent of items and 15 percent of the dollar volume. Before an inventory control system is decided on, an ABC classification usually is undertaken. Selecting the appropriate inventory control system should be based on the significance of the inventory items.

Table 12.4 shows inventory items for a discount electronics store arranged in order of decreasing dollar volume to achieve an ABC classification. In this case, two items (i.e., computers and entertainment centers) comprise 20 percent of SKUs and account for 74 percent of the total dollar volume. These are the few costly A items that require special managerial attention, because they represent a significant sales opportunity loss if they are out-of-stock. Intensive computer monitoring of inventory levels as found in the continuous review system should be used for these items.

As is common, 50 percent of the items account for a small percentage of the dollar volume inventory value (in this case, 10 percent). These are the inexpensive C items and can be managed in a more casual fashion, because a stockout does not represent a serious loss of revenue. For these items, a periodic review system might be used. The review period can be relatively long as well, which results in infrequent orders for large quantities of low-value items.

FIGURE 12.11. ABC classification of inventory items.

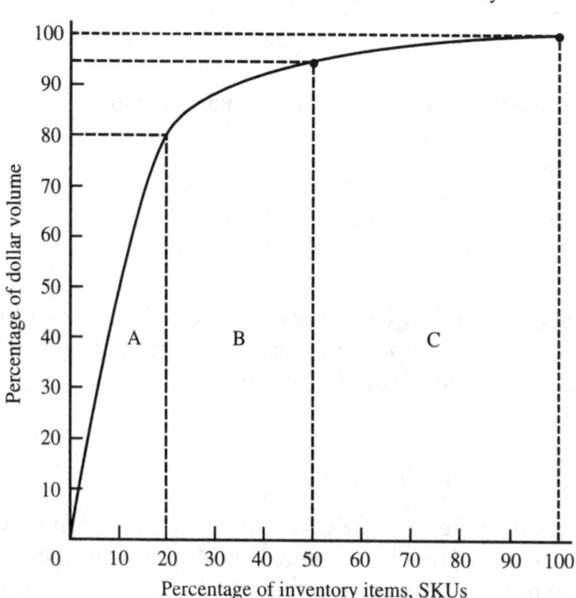

TABLE 12.4. Inventory Items Listed in Descending Order of Dollar Volume

Inventory Item	Unit Cost ($)	Monthly Sales (units)	Dollar Volume ($)	Percent of Dollar Volume	Percent of SKUs	Class
Computers	3000	50	150,000	74	20	A
Entertainment center	2500	30	75,000			
Television sets	400	60	24,000			
Refrigerators	1000	15	15,000	16	30	B
Monitors	200	50	10,000			
Stereos	150	60	9,000			
Cameras	200	40	8,000			
Software	50	100	5,000	10	50	C
Computer disks	5	1000	5,000			
CDs	20	200	4,000			
Totals			305,000	100	100	

The three B items are not so costly as to require special managerial attention, but they are not so cheap that they can be overstocked. Either a continuous review or a periodic review system could be used to manage these items.

SINGLE-PERIOD MODEL FOR PERISHABLE GOODS

Businesses sometimes accumulate an inventory in anticipation of future sales that will occur during a short period of time, after which the unsold items are drastically reduced in value. Retail examples include Christmas trees, fresh pastries, fresh fruit and vegetables, magazines, and newspapers. Given some data on past sales experience, the question to answer is how much to stock? If too small, the order quantity results in the possibility of lost sales. If the order quantity is too large, however, unsold stock represents a lost investment that may have minimal salvage value.

This decision on how much to stock will be illustrated using the classic "news vendor problem" (albeit a rather expensive newspaper). First, we begin with some notation, then follow with a distribution of expected sales including $P(D < Q)$:

D = newspapers demanded;
Q = newspapers stocked;
P = selling price of newspaper, \$10;
C = cost of newspaper, \$4;
S = salvage value of newspaper, \$2;
C_u = unit contribution from sale, $P - C$ = \$6 (opportunity cost of *under*estimating demand);
C_o = unit loss from not selling, $C - S$ = \$2 (cost of *over*estimating demand);

$P(D < Q)$ = probability of not selling all newspapers stocked; and
$P(D \geq Q)$ = probability of selling all newspapers stocked.

D	Frequency	$p(D)$	$P(D < Q)$
2	1	.028	.000
3	2	.055	.028
4	3	.083	.083
5	4	.111	.166
6	5	.139	.277
7	6	.167	.416
8	5	.139	.583
9	4	.111	.722
10	3	.083	.838
11	2	.055	.916
12	1	.028	.971

Expected Value Analysis

A payoff table is constructed to account for the financial result of each combination of actual newspapers demanded and stock level selected (for convenience, we will limit Q to values between 6 and 10). Using the probability of newspapers demanded, an expected profit will be calculated for each column of the payoff table (i.e., stock level Q). The stock level that yields the maximum expected profit will best balance the opportunity cost of lost sales and cost of investment in unsold newspapers. The payoff table is best constructed beginning with the upper left-hand cell. For cell ($D = 2$, $Q = 6$), we have the following financial result:

Sales	2($10) = $20
Salvage	(6 − 2)($2) = 8
Total revenue	$28
Less cost	6($4) = −24
Profit	$ 4

Note that as one moves across the rows, the profit decreases by $(S - C) = 2 - 4 = -\$2$, because one more unsold newspaper must be salvaged. As one moves down the columns the profit increases by $(P - S) = 10 - 2 = \$8$, because one more unsalvaged unit now is sold. This increase in profit continues until the diagonal, where $D = Q$, is reached, after which the profit remains the same as all available stock is sold and additional demand is not being satisfied.

The expected profit for each stock level Q from 6 to 10 is calculated and shown at the bottom of the table on page 371. Expected profit for $Q = 6$ is calculated by multiplying the probability of demand $p(D)$ in the first column by each payoff in column three under $Q = 6$:

$$\text{Expected profit (for } Q = 6) = .028(4) + .055(12) + .083(20) + \ldots + .055(36) + .028(36) = \$31.54$$

For this example, a stock of nine newspapers ($Q^* = 9$) will maximize expected profit at $35.99 per period.

		Stock Q				
p(D)	*D*	6	7	8	9	10
.028	2	4	2	0	−2	−4
.055	3	12	10	8	6	4
.083	4	20	18	16	14	12
.111	5	28	26	24	22	20
.139	6	36	34	32	30	28
.167	7	36	42	40	38	36
.139	8	36	42	48	46	44
.111	9	36	42	48	54	52
.083	10	36	42	48	54	60
.055	11	36	42	48	54	60
.028	12	36	42	48	54	60
Expected profit		$31.54	$34.43	$35.77	$35.99	$35.33

Incremental Analysis

Another approach to the news vendor problem uses an economic principle called *marginal analysis.* The argument is that the news vendor should continue increasing the stock (size of Q) until the expected revenue on the last unit stocked just exceeds the expected loss on the last sale. From this principle, we can derive a very useful probability called the *critical fractile:*

$$E(\text{revenue on last sale}) \geq E(\text{loss on last sale})$$

$$P(\text{revenue})(\text{unit revenue}) \geq P(\text{loss})(\text{unit loss})$$

$$P(D \geq Q)C_u \geq P(D < Q)C_o$$

$$[1 - P(D < Q)]C_u \geq P(D < Q)C_o$$

$$P(D < Q) \leq \frac{C_u}{C_u + C_o} \qquad (15)$$

where

C_u = unit contribution from newspaper sale (opportunity cost of underestimating demand),
C_o = unit loss from not selling newspaper (cost of overestimating demand),
D = demand, and
Q = newspapers stocked.

Using equation (15), we find $P(D < Q) \leq 6/(6 + 2) \leq .75$. Thus, stock $Q = 9$, because as Figure 12.12 shows, the newspaper demand from 2 through 8 sums to a cumulative probability of 0.722.

Looking back at the expected profit line in the payoff table, we find confirmation of the marginal analysis principle. Each time we increase Q, beginning

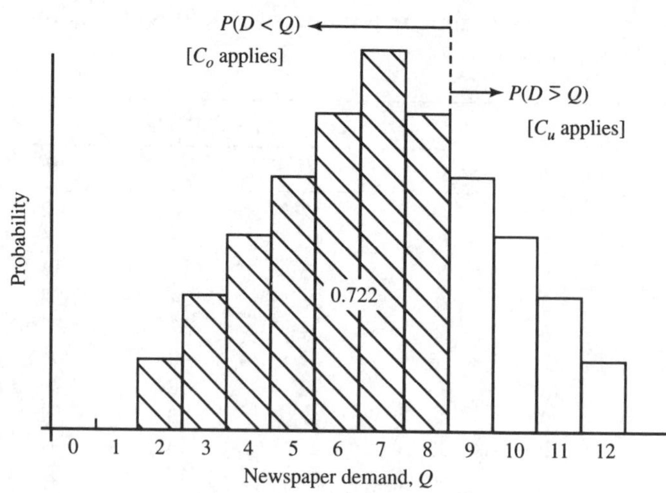

FIGURE 12.12. Critical fractile for the news vendor problem.

with a value of 6 in our abbreviated table, there is a corresponding increase in profit up to the value of 9, after which profit decreases with the 10th unit, creating an expected loss of $0.66.

RETAIL DISCOUNTING MODEL

Even with the best planning, attempting to anticipate customer demand has its risks. The sleeveless shirt that seemed to be such a great fashion statement at the Las Vegas trade show just did not catch on in Peoria. Such "dogs" end up on the shelf for months, collecting dust and depriving the retailer of shelf space for displaying new items that might sell faster. Discounting them means a loss of some profit margin, and besides, what should be an appropriate discount? In any event, the retailer surely would never sell them below cost. This dilemma can be resolved by determining the break-even discount price that will clear the inventory of "dogs" in short order and, thus, generate capital to invest in good stock that will turn rapidly. In retailing, profit is a function of mark-up multiplied by turnover. The following terms will be used for determining the discount price:

S = current selling price,
D = discount price,
P = profit margin on cost (the percent mark-up as a decimal),
Y = average number of years to sell entire stock of "dogs" at current price (total number of years to clear stock divided by 2), and
N = number of times good stock (same quantity as "dogs") turns over during the year (also calculated by dividing annual demand of good stock by number of "dogs" on hand).

The break-even discount price will be found by equating the loss per item to the gain from investing the revenue that is obtained in good stock:

$$\text{Loss per item} = \text{Gain from revenue}$$

$$S - D = D(PNY)$$

Thus, the discount price is:

$$D = \frac{S}{(1 + PNY)} \tag{16}$$

Example 12.6: Sportstown

The Graphite Princess Terminator tennis racket has not been selling well, perhaps because of its poor weight distribution. It is well made, however, and retails at \$29.95 with a 40-percent mark-up on cost. Only one sale was made last year, and there were 10 rackets remaining in stock. More popular rackets were selling at a rate of 25 per year.

The percent mark-up on cost as a decimal is $P = 0.40$, with a selling price $S = \$29.95$. With current sales of one per year, the average number of years to clear the stock of 10 rackets is $Y = 10/2 = 5$. If these "dogs" were good rackets, then $25/10 = 2.5$ lots would sell per year; thus, $N = 2.5$. Using equation (16), the discount price is:

$$D = \frac{29.95}{[1 + (0.40)(2.5)(5)]}$$
$$= \frac{29.95}{6}$$
$$= \$4.99$$

Thus, the 10 tennis rackets should be discounted immediately to sell at a price of \$4.99 each. Note that we will take an opportunity loss of $(S - D) = (\$29.95 - \$4.99) \cong \$25.00$ per item; however, the \$4.99 will be placed immediately in fast-moving stock. The \$4.99 will be marked up by 40 percent and, thus, return \$2.00 each time a good racket is sold, (0.40)(\$4.99). Good stock, however, turns over 2.5 times a year, compared with a "dog" that sells one item per year and, thus, makes 2.5(\$2.00) = \$5.00 a year. Because it will take 5 years on average to clear out the "dogs," the total revenue gain from reinvestment of profits is 5(\$5.00) = \$25.00.

In other words, we can either hold the "dogs" and eventually sell all of them at \$29.95, or we can sell them all immediately at \$4.99, put the money (i.e., \$50.00) into good stock, and regain our losses in 5 years. Note that the discount price results in a break-even in which no money is made, and we need not discount to that extreme low level. Because the wholesale price was \$29.95/1.4 = \$21.39, we might wish to discount the rackets initially to a price of \$19.95. If the rackets sell quickly, we will make money even though the selling price is below cost, because the money tied up in inventory now is moving.

SUMMARY

Inventory management can influence significantly the success of an organization. For some organizations, the extent to which their objectives are achieved is affected by the inventory system they adopt. Good inventory management is characterized by concern for inventory holding costs, inventory ordering costs, shortage costs, and the purchase price of the items. Further, the lead time for replenishment and the appropriate service level should be considered.

Because of the widespread use of bar coding, keeping track of inventory using computers is common practice. This simplifies the manipulations of large amounts of data relevant to inventory decisions.

Recalling that inventory is the price a business pays for lack of information, we will study methods of forecasting demand for services in Chapter 16.

KEY TERMS AND DEFINITIONS

Backorder a demand that is not satisfied immediately because of a stockout but is satisfied later because the customer is willing to wait until the replenishment order arrives to take delivery.

Critical fractile the cumulative probability that demand will be less than the stock level that guarantees marginal revenue just exceeds the marginal cost of the last item stocked.

Economic order quantity (*EOQ*) the reorder quantity that minimizes the total incremental cost of holding inventory and the cost of ordering replenishments.

Electronic data interchange (EDI) a computerized exchange of data between organizations that eliminates paper-based documents.

Inventory turns the number of times an inventory stock is sold per year, calculated by dividing annual demand by the average inventory held.

Point-of-sale (POS) on-line linking of sales transactions, using computerized cash registers, bar-code scanners, or credit-card readers, to a central computer allowing immediate updating of sales, inventory, and pricing information.

Replenishment lead time the time, usually in days, from an order being placed with a vendor to the delivery being made.

Reorder point level of inventory both on hand and on order when a reorder of a fixed quantity is made.

Safety stock inventory held in excess of expected demand during lead time to satisfy a desired service level.

Service level the probability that demand will be satisfied during replenishment lead time.

TOPICS FOR DISCUSSION

1. Discuss the functions of inventory for different organizations in the distribution system (i.e., manufacturing, suppliers, distributors, and retailers).
2. How would one find values for inventory management costs?
3. Compare and contrast a continuous review inventory system with a periodic review inventory system.
4. Discuss how information technology can help to create a competitive advantage through inventory management.
5. How valid are the assumptions for the simple *EOQ* model?
6. In general, how is a service level determined for most inventory items?
7. Some noninventory items (e.g., seats on an aircraft) have the same characteristics as inventories. What inventory model would apply?

Service Benchmark

Where Parts Are *the Whole*

Replacement auto parts companies live and die by their inventories. A full-line distributor carries more than 100,000 individual parts, and even a local retailer may have 10,000. Many distributors and retailers—caught between having enough parts and having too many—are asking computers to do their counting and restocking. Other industries rely on computerized inventory systems too, but few have to sort out the same number and range of items as companies that sell replacement parts.

Even in the computer age, many distributors manage their inventories by instinct and memory, guided by inventory cards attached to the parts. The results of such unsophisticated systems are apparent when the parts industry goes into a downturn. "Because distributors traditionally have been mom-and-pop types of businesses, we have seen a number go out of business anytime there is a shock to the system, like a mild winter," said Gurudutt M. Baliga, an automotive analyst with McDonald & Company Securities.

Analysts credit Genuine Parts Company with taking the industry into the computer age. Most of the 6,000 retailers, or jobbers, that buy parts from Genuine are connected by computer to one of the company's NAPA distribution warehouses. Every time a jobber sells an item, the sale is logged on a computer at the warehouse. The computer updates a list of parts to be delivered the next day to replenish the jobber's stock. Genuine Parts encourages mechanics to use rugged laptop computers to order parts electronically without leaving their service bays.

Genuine is not the only parts company to employ computers. Individual auto parts stores use computers to monitor inventories and other large distributors like Carquest Inc. have also tried to link retail stores directly with warehouses. But analysts say Genuine's system is the most successful.

"Genuine is sophisticated in the way they examine each local market and structure the inventory accordingly," said Mr. Baliga. "If they expected the wiper blade inventory to turn over three times at a particular store, and it only turned once, they send out a team of people to understand why."

Source: The New York Times, September 2, 1990, p. F4(N).

SOLVED PROBLEMS

1. Continuous Review (Q,r) System

Problem Statement

A resort hotel is planning to install a computerized inventory system to manage the complimentary guest toilet items such as soap and shampoo. The daily usage rate for bars of soap appears to be distributed normally, with a mean, $\mu = 16$, and a standard deviation, $\sigma = 3$. Once an order is placed, it takes a full week before delivery is made. The effort to place an order and receive the shipment is approximately 1 hour's time for a staff person who is paid \$10 per hour. The opportunity cost of capital is 20 percent per year. A bar of soap is valued at approximately \$0.25. The hotel is concerned about stockouts of such a basic item and, thus, desires a 94-percent service level. Recommend an order quantity (Q) and reorder point (r) for a continuous review system.

Solution

First, calculate the value of Q using equation (3) for the parameters below:

$D = (16)(365) = 5840$ per year
$S = 10$
$H = IC = (.20)(.25) = .05$

$$EOQ = \sqrt{\frac{2DS}{H}} = \sqrt{\frac{2(5840)(10)}{.05}} = 1528.4 \cong 1500$$

Second, determine the demand during lead-time distribution using equations (9) and (10):

$$d_L = \mu(LT) = (16)(7) = 112$$

$$\sigma_L = \sigma\sqrt{LT} = 3\sqrt{7} = 7.94 \cong 8$$

Third, calculate the safety stock using equation (11), and find the z value in Appendix A with .06 probability in one tail:

$$SS = z_r\sigma\sqrt{LT} = (1.555)(8) = 12.44 \cong 13(\text{round up to be conservative})$$

Finally, the reorder point is the sum of the safety stock and the mean demand during lead-time:

$$ROP = SS + d_L = 13 + 112 = 125$$

2. Periodic Review (Order-Up-To) System

Problem Statement

The resort hotel manager was not interested in continuously monitoring the usage of complementary toilet items, which he felt were better classified as low-value C items. Thus, he requested that a periodic review system be used. Recommend a review period and target inventory level for a system with a 94-percent service level.

Solution

First, calculate the review period using equation (12) based on the *EOQ* from problem 1:

$$RP = EOQ/\mu = 1500/16 = 93.75 \text{ days (or every 3 months)}$$

Second, calculate the safety stock using equation (14):

$$SS = z_r\sigma\sqrt{RP + LT} = (1.555)(3)\sqrt{94 + 7} = 46.9 \cong 47 \text{ units}$$

Finally, calculate the target inventory level using equation (13):

$$TIL = SS + \mu(RP + LT) = 47 + (16)(94 + 7) = 1663 \text{ units}$$

3. Perishable Goods

Problem Statement

A commuter airline prides itself on customer service, with features such as providing its morning passengers with a copy of *The Wall Street Journal*. The paper cost $1.50 per issue on subscription. The newsstand price is $2.50. What size subscription should be ordered if a small plane with only six seats has experienced the demand distribution below:

Passengers	2	3	4	5	6
Probability	.1	.2	.2	.3	.2

Solution

First, prepare a $P(D < Q)$ distribution as shown:

Q	2	3	4	5	6
$P(D < Q)$	0	.1	.3	.5	.8

Second, identify the cost of underestimating demand as $C_u = \$2.50$, the cost of buying a newsstand paper for the passenger without one.

Third, identify the cost of overestimating demand as $C_o = \$1.50$, the cost of a paper not used.

Finally, using equation (15), we determine the critical fractile $P(D < Q) \leq C_u/(C_u + C_o) \leq 2.5/(2.5 + 1.5) \leq .625$. Thus, buy a five-paper subscription to *The Wall Street Journal.*

EXERCISES

12.1. Annual demand for the notebook binders that Ted's Stationery Shop sells is 10,000 units. Ted operates his business on a 200-work-day year. The unit cost of a binder is $2, and the cost of placing an order with his supplier is $0.40. The cost of carrying a binder in stock for one year is 10 percent of its value.

a. What should the *EOQ* be?

b. How many orders are placed per year?

c. How many working days elapse between reorders?

12.2. Deep Six Seafood, a restaurant that is open 360 days a year and specializes in fresh Maine lobsters, is concerned about its purchase policy. Air freight charges have increased significantly, and it now costs Deep Six $48 to place an order. Because the lobsters are shipped live in a saltwater tub, the order cost is not affected by order sizes. The cost to keep a lobster alive until needed runs about $0.02 per day. The demand for lobsters during the 1-day lead time is as follows:

Lead Time Demand	Probability
0	.05
1	.10
2	.20
3	.30
4	.20
5	.10
6	.05

a. Deep Six would like to reconsider its order size. What would you recommend as an *EOQ*?

b. The Maine distributor is willing to give Deep Six a $0.50 discount on each lobster if orders are placed in lots of 360 each. Should Deep Six accept this offer?

c. If Deep Six insists on maintaining a safety stock of 2 lobsters, what is the service level?

12.3. Dutch Farms imports cheese by the case from Holland for distribution to its Texas retail outlets. During the year (360 days), Dutch Farms sells 1080 cases of cheese. Because of spoilage, Dutch Farms estimates that it costs the firm $6 per year to store a case of cheese. The cost to place an order runs about $10. The desired service level is 98 percent. The demand for cheese during the 1-day lead time is shown below.

Lead Time Demand (cases)	Probability
0	.02
1	.08
2	.20
3	.40
4	.20
5	.08
6	.02

a. Calculate the *EOQ* for Dutch Farms.

b. How many cases should Dutch Farms hold as safety stock against stockouts?

c. Dutch Farms owns a refrigerated warehouse with a capacity of 500 square feet. If each case of cheese requires 10 square feet and must be refrigerated, how much per year could Dutch Farms afford to spend on renting additional space?

12.4. The local distributor for Macho Heavy Beer is reconsidering its inventory policy now that only kegs will be sold. The sales forecast for next year (200 days) is 600 kegs. The cost to store a keg of Macho in a refrigerated warehouse is approximately $3 per year. Placing an order with the factory costs about $4. The demand for Macho during the 1-day lead time is:

Lead Time Demand (kegs)	Probability
0	.03
1	.12
2	.20
3	.30
4	.20
5	.12
6	.03

a. Recommend an *EOQ* for Macho Heavy Beer.

b. If orders are placed in carload lots of 200 kegs, the brewery is willing to give the local distributor a $0.25 discount on the wholesale price of each keg. Based on analysis of total variable inventory costs, is this offer attractive?

c. What is the recommended safety stock if Macho decides on an 85-percent service level?

12.5. Books-to-Go, Inc., has a recurring problem of clearing its shelves of hardcover books once the publisher releases the paperback edition. These books take up shelf space, and the sales are slow. More important, however, they tie up capital with which to buy new bestsellers. Typically, hardcover bestsellers initially retail for $39.95 and have sales of approximately 30 per month during the introductory period. Once the paperback becomes available, hardcover sales plummet to approximately 3 per month. The mark-up on bestsellers is 50 percent of cost.

a. If the paperback version sells for $12.95 and 15 hardbacks are in stock, recommend a discount price for the hardcover version.

b. Explain why the discount price is not influenced by the number of hardcovers in stock.

12.6. Spanish Interiors imports ceramic floor tiles from Mexico with various patterns in anticipation of contractor needs. These tiles usually are ordered a year before delivery, and the production run for each tile pattern requires a separate set-up. Therefore, the orders must be large to defray the set-up cost. Because orders are made far in advance of customer needs, the company must guess what the contractors will like and order patterns in anticipation of these demands. Occasionally, tile patterns fall out of favor, and Spanish Interiors is stuck with slow-moving stock. The mark-up is 30 percent of the tile cost, and the inventory usually turns over about three times per year. There are two slow-moving tile patterns in stock that management estimates will take 2 years each to clear. The sunburst pattern currently retails for $0.70 per square and the saguaro cactus pattern for $1.05 per square. Calculate the lowest discount price for each pattern that will clear the stock quickly.

12.7. Monthly demand for an inventory item is a normally distributed random variable with a mean of 20 units and a variance of 4. Demand follows this distribution every month, 12 months a year. When inventory reaches a predetermined level, an order for replenishment is placed. The fixed ordering cost is $60 per order. The items cost $4 per unit, and the annual inventory holding cost is 25 percent of the average value of the inventory. The replenishment lead time is exactly 4 months.

a. Determine the *EOQ*.

b. Assume that a 10-percent "all units" discount will be given if the order quantity is greater than or equal to 100 units. What order quantity would you recommend with this offer?

c. Determine the necessary reorder point and safety stock to achieve a 90-percent service level.

12.8. The daily demand for an item is distributed normally, with a mean of 5 and a variance of 2. The cost to place an order is $10, and the carrying charge per day is estimated at 10 percent of the inventory value. The supplier has offered the following purchase plan:

$$\text{cost per unit} = \begin{cases} \$15 \text{ if} & Q < 10 \\ \$14 \text{ if} & 10 \le Q < 50 \\ \$12 \text{ if} & Q \ge 50 \end{cases}$$

a. Recommend an optimal order quantity that will minimize the total inventory costs of ordering and holding plus the purchase cost of the units. Although it is not necessary, you may assume 360 days a year.

b. Determine the reorder point and safety stock that will achieve a 95-percent service level given a constant 2-day delivery lead time. Assume daily demand is an independent variable.

12.9. River City Cement Co. maintains an inventory of lime that is purchased from a local supplier. River City uses an average of 200,000 pounds of lime annually in its manufacturing operations (assume 50 operating weeks per year). The lime is purchased from the supplier at a cost of $0.10 per pound. The inventory holding cost is 30 percent of the average value of the inventory, and the cost of placing an order for replenishment is estimated to be $12 per order.

a. Assume that River City orders 10,000 pounds of lime every time it places an order for replenishment. What is the average annual cost of maintaining the inventory?

b. Determine the *EOQ*. If the forecast of annual demand is 10 percent less than actual, how much "extra" is River City paying annually because of an inaccurate forecast of demand (note that this means actual demand for lime averages 220,000 pounds)?

c. Assume that the supplier offers River City a 10-percent "all units" discount if the order quantity is 13,000 pounds or more. Also, assume that annual demand for lime averages 200,000 pounds. What is the best order quantity?

12.10. A popular item stocked by the Fair Deal Department Store has an annual demand of 600 units. The cost to purchase these units from the supplier is $20 per unit and $12 to prepare the purchase order. The annual inventory holding cost is 20 percent of the purchase cost. The manager tries to maintain the probability of stockout at 5 percent or less. Lead time demand is uniform, between 30 and 70 (i.e., the probability of lead time is $1/41 = .0244$ for demand $= 30, 31, \ldots, 70$).

a. Calculate the *EOQ*.

b. Calculate the reorder point.

c. Calculate the safety stock.

d. If we purchase 80 units or more, the unit purchase cost is reduced to $19. Calculate the *EOQ* for this quantity discount case.

12.11. The Supermart Store is about to place an order for Valentine's Day candy. The candy can be bought for $1.40 per box, and it is sold for $2.90 per box up to Valentine's Day. After Valentine's Day, any remaining boxes are sold for $1.00 each. All surplus candy can be sold at this reduced price. Demand at the regular retail price is a random variable with the following discrete probability distribution:

Demand (boxes)	Probability
8	.15
9	.15
10	.30
11	.30
12	.10

a. Determine the expected demand for boxes of candy at the regular retail price.

b. Determine the optimal number of boxes to stock using the critical fractile approach.

c. What is the expected profit for your order in **b**?

12.12. Suppose the XYZ Company, which has an annual demand of 12,000 units per year, order cost of $25, and annual holding cost per unit of $0.50, decides to operate with a planned shortage inventory policy with the backorder cost estimated as $5 per unit per year.

a. Determine the *EOQ*.

b. Determine the maximum number of backorders.

c. Determine the maximum inventory level.
d. Determine the cycle time in work days (assume 250 work days per year).
e. Determine the total inventory cost per year.

12.13. The A & M Hobby Shop carries a line of radio-controlled model racing cars. Demand for these cars is assumed to be a constant rate of 40 cars per month. The cars cost $60 each, and ordering costs are approximately $15 per order regardless of the order size. Inventory carrying costs are 20 percent annually.
a. Determine the *EOQ* and total annual costs under the assumption that no backorders are permitted.
b. Using a $45-per-unit-per-year backorder cost, determine the minimum cost inventory policy and total annual cost.
c. What is the maximum number of days a customer would have to wait for a backorder under the policy in part **b**? Assume the Hobby Shop is open for business 300 days per year.
d. Would you recommend a no-backorder or a backorder inventory policy for this product? Explain.
e. If the lead time is 6 days, what is the reorder point in terms of on-hand inventory for both the no-backorder and the backorder inventory policies?

12.14. The J & B Card Shop sells calendars with different coral reef pictures shown for each month. The once-a-year order for each year's calendar arrives in September. From past experience, the September-to-July demand for these calendars can be approximated by a normal distribution with mean of 500 and standard deviation of 120. The calendars cost $1.50 each, and J & B sells them for $3 each.
a. If J & B throws out all unsold calendars at the end of July (i.e., salvage value is zero), how many calendars should be ordered?
b. If J & B reduces the calendar price to $1 at the end of July and can sell all surplus calendars at this price, how many calendars should be ordered?

12.15. The Gilbert Air Conditioning Company is considering purchase of a special shipment of portable air conditioners from Japan. Each unit will cost Gilbert $80 and be sold for $125. Gilbert does not want to carry over surplus air conditioners to the following year. Thus, all supplies will be sold to a wholesaler who has agreed to take all surplus units for $50 per unit. Given the probability distribution for air conditioners shown below, recommend an order quantity and the anticipated profit using expected value analysis:

Demand	Estimated Probability
0	.30
1	.35
2	.20
3	.10
4	.05

12.16. To limit dependence on imported oil, the Four Corners Power Company has decided to cover a fixed part of the regional demand for electricity by using coal. The annual demand for coal is estimated to be 500,000 tons, which are used uniformly throughout the year. The coal can be strip-mined near the power-generating plant and delivered with a set-up requiring 2 days for a cost of $2000 per mining run. Holding coal in inventory costs approximately $3.00 per ton per year.

a. Determine the economic order quantity for coal assuming 250 work days per year.

b. Assume the daily demand for coal is distributed normally, with mean of 2000 tons and standard deviation of 500 tons. What quantity should be set as safety stock to guarantee a 99-percent service level?

c. If the coal were mined in quantities of 50,000 tons per order, a savings of $0.01 per ton could be passed along to the power company. Should Four Corners Power Company reconsider its coal production quantity as calculated in **a**?

d. What would be the basis for determining the cost of a coal stockout for Four Corners Power Company?

12.17. A wholesaler encounters a constant demand of 200 cases of one brand and box size of soap flakes per week from his retail accounts. He obtains the soap flakes from the manufacturer at $10 per case after paying the transportation costs. The average cost of each order placed is $5, and he computes his inventory carrying charges as 20 percent of the average inventory value on hand over a 1-year period.

a. Compute the *EOQ* for this product.

b. Assuming a constant lead time of 5 days for this product, what is the minimum reorder point that will allow the wholesaler to provide 100-percent customer service? Assume 5 operating days per week.

c. Determine the wholesaler's total cost per year for this product.

d. The manufacturer offers the wholesaler a quantity discount of $1 per case for purchasing in quantities of 400 cases or more. Should the wholesaler take advantage of this quantity discount?

12.18. Leapyear Tire is interested in carrying insufficient numbers of budget tires deliberately. If a customer finds a budget tire is not available, a salesperson will try to sell a more expensive substitute tire, but if this strategy fails, the customer is placed on a waiting list and notified when the next order arrives from the distributor. Leapyear Tire wishes to design an ordering system that will allow backorders to accumulate to a number approximately one-tenth the size of the replenishment order quantity at the time the delivery arrives from the distributor. The cost to hold a tire in stock for a year is $2 and the cost to place an order with the distributor is $9.

a. What is the implied cost of backordering a customer?

b. What would be the recommended order quantity for a 195HR14 tire with an annual demand of 1000?

CASE: ELYSIAN CYCLES[3]

Located in a major southwestern U.S. city, Elysian Cycles (EC) is a wholesale distributor of bicycles and bicycle parts. Its primary retail outlets are located in eight cities within a 400-mile radius of the distribution center. These retail outlets generally depend on receiving orders for additional stock within 2 days after notifying the distribution center (if the stock is available). The company's management feels this is a valuable marketing tool that aids its survival in a highly competitive industry.

EC distributes a wide variety of finished bicycles, but all are based on five different frame designs, each of which may be available in several sizes. Table 12.5 gives a breakdown of product options that are available to the retail outlets.

[3]Prepared by James H. Vance under the supervision of Professor James A. Fitzsimmons.

EC receives these different styles from a single manufacturer overseas, and shipments may take as long as 4 weeks from the time an order is made by telephone or telex. Including the costs of communication, paperwork, and customs clearance, EC estimates that it incurs a cost of $65 each time an order is placed. The cost per bicycle is roughly 60 percent of the suggested list price for any of the styles available.

Demand for these bicycles is somewhat seasonal in nature, being heavier in spring and early summer and tapering off through fall and winter (except for a heavy surge in the 6 weeks before Christmas). A breakdown of the previous year's business with the retail outlets usually forms the basis for EC's yearly operations plan. A growth factor (either positive or negative) is used to refine further the demand estimate by reflecting the upcoming yearly market. By developing a yearly plan and updating it when appropriate, EC can establish a

TABLE 12.5 Prices and Options of Available Bicycles

Frame Style	Available Sizes (in)	Gears (n)	Suggested List Price ($)
A	18, 21, 23	3	99.95
B	18, 21, 23	10	124.95
C	18, 21, 23, 24.5	10	169.95
D	21, 23, 24.5	10	219.95
E	21, 23, 24.5	10 or 15	349.95

TABLE 12.6 Monthly Bicycle Demand

	Frame Style					
Month	A	B	C	D	E	Total
January	0	3	5	2	0	10
February	2	8	10	3	1	24
March	4	15	21	12	2	54
April	4	35	40	21	3	103
May	3	43	65	37	3	151
June	3	27	41	18	2	91
July	2	13	26	11	1	53
August	1	10	16	9	1	37
September	1	9	11	7	1	29
October	1	8	10	7	2	28
November	2	15	19	12	3	51
December	3	30	33	19	4	89
Total	26	216	297	158	23	720

reasonable basis for obtaining any necessary financing from the bank. Last year's monthly demand for the different bicycle styles that EC distributes is shown in Table 12.6.

Because of the increasing popularity of bicycles for recreational purposes and for supplanting some automobile usage, EC believes that its market may grow by as much as 25 percent in the upcoming year. There have been years when the full amount of expected growth did not materialize, however, so EC has decided to base its plan on a more conservative 15-percent growth factor to allow for variations in consumer buying habits and to ensure that it is not excessively overstocked if the expected market does not occur. Holding costs that are associated with inventory of any bicycle style are estimated to be about 0.75 percent of the unit cost of a bicycle per month.

Assignment

Develop an inventory control plan for EC to use as the basis for its upcoming annual plan. Justify your reasons for choosing a particular type (or combination of types) of inventory system(s). On the basis of your particular plan, specify the safety stock requirements if EC institutes a policy of maintaining a 95-percent service level.

SELECTED BIBLIOGRAPHY

CHIANG, W., J. A. FITZSIMMONS, Z. HUANG, and S. X. LI: "A Game-Theoretic Approach to Quantity Discount Problems," *Decision Sciences,* vol. 25, no. 1, January–February 1994, pp. 153–168.

HESS, RICK, and GENE WOOLSEY: *Applied Management Science: A Quick & Dirty Approach,* Science Research Associates, Chicago, 1974.

SILVER, E. A., and R. PETERSON: *Decision Systems for Inventory Management and Production Planning,* 2nd ed., Wiley, New York, 1985.

TEDLOW, RICHARD S.: *New and Improved: The Story of Mass Marketing in America,* Harvard Business School, Boston, 1996.

TERSINE, RICHARD J.: *Principles of Inventory and Materials Management,* Elsevier North-Holland, New York, 1987.

VOLLMANN, T. E., W. L. BERRY, and D. C. WHYBARK: *Manufacturing Planning and Control Systems,* 3rd ed., Irwin, Homewood, Ill., 1991.

CHAPTER 13

Managing Capacity and Demand

LEARNING OBJECTIVES

After completing this chapter, you should be able to:

1. Describe the strategies for matching supply and demand for services.
2. Determine the overbooking strategy for a service that minimizes expected loss.
3. Use a Linear Programming model to prepare a weekly workshift schedule with two consecutive days off for each employee.
4. Prepare a work schedule for part-time employees.
5. Use yield management to establish the inventory level of a perishable resource to reserve for customers who are willing to pay a premium.

After fixed capacity investment decisions have been made (e.g., number of hotel rooms to be built or aircraft to be purchased) using the approaches described in Chapter 17, "Queuing Models and Capacity Planning," the hotel beds must be filled or airline seats sold to make the daily operations profitable. The subject of this chapter is the challenge that is faced by managers of matching service supply with customer demand on a daily basis in a dynamic environment.

Service capacity is a perishable commodity. For example, a plane flying with empty seats has lost forever the revenue opportunity of carrying those additional passengers. American Airlines was the first in its industry to address this problem and to realize the potential of using what now is called *yield management,* which was discussed briefly in Chapter 4 and will be addressed in more detail here. Use of information technology to support yield management was not lost on Mr. Donald Burr, CEO of People Express, whose failing airline was bought by Texas Air in 1986. He is quoted as saying, "I'm the world's leading example of a guy killed by a computer chip."[1]

Unlike products that are stored in warehouses for future consumption, a service is an intangible personal experience that cannot be transferred from one person to another. Instead, a service is produced and consumed simultaneously. Whenever demand for a service falls short of the capacity to serve, the results are idle servers and facilities. Further, the variability in service demand is quite pronounced, and in fact, our culture and habits contribute to these fluctuations. For example, most of us eat our meals at the same hours and take our vacations in July and August, and studies of hospitals indicate low utilization in the summer and fall months. These natural variations in service demand create periods of idle service at some times and of consumer waiting at others.

CHAPTER PREVIEW

In this chapter, we shall explore operating strategies that can increase capacity utilization by better matching the supply of and demand for services. We begin with a discussion of marketing-oriented strategies that can alter and smooth customer demand, such as using price incentives and promotion to stimulate off-peak utilization. Another common strategy is creating complementary services to balance the total demand among several services. In addition, the controversial practice of *overbooking* is examined in the context of making better use of perishable service capacity.

We also will look at operations-oriented strategies to control the level of service supply, such as scheduling workshifts, using part-time employees, and cross-training customer contact personnel to be more flexible in response to changes in customer demand. In conclusion, the new concept of yield management as pioneered by the airline industry will be explored as a comprehensive approach using many of these strategies in a sophisticated on-line information system.

[1]R. L. Rose and J. Dahl, "Skies Are Deregulated, but Just Try Starting a Sizable New Airline," *The Wall Street Journal,* July 19, 1989, p. 1.

STRATEGIES FOR MANAGING DEMAND

Excessive fluctuations in demand for service need not be accepted as inevitable. Service systems can smooth their demand by using both active and passive measures. With *smoothed demand,* the cyclical variation has been reduced. While the arrival of consumers will continue to occur at random intervals, the average rate of arrivals will be more stable over time. We shall discuss several strategies for smoothing demand, and Figure 13.1 summarizes those that commonly are used to manage service capacity.

Partitioning Demand

Demand for a service seldom derives from a homogeneous source. For example, airlines differentiate between weekday business travelers and weekend pleasure travelers. Demand often is grouped into random arrivals and planned arrivals. For example, a drive-in bank can expect visits from its commercial account holders on a regular, daily basis and at approximately the same time; it also can expect visits from its personal account holders on a random basis.

An analysis of health clinic demand by E. J. Rising, R. Baron, and B. Averill showed that the greatest number of walk-in patients arrived on Monday and

FIGURE 13.1. Strategies for matching supply of and demand for services.

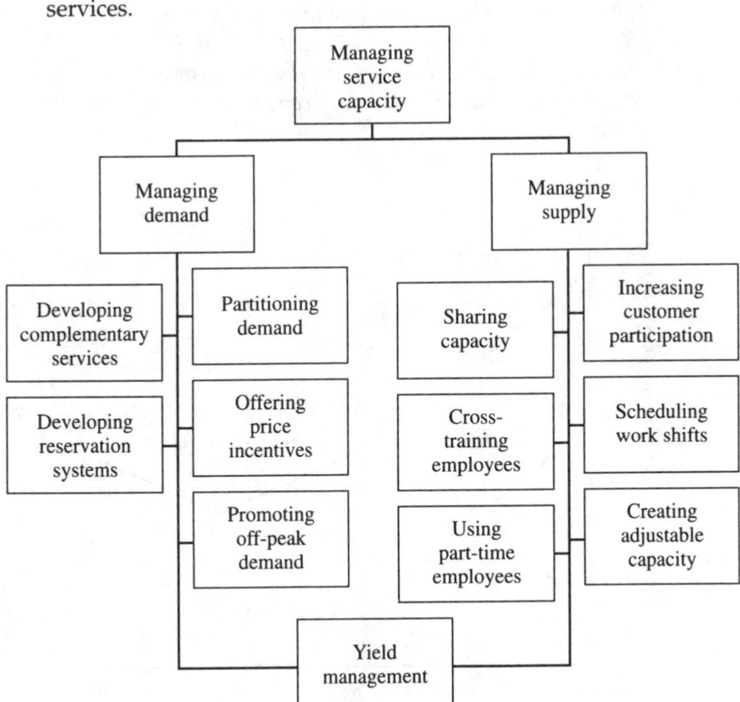

fewer during the remaining weekdays.[2] While walk-in demand is not controllable, appointments are. Therefore, why not make appointments in the latter part of the week to level demand? Using data for the same week in the previous year, these researchers noted the number of walk-in patients for each weekday. Subtracting these walk-in patients from daily physician capacity gives the number of appointment patients who are needed each day to smooth demand. For the sample week shown in Figure 13.2, this procedure yielded the number of appointment periods per day shown in Table 13.1.

The daily smoothing of demand was refined further by scheduling appointments at appropriate times during the day. After a 2-month shakedown period, smoothing demand yielded the following benefits:

1. The number of patients seen increased by 13.4 percent.
2. This increase in patient demand was met, even though 5.1 percent fewer physician hours were scheduled.
3. The overall time physicians spent with patients increased 5.0 percent because of the increased number of appointments.

[2]E. J. Rising, R. Baron, and B. Averill, "A Systems Analysis of a University Health-Service Outpatient Clinic," *Operations Research,* vol. 21, no. 5, September 1973, pp. 1030–1947.

FIGURE 13.2. Effect of smoothing physician visits. *(E. J. Rising, R. Baron, and B. Averill, "A Systems Analysis of a University Health-Service Outpatient Clinic." Reprinted with permission from* Operations Research, *vol. 21, no. 5, Sept.–Oct. 1973, p. 1035, Operations Research Society of America. No further reproduction permitted without the consent of the copyright owner.)*

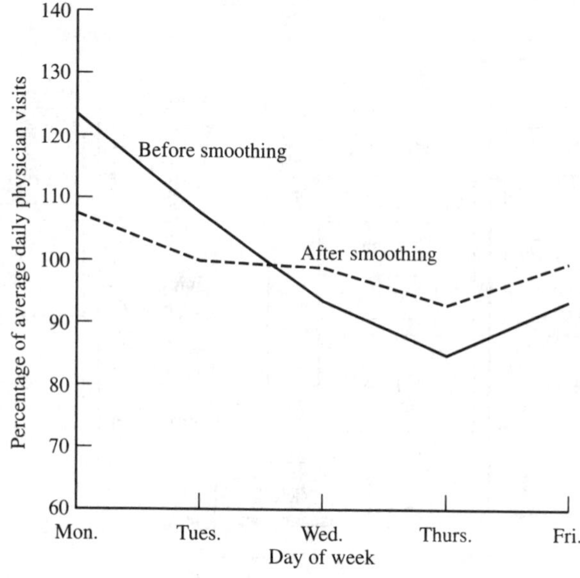

TABLE 13.1. Smoothing Demand by Appointment Scheduling

Day	Appointments (n)
Monday	84
Tuesday	89
Wednesday	124
Thursday	129
Friday	114

4. The average waiting time for patients remained the same.
5. A team of sociologists concluded that physician morale increased.

Offering Price Incentives

There are many examples of differential pricing. Consider the following:

1. Weekend and night rates for long-distance telephone calls.
2. Matinee or reduced prices before 6 PM at movie theaters.
3. Off-season hotel rates at resort locations.
4. Peak-load pricing by utility companies.

Differential pricing has been suggested for federal campsites to encourage better use of this scarce resource. For example, J. C. Nautiyal and R. L. Chowdhary developed a discriminatory pricing system to ensure that camping fees accurately reflect the marginal benefit of the last campsite on any given day.[3]

They identified four different camping experiences on the basis of days and weeks of the camping season. Table 13.2 contains a schedule of daily fees by experience type.

[3]J. C. Nautiyal and R. L. Chowdhary, "A Suggested Basis for Pricing Campsites: Demand Estimation in an Ontario Park," *Journal of Leisure Research*, vol. 7, no. 2, 1975, pp. 95–107.

TABLE 13.2. Suggested Discriminatory Fee Schedule

Experience Type	Days and Weeks of Camping Season	Days (n)	Daily Fee ($)
1	Saturdays and Sundays of weeks 10 to 15, plus Dominion Day and civic holidays	14	6.00
2	Saturdays and Sundays of weeks 3 to 9 and 15 to 19, plus Victoria Day	23	2.50
3	Fridays of weeks 3 to 15, plus all other days of weeks 9 to 15 that are not in experience type 1 or 2	43	0.50
4	Rest of camping season	78	Free

These experience groupings were made on the basis of total daily occupancy in the park under the assumption that occupancy is directly affected by available leisure time and climate. Campers in each experience group were interviewed to determine their travel costs. The marginal visitor was assumed to be the camper who incurred the highest cost in coming to the recreation site. This information was used to develop a demand curve for each experience type, and given the available number of campsites, the campsite fee was determined by means of these demand curves. Table 13.3 compares revenues generated under the existing system with those estimated when using discriminatory fees. Note that under the proposal, more campers are attracted, but with a corresponding reduction in total revenue. During the 78 days of free camping, however, a savings in labor cost is possible, because no ranger is needed to collect fees at the campsite. Even so, for the arrangement to work effectively in altering demand, it must be well advertised and include an advance booking system for campsites.

Note the projected increase in demand for experience type 3 because of the substantially reduced fee. The result of off-peak pricing is to tap a latent demand for campsites instead of redistributing peak demand to off-peak times. Thus, discriminatory pricing fills in the valleys (i.e., periods of low demand) instead of leveling off the peaks. The result is better overall utilization of a scarce resource and, for a private-sector firm, the potential for increased profit (assuming that fees cover variable costs). Private firms, however, also would want to avoid directing high-paying customers to low-rate schedules. For example, airlines exclude the business traveler from discount fares through restrictions such as requiring passengers to remain at their destination over a weekend.

Promoting Off-Peak Demand

Creative use of off-peak capacity results from seeking different sources of demand. One example is use of a resort hotel during the off-season as a retreat location for business or professional groups. Another is a mountain ski resort that becomes a staging area for backpacking during the summer. Telephone companies offer lower rates to encourage long-distance dialing at night or on weekends,

TABLE 13.3. Comparison of Existing Revenue and Projected Revenue from Discriminatory Pricing

	Existing Fee of $2.50		*Discriminatory Fee*	
Experience Type	Campsites Occupied	Revenue ($)	Campsites Occupied (est.)	Revenue ($)
1	5,891	14,727	5,000	30,000
2	8,978	22,445	8,500	21,250
3	6,129	15,322	15,500	7,750
4	4,979	12,447	....	....
Total	25,977	$64,941	29,000	$59,000

	Monday	Tuesday	Wednesday	Thursday	Friday	Saturday	Sunday
8 AM–5 PM							
5 PM–11 PM							
11 PM–8 AM							

Day Rate	Evening Rate	Night/Weekend Rate
Plus additional volume discounts of 10%	Plus additional volume discounts of 20%–30%	Plus additional volume discounts of 20%–30%

FIGURE 13.3. Rate schedule for Sprint PLUS.

when switching equipment is underutilized. Figure 13.3 shows such a schedule for one such long-distance carrier.

The strategy of promoting off-peak demand can be used to discourage overtaxing the facility at other times. A department store's appeal to "shop early and avoid the Christmas rush" as well as a supermarket's offer of double coupons on Wednesdays are examples.

Developing Complementary Services

Restaurants have discovered the benefits of complementary services by adding a bar. Diverting waiting customers into the lounge during busy periods can be profitable for the restaurant as well as soothing to anxious consumers. Movie theaters traditionally have sold popcorn and soft drinks, but now they also include video games in their lobbies. These examples illustrate complementary services being offered to occupy waiting consumers.

Convenience stores have expanded their services to include self-service gas pumps and fast-food meals. The concept of holistic medicine, which combines traditional medical attention with nutritional and psychiatric care, is a further example. Developing complementary services is a natural way to expand one's market, and it is particularly attractive if the new demands for service are contracyclical and result in a more uniform aggregate demand (i.e., when the new service demand is high, the original service demand is low). This explains why nearly all heating contractors also perform air-conditioning services.

Using Reservation Systems and Handling the Overbooking Problem

Taking reservations presells the potential service. As reservations are made, additional demand is deflected to other time slots at the same facility or to other facilities within the same organization. Hotel chains with national reservation systems regularly book customers in nearby hotels owned by their chain when the customer's first choice is not available.

Reservations also benefit consumers by reducing waiting and guaranteeing service availability. Problems do arise, however, when customers fail to honor their reservations. (These customers are referred to as *no-shows*.) Usually, customers are not held financially liable for their unkept reservations. This can lead to undesirable behavior, such as when passengers make several flight reservations to cover contingencies. This was a common practice of business passengers who did not know exactly when they would be able to depart; with multiple reservations, they would be assured of a flight out as soon as they were able to leave. All unused reservations result in empty seats, however, unless the airline is notified of the cancellations in advance. To control no-shows among discount flyers, airlines now issue nonrefundable tickets.

Faced with flying empty seats because of the no-shows, airlines adopted a strategy of *overbooking*. By accepting reservations for more than the available seats, airlines hedge against significant numbers of no-shows; however, the airlines risk turning away passengers with reservations if they overbook too many seats. Because of overbooking abuses, the U.S. Federal Aviation Administration instituted regulations requiring airlines to reimburse overbooked passengers and to find them space on the next available flight. Similarly, many hotels place their overbooked guests in a nearby hotel of equal quality at no expense to the guests. A good overbooking strategy should minimize the expected opportunity cost of idle service capacity as well as the expected cost of turning away reservations. Thus, adopting an overbooking strategy requires training front-line personnel (e.g., front-desk clerks at a hotel) to handle graciously guests whose reservations cannot be honored. At a minimum, a courtesy van should be available to transport the customer to a competitor's hotel after making arrangements for an equivalent room.

Example 13.1: Surfside Hotel

During the past tourist season, Surfside Hotel did not achieve very high occupancy despite a reservation system that was designed to keep the hotel fully booked. Apparently, prospective guests were making reservations that, for one reason or another, they failed to honor. A review of front-desk records during the current peak period, when the hotel was fully booked, revealed the record of no-shows given in Table 13.4.

TABLE 13.4. Surfside Hotel No-Show Experience

No-shows (d)	Probability ($P[d]$)	Cumulative Probability ($P[d < x]$)
0	.07	.00
1	.19	.07
2	.22	.26
3	.16	.48
4	.12	.64
5	.10	.76
6	.07	.86
7	.04	.93
8	.02	.97
9	.01	.99

A room that remains vacant because of a no-show results in an opportunity loss of the $40 room contribution. The expected number of no-shows is calculated from Table 13.4 as:

$$0(.07) + 1(.19) + 2(.22) + \cdots + 8(.02) + 9(.01) = 3.04$$

This yields an expected opportunity loss of 3.04 × $40, or $121.60, per night. To avoid some of this loss, management is considering an overbooking policy; however, if a guest holding a reservation is turned away owing to overbooking, then other costs are incurred. Surfside has made arrangements with a nearby hotel to pay for the rooms of guests who it cannot accommodate. Further, a penalty is associated with the loss of customer goodwill and the impact this has on future business. Management estimates this total loss to be approximately $100 per guest "walked" (a term used by the hotel industry). A good overbooking strategy should strike a balance between the opportunity cost of a vacant room and the cost of not honoring a reservation; the best overbooking strategy should minimize the expected cost in the long run.

Table 13.5 displays the loss that is associated with each possible overbooking alternative. Note that no costs are incurred along the diagonal of the table, because in each case, the number of reservations that were overbooked exactly matched the no-shows for that day (e.g., if 4 reservations were overbooked and 4 guests failed to arrive, then every guest who did arrive would be accommodated and, further, the hotel is fully occupied, which is a win-win situation). The values above the diagonal are determined by moving across each row and increasing the cost by a multiple of $100 for each reservation that could not be honored, because fewer no-shows occurred than anticipated. For example, consider the first row, which is associated with zero no-shows occurring, and note that a $100 loss is associated with overbooking by one reservation. The values below the diagonal are shown as increasing by multiples of $40 as we move down each column, because more no-shows occurred than expected, which resulted in vacant rooms for the night. For example, consider the first column that is associated with not implementing an overbooking strategy, and note the increasing cost implications of trusting guests to honor their reservations.

For each overbooking reservation strategy, the expected loss is calculated by multiplying the loss for each no-show possibility by its probability of occurrence and then adding the products. For example, the expected loss of overbooking by two reservations is calculated by multiplying the probabilities in column 2 (i.e., Probability) by the losses in column 5 (i.e., 2 Reservations Overbooked) as follows:

$$.07(\$200) + .19(\$100) + .22(\$0) + .16(\$40) + .12(\$80) + .10(\$120)$$
$$+ .07(\$160) + .04(\$200) + .02(\$240) + .01(\$280) = \$87.80$$

Table 13.5 indicates that a policy of overbooking by two rooms will minimize the expected loss in the long run. If this policy is adopted, we can realize a gain of $33.80 per night from overbooking. That is the difference in

TABLE 13.5. Overbooking Loss Table

		Reservations Overbooked									
No-shows	Probability	0	1	2	3	4	5	6	7	8	9
0	.07	0	100	200	300	400	500	600	700	800	900
1	.19	40	0	100	200	300	400	500	600	700	800
2	.22	80	40	0	100	200	300	400	500	600	700
3	.16	120	80	40	0	100	200	300	400	500	600
4	.12	160	120	80	40	0	100	200	300	400	500
5	.10	200	160	120	80	40	0	100	200	300	400
6	.07	240	200	160	120	80	40	0	100	200	300
7	.04	280	240	200	160	120	80	40	0	100	200
8	.02	320	280	240	200	160	120	80	40	0	100
9	.01	360	320	280	240	200	160	120	80	40	0
Expected loss ($)	. . .	121.60	91.40	87.80	115.00	164.60	231.00	311.40	401.60	497.40	560.00

the expected loss between not overbooking of $121.60 and the expected loss from overbooking by two rooms of $87.80. This substantial amount explains why overbooking is a popular strategy for capacity-constrained service firms such as airlines and hotels.

In Chapter 12, "Managing Facilitating Goods," the *critical fractile* criterion was derived:

$$P(d < x) \leq \frac{C_u}{C_u + C_o} \tag{1}$$

where C_u = the $40 room contribution that is lost when a reservation is not honored (i.e., the number of no-shows is *under*estimated),
C_o = the $100 opportunity loss associated with not having a room available for an overbooked guest (i.e., the number of no-shows is *over*estimated),
d = the number of no-shows based on past experience, and
x = the number of rooms overbooked.

This critical probability, which is based on marginal analysis, also can be used to identify the best overbooking strategy. Thus, the number of rooms overbooked should just cover the cumulative probability of no-shows and no more, as calculated below:

$$P(d < x) \leq \frac{\$40}{\$40 + \$100}$$

$$\leq 28.6$$

From Table 13.4, a strategy of overbooking by two rooms satisfies the critical fractile criterion, because the cumulative probability $P(d < x) = .26$ and, thus, confirms the earlier decision based on minimizing the expected overbooking loss.

STRATEGIES FOR MANAGING SUPPLY

For many services, demand cannot be smoothed very effectively. Consider, for example, the demand for telephone operators as shown in Figure 13.4. These data are the half-hourly call rates during a typical 24-hour day for a metropolitan telephone company. We see that peak volume (2500 calls) occurs at 10:30 AM and minimum volume (20 calls) occurs at 5:30 AM. The peak-to-valley variation is 125 to 1. No inducements are likely to change this demand pattern substantially; therefore, control must come from adjusting service supply to match demand. Several strategies can be used to achieve this goal.

Using Daily Workshift Scheduling

By scheduling workshifts carefully during the day, the profile of service supply can be made to approximate demand. Workshift scheduling is an important staffing problem for many service organizations that face cyclical demand, such as telephone companies, hospitals, banks, and police departments.

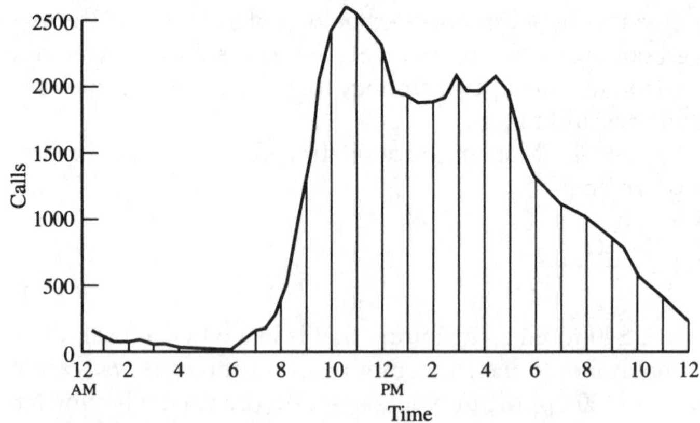

FIGURE 13.4. Daily demand for telephone operators.
(E. S. Buffa, M. J. Cosgrove, and B. J. Luce, "An Integrated Work Shift Scheduling System," Decision Sciences, *vol. 7, no. 4, October 1976, p. 622. Reprinted with permission from Decision Sciences Institute, Georgia State University.)*

The general approach begins with a forecast of demand by hour, which is converted to hourly service staffing requirements. The time interval could be less than an hour; for example, 15-minute intervals are used by fast-food restaurants to schedule work during meal periods. Next, a schedule of tours, or shifts, is developed to match the staffing requirements profile as closely as possible. Finally, specific service personnel are assigned to tours, or shifts. The telephone-operator staffing problem will be used to demonstrate the analysis required for each step; however, the approach can be generalized to any service organization.

Forecast Demand

Daily demand is forecast in half-hour intervals, as shown in Figure 13.4, and must account for both weekday and weekend variations as well as seasonal adjustments. The Saturday and Sunday call load was found to be approximately 55 percent of the typical weekday load. Summer months were found to be generally lower in demand. Special high-demand days, such as Mother's Day and Christmas, were taken into account.

Convert to Operator Requirements

A profile of half-hour operator requirements is developed on the basis of the forecast daily demand and call distribution. A standard service level, which is defined by the Public Utilities Commission, requires that 89 percent of the time, an incoming call must be answered within 10 seconds. The half-hour operator requirements thus are determined through a conventional queuing model to ensure that the service level is achieved for each half-hour.[4] The result is a profile of operators required by the half-hour, as shown in Figure 13.5.

[4]The $M/M/c$ queuing model as described in Chapter 17 is used. This model permits the calculation of probabilities of a telephone caller having to wait for different numbers of operators.

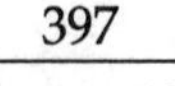

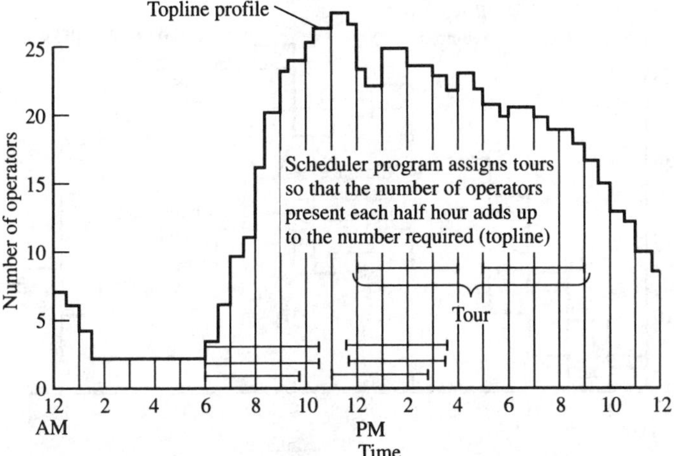

FIGURE 13.5. Profile of operator requirements and tour assignments.
(E. S. Buffa, M. J. Cosgrove, and B. J. Luce, "An Integrated Work Shift Scheduling System," Decision Sciences, *vol. 7, no. 4, October 1976, p. 626. Reprinted with permission from Decision Sciences Institute, Georgia State University.)*

Schedule Shifts

Tours, representing various start and end times of work, need to be assigned so that they aggregate to the top-line profile, shown in Figure 13.5. Each tour consists of two working sessions separated by a rest pause or meal period (e.g., 9 AM–1 PM, lunch break, 2 PM–6 PM). The set of possible tours is defined by state and federal laws, union agreements, and company policy. A heuristic computer program prepared especially for this problem chooses tours from the permissible set such that the absolute difference between operator requirements and operators assigned is minimized when summed over all "n" half-hour periods. If R_i is the number of operators required in period i and W_i is the number of operators assigned in period i, then the objective can be stated as follows:

$$\text{Minimize} \sum_{i=1}^{n} |R_i - W_i| \qquad (2)$$

The schedule-building process is shown schematically in Figure 13.6. At each iteration, one tour at a time is selected from all possible tours. The tour selected at each step is the one that best meets the criterion stated in equation (2). Because this procedure favors shorter tours, the different shift lengths are weighted in the calculation to avoid this bias. The result is a list of tours required to meet the forecast demand, as well as a schedule of lunch and rest periods during those tours.

Assign Operators to Shifts

Given the set of tours required, the assignment of operators to these tours is complicated because of the 24-hour, 7-days-per-week operation. Questions of equity arise regarding the timing of days off and the assignment of overtime work, which involves extra pay. Another computer program makes operator assign-

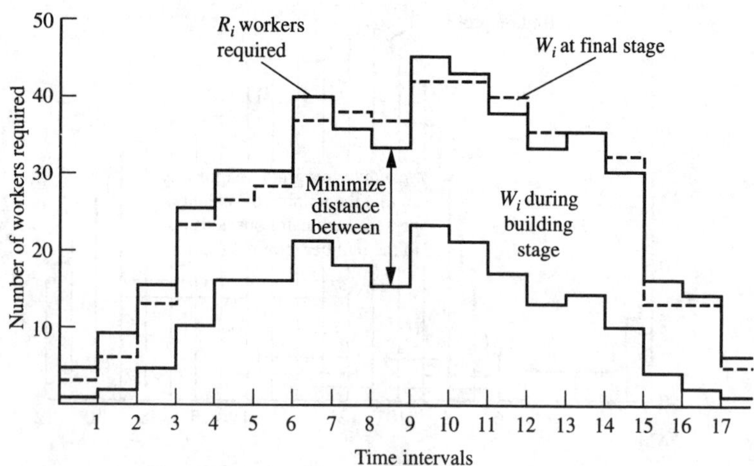

FIGURE 13.6. The schedule-building process.
(E. S. Buffa, M. J. Cosgrove, and B. J. Luce, "An Integrated Work Shift Scheduling System," Decision Sciences, *vol. 7, no. 4, October 1976, p. 622. Reprinted with permission from Decision Sciences Institute, Georgia State University.)*

ments according to policies such as "give at least 1 day off per week and maximize consecutive days off." The actual assignment of operators to shifts also accounts for employee shift preferences. The result of this final step is a feasible schedule of employees assigned to tours.

Using Weekly Workshift Scheduling with Days-Off Constraint

As noted, developing tours to match the profile of daily demand is only part of the problem. Many public services such as police, fire protection, and emergency hospital care must be available 24 hours a day, every day of the week. For these organizations, a typical employee works 5 days a week with 2 consecutive days off each week, but not necessarily Saturday and Sunday. Management is interested in developing work schedules and meeting the varying employee requirements for weekdays and weekends with the smallest number of staff members possible.

This problem can be formulated as an integer linear programming (ILP) model. To begin, the desired staffing levels are determined for each day in the week. The problem then becomes one of determining the minimum number of employees required for assignment to each of seven possible tours. Each tour consists of 5 days on and 2 consecutive days off; each will begin on a different day of the week and last for 5 consecutive working days. Consider the following general formulation of this problem as an ILP model.

Variable definitions:

x_i = number of employees assigned to tour i, where day i begins 2 consecutive days off (e.g., employees assigned to x_1 have Sunday and Monday off), and

b_j = desired staffing level for day j

Objective function:

$$\text{Minimize} \quad x_1 + x_2 + x_3 + x_4 + x_5 + x_6 + x_7$$

Constraints:

$$\begin{array}{lrcl}
\text{Sunday} & x_2 + x_3 + x_4 + x_5 + x_6 & \geq & b_1 \\
\text{Monday} & x_3 + x_4 + x_5 + x_6 + x_7 & \geq & b_2 \\
\text{Tuesday} & x_1 + x_4 + x_5 + x_6 + x_7 & \geq & b_3 \\
\text{Wednesday} & x_1 + x_2 + x_5 + x_6 + x_7 & \geq & b_4 \\
\text{Thursday} & x_1 + x_2 + x_3 + x_6 + x_7 & \geq & b_5 \\
\text{Friday} & x_1 + x_2 + x_3 + x_4 + x_7 & \geq & b_6 \\
\text{Saturday} & x_1 + x_2 + x_3 + x_4 + x_5 & \geq & b_7 \\
 & x_i \geq 0 \text{ and integer} & &
\end{array}$$

Example 13.2: Hospital Emergency Room

The emergency room is operated on a 24-hour, 7-days-per-week schedule. The day is divided into three 8-hour shifts. The total number of nurses required during the day shift is:

Day	Su	M	Tu	W	Th	F	Sa
Nurses	3	6	5	6	5	5	5

The emergency room director is interested in developing a workforce schedule that will minimize the number of nurses required to staff the facility. Nurses work 5 days a week and are entitled to 2 consecutive days off each week.

The ILP model above is formulated with the appropriate right-hand-side constraint values (i.e., $b_1 = 3, b_2 = 6, \ldots b_6 = 5, b_7 = 5$), and the solution yields the following results: $x_1 = 1, x_2 = 1, x_3 = 2, x_4 = 0, x_5 = 3, x_6 = 0, x_7 = 1$. This means we have one tour with Sunday and Monday off, one tour with Monday and Tuesday off, two tours with Tuesday and Wednesday off, three tours with Thursday and Friday off, and one tour with Saturday and Sunday off. The corresponding staffing schedule is shown in Table 13.6 with excess staff occurring only on Sunday and Saturday.

These scheduling problems typically result in multiple optimal solutions. For example, in this case the solution $x_1 = 1, x_2 = 1, x_3 = 1, x_4 = 1, x_5 = 1, x_6 = 1, x_7 = 2$ is feasible and also requires eight nurses. Why might this second solution be preferred to the schedule shown in Table 13.6?

Increasing Customer Participation

The strategy of increasing customer participation is illustrated best by the fast-food restaurants that have eliminated personnel who serve food and clear tables. The customer (now a coproducer) not only places the order directly from a limited menu but also clears the table after the meal. Naturally, the customer expects faster service and less-expensive meals to compensate for this help; however, the service provider benefits in many subtle ways. Of course, there are fewer personnel to supervise and to pay, but more important, the customer as a coproducer

TABLE 13.6. Weekly Nurse Staffing Schedule, × = workday

Nurse	Su	M	Tu	W	Th	F	Sa
A	...	...	×	×	×	×	×
B	×	...	...	×	×	×	×
C	×	×	...	...	×	×	×
D	×	×	...	...	×	×	×
E	×	×	×	×	...	...	×
F	×	×	×	×	...	...	×
G	×	×	×	×	...	...	×
H	...	×	×	×	×	×	...
Total	6	6	5	6	5	5	7
Required	3	6	5	6	5	5	5
Excess	3	0	0	0	0	0	2

provides labor just at the moment it is required. Thus, capacity to serve varies more directly with demand rather than being fixed.

Some drawbacks to self-service do exist, because the quality of labor is not completely under the service manager's control. A self-service gas customer may fail to check the tire pressure and oil level regularly, which eventually can lead to problems. Self-service of "bulk" foods (e.g., cereals, grains, honey, peanut butter) in markets can lead both to contamination of the product in the bulk container and to waste because of spillage.

Creating Adjustable Capacity

Through design, a portion of capacity can be made variable. Airlines routinely move the partition between first class and coach to meet the changing mix of passengers. An innovative restaurant, Benihana of Tokyo, arranged its floor plan to accommodate eating areas serving two tables of eight diners each. Chefs are assigned to each area, and they prepare the meal at the table in a theatrical manner, with flashing knives and animated movements. Thus, the restaurant can adjust its capacity effectively by having only the number of chefs on duty that is needed.

Capacity at peak periods can be expanded by the effective use of slack times. Performing supportive tasks during slower periods of demand allows employees to concentrate on essential tasks during rush periods. This strategy requires some cross-training of employees to allow performance of noncustomer-contact tasks during slow-demand periods. For example, servers at a restaurant can wrap silverware in napkins or clean the premises when demand is low; thus, they are free of these tasks during the rush period.

Sharing Capacity

A service delivery system often requires a large investment in equipment and facilities. During periods of underutilization, it may be possible to find other uses for this capacity. Airlines have cooperated in this manner for years. At small airports, airlines share the same gates, ramps, baggage-handling equipment, and ground personnel. It also is common for some airlines to lease their aircraft to others during the off-season; the lease agreement includes painting on the appropriate insignia and refurbishing the interior.

Cross-Training Employees

Some service systems are made up of several operations. When one operation is busy, another operation sometimes may be idle. Cross-training employees to perform tasks in several operations creates flexible capacity to meet localized peaks in demand.

The gains from cross-training employees can be seen at supermarkets. When queues develop at the cash registers, the manager calls on stockers to operate registers until the surge is over. Likewise, during slow periods, some of the cashiers are busy stocking shelves. This approach also can help to build an esprit de corps and give employees relief from monotony. In fast-food restaurants, cross-trained employees create capacity flexibility, because tasks can be reassigned to fewer employees during slow periods (temporarily enlarging the job) and become more specialized during busy periods (division of labor).

Using Part-Time Employees

When peaks of activity are persistent and predictable, such as at mealtimes in restaurants or paydays in banks, part-time help can supplement regular employees. If the required skills and training are minimal, then a ready part-time labor pool is available from high school and college students as well as others who are interested in supplementing their primary source of income.

Another source of part-time help is off-duty personnel who are placed on standby. Airlines and hospitals often pay their personnel some nominal fee to restrict their activities and be ready for work if they are needed.

Scheduling Part-Time Tellers at a Drive-In Bank[5]

Drive-in banks experience predictable variations in activity on different days of the week. Figure 13.7 shows the teller requirements for a typical week based on customer demand variations. This bank usually employed enough tellers to meet peak demands on Friday; however, the policy created considerable idle teller time on the low-demand days, particularly Tuesday and Thursday. To reduce teller costs, management decided to employ part-time tellers and to reduce their full-time staff to a level that just meets the demand for Tuesday. Further, to provide equity in hours worked, it was decided that a part-time teller should work at least 2, but no more than 3, days in a week.

A primary objective of scheduling part-time workers is to meet the requirements with the minimum number of teller-days. A secondary objective is to have a minimum number of part-time tellers. This approach is illustrated here using bank tellers, but the same procedure can be used for scheduling part-time employees in many other services.

[5]From V. A. Mabert and A. R. Raedels. "The Detail Scheduling of a Part-Time Work Force: A Case Study of Teller Staffing," *Decision Sciences*, vol. 8, no. 1, January 1977, pp. 109–120.

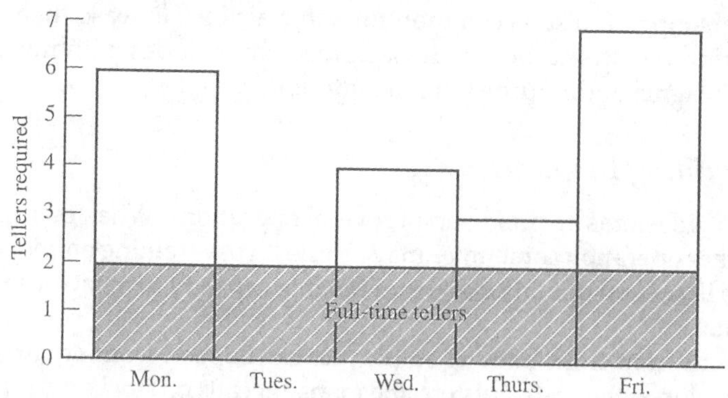

FIGURE 13.7. Teller requirements.

Determine the Minimum Number of Part-Time Tellers Needed

Figure 13.7 shows that with two full-time tellers, 12 teller-days remain to be covered during the week. Using 3-day schedules, we see that five tellers on Friday determines the feasible minimum in this case.

Develop a Decreasing-Demand Histogram

From Figure 13.7, note the daily part-time teller requirements. Resequence the days in order of decreasing demand, as shown in Figure 13.8.

Assign Tellers to the Histogram

Starting with the first part-time teller, assign that individual in Figure 13.8 to the first block on Friday, the second teller to block two, and so forth. Repeat the sequence with Monday, and carry over the remaining tellers into Wednesday. Table 13.7 summarizes the resulting daily part-time work schedule, which consists of two 3-day work assignments for Tellers 1 and 2 and three 2-day work assignments for Tellers 3, 4, and 5.

FIGURE 13.8. Histogram of decreasing part-time teller demand.

TABLE 13.7. Daily Part-Time Work Schedule, × = Workday

Teller	Mon.	Tues.	Wed.	Thurs.	Fri.
1	×	...	×	...	×
2	×	...	...	×	×
3, 4	×	...	...	...	×
5	...	...	×	...	×

YIELD MANAGEMENT[6]

Since deregulation permitted airlines to set their own prices, a new approach to revenue maximization called *yield management*—has emerged. Yield management actually is a comprehensive system that incorporates many of the strategies discussed earlier in this chapter (e.g., reservation systems, overbooking, and partitioning demand).

Because of the perishable nature of airline seats (i.e., once a flight has departed, the potential revenue from an empty seat is lost forever), offering a discount on fares to fill the aircraft became attractive. Selling all seats at a discount, however, would preclude the possibility of selling some at full price. Yield management attempts to allocate the fixed capacity of seats on a flight to match the potential demand in various market segments (e.g., coach, tourist, and supersaver) in the most profitable manner. Although airlines were the first to develop yield management, other capacity-constrained service industries (e.g., hotels, rental-car firms, and cruise lines) also are adopting this practice.

Yield management is most appropriate for service firms that exhibit the following characteristics:

Relatively fixed capacity. Service firms with a substantial investment in facilities (e.g., hotels and airlines) can be considered as being capacity-constrained. Once all the seats on a flight are sold, further demand can be met only by booking passengers on a later flight. Motel chains with multiple inns in the same city, however, have some capacity flexibility, because guests attempting to find room at one site can be diverted to another location within the same company.

Ability to segment markets. For yield management to be effective, the service firm must be able to segment its market into different customer classes. By requiring a Saturday-night stay for a discounted fare, airlines can discriminate between a time-sensitive business traveler and a price-sensitive customer. Developing various price-sensitive classes of service is a major marketing challenge for a firm using yield management. Figure 13.9 shows how a resort hotel might segment its market into three customer classes and adjust the allocation of available rooms to each class on the basis of the seasons of the year.

Perishable inventory. For capacity-constrained service firms, each room or seat is referred to as a *unit* of inventory to be sold (actually, to be rented). As noted for the airlines, revenue from an unsold seat is lost forever. Airlines attempt to minimize this spoiled inventory by encouraging standby passengers. Given this time-perishable nature of an airline seat, what is the cost to the airline when a passenger is awarded a free ticket on a flight that has at least one empty seat?

Product sold in advance. Reservation systems are adopted by service firms to sell capacity in advance of use; however, managers are faced with the uncertainty of whether to accept an early reservation at a discount price or to wait and hope to sell the inventory unit to a higher-paying customer. In Figure 13.10, a demand-control chart (recall quality-control charts from Chapter 10) is drawn for a hotel on the basis of past bookings for a particular day

[6]From Sheryl E. Kimes, "Yield Management: A Tool for Capacity-Constrained Service Firms," *Journal of Operations Management*, vol. 8, no. 4, October 1989, pp. 348–363.

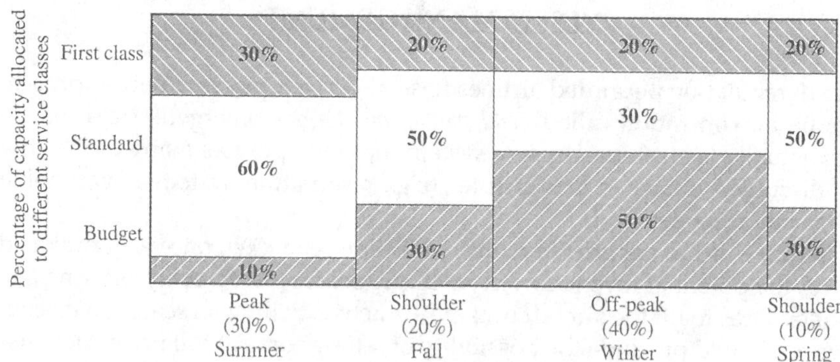

FIGURE 13.9. Seasonal allocation of rooms by service class for a resort hotel. *(After Christopher H. Lovelock, "Strategies for Managing Demand in Capacity-Constrained Service Organizations,"* Service Industries Journal, *vol. 4, no. 3, November 1984, p. 23.)*

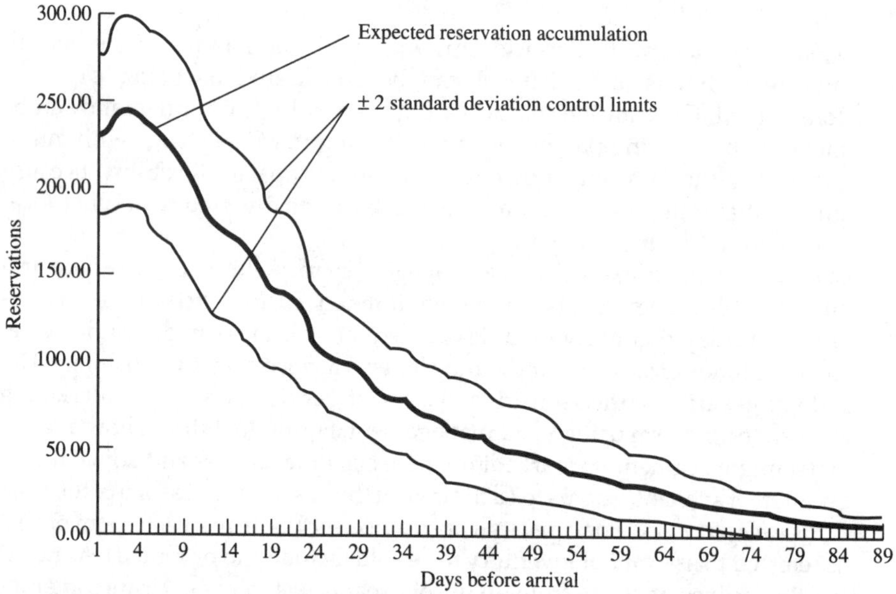

FIGURE 13.10. Demand control chart for a hotel. *(Adapted from Sheryl E. Kimes, "Yield Management: A Tool for Capacity-Constrained Service Firms,"* Journal of Operations Management, *vol. 8, no. 4, October 1989, p. 359. Reprinted with permission, The American Production and Inventory Society.)*

of the week and season of the year. Because some variation in demand is expected, an acceptable range (in this case, ± 2 standard deviations) is drawn around the expected reservation accumulation curve. If demand is higher than expected, budget-rate classes are closed and only reservations at standard rates accepted. If the accumulation of reservations falls below the acceptable range, then reservations for rooms at budget rates are accepted.

Fluctuating demand. Using demand forecasting, yield management allows managers to increase utilization during periods of slow demand and to increase revenue during periods of high demand. By controlling the availability of budget rates, managers can maximize total revenue for the constrained service. Yield management is implemented in real time by opening and/or closing reserved sections—even on an hourly basis if desired.

Low marginal sales costs and high marginal capacity change costs. The cost of selling an additional unit of inventory must be low, such as the negligible cost of a snack for an airline passenger. The marginal cost of capacity additions is large, however, because of the necessary lumpy facility investment (i.e., a hotel addition must be at least an increment of 100 rooms).

Example 13.3: Blackjack Airline

During the recent economic slump, Blackjack Airline discovered that airplanes on its Los Angeles–to–Las Vegas route have been flying with more empty seats than usual. To stimulate demand, it has decided to offer a special, nonrefundable, 14-day advance-purchase "gamblers fare" for only $49 one-way based on a round-trip ticket. The regular full-fare coach ticket costs $69 one-way. The Boeing 737 used by Blackjack, as shown in Figure 13.11, has a capacity of 95 passengers in coach, and management wants to limit the number of seats that are sold at the discount fare in order to sell full-fare tickets to passengers who have not made advance travel plans. Considering recent experience, the demand for full-fare tickets appears to have a normal distribution, with a mean of 60 and a standard deviation of 15.

Phillip E. Pfeifer observed that this yield management problem can be analyzed with the critical fractile model used earlier in the chapter [equation (1)] for analyzing the overbooking problem.[7]

$$P(d < x) \leq \frac{C_u}{C_u + C_o}$$

where

x = seats reserved for full-fare passengers.
d = demand for full-fare tickets.
C_u = lost revenue associated with reserving too few seats at full fare (i.e., underestimated demand). The lost opportunity is the difference between the fares ($69 – $49 = $20), because we assume that the nonshopper passenger, who is willing to pay full fare, purchased a seat at the discount price.
C_o = cost of reserving one-too-many seats for sale at full fare (i.e., overestimated demand). We assume that the empty full-fare seat could have been sold at the discount price. However, C_o takes on two values, depending on the buying behavior of the passenger who would have purchased the seat if not reserved for full fare.

$$C_o = \begin{cases} \$49 & \text{if passenger is a shopper.} \\ -(\$69 - \$49) & \text{if passenger is a nonshopper.} \end{cases}$$

[7] Phillip E. Pfeifer, "The Airline Discount Fare Allocation Problem," *Decision Sciences*, vol. 20, Winter 1989, p. 155.

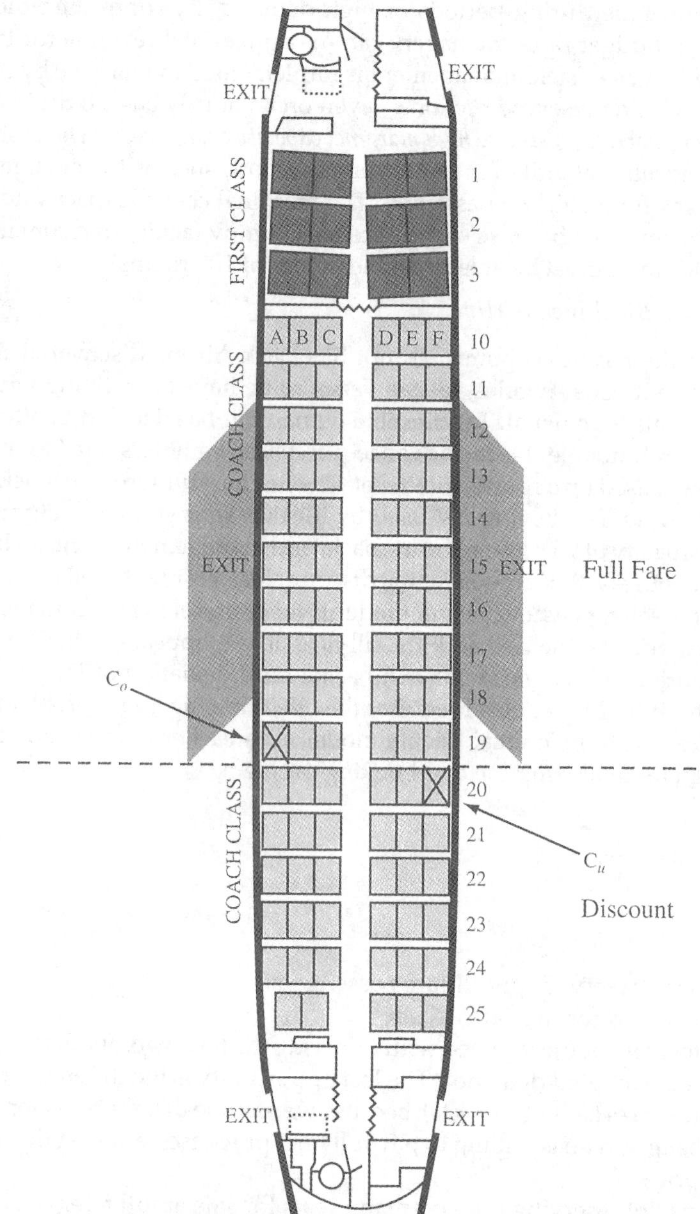

FIGURE 13.11. The Boeing 737 cabin.

For the nonshopper case, the cost is reduced by the difference between the fares, because the airline profits from the nonshopper, who did not make the purchase, paying the full rather than the discount fare. To establish an expected value for C_o, however, we need the proportion p of passengers who are shoppers. In this case, market research determined that approximately

90 percent of passengers are discount seekers; thus, the expected value for the cost of overage becomes:

$$C_o = (0.9)(\$49) - (1 - 0.9)(\$69 - \$49)$$
$$= \$42.10$$

The critical fractile value, as illustrated in Figure 13.12, $P(d < x) = \$20/(\$20 + \$42.10) = .32$. From Appendix A, Areas of a Standard Normal Distribution, the z value for a cumulative probability of .32 is −.47. Thus, the number of full-fare seats to reserve is found as follows:

$$\text{Reserved full-fare seats} = \mu + z\sigma$$
$$= 60 + (-.47)(15)$$
$$= 53$$

Substituting symbols for the values used in the example above, we can derive a simple expression for determining the number of full-fare seats to reserve:

$$P(d < x) \leq \frac{(F - D)}{p \cdot F} \qquad (3)$$

where

x = seats reserved for full-fare passengers,
d = demand for full-fare tickets,
F = price of full fare,
D = price of discount fare, and
p = probability that a passenger is a shopper.

FIGURE 13.12. Critical fractile for Blackjack Airline.

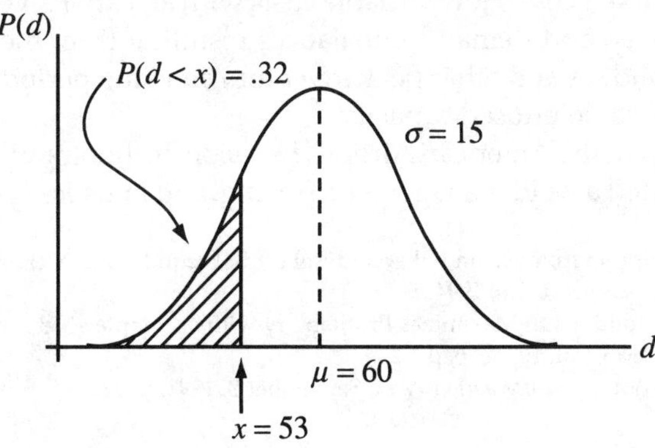

Yield Management Applications[8]

The following discussion provides a sampling of how yield management is used by other companies that face high fixed costs/low variable costs, spoilage, and temporary demand imbalances to accomplish the same goals that airline pricing and yield management systems achieve.

Holiday Inn Reservation Optimization (HIRO)[9]

The hotel industry is similar to the airline industry, because hotels have extremely high costs invested in real estate and maintenance, temporary capacity, and demand imbalances. Imbalances such as varying, peak and low seasons, spoilage, and rooms not rented out for a night all represent lost revenue opportunities. Holiday Inn has recognized these classic management problems and uses both demand and capacity management to maximize revenues.

To achieve Holiday Inn's corporate objectives of ensuring that maximum occupancy and revenue are realized in each hotel and that guests, franchises, and internal staff are experiencing the highest level of customer satisfaction, Holiday Inn installed HIRO. The goal of maximizing occupancy and revenue means renting as many rooms as possible for the best price that the market will bear. With more than 500,000 rooms in the equation, a yield management optimization system could increase revenue tremendously.

HIRO, which is similar to American Airlines' SABRE, uses historical and current booking behavior to analyze room requests for each hotel. The yield management optimization equation includes seasonal occupancy patterns, local events, weekly cycles, and current trends to develop a hurdle price (i.e., the lowest point at which rooms should be booked at that particular hotel). The system predicts full occupancy at hotels and "filters out" discounted requests. HIRO even uses overbooking to account for cancellations and no-shows. As with any yield management system in the service industry, HIRO helps the hotel manager to balance the ability to charge full price for a room and still maintain satisfaction from its loyal customer base.

Ryder's RyderFirst[10]

Ryder must manage the same logistical problems that are faced by any transportation company, and the shipping and trucking industry can use yield management to maximize revenue very effectively. Again, we see the classic business problem of high fixed costs/low variable costs with an expansive fleet of trucks, temporary capacity, and demand imbalances resulting from the seasonality of shipping (i.e., holidays and other peak inventory stocking periods), the threat of spoilage, and valuable unused capacity.

With the help of the American Airlines Decision Technology Group (AADT), Ryder implemented a yield management, pricing, and logistics system that helps

[8]Adapted with permission from Kevin Baker and Robert B. Freund, "The Yield Management Analyst," University of Texas at Austin, 1994.

[9]Lenny Leibmann, "Holiday Inn Maximizes Profitability with a Complex Network Infrastructure," *LAN Magazine*, June 1995, vol. 10, no. 6, p. 123.

[10]"On the Road to Rebound," *Information Week*, September 3, 1991, p. 32.

it to react quickly to competition and take advantage of the price elasticities of its different customer segments. The yield management system allows Ryder to move its truck capacity from areas of surplus to areas of demand by modeling the historical utilization patterns in each market.

Restaurant Catering Software[11]

Yield management techniques are being incorporated into software for use in the restaurant catering industry to ensure efficient utilization of expensive kitchens. Yield management software alerts operators to the potential for increased off-premise or catering bookings during anticipated low in-store demand days, thus enhancing overall profitability. Computer modeling also includes the manipulation of prices based on demand fluctuations. For example, a restaurant may reduce its menu item prices to increase customer count and overall revenue. Similarly, in peak demand periods, item prices may be increased to increase the average check revenue. Yield management helps to smooth the fluctuating demand patterns in the catering industry by anticipating when temporary demand and capacity imbalances will occur.

Amtrak[12]

As far back as 1988, Amtrak introduced a pricing and yield management system identical to that of airlines. This yield management system utilizes a tiered-fare structure, overbooking, discount allocation, and traffic management to maximize yields and capacity utilization. Like the airlines, Amtrak uses the yield management market information to decide what routes to enter and how much capacity is necessary to satisfy demand. Amtrak's flexible capacity allows it to make last-minute capacity adjustments much more easily than in the airline industry by attaching and detaching different classes of rail cars.

SUMMARY

The inherent variability of demand creates a challenge for managers trying to make the best use of service capacity. The problem can be approached from two perspectives. One focuses on smoothing consumer demand, permitting fuller utilization of a fixed service capacity. Various alternatives for managing demand are available, such as partitioning demand, offering price incentives, promoting off-peak use, and developing complementary services and reservation systems.

Another strategy considers the problem from the supply side, and many alternatives have been proposed to adjust service capacity to match demand. Elaborate procedures for workshift scheduling have been developed to adjust capacity to demand. When possible, part-time employees can be used to create

[11]Michael Kasavana, "Catering Software: Problems for Off-Premise Bookings Can Greatly Increase Operational Efficiency," *Restaurant Business*, vol. 90, no. 13, September 1, 1991, p. 90.
[12]"Travel Advisory: Amtrak Adopts Fare System of Airlines," *The New York Times*, December 4, 1989, Section 3, p. 3.

variable capacity. Increasing consumer participation in the service process shifts some tasks to the consumer and reduces part of the burden during peak-demand periods. Other possibilities include sharing capacity with others, as airlines do by leasing aircraft during off-season periods. Occasionally, capacity can be adjusted—for example, by opening and closing dining areas in a restaurant. Cross-training employees also can provide flexible capacity by enabling employees to assist one another during busy periods.

The strategies are presented as two separate views of the same problem, one from the demand side and the other from the supply side. Of course, this should not preclude the use of mixed strategies to mediate the problem from both perspectives. Yield management as practiced by American Airlines is considered just such a mixed strategy, because the company integrates supply and demand management using the power of information contained in its computer reservation system. The result is the real-time ability to sell a class of service to the right customer at the appropriate time and the most competitive price.

KEY TERMS AND DEFINITIONS

Critical fractile the cumulative probability of demand formed by the ratio of the cost of *under*estimating demand divided by the sum of the costs of *under*estimating demand and *over*estimating demand.

Overbooking taking reservations in excess of available capacity in anticipation of customer no-shows.

Yield management a comprehensive system to maximize revenue for capacity-constrained services using reservation systems, overbooking, and partitioning demand.

TOPICS FOR DISCUSSION

1. Explain, from a consumer-participation point of view, why airlines find it profitable to offer reduced fares for standby passengers.
2. What noneconomic incentives might encourage banking customers to use the drive-in window at off-peak times?
3. It has been suggested that the price of airline tickets should be variable, with the cost becoming higher as the time of departure approaches. Comment.
4. What organizational problems can arise from the use of part-time employees?
5. How can computer-based reservation systems increase service capacity utilization?
6. Illustrate how a particular service has implemented successful strategies for managing both demand and supply.
7. What possible dangers are associated with developing complementary services?

Service Benchmark

Yield Management at American Airlines

In its 1987 annual report, American Airlines broadly described the function of yield management as "selling the right seats to the right customers at the right prices." While this statement oversimplified yield management, it does capture the basic motivation behind the strategy. A better description of yield management as it applies to airlines is the control and management of reservations inventory in a way that increases (maximizes, if possible) company profitability, given the flight schedule and fare structure.

The role of yield management at American is analogous to the inventory control function for a manufacturing company. Planning departments determine the airline's flight schedule and fares. The combination of schedule and fares defines the products to be offered to the public. Yield management then determines how much of each product to put on the shelf (make available for sale). American's "store front" is the computerized reservations system. SABRE* (semi-automated business research environment). All sale and cancellation transactions, whether from American Airlines reservations agents or travel agents, pass through SABRE, updating reservations inventory for all affected flights. New reservations are accepted only if yield management controls permit.

Although there is some interaction, the American Airlines yield management system is typically divided into three major functions:

(1) *Overbooking* is the practice of intentionally selling more reservations for a flight than there are actual seats on the aircraft. Airlines use overbooking to offset the effects of passenger cancellations and no-shows. Without overbooking, about 15 percent of seats would be unused on flights sold out at departure. Even more seats would be unused for flights sold out prior to departure.

(2) *Discount allocation* is the process of determining the number of discount fares to offer on a flight. Airlines offer discount fares to stimulate demand and fill seats that would otherwise be empty. The availability of discount fares must be limited on popular flights to preserve space for late-booking, higher-revenue passengers. Therefore, airlines treat reservation space as a scarce resource that must be intelligently allocated to various discount fares.

(3) *Traffic management* is the process of controlling reservations by passenger origin and destination to provide the mix of markets (multiple-flight connecting markets versus single-flight markets) that maximizes revenue. A passenger flying into Dallas/Fort Worth can connect and continue on to any of several final destinations on a second flight. Therefore, to maximize revenue across the entire system of flights, reservation inventory controls for one flight must consider the passenger demand on connecting flights.

The nature of today's marketplace in the airline industry makes yield management absolutely essential to profitable operations. At large airlines, such as American, the number of inventory controls and the frequency of updates requires an automated decision-making system. American's current yield management system, DINAMO (dynamic inventory and maintenance optimizer), was fully implemented in 1988. DINAMO is the latest step of a development process that spans the last 25 years, responding to changes in the airline industry and taking advantage of innovations in computer technology. Three major changes motivated and shaped yield management development:

—The implementation of a computer reservations system (SABRE) in 1966, which had the capability of controlling reservations inventory;

—The introduction of super-saver discount fares in 1977; and

—The deregulation of airline schedules and prices in 1979.

Prior to the implementation of SABRE, American had no centralized methods for reviewing or controlling reservation activity. Reservation offices, established in major cities, acted independently in making inventory decisions. Without the data on passenger behavior needed to do more sophisticated yield management, reservations control was limited to rudimentary overbooking.

SABRE provided a central point from which to collect data. SABRE also provided the centralized control needed to coordinate and enforce these new decisions. In 1968, American Airlines implemented

*Since the original publication of this article, American Airlines, Inc., and the SABRE Group have become separate subsidiaries of AMR, Inc.

an automated overbooking process, the flight load predictor, which determined overbooking levels based on management specified service levels. In 1976, this system was replaced by a different approach to overbooking. The new system, RIPACS (reservations inventory planning and control system), attempted to maximize overbooking profitability by explicitly accounting for the revenue and costs associated with the decision. The current overbooking model, implemented in 1987, makes better use of information on costs and benefits.

With the introduction of super-saver discount fares in 1977, the role of yield management expanded to include allocating reservations inventory to different classes of passengers who compete for space on the same flights. Super-saver fares introduced new pricing controls to the industry and enabled airlines to effectively divide passengers into business travelers and personal and pleasure travelers. Turning super-saver availability on and off resulted in an early form of demand-responsive pricing. The objective of this type of pricing is to adjust the demand to match the supply of seats. American offered cheaper fares to stimulate demand in a controlled manner on low demand flights while maintaining higher profits on popular flights by limiting the number of super-saver fares offered. Allowing the sale of too many discount fares causes the displacement of higher revenue passengers, while allowing too few discount sales results in empty seats on the plane. In 1982, Decision Technologies developed an optimization model to determine the appropriate number of reservations to allocate to each fare type.

Airline deregulation in 1979 led to additional complexity in the practice of yield management. Two major changes took place. First, the number and variety of discount fares increased. Second, airlines began offering connecting service, using centrally located airports as hubs, to serve more of the traveling public and provide national service. For example, a single American Airlines flight from Dallas/Fort Worth to Denver may serve passengers from over 40 different eastern cities who are connecting to the Denver flight. The resulting airline environment is very complex. Many different passenger itineraries are possible, all with many different fares. Also, prices change rapidly, with up to 50,000 fare changes made daily.

Yield management has played a key role in allowing American Airlines to compete and succeed in an environment of stiff price competition. Some of the benefits are difficult to measure, such as increasing American Airlines' ability to survive price wars. Overall, yield management has provided quantifiable benefits of over $1.4 billion for the last three years. To put these increased revenues in perspective, AMR (the holding company for American Airlines) had net profit (after all expenses and taxes) of $892 million for the same three year period. As the airline grows and yield-management models become more sophisticated, the annual revenue benefit will increase.

Source: Barry C. Smith, John F. Leimkuhler, and Ross M. Darrow, "Yield Management at American Airlines." *Interfaces,* Vol. 22, No. 1, January–February 1992, pp. 8–31.

SOLVED PROBLEMS

1. Overbooking Problem

Problem Statement

A family-run inn is considering the use of overbooking, because the frequency of no-shows listed below has left many rooms vacant during the past summer season. An empty room represents an opportunity cost of $69, which is the average room rate. Accommodating an overbooked guest is expensive, however, because the nearby resort rooms average $119 and the inn must pay the difference. What would be the expected gain per night from overbooking?

No-shows	0	1	2	3
Frequency	4	3	2	1

Solution

First, create an overbooking loss table using $69 as the cost of an empty room and $119 – $69 = $50 as the cost of "walking" a guest.

No-Shows	Probability	*Reservations Overbooked* 0	1	2	3
0	.4	0	50	100	150
1	.3	69	0	50	100
2	.2	138	69	0	50
3	.1	207	138	69	0
Expected Loss		69.00	47.60	61.90	100.00

Second, calculate the expected loss by multiplying each overbooking column by the corresponding probability of no-shows and then adding each term. For 0 reservations overbooked, this yields:

$$(0)(.4) + (69)(.3) + (138)(.2) + (207)(.1) = 69$$

Looking across the expected-loss row, we find that overbooking by one reservation will minimize the expected loss and result in an expected nightly gain from overbooking of $69.00 – $47.60 = $21.40.

2. Weekly Workshift Scheduling

Problem Statement

The telephone reservation department for a major car-rental firm has the daily shift requirements for operators below:

Day	Sun.	Mon.	Tues.	Wed.	Thurs.	Fri.	Sat.
Operators	4	8	8	7	7	6	5

Prepare a weekly workshift schedule with 2 consecutive days off.

Solution

Formulate the problem as an integer linear programming model, and solve using Excel Solver.

Objective function:

Minimize $x_1 + x_2 + x_3 + x_4 + x_5 + x_6 + x_7$

Constraints:

Sunday	$x_2 + x_3 + x_4 + x_5 + x_6 \geq 4$
Monday	$x_3 + x_4 + x_5 + x_6 + x_7 \geq 8$
Tuesday	$x_1 + x_4 + x_5 + x_6 + x_7 \geq 8$
Wednesday	$x_1 + x_2 + x_5 + x_6 + x_7 \geq 7$
Thursday	$x_1 + x_2 + x_3 + x_6 + x_7 \geq 7$
Friday	$x_1 + x_2 + x_3 + x_4 + x_7 \geq 6$
Saturday	$x_1 + x_2 + x_3 + x_4 + x_5 \geq 5$

$x_i \geq 0$ and integer

Using Excel Solver yields the following: $x_1 = 2$, $x_2 = 0$, $x_3 = 0$, $x_4 = 0$, $x_5 = 3$, $x_6 = 1$, and $x_7 = 4$.

The corresponding weekly workshift schedule is:

	Schedule Matrix, × = Workday						
Operator	Su	M	Tu	W	Th	F	Sa
A	...	...	×	×	×	×	×
B	...	...	×	×	×	×	×
C	×	×	×	×	...	...	×
D	×	×	×	×	...	...	×
E	×	×	×	×	...	...	×
F	×	×	×	×	×	...	...
G	...	×	×	×	×	×	...
H	...	×	×	×	×	×	...
I	...	×	×	×	×	×	...
J	...	×	×	×	×	×	...
Total	4	8	10	10	7	6	5
Required	4	8	8	7	7	6	5
Excess	0	0	2	3	0	0	0

3. Yield Management

Problem Statement

A ski resort is planning a year-end promotion by offering a weekend special for $159 per person based on double occupancy. The high season rate for these rooms, which includes lift tickets, normally is $299. Management wants to hold some rooms for late arrivals who are willing to pay the season rate. If the proportion of skiers who are willing to pay full rate is approximately 20 percent and their average weekend demand has a normal distribution with a mean of 50 and a standard deviation of 10, how many rooms should be set aside for full-paying skiers?

Solution

Using equation (3), we can determine the critical fractile as follows:

$$P(d < x) \leq \frac{(F - D)}{p \cdot F} = \frac{(299 - 159)}{(0.8)(299)} \leq .58$$

Turning to areas of a Standard Normal Distribution in Appendix A, the z value for a cumulative probability of .58 is .0319. Thus, the number of rooms to protect for full-paying skiers is:

$$\begin{aligned} \mu + z\sigma &= 50 + (.3019)(10) \\ &= 53 \text{ rooms} \end{aligned}$$

EXERCISES

13.1. An outpatient clinic has kept a record of walk-in patients during the past year. The table below shows the expected number of walk-ins by day of the week:

Day	Mon.	Tues.	Wed.	Thurs.	Fri.
Walk-ins	50	30	40	35	40

The clinic has a staff of five physicians, and each can examine 15 patients a day on average.

a. What is the maximum number of appointments that should be scheduled for each day if it is desirable to smooth out the demand for the week?

b. Why would you recommend against scheduling appointments at their maximum level?

c. If most walk-ins arrive in the morning, when should the appointments be made to avoid excessive waiting?

13.2. Reconsider Example 13.1 (Surfside Hotel), because rising costs now have resulted in a $100 opportunity loss from a no-show. Assume that the no-show experience has not significantly changed and that the resulting loss when a guest is overbooked still is $100. Should Surfside revise its no-show policy?

13.3. A commuter airline overbooks all its flights by one passenger (i.e., the ticket agent will take seven reservations for an airplane that only has six seats). The no-show experience for the past 20 days is shown below:

No-shows	0	1	2	3	4
Frequency	6	5	4	3	2

Using the critical fractile $P(d < x) \leq C_u/(C_u + C_o)$, find the maximum implied overbooking opportunity loss C_o if the revenue C_u from a passenger is $20.

13.4. Crazy Joe operates a canoe rental service on the Guadalupe River. He currently leases 15 canoes from a dealer in a nearby city at a cost of $10 per day. On weekends, when the water is high, he picks up the canoes and drives to a launching point on the river, where he rents canoes to white-water enthusiasts for $30 per day. Lately, canoeists have complained about the unavailability of canoes, so Crazy Joe has recorded the demand for canoes and found the experience below for the past 20 days:

Daily demand	10	11	12	13	14	15	16	17	18	19	20
Frequency	1	1	2	2	2	3	3	2	2	1	1

Recommend an appropriate number of canoes to lease.

13.5. An airline serving Denver's Stapleton Airport and Steamboat Springs, Colorado, is considering overbooking its flights to avoid flying with empty seats. For example, the ticket agent is thinking of taking seven reservations for an airplane that has only six seats. During the past month, the no-show experience has been:

No-shows	0	1	2	3	4
Percentage	30	25	20	15	10

The operating costs associated with each flight are: pilot, $150; first officer, $100; fuel, $30; and landing fee, $20.

What would be your recommendation for overbooking if a one-way ticket sells for $80 and the cost of not honoring a reservation is a free lift ticket worth $50 plus a seat on the next flight? What is the expected profit per flight for your overbooking choice?

13.6. Reconsider Example 13.2 (Hospital Emergency Room) to determine if additional nurses will be required to staff the revised daily shift requirements shown below:

Day	Sun.	Mon.	Tues.	Wed.	Thurs.	Fri.	Sat.
Nurses	3	6	5	6	6	6	5

Develop a weekly workshift schedule providing 2 consecutive days off per week for each nurse. Formulate the problem as an integer linear programming model to minimize the number of nurses needed, and solve using Excel Solver. If more nurses are required than the existing staff of eight, suggest an alternative to hiring full-time nurses.

13.7. The sheriff has been asked by the county commissioners to increase weekend patrols in the lake region during the summer months. The sheriff has proposed the following weekly schedule, shifting deputies from weekday assignments to weekends:

Day	Sun.	Mon.	Tues.	Wed.	Thurs.	Fri.	Sat.
Assignments	6	4	4	4	5	5	6

Develop a weekly workshift schedule of duty tours, providing 2 consecutive days off per week for each officer. Formulate the problem as an integer linear programming model to minimize the number of officers needed, and solve using Excel Solver.

13.8. Reconsider Example 13.3 (Blackjack Airline). After initial success with the Los Angeles–to–Las Vegas route, Blackjack Airline's demand for full-fare tickets has increased to an average of 75, with the standard deviation remaining at 15. This early experience has allowed Blackjack to make a better estimate of the percentage of discount-seeking passengers, which appears to be 80 percent. Consequently, Blackjack has decided to raise all ticket prices by $10. Under these new conditions, how many full-fare seats should Blackjack reserve?

13.9. Town and Country has experienced a substantial increase in business volume because of recent fare wars between the major air carriers. Town and Country operates a single office at a major international airport, with a fleet of 60 compact and 30 midsize cars. Recent developments have prompted management to rethink the company's reservation policy. The table below contains data on the rental experience of Town and Country:

Car	Rental rate ($)	Discount rate ($)	Discount seekers (%)	Daily demand	Standard deviation
Compact	30	20	80	50	15
Midsize	40	30	60	30	10

The daily demand appears to follow a normal distribution; however, it has been observed that midsize-car customers do not choose to rent a compact when no midsize car is available. The discount rate is available to persons who are willing to reserve a car at least 14 days in advance and agree to pick up that car within 2 hours after their flight arrives. Otherwise, a nonrefundable deposit against their credit card will be forfeited. The current reservation policy is: 40 compact cars are held for customers who are willing to pay the full rate, and 25 midsize cars are held for full rate–paying customers.

a. Using yield management, determine the optimal number of compact and midsize cars to be held for customers paying the full rate.

b. Given your optimal reservation policy determined here, would you consider a fleet expansion?

CASE: RIVER CITY NATIONAL BANK

River City National Bank has been in business for 10 years and is a fast-growing community bank. Its president, Gary Miller, took over his position 5 years ago in an effort to get the bank on its feet. He is one of the youngest bank presidents in the southwest, and his energy and enthusiasm explain his rapid advancement. Mr. Miller has been the key factor behind the bank's increased status and maintenance of high standards. One reason for this is that the customers come first in Mr. Miller's eyes; to him, one of the bank's main objectives is to serve its customers better.

The main bank lobby has one commercial teller and three paying-and-receiving teller booths. The lobby is designed to have room for long lines should they occur. Attached to the main bank are six drive-in lanes (one is commercial only) and one walk-up window to the side of the drive-in. Because of the bank's rapid growth, the drive-in lanes and lobby have been constantly overcrowded, although the bank has some of the longest hours in town. The lobby is open from 9 AM until 2 PM, Monday through Saturday, and reopens from 4 to 6 PM on Friday. The drive-in is open from 7 AM until midnight, Monday through Friday, and on Saturday from 7 AM until 7 PM. Several old and good customers have complained, however. They did not like the long wait in line and also felt that the tellers were becoming quite surly.

This was very disheartening to Mr. Miller, despite the cause of the problem being the increased business. Thus, it was with his strong recommendation that the board of directors finally approved the building of a remote drive-in bank just down the street. As Figure 13.13 shows, this drive-in can be approached from two directions and has four lanes on either side. The first lane on either side is commercial only, and the last lane on each side has been built but is not yet operational. Hours for this facility are 7 AM to 7 PM, Monday through Saturday.

The bank employs both full-time and part-time tellers. The lobby tellers and the morning tellers (7 AM to 2 PM) are considered to be full-time employees, whereas the drive-in tellers on the afternoon shift (2 PM to 7 PM) and the night-owl shift (7 PM to midnight) are considered to be part-time. The tellers perform normal banking services: cashing checks, receiving deposits, verifying deposit balances, selling money orders and traveler's checks, and cashing government savings bonds.

At present, overcrowding for the most part has been eliminated. The hardest problem in resolving the situation was making customers aware of the new facility. After 6 months, tellers at the remote drive-in still hear customers say, "I didn't realize ya'll were over here. I'm going to start coming here more often!"

Now, instead of facing an overcrowding situation, the bank is finding problems with fluctuating demand. River City National rarely experienced this problem until the extra capacity of tellers and drive-in lanes was added at the new remote facility.

Two full- and four part-time tellers are employed at the remote drive-in Monday through Friday. Scheduling on Saturdays is no problem, because all six tellers take turns rotating, with most working every other Saturday. On paydays and Fridays, the lanes at the remote drive-in have cars lined up out to the street. A high demand for money and service from the bank

FIGURE 13.13. Layout of remote drive-in.

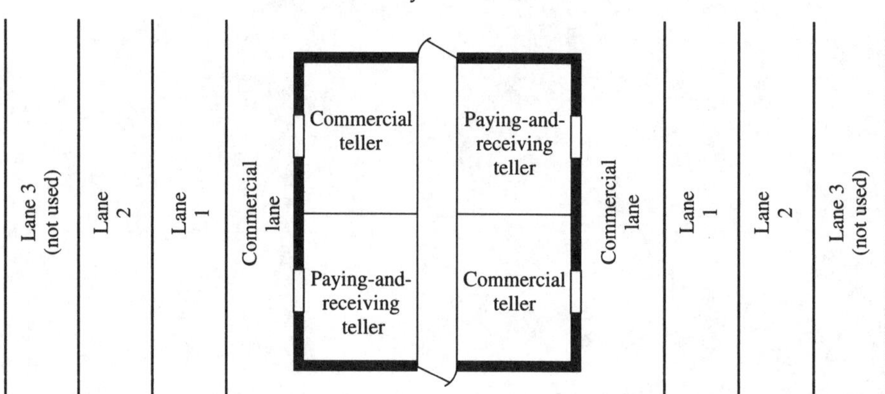

TABLE 13.8. Transactions for Typical Month at Remote Drive-In

	First Week		*Second Week*	
Day of Week	Morning Shift	Afternoon Shift	Morning Shift	Afternoon Shift
Monday	...	...	175	133
Tuesday	...	...	120	85
Wednesday	200	195	122	115
Thursday	156	113	111	100
Friday	223*	210	236*	225
Saturday	142	127	103	98

	Third Week		*Fourth Week*	
Day of Week	Morning Shift	Afternoon Shift	Morning Shift	Afternoon Shift
Monday	149	120	182	171
Tuesday	136	77	159	137
Wednesday	182	186	143	103
Thursday	172	152	118	99
Friday	215*	230	206*	197
Saturday	147	150	170	156

	Fifth Week	
Day of Week	Morning Shift	Afternoon Shift
Monday	169	111
Tuesday	112	89
Wednesday	92	95
Thursday	147	163
Friday	259*	298

*Most of these transactions occurred after 10 AM

is the main reason for this dilemma, but certainly not the only one. Many customers are not ready when they get to the bank. They need a pen or a deposit slip, or they do not have their check filled out or endorsed yet. Of course, this creates idle time for the tellers. There also are other problems with customers that take time, such as explaining that their accounts are overdrawn and their payroll checks therefore must be deposited instead of cashed. In addition, there usually is a handful of noncustomers who are trying to cash payroll or personal checks. These people can become quite obstinate and take up a lot of time when they find that their checks cannot be cashed. Transactions take 30 seconds on average; transaction times range from 10 seconds for a straight deposit to 90 seconds for cashing a bond to about 3 minutes for making out traveler's checks. (The latter occurs very rarely.)

Compared with the peak banking days, the rest of the week is very quiet. The main bank stays busy but is not crowded. On the other hand, business at the remote drive-in is unusually slow. Mr. Miller's drive-in supervisor, Ms. Shang-ling Chen, studied the number of transactions that tellers at the remote facility made on the average. The figures for a typical month are shown in Table 13.8.

Once again, customers are complaining. When tellers at the remote drive-in close out at 7 PM on Fridays, they are always turning people away while they are in the process of balancing. These customers have asked Mr. Miller to keep the new drive-in open at least until 9 PM on Friday. The tellers are very much against the idea, but the board of directors is beginning to favor it. Mr. Miller wants to keep his customers happy but feels there must be some other way to resolve the situation. Therefore, he calls in Ms. Chen and requests that she look into the problem and make some recommendations for a solution.

Assignment

As Ms. Chen's top aide, you are assigned the task of analyzing the situation and recommending a solution. This is your opportunity to serve your company and community as well as to make yourself "look good" and earn points toward your raise and promotion.

CASE: GATEWAY INTERNATIONAL AIRPORT[13]

Gateway International Airport (GIA) has experienced substantial growth in both commercial and general aviation operations during the past several years. (An *operation* is a landing or takeoff.) Because of the initiation of new commercial service at the airport, which is scheduled for several months in the future, the Federal Aviation Administration (FAA) has concluded that the increased operations and associated change in the hourly distribution of takeoffs and landings will require an entirely new work schedule for the current air traffic control (ATC) staff. The FAA feels that GIA may need to hire additional ATC personnel, because the present staff of five probably will not be enough to handle the expected demand.

After examining the various service plans that each commercial airline submitted for the next 6-month period, the FAA developed an average hourly demand forecast of total operations (Figure 13.14) and a weekly forecast of variation from the average daily demand (Figure 13.15). An assistant to the manager for operations has been delegated the task of developing workforce requirements and schedules for the ATC staff to maintain an adequate level of operational safety with a minimum of excess ATC "capacity."

The various constraints are:

1. Each controller will work a continuous, 8-hour shift (ignoring any lunch break), which always will begin at the start of an hour at any time during the day (i.e., any and all shifts begin at X:00), and the controller must have at least 16 hours off before resuming duty.
2. Each controller will work exactly 5 days per week.

[13]Prepared by James H. Vance under the supervision of Professor James A. Fitzsimmons.

FIGURE 13.14. Hourly demand for operations.

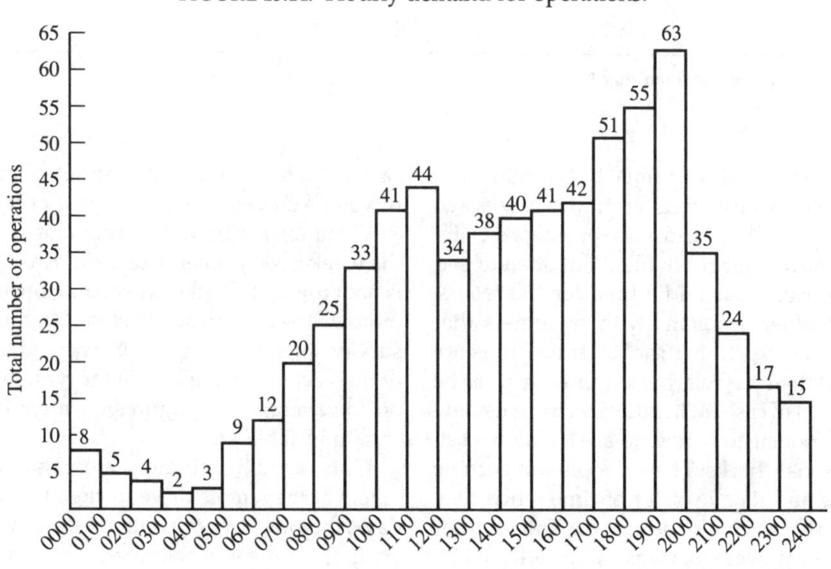

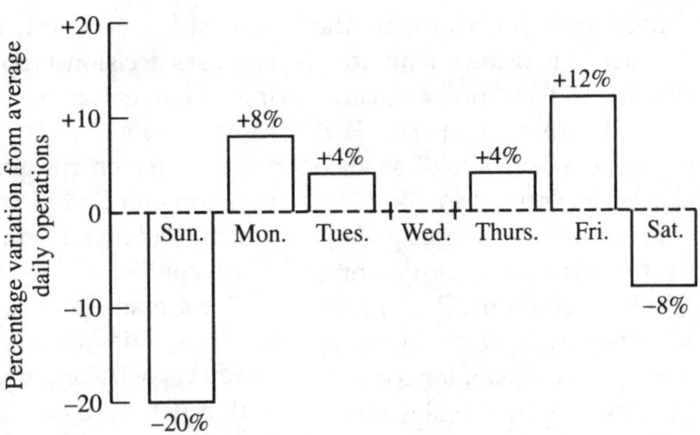

FIGURE 13.15. Daily demand variation from average.

3. Each controller is entitled to 2 consecutive days off, with any consecutive pair of days being eligible.
4. FAA guidelines will govern GIA's workforce requirements so that the ratio of total operations to the number of available controllers in any hourly period cannot exceed 16.

Questions

1. Assume that you are the assistant to the manager for operations at the FAA. Use the techniques of workshift scheduling to analyze the total workforce requirements and days-off schedule. For the primary analysis, you may assume that:

a. Operator requirements will be based on a shift profile of demand (i.e., 8 hours).

b. There will be exactly three separate shifts each day, with no overlapping of shifts.

c. The distribution of hourly demand in Figure 13.14 is constant for each day of the week, but the levels of hourly demand vary during the week as shown in Figure 13.15.

2. On the basis of your primary analysis, discuss the potential implications for workforce requirements and days-off scheduling if assumptions **a** and **b** above are relaxed so that the analysis can be based on hourly demand without the constraints of a preset number of shifts and no overlapping of shifts. In other words, discuss the effects of analyzing hourly demand requirements on the basis of each ATC position essentially having its own shift, which can overlap with any other ATC shift to meet that demand.

3. Do you feel this would result in a larger or smaller degree of difficulty in meeting the four general constraints? Why?

4. What additional suggestions could you make to the manager of operations to minimize the workforce requirements level and days-off scheduling difficulty?

CASE: THE YIELD MANAGEMENT ANALYST[14]

On the morning of November 10, 1992, Jon Thomas, market analyst for the Mexico Leisure markets, canceled more than 300 seats "illegally" reserved on two flights to Acapulco. All the seats on Jon's Acapulco flights were booked by the same sales representative under a corporate name, Uniden Corporation. Jon could tell that the sales representative reserved space one passenger at a time using the relevant available fare; some seats were reserved at round-trip fares of more than $2000 per person. By using a special corporate name field, the sales representative used a common gaming technique to suspend auto cancellation and instant purchase payment programs that are required for all individual bookings by SABRE (Semi-*A*utomated *B*usiness *R*esearch *E*nvironment), American Airlines' (AA's) customer reservation system. Jon felt justified in canceling this space, because he previously had denied the group-space request and the sales representative subsequently violated established rules regarding the reservation of space for large groups.

[14]Adapted with permission from Kevin Baker and Robert B. Freund. *The Yield Management Analyst*, University of Texas at Austin, 1994.

No more than 24 hours after Jon canceled the Uniden Corporation's space, he received an irate phone call from Patty Dial, the Dallas–Fort Worth area regional sales manager. Uniden, a local Fort Worth–based company, needed more than 300 seats to Acapulco for its annual sales incentive trip. Jon faces the conflict of whether to accept or deny large groups each day, and he realizes that his market judgment is all part of managing yield for each flight. The Uniden group issue escalated to higher levels of management when Uniden, a major corporate customer for AA, found out that space promised by AA's sales representative had been canceled. With the customer relations issue in mind, Jon entered a negotiation process with Patty to reallocate space.

Normal group reservation procedure requires the sales representative to send an electronic message to the yield management analyst to request a block of space on a flight. It is the yield management analyst's prerogative to approve the request and block space for the group or to deny that request. The yield management analyst uses a variety of decision support systems based on historical market activity to make this decision. From the sales representative's perspective, capturing this group is a clear victory, because it drives market share through increased sales volume for their region. From the yield manager's perspective, filling the plane with one group at the same fare on a peak-period flight is a wasted opportunity to use excess demand and the market's limited capacity to maximize revenue per passenger. Unfortunately, sales representatives can fool SABRE into accepting group reservations without the yield manager's approval. As in Jon's case, a sales representative may book seats in blocks of fewer than 10 passengers, set up a corporate name field in the reservation that suspends all autocancellation programs, establish a sales contract, and negotiate a special off-tariff price for the group regardless of the fares listed in each reservation.

Conflicting corporate objectives for sales representatives and yield managers is a major source of frustration for a yield management analyst. AA's sales representatives establish monthly revenue and passenger goals to meet progressively higher market share objectives. Sales representatives maintain relationships with large corporate clients and travel agencies, and they implement volume- and revenue-based discount programs for large corporate accounts and travel agencies. AA's yield management analyst attempts to maximize aircraft utilization (revenue per passenger and load factor at the same time) to improve overall market revenue. The yield management analyst has very little contact with the end customer and uses decision support systems to manipulate pricing and inventory allocation programs. The sales representative's goal is stimulation of sales, while the yield management analyst's goal is sales optimization. Jon and Patty's conflict highlights a situation in which yield management and sales objectives come in direct conflict and the system breaks down.

Yield management is an ideal operating strategy for companies that face temporary imbalances between capacity and demand, spoilage (i.e., a product that must be used immediately), and high fixed costs/low variable costs. Yield management enables companies to maximize use of constrained productive capacity with a discriminating eye on product yield. Each day, Jon faces the decision of whether to fill a plane early with lower fares or to save space for higher-revenue passengers.

Yield Management in the Airline Industry

Passenger demand often outpaces capacity during peak seasons, days, or other times, as in Jon's Acapulco market. In essence, airlines face temporary imbalances between capacity and demand on a daily basis. In the situation that Jon faces, only Aeromexico, Mexicana, and AA have direct flights to Mexico from Dallas. During low season periods, it is difficult to fill these planes, whereas in high season, there is more demand than the total market capacity can handle. Clearly, AA faces high fixed costs and low variable costs, because adding one more passenger to a flight costs very little compared with the fixed costs of providing and maintaining the scheduled aircraft service. Finally, once the airplane pulls away from the gate, all the empty seats can never be sold, and this results in spoilage. When faced with excess demand and limited capacity, the yield management analyst may "choose" what traffic is most desirable to optimize the total revenue on each flight. The different levels of yield management sophistication between airlines is the source of a competitive advantage in some highly competitive markets.

From mid-November through the end of May, Jon's Mexico leisure market enters its peak season and provides an excellent opportunity for textbook yield management strategies. During the time that this case covers, AA has a total of nine daily round-trip flights to Acapulco, Cancun, and Puerto Vallerta. Jon is in charge of setting all the fares connecting Mexico with the rest of the world as well as managing the inventory control. Each origin–destination market, such as Dallas–Cancun, has more than 30 fares to maintain. In general, all airlines use price discrimination and yield management to maximize revenue. By maintaining a tiered-fare structure, the yield management analyst can force passengers to pay higher prices in times of greater demand.

Jon helps AA to maintain a tiered, market–based fare structure that leverages the price sensitivities and flexibility of its business and leisure customer segments. Fare rules and prices are differentiated based on the time and date of the flight, origin of the passenger, and historical demand patterns in that market. Table 13.9 outlines the different behavior of the two passenger segments.

Facing spoilage, high fixed costs/low variable costs, and temporary demand imbalances, airlines use *both* demand and capacity management to maximize revenue. Airlines use three yield management tools to maximize revenue and sell the "right" fares to the "right" passengers: "overbooking, discount allocation, and traffic management."[15] Tiered-price structure or price discrimination provides the ability or foundation to force passengers to pay more or "sell-up." To execute price discrimination with a tiered-fare structure, the airplane capacity is divided into different sections, regardless of where the passenger sits (unless the passenger is in business or first class). The yield management analyst spreads the available fares over the sections (i.e., discount allocation) and uses overbooking and traffic management strategies to maximize revenue.

[15]Quoted from Barbara Amster, former vice president of the American Airlines Pricing and Yield Management department and current vice president of Canadian Pacific Airlines Pricing and Yield Management department.

Taking passenger reservations beyond the true capacity of the airplane to ensure a full flight is referred to as *overbooking*. This strategy accounts for expected no-shows, last-minute cancellations, and missed connections based on seasonally adjusted historical data. Overbooking generates a tremendous amount of incremental revenue for the airline, and it provides airline travelers with greater choice. More flights and fares are made available to a greater number of passengers. In Jon's Mexico leisure markets, levels of overbooking average approximately 25 percent more than capacity and can reach as high as 50 percent. The overbooking level typically starts off high 6 months before departure of a flight and slowly declines as bookings turn over, restrict excess sales, and force "selling-up" during periods closer to departure.

Discount allocation works together with traffic management to spread the tiered-fare structure over the different inventory sections of a plane. Discount allocation attempts to save seats for higher-valued, last-minute business customers who are willing to pay more than the discounted price. AA's Boeing 727, which is the aircraft used in Jon's Mexico markets, holds 150 passengers: 12 in first class and 138 in coach. On a typical flight, Jon may have two or three separate fares for first-class passengers and 25 different fares for coach passengers. AA's traffic management or indexing system automatically spreads Jon's fares over the plane's inventory sections to provide more inventory for higher-paying and less inventory for lower-paying passengers when faced with excess demand. Traffic management or AA's indexing system also values long-haul, higher-paying passengers more than short-haul passengers, and it provides increased inventory availability for the higher fares.

Overbooking and discount allocation levels are set differently based on historical demand patterns for

TABLE 13.9. Behavior of Airline Passenger Segments

Leisure Passenger	Business Passenger
Price-sensitive	Price-insensitive
Advance booking	Last minute booking
Flexible day and time	Inflexible on day and time
Long trips	Short trips
Discretionary travel	Time-dependent travel
Consults travel agents	Frequent flyer and knows destination
Travels over weekends	Weekday travel only
Seasonal travel	Less seasonal
Little loyalty	Loyalty based on frequent flyer credit

the particular flight's departure time, day of week, days until departure, and season of departure. The levels change daily for each flight in AA's expansive system based on fluctuating demand. Jon is responsible for overriding system decisions and implementing different and new discount allocation and traffic management strategies to improve the average revenue per passenger and the load factor of his market. Specifically, Jon decides what fares to file for each passenger group, what restrictions to apply to each fare, how many seats to save between higher- and lower-valued fares, increased availability for longer-haul and high-demand markets, and inventory restriction for lower-valued fares.

SABRE opens flights for sale more than 300 days before departure. Maintaining yield in a volatile market, such as Jon's Mexico leisure market, adds increased uncertainty because of the large fluctuation and less predictable nature of the historical demand patterns. Jon's Mexico leisure markets are especially unpredictable, because frequent yet dispersed group movements distort decision support system inventory projections, average demand, overbooking levels, and discounted seat allocation.

Assignment

Your instructor will supply you with instructions and a revenue tally sheet for playing "The Yield Management Game." The game gives you an opportunity to step into Jon's shoes and maximize total revenue for one flight.

SELECTED BIBLIOGRAPHY

ANTLE, D. W., and R. A. REID: "Managing Service Capacity in an Ambulatory Care Clinic," *Hospital & Health Services Administration,* vol. 33, no. 2, Summer 1988, pp. 201–211.

BAKER, K. R., and M. J. MAGAZINE: "Workforce Scheduling with Cyclic Demands and Day-Off Constraints," *Management Science,* vol. 24, no. 2, October 1977, pp. 161–167.

BECHTOLD, S. E.: "Implicit Optimal and Heuristic Labor Staffing in a Multiobjective, Multilocation Environment," *Decision Sciences,* vol. 19, no. 2, Spring 1988, pp. 353–372.

——— and M. J. SHOWALTER: "A Methodology for Labor Scheduling in a Service Operating System," *Decision Sciences,* vol. 18, no. 1, Winter 1987, pp. 89–107.

BELOBABA, PETER P.: "Application of a Probabilistic Decision Model to Airline Seat Inventory Control," *Operations Research,* vol. 37, no. 2, March–April 1989, pp. 183–197.

BITRAN, G. R., and S. V. MONDSCHEIN: "An Application of Yield Management to the Hotel Industry Considering Multiple Day Stays," *Operations Research,* vol. 43, no. 3, May–June 1995, pp. 427–443.

COLLIER, D. A.: "A Managerial Guide for the Service Capacity-Scheduling Decision," *Service Management: Operating Decisions,* Prentice-Hall, Englewood Cliffs, NJ., 1987, pp. 51–55.

GLOVER, F., R. GLOVER, J. LORENZO, and C. MCMILLAN: "The Passenger-Mix Problem in the Scheduled Airlines," *Interfaces,* vol. 12, no. 3, June 1982, pp. 73–80.

KIMES, SHERYL E.: "Yield Management: A Tool for Capacity-Constrained Service Firms," *Journal of Operations Management,* vol. 8, no. 4, October 1989, pp. 348–363.

———: "The Basics of Yield Management," *The Cornell H.R.A. Quarterly,* November 1989, pp. 14–19.

LOVELOCK, C. H.: "Strategies for Managing Demand in Capacity-Constrained Service Organizations," *Service Industries Journal,* vol. 4, no. 3, November 1984, pp. 12–30.

NORTHCRAFT, G. B., and R. B. CHASE: "Managing Service Demand at the Points of Delivery," *Academy of Management Review,* vol. 10, no. 1, 1985, pp. 66–75.

PFEIFER, PHILLIP E.: "The Airline Discount Fare Allocation Problem," *Decision Sciences,* vol. 20, Winter 1989, pp. 149–157.

RELIHAN, WALTER J. III: "The Yield-Management Approach to Hotel-Room Pricing," *The Cornell H.R.A. Quarterly,* May 1989, pp. 40–45.

THOMPSON, GARY M.: "Shift Scheduling in Services When Employees Have Limited Availability: An L.P. Approach," *Journal of Operations Management*, vol. 9, no. 3, August 1990, pp. 352–370.

SASSER, W. EARL: "Match Supply and Demand in Service Industries," *Harvard Business Review*, November–December 1976, pp. 133–140.

SHEMWELL, D. J., and J. J. CRONIN: "Services Marketing Strategies for Coping with Demand/Supply Imbalances," *Journal of Services Marketing*, vol. 8, no. 4, 1994, pp. 14–24.

SMITH, B. C., J. F. LEIMKUHLER, and R. M. DARROW: "Yield Management at American Airlines," *Interfaces*, vol. 22, no. 1, January/February 1992, pp. 8–31.

WILLIAMS, FRED E.: "Decision Theory and the Innkeeper: An Approach for Setting Hotel Reservation Policy," *Interfaces*, vol. 7, no. 4, August 1977, pp. 18–30.

PART FIVE

Toward World-Class Service

Competition in services has become global, as Federal Express discovered during its attempt to expand overseas. The danger of services following the decline in competitiveness that has been experienced by manufacturing is possible, because no market is isolated in today's global economy. A service firm can reach, and sustain, a competitive position by promoting a culture of continuous improvement in productivity and quality. In this regard, the application of Deming's philosophy of continuous service process improvement is recalled from Chapter 10, Service Quality, and explored further. A technique called *data envelopment analysis (DEA)* will be used to measure productivity of a service unit as the ratio of resource inputs to service outputs.

Service expansion strategies can be described in the context of being multisite or multiservice. The traditional multisite service expansion strategy of franchising is explored, with a discussion of the issues that arise between franchisee and franchiser. For services considering multinational expansion, additional considerations such as cultural transferability and host-government policies arise.

CHAPTER 14

Productivity and Quality Improvement

LEARNING OBJECTIVES

After completing this chapter, you should be able to:

1. Categorize a service firm according to its stage of competitiveness.
2. Discuss the analogous roles that inventory plays in manufacturing and queuing plays in services.
3. Discuss the organizational implications of following a strategy of continuous improvement.
4. Apply the Deming philosophy of continual improvement to a service.
5. Conduct a data envelopment analysis.

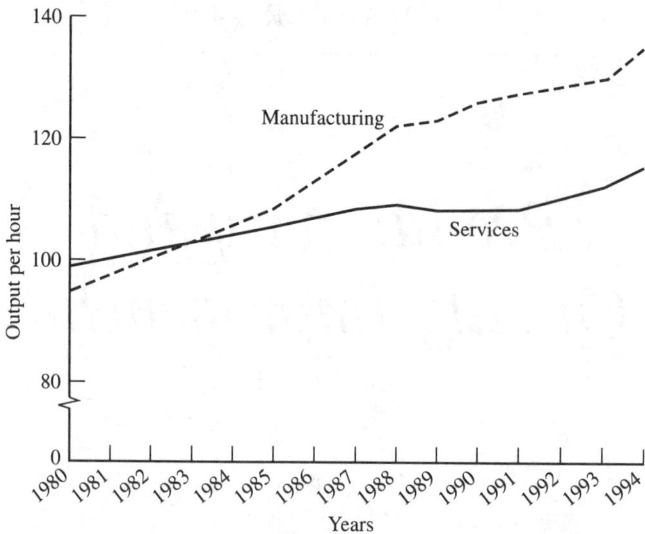

FIGURE 14.1. Productivity in manufacturing and services. *[After "Productivity and Related Measures: 1970 to 1994," Statistical Abstract of the U.S., U.S. Department of Commerce, Economics and Statistics Administration, Bureau of the Census, 1995, table no. 670, p. 430.]*

Increasing productivity is important if a nation's standard of living is to rise. For a company to remain competitive in the global economy, wages can be raised only if they are matched by increased productivity. As Figure 14.1 shows, productivity as measured by output per hour has steadily increased in the past decade for manufacturing, whereas the output per hour for services has remained relatively flat. Many explanations are given for this lack of productivity improvement: the service sector was absorbing the baby boomers entering the labor force, thus workers were young and inexperienced; capital investment per worker was (and still is) much lower in services than in manufacturing; automation was displacing workers in the manufacturing sector; service output was (and remains) difficult to quantify; and training of service workers was neglected.

Changing demographics in the 1990s and the anticipated future labor shortage will force services to become more productivity-conscious. Consider the labor-saving ideas that have been incorporated by the new Sleep Inn chain to reduce the labor costs of operating a hotel unit. For example, clothes washers and dryers are located behind the front desk, so the night clerk can load and unload laundry while on duty. To help reduce housekeeping chores, nightstands are bolted to the wall so that maids need not vacuum around legs, and the shower stall is round to prevent dirt from collecting in corners. In addition, the computerized electronic security system has eliminated room keys: guests use their own credit cards to enter their rooms. Also, to reduce energy costs, heat or air-conditioning is turned on or off automatically when the guest checks in or out. In addition, the computer records the time that maids spend cleaning each room.

Thus, creative facility design, effective use of labor, and innovative use of computers can have a major impact on increasing service productivity.[1]

CHAPTER PREVIEW

The focus of this chapter is on continuous improvement in service organizations through productivity and quality initiatives. Productivity is more than a design issue; it represents an on-going commitment to improving operations and customer service. Because of customer participation in the service delivery process, any changes in this raise the issue of customer acceptance, which is even more critical when the automation of services extends from the back office to the front desk.

Continuous improvement is a way of thinking that must be incorporated into the firm's culture. Continuous improvement can be demonstrated by the analogy of queue reduction in services and inventory reduction in manufacturing using the just-in-time philosophy. The Deming philosophy of continuous improvement also will be presented through the experience of Florida Power and Light, the first non-Japanese firm to win the prestigious Deming Prize.

Finally, a linear programming model referred to as *data envelopment analysis (DEA)* will be introduced as a method to measure the efficiency of service delivery units. The comparative analysis of unit performance using DEA provides an opportunity to promote continuous improvement through shared learning.

We begin our discussion with a framework that categorizes service firms according to their level of competitiveness with respect to key operational dimensions, all of which are sources of both productivity and quality innovations.

STAGES IN SERVICE FIRM COMPETITIVENESS[2]

If a service firm is to remain competitive, continual improvement in productivity and quality must be part of its strategy and corporate culture. The framework shown in Table 14.1 was developed by Chase and Hayes to describe the role of operations in the strategic development of service firms. This framework also is useful as an illustration of the many sources of productivity and quality improvement (i.e., new technology is only one source). In addition, the framework provides a way to measure and evaluate a firm's progress in the development of its service delivery system. It organizes service firms into four different stages of development according to their competitiveness in service delivery, and for each stage, the management practices and attitudes of the firm are compared across key operational dimensions.

It should be noted that services need not start at stage 1, but during their life cycle, they could revert to stage 1 out of neglect. For example, one might argue that Federal Express began service as a stage 3 competitor because of its innovative hub-and-spoke network concept, whereby all sorting is accomplished at the single Memphis hub (thus guaranteeing overnight delivery).

[1]From David Wessel, "With Labor Scarce, Service Firms Strive to Raise Productivity," *The Wall Street Journal*, June 1, 1989, p. 1.

[2]Adapted from R. B. Chase and R. H. Hayes, "Operations' Role in Service Firm Competitiveness," *Sloan Management Review*, vol. 33, no. 1, Fall 1991, pp. 1526.

TABLE 14.1. Four Stages of Service Firm Competitiveness

	1. Available for Service	2. Journeyman	3. Distinctive Competence Achieved	4. World-Class Service Delivery
	Customers patronize service firm for reasons other than performance.	Customers neither seek out nor avoid the firm.	Customers seek out the firm on the basis of its sustained reputation for meeting customer expectations.	The company's name is synonymous with service excellence. Its service doesn't just satisfy customers; it *delights* them and, thereby, expands customer expectations to levels its competitors are unable to fulfill.
	Operations is reactive at best.	Operations functions in a mediocre, uninspired fashion.	Operations continually excels, reinforced by personnel management and systems that support an intense customer focus.	Operations is a quick learner and fast innovator; it masters every step of the service delivery process and provides capabilities superior to competitors.
Service quality	Is subsidiary to cost and highly variable.	Meets some customer expectations; consistent on one or two key dimensions.	Exceeds customer expectations; consistent on multiple dimensions.	Raises customer expectations and seeks challenges; improves continuously.
Back office	Counting room.	Contributes to service, plays an important role in the total service, is given attention, but still a separate role.	Is equally valued with front office; plays integral role.	Is proactive, develops its own capabilities, and generates opportunities.

TABLE 14.1. (*Continued*)

	1. Available for Service	2. Journeyman	3. Distinctive Competence Achieved	4. World-Class Service Delivery
Customer	Unspecified, to be satisfied at minimum cost.	A market segment whose basic needs are understood.	A collection of individuals whose variation in needs is understood.	A source of stimulation, ideas, and opportunity.
Introduction of new technology	When necessary for survival under duress.	When justified by cost savings.	When promises to enhance service.	Source of first-mover advantages, creating ability to do things competitors cannot.
Workforce	Negative constraint.	Efficient resource; disciplined; follows procedures.	Permitted to select among alternative procedures.	Innovative; creates procedures.
First-line management	Controls workers.	Controls the process.	Listens to customers; coaches and facilitates workers.	Is listened to by top management as a source of new ideas. Mentors workers to enhance their career growth.

Source: Reprinted from "Operations' Role in Service Firm Competitiveness," by R.B. Chase and R.H. Hayes, *Sloan Management Review*, vol. 33, no. 1, Fall 1991, p. 17, by permission of publisher.

Available for Service

Some service firms—and, often, government services in particular—fall into this category, because they view operations as a necessary evil to be performed at minimum cost. There is little motivation to seek improvements in quality, because the customers often have no alternatives. Workers require direct supervision because of their limited skills and the potential for poor performance that results from minimal investment in training. Investment in new technology is avoided until it is necessary for survival (e.g., consider the long-overdue adoption of Doppler radar by the Federal Aviation Administration for air traffic control). These firms are essentially noncompetitive, and they only exist in this stage until they are challenged by competition.

Journeyman

After maintaining a sheltered existence in stage 1, a service firm may face competition and, thus, may be forced to reevaluate its delivery system. Operations managers then must adopt industry practices to maintain parity with its new competitors and avoid a significant loss of market share. For example, if all successful airlines used the same kind of plane, then a fledgling airline just entering the market also might be inclined to use that same aircraft. The contribution of operations in this hypothetical situation becomes competitive-neutral, because all the firms in the industry have adopted similar practices and even look like each other (because they have purchased equipment from the same supplier).

When firms do not compete on operations effectiveness, they often are creative in competing along other dimensions (e.g., breadth of product line, peripheral services, advertising). The workforce is disciplined to follow standard procedures and is not expected to take any initiative when unusual circumstances arise. These firms have not yet recognized the potential contribution of operations to a firm's competitiveness.

Distinctive Competence Achieved

Firms in stage 3 are fortunate to have senior managers with a vision of what creates value for the customer and who understand the role that operations managers must play in delivering the service. For example, Jan Carlzon, CEO of Scandinavian Airlines (SAS), realized that recapturing the business-traveler market, which had been lost to aggressive competition, required improving on-time departure performance. To achieve this goal, he had to provide a leadership role that fostered operations innovations, which then would improve the delivery system.[3]

Operations managers are the typical advocates of total quality management (TQM) in their firms and take the lead in instituting service guarantees, worker empowerment, and service-enhancing technologies. Workers in these organizations often are cross-trained and encouraged to take the initiative when necessary to achieve operational goals that are stated clearly (e.g., overnight delivery for Federal Express). Firms in this category implement management strategies to achieve the corporate vision and, thereby, differentiate themselves from their competition.

World-Class Service Delivery

Not satisfied with just meeting customer expectations, world-class firms expand on these expectations to levels that competitors find difficult to meet. Management is proactive in promoting higher standards of performance and identifying new business opportunities by listening to customers. World-class service firms such as Disney, Marriott, and American Airlines define the quality standards by which others are judged.

New technology no longer is viewed only as a means to reduce costs; it is considered to be a competitive advantage that is not easily duplicated. For example, Federal Express developed COSMOS (Customer Operations Service Master On-line System) to provide a system that tracks packages from pick-up to delivery. Customers can call at any time and receive information on the exact location of their packages. This system also can be used to tell a driver en route to make customer pick-ups.

[3]Jan Carlzon, *Moments of Truth,* Ballinger Publishing, Cambridge, Mass., 1987.

Working at a world-class firm is considered to be something special, and employees are encouraged to identify with the firm and its mission. For example, a Disney trash collector is considered to be a "cast member" who helps visitors to enjoy the experience.

Sustaining superior performance throughout the delivery system is a major challenge. Duplicating the service at multiple sites, however, and in particular overseas, is the true test of a world-class competitor.

MAKING CONTINUAL IMPROVEMENT A COMPETITIVE STRATEGY[4]

The history of economic development has been based on learning from experience and then applying this knowledge to improve productivity. For example, Henry Ford is credited with discovering the revolutionary concept of the moving assembly line, on which material is moved past workstations in a factory; however, this idea could have originated from an agricultural analogy, in which equipment is moved through stationary fields for planting and harvesting. This analogy also could be extended to service firms, in which customers are moved to or through a process at a fixed facility. Thus, with proper translation, it is possible for a productivity improvement in one sector of the economy to be useful in another.

For the past decade, we all have been students of the Japanese manufacturing philosophy. First, we observed the use of the Kanban card and concluded that this novel method of shop-floor control must be the secret of success. Further study revealed the emphasis on inventory reduction, however, and we coined the phrase *just-in-time (JIT)* to describe the process of production with zero inventories. Our understanding of JIT led to an appreciation of its effect on quality improvement. Then, to our surprise, we discovered a method of organizing production that yielded high-quality products at low cost. This realization shattered our long-held assumption of a tradeoff between quality and cost. The production function itself now has become a strategic competitive weapon. The success of Japanese penetration into foreign markets proves the effectiveness of this competitive strategy.

Identifying inventory as undesirable because it hides mistakes and decouples workers allows us to see its most serious fault. With inventory buffers, management and, more important, workers are not motivated to engage in problem solving. When inventory is reduced, problems no longer can be buried or sent to a rework area; instead, they must be faced immediately by the workers themselves. A manufacturing culture is established in which everyone is responsible for process and quality improvement. Reliance on a staff of industrial and manufacturing engineers to provide ideas for process improvements is not necessary; instead, the workers dealing with the process on a daily basis are asked to use their minds as well as their hands. The competitive implications of the experience curve are well-known, and the leading Japanese manufacturing firms have institutionalized this concept in their organizations through use of JIT.

[4]From James A. Fitzsimmons, "Making Continual Improvement a Competitive Strategy for Service Firms," in *Service Management Effectiveness*, Bowen, Chase, Cummings and Associates, Jossey-Bass Publishers, San Francisco, 1990, pp. 284–295.

The concept of making continual improvements in the production process is central to a firm's competitive strength and a nation's productive growth. Approximately 70 percent of the gross national product of the world's leading economic nations is generated by the service sector; thus, an ethic of productivity improvement for services is imperative to assure future prosperity.

Inventory and Waiting Line Analogy

In *manufacturing*, the focus of attention is on *material* resources. JIT views idle material resources or inventory as an "evil" to be eliminated, or at least reduced. In *services*, the focus of our attention is on *human* resources. The "evils" to be eliminated or reduced in this case are customer waiting lines and idle staff. Thus, an analogy between inventory in manufacturing and waiting lines in services can be made.

As Table 14.2 shows, inventory and waiting lines share some common features. The cost of a customer waiting in line is a forgone opportunity, which generally is difficult to quantify. Unlike investment in inventory, which can be quantified in financial terms, the cost of keeping customers waiting for service is subjective, but it can be very high. For example, one business executive who was kept waiting in his doctor's office sued the physician for lost time—and won the case. Thus, real costs can be associated with customer waiting, the most important being loss of future business. Storing inventory requires space and the associated investment in a protective facility. Waiting lines also create the need for otherwise unproductive space, which should, in addition, be attractively furnished. Banks have been known to devote one-half of their expensive real estate to drive-in banking facilities, with most of the area being used for a driveway.

Inventory is an excellent place to hide poor quality. The intangibility of services makes it difficult for customers to judge quality. Thus, they use surrogates such as the length of time they are kept waiting in line to evaluate service performance. As noted in Chapter 11, Managing Queues, excessive waiting can be considered psychological punishment, and the significant negative impression that it creates is difficult for the service to overcome.

Waiting lines also perform some of the same functions in the management of services that inventory did for manufacturing before the advent of JIT. For years, the decoupling function of inventory has been used to simplify the man-

TABLE 14.2. Inventory and Waiting Line Analogy

Feature	Inventory	Waiting Line
Costs	Opportunity cost of capital	Opportunity cost of time
Space	Warehouse	Waiting area
Quality	Poor quality is hidden	Negative impression
Decoupling	Promotes independence of production stages	Allows division of labor and specialization
Utilization	Work-in-process keeps machines busy	Waiting customers keep servers busy
Coordination	Detailed scheduling not necessary	Avoids matching supply and demand

agement of production operations. Work-in-process inventory allows management to divide the production process into independent departments, or stages, that can be managed in a decentralized fashion, with supervisors and other work leaders having centralized production control. Waiting lines serve a similar decoupling function by permitting division of labor and specialization. For example, lines for a commercial teller at a bank cannot be served by idle retail tellers or, heaven forbid, by a loan officer. Thus, management is able to create different job classifications and pay according to the skills that are required, with high-customer-contact tellers being paid entry-level wages. This division of labor has its price in loss of flexibility to respond to customer demands.

In manufacturing, work-in-process inventory traditionally has been used to reduce, or even eliminate, machine or operator idle time. Keeping an inventory of inputs before an operation would ensure high labor and equipment utilization. Waiting customers are used in a similar role to keep service personnel busy and under pressure to work at a productive rate. The U.S. Post Office is notorious for employing this strategy as a cost-saving measure, but physicians also keep their waiting rooms full to avoid being idle themselves. In job shops, the level of inventory is quite high, which reflects the complex nature of coordinating the operation. Detailed scheduling of the operation as a whole is impossible, and inventory is used to decentralize the scheduling and allow individual machine centers to focus on selecting jobs from their queue. For service managers, waiting lines are used to store excess demand when it is impossible to adjust service capacity. Restaurants traditionally have used the bar as a holding area for customers who walk in without reservations.

The presence of excessive inventory in a factory or of long waiting lines at a service is an indictment of poor management. This reliance on idle resources (i.e., queues of people or material) to create a smooth operation reveals a lazy management that is unwilling to assume the responsibility of continual process and quality improvement. Organizations without such a competitive operations strategy will be handicapped in the marketplace.

Continual Improvement as Part of the Service Organization Culture

How can continual improvement in productivity and quality be made a part of the service organization culture? What is needed is a clear and visible signal that problem solving is required. An excessively long waiting line of customers or idle servers is an obvious indication that the service is not being deployed effectively. Depending on the circumstance, a variety of responses is possible:

- Ask back-office personnel to come forward and open additional service stations in parallel. For example, have platform personnel at a bank open additional teller windows.
- Ask back-office personnel to assist in performing the service. For example, have stockers assist checkout clerks in bagging groceries in a supermarket.

In response to periods of front-office idleness, customer-contact personnel can help in the back office. For example, in banking, tellers can help to prepare customer account statements for mailing. For a supermarket, checkout clerks can help to stock shelves during slow periods. In general, the response is a redeployment of personnel to serve the customer better while maintaining high utilization of human resources.

What can be learned from these experiences to improve the service process? If customer queues develop at the same time each day, then redeployment can be instituted before the lines form instead of in reaction to them. Other ideas could follow, such as instituting an express lane during these busy periods or having the manager preapprove checks to avoid delays. Ideas should flow naturally, because service employees themselves are service customers and know instinctively what solutions should guarantee reasonable results. In banking, instead of opening express lanes, a better approach might be to staff special desks for the time-consuming services (e.g., selling traveler's checks and CDs). A host or hostess, or even a sign, could direct arriving customers to the appropriate server. In this way, the large number of short transactions is expedited and the congestion eliminated quickly. Customers with minor requests, and who often are in a hurry, will be served promptly. Customers with more demanding requirements usually are more willing to wait, because the ratio of service time to wait time meets their expectations.

This example illustrates the need for improved real-time communication among personnel. In the JIT environment, this is accomplished by use of cards (the Japanese term is *Kanban*) and other simple devices. We are convinced that service employees can create innovative methods to alert coworkers to changing levels of customer demands and, thus, to initiate the necessary redeployment of resources. The resulting interconnectedness will promote a team approach to customer service.

A major distinction between the traditional manufacturing organization and JIT is the source (i.e., direction) of production control. Traditionally, work was released to the first stage of the production process and then *pushed* through the plant from one station to the next. In the JIT system, production orders originate at the final assembly station, and work is *pulled* from the upstream stages as needed. Thus, the entire production system becomes interconnected, and work focuses on meeting the final demand. Each workstation is both a customer for upstream stations and a server for downstream stations. The result is a chain of workers acting as one team. For services, the process flow is seldom as well-defined as that in manufacturing; thus, there is a greater need for an innovative communication linkage between servers. In services, upstream stations such as the receptionist are the first to experience customer demand, unlike the situation in JIT manufacturing (where work is pulled by the final assembly station from upstream stations). Thus, these stations are in a position to provide advance warning to downstream stations to prepare for arriving customers. Ideally, when a customer enters a service system, a "greeter" identifies the particular needs and uses an internal communication system (i.e., Kanban) to alert the downstream service providers. Just as in the JIT manufacturing system, the customer "pulls" resources into play as they are needed.

Examples of this approach already exist. When a long line develops at a Burger King or Wendy's, a service person walks up the line and takes orders to speed the transaction time at the counter and, possibly, to deter customer reneging. At a motor vehicle license and registration office, a greeter is stationed just inside the entry to provide customers with forms and directions to the appropriate service counter. The most comprehensive example is found at The Limited retail clothing stores. Sales trends are collected immediately by electronic cash registers and sent directly to the huge Columbus, Ohio, warehouse for distribution; at the same time, factory orders are placed worldwide on the basis of demand, which is being monitored in real time.

The customer automatically becomes the focus of attention when service employees redeploy their efforts to reduce the waiting lines. Thus, even if new ways to improve service are not immediately discovered, at least the customer is aware that special efforts are being made on her or his behalf.

Management Implications

Allowing service employees the discretion to react to customer waiting lines in creative ways has many implications for management. Table 14.3 compares the work environment and dimensions of organizational structure for traditional and world-class service organizations.

We begin with the assumption that a service organization operates as an open system in its environment. This does not suggest that some back-room activities cannot be treated as a buffered core (i.e., isolated from direct customer contact). For the customer-contact personnel, however, we premise their job design on the need for flexibility. Adam Smith's concept of "division of labor," although appropriate for the closed systems in manufacturing, can be counterproductive in an open service environment, in which servers are in direct contact with customers. Flexibility for service jobs means cross-training, with the ability either to step in and perform another's task or to help facilitate the activities of another employee. Cross-training implies an increased organizational commitment to its personnel and, thus, a change in attitude about the desirability of high turnover and use of minimum-wage labor. This should translate into improved employee relations, because workers are treated with the same respect as the customers.

The organizational structure must be fluid to permit the redeployment of all personnel to meet fluctuations in customer demand. On occasion, back-office personnel must share the task of serving customers directly. If restrictive union

TABLE 14.3. Organizational Structure and Work Environment of Traditional and World-Class Service Organizations

Dimension	Traditional	World-Class
System assumption	Closed system	Open system
Job design premise	Division of labor	Flexibility
Structure	Rigid	Fluid
Relation to others	Individual	Team player
Employee orientation	Task	Customer
Management	Supervisor	Coach and facilitator
Technology	Replace human effort	Assist service delivery
Information	Efficiency	Effectiveness

work rules such as those found in manufacturing were applied to services, however, they would prevent realization of the competitive advantage of this operations strategy of fluidity. With this strategy, working as a team becomes the norm, and attention is focused on serving the customer instead of simply completing a task. In addition, the role of management changes from that of a traditional supervisor or checker to a coach and team builder.

Technology becomes more important as a method to assist delivery of the service rather than to replace human contact. An exception to this approach is the promotion of self-service through devices such as automated teller machines or airline ticket machines. For example, Southwest Airlines offers a free cocktail to customers who use their credit cards to purchase tickets at a self-service machine. This role of the customer as participant in the service process to increase productivity is an important feature of services, and computerized information processing will play a central role in high-tech, high-touch service delivery systems. The creative use of information is central to the effective delivery of a service by acting as the Kanban to permit prepositioning of service delivery activities in a "pull" work-scheduling environment.

It is interesting to note the implications of a service "pull" philosophy that is based on corporate flexibility and real-time information processing, as well as the implications of the traditional mass-marketing "push" philosophy practiced by most manufacturers (e.g., automobile firms). In a service "pull" environment, the operations function becomes critical instead of being taken for granted as in the "push" environment, in which marketing is critical. With the exception of some group services such as lectures, sports events, or the theater, services are not batched; instead, they are performed on the individual. Thus, there is no set-up as in manufacturing. Consequently, a service "pull" system can be implemented with ease. Customer experience with service "pull" systems will provide the incentive for manufacturers to adopt a more service-oriented approach. Eventually, we should witness the transformation from a *push* economy to a *pull* economy.

AN APPLICATION OF DEMING'S PHILOSOPHY OF CONTINUAL IMPROVEMENT: THE CASE OF FLORIDA POWER AND LIGHT[5]

In 1985, John Hudiburg, CEO and chairman of the board of Florida Power and Light (FPL), announced a company-wide effort to win the Deming Prize. A bronze medal, the Deming Prize, is named after W. Edwards Deming, a U.S. statistician whose pioneering ideas about quality control were adopted eagerly by the Japanese when Deming fixed their fouled-up telephone service after World War II. In the spring of 1990, FPL was the first non-Japanese company to win the prestigious prize created by the Japanese several decades ago in Deming's honor.

[5]Adapted from Gary Dessler and D. L. Farrow, "Implementing a Successful Quality Improvement Programme in a Service Company: Winning the Deming Prize," *International Journal of Service Industry Management*, vol. 1, no. 2, 1990, pp. 45–53.

Foundations of the Quality-Improvement Program

As noted, the quality-improvement program at FPL was based on the teachings and philosophy of W. Edwards Deming. The foundations of this program consisted of four principles: customer satisfaction, management by facts, Deming's wheel, and respect for people.

Customer Satisfaction

The entire program is focused on satisfying customer needs. This requires an attitude of putting the customer first and a belief that this principle is the object of one's work.

Management by Facts

Objective data must be collected and presented to management for decision making. This approach requires formal data gathering and statistical analysis of those data by the company's quality-improvement teams.

Deming's Wheel

Deming's approach to quality emphasizes that checking or inspecting for quality is just one stage in the quality-improvement process. Deming's approach consists of four steps: (1) *plan* what to do; (2) *do*, or carry out, the plan; (3) *check* what was done; and (4) *act* to prevent error or improve the process. As Figure 14.2 shows, the Deming wheel is a repetitive cycle that consists of these four steps: plan, do, check, act (PDCA). Implicit in the Deming PDCA approach is that improvements in quality result from continuous, incremental turns of the wheel.

Respect for People

A company-wide quality-improvement program assumes that all employees have the capacity for self-motivation and creative thought. Employees are given support, and their ideas are solicited in an environment of mutual self-respect.

FIGURE 14.2. Deming's quality-improvement wheel.

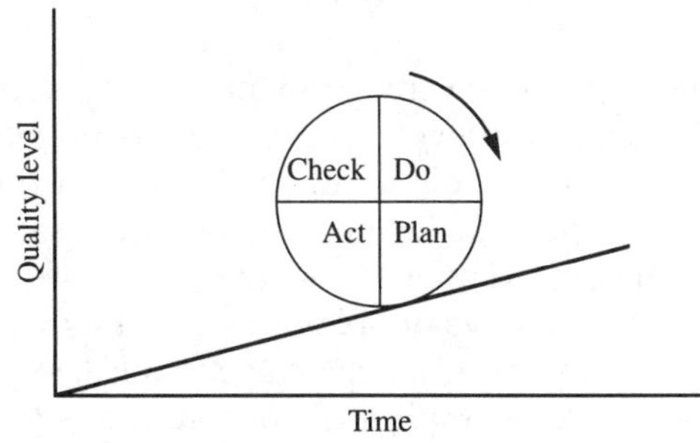

Phases of the Quality-Improvement Program

The quality-improvement program at FPL was implemented in three phases: (1) policy deployment, (2) development of quality-improvement teams, and (3) instituting a quality-in-daily-work program for individual employees.

Policy Deployment

A policy deployment process was initiated by top management to concentrate FPL's resources on a few priority issues. The motivation was a recognition that changes were occurring in the marketplace that eventually could undermine the company's performance. Objectives that emerged from the customer-needs assessment included: (1) reduce the number of complaints to the Florida Public Service Commission, and (2) strengthen fossil unit reliability. These objectives were translated into more measurable terms and then distributed to all employees to provide direction in their quality-improvement efforts.

Quality-Improvement Teams

Key team members underwent extensive training in statistical quality-control methods, PDCA cycle philosophy, and group decision-making techniques. The concept of the "customer-next process" was introduced to help focus the working group on who their customers were, whether inside or outside the company.

The teams were taught to present their quality-improvement suggestions in a seven-step "story": (1) reason for improvement; (2) current situation, including data collected; (3) analysis using fishbone charts and Pareto diagrams; (4) countermeasures, including analyses of barriers and aids; (5) results of meeting the target; (6) standardization of countermeasures for replication in other departments; and (7) future plans.

Quality in Daily Work

In the final phase of the quality-improvement program, the team approach was extended to individual workers, who were encouraged to take a quality-improvement approach to their work. For example, using this approach, meter readers were able to reduce reading errors by 50 percent.

SUMMARY

Productivity and quality improvement are an important part of an organization's development and determine the level of a firm's competitiveness. Technological innovation plays an important role in advancing a firm through the various stages of competitiveness. Introducing new technology in services is a challenge, however, because both employees and customers often are affected personally by the need to adapt to new ways of doing things. Automation of services has followed the lead of manufacturing in replacing manual tasks with machines but also has gone further, as in the application of computers to assist in problem-solving and decision-making tasks.

Making continual improvement a competitive strategy was explored by considering an analogy between JIT in manufacturing and reduction of queues in services. Finally, an application of Deming's philosophy of continual improvement was illustrated by the FLP experience.

In Chapter 15, we will consider another challenge that services face in the global market: growth and expansion.

KEY TERMS AND DEFINITIONS

Automation the application of technology, both hard (i.e., machines) and soft (i.e., information), to achieve productivity gains.

Data envelopment analysis (DEA) the use of a linear programming model to identify efficient and inefficient units in a multisite service operation.

Just-in-time (JIT) a production process emphasizing operating with minimal levels of inventory and resulting attention to quality.

Kanban the Japanese term for a card used to communicate the specifications for material or parts from an upstream or prior station in an assembly process.

TOPICS FOR DISCUSSION

1. Could firms in the "world-class service delivery" stage of competitiveness be described as "learning organizations?"
2. What emerging technologies will have a significant effect on the delivery of services in the future?
3. Contrast the philosophies of "continuous improvement" and "process reengineering." Is there a role for both points of view in service firms?

Service Benchmark

Shoppers Act as Their Own Cashiers at Some Stores

Your shopping cart is loaded with bread and toilet paper and eggplant, and you're ready for the checkout line.

Instead of looking for the speediest checker, you head toward the lane with only a computer screen and an empty bag. You scan your groceries, bag them and pay with a bank card.

If you stick an unscanned bottle of antacid into your bag, a face comes on the computer screen and points out your—ahem—mistake.

This scenario is being played out throughout the country at grocery and drug stores experimenting with self-service checkout.

"The customer feels it's faster because they walk up and do the scanning themselves," said Jonathan Hayward, vice president and chief engineer at Stores Automated Systems, Inc., in Bristol, which recently introduced a self-scan checkout system.

Stores can save money by replacing some cashiers, even though a flesh and blood clerk must be stationed at the junction of three checkout lanes to assist shoppers using SASI's system, Hayward said.

Rite Aid, the drug store chain with 2,771 stores in 21 states and Washington, D.C., is testing SASI's new system, eXPRESS, at two Philadelphia-area stores this summer.

A sensitive scale under the customer's bag detects any unscanned items. Customers using coupons or paying with cash still need the help of the clerk, as will anyone who bags an unscanned item.

"We are a very convenience-oriented chain, and this is basically one additional possible service that we could provide to assist in the convenience of our shoppers," Rite Aid spokesman Craig Muckle said.

After a six-month test, Rite Aid will decide whether to place the system in other stores.

Several grocery chains have been experimenting with self-scanning stations produced by Optimal Robotics of Plattsburgh, N.Y. Store employees monitoring the checkouts over a closed-circuit television are available to help any customers stymied by the system, U-Scan Express.

Joanne Gage, spokeswoman for Price Chopper of Schenectady, N.Y., said the company has made modifications to Optimal's system while testing it at a Clifton Park, N.Y., grocery the past three years.

"It's used more like an express lane. People tend not to use it for big orders . . ." she said. "There are some customers that never want to use it."

Shoplifting has not been a problem, said Gage, who called the system foolproof.

"There is some supervision. There is a person there who helps to identify produce. One person can man four stations, so it's a great labor-saving device," she said.

Price Chopper will install the system in one store but has no plans to expand to its 90 other groceries.

A Lakewood, Ohio, Finast supermarket has been testing a hand-held scanner, the Personal Shopper System, which allows shoppers approved by the store to register their selections as they roll their carts through the aisles.

The store initially tested the portable scanners with 100 shoppers, has extended it to 300, and plans to have 1,000 customers using the system by the end of summer, according to Nancy Tully, spokeswoman for scanner developer Symbol Technologies Inc. of Holtsville, N.Y.

The portable scanner, first used in the Netherlands, has been installed in 24 stores in a British chain that plans to introduce it to 36 more markets this summer. Another dozen U.S. grocery and discount stores are planning to test the system as well, Tully said.

When customers return their scanners, they receive a bar-coded ticket that they take to the clerk in a special express lane.

The portable system costs $200,000 to $300,000. Grocers report shoppers are spending more and shoplifting has declined, said Tully.

Wendell Young III, president of United Food and Commercial Workers Union Local 1776 in Philadelphia, said he was more concerned about the effect the machines will have on employees.

"One person handling three machines, especially in a food store, it's just not humanly possible. I don't see it working because so far it hasn't worked. I don't see it's going to be revolutionary and replace people," Young said.

Young said customers still want personal interaction with a clerk.

"It's like being served a beer by a robot in a pub," he said.

Source: Dinah Wisenberg Brin, "Shoppers Act as Their Own Cashiers at Some Stores," *Austin American Statesman,* August 12, 1996, p. D3.

CASE: MEGA BYTES RESTAURANT[6]

Mega Bytes is a restaurant that caters to business travelers and has a self-service breakfast buffet. To measure customer satisfaction, the manager constructs a survey and distributes it to diners during a 3-month period. The results, as summarized by the Pareto chart in Figure 14.3, indicate that the restaurant's major problem is customers waiting too long to be seated.

A team of employees is formed to work on resolving this problem. The team members decide to use the Seven-Step Method (SSM), which is a structured approach to problem solving and process improvement originally developed by Joiner Associates, Inc., of Madison, Wisconsin. The SSM leads a team through a logical sequence of steps that force a thorough analysis of the problem, its potential causes, and its possible solutions. The structure imposed by the SSM helps the team to focus on the correct issues and avoid diffusing its energy on tangential or counterproductive efforts. The SSM is directed at analytic rather than enumerative studies. In general, analytic studies are interested in cause and effect and in making predictions, whereas enumerative studies are focused on an existing population.

The steps in this method are shown in Table 14.4 and applied here to the case of Mega Bytes:

Step 1: Define the project. The results of the Mega Bytes survey indicate that customers wait too long to be seated. Most customers are business travelers who want to be served promptly or an opportunity to discuss business during their meal. The team considers several questions such as "When does the wait start? When does it end? How is it measured?" and then arrives at an operational definition of the problem it must solve as "waiting to be seated."

Step 2: Study the current situation. The team collects baseline data and plots them as shown in Figure 14.4. At the same time, a flowchart for seating a party is developed, and the team also diagrams the floor plan of Mega Bytes as shown in Figure 14.5.

The baseline data indicate that the percentage of people who must wait is higher early in the week than it is late in the week. This finding is to be expected, however, because most Mega Bytes customers are business travelers. The size of the party does not appear to be a factor, and no surprises were found when a histogram of the number of people waiting in excess of 1 minute was plotted against the time of the morning: more people wait during the busy hours than during the slow hours.

The reason for the waiting, however, is interesting. Most people are kept waiting either because no table is available or no table in the area of their preference is available. Customers seldom have to wait because a host or hostess is not available to seat them or others in their party have not yet arrived. At this point, it would be easy to jump to the conclusion that the problem could be solved

[6]Reprinted and selectively adapted with permission from M. Gaudard, R. Coates, and L. Freeman, "Accelerating Improvement," *Quality Progress,* vol. 24, no. 10, October 1991, pp. 81–88.

FIGURE 14.3. Pareto chart of complaints.
(Reprinted with permission from M. Gaudard, R. Coates, and L. Freeman, "Accelerating Improvement," Quality Progress, *vol. 24, no. 10, October 1991, p. 83.)*

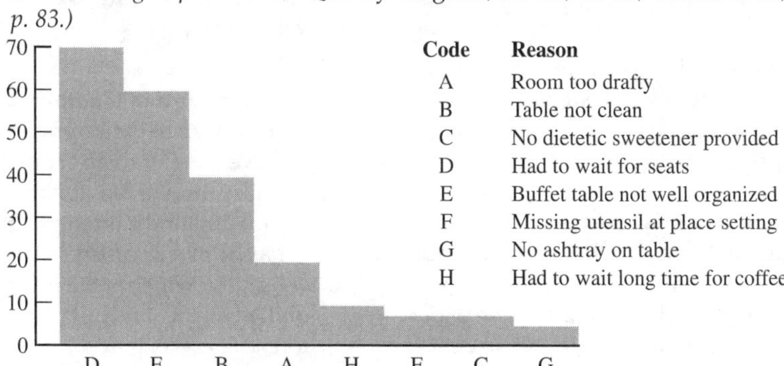

TABLE 14.4. The Seven-Step Method

Step 1 Define the project.

1. Define the problem in terms of a gap between what is and what should be. (For example, "Customers report an excessive number of errors. The team's objective is to reduce the number of errors.")
2. Document why it is important to be working on this particular problem:
   - Explain how you know it is a problem, providing any data you might have that support this.
   - List the customer's key quality characteristics. State how closing the gap will benefit the customer in terms of these characteristics.
3. Determine what data you will use to measure progress:
   - Decide what data you will use to provide a baseline against which improvement can be measured.
   - Develop any operational definitions you will need to collect the data.

Step 2 Study the current situation.

1. Collect the baseline data and plot them. (Sometimes historical data can be used for this purpose.) A run chart or control chart is usually used to exhibit baseline data. Decide how you will exhibit these data on the run chart. Decide how you will label your axes.
2. Develop flowcharts of the processes.
3. Provide any helpful sketches or visual aids.
4. Identify any variables that might have a bearing on the problem. Consider the variables of what, where, to what extent, and who. Data will be gathered on these variables to localize the problem.
5. Design data collection instruments.
6. Collect the data and summarize what you have learned about the variables' effects on the problem.
7. Determine what additional information would be helpful at this time. Repeat substeps 2 through 7 until there is no additional information that would be helpful at this time.

Step 3 Analyze the potential causes.

1. Determine potential causes of the current conditions:
   - Use the data collected in step 2 and the experience of the people who work in the process to identify conditions that might lead to the problem.
   - Construct cause-and-effect diagrams for these conditions of interest.
   - Decide on most likely causes by checking against the data from step 2 and the experience of the people working in the process.
2. Determine whether more data are needed. If so, repeat substeps 2 through 7 of step 2.
3. If possible, verify the causes through observation or by directly controlling variables.

Step 4 Implement a solution.

1. Develop a list of solutions to be considered. Be creative.
2. Decide which solutions should be tried:
   - Carefully assess the feasibility of each solution, the likelihood of success, and potential adverse consequences.
   - Clearly indicate why you are choosing a particular solution.
3. Determine how the preferred solution will be implemented. Will there be a pilot project? Who will be responsible for the implementation? Who will train those involved?
4. Implement the preferred solution.

Step 5 Check the results.

1. Determine whether the actions in step 4 were effective:
   - Collect more data on the baseline measure from step 1.
   - Collect any other data related to the conditions at the start that might be relevant.
   - Analyze the results. Determine whether the solution tested was effective. Repeat prior steps as necessary.
2. Describe any deviations from the plan and what was learned.

Step 6 Standardize the improvement.

1. Institutionalize the improvement:
   - Develop a strategy for institutionalizing the improvement and assign responsibilities.
   - Implement the strategy and check to see that it has been successful.
2. Determine whether the improvement should be applied elsewhere and plan for its implementation.

TABLE 14.4. (*Continued*)

Step 7 Establish future plans.

1. Determine your plans for the future:
   - Decide whether the gap should be narrowed further and, if so, how another project should be approached and who should be involved.
   - Identify related problems that should be addressed.
2. Summarize what you learned about the project team experience and make recommendations for future project teams.

Source: Reprinted with permission from M. Gaudard, R. Coates, and L. Freeman, "Accelerating Improvement," *Quality Progress,* vol. 24, no. 10, October 1991, p. 82.

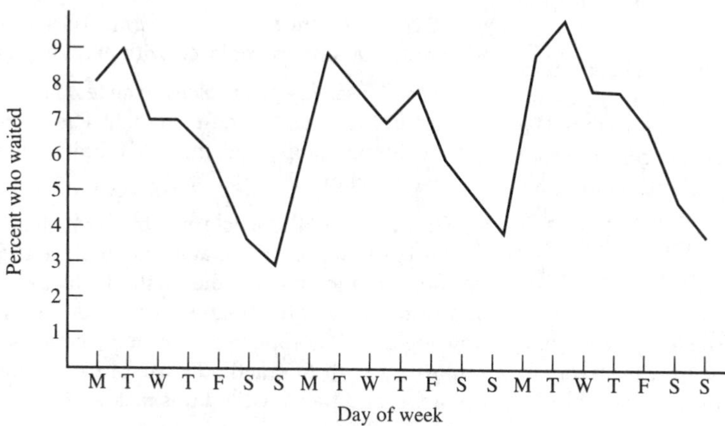

FIGURE 14.4. Run chart of percent of customers waiting more than one minute to be seated.
(Reprinted with permission from M. Gaudard, R. Coates, and L. Freeman, "Accelerating Improvement," Quality Progress, *vol. 24, no. 10, October 1991, p. 83.)*

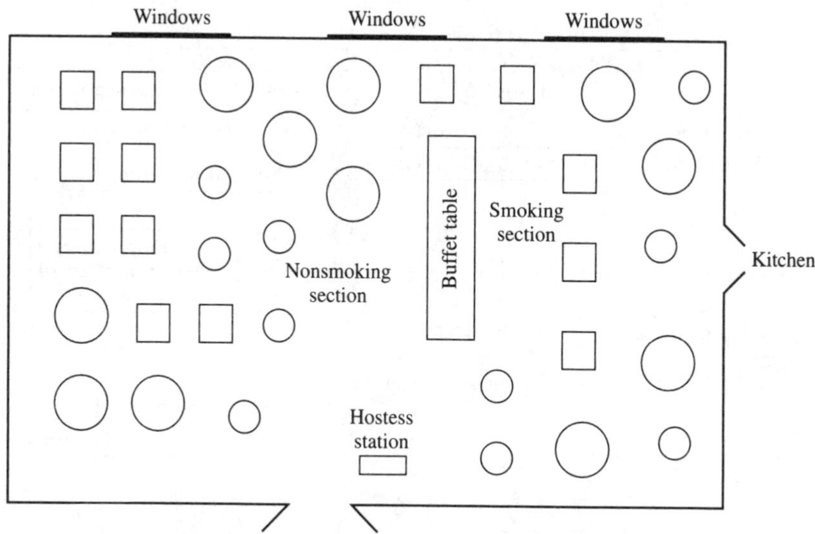

FIGURE 14.5. Restaurant floor plan.
(Reprinted with permission from M. Gaudard, R. Coates, and L. Freeman, "Accelerating Improvement," Quality Progress, *vol. 24, no. 10, October 1991, p. 83.)*

just by adding more staff early in the week and during the busy hours.

The team members decide, however, that they need additional information on why these tables are not available and how seating preferences affect the waiting time. Subsequent data indicate that "unavailable" tables usually are unavailable because they need to be cleared, not because they are occupied by diners. The data also show that most people who wait have a preference for the nonsmoking section.

Step 3: Analyze the potential causes. A cause-and-effect diagram is constructed for "why tables are not cleared quickly," as shown in Figure 14.6. The team concludes that the most likely cause of both problems (i.e., uncleared tables and waiting for nonsmoking tables) may be attributed to the distance between the tables and the kitchen and, perhaps, to the current ratio of smoking-to-nonsmoking tables.

Step 4: Implement a solution. The team develops a list of possible solutions. Because the team cannot verify its conclusion by controlling variables, it chooses a solution that can be tested easily: set up temporary work stations in the nonsmoking area. No other changes are made, and data on the percentage of people now waiting longer than 1 minute to be seated are collected.

Step 5: Check the results. The team analyzes the results of data collected for 1 month in step 4 of the study. As Figure 14.7 shows, the improvement is dramatic.

Step 6: Standardize the improvement. The temporary work stations are replaced with permanent ones.

Step 7: Establish future plans. The team decides to address the next highest bar in the Pareto chart of customer complaints; that the buffet table is not well organized.

The authors of the article on which our Mega Bytes case is based report that managers who used SSM in various situations found the method's focus and restraint to be valuable because it provided organization, logic, and thoroughness. The managers also were impressed with the method's use of data instead of opinions, and they credited this factor with reducing

FIGURE 14.6. Cause-and-effect diagram describing why tables are not cleared quickly. *(Reprinted with permission from M. Gaudard, R. Coates, and L. Freeman, "Accelerating Improvement,"* Quality Progress, *vol. 24, no. 10, October 1991, p. 84.)*

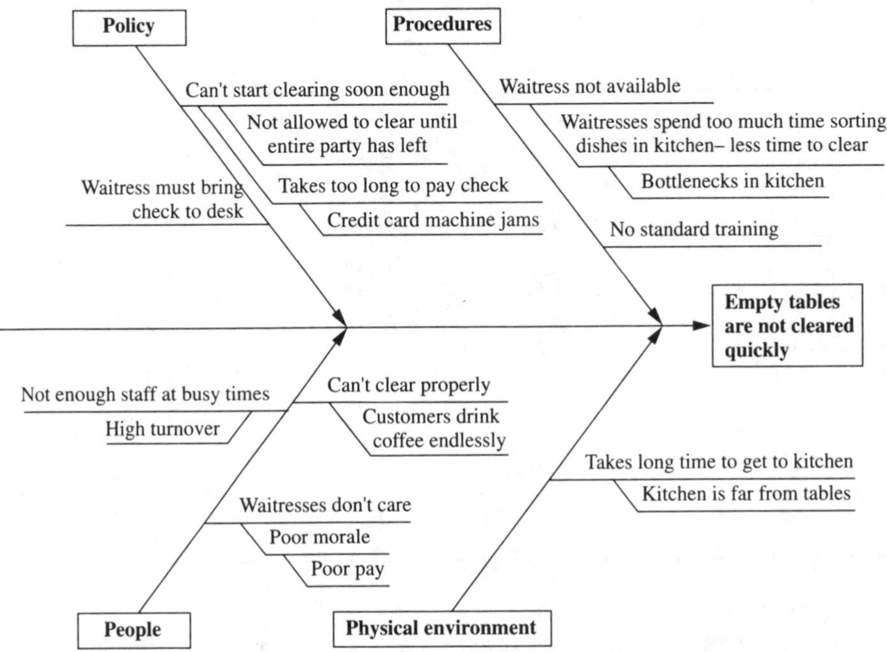

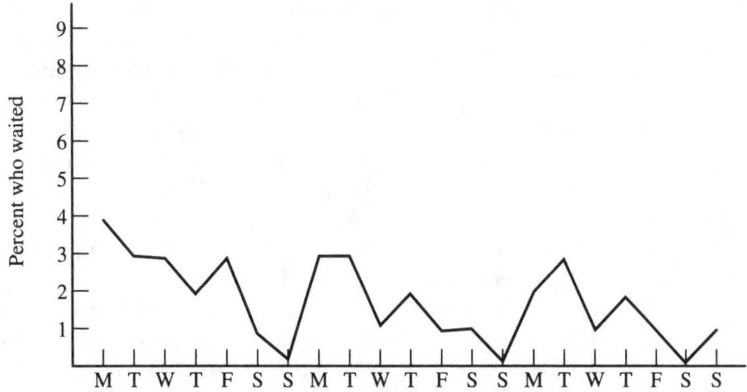

FIGURE 14.7. Run chart of percent of customers waiting more than one minute to be seated after implementation of solution. *(Reprinted with permission from M. Gaudard, R. Coates, and L. Freeman, "Accelerating Improvement,"* Quality Progress, *vol. 24, no. 10, October 1991, p. 85.)*

territorial squabbles and promoting both cooperation and trust among team members.

While very valuable, SSM does entail some difficulties. For example, project teams have found several concepts in the first two steps very difficult to formulate. In particular, a team may have trouble developing a problem statement, because the tendency is to frame a solution as a problem. In the case of Mega Bytes, the team had to avoid identifying the problem as "There are too few servers," "There aren't enough tables," or "The servers need to work faster." The real problem was identified correctly as "The customers must wait too long."

Another concept that has been difficult for study teams is localization, which is a process of focusing on smaller and smaller vital pieces of the problem. This concept initially proved difficult because team members had not yet internalized the idea that improvement should be driven by customer requirements.

Some study teams have experienced an assortment of other difficulties. Occasionally, team members could not see the benefit of collecting data accurately, or they did not understand how baseline data would be used to validate a solution. Some members had trouble keeping an open mind and, consequently, resisted investigating the effects of variables they felt to be irrelevant. In some cases, members had to learn new skills, such as how to obtain information in a nonthreatening way from workers in the system. Finally, organizational problems such as arranging meeting times and getting support from coworkers had to be resolved as well.

Questions

1. How is SSM different from Deming's PDCA cycle?

2. Prepare a cause-and-effect or fishbone diagram for a problem such as "Why customers have long waits for coffee." Your fishbone diagram should be similar to that in Figure 14.6, using the main sources of cause: policy, procedure, people, and physical environment.

3. How would you resolve the difficulties that study teams have experienced when applying SSM?

SELECTED BIBLIOGRAPHY

Baker, Edward M., and H. L. Artinian: "The Deming Philosophy of Continuing Improvement in a Service Organization: The Case of Windsor Export Supply," *Quality Progress*, vol. 18, no. 6, June 1985, pp. 61–69.

BANKER, RAJIV D.: "Maximum Likelihood, Consistency and DEA: Statistical Foundation," *Management Science*, vol. 39, no. 10, October 1993, pp. 1265–1273.

———, A. CHARNES, and W. W. COOPER: "Some Models for Estimating Technical and Scale Inefficiencies in Data Envelopment Analysis," *Management Science*, vol. 30, no. 9, September 1984, pp. 1078–1092. (The "BCC" Model)

———, ———, ———, J. SWARTS, and D. A. THOMAS: "An Introduction to Data Envelopment Analysis with Some of Its Models and Their Use," *Research in Government and Nonprofit Accounting*, vol. 5, 1989, pp. 125–163.

———, R. B. CONRAD, and R. P. STRAUSS: "A Comparative Application of Data Envelopment Analysis and Translog Methods: An Illustration Study of Hospital Production," *Management Science*, vol. 32, no. 1, January 1986, pp. 30–44.

———, and R. C. MOREY: "Efficiency Analysis for Exogenously Fixed Inputs and Outputs," *Operations Research*, vol. 34, no. 4, July–August 1986, pp. 513–521.

BERG, SANFORD V.: "Determinants of Technological Change in the Service Industries," *Technological Forecasting and Social Change*, vol. 5, no. 3, 1973, pp. 407–421.

BERRY, L. L., V. A. ZEITHAML, and A. PARASURAMAN: "Five Imperatives for Improving Service Quality," *Sloan Management Review*, vol. 31, no. 4, Summer 1990, pp. 29–38.

CHARNES, A., W. W. COOPER, and E. RHODES: "Evaluating Program and Managerial Efficiency: An Application of Data Envelopment Analysis to Program Follow Through," *Management Science*, vol. 27, no. 6, June 1981, pp. 668–697.

———: "Measuring the Efficiency of Decision Making Units," *European Journal of Operations Research*, vol. 2, no. 6, November 1978, pp. 429–444. (The "CCR" Model)

DESSLER, GARY, and D. L. FARROW: "Implementing a Successful Quality Improvement Programme in a Service Company: Winning the Deming Prize," *International Journal of Service Industry Management*, vol. 1, no. 2, 1990, pp. 45–53.

FITZSIMMONS, JAMES A.: "Making Continual Improvement a Competitive Strategy for Service Firms," *Service Management Effectiveness*, Bowen, Chase, Cummings and Associates, Jossey-Bass Publishers, San Francisco, 1990, pp. 284–295.

LEWIN, ARIE Y., R. C. MOREY, and T. J. COOK: "Evaluating the Administrative Efficiency of Courts," *OMEGA*, vol. 10, no. 4, 1982, pp. 401–411.

MCLAUGHLIN, CURTIS P., and SYDNEY COFFY: "Measuring Productivity in Services," *International Journal of Service Industry Management*, vol. 1, no. 1, 1990, pp. 46–64.

MEHRA, S., and R. A. INMAN: "JIT Implementation within a Service Industry: A Case Study," *International Journal of Service Industry Management*, vol. 1, no. 3, 1990, pp. 53–61.

QUINN, JAMES BRIAN, J. J. BARUCH, and P. C. PAQUETTE: "Technology in Services," *Scientific American*, vol. 257, no. 6, December 1987, pp. 50–58.

ROACH, STEPHEN S.: "Services under Siege—The Restructuring Imperative," *Harvard Business Review*, September–October 1991, pp. 82–91.

SEIFORD, LAWRENCE M.: *A Bibliography of Data Envelopment Analysis (1978–1990)*, Dept. of IE and OR, University of Massachusetts, Amherst, Mass., April 1990.

SHERMAN, DAVID H.: "Improving the Productivity of Service Business," *Sloan Management Review*, vol. 25, no. 3, Spring 1984, pp. 11–23.

CHAPTER 14 SUPPLEMENT: Data Envelopment Analysis (DEA)

How can corporate management evaluate the productivity of a fast-food outlet, a branch bank, a health clinic, or an elementary school? The difficulties in measuring productivity are threefold. First, what are the appropriate inputs to the system (e.g., labor hours, material dollars) and the measures of those inputs? Second, what are the appropriate outputs of the system (e.g., checks cashed, certificate of deposits) and the measures of those outputs? Third, what are the appropriate ways of measuring the relationship between these inputs and outputs?

Measuring Service Productivity

The measure of an organization's productivity, if viewed from an engineering perspective, is similar to the measure of a system's efficiency. It can be stated as a ratio of outputs to inputs (e.g., miles per gallon for an automobile).

To evaluate the operational efficiency of a branch bank, for example, an accounting ratio such as cost per teller transaction might be used. A branch with a high ratio in comparison with those of other branches would be considered less efficient, but the higher ratio could result from a more complex mix of transactions. For example, a branch opening new accounts and selling CDs would require more time per transaction than another branch engaged only in simple transactions such as accepting deposits and cashing checks. The problem with using simple ratios is that the mix of outputs is not considered explicitly. This same criticism also can be made concerning the mix of inputs. For example, some branches may have automated teller machines in addition to live tellers, and this use of technology could affect the cost per teller transaction.

Broad-based measures such as profitability or return on investment are highly relevant as overall performance measures, but they are not sufficient to evaluate the operating efficiency of a service unit. For instance, one could not conclude that a profitable branch bank is necessarily efficient in its use of personnel and other inputs. A higher-than-average proportion of revenue-generating transactions could be the explanation rather than the cost-efficient use of resources.

The DEA Model

Fortunately, a technique has been developed with the ability to compare the efficiency of multiple service units that provide similar services by explicitly considering their use of multiple inputs (i.e., resources) to produce multiple outputs (i.e., services). The technique, which is referred to as *data envelopment analysis (DEA),* circumvents the need to develop standard costs for each service, because it can incorporate multiple inputs and multiple outputs into both the numerator and the denominator of the efficiency ratio without the need for conversion to a common dollar basis. Thus, the DEA measure of efficiency explicitly accounts for the mix of inputs and outputs and, consequently, is more comprehensive and reliable than a set of operating ratios or profit measures.[7]

DEA is a linear programming model that attempts to maximize a service unit's efficiency, expressed as a ratio of outputs to inputs, by comparing a particular unit's efficiency with the performance of a group of similar service units that are delivering the same service. In the process, some units achieve 100-percent efficiency and are referred to as the *relatively efficient units,* whereas other units with efficiency ratings of less than 100 percent are referred to as *inefficient units.*

Corporate management thus can use DEA to compare a group of service units to identify relatively inefficient units, measure the magnitude of the inefficiencies, and by comparing the inefficient with the efficient ones, discover ways to reduce those inefficiencies.

The DEA linear programming model is formulated as follows.

Definition of Variables

Let E_k, with $k = 1, 2, \dots, K$, be the efficiency ratio of unit k, where K is the total number of units being evaluated.

Let u_j, with $j = 1, 2, \dots, M$, be a coefficient for output j, where M is the total number of output types being considered. The variable u_j is a measure of the

[7]A. Charnes, W. W. Cooper, and E. Rhodes, "Measuring the Efficiency of Decision Making Units," *European Journal of Operations Research,* November 1978, pp. 429–444.

relative decrease in efficiency with each unit reduction of output value.

Let v_i, with $i = 1, 2, \ldots, N$, be a coefficient for input i, where N is the total number of input types being considered. The variable v_i is a measure of the relative increase in efficiency with each unit reduction of input value.

Let O_{jk} be the number of observed units of output j generated by service unit k during one time period.

Let I_{ik} be the number of actual units of input i used by service unit k during one time period.

Objective Function

The objective is to find the set of coefficient u's associated with each output and of v's associated with each input that will give the service unit being evaluated the highest possible efficiency.

$$\max E_e = \frac{u_1 O_{1e} + u_2 O_{2e} + \cdots + u_M O_{Me}}{v_1 I_{1e} + v_2 I_{2e} + \cdots + v_N I_{Ne}} \qquad (1)$$

where e is the index of the unit being evaluated.

This function is subject to the constraint that when the same set of input and output coefficients (u_j's and v_i's) is applied to all other service units being compared, no service unit will exceed 100-percent efficiency or a ratio of 1.0.

Constraints

$$\frac{u_1 O_{1k} + u_2 O_{2k} + \cdots + u_M O_{Mk}}{v_1 I_{1k} + v_2 I_{2k} + \cdots + v_N I_{Nk}} \le 1.0$$

$$k = 1, 2, \cdots, K \qquad (2)$$

where all coefficient values are positive and nonzero.

To solve this fractional linear programming model using standard linear programming software requires a reformulation. Note that both the objective function and all constraints are ratios rather than linear functions. The objective function in equation (1) is restated as a linear function by arbitrarily scaling the inputs for the unit under evaluation to a sum of 1.0.

$$\max E_e = u_1 O_{1e} + u_2 O_{2e} + \cdots + u_M O_{Me} \qquad (3)$$

subject to the constraint that

$$v_1 I_{1e} + v_2 I_{2e} + \cdots + v_N I_{Ne} = 1 \qquad (4)$$

For each service unit, the constraints in equation (2) are similarly reformulated;

$$u_1 O_{1k} + u_2 O_{2k} + \cdots + u_M O_{Mk} - (v_1 I_{1k} + v_2 I_{2k} + \cdots + v_N I_{Nk}) \le 0 \qquad k = 1, 2, \cdots, K \qquad (5)$$

where:

$u_j \ge 0 \qquad j = 1, 2, \ldots, M$

$v_i \ge 0 \qquad i = 1, 2, \ldots, N$

A question of sample size often is raised concerning the number of service units that are required compared with the number of input and output variables selected in the analysis. The following relationship relating the number of service units K used in the analysis and the number of input N and output M types being considered is based on empirical findings and the experience of DEA practitioners:

$$K \ge 2(N + M) \qquad (6)$$

Example 14.1: Burger Palace

An innovative drive-in-only burger chain has established six units in several different cities. Each unit is located in a strip shopping center parking lot. Only a standard meal consisting of a burger, fries, and a drink is available. Management has decided to use DEA to improve productivity by identifying which units are using their resources most efficiently and then sharing their experience and knowledge with the less efficient locations. Table 14.5 summarizes data for two inputs: labor-hours and material dollars consumed during a typical lunch-hour period to generate an output of 100 meals sold. Normally, output will vary among the service units, but in this example, we have made the outputs equal to allow for a graphical presentation of the units' productivity. As Figure 14.8 shows, service units S_1, S_3, and S_6 have been joined to form an efficient-production frontier of alternative methods of using labor-hours and material resources to generate 100 meals. As can be seen, these efficient units have defined an envelope that contains all the inefficient units—thus the reason for calling the process "data envelopment analysis."

For this simple example, we can identify efficient units by inspection and see the excess inputs being used by inefficient units (e.g., S_2 would be as efficient as S_3 if it used \$50 less in materials). To gain an understanding of DEA, however, we

TABLE 14.5. Summary of Outputs and Inputs for Burger Palace

Service Unit	Meals Sold	Labor-Hours	Material Dollars
1	100	2	200
2	100	4	150
3	100	4	100
4	100	6	100
5	100	8	80
6	100	10	50

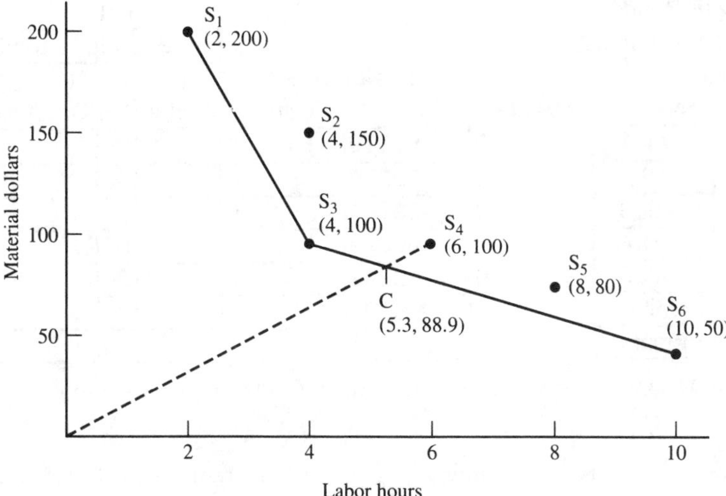

FIGURE 14.8. Productivity frontier for Burger Palace.

will proceed to formulate the linear programming problems for each unit, then solve each of them to determine efficiency ratings and other information.

We begin by illustrating the LP formulation for the first service unit, S_1, using equations (3), (4), and (5).

$$\begin{aligned}
&\max E(S_1) = u_1 100 \\
&\text{subject to:} \\
&u_1 100 - v_1 2 - v_2 200 \le 0 \\
&u_1 100 - v_1 4 - v_2 150 \le 0 \\
&u_1 100 - v_1 4 - v_2 100 \le 0 \\
&u_1 100 - v_1 6 - v_2 100 \le 0 \\
&u_1 100 - v_1 8 - v_2 80 \le 0 \\
&u_1 100 - v_1 10 - v_2 50 \le 0 \\
&\qquad v_1 2 + v_2 200 = 1 \\
&\qquad\quad u_1, v_1, v_2 \ge 0
\end{aligned}$$

Similar linear programming problems are formulated (or, better yet, the S_1 linear programming problem is edited) and solved for the other service units by substituting the appropriate output function for the objective function and substituting the appropriate input function for the last constraint. Constraints 1 through 6, which restrict all units to no more than 100-percent efficiency, remain the same in all problems.

This set of six linear programming problems was solved with Excel Solver 7.0 in fewer than 5 minutes by editing the data file between each run. Because the output is 100 meals for all units, only the last constraint must be edited by substituting the appropriate labor and material input values from Table 14.5 for the unit being evaluated.

The data file for unit 1 of Burger Palace using a Linear Programming Excel Add-in is shown in Figure 14.9.[8] The linear programming results for

[8]Paul A. Jensen, *Operations Research Add-ins for Microsoft Excel*, Operations Research Group, Dept. of Mechanical Engineering, University of Texas at Austin, 1996.

Linear Model

Name:	Unit 1
Type:	LP
No. Var.:	3
Int. Var.:	0
No. Con.:	7
Nonlinear:	0

Objective Value

0

Model	Variables		1	2	3
	Num.		1	2	3
	Name		u1	v1	v2
0	Values		0	0	0
3	Linear Obj. Coef.		100	0	0
TRUE	Lower Bounds		0	0	0
TRUE	Upper Bounds		99999	99999	99999
TRUE	Constraints				
TRUE					
100					

Constraints Num.	Name	Value	Constraint Bounds Lower	Upper	Constraint Coefficients		
1	Unit 1	0	-99999	0	100	-2	-200
2	Unit 2	0	-99999	0	100	-4	-150
3	Unit 3	0	-99999	0	100	-4	-100
4	Unit 4	0	-99999	0	100	-6	-100
5	Unit 5	0	-99999	0	100	-8	-80
6	Unit 6	0	-99999	0	100	-10	-50
7	Inputs	0	1	1	0	2	200

FIGURE 14.9. Excel data file for DEA analysis of Burger Palace unit 1.

each unit are shown in Table 14.6 and summarized in Table 14.7.

In Table 14.7, we find that DEA has identified the same units shown as being efficient in Figure 14.8. Units S_2, S_4, and S_5 all are inefficient in varying degrees. Also shown in Table 14.7 and associated with each inefficient unit is an *efficiency reference set*. Each inefficient unit will have a set of efficient units associated with it that defines its productivity. As Figure 14.8 shows for inefficient unit S_4, the efficient units S_3 and S_6 have been joined with a line defining the efficiency frontier. A dashed line drawn from the origin to inefficient unit S_4 cuts through this frontier and, thus, defines unit S_4 as inefficient. In Table 14.7, the value in parentheses that is associated with each member of the efficiency reference set (i.e., .7778 for S_3 and .2222 for S_6) represents the relative weight assigned to that efficient unit in calculating the efficiency rating for S_4. These relative weights are the shadow prices that are associated with the respective efficient-unit constraints in the linear programming solution. (Note in Table 14.6 that for unit 4, these weights appear as opportunity costs for S_3 and S_6.)

The values for v_1 and v_2 that are associated with the inputs of labor-hours and materials, respectively, measure the relative increase in efficiency with each unit reduction of input value. For unit S_4, each unit decrease in labor-hours results in an efficiency increase of 0.0555. For unit S_4 to become efficient, it must increase its efficiency rating by 0.111 points. This can be accomplished by reducing labor used by 2 hours (i.e., 2 hours × 0.0555 = 0.111). Note that with this reduction in labor-hours, unit S_4 becomes identical to efficient unit S_3. An alternative approach would be a reduction in materials used by \$16.57 (i.e., 0.111/0.0067 = 16.57). Any linear combination of these two measures also would move unit S_4 to the productivity frontier defined by the line segment joining efficient units S_3 and S_6.

Table 14.8 contains the calculations for a hypothetical unit C, which is a composite reference unit defined by the weighted inputs of the reference set S_3 and S_6. As Figure 14.8 shows, this composite unit C is located at the intersection of the productivity frontier and the dashed line drawn from the origin to unit S_4. Thus, compared with this reference unit C, inefficient unit S_4 is using excess inputs in the amounts of 0.7 labor-hours and 11.1 material dollars.

DEA offers many opportunities for an ineffi-

TABLE 14.6 LP Solutions for DEA Study of Burger Palace

Summarized results for unit 1 — Page : 1

Variables No.	Variables Names	Solutions	Opportunity costs	Variables No.	Variables Names	Solutions	Opportunity costs
1	U1	+1.0000000	0	6	S3	0	0
2	V1	+.16666667	0	7	S4	+33.333336	0
3	V2	+.00333333	0	8	S5	+60.000000	0
4	S1	0	+1.0000000	9	S6	+83.333336	0
5	S2	+16.666670	0	10	A7	0	+100.00000

Maximized objective function = 100 Iterations = 4

Summarized results for unit 2 — Page : 1

Variables No.	Variables Names	Solutions	Opportunity costs	Variables No.	Variables Names	Solutions	Opportunity costs
1	U1	+.85714287	0	6	S3	0	+.71428573
2	V1	+.14285715	0	7	S4	+28.571430	0
3	V2	+.00285714	0	8	S5	+51.428574	0
4	S1	0	+.28571430	9	S6	+71.428574	0
5	S2	+14.285717	0	10	A7	0	+85.714287

Maximized objective function = 85.71429 Iterations = 4

Summarized results for unit 3 — Page : 1

Variables No.	Variables Names	Solutions	Opportunity costs	Variables No.	Variables Names	Solutions	Opportunity costs
1	U1	+1.0000000	0	6	S3	0	+1.0000000
2	V1	+.06250000	0	7	S4	+12.500000	0
3	V2	+.00750000	0	8	S5	+10.000001	0
4	S1	+62.500000	0	9	S6	0	0
5	S2	+37.500008	0	10	A7	0	+100.00000

Maximized objective function = 100 Iterations = 3

cient unit to become efficient regarding its reference set of efficient units. In practice, management would choose a particular approach on the basis of an evaluation of its cost, practicality, and feasibility; however, the motivation for change is clear (i.e., other units actually are able to achieve similar outputs with fewer resources).

DEA and Strategic Planning

When combined with profitability, DEA efficiency analysis can be useful in strategic planning for services that are delivered through multiple sites (e.g., hotel chains). Figure 14.10 presents a matrix of four possibilities that arise from combining efficiency and profitability.

Considering the top-left quadrant of this matrix (i.e., underperforming potential stars) reveals that units operating at a high profit may be operating inefficiently and, thus, have unrealized potential. Comparing these with similar, efficient units could suggest measures that would lead to even greater profit through more efficient operations.

Star performers can be found in the top-right quadrant (i.e., benchmark group). These efficient units also are highly profitable and, thus, serve as examples

TABLE 14.6 (*Continued*)

Summarized results for unit 4 Page : 1

Variables No.	Names	Solutions	Opportunity costs	Variables No.	Names	Solutions	Opportunity costs
1	U1	+.88888890	0	6	S3	0	+.77777779
2	V1	+.05555556	0	7	S4	+11.111112	0
3	V2	+.00666667	0	8	S5	+8.8888893	0
4	S1	+55.555553	0	9	S6	0	+.22222224
5	S2	+33.333340	0	10	A7	0	+88.888885

Maximized objective function = 88.88889 Iterations = 3

Summarized results for unit 5 Page : 1

Variables No.	Names	Solutions	Opportunity costs	Variables No.	Names	Solutions	Opportunity costs
1	U1	+.90909088	0	6	S3	0	+.45454547
2	V1	+.05681818	0	7	S4	+11.363637	0
3	V2	+.00681818	0	8	S5	+9.0909100	0
4	S1	+56.818180	0	9	S6	0	+.54545450
5	S2	+34.090916	0	10	A7	0	+90.909088

Maximized objective function = 90.90909 Iterations = 4

Summarized results for unit 6 Page : 1

Variables No.	Names	Solutions	Opportunity costs	Variables No.	Names	Solutions	Opportunity costs
1	U1	+1.0000000	0	6	S3	0	0
2	V1	+.06250000	0	7	S4	+12.500000	0
3	V2	+.00750000	0	8	S5	+10.000001	0
4	S1	+62.500000	0	9	S6	0	+1.0000000
5	S2	+37.500008	0	10	A7	0	+100.00000

Maximized objective function = 100 Iterations = 4

for others to emulate both in operations efficiency and marketing success in generating high revenues.

The lower-right quadrant (i.e., candidates for divestiture) contains efficient but unprofitable units. These units are limited in profit potential, perhaps because of a poor location, and should be sold to generate capital for expansion in new territories.

It is not clear which strategy to employ with the lower-left quadrant units (i.e., problem branches). If profit potential is limited, investments in efficient operations might lead to a future candidate for divestiture.

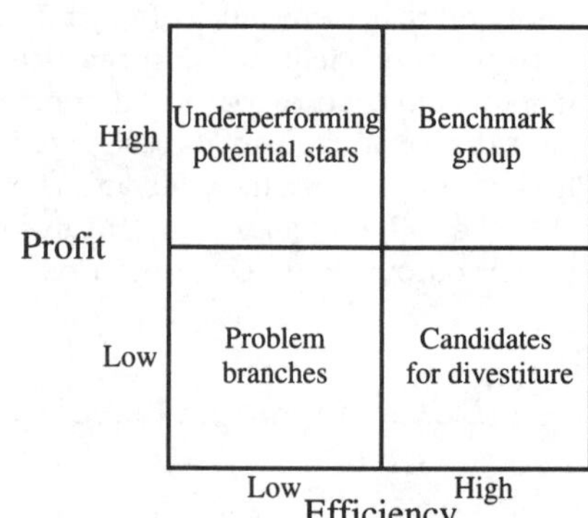

FIGURE 14.10. DEA strategic matrix.

TABLE 14.7. Summary of DEA Results

Service Unit	Efficiency Rating (E)	Efficiency Reference Set	Relative Labor-Hour Value (v_1)	Relative Material Value (v_2)
S_1	1.000	—	.1667	.0033
S_2	0.857	S_1 (.2857) S_3 (.7143)	.1428	.0028
S_3	1.000	—	.0625	.0075
S_4	0.889	S_3 (.7778) S_6 (.2222)	.0555	.0067
S_5	0.901	S_3 (.4545) S_6 (.5454)	.0568	.0068
S_6	1.000	—	.0625	.0075

TABLE 14.8. Calculation of Excess Inputs Used by Unit S_4

Outputs and Inputs	*Reference Set* S_3	*Reference Set* S_6	Composite Reference Unit C	S_4	Excess Inputs Used
Meals	(.7778) × 100 +	(.2222) × 100 =	100	100	0
Labor-hours	(.7778) × 4 +	(.2222) × 10 =	5.3	6	0.7
Material ($)	(.7778) × 100 +	(.2222) × 50 =	88.9	100	11.1

Exercises

14.1. For the Burger Palace example, perform a complete analysis of efficiency improvement alternatives for unit S_2, including determination of a composite reference unit.

14.2. For the Burger Palace example, perform a complete analysis of efficiency improvement alternatives for unit S_5, including determination of a composite reference unit.

14.3. For the Burger Palace example, what is the effect of removing an inefficient unit from the analysis (e.g., S_2)?

14.4. For the Burger Palace example, what is the effect of removing an efficient unit from the analysis (e.g., S_6)?

CASE: MID-ATLANTIC BUS LINES

Mid-Atlantic Bus Lines was founded by a group of managers from Trailways when that company was acquired by Greyhound. They launched a first-class, express bus service operating between the major coastal cities from Philadelphia, Pennsylvania, to Jacksonville, Florida. By hiring laid-off Trailways drivers and leasing buses, they established franchises in each city with local entrepreneurs, who were given the right to operate a Mid-Atlantic bus terminal. A percentage of the passenger ticket sales and freight sales would be kept by the terminal operator to cover his or her costs and profit.

After several months of operation, some franchisees complained about inadequate profits and threatened to close their terminals. Because other franchisees were pleased with their experiences, however,

TABLE 14.9. Outputs and Inputs for Mid-Atlantic Bus Lines

Bus Depot	City Served	Ticket Sales	Freight Sales	Labor-Hours	Facility Dollars
1	Philadelphia, Pa.	700	300	40	500
2	Baltimore, Md.	300	600	50	500
3	Washington, D.C.	200	700	50	400
4	Richmond, Va.	400	600	50	500
5	Raleigh, N.C.	500	400	40	400
6	Charleston, S.C.	500	500	50	500
7	Savannah, Ga.	800	500	40	600
8	Jacksonville, Fl.	300	200	30	400

a study of all terminal operations in the system was undertaken. The information in Table 14.9 was collected over several weeks and represents a typical day's operation.

Questions

1. Use DEA to identify efficient and inefficient terminal operations. Formulate the problem as a linear programming model, and solve using computer software such as Excel Solver that permits input file editing between runs.

2. Using the appropriate reference set of efficient terminals, make recommendations for changes in resource inputs for each inefficient terminal.

3. What recommendations would you have for the one seriously inefficient terminal in regard to increasing its outputs?

4. Discuss any shortcomings in the application of DEA to Mid-Atlantic Bus Lines.

CHAPTER 15

Growth and Expansion

LEARNING OBJECTIVES

After completing this chapter, you should be able to:

1. Identify the expansion strategy that a service firm is using.
2. Discuss the nature of franchising from the the franchiser and franchisee points of view.
3. Discuss the factors to be considered in multinational development.
4. Describe and contrast the global service strategies.

In June 1991, a guest and an employee were found electrocuted by a faulty underwater light in the swimming pool of a Days Inn in Orange, Texas.[1] This tragic incident is part of the story of a once-successful motel chain that was taken over in a leveraged buyout in 1984. Cecil B. Day founded the chain in 1970 and operated it for years on the principle of strict adherence to exacting standards of excellence. A high-minded man, Day prohibited the sale of alcohol on his properties, kept a chaplain on call 24 hours a day at each unit, and established a security department that was the envy of the industry. To maintain standards and consistency, the company owned at least half of its motels and granted franchises sparingly, rejecting more than 90 percent of applicants.

Twenty-two years after its founding, Days Inn does not own a single motel. After the 1984 leveraged buyout, Days Inn became an organization that merely sells its sign and its reservation and marketing services—and claims to be the fastest-growing motel chain. Franchise revenue became all that mattered, with each inn paying Days Inn 6 to 10 percent of its sales revenue. Lack of attention to the properties has resulted in stained walls, worn furniture, and broken air conditioners. More important, guests now appear to be at some risk from lax security and deferred maintenance, as illustrated by the electrocution incident.

Unlike competitors that require a new franchisee to build an inn from the ground up to exacting specifications, the post-takeover Days Inn would erect its sign on a franchisee's existing property and ask for compliance later. This practice has resulted in inconsistent quality throughout the chain. Note that a major selling point of most motel chains is consistent quality, and Days Inn's willingness to accept any existing motel as part of its chain has not been lost on Red Roof Inns, which advertises that its competition has "no two . . . alike" while touting its own inns as being corporate-owned and -operated. By selling off all company-owned units, Days Inn also deviated from accepted franchising practice. Without daily involvement in operations, a franchiser generally is believed to be less effective in dealing with franchisee problems. Former company insiders and industry experts point to Days Inn as an example of the dangers of rapid franchising.

CHAPTER PREVIEW

This chapter begins with a look at service growth and expansion in the context of multisite and multiservice expansion strategies. Using these dimensions, we put services into four classifications: focused service, focused network, clustered service, and diversified network.

Franchising can be an effective multisite expansion strategy for a well-defined service concept. We will explore benefits to the franchisee and responsibilities of the franchiser in an organizational arrangement held together by a contract.

Because our world has become "borderless," service expansion no longer can end with development of the domestic market alone. Expansion overseas presents unique challenges, however, such as the cultural transferability of the ser-

[1]From Kevin Helliker, "How a Motel Chain Lost Its Moorings after 1980's Buy-Out," *The Wall Street Journal*, May 26, 1992, p. 1.

vice and discriminatory practices of foreign governments to protect their own domestic services from competition.

GROWTH AND EXPANSION STRATEGIES

The expectation of an entrepreneurial innovation is initial acceptance of the service concept followed by increasing customer demand. The need to expand a successful innovative service often is thrust on the owner by the pressure of market potential and the desire to protect the service concept from competitors through building barriers to entry. To understand better the various ways in which a firm can expand its concept, consider Figure 15.1, which shows the fundamental expansion strategies that are available to service firms. We shall explore each of these strategies in turn with a discussion of the risks involved and the implications for management.

Focused Service

Typically, a service innovation begins at a single location with an initial service concept. This initial service concept usually is a well-defined vision focused on delivering a new and unique service. For example, Fred Smith's vision for Federal Express was use of a single hub-and-spoke network to guarantee overnight delivery of packages.

Success leads to increased demand, which requires capacity expansion at the site. Typically, the facility is expanded and personnel added.

The successful firm also will attract competition and need to build a preferred position among as many customers as possible in the local market area. Adding peripheral services is one approach to penetrating the market or holding market share against the competition. Examples of peripheral services for a restaurant would include a salad bar or drive-through window. The core service for a successful restaurant, however, usually is excellent cuisine.

Risks that are associated with a single service location include being captive to the future economic growth of that area and being vulnerable to competition that can move in and capture market share. Management and control of the enterprise, however, are much simpler than in any of the other growth strategies.

FIGURE 15.1. Multisite and multiservice expansion strategies.

	Single Service	Multiservice
Single Location	*Focused service:* • Dental practice • Retail store • Family restaurant	*Clustered service:* • Stanford University • Mayo Clinic • USAA Insurance
Multisite	*Focused network:* • Federal Express • McDonald's • Red Roof Inns	*Diversified network:* • Nations Bank • American Express • Arthur Andersen

Many examples of successful focused services exist. Consider fine restaurants in particular, such as Chez Panisse in Berkeley or Antoine's in New Orleans. A *focused service* often is limited to a single site because of talented personnel, such as an award-winning chef or a nationally recognized heart surgeon. If the site is a key element of the service, such as a sheltered cove for a marina, it may not be duplicated easily elsewhere.

Focused Network

A service firm that must be readily accessible to customers (e.g., a fast-food restaurant) must consider adding sites to achieve significant growth. For firms such as McDonald's, a *focused network* allows management to maintain control, which ensures consistency of service across all locations. For services such as Federal Express and other transportation or communications firms, the existence of a network is required merely to enable the service to function. Also, an entrepreneurial firm that has a successful, well-defined service concept and wants to reach a mass market can prevent imitation from competitors by capturing premium locations in different geographic areas.

The service concept must be well focused, however, thus being easy to duplicate with rigorous control of service quality and costs. Frequently, the "cookie-cutter" concept of replicating service units is employed in facility construction, operating manuals, and personnel training. Franchising often is used to achieve the objective of rapid growth, with investment capital from franchisees and the motivation of independent operators. A more complete discussion of franchising is found later in this chapter.

For a single site, the founder is physically present to manage the firm's resources, market the service, train personnel, and ensure the integrity of the service concept. Especially in the beginning, expansion can occur on an incremental basis. Initially, as the number of locations grows, managerial control slowly shifts from being informal to being formal so that the owner can control operations effectively even though he or she is absent from the additional sites.

Managing a network of service locations requires different management skills, however, and it involves the challenges of using sophisticated communications and control. Above all, the service concept must be rationalized and communicated to unit managers and staff, who then must execute the service consistently on a daily basis. Much planning must precede a multisite expansion, such as preparing training and operations manuals, branding the concept, and launching a national marketing effort.

Service growth using the multisite strategy is very attractive because of its ability to reach the mass market quickly, but the risks of overexpansion and loss of control have resulted in many failures. Even so, the miles of "franchise rows" that are found in almost every city attest to the success of delivering a focused service through a multisite network.

Finally, having multiple sites in different geographic locations reduces the financial risk to the firm from severe, localized economic downturns. A longitudinal study of occupancy at La Quinta Motor Inns during the 1980s dramatically illustrates the benefit of geographic risk containment. Founded in Texas, La Quinta Motor Inns became a major presence in the state, with inns in all the major Texas cities by 1980. During the oil and gas boom of the early 1980s, La Quinta began an expansion strategy of following the exploration activity into the oil-producing states of Colorado, Louisiana, Oklahoma, and Wyoming. When the oil and gas boom ended in the mid-1980s, the occupancy of many of the new inns, and even some of the inns in Texas, plummeted. A financial disaster for the firm was avoided, however, because other La Quinta inns that were not associated with the oil and gas industry continued to prosper.[2]

Clustered Service

Service firms with large fixed facilities often decide to grow by diversifying the service they offer. For example, during the 1970s, many small colleges expanded into 4-year regional universities to accommodate the increasing demand for a university degree. Another example is United Services Automobile Association (USAA), which originally was founded to provide automobile insurance for military officers by direct mail. Located in San Antonio, Texas, USAA now is a major employer, and the physical facility is situated in a campus-like setting of several acres. Today, the services offered by USAA have been expanded to include banking, mutual funds, auto and homeowners' insurance, travel services, and a buying service. Large medical complexes such as the Mayo Clinic, M.D. Anderson, and Massachusetts General Hospital are examples of classic multiservice, single-site facilities, or *clustered service.* All these examples share the common feature that their service market is not defined by their location. For some, such as medical centers and colleges, customers are willing to travel to the service location and spend considerable time at the facility (even years in the case of college students). For others, such as USAA, travel is unnecessary, because business is conducted without the need for physical interaction with a customer.

A major risk of service diversification is potential loss of focus and neglect of the core service. For example, a ski resort may decide to use idle facilities during the summer by attracting conference business; however, the accommodations, food, and beverage facilities that are suitable for skiers may be inadequate for hosting such meetings. One saving grace in this situation is that at least the different market segments are separated by the seasons. Facility management becomes extremely complex when an attempt is made to serve more than one market segment concurrently. For example, hotels serving both tourists and business customers may have difficulty satisfying both markets.

To avoid losing focus, a strategy of "concentric diversification" has been advocated.[3] Concentric diversification limits expansion to services with synergistic logic around the core service. The evolution of the convenience store is an excellent example. Beginning with a limited selection of convenience items that could be purchased in a hurry, these stores have added self-serve gasoline, video rentals, an automatic car wash, and self-serve microwave lunches. Concentric diversification creates economies of scale, because the additional services require only marginal increases in variable costs (e.g., no additional cashier is needed).

[2]S. E. Kimes and J. A. Fitzsimmons, "Selecting Profitable Hotel Sites at La Quinta Motor Inns," *Interfaces,* vol. 20, no. 2, March 1990, pp. 12–20.

[3]M. Carman and Eric Langeard, "Growth Strategies for Service Firms," *Strategic Management Journal,* vol. 1, no. 1, January–March 1980, p. 19.

Diversified Network

Service firms that grow through acquisition often find themselves combining both the multisite and the multiservice strategies. Several years ago, United Airlines acquired hotels and car-rental agencies in the belief that sufficient synergy existed through use of its Apollo reservation system to direct the traveling customer to its several businesses. Anticipated revenues never materialized, however, so United sold off the peripheral services and returned to its core airline business. Managing a *diversified network* is a very complex task, as United Airlines and many other firms have learned.

Success more often is realized when the services are offered under one brand name that establishes a broad marketing image. American Express has been particularly successful managing a global service network that offers financial and travel services with real synergy.

FRANCHISING

Franchising is an alternative to expanding through use of internally generated profits or by seeking funds in the capital markets. Recall from Chapter 4, Service and Information Technology, that Mrs. Fields's Cookies did not use franchising as a method of expansion until very recently. Franchising is a common vehicle, however, for duplicating a service geographically by attracting investors who become independent owner-operators bound by a contractual agreement. For multisite services, incorporation of conformance quality into the service concept has been the hallmark of the franchising agreement. The franchiser guarantees a consistent service, because the concept is standardized in design, operation, and pricing. Just as they make no distinction between products of the same brand, customers expect identical service from any franchise outlet. All outlets benefit from this consistency in service, because customers develop a brand loyalty that is not bound by geography. For example, a U.S. tourist in Germany is treated to a McDonald's french fries, burger, and Coke meal that is identical to that served in San Francisco, Tokyo, and now, Moscow.

The Nature of Franchising

The International Franchise Association defines franchising as a system by which a firm (i.e., the franchiser) grants to others (i.e., the franchisees) the right and license (i.e., franchise) to sell a product or service and, possibly, use the business system developed by the firm.

The franchisee owns the business through payment of a franchise fee and purchase of the facility and equipment, and he or she assumes responsibility for all normal operating activities, including hiring employees, making daily decisions, and determining local advertising. The initial investment will vary depending on capital requirements. For example, an H & R Block franchise may cost only $5000, but a McDonald's franchise could require $500,000. The service franchisee usually is granted an exclusive right or license to deliver the service in a specific market region to protect the franchisee against dilution of sales from other franchisees of the same brand. For example, Hardee's, a fast-food restaurant, agrees not to license another Hardee's franchisee within 1½ miles of existing locations.

The franchiser retains the right to dictate conditions. Standard operating procedures must be followed. Materials must be purchased from either the franchiser or an approved supplier. No deviation from the product line is permitted, training sessions must be attended, and continuing royalty fees (e.g., 4 percent of gross sales for Wendy's) must be paid.

Benefits to the Franchisee

As a franchisee, the owner relinquishes some personal independence and control in return for a relationship based on the expectation of greater gains through group membership. The franchisee is given the opportunity to own a small business that carries a lower-than-normal risk of failure because of the identification with an established service brand. Membership in the franchiser organization also includes many additional benefits.

Management Training

Before opening a new outlet, many franchisers provide an extensive training program. For example, McDonald's franchisees must spend 2 weeks at Hamburger University in suburban Chicago learning the McDonald's way of food preparation and customer service. This training accomplishes two objectives. First, the franchisee becomes prepared to operate a business profitably; second, McDonald's ensures that its procedures will be followed to guarantee consistency across units. Subsequent training often is offered through videotapes and traveling consultants.

Brand Name

The franchisee gains immediate customer recognition from the nationally known and advertised brand name. The result is more-immediate increased customer draw; thus, the break-even point is reached sooner than in a traditional new-business venture.

National Advertising

Although the franchisee usually must contribute approximately 1 percent of gross sales to the franchiser for national advertising, the results benefit all operations. Further, for businesses such as fast-food restaurants and motels in particular, a significant proportion of sales are to customers arriving from outside the immediate geographic region.

Acquisition of a Proven Business

Traditionally, independent owners face a high rate of failure, which a franchisee can expect to avoid. The franchiser has a track record of selecting appropriate sites, operating a reliable accounting system, and most important, delivering a service concept that already is accepted by the public.

Economies of Scale

As a member of the franchiser network, the franchisee benefits from centralized purchasing and savings on the cost of materials and equipment that are unavailable to an independent owner.

Issues for the Franchiser

Franchising is an alternative to internally generated expansion for a firm seeking to develop a focused network of geographically dispersed units. Franchising allows the firm to expand rapidly with minimal capital requirements by selling the business concept to prospective entrepreneurs. Thus, franchising relies heavily on the motivation of investor-owners, and it allows the firm to grow without the cost of developing key managers. Of course, the process of screening potential franchisees must go beyond the minimum requirement of simply having the necessary capital. For example, Benihana of Tokyo found that many early franchisees were unqualified to manage an authentic Japanese-theme restaurant.

Other issues include decisions on the degree of franchisee autonomy, the nature of the franchise contract, and a process for conflict resolution.

Franchisee Autonomy

A franchisee's autonomy is the amount of freedom that is permitted in the operation of the unit. The degree of autonomy is a function of the extent of operations programming dictated in the franchise contract and of the success of "branding" the national advertising achieves.

The extent of operations programming is important to guarantee compliance with uniform standards of quality and service throughout the entire chain. If some franchisees were allowed to operate at substandard levels, the image of the entire chain would suffer, as occurred in the Days Inn example. A highly programmed operation might include:

1. Franchiser specifications such as day-to-day operating procedures, site selection, facility design, accounting system, supplies used and their sources, pricing, and menu items for the restaurant.
2. Frequent inspections of the facility.
3. The right to repurchase the outlet for noncompliance.

Branding reinforces operations programming by establishing rather clear customer expectations from which it is difficult for the individual franchisee to deviate. In addition, successful branding should lead to a greater profit potential, reduced risk, and a more sought-after investment opportunity.

Franchise Contract

Control and power tend to concentrate in the hands of the franchiser, and this raises questions concerning the relationship between franchiser and franchisee as well as the misuse of power. The franchise contract is the vehicle for providing this relationship on a continuing basis. Very often, these contracts include specific obligations on the part of the franchisee but are ambiguous regarding the responsibilities of the franchiser, and often, no attention is given to the rights of the franchisee. For example, litigation has arisen from contract stipulations regarding establishment of the resale value of the franchise and binding agreements requiring the purchase of supplies from the franchiser.

The objective in writing franchise contracts should be to avoid future litigation that might prevent a cooperative relationship from developing. Franchise contracts should be prepared to protect both parties and preserve the competitive strength of the entire franchise organization.

Conflict Resolution

An intelligent and fair franchise contract will be the most effective means to reduce potential conflict. Conflict frequently arises, however, over the following issues because of differing objectives of the franchiser and franchisee:

1. How should fees be established and profits distributed?
2. When should franchisee facilities be upgraded, and how are the costs to be shared?
3. How far should the franchiser go in saturating a single market area with outlets?

The franchise system is a superorganization requiring interorganizational management. Thus, a critical task of the franchiser is the development of policy and procedures to handle conflict before it becomes divisive and impairs the entire system.

MULTINATIONAL DEVELOPMENT

Because its customers increasingly wanted to send packages to Europe and Asia, Federal Express decided in 1988 to duplicate its service overseas, and these overseas operations have been drawing red ink ever since, resulting in a first-ever quarterly operating loss for the company in 1991. Unfortunately, Federal Express arrived well after the competition, DHL and TNT, which having imitated the Federal Express concept in the late 1970s, had been providing express service to this region for about a decade. Also, Federal Express was unprepared for the government regulations and bureaucratic red tape that are used to protect established firms. For example, it took 3 years to get permission from Japan to make direct flights from the Memphis hub to Tokyo, a key link in the overseas system. Just days before that service was to begin, however, Federal Express was notified that no packages weighing more than 70 pounds could pass through Tokyo; this was a provision to protect local transport businesses.

The company's obsession with tight central control also contributed to the problems. Until recently, all shipping bills were printed in English, and the cutoff time for package pick-ups was 5 PM, as is the practice in the United States. The Spanish, however, typically work until 8 PM after a lengthy midday break. Federal Express now is relaxing its go-it-alone, centralized-control method of business that has been successful in the United States. Pick-up times, weight standards, and technology now will vary from country to country, and joint ventures with local firms are being sought to handle deliveries and marketing.[4]

Another issue is the frequent lack of supporting infrastructure, something we take for granted in the United States, in some foreign countries. For example, the opening of the first McDonald's in Moscow required substantial supplier development. Management not only had to build a commissary to prepare all products for the restaurant but also had to show farmers how to plant and harvest the crops that were needed (e.g., potatoes and lettuce).

[4]From Daniel Pearl, "Federal Express Finds Its Pioneering Formula Falls Flat Overseas," *The Wall Street Journal*, April 15, 1991, p. 1.

The Nature of the Borderless World[5]

Kenichi Ohmae, who has written extensively on strategic management, argues that we now live in a borderless world, where customers worldwide are aware of the best products and services and expect to purchase them with no concern over their national origin. In his strategic view, all firms compete in an interlinked world economy, and to be effective, they must balance the five C's of strategic planning: *c*ustomers, *c*ompetitors, *c*ompany, *c*urrency, and *c*ountry.

Customers

When people vote with their pocketbooks, they are interested in quality, price, design, value, and personal appeal. Brand labels such as the "golden arches" are spreading all over the world, and news of performance is hard to suppress. The availability of information, particularly in the industrialized "Triad" markets of North America, Europe, and Japan, has empowered customers and stimulated competition.

Competitors

Nothing stays proprietary for long. Equipment and software vendors supply their products and services to a wide range of customers, and the result is rapid dispersion of the technology available to all firms. Two factors, time and being the first mover, now have become more critical as elements of strategy. Further, a single firm cannot be on the cutting edge of all technologies. Thus, operating globally means operating with partners, a lesson that Federal Express has learned.

Company

Automation during the recent past has moved firms from a variable-cost to a fixed-cost environment. Management focus thus has changed from boosting profits by reducing material and labor costs to increasing sales to cover fixed costs. This is particularly true for many service firms (e.g., airlines and communications businesses), which to a large extent are fixed-cost activities with huge investments in facilities and equipment. The search for a larger market has driven these firms toward globalization.

The nature of a firm's corporate culture, however, may determine how effectively its service will travel overseas. The domestic success of Federal Express was built on a go-it-alone attitude, on rewards for nonunion employees who propose cost-cutting ideas, and on direct access to the CEO, Fred Smith, with any complaints. In contrast, UPS, which works with a union labor force and strict work standards, has moved overseas with fewer problems.

Currency

Global companies have tried to neutralize their exposure to fluctuating currency exchange rates by matching costs to revenues and becoming strong in all regions of the Triad so that if one region is negative, it may be offset by others that are positive. Companies also have employed international finance techniques such as hedging and options. Thus, to become currency-neutral, a firm is forced into global expansion.

[5]From Kenichi Ohmae, *The Borderless World*, Harper Business, New York, 1990, p. 19.

Country

Having a strong presence in all Triad regions provides additional strategic benefits beyond currency considerations. First, as noted, exposure to economic downturns in one region may be offset by operations in other economies. Second, selling in your competitor's domestic market neutralizes that competitor's option to employ a strategy of using excessive profits earned in a protected domestic market for expansion overseas. For example, with government cooperation, Japanese companies have exploited this strategy and recently been criticized for this by their trading partners.

Only truly global companies, however, can achieve "global localization" (a term coined by Akio Morita of Sony) and, thereby, be accepted as a local company while maintaining the benefits of worldwide operations. To reach this level, a firm must become close to the customers in the foreign country and accommodate their unique service needs. For fast-food restaurants, discovering the drinking and eating habits of the host country is critical for success; thus, instead of expecting the Germans to enjoy a Big Mac with a Coke, McDonald's added beer to the menu. Permitting local management to modify the service within limits to accommodate local tastes should be encouraged, even at the risk of introducing some inconsistency across locations. An extreme example is Mr. Donut's in Japan, which changed everything about its product and service except the logo.

Considerations in Planning Multinational Operations[6]

In true services, which exclude receipts and payments on investments and government transactions, the United States has been maintaining a trade surplus for the past 20 years. Leadership in "knowledge-based" services such as software, telecommunications, and information services has proved to be very mobile. Not all services travel equally well, however, and considerations of cultural transferability, network development, and host-government policy must be considered.

Cultural Transferability

Commercial banking would seem to be culturally neutral, because financial needs and associated business transactions are relatively homogeneous worldwide. Of course, the exception is the Middle East, where paying interest on a loan is not recognized by the Muslim faith; thus, banks must adjust by creating service charges that include, but do not mention, interest costs. Customer services also are faced with the obvious language barrier and behavioral customs that might affect the service delivery (e.g., the need for nonsmoking areas in U.S. restaurants).

In food service, however, the desire often is to emulate the cultural experience of a foreign land. The success of Benihana of Tokyo in the United States partly results from creating the illusion of a Japanese dining experience while still serving familiar food. Likewise, for many non-Americans, eating at McDonald's and drinking a Coke is an opportunity to experience something "American."

[6]From James L. Heskett, "The Multinational Development of Service Industries," *Managing in the Service Economy,* Harvard Business School Press, Boston, 1986, pp. 140–152.

Network Development

As in the case of Federal Express, many service firms reluctantly expand into global operations, forced by the desires of their customers. In the case of VISA and MasterCard, customers expected to be able to use their credit cards wherever they traveled. In both cases, the original concept was designed for a domestic market, but the customers eventually insisted on a global network. Maintaining operations control and standards of quality becomes difficult, however, because staffing usually is accomplished with nationals of the host country and, thus, entails inherent language and cultural differences.

Host-Government Policy

Governments around the world have played a significant role in restricting the growth of multinational services. This includes, but is not limited to, making it difficult to repatriate funds (i.e., to take profits out of the host country). Discrimination has taken a number of creative forms, such as banning the sale of insurance by foreign firms, giving preferential treatment to local shippers, placing restrictions on the international flow of information, and creating delays in the processing of licensing agreements. A major reason for this situation is the continuing refusal of countries (with the exception of the United States) to recognize the importance of services in international trade.

In November 1982, for the first time, trade barriers on services were placed on the agenda at a meeting of the General Agreement on Tariffs and Trade (GATT), a group of 88 trading nations that for decades has been establishing codes of conduct for trading goods. In 1993, the GATT agreement considering financial services was held hostage by several Asian countries that wished to protect their domestic firms from global competition. For example, Korea prohibits outright foreigners selling mutual funds to local investors, and Japan requires a multiyear application process with no clear objective criteria for approval.[7] In 1994, the Uruguay round of trade negotiations produced new rules to help liberalize trade in services such as tourism.

GLOBAL SERVICE STRATEGIES[8]

Firms and industries must pay attention to the need for global competitive strategies for their services. The biggest factor in a service operations globalization decision should be whether it fits with the firm's global strategy. The service company that responds to heightened competition will look very different from its predecessors. Because it will be focused strategically, it will have an efficient delivery system, a high-quality product, and a flexible cost structure.

Five basic globalization strategies can be identified: (1) multicountry expansion, (2) importing customers, (3) following your customers, (4) service unbundling, and (5) beating-the-clock. These strategies are not all mutually exclu-

[7]From Robert C. Pozen, "Is America Being Shut Out Again?" *The New York Times,* January 10, 1993, p. 13.

[8]From Curtis P. McLaughlin and James A. Fitzsimmons, "Strategies for Globalizing Service Operations," *International Journal of Service Industry Management*, vol. 7, no. 4, 1996, pp. 45–59.

sive, however. One can think of a number of ways to combine strategies (e.g., combining multicountry expansion with beating-the-clock).

Table 15.1 shows how each globalization strategy is affected by the globalization factors faced by multinational service firms. Using this table, managers can consider how these factors affect the implementation of various candidate strategies and their likelihood of success for a specific business in a target country or region. Table 15.1 also summarizes key opportunities and potential problems that each globalization factor contributes to each global service strategy. The service strategy and management implications for service globalization are discussed, beginning with the multicountry expansion strategy.

Multicountry Expansion

Multisite expansion commonly has been accomplished using franchising to attract investors and a "cookie-cutter" approach to clone the service rapidly in multiple locations. This expansion strategy is necessary when the service market is defined by the need for customers to travel physically to the service facility. Exporting a successful service to another country without modification, however,

TABLE 15.1. Considerations in Selecting a Global Service Strategy

	Global Service Strategies				
Globalization Factors	Multicountry Expansion	Importing Customers	Follow Your Customers	Service Unbundling	Beating-the-Clock
Customer contact	Train local workers	Develop foreign language and cultural sensitivity skills	Develop foreign customers	Specialize in front- or back-office service components	Provide extended hours of service
Customization	Usually a standard service	Strategic opportunity	Reprototype locally	Meet segments' needs better	More need for reliability and coordination
Complexity	Usually routine	Strategic opportunity	Modify operations	Opportunity for focus	Time compression
Information intensity	Satellite network	On-site advantage	Move experienced managers	May require heavy capital investments	Exploit opportunity
Cultural adaptation	Modify service	Accommodate foreign guests	Could be necessary to achieve scale	Manage worker diversity	Common language necessary
Labor intensity	Reduced labor costs	Increased labor costs	Hire local personnel	Reduced labor costs	Reduced labor costs
Other	Government restrictions	Logistics management	Inadequate infrastructure	Merchandise unbundled component	Capital investments

Source: Adapted from Curtis P. McLaughlin and James A. Fitzsimmons, "Strategies for Globalizing Service Operations," *International Journal of Service Industry Management*, vol. 7, no. 4, 1996, pp. 45–59.

can capitalize on selling "a country's cultural experience," as illustrated by the success of McDonald's in Europe, and especially by its experience in Moscow. Cultural adaptation often requires some modification of the service concept, however, as seen in the availability of beer in German McDonald's. Federal Express faced a different cultural adaptation problem in Spain, where the standard 5:00 PM pickup was not workable because of the mid-day siesta and business hours extending into the evening.

Many strategic issues are involved in moving a service operation out and around the world, or *multicountry expansion.* Duplicating a service worldwide is best accomplished when routine services are involved, such as in the example of McDonald's. The customer contact or front-office operations require sensitivity to the local culture, however. The best approach would appear to be hiring and training locals to handle that part of the process in consultation with those who know the approaches that have been successful in other countries.

With the exception of professional services, customization and complexity are not important issues considering the routine nature of many multisite consumer services (e.g., fast foods). Information intensity is not an important consideration either, but managing a global network of service sites might require communications by satellite.

Cultural adaptation, however, is a major issue in service design. Should it be centralized or managed country by country? These questions were addressed by Kentucky Fried Chicken, as noted by the following quote explaining the situation in the late 1960s with which successive sets of professional managers at Heublein and RJ Reynolds (now RJR Nabisco Holdings Corporation) struggled for another twenty years[9]:

> The country managers were like Roman governors sent to govern distant provinces with nothing more than an exhortation to maintain Rome's imperial power and reputation. Few had any operating expertise, they were offered little staff support and the only attention paid to operations was Colonel Sanders' personal efforts to maintain the quality of his original product. Each country manager was on his own to make a success of his venture, and most had to learn the business from scratch.

Unfortunately, the corporate staff seemed to have had little to offer, except to try making the foreign operation conform to the U.S. template. After all, the raison d'être of franchising collapses in the face of local cultural adaptation. The country managers were well aware, however, that the cookie-cutter approach also would not work.

Importing Customers

For the multiservice single-site strategy to be successful internationally, customers must be willing to travel a long distance and stay for an extended time, or telecommunications must be substituted for physical travel. Many services such as prestigious colleges and universities, medical centers (e.g., Mayo Clinic), and tourist attractions (e.g., Disney World) meet these stipulations. Because of a

[9]Kentucky Fried Chicken (Japan) Limited, case no. 9-387-043, *Harvard Business School,* Boston, 1993, p. 1.

unique tourist attraction at a particular location (e.g., Mt. Crested Butte in Colorado), a service evolves that is focused on that attraction, such as catering to skiers in the winter and mountain bikers in the summer. Rather than exporting the service as in a multisite strategy, the multiservice strategy involves *importing customers.*

A service that decides to retain its location and attract customers from around the world will be faced with developing the foreign-language skill and cultural sensitivity of its customer-contact employees. It may have to pay more to get those skills. The unique features of the location (e.g., tourist attraction or reputation of service personnel) will dictate the selection of this strategy. Differentiation will occur through customization and complexity of the service, and transportation infrastructure and logistics management will be required to accommodate the visiting customers. For example, the Netherlands island of Bonaire, off the coast of Venezuela, caters to scuba divers and is served once a week by a direct KLM flight from Amsterdam.

Follow Your Customers

Many service companies open offices overseas not to serve the local markets but to follow their corporate clients overseas and continue to serve them. Attracting local business many require modifications in the service package, however, as well as employment of people who are familiar with local business practices.

To implement this strategy, one of the largest business-travel agencies has formed partnerships in almost every area of the world. Its corporate customers want their people served adequately wherever they go. For example, the local representative on the Arabian peninsula was able to extricate travelers from Kuwait during the Iraqi invasion.

Just as law firms expanded into multiple cities to align themselves with their corporate accounts, service companies are pushed to operate in the same countries as their clients. The truly global company wants and demands truly global service from its travel agents, auditors, consultants, and others.

The weakness of this strategy for a company already committed to overseas operations is that it ignores the vast markets represented by the rapidly growing middle classes of many countries. It also leaves the companies that serve these populations free to grow without competition until they reach sufficient quality and scale to become a threat internationally.

Usually, the sales volume that is available from visitors or expatriates in a foreign country is small. This leaves the service manager with interesting choices—should I design my service to follow my customers and their needs, design it to adapt to the local culture, or make a compromise between the two and hope to straddle them both successfully? Everything that operations managers know about services would seem to argue against the likelihood of a successful straddle. Therefore, managers have interesting focus and scale issues to contend with in terms of whether to serve expatriates and visitors or cater to local customers. Where expatriate markets are small and the local market requires considerable adaptation, partnering with local organizations would seem to be an attractive alternative. Even when a new service prototype is not needed for the front office, it may be necessary to adapt operations to the local environment and bring in experienced and flexible managers to make the transplantation work in the face of local infrastructure and social system complexities.

Service Unbundling

Service unbundling involves separating pieces of the value-added chain and focusing on those parts not requiring face-to-face interactions. Discount brokerage is an example: the routinized market transaction activities in the back office are separated from customized professional advising activities and made into a distinct and viable business. When creating global service operations, unbundling can lead to many of the benefits of a focused strategy being achieved.

Complexity seems to be less and less of a problem as managers find more and more ways of unbundling service components and moving those that are information-intensive globally. In the long run, complexity probably will prove to be no more of a barrier to globalization in services than it has been in manufacturing. Many countries have large pools of unemployed and underemployed educated persons, many of whom have high levels of technical training. They are looking for any level of work but readily adapt to higher levels, especially those who have quantitative skills.

All managers should be aware of the distinction between the physical and the informational parts of a process, and they should recognize that today, the informational work can be done almost anywhere in the world. New overseas operations may offer opportunities to install prototype reengineered systems without concern for existing capital investments and employee work rules or habits. This phenomenon is important, for example, in international banking, in which newcomers have major advantages over existing, and often over-staffed, domestic financial services firms. This is especially true for new competitors in countries where automation may have taken place to offset inflationary uncertainties but labor laws or syndicates have restricted downsizing.

Labor intensity often is a factor in choices that are made concerning the globalization of services, but it is not always the same labor-intensity issue that the operations management literature has emphasized. Labor intensity has tended to be associated with customer contact. Managers should examine the labor intensity of an operation when considering alternatives for globalization, but they also should study the interaction of labor intensity with information intensity.

If management chooses to unbundle the service and focus on only part of the former value-added chain, then the customer segments involved will have to accept the new service concept. The unbundled operations must meet those segments better than before, which may require heavy capital investments in information processing and telecommunications facilities to upgrade and enhance the service globally.

Beating-the-Clock

Beating-the-clock describes the competitive advantages gained from the fact that one can bypass the constraints of the clock and domestic time zones, including time-based domestic work rules and regulations. Companies in the United States long have known that combining the demand from multiple time zones could improve the productivity of reservation clerks and telemarketers. Quarterdeck, a California software company, provides technical support to its more easterly U.S. customers by transferring their early morning telephone inquiries to Quarterdeck's European technical support center in Ireland. The advantage derives from supplying service to East Coast customers at hours when the California office would be closed. The advantage of being able to give 24-hour service despite local work norms or government regulations on market closings has helped to produce the true globalization of securities markets.

Projects can be expedited by taking advantage of coordinated activities around the globe. For example, a North Carolina bank is having its loan record systems expanded and reprogrammed by an Indian firm. Indian personnel in the United States communicate daily with programmers in India via satellite. The bank management is delighted because the work goes quickly as workers at the Indian site do programming for one half of the clock and workers at the North Carolina site do testing and debugging during the other half.

The advantages from time compression of the software development process are not likely to go unnoticed in a number of settings. Time-based competition is a widely accepted strategy in manufacturing. In the real-time world of services, there is every reason to expect new innovations to use the speed of light to beat the clock around the world and gain a competitive advantage.

Managers should look at their service processes to find ways in which electronic means can be used to beat the clock. Once these are identified, managers should begin to develop either offensive or defensive strategies. This analysis should include consideration of the potential impact of time-zone shifts on marketing, operations, or human resource aspects of the service. Can such shifts: (1) result in economies of operation, (2) provide better access for foreign and domestic customers, (3) support time-based competition in operations, or (4) add to the creativity available in the process without slowing it down? Defensive strategies would involve forming strategic alliances in other time zones. Offensive activities might involve moving to or modifying operations in nondomestic time zones to tap new markets or improve existing ones to beat the competition by beating-the-clock.

The need for greater reliability and coordination among locations and time zones may require substantial additional investments in training, methods of operation, and telecommunications. Telecommunications certainly will be necessary to make the shift in location transparent to the customer and to realize the full value from the time advantage.

SUMMARY

A successful service innovation can grow in two fundamental ways: (1) duplication of the service in different geographic locations with a multisite strategy of becoming a "focused network," or (2) incorporation of different services at the original site using a multiservice strategy, thereby becoming a "clustered service." Although it is not necessarily a desirable objective, some mature service firms combine both strategies and become a "diversified network."

Franchising has become the most common method to implement a multisite strategy in a very rapid manner, using capital that is furnished by investor-owners. Franchising is attractive to prospective entrepreneurs because of the many advantages of buying into a proven concept, but most important, the risk of failure is diminished.

We now live in a "borderless world," with information on products and services available to customers worldwide. For many services, a global presence no longer is an option but a necessity if they wish to continue to serve their customers. Overseas expansion has its risks and challenges depending on the cultural transferability of the service, network development in a foreign land, and government discrimination against foreign services.

Chapter 16 begins Part VI, which includes several quantitative methods that can be applied to service situations, and will look at ways of forecasting demand.

KEY TERMS AND DEFINITIONS

Beating-the-clock using service locations around the globe to achieve 24-hour service availability.

Clustered service a situation in which many services are offered at a single location (e.g., a hospital).

Diversified network a situation in which many services are offered at multiple locations (e.g., branch banks).

Franchising a method of duplicating a service concept by attracting investors who become owner-operators bound by a contractual agreement to offer the service in a consistent manner.

Focused network a single service offered at multiple sites, often by use of franchising (e.g., a motel chain).

Focused service a single service offered at a single location (e.g., a family restaurant).

Follow your customers a concept involving expansion overseas to service existing customers who already have established multinational operations.

Importing customers an approach to growth that attracts customers to an existing site rather than building sites overseas.

Multicountry expansion a growth strategy in which a service is duplicated in more than one country using a franchising formula with little adaptation to the local culture.

Service unbundling a separation of the front- and back-office activities to permit a focused strategy, such as outsourcing the back-office activities to an offshore site.

TOPICS FOR DISCUSSION

1. For service firms, how does the operations strategy differ from the marketing strategy?
2. Is the competitive role of operations more important for a service firm than a manufacturing firm?
3. Do you agree that the effect of learning and experience on total unit cost (i.e., the learning curve) has not been demonstrated in a service situation?
4. Manufacturing firms often grow through product innovation. Are there examples of service firms that practice the equivalent strategy?
5. What is your assessment of the multinational competition in services?

Service Benchmark

Is America Being Shut Out Again?

The world's trade negotiators, having reached a tentative agreement on agriculture, are pushing to conclude an agreement on other sectors by next month, when the Uruguay Round of the General Agreement on Tariffs and Trade is slated to be completed. For the American financial services sector, however, a quick completion of the Uruguay Round threatens to cast in concrete the current one-way street: American financial markets would remain open to all comers, while Asian markets would continue to restrict access.

Under the ground rules for service agreements, GATT does not grant foreigners the right to compete in domestic markets unless that right is included in a country's GATT service schedules. This creates a disadvantage for American and European financial institutions, whose markets are open to foreign banks and brokers that meet the regulatory standards of domestic institutions.

By contrast Asian countries generally impose special restrictions on foreign access to their financial markets. For example, Korea has an outright prohibition on foreigners selling mutual funds to local investors, while Japan requires foreign fund companies to go through a multi-year application process without clear objective criteria for approval. Most Asian countries limit the number of foreign banks and/or the scope of their local activities, while many Asian countries have only recently begun to allow the entry of foreign securities dealers on any conditions.

Given these existing disparities, Americans and Europeans can improve their relative market access through the GATT negotiations only if the Asians make substantial commitments to open up their financial markets to foreigners. However, such commitments to date have been very thin.

For example, Korea has even refused to guarantee that it would maintain the limited market access it currently affords to foreign banks and securities firms. Other Asian countries with significant exports are trying to position themselves as third world economies in need of protection for local financial markets. Singapore and Thailand, despite having advanced financial centers, exclude virtually all of their domestic banking sectors and the dealer portions of their local securities markets.

If the Asian commitments on financial services do not substantially improve, the United States would be locking in current disparities by signing the Uruguay Round. It would be prohibited from using access to its financial markets as a basis for reciprocal negotiations with Asian countries. Any special limits on Asian access to American financial markets would violate the most favored nation provision of GATT—a requirement to all signatories with the best market access afforded to any signatory. Thus, the most-favored-nation requirement would eliminate nearly all American leverage in bilateral negotiations with the Asians.

What should be done? If the Asian countries do not make reasonable commitments to open their financial markets within the next month, the United States and Europe should claim a most favored nation exemption for financial services. At the same time, they should agree to maintain the current openness of their financial markets between themselves.

The United States would then be free to adopt a reciprocity statue like the Fair Trade in Financial Services Act, which last year passed the Senate, but not the House. Under this act, the Treasury would be required to evaluate whether American firms were being given fair access to Asian financial markets. If not, the United States could deny or condition licenses to Asian firms doing business in the American financial markets.

Although the United States negotiators are under intense international pressure to complete the Uruguay Round without taking major exceptions in any service sector, they should not allow Asia to become a "free rider" on the GATT agreement for financial services. By taking a most favored nation exemption for financial services, the United States would pave the way for tough bilateral negotiations based on true reciprocity—the only viable method for getting equal access to Asian financial markets.

Source: Robert C. Pozen, "Is America Being Shut Out Again?" *The New York Times,* January 10, 1993, p. F13.

CASE: FEDERAL EXPRESS: TIGER INTERNATIONAL ACQUISITION[10]

What has become one of America's great success stories began operations almost two decades ago in Memphis, Tennessee. At that time, those who knew of Fred Smith's idea did not realize that his small company was about to revolutionize the air-cargo industry.

In 1972, the Civil Aeronautics Board ruled that operators flying aircraft with an "all-up" weight of less than 75,000 pounds could be classified as an "air taxi" and would not be required to obtain a certificate of "public convenience and necessity" to operate. This made it possible for Federal Express (FedEx) to penetrate the heavily entrenched air-freight industry. FedEx ordered a fleet of 33 Dassault Falcon fan-jets in 1972 and commenced operations a year later. On April 17, 1973, the company delivered 18 packages, becoming the first to offer nationwide overnight delivery.

One of FedEx's fundamental principles was use of the hub-and-spoke system, in which all packages were flown to Memphis first, sorted during the night, and then shipped to their destinations the following morning. This system allowed FedEx to serve a large number of cities with a minimum number of aircraft. It also provided tight control and efficiency of ground operations and soon became increasingly important as package-tracking systems were installed.

[10]Prepared by Garland Wilkinson under the supervision of Professor James A. Fitzsimmons.

During the first 2 years of operations, FedEx lost money, but revenues surpassed the $5 billion mark in fiscal year 1989, partly because of the acquisition of Tiger International.

As Table 15.2 shows, FedEx began global expansion in 1984, when it purchased Gelco International. FedEx followed that expansion with its first scheduled flight to Europe in 1985, and it established a European headquarters in Brussels, Belgium, that same year.

Domestic operations were expanded as well. In 1986, regional hubs were established in Oakland, California, and in Newark, New Jersey. In 1987, a sorting facility was opened in Indianapolis, and Honolulu was chosen for the Far East headquarters. That same year, FedEx was granted the rights to a small-cargo route to Japan, and the following year the company was making regularly scheduled flights to Asia.

International expansion did not result in immediate international success, however. In Asia, its planes were flying at half their capacity because of treaty restrictions, and a lack of back-up planes in its South American operations jeopardized guaranteed delivery

TABLE 15.2. Federal Express Corporation Timeline

1973	Began service with Falcon fan-jets from Memphis to 25 cities in April.
1977	Air-cargo industry deregulated.
1978	Purchased its first Boeing 727 and became a publicly held corporation.
1980	Took delivery of first McDonnell-Douglas DC10 and implemented computerized tracking system.
1981	Introduced Overnight Letter, a lower-cost document service. Opened greatly expanded Superhub in Memphis.
1982	Shortened overnight delivery commitment to 10:30 AM in all major markets.
1983	Opened first Business Service Center. Became first company to achieve annual revenues of $1 billion in 10 years.
1984	Purchased Gelco International and made first scheduled trans-Atlantic flight to Europe. Established European headquarters in Brussels.
1986	Enhanced tracking and informational capabilities with introduction of SuperTracker. Acquired Lex Wilkinson Ltd. of United Kingdom and Cansica of Canada.
1987	Acquired Indianapolis hub. Was granted exclusive small-cargo route to Japan.
1988	Scheduled first trans-Pacific flight to Japan. Acquired nine offshore transportation companies. Announced plan to purchase Tiger International.
1989	Completed purchase of Tiger International and merged Flying Tigers into system, becoming the world's largest full-service all-cargo airline.

when regular aircraft were grounded. Even worse, many managers of the companies acquired in Europe had quit.

As a solution to these international bottlenecks, FedEx made a dramatic move in December of 1988, announcing plans to purchase Tiger International, the parent company of Flying Tigers, the world's largest heavy-cargo airline. The purchase price was about $880 million.

This action catapulted FedEx to the forefront of the international cargo market, giving it landing rights in 21 additional countries; however, the addition of Tigers was not without challenges. For example, the leveraged acquisition more than doubled FedEx's long-term debt, to approximately $2 billion. Moreover, FedEx had bought into the business of delivering heavy cargo, much of which was not sent overnight, which represented a significant departure from FedEx's traditional market niche. One of the largest dilemmas facing FedEx following the merger was how to integrate the two workforces.

Major Players in the Domestic Air-Cargo Industry

Federal Express is the nation's largest overnight carrier, with more than 40 percent of the domestic market. United Parcel Service (UPS), Emery Air Freight, Airborne Express, DHL (an international carrier based in Brussels), and a few other carriers account for the remaining market share. FedEx had revenues of $3.9 billion and a net income of $188 million in 1988.[11] FedEx had lost approximately $74 million on its international business since 1985, however, prompting the carrier to purchase Tiger International. That acquisition, which gained U.S. government approval on January 31, 1989, gave FedEx a strong entry position into heavy cargo as well as access to 21 additional countries.

Price wars, which began with UPS's entry into the overnight business, have decreased FedEx's revenues per package by 15 percent since 1984. Another setback to FedEx was its $350 million loss on Zapmail, which it dropped in 1986. A document transmission service that relayed information via satellite, Zapmail was quickly made obsolete by facsimile machines.

FedEx does offer its customers several other benefits not matched by its competitors, however. For example, it offers a 1-hour "on-call" pick-up service, and through use of its data base information system, COSMOS, FedEx guarantees that it can locate any package in its possession within 30 minutes. FedEx has found that this type of customer security helps to ensure continued growth.[12]

The Nature of the Competition

The air-cargo industry has undergone a series of mergers resulting from the recent price wars that rocked the industry. Also, marketing alliances have been formed between domestic and foreign carriers to take better advantage of international trade and to create new routes and services (e.g., package tracking).

When UPS entered the overnight-package market in 1982, competition rose substantially, starting the series of price wars that have hurt all air-cargo players. FedEx's average revenue per package declined by 30.3 percent between 1983 and 1988.

Fortunately, it appears that the price-cutting strategy may have finally run its course. When UPS, which created the price wars, announced another price cut in October of 1988, its competitors refused to follow, and in January 1993, UPS announced its first price increase in almost 6 years, a 5-percent increase in charges for next-day service. Several factors such as continued overcapacity, low switching costs, and high exit barriers, however, will continue to make the air-cargo industry extremely competitive.

Conclusions on the Air-Cargo Environment

Although the situation may be improving, intraindustry competition and rivalry remain the main deterrent to the air-cargo industry. With overcapacity in the industry, firms, which are desperate to fill planes, continue to realize declining yields on the packages they ship. Moreover, passenger airlines are reentering the air-cargo market with increased vigor, which also does not help the capacity situation. All these factors are leading current players to consolidate their operations in hope of achieving increased economies of scale.

Technology is acting as both friend and foe of the air-cargo industry. Facsimile machines have carved a large niche from the overnight-document segment; on

[11]Dean Foust, "Mr. Smith Goes Global," *BusinessWeek*, February 13, 1989, pp. 66–72.

[12]David A. Clancy, "Air Cargo Takes Off," *Transportation and Distribution*, January 1989, pp. 32–36.

the other hand, improved data bases are enabling companies to provide their clients with another valuable service: improved tracking information on the status of important shipments.

Until now, the large number of shippers has enabled buyers to enjoy low rates, but because of their wide dispersion, buyers are not able to control effectively the air-cargo companies. Likewise, air-cargo companies continue to have an advantage over their suppliers. The ability to purchase older planes keeps firms less dependent on aircraft manufacturers, and a large, unskilled labor pool helps to keep hub labor costs down. A lack of available airport facilities, however, presents a serious problem to the commercial air-freight industry. Not only is the lack of landing slots a problem in the United States, but acquiring government-controlled access to crowded international hubs can present a formidable challenge.

Worldwide Distribution

As the globe continues to shrink and economies grow more interdependent, customers are demanding new services to facilitate revamped production processes. One of the most publicized is the just-in-time (JIT) system that many U.S. firms have borrowed from their Japanese competitors. JIT systems argue for elimination of the traditional inventory stockpiles common to manufacturing, including the raw material, work-in-process, and finished-goods inventories. Without question, such a scheme relies on having the right part at the right place at the right time.

Air express has been able to play a reliable role in delivering these needed materials on time. FedEx and its competitors have succeeded in contracting with manufacturers to supply the needed logistical expertise to support its JIT framework. Essentially, the planes have become flying warehouses. As this area grows, the Tiger addition to FedEx should reap large yields with its ability to handle the heavier shipments that are associated with international manufacturing. For example, an increasing amount of parts made in Asia are being shipped to the United States for final assembly.

Powership

To facilitate further penetration into a customer's business, FedEx developed Powership, which is a program that locates terminals on a client's premises and, thus, enables FedEx to stay abreast of the firm's needs. In simplifying the daily shipping process, an automated program tracks shipments, provides pricing information, and prints invoices. Such a device helps to eliminate the administrative need of reconciling manifests with invoices. Currently, more than 7000 of FedEx's highest-volume customers are integrated into the Powership system.

At Federal Express, customer automation is expected to play an increasingly significant role. By tying technological innovations with reliable on-time delivery, FedEx is achieving its goal of getting closer to the customer.

Corporate Culture

Many believe that FedEx could not have grown to its current magnitude had it been forced to deal with the added pressure of negotiating with a unionized workforce. FedEx has never employed organized labor, although attempts at unionization have been made. In 1976, the International Association of Machinists and Aerospace Workers tried to organize the company's mechanics, who rejected the offer. Likewise, FedEx's pilots rejected an offer by the Airline Pilots Association during that same period. In 1978, the Teamsters attempted to organize the hub sorters but could not get enough signatures for a vote.

Despite an admirable human resource track record, the outlook for FedEx to continue its past performance is hazy. Because of the Tiger International acquisition, FedEx had to merge the unionized Flying Tigers workforce with its own union-free environment. Previously, the willingness of FedEx workers to go above and beyond in performing their duties had given the company a marked advantage over UPS, the nation's largest employer of United Brotherhood of Teamsters members. As the FedEx–Tiger merger progressed, however, many questions remained to be answered.

Acquisition of Tiger International

In December 1988, FedEx announced its intent to purchase Flying Tigers, and in early 1989, more than 40 years of air-cargo experience were merged with FedEx. Besides giving FedEx entry into an additional 21 nations, the Tigers merger possessed several other advantages for the aggressive company. Almost overnight, FedEx became owner of the world's largest full-service, all-cargo airline, nearly three times the size of its nearest competitor. Because FedEx could use this large fleet on its newly acquired routes, it no longer would be forced into the position of contracting out to other freight carriers in markets not served previously.

The addition of heavy freight to the FedEx service mix was viewed as a boost to its traditional express package-delivery business. The merger fit in neatly with the company's plans to focus on the higher-margin box business while shifting away from document service. During the preceding 2 years, box shipments had increased by 53 percent, generating as much as 80 percent of revenues and an estimated 90 percent of profits.

On the downside, as noted earlier, the $2 billion debt that was incurred by the merger and the capital intensiveness of the heavy-cargo business made the company more vulnerable to economic swings. Although the merger meshed well into its plans, FedEx still was a newcomer to the heavy-cargo market.

Another hurdle was that many premerger Flying Tigers customers were competitors that used Tigers to reach markets where they, like FedEx, had no service or could not establish service.

Finally, FedEx had to integrate the 6500 unionized Tigers workers into a union-free company. Although Flying Tigers was founded with much the same type of entrepreneurial spirit that was cherished at Federal Express, the carrier had seen its workforce become members of organized labor early in its existence.

At the time of the merger, the Tigers union ties were severed. FedEx promised to find positions for all employees, but critics felt that the union background of Tigers workers would dilute the corporate culture at Federal Express. Whether FedEx could continue its success story appeared to hinge on its ability to impart its way of life to the Tigers workers, not vice versa.

Questions

1. Describe the growth strategy of Federal Express. How has this strategy differed from those of its competitors?

2. What risks are involved in the acquisition of Tiger International?

3. In addition to the question of merging FedEx and Flying Tiger pilots, what other problems could be anticipated in accomplishing this merger?

4. Suggest a plan of action that Fred Smith could have used to address the potential acquisition problems given in your answer to the previous question.

SELECTED BIBLIOGRAPHY

CARMAN, J. M., and E. LANGEARD: "Growth Strategies for Service Firms," *Strategic Management Journal,* vol. 1, no. 1, January–March 1980, pp. 7–22.

CHASE, R. B., and R. H. HAYES: "Operations' Role in Service Firm Competitiveness," *Sloan Management Review,* vol. 33, no. 1, Fall 1991, pp. 15–26.

COWELL, DONALD: "Service Product Planning and Development," *The Marketing of Services,* Heinemann, London, 1984, pp. 115–146.

HAYWOOD-FARMER, J., and J. GARCELON: "The Theoretical Issues Propagated by International Trade in Services," *Operations Management Review,* vol. 9, no. 1, 1992, pp. 18–27.

———, and J. NOLLET: "Growth and Strategy," *Services PLUS,* G. Morin Publisher Ltd., Boucherville, Quebec, Canada, 1991, pp. 119–136.

HESKETT, J. L.: "The Multinational Development of Service Industries," *Managing in the Service Economy,* Harvard Business School Press, Boston, 1986, pp. 135–152.

MCLAUGHLIN, C. P., and J. A. FITZSIMMONS: "Strategies for Globalizing Service Operations," *International Journal of Service Industry Management,* vol. 7, no. 4, 1996, pp. 45–59.

OHMAE, KENICHI: *The Borderless World,* Harper Business, New York, 1990.

PORTER, MICHAEL E.: "Competitive Strategy in Fragmented Industries," *Competitive Strategy,* Free Press, New York, 1980, pp. 191–215.

SASSER, W. E., R. P. OLSEN, and D. D. WYCKOFF: "The Multi-Site Service Firm Life Cycle," *Management of Service Operations,* Allyn and Bacon, Boston, 1978, pp. 534–566.

SHAW, JOHN C.: "Competitive Strategy in Service Industries," *The Services Bulletin*, vol. 3, January 1987, pp. 3–4.

———: *The Service Focus*, Dow Jones–Irwin, Homewood, Ill., 1990.

STEPHENSON, P. R., and R. G. HOUSE: "Perspective on Franchising," *Business Horizons*, vol. 14, no. 4, August 1971, pp. 35–42.

THOMAS, DAN R. E.: "Strategy Is Different in Service Business," *Harvard Business Review*, July–August 1978, pp. 158–165.

PART SIX

Quantitative Models with Service Applications

This concluding part of the book contains a selection of quantitative and qualitative models with applications in service management. A forecast of service demand is essential for planning new ventures as well as for planning the hourly, daily, and even long-range activities of a service operation. In Chapter 16, we will look at several tools for making forecasts, including subjective, causal, and time series models.

Because some customer waiting is unavoidable in a service delivery system, the ability to predict the waiting experience of customers under various conditions is useful in the planning capacity needs. Chapter 17 reviews the various analytical queuing models, with service illustrations and applications to service capacity planning under different system performance criteria.

Finally, Chapter 18 introduces linear programming models with service applications and solutions using the personal-computer software Excel Solver.

CHAPTER 16

Forecasting Demand for Services

LEARNING OBJECTIVES

After completing this chapter, you should be able to:

1. Recommend the appropriate forecasting model for a given situation.
2. Conduct a Delphi forecasting exercise.
3. Describe the features of exponential smoothing that make it an attractive model for time series forecasting.
4. Conduct time series forecasting using the exponential smoothing model with trend and seasonal adjustments.

Forecasting techniques allow us to translate the multitude of information available from data bases into strategies that can give a service a competitive advantage. The particular techniques we will describe are classified into three basic models: subjective, causal, and time series. It must be noted, however, that whereas some services may use only one or another of these models, others will use two or more depending on the application. For example, a fast-food restaurant may be interested in using a time series model to forecast the daily demand for menu items. The demand for hotel services, however, has both temporal and spatial characteristics, which will require the use of both time series and causal models. On occasion, service firms may use subjective models to assess the future impact of changing demographics, such as the aging of the general population. Overall, as we move from subjective to causal to time series models, the forecast time horizon becomes shorter. The models, their characteristics, and their possible applications are shown in Table 16.1.

CHAPTER PREVIEW

This chapter begins with subjective models, because these methods are useful at the initial planning stage for service delivery systems when a long-term horizon is being considered. The Delphi technique is illustrated with an application to government policy planning for nuclear power. Causal models use regression analysis to form a linear relationship between independent variables and a dependent variable of interest. The site-selection problem facing motel chains is

TABLE 16.1. Characteristics of Forecasting Methods

Method	Data Required	Relative Cost	Forecast Horizon	Application
Subjective models				
Delphi method	Survey results	High	Long term	Technological forecasting
Cross-impact analysis	Correlations between events	High	Long term	Technological forecasting
Historical analogy	Several years of data for a similar situation	High	Medium to long term	Life-cycle demand projection
Causal models				
Regression	All past data for all variables	Moderate	Medium term	Demand forecasting
Econometric	All past data for all variables	Moderate to high	Medium to long term	Economic conditions
Time series models				
Moving average	N most recent observations	Very low	Short term	Demand forecasting
Exponential smoothing	Previous smoothed value and most recent observation	Very low	Short term	Demand forecasting

used to illustrate the causal modeling approach to forecasting future occupancy of alternative sites.

The discussion of time series models begins with the common *N*-period moving average. A more sophisticated time series model, called *exponential smoothing,* then is introduced and shown to accommodate trends and seasonal data.

SUBJECTIVE MODELS

Most forecasting techniques, such as time series and causal models, are based on data whose pattern is relatively stable over time, so we can expect to make reasonably useful forecasts. In some cases, however, we may have few or no data with which to work, or we may have data that exhibit patterns and relationships only over the short run and, therefore, are not useful for long-range forecasts.

When we lack sufficient or appropriate data, we must resort to forecast methods that are subjective or qualitative in nature. These include the Delphi method, cross-impact analysis, and historical analogy.

Delphi Method

Developed at the Rand Corporation by Olaf Helmer, the *Delphi method* is based on expert opinion. In its simplest form, persons with expertise in a given area are asked questions, and these individuals are not permitted to interact with each other. Typically, the participants are asked to make numerical estimates. For example, they might be asked to predict the highest Dow Jones average for the coming year.

The test administrator tabulates the results into quartiles and supplies these findings to the experts, who then are asked to reconsider their answers in light of the new information. Additionally, those whose opinions fall in the two outside quartiles are asked to justify their opinions. All the information from this round of questioning is tabulated and once again returned to the participants. On this occasion, each participant who remains outside the middle two quartiles (i.e., the interquartile range) may be asked to provide an argument as to why he or she believes those at the opposite extreme are incorrect.

The process may continue through several more iterations, with the intent of eventually having the experts arrive at a consensus that can be used for future planning. This method is very labor-intensive and requires input from persons with expert knowledge. Obviously, Delphi is a very expensive, time-consuming method and is practical only for long-term forecasting.

An example of the Delphi method can be seen in a study of the nuclear power industry.[1] Ninety-eight persons agreed to participate in this study. These people occupied key upper-level positions with architect-engineering firms, reactor manufacturers, and utility companies in the industrial sector concerned with nuclear power as well as with state regulatory agencies, state energy commissions, congressional staffs, and nuclear regulatory agencies in the public sector.

[1]C. H. Davis and J. A. Fitzsimmons, "The Future of Nuclear Power in the United States," *Technological Forecasting and Social Change,* vol. 40, no. 2, September 1991, pp. 151–164.

The round 1 questionnaire contained 37 questions, 11 concerning the past evolution of the nuclear industry and 26 concerning the future. These questions were to be answered on a seven-point Likert scale, ranging from "strongly agree" to "uncertain" to "strongly disagree," as shown below:

It is desirable *that utilities be permitted to integrate capital investment costs more aggressively into rate structures.*

______	______	______	______	______	______	______	______
No jdgmt.	Strong. disagr.	Disagr.	Disagr. somewh.	Uncert.	Agree somewh.	Agree	Strong. agree

The questionnaire also asked for open-ended comments.

For round 2 of this study, the administrator provided a comprehensive summary of the first-round responses to the 11 questions concerning the past and a summary of the open-ended comments concerning the future. The number of responses to the question above are noted below, with the median (*M*) and interquartile range (designated by the vertical bars) shown below the responses:

	1	6	5	6	15	35	8
No jdgmt.	Strong. disagr.	Disagr.	Disagr. somewh.	Uncert.	Agree somewh.	Agree	Strong. agree
			|--------------	---------------	---------------	--*M*--|	

The 11 questions concerning the past were dropped from the round 2 questionnaire, and 11 new questions prompted by the open-ended comments from round 1 were added. The participants were invited to "defend" their positions with supporting comments if their opinions fell outside the interquartile range.

For round 3, which was the final round in this study, the administrator once again supplied the participants with feedback, this time from round 2, and invited the participants to "vote" again on the same questions. The following illustration of the resulting median and interquartile range after each round of voting demonstrates how the opinions shifted and finally arrived at a consensus for this particular question:

	No jdgmt.	Strong. disagr.	Disagr.	Disagr. somewh.	Uncert.	Agree somewh.	Agree	Strong. agree
Round 1				|--------------	---------------	---------------	--*M*--|	
Round 2					|--------------	--*M*----------	-------|	
Round 3						|--------------	--*M*--|	

As noted, some of the questions asked for assessments of where the industry has been and where it stands today. Other questions not only asked the experts where they thought it should be headed but also to address issues such as resource allocation and the political realities affecting the future of nuclear power. As shown, the Delphi method is a useful tool in addressing situations for which quantifiable data are not available.

Cross-Impact Analysis

Cross-impact analysis assumes that some future event is related to the occurrence of an earlier event. As in the Delphi method, a panel of experts study a set of correlations between events presented in a matrix. These correlations form the basis for estimating the likelihood of a future event occurring.

For example, consider a forecast conducted in 1997 that assumes $3-per-gallon gasoline prices by 2000 (event A) and the corresponding doubling of ridership on mass transit by 2005 (event B). By initial consensus, it might be determined that given A, the conditional probability of B is .7, and that given B, the conditional probability of A is .6. These probabilities are shown in the matrix below:

	Probability of Event	
Given event	A	B
A	—	.7
B	.6	—

Assume that the forecasted unconditional probability for doubling mass transit ridership by 2005 is 1.0, and that the forecasted unconditional probability of $3 per gallon for gasoline by 2000 is .8. These new values are statistically inconsistent with the values in the matrix. The inconsistencies would be pointed out to the experts on the panel, who then would revise their estimates in a series of iterations. As with the Delphi method, an experienced administrator is needed to arrive at a satisfactory conditional probability matrix that can be used for generating a forecast.

Historical Analogy

Historical analogy assumes that the introduction and growth pattern of a new service will mimic the pattern of a similar concept for which data are available. Historical analogy frequently is used to forecast the market penetration or life cycle of a new service. The concept of a product life cycle as used in marketing involves stages, such as introduction, growth, maturity, and decline.

A famous use of historical analogy was the prediction of the market penetration by color television based on the experience with black-and-white television only a few years earlier. Of course, the appropriate analogy is not always so obvious. For example, growth in the demand for housekeeping services could follow the growth curve for child-care services. Because the pattern of previous data can have many interpretations and the analogy can be questioned, the credibility of any forecast using this method often is suspect. The acceptance of historical analogy forecasts depends on making a convincing analogy.

CAUSAL MODELS

It is fairly easy to make short-term forecasts when we are presented with uncomplicated data. On occasion, however, a competitive service organization must deal with a wealth of statistical information, some of which may be relevant to making profitable forecasts and some of which may be extraneous. In these situations, it also is more likely that the forecasts must be made for the next year—or for the next decade—rather than just for the next day, week, or month. Obviously, a long-term forecast has the potential of spelling success or devastation for the organization. Therefore, we need a way of separating out the critical information and processing it to help us make an appropriate forecast.

Causal models make assumptions that are similar to those of time series models (which we will consider later): that the data follow an identifiable pattern over time, and that an identifiable relationship exists between the information we wish to forecast and other factors. These models range from very simple ones, in which the forecast is based on a technique called *regression analysis,* to those known as *econometric models,* which use a system of equations.

Regression Models

A regression model is a relationship between the factor being forecasted, which is designated as the *dependent variable* (or Y), and the factors that determine the value of Y, which are designated as the *independent variables* or (X_i). If there are n independent variables, then the relationship between the dependent variable Y and the independent variables X is expressed as:

$$Y = a_0 + a_1X_1 + a_2X_2 + \cdots + a_nX_n \tag{1}$$

The values $a_0, a_1, a_2, \ldots, a_n$ are constant coefficients, which are determined by the computer program being used. If calculations are done by hand, values are determined by using regression equations found in elementary statistics texts.

As an example, the management of La Quinta Inn, a national chain of hotels, commissioned a study to determine the direction of its expansion efforts.[2] It wanted to know which factors determined a profitable hotel location and, thus, would allow management to screen available real estate for new hotel sites. Investigators collected data on many factors at existing locations, such as traffic count, number of competitive rooms nearby, visibility of signs, local airport traffic, types of neighboring businesses, and distance to the central business district. In all, 35 factors, or independent variables, were considered, as shown in Table 16.2.

A preliminary statistical evaluation of the data for all those variables then allowed the investigators to identify four critical factors—STATE, PRICE, INCOME, and COLLEGE—to be used in the forecast model.

The firm's operating margin, obtained by adding depreciation and interest expenses to the profit and then dividing by the total revenue, was chosen as the most reliable measure, or dependent variable Y, on which to base a forecast. For this case, the constant coefficients were calculated as $a_0 = 39.05$, $a_1 = -5.41$, $a_2 = +5.86$, $a_3 = -3.09$, and $a_4 = +1.75$. Substituting these coefficient values and the in-

[2]S. E. Kimes and J. A. Fitzsimmons, "Selecting Profitable Hotel Sites at La Quinta Motor Inns," *Interfaces,* vol. 20, no. 2, March–April 1990, pp. 12–20.

TABLE 16.2. Independent Variables for Hotel Location

Name	Description
	Competitive Factors
INNRATE	Inn price
PRICE	Room rate for the inn
RATE	Average competitive room rate
RMS1	Hotel rooms within 1 mile
RMSTOTAL	Hotel rooms within 3 miles
ROOMSINN	Inn rooms
	Demand Generators
CIVILIAN	Civilian personnel on base
COLLEGE	College enrollment
HOSP1	Hospital beds within 1 mile
HOSPTOTL	Hospital beds within 4 miles
HVYIND	Heavy industrial employment
LGTIND	Light industrial acreage
MALLS	Shopping mall square footage
MILBLKD	Military base blocked
MILITARY	Military personnel
MILTOT	MILITARY + CIVILIAN
OFC1	Office space within 1 mile
OFCTOTAL	Office space within 4 miles
OFCCBD	Office space in central business district
PASSENGR	Airport passengers enplaned
RETAIL	Scale ranking of retail activity
TOURISTS	Annual tourists
TRAFFIC	Traffic count
VAN	Airport van
	Area Demographics
EMPLYPCT	Unemployment percentage
INCOME	Average family income
POPULACE	Residential population
	Market Awareness
AGE	Years inn has been open
NEAREST	Distance to nearest inn
STATE	State population per inn
URBAN	Urban population per inn
	Physical Attributes
ACCESS	Accessibility
ARTERY	Major traffic artery
DISTCBD	Distance to downtown
SIGNVIS	Sign visibility

Source: Reprinted by permission, "Selecting Profitable Hotel Sites at La Quinta Motor Inns," S. E. Kimes and J. A. Fitzsimmons, *Interfaces*, vol. 20, no. 2, March–April 1990, p. 14.

dependent variables into equation (1) yields the following regression forecasting model:

$$\text{Operating margin } Y = 39.05 + (-5.41)\text{STATE} + (5.86)\text{PRICE} + (-3.09)\text{INCOME} + (1.75)\text{COLLEGE}$$

By collecting data on the independent variables at a proposed hotel site and making appropriate transformations as needed, the operating margin can be forecasted. The results of this study proved the model to be very good in predicting the likelihood of success for a new inn at a proposed location.

As shown, development of a regression model requires an extensive data collection effort to meet the needs of the individual organization, which often involves considerable time and expense. It also requires expertise in the selection of independent and dependent variables to ensure a relationship that has a logical and meaningful interpretation. For these reasons, regression models are appropriate for making medium- and long-term forecasts.

Econometric Models

Econometric models are versions of regression models that involve a system of equations. The equations are related to each other, and the coefficients are determined as in the simpler regression models. An econometric model consists of a set of simultaneous equations expressing a dependent variable in terms of several different independent variables. Econometric models require extensive data collection and sophisticated analysis to create; thus, they generally are used for long-range forecasts.

TIME SERIES MODELS

Time series models are applicable for making short-term forecasts when the values of observations occur in an identifiable pattern over time. These models range from the simple *N-period moving average* model to the more sophisticated and useful *exponential smoothing* models.

N-*Period Moving Average*

Sometimes, observations that are made over a period of time appear to have a random pattern; consequently, we do not feel confident in basing forecasts on them. Consider the data in Table 16.3 for a 100-room hotel in a college town. We have decided to forecast only Saturday occupany, because the demand for each day of the week is influenced by different forces. For example, on weekdays, demand is generated by business travelers, but weekend guests often are people on vacation or visiting friends. Selection of the forecasting period is an important consideration and should be based on the nature of the demand and the ability to use that information. For example, fast-food restaurants forecast demand by the hour of the day.

TABLE 16.3. Saturday Occupancy at a 100-Room Hotel

Saturday	Period	Occupancy	Three-Period Moving Average	Forecast
Aug. 1	1	79		
8	2	84		
15	3	83	82	
22	4	81	83	82
29	5	98	87	83
Sept. 5	6	100	93	87
12	7			93

The hotel owner has noted increased occupancy for the last two Saturdays and wishes to prepare for the coming weekend (i.e., September 12), perhaps by discontinuing the practice of offering discount rates. Do the higher occupancy figures indicate a change in the underlying average occupancy? To answer this question, we need a way of taking out the "noise" of occasional blips in the pattern so that we do not overreact to a change that is random rather than permanent and significant.

The N-period moving-average method may be used in this simple example to smooth out random variations and produce a reliable estimate of the underlying average occupancy. The method calculates a moving average MA_t for period t on the basis of selecting N of the most recent actual observations A_t, as shown in equation (2):

$$MA_t = \frac{A_t + A_{t-1} + A_{t-2} + \cdots + A_{t-N+1}}{N} \tag{2}$$

If we select N equal to 3, then we cannot begin our calculation until period 3 (i.e., August 15), at which time we add the occupancy figures for the three most recent Saturdays (i.e., August 1, 8, and 15) and divide the sum by 3 to arrive at a three-period moving average of $[(83+84+79)/3]=82$. We use this value to forecast occupancy for the following Saturday (i.e., August 22). The moving-average forecast has smoothed out the random fluctuations to track better the average occupancy, which then is used to forecast the next period. Each three-period moving-average forecast thus involves simply adding the three most recent occupancy values and dividing by 3. For example, to arrive at the moving average for August 22, we drop the value for August 1, add the value for August 22, and recalculate the average, getting 83. Continuing this iterative process for the remaining data, we see how the moving-average occupancy of approximately 82 percent for Saturdays in August has increased recently, reflecting the near-capacity occupancy of the past two weekends. If the local college football team, after playing two consecutive home games, is scheduled for an away game on September 12, how confident are you in forecasting next Saturday's occupancy at 93 percent?

Although our N-period moving average has identified a change in the underlying average occupancy, this method is slow to react, because old data are given the same weight (i.e., $1/N$) as new data in calculating the averages. More recent data may be better indicators of change; therefore, we may wish to assign more weight to recent observations. Rather than arbitrarily assigning weights to our moving-average data to fix this shortcoming, we instead will use a more sophisticated forecasting method that systematically ages the data. Our next topic, exponential smoothing, also can accommodate trends and seasonality in the data.

Simple Exponential Smoothing

Simple exponential smoothing is the time series method most frequently used for demand forecasting. Simple exponential smoothing also "smooths out" blips in the data, but its power over the N-period moving average is threefold: (1) old data are never dropped or lost, (2) older data are given progressively less weight, and (3) the calculation is simple and requires only the most recent data.

Simple exponential smoothing is based on the concept of feeding back the forecast error to correct the previous smoothed value. In equation (3) below, S_t is the smoothed value for period t, A_t is the actual observed value for period t, and α is a smoothing constant that usually is assigned a value between 0.1 and 0.5.

$$S_t = S_{t-1} + \alpha(A_t - S_{t-1}) \tag{3}$$

The term $(A_t - S_{t-1})$ represents the forecast error, because it is the difference between the actual observation and the smoothed value that was calculated in the prior period. A fraction α of this forecast error is added to the previous smoothed value to obtain the new smoothed value S_t. Note how self-correcting this method is when you consider that forecast errors can be either positive or negative.

Our moving-average analysis of the occupancy data in Table 16.3 indicated an actual increase in average occupancy over the two most recent Saturdays. These same occupancy data are repeated in Table 16.4, with the actual value for each period (A_t) shown in the third column. Using simple exponential smoothing, we will demonstrate again that a significant change in the mean occupancy has occurred.

Because we must start somewhere, let the first observed, or actual, value A_t in a series of data equal the first smoothed value S_t. Therefore, as Table 16.4

TABLE 16.4. Simple Exponential Smoothing
(Saturday hotel occupancy [a = 0.5])

Saturday	Period (t)	Actual Occupancy (A_t)	Smoothed Value (S_t)	Forecast (F_t)	Forecast Error $\lvert A_t - F_t \rvert$
Aug. 1	1	79	79.00		
8	2	84	81.50	79	5
15	3	83	82.25	82	1
22	4	81	81.63	82	1
29	5	98	89.81	82	16
Sept. 5	6	100	94.91	90	10

shows, S_1 for August 1 equals A_1 for August 1, or 79.00. The smoothed value for August 8 (S_2) then may be derived from the actual value for August 8 (A_2) and the previous smoothed value for August 1 (S_1) according to equation (3). We have selected an α equal to 0.5, because as will be shown later, this results in a forecast that is similar to the one obtained using a three-period moving average. For August 8:

$$\begin{aligned} S_2 &= S_1 + \alpha(A_2 - S_1) \\ &= 79.00 + 0.5(84 - 79.00) \\ &= 81.50 \end{aligned}$$

Similar calculations then are made to determine the smoothed values (S_3, S_4, S_5, S_6) for successive periods.

Simple exponential smoothing assumes that the pattern of data is distributed about a constant mean. Thus, the smoothed value calculated in period t is used as the forecast for period $(t + 1)$ rounded to an integer, as shown below:

$$F_{t+1} = S_t \tag{4}$$

Our best estimate for August 15 occupancy will be 81.50, the most recent smoothed value at the end of August 8. Note that the forecast error (84 – 79) was a positive 5 (i.e., we underestimated demand by 5), and that one-half of this error was added to the previous smoothed value to increase the new estimate of average occupancy. This concept of error feedback to correct an earlier estimate is an idea borrowed from control theory.

The smoothed values shown in Table 16.4 were calculated using an α value of 0.5. As noted, however, if we wish to make the smoothed values less responsive to the latest data, we can assign a smaller value to α. Figure 16.1 demon-

FIGURE 16.1. Simple exponential smoothing: Saturday hotel occupancy.

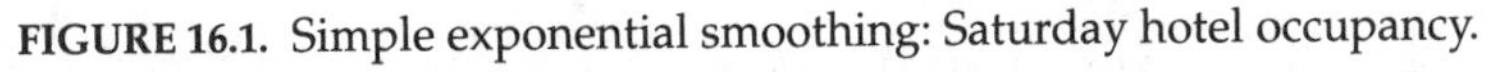

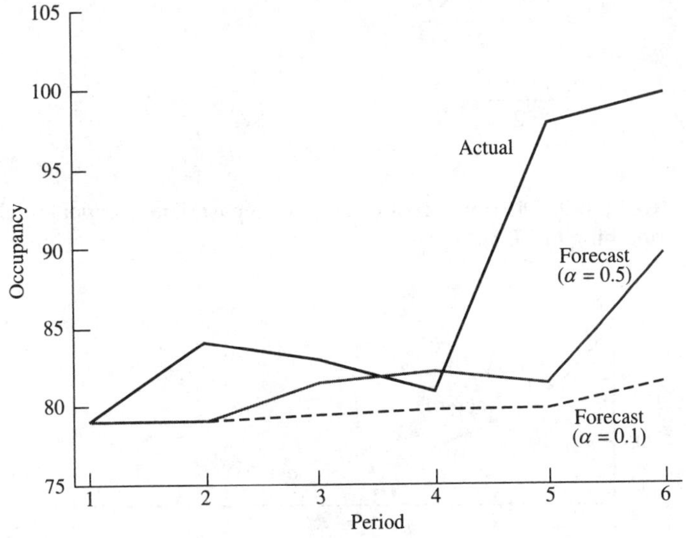

strates graphically how an α of 0.1 and of 0.5 smooth the curve of the actual values. It is easily seen in this figure that the smoothed curve, particularly with an α of 0.5, has reduced the extremes (i.e., the dips and peak) and responded to the increased occupancy in the last two Saturdays. Therefore, basing forecasts on smoothed data helps to prevent overreacting to the extremes in the actual observed values.

Equation (3) may be rewritten as follows:

$$S_t = \alpha(A_t) + (1 - \alpha)S_{t-1} \tag{5}$$

The basis for the name "exponential smoothing" can be observed in the weights that are given past data in equation (5). We see that A_t is given a weight α in determining S_t, and we easily can show by substitution that A_{t-1} is given a weight $\alpha(1 - \alpha)$. In general, actual value A_{t-n} is given a weight $\alpha(1 - \alpha)^n$, as Figure 16.2 shows by graphing the exponential decay of weights given a series of observations over time. Note that older observations never disappear entirely from the calculation of S_t as they would when the N-period moving average is used, but they do assume progressively decreasing importance.

Relationship between α *and* N

Selecting the value for α is a matter of judgment, often based on the pattern of historical data, with large values giving much weight to recent data in anticipation of changes. To help select α, a relationship can be made between the number of periods N in the moving-average method and the exponential smoothing constant α. If we assume that the two methods are similar when the average ages of past data are equal, then the following relationship results:

Moving average:

$$\begin{aligned} \text{Average age} &= \frac{(0 + 1 + 2 + \cdots + N - 1)}{N} \\ &= \frac{(N - 1)(N/2)}{N} \\ &= \frac{N - 1}{2} \end{aligned}$$

FIGURE 16.2. Distribution of weight given past data in exponential smoothing ($\alpha = 0.3$).

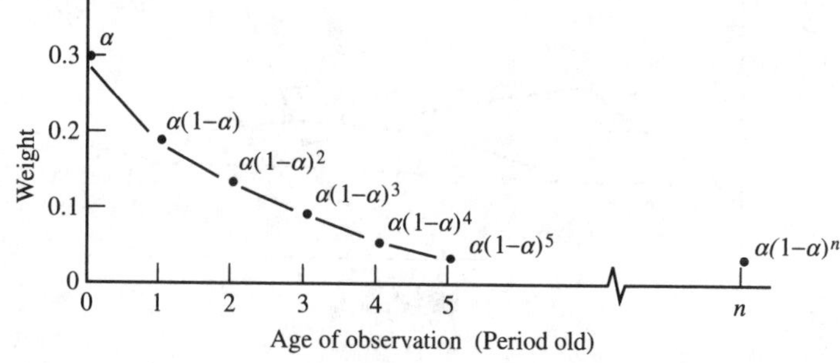

Exponential smoothing:

$$\text{Average age} = 0(\alpha) + 1(\alpha)(1-\alpha) + 2(\alpha)(1-\alpha)^2 + \cdots$$
$$= \frac{(1-\alpha)}{\alpha}$$

The calculation above is a geometric series with the sum equal to:

$$\frac{ar}{(1-r)^2} \quad \text{for } a = \alpha \text{ and } r = 1 - \alpha$$

When the average ages are equated, the result is:

$$\alpha = \frac{2}{(N+1)} \quad \text{or} \quad N = \frac{(2-\alpha)}{\alpha}$$

Using this relationship results in the following sample values for equating α and N:

α	0.05	0.1	0.2	0.3	0.4	0.5	0.667
N	39	19	9	5.7	4	3	2

As shown, the usual assignment of a smoothing value between 0.1 and 0.5 is reasonable when compared with the number of periods in an equivalent moving-average forecast. The particular value assigned to α is a tradeoff between overreacting to random fluctuations about a constant mean and detecting a change in the mean value. Higher values of α are more responsive to change because of the greater weight that is given to recent data. In practice, the value of α often is selected on the basis of minimizing the forecast error as measured by the mean absolute deviation (MAD).

Forecast Error

Although it is obvious in Figure 16.1 that the smoothed curves have evened out the peaks and valleys of the actual curve, how do we measure the accuracy of forecasts? One common method is calculating the *mean absolute deviation (MAD)*. This is the calculation of the average value for the *absolute* values of forecast errors $|A_t - F_t|$ shown in Table 16.4. To calculate the MAD for this example, total the absolute differences and then divide by the number of observations. For this case, MAD = (5 + 1 + 1 + 16 + 10)/5 = 6.6.

Recall that the forecast values in this example were derived from smoothed values calculated with $\alpha = 0.5$, because this method is similar to a three-period moving-average method. For the three-period moving-average forecast developed earlier, the MAD value is 9.7. In this case, simple exponential smoothing resulted in more accurate forecasts than the corresponding three-period moving-average method. If an α of 0.1 is used, however, the MAD value is 8.8, reflecting the unresponsiveness to change of a small smoothing constant. It should be noted that selecting an α to minimize MAD for a set of data can be accomplished using Excel Solver.

In any event, we desire an unbiased forecast with respect to its tracking of the actual mean for the data. Thus, the sum of the forecast errors should tend toward zero, taking into account both positive and negative differences. If it does not, then we should look for underlying trends or seasonality and account for them explicitly. For the results shown in Table 16.4, the sum of forecast errors is calculated as:

$$\sum (A_t + F_t) = 5 + 1 - 1 + 16 + 10 = 31$$

This high positive sum suggests that an upward trend exists in the data, and that our simple exponential smoothing forecasts are falling short of actual hotel occupancy. Thus, we must incorporate a trend adjustment into our forecast.

Exponential Smoothing with Trend Adjustment

The *trend* in a set of data is the average rate at which the observed values change from one period to the next over time. The changes created by the trend can be treated using an extension of simple exponential smoothing.

Table 16.5 follows the experience of a new commuter airline during its first 8 weeks of business. The average weekly load factors (i.e., percentages of seats sold) show a steady increase, from approximately 30 percent for week 1 to approximately 70 percent for week 8. In this example the smoothed value S_t is calculated using equation (6), which is equation (5) modified by the addition of a trend value T_{t-1} to the previous smoothed value S_{t-1} to account for the weekly rate of increase in load factor.

$$S_t = \alpha(A_t) + (1 - \alpha)(S_{t-1} + T_{t-1}) \tag{6}$$

To incorporate a trend adjustment in our calculation, we will use β as a smoothing constant. This constant usually is assigned a value between 0.1 and 0.5 and may be the same as, or different from, α. The trend for a given period t is defined by $(S_t - S_{t-1})$, the rate of change in smoothed value from one period to the next (i.e., the slope of the demand curve). The smoothed trend T_t then is

TABLE 16.5. Exponential Smoothing with Trend Adjustment
(Commuter airline load factor [$\alpha = 0.5$, $\beta = 0.3$])

Week t	Actual Load Factor (A_t)	Smoothed Value (S_t)	Smoothed Trend (T_t)	Forecast (F_t)	Forecast Error $\lvert A_t - F_t \rvert$
1	31	31.00	0.00		
2	40	35.50	1.35	31	9
3	43	39.93	2.27	37	6
4	52	47.10	3.74	42	10
5	49	49.92	3.47	51	2
6	64	58.69	5.06	53	11
7	58	60.88	4.20	64	6
8	68	66.54	4.63	65	3
					MAD 6.7

calculated at period t using equation (7), which is a modification of the basic exponential smoothing equation—equation (5)—with the observed trend $(S_t - S_{t-1})$ used in place of A_t.

$$T_t = \beta(S_t - S_{t-1}) + (1 - \beta)T_{t-1} \tag{7}$$

To anticipate cash flows during the business start-up period, the commuter airline owners are interested in forecasting future weekly load factors. After observing the first two weeks of activity, you are asked to provide a forecast for week 3. The smoothed values, trend figures, and forecasts in Table 16.5 are calculated in a stepwise manner. For the first observation in a series, week 1 in this instance, the smoothed value S_1 is equal to the actual value A_1, and the trend T_1 is set equal to 0.00. The forecast for week 2 is calculated using equation (8). In this case, $F_2 = 31 + 0.00 = 31.00$.

$$F_{t+1} = S_t + T_t \tag{8}$$

To compute the figures for week 2 and a forecast for week 3, we will use $\alpha = 0.5$ and $\beta = 0.3$. First, the smoothed value S_2 for week 2 is calculated using equation (6):

$$\begin{aligned} S_2 &= (0.5)(40) + (1 - 0.5)(31 + 0.00) \\ &= 35.50 \end{aligned}$$

Now, we calculate the trend for week 2 with equation (7):

$$\begin{aligned} T_2 &= (0.3)(35.50 - 31.00) + (1 - 0.3)0.00 \\ &= 1.35 \end{aligned}$$

The final step is to make a forecast for week 3 according to equation (8):

$$F_3 = 35.5 + 1.35 = 36.85 \cong 37$$

When the actual data for the following weeks are received, similar calculations can be made for the smoothed value, the trend, the forecast, and the forecast error. For all the forecasts shown in Table 16.5, the MAD is 6.7.

The sum of the forecast error values (both positive and negative) is a measure of forecast bias. For this example $\Sigma\,(A_t - F_t) = 9 + 6 + 10 - 2 + 11 - 6 + 3 = 31$. The sum of forecast errors for an unbiased forecast should approach zero (i.e., the positive and negative errors cancel out each other).

In Figure 16.3, the actual load factors are plotted against the forecasts to illustrate the tracking ability of exponential smoothing with a trend adjustment.

Exponential Smoothing with Seasonal Adjustment

To account for seasonal effects on a set of data, we can use another extension of simple exponential smoothing. In simplest terms, we first remove the seasonal-

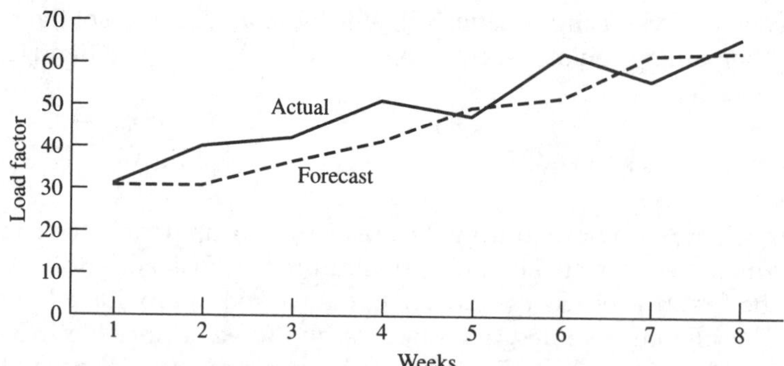

FIGURE 16.3. Exponential smoothing with trend adjustment: commuter airline load factors ($\alpha = 0.5, \beta = 0.3$).

ity from the data and then smooth those data as we already have learned; finally, we put the seasonality back in to determine a forecast.

We will apply this seasonal adjustment to the data in Table 16.6, which reports the number of passengers per month taking a ferry to a resort island in the Caribbean for the years 1995 and 1996. In general, we denote a cycle, L, as the length of one season. L may be any length of time, even the 24 hours of a day, but frequently, as in this case, it is 12 months. Note that we must have actual data for at least one full season before we can begin smoothing and forecasting calculations.

A *seasonality index* I_t is used to deseasonalize the data in a given cycle L. Initially, I_t is estimated by calculating a ratio of the actual value for period t, A_t, divided by the average value $\bar{A}$ for all periods in cycle L as shown in equation (9):

$$I_t = \frac{A_t}{\bar{A}} \tag{9}$$

where

$$\bar{A} = (A_1 + A_2 + \cdots + A_L)/L$$

In our passenger ferry example, $\bar{A} = 1971.83$, and by substituting this value into equation (9), we can calculate the index I_t for each period in the first season of L periods. The resulting indices for the months of 1995, which are shown in column 5 of Table 16.6, then are used to deseasonalize the data for the corresponding months in 1996 according to equation (10), which is a minor modification of our basic exponential smoothing equation—equation (5)—with A_t adjusted to account for seasonality using index I_{t-L}.

$$S_t = \alpha \frac{A_t}{I_{t-L}} + (1 - \alpha) S_{t-1} \tag{10}$$

For this example, data for the 12 months in 1995 are used to give initial estimates of the seasonality indices. Therefore, we cannot begin to calculate new smoothed data until period 13 (i.e., January 1996). To begin the process, we assume that S_{12} equals A_{12}, as shown in Table 16.6 with a value of 1794. The

TABLE 16.6. Exponential Smoothing with Seasonal Adjustment
(Ferry passengers taken to a resort island [$\alpha = 0.2, \gamma = 0.3$])

Period	t	Actual Passengers (A_t)	Smoothed Value (S_t)	Index (I_t)	Forecast (F_t)	Forecast Error $\lvert A_t - F_t \rvert$
			1995			
January	1	1651	....	0.837	....	
February	2	1305	....	0.662	....	
March	3	1617	....	0.820	....	
April	4	1721	....	0.873	....	
May	5	2015	....	1.022	....	
June	6	2297	....	1.165	....	
July	7	2606	....	1.322	....	
August	8	2687	....	1.363	....	
September	9	2292	....	1.162	....	
October	10	1981	....	1.005	....	
November	11	1696	....	0.860	....	
December	12	1794	1794.00	0.910	....	
			1996			
January	13	1806	1866.74	0.876	....	....
February	14	1731	2016.35	0.721	1236	495
March	15	1733	2035.76	0.829	1653	80
April	16	1904	2064.81	0.888	1777	127
May	17	2036	2050.28	1.013	2110	74
June	18	2560	2079.71	1.185	2389	171
July	19	2679	2069.06	1.314	2749	70
August	20	2821	2069.19	1.363	2820	1
September	21	2359	2061.38	1.157	2404	45
October	22	2160	2078.95	1.015	2072	88
November	23	1802	2082.23	0.862	1788	14
December	24	1853	2073.04	0.905	1895	42
						MAD 110

smoothed value for January 1996 now can be calculated using equation (10), with $I_{t-L} = 0.837$ (i.e., the index I_t of 12 months ago for January 1995) and $\alpha = 0.2$:

$$S_{13} = (0.2)\frac{1806}{0.837} + (1 - 0.2)1794$$
$$= 1866.74$$

The forecast for February (period $t + 1$) then is made by seasonalizing the smoothed value for January according to the following formula:

$$F_{t+1} = (S_t)(I_{t-L+1}) \qquad (11)$$

Note that the seasonalizing factor I_{t-L+1} in this case is the index I_t for February 1995. Therefore, our forecast for February 1996 is:

$$F_{14} = (1866.74)(0.662)$$
$$= 1235.78 \cong 1236$$

If the seasonality indices are stable, forecasts that are based on only one cycle, L, will be reliable. If, however, the indices are not stable, they can be adjusted, or smoothed, as new data become available. After calculating the smoothed value S_t for an actual value A_t at the most recent period t, we can denote a new observation for a seasonality index at period t as (A_t/S_t). To apply the concept of exponential smoothing to the index, we use a new constant, γ, which usually is assigned a value between 0.1 and 0.5. The smoothed estimate of the seasonality index then is calculated from the following formula:

$$I_t = \gamma \frac{A_t}{S_t} + (1 - \gamma)I_{t-L} \tag{12}$$

Now, we can continue the calculations for 1996 in Table 16.6 by using equation (12) to update the seasonality indices for each month for future use. Remember, however, that in actual practice, smoothed values, indices, and forecasts for each period (i.e., month) in this new season of L periods would be calculated on a month-to-month basis as the most recent actual values became available. Here, according to equation (12), the new smoothed seasonality index for January 1996, I_{13}, using $\gamma = 0.3$ is:

$$\begin{aligned} I_{13} &= 0.3 \frac{1806}{1866.74} + (1 - 0.3)0.837 \\ &= 0.876 \end{aligned}$$

The MAD for February through December 1996 is 110, which indicates a very good fit of forecasts to actual data that exhibit a definite seasonality. Is it possible, however, to make even more accurate forecasts?

Exponential Smoothing with Trend and Seasonal Adjustments

The answer to the earlier question—Is it possible to make even more accurate forecasts?—is yes (sometimes). In some cases, adjusting only for trend or seasonality will provide the current best estimate of the average; at others, the forecast can be improved by considering all factors together. We can include *both* trend and seasonal adjustments in exponential smoothing by weighting a *base* smoothed value with trend and seasonal indices to forecast the following period. The appropriate equations are:

$$S_t = \alpha \frac{A_t}{I_{t-L}} + (1 - \alpha)(S_{t-1} + T_{t-1}) \tag{13}$$

$$T_t = \beta(S_t - S_{t-1}) + (1 - \beta)T_{t-1} \tag{14}$$

$$I_t = \gamma \frac{A_t}{S_t} + (1 - \gamma)I_{t-L} \tag{15}$$

$$F_{t+1} = (S_t + T_t)I_{t-L+1} \tag{16}$$

These equations can be applied to the data in Table 16.7, and the resulting MAD of 160 for February through December 1996 tells us that in this case, we have not gained anything by adding a trend adjustment to the seasonal adjustment. Figure 16.4 demonstrates graphically the results of treating the actual data with a seasonal adjustment only and with both seasonal and trend adjustments.

Summary of Exponential Smoothing

Exponential smoothing is a relatively easy and straightforward way to make short-term forecasts. It has many attributes, including:

- All past data are considered in the smoothing process.
- Recent data are assigned more weight than older data.
- Only the most recent data are required to update a forecast.

TABLE 16.7. Exponential Smoothing with Seasonal and Trend Adjustments
(Ferry passengers taken to a resort island [$\alpha = 0.2, \beta = 0.2, \gamma = 0.3$])

Period	t	Actual Passengers (A_t)	Smoothed Value (S_t)	Trend (T_t)	Index (I_t)	Forecast (F_t)	Forecast Error $\lvert A_t - F_t \rvert$
			1995				
January	1	1651	....	....	0.837	....	
February	2	1305	....	....	0.662	....	
March	3	1617	....	....	0.820	....	
April	4	1721	....	....	0.873	....	
May	5	2015	....	....	1.022	....	
June	6	2297	....	....	1.165	....	
July	7	2606	....	....	1.322	....	
August	8	2687	....	....	1.363	....	
September	9	2292	....	....	1.162	....	
October	10	1981	....	....	1.005	....	
November	11	1696	....	....	0.860	....	
December	12	1794	1794.00	0.00	0.910	....	
			1996				
January	13	1806	1866.59	14.52	0.876	....	
February	14	1731	2027.99	43.89	0.719	1245	486
March	15	1733	2080.17	45.55	0.824	1699	34
April	16	1904	2136.87	47.78	0.878	1855	49
May	17	2036	2146.20	40.09	1.000	2232	196
June	18	2560	2188.55	40.54	1.166	2547	13
July	19	2679	2188.69	32.46	1.292	2946	267
August	20	2821	2190.96	26.42	1.340	3027	206
September	21	2359	2179.80	18.91	1.138	2577	218
October	22	2160	2188.97	16.96	0.999	2209	49
November	23	1802	2183.75	12.53	0.850	1897	95
December	24	1853	2164.36	6.14	0.894	1998	145
							MAD 160

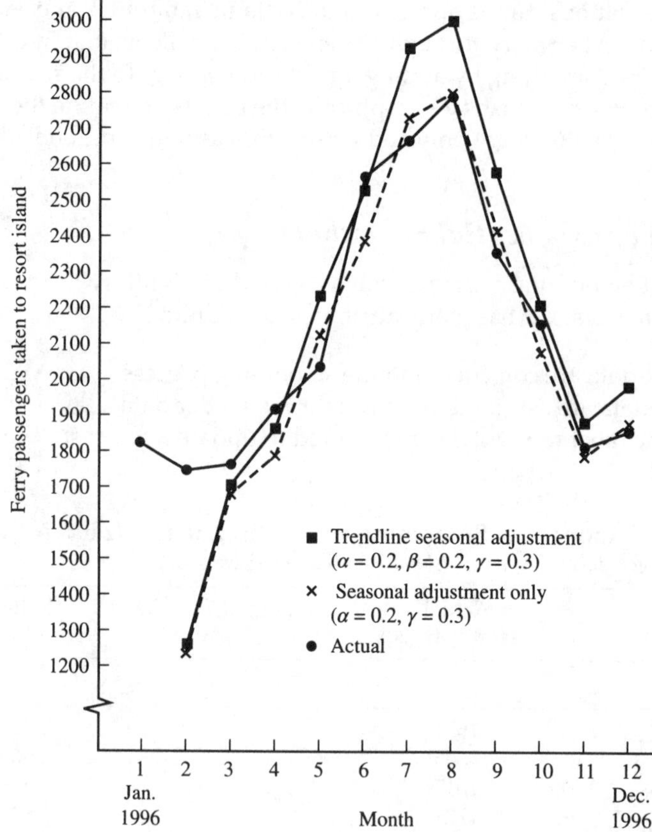

FIGURE 16.4. Exponential smoothing with seasonal adjustment.

- The model is easy to implement on a personal computer using spreadsheet software.
- Smoothing constants allows us to alter the rate at which the model responds to changes in the underlying pattern in the data.

SUMMARY

Decisions to embark on a new service concept often require subjective judgments about the future needs of customers. Subjective models like the Delphi method allow a panel of experts to defend their positions concerning the future, and through a number of iterations, these experts approach a consensus. Regression models have found application in service location analysis because of the need to account for several independent variables that contribute to demand generation. We ended our discussion of forecasting with an examination of time series models. Although the moving-average method is straightforward, we discovered that exponential smoothing has many superior qualities and has found wide acceptance in practice. Accounting for trends and seasonality is an important feature in forecasting service demand and is accommodated easily by means of exponential smoothing.

KEY TERMS AND DEFINITIONS

Cross-impact analysis a technological forecasting method that assumes some future event is related to an earlier event with an estimated probability.

Delphi method a technological forecasting method that uses a group of experts to arrive at a consensus about the future.

Exponential smoothing a time series forecast based on the concept of adjusting a previous forecast by feeding back a percentage of the forecast error.

Forecast error the difference between the actual observation and the forecasted value.

Mean absolute deviation (MAD) a measure of forecasting accuracy calculated as the average absolute forecast error.

Moving-average forecast a simple time series forecast formed by adding together the most recent data and dividing by the number of observations.

TOPICS FOR DISCUSSION

1. What characteristics of service organizations make forecast accuracy important?
2. For each of the three forecasting methods (i.e., time series, causal, and subjective), what costs are associated with the development and use of the forecast model? What costs are associated with forecast error?
3. The number of customers at a bank likely will vary by the hour of the day and by the day of the month. What are the implications of this for choosing a forecasting model?
4. Compare *N*-period moving-average models with exponential smoothing models.
5. Suggest a number of independent variables for a regression model to predict the potential sales volume of a given location for a retail store (e.g., a video rental store).
6. Suggest how the Delphi method can be incorporated into a cross-impact analysis.

Service Benchmark

L. L. Bean Improves Call-Center Forecasting

Two forecasting models are developed for use at L. L. Bean, Inc., a widely known retailer of high-quality outdoor goods and apparel. The models forecast customer telephone call volumes incoming to L. L. Bean's call-center which are used to produce weekly staffing schedules. The majority of L. L. Bean's sales are generated through telephone orders via 800-service, which was introduced in 1986. Ten percent of the 870 million dollars in 1993 sales was derived through store transactions and 18 percent ordered through the mail. However, 72 percent of the total sales volume was generated through orders taken at the company's call center.

Calls to L. L. Bean's call center fit into two major classifications, telemarketing (TM) and telephone-inquiry (TI), each with its own 800-number. TM calls are primarily the order-placing calls that generate the vast majority of the company's sales. TI callers are mainly customers who ask about the status of their orders, report problems regarding orders they have received, or inquire about a number of other issues.

The volume and average duration are quite different for these two classes of incoming calls. Annual call volumes for TM are many times higher than those of TI, but the average length of a TM call is much less than that of a TI call. TI agents are responsible for customer inquiries in a variety of areas, including order information, back orders, catalog requests, returns and exchanges, product questions, address corrections, and billing. Not surprisingly, with all this added complexity, TI agents require special training. Thus, it is important to forecast accurately the incoming call volumes for TI and TM separately to properly schedule these two distinct server groups.

Schedulers use the two forecasting models to predict daily call volumes for the next three weeks so that they can create week-long staffing schedules. However, with a two-week scheduling lead-time, the real focus of these predictions is on the third week ahead. That is, every Monday, on the first day of the 21-day planning horizon, the TI and TM schedules each loads a seven day forecast of daily call volumes for Monday (the 15th day) through Sunday (the 21st day) into their automated staff scheduling system. This allows them to post agent work schedules for work weeks (Monday–Sunday) two weeks in advance.

Inaccurate forecasts are very costly to L. L. Bean because they result in a mismatch of supply and demand. Understaffing of TM agents increases opportunity costs due to diminished revenues from lost orders—since a percentage of the customers who do not get through immediately will abandon and never return. Understaffing of TI agents decreases overall customer satisfaction, which erodes patron loyalty and the likelihood of repeat business. Furthermore, understaffing in either server group leads to excessive queue times, which cause telephone-connect charges to increase dramatically. On the other hand, overstaffing of TI or TM agents incurs the obvious penalty of excessive direct labor costs for the underutilized pool of telephone agents on duty.

These staffing decisions would be quite routine were it not for the erratic nature and extreme seasonality of L. L. Bean's business as shown in the figure. The three-week peak period just before Christmas can make or break the year: the company accepts nearly 20 percent of its annual calls during these three weeks. For the peak season, L. L. Bean will typically more than double the number of agents and almost quadruple the quantity of the telephone lines. Following this rapid build up for the peak season, management must shift its focus to the opposite extreme—the build-down process.

The forecasting models used the autoregressive/integrated/moving average (ARIMA) methodology put forth by Box and Jenkins.[3] Autoregressive (AR) terms, which are lagged values of the dependent variable, serve as independent variables in the model. Moving average (MA) terms are lagged values of the errors between past actual values and their predicted values and also serve as independent variables. Integrated (I) refers to the practice of differencing, which transforms a time series by subtracting past values of itself.

DATA DESCRIPTION

As seen in the figure, plots of these daily call data reveal the presence of strong day-of-week patterns. Monday generally has the highest call volume, with each successive day decreasing monotonically to the weekly low on Sunday. As noted, TI and TM both exhibit strong seasonal patterns for the year. Call volumes are reasonably stable through the second and third quarters of each year. TI and TM volumes begin to steadily ramp up during the fourth quarter and then virtually explode in the last month of the year. Then they drop down to their stable level during the first quarter of the next year. Weekly TI call volumes usually rise and fall without a break in the uptrend or downtrend until they reach a trend turning point, while weekly TM volumes seem much more volatile. Also, TM ramps more steeply up to and down from its Christmas peak than does TI. Lastly, TI consistently peaks two to three weeks later than TM.

Two four-year time series plots show that these seasonal patterns recur from year to year for both TI and TM. Unfortunately, the repetition is not exact. Although call volumes do not show an overwhelming pattern for Bean's off-season, the busy-season peaks and total annual volumes generally have been increasing each year for both TI and TM. Coinciding with this, it appears that their within-year variability has been increasing in recent years.

[3]G. E. P. Box and G. M. Jenkins, *Time Series Models for Forecasting and Control.* Holden Day, San Francisco, CA, 1976.

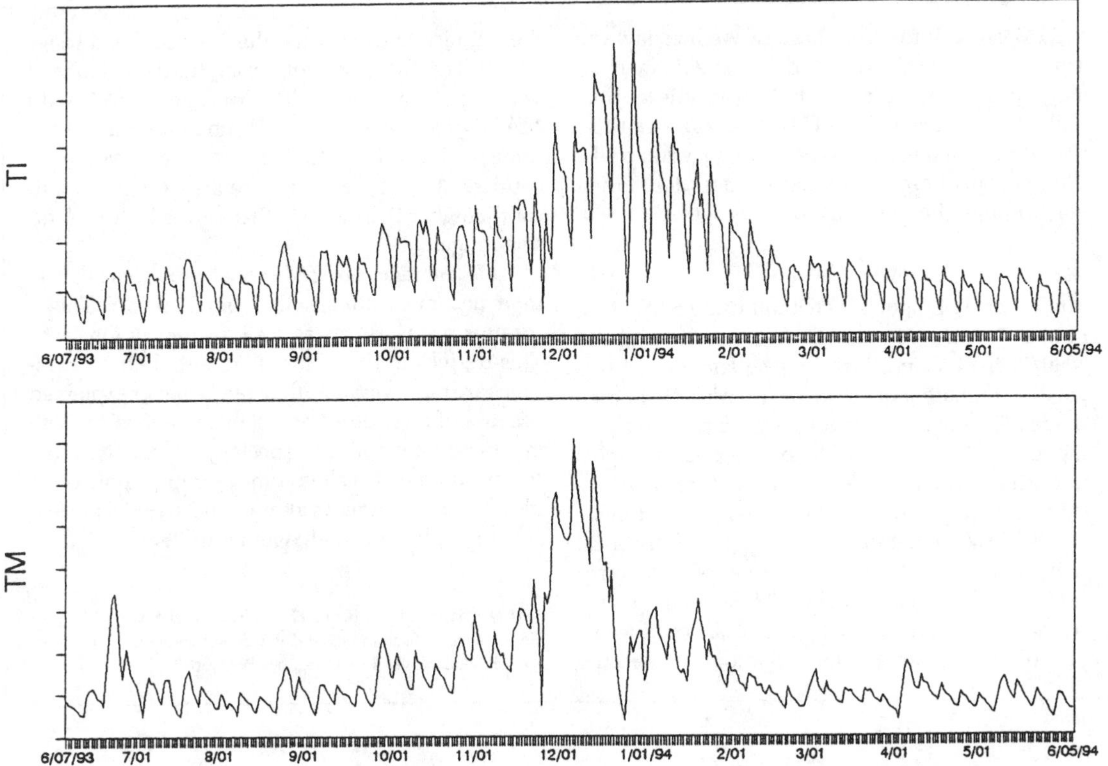

L.L. Bean time series plot of TI and TM daily call volume for the full-year period from June 7, 1993 to June 5, 1994.

TM and TI call volumes are both driven by orders, but in different ways. For TM, the relationship is direct and immediate. That is, today's orders calls produce today's orders. The connection for TI is more complicated. When an order is taken on a TI 800-line, the relationship is immediate here too. More often, however, the response is lagged and occurs when a customer subsequently calls to inquire about the status of an outstanding order or to report a problem with a recently received order. To further complicate matters, some TI calls are for such purposes as address corrections, which are not related to orders at all.

In many weeks, the normal, declining day-of-week pattern does not hold. Most of these disruptions coincide with the occurrence of holidays or catalog mailings. Call volumes are generally much lower on holidays than would otherwise be expected. Usually, one or two days before a holiday call volumes decrease. After a holiday, call volumes calls increase over normal levels as customers make up for the lack of ordering over the previous days. The magnitudes of these decreases and increases and the number of days affected depend upon the importance of the holiday. For example, the Fourth of July causes a larger and longer decrease than President's Day.

Catalogs are the primary medium through which L. L. Bean advertises and stimulates customer calling. The company mails out millions of copies of 20 to 25 different catalogs a year, each offering different merchandise depending upon the season and the target customers. L. L. Bean times most catalog mailings, or "drops," so that the bulk of the catalogs arrive around Tuesday. Many eager customers order immediately from their new catalogs. This results in high weekly order and call volumes, and it also causes the day-of-week pattern to deviate greatly from what occurs in a week without a catalog drop. For example, many catalogs cause the TM call volumes for Tuesday, Wednesday, and Thursday to rise above Monday's level. Other catalogs yield less dramatic shifts from the normal daily distribution. On the TI side, catalogs can also distort the usual pattern as heavy congestion on the TM lines encourage customers to "backdoor" their way through the TI lines to place orders.

MODEL RESULTS

The TI and TM models were built using SAS's Economic Time Series package on a mainframe IBM 3090/200J-VF. Conditional least squares option was used to estimate more than 100 coefficients in each model. The extensive exploratory efforts during the model-construction phase and subsequent ex-post forecasting evaluations led to hundreds of SAS runs, each averaging about three minutes of CPU time.

The TM model fit over five years of historical daily data with a mean absolute percent error (MAPE) of 7.4 percent, and the TI model fit its time series with a MAPE of 11.4 percent. We produced a year of ex-post forecasts for each model to measure their ability to predict the third week ahead (days 15–21). The TM model forecasted third-week-ahead volumes, from June 7, 1993 to June 3, 1994, with MAPE of 9.8 percent. The TI model forecasted the same period with a MAPE of 12.0 percent. We are encouraged by these results since they are not significantly higher than the MAPEs for the historical fitting ranges.

On average, our TM model produces slightly more accurate estimates than our TI model. This is true for historical fits as well as ex-post forecasts. This derives from the fact that, although TM volumes are more variable, they can be better explained because of their direct and stable relationship with independent variables, especially orders. Since the composition of TI call volumes is much more complex, the independent variables in its model are less able to predict their behavior accurately.

Source: Adapted from Bruce H. Andrews and Shawn M. Cunningham, "L. L. Bean Improves Call-Center Forecasting," *Interfaces*, vol. 25, no. 6, November–December 1995, pp. 1–13.

SOLVED PROBLEMS

1. Simple Exponential Smoothing

Problem Statement

The second week demand for a new barbecue burger is:

Day	Demand, units
Monday	22
Tuesday	27
Wednesday	38
Thursday	32
Friday	29

What is the forecast demand for next Monday using a smoothing constant $\alpha = 0.3$?

Solution

Using equation (5) with $\alpha = 0.3$ yields the simple exponential smoothing model, $S_t = 0.3(A_t) + 0.7\ (S_{t-1})$ with $F_{t+1} = S_t$. The calculations are shown in the worktable below:

Day	Period (t)	Actual (A_t)	Smoothed (S_t)	Forecast (F_t)	Error $\lvert A_t - F_t \rvert$
Mon.	1	22	22	–	–
Tu.	2	27	23.5	22	5
Wed.	3	38	27.85	24	14
Th.	4	32	29.095	28	4
Fri.	5	34	29.9665	29	5
Mon.				30	MAD = 7.0

2. Exponential Smoothing with Trend

Problem Statement

Recalculate the forecast for next Monday using a trend adjustment with $\beta = 0.2$. Using the MAD measure, compare the quality of this trend-adjusted forecast with the simple exponential smoothing in problem 1.

Solution

Using equations (6), (7), and (8) with $\alpha = 0.3$ and $\beta = 0.2$, we get the following exponential smoothing model with trend adjustment. The calculations are shown in the worktable below:

$$S_t = .3(A_t) + .7(S_{t-1} + T_{t-1})$$
$$T_t = .2(S_t - S_{t-1}) + .8(T_{t-1})$$
$$F_{t+1} = S_t + T_t$$

Day	Period (t)	Actual (A_t)	Smoothed (S_t)	Trend (T_t)	Forecast (F_t)	Error $\lvert A_t - F_t \rvert$
Mon.	1	22	22	0	—	—
Tu.	2	27	23.5	0.3	22	5
Wed.	3	38	28.06	1.15	23.8 ≅ 24	14
Th.	4	32	30.047	1.3174	29.21 ≅ 29	3
Fri.	5	34	31.55508	1.355536	31.3644 ≅ 31	3
Mon.					32.9106 ≅ 33	MAD = 6.25

3. Exponential Smoothing with Seasonal Adjustment

Problem Statement

Given the data below from the second week, there appears to be a cycle during the week peaking on Wednesday. Recalculate the forecast for Monday of the following week using a seasonal adjustment with $\gamma = 0.3$.

Day	Demand (burgers)
Monday	25
Tuesday	31
Wednesday	42
Thursday	34
Friday	32

Solution

Using Equations (9), (10), (11), and (12) with $\alpha = 0.3$ and $\gamma = 0.2$ yields the following exponential smoothing model with seasonal adjustment. Results are shown in the worktable below.

$$I_t = \frac{A_t}{\overline{A}}$$

$$S_t = .3\frac{A_t}{I_{t-L}} + .7(S_{t-l})$$

$$F_{t+1} = (S_t)(I_{t-L+1})$$

$$I_t = .2\frac{A_t}{S_t} + .8(I_{t-L})$$

First, the average value $\overline{A}$ for the first week is calculated and then used in formula (9) to calculate the initial seasonality indexes.

$$\overline{A} = (22 + 27 + 38 + 32 + 34)/5 = 30.6$$

Second, using formula (9), the initial seasonality indexes are calculated as shown in the worktable below for the first week:

Day	Period (t)	Actual (A_t)	Smoothed (S_t)	Index (I_t)
Mon.	1	22	—	0.72
Tu.	2	27	—	0.88
Wed.	3	38	—	1.24
Th.	4	32	—	1.05
Fri.	5	34	34	1.11

Third, the smoothed values, undated seasonal index, and forecast are made using formulas (10), (11), and (12) as shown in the worktable below:

Day	Period (t)	Actual (A_t)	Smoothed (S_t)	Index (I_t)	Forecast (F_t)	Error $\lvert A_t - F_t \rvert$
Mon.	6	25	34.217	0.74	—	—
Tu.	7	31	34.520	0.88	$30.11 \cong 30$	1
Wed.	8	42	34.325	1.24	$42.80 \cong 43$	1
Th.	9	34	33.742	1.04	$36.04 \cong 36$	2
Fri.	10	32	32.268	1.09	$37.45 \cong 37$	5
Mon.	11				$23.88 \cong 24$	MAD = 2.25

EXERCISES

16.1. In September 1996, there were 1035 checking-account customers at a neighborhood bank. The forecast for September, which was made in August, was for 1065 checking-account customers. Use an α of 0.1 to update the forecast for October.

16.2. During the noon hour this past Wednesday at a fast-food restaurant, 72 hamburgers were sold. The smoothed value calculated the week before was 67. Update the forecast for next Wednesday using simple exponential smoothing and an α of 0.1.

16.3. For the data in exercise 16.2, update the fast-food restaurant forecast if a trend value of 1.4 was calculated for the previous week. Use a β of 0.3 to update the trend for this week, and determine the forecast for next Wednesday using exponential smoothing with trend adjustment.

16.4. The demand for a certain drug in a hospital has been increasing. For the past 6 months, the following demand has been observed:
Use a 3-month moving average to make a forecast for July.

Month	Demand (units)
January	15
February	18
March	22
April	23
May	27
June	26

16.5. For the data in exercise 16.4, use an α of 0.1 to make a forecast for July.

16.6. For the data in exercise 16.4, use an α of 0.1 and β of 0.2 to make a forecast for July and August. Calculate the MAD for your January through June forecasts.

16.7. Prepare a spreadsheet model for the Saturday hotel occupancy data in Table 16.4, and recalculate the forecasts using an α of 0.3. What is the new MAD?

16.8. Prepare a spreadsheet model for the commuter airline's weekly load factor data in Table 16.5, and recalculate the forecasts using an α of 0.2 and β of 0.2. Have you improved on the original MAD?

16.9. Prepare a spreadsheet model for the ferry passenger data in Table 16.6, and recalculate the forecasts using an α of 0.3 and γ of 0.2. Has this change in the smoothing constants improved the MAD?

16.10. Prepare a spreadsheet model for the ferry passenger data in Table 16.7, and recalculate the forecasts using an α of 0.3, β of 0.1, and γ of 0.2. Has this change in the smoothing constants improved the MAD?

CASE: OAK HOLLOW EVALUATION CENTER[4]

Oak Hollow Medical Evaluation Center is a nonprofit agency offering multidisciplinary diagnostic services to study children with disabilities or developmental delays. The center can test each patient for physical, psychological, or social problems. Fees for services are based on an ability-to-pay schedule.

The evaluation center exists in a highly competitive environment. Many public-spirited organizations are competing for shrinking funds (i.e., Proposition 13 syndrome), and many groups such as private physicians, private and school psychologists, and social service organizations also are "competing" for the same patients. As a result of this situation, the center finds itself in an increasingly vulnerable financial position.

Mr. Abel, the director of the center, is becoming increasingly concerned with the center's ability to attract adequate funding and serve community needs. Mr. Abel now must develop an accurate estimate of the future patient load, staffing requirements, and operating expenses as part of his effort to attract funding. To this end, the director has approached an operations management professor at the local university for assistance in preparing a patient, staffing, and budget forecast for the coming year. The professor has asked you to aid her in this project. Tables 16.8 through 16.11 give you some pertinent information.

[4]Prepared by Frank Krafka under the supervision of Professor James A. Fitzsimmons.

TABLE 16.8. Annual Number of Patient Tests Performed*

Test	1992	1993	1994	1995	1996
Physical exam	390	468	509	490	582
Speech and hearing screening	102	124	180	148	204
Psychological testing	168	312	376	386	437
Social-worker interview	106	188	184	222	244

*All entering patients are given a physical examination. Patients then are scheduled for additional testing deemed appropriate.

TABLE 16.9. Annual Expenses ($)

Area	1992	1993	1994	1995	1996
Physical and neurological exams	18,200	24,960	32,760	31,500	41,600
Speech and hearing tests	2,040	2,074	3,960	3,950	4,850
Psychological testing	6,720	12,480	16,450	16,870	20,202
Social-worker interview	3,320	3,948	4,416	5,550	7,592
Subtotal	30,280	43,462	57,586	57,870	74,244
Other expenses	46,559	48,887	51,820	55,447	59,883
Total	76,839	92,349	109,406	113,317	134,127

TABLE 16.10. Monthly Patient Demand, September 1995–December 1996

	Physical Exam	Speech and Hearing Tests	Psychological Testing	Social-Worker Interview
		1995		
September	54	16	42	24
October	67	21	54	31
November	74	22	48	33
December	29	9	23	13
		1996		
January	58	20	44	24
February	52	18	39	22
March	47	16	35	20
April	41	14	31	17
May	35	12	26	15
June	29	10	22	12
July	23	8	17	10
August	29	10	22	12
September	65	24	48	27
October	81	29	61	34
November	87	31	66	37
December	35	12	26	14

TABLE 16.11. Current Staffing Levels*

Physicians	2 part-time, 18 hours per week
Speech and hearing clinicians	1 part-time, 20 hours per week
Psychologists	1 full-time, 38 hours per week
	1 part-time, 16 hours per week
Social workers	1 full-time, 40 hours per week

*The Oak Hollow Evaluation Center operates on a 50-week year.

Assignments

1. Given the information available and your knowledge of different forecasting techniques, recommend a specific forecasting technique for this study. Consider the advantages and disadvantages of your preferred technique, and identify what additional information, if any, Mr. Abel would need.

2. Develop forecasts for patient, staffing, and budget levels for next year.

CASE: GNOMIAL FUNCTIONS, INC.[5]

Gnomial Functions, Inc. (GFI), is a medium-sized consulting firm in San Francisco that specializes in developing various forecasts of product demand, sales, consumption, or other information for its clients. To a lesser degree, it also has developed on-going models for internal use by its clients. When contacted by a potential client, GFI usually establishes a basic work agreement with the firm's top management that sets out the general goals of the end product, primary contact personnel in both firms, and an outline of the project's overall scope (including any necessary time constraints for intermediate and final completion and a rough price estimate for the contract). Following this step, a team of GFI personnel is assembled to determine the most appropriate forecasting technique and develop a more detailed work program to be used as the basis for final contract negotiations. This team, which may vary in size according to the scope of the project and the client's needs, will perform the tasks that are established by the work program in conjunction with any personnel from the client firm who would be included in the team.

Recently, GFI was contacted by a rapidly growing regional firm that manufactures, sells, and installs active solar water-heating equipment for commercial and residential applications. DynaSol Industries has seen its sales increase by more than 200 percent during the past 18 months, and it wishes to obtain a reliable estimate of its sales during the next 18 months. The company management expects that sales should increase substantially because of competing energy costs, tax-credit availability, and fundamental shifts in the attitudes of the regional population toward so-called exotic solar systems. The company also faces increasing competition within this burgeoning market. This situation requires major strategic decisions concerning the company's future. When GFI was contacted, DynaSol had almost reached the manufacturing capacity of its present facility, and if it wishes to continue growing with the market, it must expand either by relocating to a new facility entirely or by developing a second manufacturing location. Each involves certain known costs, and each has its advantages and disadvantages. The major unknown factors as far as management is concerned are growth of the overall market for this type of product and how large a market share the company would be able to capture.

Table 16.12 contains the preliminary information available to GFI on DynaSol's past sales.

[5]Prepared by Frank Krafka under the supervision of Professor James A. Fitzsimmons.

Assignments

1. Given the information available and your knowledge of different forecasting techniques, develop a recommendation for utilizing a specific forecasting technique in the subsequent study. The final contract negotiations are pending, and so it is essential that you account for the advantages and disadvantages of your preferred technique as they would apply to the problem at hand and point out any additional information you would like to have.

2. Assume that you are a member of DynaSol's small marketing department and that the contract ne-

TABLE 16.12. DynaSol Monthly Sales for Period September 1994–February 1996

Month	DynaSol Industries Sales, Units	Sales ($)	Regional Market Sales, Units	Sales ($)
		1994		
September	24	44,736	223	396,048
October	28	52,192	228	404,928
November	31	59,517	230	408,480
December	32	61,437	231	422,564
		1995		
January	30	57,998	229	418,905
February	35	67,197	235	429,881
March	39	78,621	240	439,027
April	40	80,637	265	484,759
May	43	86,684	281	529,449
June	47	94,748	298	561,479
July	51	110,009	314	680,332
August	54	116,480	354	747,596
September	59	127,265	389	809,095
October	62	137,748	421	931,401
November	67	148,857	466	1,001,356
December	69	153,300	501	1,057,320
		1996		
January	74	161,121	529	1,057,320
February	79	172,007	573	1,145,264

gotiations with GFI have fallen through irrevocably. The company's top management has decided to use your expertise to develop a forecast for the next 6 months (and, perhaps, for the 6-month period following that one as well), because it must have some information on which to base a decision about expanding its operations. Develop such a forecast, and for the benefit of top management, note any reservations or qualifications you feel are vital to its understanding and use of the information.

SELECTED BIBLIOGRAPHY

BOX, G. E. P., and G. M. JENKINS: *Time Series Analysis: Forecasting and Control,* Holden-Day, San Francisco, 1976.

CHAMBERS, J. C., S. K. MULLICK, and D. D. SMITH: "How to Choose the Right Forecasting Technique," *Harvard Business Review,* July–August 1971, pp. 45–74.

CRYER, J.: *Time Series Forecasting,* Duxbury, Boston, 1986.

DAVIS, C. H., and J. A. FITZSIMMONS: "The Future of Nuclear Power in the United States," *Technological Forecasting and Social Change,* vol. 40, no. 2, September 1991, pp. 151–164.

KIMES, S. E., and J. A. FITZSIMMONS: "Selecting Profitable Hotel Sites at La Quinta Motor Inns," *Interfaces,* vol. 20, no. 2, March–April 1990, pp. 12–20.

MAKRIDAKIS, SPYROS, and STEVEN C. WHEELWRIGHT, editors: *The Handbook of Forecasting: A Manager's Guide,* Wiley, New York, 1982.

NETER, JOHN, WILLIAM WASSERMAN, and MICHAEL H. KUTNER: *Applied Linear Regression Models,* Irwin, Homewood, Ill., 1989.

WILSON, J. HOLTON, and BARRY KEATING: *Business Forecasting,* Irwin, Homewood, Ill., 1990.

CHAPTER 17

Queuing Models and Capacity Planning

LEARNING OBJECTIVES

After completing this chapter, you should be able to:

1. Describe a queuing model using the $A/B/C$ notation.
2. Use queuing models to calculate system performance measures.
3. Describe the relationships between queuing system characteristics.
4. Perform capacity planning using queuing models and various decision criteria.

The capacity planning decision involves a tradeoff between the cost of providing a service and the cost or inconvenience of customer waiting. The cost of service capacity is determined by the number of servers on duty, whereas customer inconvenience is measured by waiting time. Figure 17.1 illustrates this tradeoff, assuming that a monetary cost can be attributed to waiting. Increasing service capacity typically results in lower waiting costs and higher service costs. If the combined cost to the firm constitutes our planning criterion, then an optimal service capacity minimizes these service-versus-waiting costs.

Xerox Corporation faced precisely this dilemma when it introduced the Model 9200 Duplicating System.[1] Its existing service and maintenance operation, which consisted of individual technical representatives serving individual territories, no longer was able to provide the level of service that gave the company its decisive competitive advantage. Compromising the level of service meant that customers would have to wait, which would translate in this case into lost revenue for the customer (and, indirectly, for Xerox). Consequently, Xerox performed a queuing analysis to determine the best way to resolve its dilemma. Initial constraints, primarily involving human factors such as some loss of autonomy by the technical representatives and perceptions by the customer of less "personal" attention, led the company to consider establishing miniteams of service people who could provide faster service for more customers.

The cost to the Xerox customer was straightforward, because the Model 9200 was being used to replace a printer's previous offset system. Thus, a Xerox machine that was "down" meant lost income.

The problem Xerox faced at this point was to determine the appropriate number of members to assign to each team. The company used queuing analysis to minimize both the customer waiting cost and the Xerox service cost, and they arrived at an optimum result of three representatives per team.

The monetary cost of delaying a customer usually is more difficult to calculate than in this example, and it sometimes is impossible to determine. In a hospital, the cost of keeping a surgical team waiting for a pathologist's report could be the combined salaries of the team members plus the operating room cost. The cost of keeping a patient waiting in the reception room for a physician, however,

[1]W. H. Bleuel, "Management Science's Impact on Service Strategy," *Interfaces*, vol. 6, no. 1, November 1975, part 2, pp. 4–12.

FIGURE 17.1. Economic tradeoff in capacity planning.

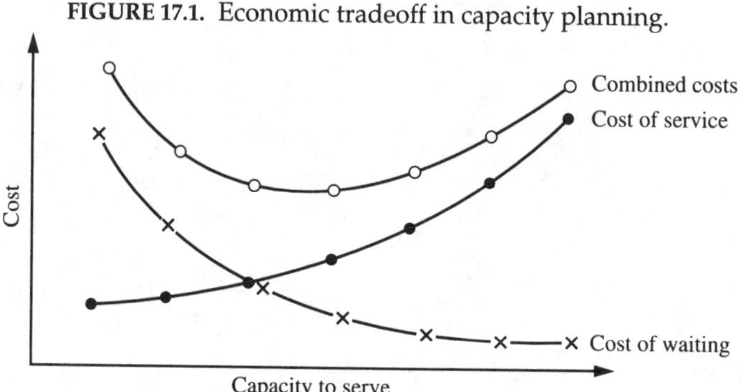

is not easily calculated. Further, as noted in Chapter 11, Managing Queues, circumstances affect the customer's perception of waiting.

The tradeoff between customer waiting and service capacity can be seen daily. For example, an emergency ambulance seldom is busy more than 30 percent of the time. Such low utilization is required in exchange for the ability to provide assistance on a moment's notice. Excess ambulance capacity is necessary, because the implicit cost of waiting for this particular service may be exorbitant in terms of human lives. The usual scene at a post office, however, is lines of impatient people waiting for service. Here, a judgment has been made that the implicit cost of waiting is not critical—and certainly not life-threatening—and besides, customers have few alternatives. Another result of this strategy is harried postal employees, who may not be able to provide the best possible service under the pressure of demanding customers! The desire of customers to avoid waiting has not been lost on the Travis County, Texas, Tax Collector/Assessor's office; for an extra dollar, an automobile owner has the option of renewing his or her annual auto registration by mail, thus avoiding the necessity of appearing in person.

CHAPTER PREVIEW

It is necessary to predict the degree of customer waiting that is associated with different levels of capacity. This chapter presents a number of analytical queuing models for use in making these waiting-time predictions. The models are analytical in that, for each case, a number of equations have been derived. Given a minimal amount of data—in particular, the mean arrival and mean service rates—these equations can generate the characteristics of a given system, such as the average customer waiting time. From these calculations, capacity planning decisions (e.g., determining the size of a parking lot) can be made using a number of different criteria. In addition, the queuing models help to explain the queuing phenomenon. For example, these models can predict the results of adding servers to a multiple-server system, as shown in the Xerox example, or they can show the effect of reducing service time variation on waiting time.

Equations for selected queuing models are listed at the end of this chapter. One should be neither dismayed nor awed by these models. They are merely useful tools for the effective management of services, and they can be used easily, even scratched out "on the spot" on the back of an envelope—often to the amazement of those looking to you for answers to their situations.

ANALYTICAL QUEUING MODELS

On the basis of our discussion of queues in Chapter 11, "Managing Queues," it is evident that many different queuing models exist. A popular system proposed by D. G. Kendall classifies parallel-server queuing models and uses the following notation in which three features are identified: $A/B/C$. A represents the distribution of time between arrivals, B the distribution of service times, and C the number of parallel servers. The descriptive symbols used for the arrival and service distributions include:

M = exponential interarrival or service time distribution (or the equivalent Poisson distribution of arrival or service rate),
D = deterministic or constant interarrival or service time,
E_k = Erlang distribution with shape parameter k (if $k = 1$, then Erlang is equivalent to exponential, and if $k = \infty$, then Erlang is equivalent to deterministic), and
G = general distribution with mean and variance (e.g., normal, uniform, or any empirical distribution).

Thus, $M/M/1$ designates a single-server queuing model with Poisson arrival rate and exponential service time distribution. The Kendall notation will be used here to define the class to which a queuing model belongs. Further considerations that are particular to the model in question, such as if the queue length is finite because of little space (e.g., parking lot) or a small number of potential customers (e.g., an office cafeteria), will be noted. Figure 17.2 classifies the six analytical queuing models that we will study in this chapter according to these features using the Kendall notation. Each queuing model (e.g., $M/M/1$) also is given a roman numeral (e.g., I, II, III) to designate a set of equations for that model. These equations are repeated at the end of the chapter for quick reference.

A final consideration involves the concepts of *transient state* and *steady state.* In a transient state, the values of the operating characteristics of a system depend on time. In a steady state, the system characteristics are independent of time, and the system is considered to be in statistical equilibrium. Because of their dependence on initial conditions, system characteristics usually are transient during the early stages of operation. For example, compare the initial conditions for a department store at opening time on a normal business day and on an end-of-year-sale day, when crowds overwhelm the clerks. The number in queue initially will be quite large, but given a long enough period of time, the system eventually will settle down. Once normal conditions have been reached, a statistical equilibrium is achieved in which the number in queue assumes a distribution

FIGURE 17.2. Classification of queuing models.

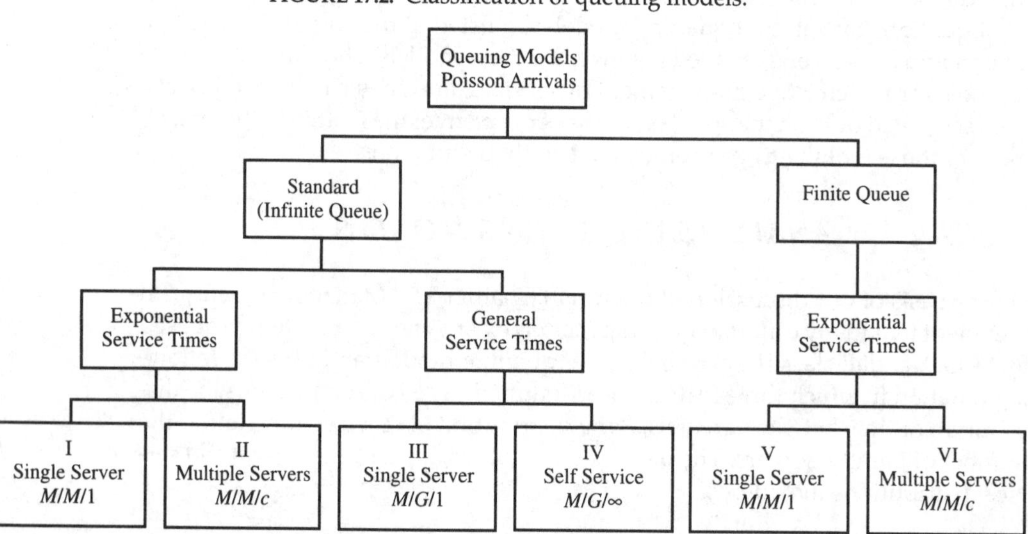

that is independent of the starting condition. All the queuing model equations given at the end of this chapter assume that a steady state has been reached. As noted in Chapter 11, most service systems operate in a dynamic environment, with arrival rates sometimes changing every hour; thus, a steady state seldom is achieved. However, steady-state models can provide useful system performance projections for long-range capacity planning decisions.

For each queuing model, the assumptions underlying its derivation are noted. The usefulness of an analytical model for a particular situation is limited by these assumptions. If the assumptions are invalid for a particular application, then one typically resorts to a computer-simulation approach.

Applications of these queuing models to decision-making situations use the equations listed at the end of the chapter and in Appendix B, "Values of L_q for the $M/M/c$ Queuing Model." The symbols used in these models and their definitions are:

n = number of customers in the system,
λ = [lambda] mean arrival rate (e.g., customer arrivals per hour),
μ = [mu] mean service rate per busy server (e.g., service capacity in customers per hour),
ρ = [rho] traffic intensity (λ/μ),
N = maximum number of customers allowed in the system,
c = number of servers,
P_n = probability of exactly n customers in the system,
L_s = mean number of customers in the system,
L_q = mean number of customers in queue,
L_b = mean number of customers in queue for a busy system,
W_s = mean time customer spends in the system,
W_q = mean time customer spends in the queue, and
W_b = mean time customer spends in queue for a busy system.

Standard M/M/1 *Model*

Every queuing model requires specific assumptions regarding the queuing system features as discussed in Chapter 11 (i.e., calling population, arrival process, queue configuration, queue discipline, and service process). The application of any queuing model, therefore, should include validation with respect to these assumptions. The derivation of the standard $M/M/1$ model requires the following set of assumptions about the queuing system:

1. *Calling population.* An infinite or very large population of callers arriving. The callers are independent of each other and not influenced by the queuing system (e.g., an appointment is not required).
2. *Arrival process.* Negative exponential distribution of interarrival times or Poisson distribution of arrival rate.
3. *Queue configuration.* Single waiting line with no restrictions on length and no balking or reneging.
4. *Queue discipline.* First-come, first-served (FCFS).
5. *Service process.* One server with negative exponential distribution of service times.

The selected equations at the end of this chapter can be used to calculate performance characteristics on the basis of only the mean arrival rate λ and the mean service rate per server μ. These equations clearly indicate why the mean arrival rate λ always must be *less* than the mean service rate μ for a single-server model. If this condition were not true and λ were equal to μ, the mean values for the operating characteristics would be undefined, because all the equations for mean values have the denominator $(\mu - \lambda)$. Theoretically, the system would never reach a steady state. In general, the system's capacity to serve, which is represented by $c\mu$ (i.e., number of servers times service rate per server), always must exceed the demand rate λ.

Example 17.1: Boat Ramp

Lake Travis has one launching ramp near the dam for people who trailer their small boats to the recreational site. A study of cars arriving with boats in tow indicates a Poisson distribution with a mean rate of $\lambda = 6$ boats per hour during the morning launch. A test of the data collected on launch times suggests that an exponential distribution with a mean of 6 minutes per boat (equivalent service rate $\mu = 10$ boats launched per hour) is a good fit. If the other assumptions for an $M/M/1$ model apply (i.e., infinite calling population, no queue length restrictions, no balking or reneging, and FCFS queue discipline), then the equations at the end of this chapter (and repeated here) may be used to calculate the system characteristics.
(Note: $\rho = \lambda/\mu = 6/10 = 0.6$.)

Probability that an arriving customer waits (i.e., $k = 1$):

$$P(n \geq 1) = \rho^1 = 0.6^1 = 0.6 \tag{I.2}$$

Probability of finding the ramp idle:

$$P_0 = 1 - \rho = 0.4 \tag{I.1}$$

Mean number of boats in the system:

$$L_s = \frac{\lambda}{\mu - \lambda} = \frac{6}{10 - 6} = 1.5 \text{ boats} \tag{I.4}$$

Mean number of boats in queue:

$$L_q = \frac{\rho\lambda}{\mu - \lambda} = \frac{(0.6)(6)}{10 - 6} = 0.9 \text{ boat} \tag{I.5}$$

Mean time in system:

$$W_s = \frac{1}{\mu - \lambda} = \frac{1}{10 - 6} = 0.25 \text{ hour (15 min.)} \tag{I.7}$$

Mean time in queue:

$$W_q = \frac{\rho}{\mu - \lambda} = \frac{0.6}{10 - 6} = 0.15 \text{ hour (9 min.)} \quad \text{(I.8)}$$

From our calculations, we find that the boat ramp is busy 60 percent of the time. Thus, arrivals can expect immediate access to the ramp without delay 40 percent of the time (i.e., when the ramp is idle). The calculations are internally consistent, because the mean time in system (W_s) of 15 minutes is the sum of the mean time in queue (W_q) of 9 minutes and the mean service time of 6 minutes. Arrivals can expect to find the number in the system (L_s) to be 1.5 boats and the expected number in queue (L_q) to be 0.9 boat. The expected number of boats in queue plus the expected number being launched should sum to the expected number of boats in the system. The expected number of boats being launched is not 1, the number of servers, however, but instead is calculated as:

$$\begin{aligned} \text{Expected number being served} &= \text{expected number when idle} + \text{expected number when busy} \\ &= P_0(0) \qquad + P(n > 0)(1) \\ &= (1 - \rho)(0) \qquad + \rho(1) \\ &= \rho \end{aligned}$$

Adding $\rho = 0.6$ person in the process of launching a boat and 0.9 boat on the average in queue, we get the expected 1.5 boats in the system.

Note that the number of customers in the system, n, is a random variable with a probability distribution given by equation (I.3), which is listed at the end of the chapter and repeated here in different form:

$$P_n = (1 - \rho)\rho^n \quad \text{(I.3)}$$

The number of customers in the system also can be used to identify system states. For example, when $n = 0$, the system is idle. When $n = 1$, the server is busy but no queue exists; when $n = 2$, the server is busy and a queue of 1 has formed. The probability distribution for n can be very useful in determining the proper size of a waiting room (i.e., the number of chairs) to accommodate arriving customers with a certain probability of assurance that each will find a vacant chair.

For the boat ramp example, determine the number of parking spaces needed to ensure that 90 percent of the time, a person arriving at the boat ramp will find a space to park while waiting to launch. Repeatedly using the probability distribution for system states for increasing values of n, we accumulate the system-state probabilities until 90 percent assurance is exceeded. Table 17.1 contains these calculations and indicates that a system state of $n = 4$ or less will occur 92 percent of the time. This suggests that room for four boat trailers should be provided, because 92 percent of the time, ar-

TABLE 17.1. Determining Required Number of Parking Spaces

n	P_n	P(number of customers $\leq n$)
0	$(0.4)(0.6)^0 = 0.4$	0.4
1	$(0.4)(0.6)^1 = 0.24$	0.64
2	$(0.4)(0.6)^2 = 0.144$	0.784
3	$(0.4)(0.6)^3 = 0.0864$	0.8704
4	$(0.4)(0.6)^4 = 0.05184$	0.92224

rivals will find three (i.e., four minus the one being served) or fewer people waiting in queue to launch.

Finite-Queue M/M/1 *Model*

A modification of the standard $M/M/1$ model can be made by introducing a restriction on the allowable number of customers in the system. Suppose that N represents the maximum number of customers allowed, or, in a single-server model, that $N - 1$ indicates the maximum number of customers in the queue. Thus, if a customer arrives at a point in time when N customers already are in the system, then the arrival departs without seeking service. An example of this type of *finite queue* is a telephone exchange in which callers are put on hold until all the trunk lines are in use; then, any further callers receive a busy signal. Except for this one characteristic of finite capacity, all the assumptions of the standard $M/M/1$ model still hold. Note that the traffic intensity ρ now may exceed unity. Further, P_N represents the probability of not joining the system, and λP_N is the expected number of customers who are lost.

This particular model is very useful in estimating lost sales to be expected from an inadequate waiting area or excessive queue length. In the boat ramp example, assume that the waiting area can accommodate only two boat trailers; thus, $N = 3$ for the system. Using equations (V.1) and (V.3) at the end of the chapter and repeated here, we can calculate the probabilities of 0, 1, 2, and 3 customers being in the system when $N = 3$ and $\rho = 0.6$:

$$P_0 = \frac{1-\rho}{1-\rho^{N+1}} \qquad \text{for } \lambda \neq \mu \tag{V.1}$$

$$P_n = P_0\rho^n \qquad \text{for } n \leq N \tag{V.3}$$

n	Calculation	P_n
0	$\frac{1-0.6}{1-0.6^4}(0.6)^0$	0.46
1	$(0.46)(0.6)^1$	0.27
2	$(0.46)(0.6)^2$	0.17
3	$(0.46)(0.6)^3$	0.10
		1.00

Note that this distribution totals 1.00, which indicates that we have accounted for all possible system states. System state $n = 3$ occurs 10 percent of the time. With an arrival rate of 6 people per hour, 0.6 person per hour (6×0.10) will find inadequate waiting space and look elsewhere for a launching site. Using equation (V.4), which is repeated here, we can calculate the expected number in the system (L_s): 0.9. This figure is much smaller than that in the unlimited-queue case, because on average, only 90 percent of the arrivals are processed.

$$L_s = \frac{\rho}{1-\rho} - \frac{(N+1)\rho^{N+1}}{1-\rho^{N+1}} \quad \text{for } \lambda \neq \mu \tag{V.4}$$

$$= \frac{0.6}{1-0.6} - \frac{4(0.6)^4}{1-(0.6)^4}$$

$$= 1.5 - 0.6$$

$$= 0.9$$

M/G/1 Model

For the $M/G/1$ model, any general service time distribution with mean $E(t)$ and variance $V(t)$ may be used. The condition that ρ be less than 1 still applies for the steady state, where ρ now equals $\lambda E(t)$. Except for the generality of the service time distribution, all the assumptions for the standard $M/M/1$ model apply. Unfortunately, an equation does not exist for determining the system-state probabilities; however, the list of equations at the end of the chapter does contain equations for L_s, L_q, W_s, and W_q. Equation (III.2) is repeated here, because the appearance of the service time variance term $V(t)$ provides some interesting insights:

$$L_q = \frac{\rho^2 + \lambda^2 V(t)}{2(1-\rho)} \tag{III.2}$$

Clearly, the expected number of customers waiting for service directly relates to the variability of service times. This suggests that customer waiting can be reduced by controlling the variability in service times. For example, the limited menu of fast-food restaurants contributes to their success, because such reduction in the variety of offered meals allows for standardization of service.

Recall from Chapter 11, Managing Queues, that the variance of the exponential distribution is $1/\mu^2$, and note that substituting this value for $V(t)$ in equation (III.2) yields $L_q = \rho^2/(1-\rho)$, which is equivalent to equation (I.5) for the standard $M/M/1$ model. Now consider the $M/D/1$ model, with a deterministic service time and zero variance. Again, according to equation (III.2), when $V(t) = 0$, then $L_q = \rho^2/[2(1-\rho)]$. Thus, one-half the congestion measured by L_q is explained by the variation in service times. This implies that the variability in time between arrivals accounts for the remaining congestion. Thus, considerable potential exists for reducing congestion simply by using appointments or reservations to control the variability in arrivals. Congestion in a queuing system is caused equally by variability in service times and interarrival times; therefore, strategies for controlling congestion should address both sources.

Standard **M/M/c** *Model*

The assumptions for the standard $M/M/c$ model are the same as those for the standard $M/M/1$ model, with the stipulation that service rates across channels be independent and equal (i.e., all servers are considered to be identical). As before, $\rho = \lambda/\mu$; however, ρ now must be less than c, the number of servers, for steady-state results to occur. If we define the system utilization factor as $\lambda/c\mu$, then for any steady-state system, the utilization factor must range between 0 and 1. Figure 17.3 illustrates the characteristic curves for L_s as a function of the utilization factor and c, the number of parallel servers. These curves graphically demonstrate the excessive congestion that occurs as one attempts to gain full utilization of service capacity.

The curves also can be used to demonstrate the disproportional gain that occurs when congestion is reduced by adding parallel servers. For example, consider a single-server system ($c = 1$) with a utilization factor of 0.8. From Figure 17.3, the value of L_s is 4. By adding another identical server, a two-channel system is created, and the utilization factor is reduced by one-half to 0.4. Figure 17.3 gives $L_s \approx 1$, and a 400-percent reduction in congestion is achieved just by doubling the number of servers.

Now, instead of creating a two-channel system, double the service rate of the single-server system and, thus, reduce the utilization factor to 0.4. Figure 17.3 gives $L_s \approx 0.67$ for this superserver system; however, this additional gain in reducing L_s is obtained at the cost of increasing the expected number in queue (from $L_q = 0.15$ to 0.27), as seen in Table 17.2. This is not surprising, because a single-server system would require more people to wait in line. In a multiple-server system of equal capacity, more people are able to be in service; thus, fewer wait in line. Therefore, the decision to use one superserver or the equiv-

FIGURE 17.3. $M/M/c$ model curves for L_s.

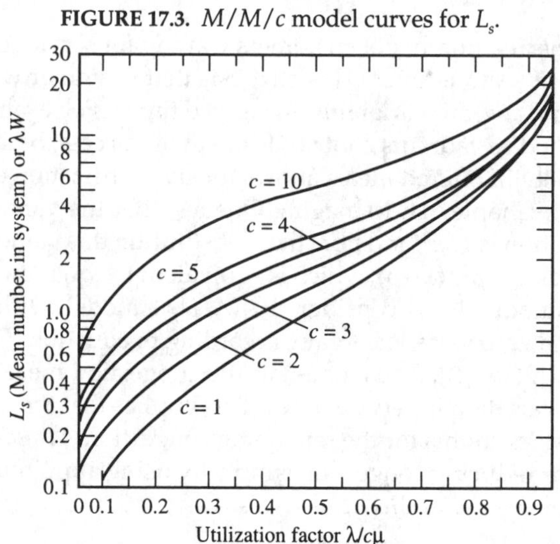

TABLE 17.2. Effects of Doubling Service Capacity

System Characteristic	Single-Server Baseline System	Two-Server System	Single-Superserver System
ρ	0.8	0.8	0.4
$(\lambda/c\mu)$*	0.8	0.4	0.4
L_s	4.0	0.95	0.67
L_q	3.2	0.15	0.27

*Utilization factor.

alent capacity with several servers in parallel depends on concern for the expected waiting time in queue (L_q/λ) or the expected time in system (L_s/λ). As noted in Chapter 11, a concern for reducing the waiting time in queue usually is advisable, particularly if people must physically wait in line. Further, once service begins, the customer's attitude toward time changes, because now the customer is the center of attention. The concept of using one large computer system to serve an entire university community often is justified, however, because short turnaround time (i.e., time in system) and large memory are of primary importance.

Consolidating the entire service capacity into a single superserver is one approach to achieving economies of scale in services. Another is the concept of pooling services, which is accomplished by gathering together independent servers at one central location to form a single service facility with multiple servers.

Example 17.2: The Secretarial Pool

A small business school has assigned a secretary to each of its four departments: accounting, finance, marketing, and management. The secretaries type class materials and correspondence only for their own departmental faculty. The dean has received complaints from the faculty, however, and particularly from the accounting faculty, about delays in getting work accomplished. The dean assigns an assistant to collect data on arrival rates and service times. After analyzing these data, the assistant reports that secretarial work arrives with a Poisson distribution at an average rate of $\lambda = 2$ requests per hour for all departments except accounting, which has an average rate of $\lambda = 3$ requests per hour. The average time to complete a piece of work is 15 minutes regardless of its source, and the service times are distributed exponentially.

Because of budget limitations, no additional secretaries can be hired. The dean believes, however, that service could be improved if all the secretaries were pooled and instructed to receive work from the entire business school faculty. All work requests would be received at one central location and processed on a first-come, first-served basis by the first secretary who became available, regardless of his or her departmental affiliation. Before proposing the plan to the faculty, the dean asks the assistant who collected the data to analyze the performance of the existing system and compare it with the pooling alternative.

The present system is essentially four $M/M/1$ independent, single-channel queuing systems, each with a service rate of $\mu = 4$ requests per hour. The appropriate measure of system performance is the expected time in the system—or turnaround time, from the faculty viewpoint. The difference in arrival rates should explain why the accounting faculty is particularly concerned about delays. Using the $M/M/1$ equation $W_s = 1/(\mu - \lambda)$, we find for the present system of independent departmental secretaries that accounting faculty members experience an average turnaround time of $W_s = 1/(4-3) =$ 1.0 hour, or 60 minutes, and the faculty members in the other departments experience an average turnaround time of $W_s = 1/(4-2) = 0.5$ hour, or 30 minutes.

The proposal to pool the secretarial staff creates a multiple-channel, single-queue system, or an $M/M/4$ system in this case. The arrival rate is the combined arrivals $(2+2+2+3)$ from all departments, or $\lambda = 9$ requests per hour. Equation (II.1), which is repeated here with $c = 4$ and $\rho = 9/4$, is used to calculate the value of P_0:

$$P_0 = \frac{1}{\left(\sum_{i=0}^{c-1} \frac{\rho^i}{i!}\right) + \frac{\rho^c}{c!(1-\rho/c)}} \tag{II.1}$$

$$\begin{aligned} P_0 &= \frac{1}{\frac{(9/4)^0}{0!} + \frac{(9/4)^1}{1!} + \frac{(9/4)^2}{2!} + \frac{(9/4)^3}{3!} + \frac{(9/4)^4}{4!(1-9/16)}} \\ &= \frac{1}{1 + 9/4 + \frac{81/16}{2} + \frac{729/64}{6} + \frac{6561/256}{24(7/16)}} \\ &= \frac{1}{7.68 + 2.44} \\ &= 0.098 \end{aligned}$$

Equation (II.4), which is repeated here, is used to calculate the value of L_s:

$$L_s = \frac{\rho^{c+1}}{(c-1)!(c-\rho)^2} P_0 + \rho \tag{II.4}$$

$$\begin{aligned} &= \frac{(9/4)^5}{(4-1)!(4-9/4)^2}(0.098) + 9/4 \\ &= \frac{59{,}049/1024}{6(1.75)^2}(0.098) + 2.25 \\ &= 0.31 + 2.25 \\ &= 2.56 \end{aligned}$$

$$W_s = \frac{L_s}{\lambda} = \frac{2.56}{9} = 0.28 \text{ hour, or 17 minutes}$$

The substantial reduction in expected turnaround time from 30 minutes (60 minutes for the accounting faculty) to 17 minutes should easily win faculty approval.

The benefits from pooling are achieved through better utilization of idle secretaries. Under the departmental system, four independent queues existed, which allowed situations to develop in which a secretary in one department could be burdened with a long waiting line of work whereas a secretary in another department was idle. If a waiting request could be transferred to the idle secretary, then it would be processed immediately. Switching to a single queue avoids the utilization problem by not allowing a secretary to become idle until the waiting line of requests is empty.

Because calculations for the $M/M/c$ model are so tedious, we tyically use Appendix B, Values of L_q for the $M/M/c$ Queuing Model, to solve for L_q. For this problem, in which $c = 4$ and $\rho = 2.25$, we find $L_q = 0.31$ by interpolation and, thus, $L_s = L_q + \rho = 2.56$.

The success of pooling service resources comes from realizing that congestion results from variation in the rate of arrivals and service times. If a total systems perspective of the process is taken, temporary idleness at one location can be used to reduce congestion at another that has been caused by a temporary surge in demand or time-consuming requests. Further, server idleness that can be put to use but is not represents lost service capacity and results in a deterioration of service quality as measured by customer waiting. The concept of pooling need not apply only to servers who are at different locations. The common practice in banks and post offices of having customers form a single queue rather than line up in front of the individual windows represents an application of the pooling concept. Theoretically, the average waiting time is reduced from that of multiple queues; however, the single long line may give arriving customers the impression of long waits. This is the reason McDonald's gave for abandoning the idea: it was feared that customers would balk on seeing a long line.

Pooling service resources at one location should be undertaken with some caution if customers must travel to that facility. In this case, the expected travel time to the facility should be included with the expected waiting time in queue when the proposal is evaluated. For emergency services, dispersing servers throughout the service area generally is preferred to assigning all services to one central location. An emergency ambulance system is a particularly good example of this need for physically dispersed servers to minimize response time.

Finite-Queue M/M/c *Model*

This finite-queue $M/M/c$ model is similar to the finite-queue $M/M/1$ model, with the exception that N, the maximum number in the system, must be equal to or greater than c, the number of servers. An arriving customer is rejected if the number in the system equals N or the length of the queue is $N - c$. All other assumptions for the standard $M/M/c$ model hold, except that ρ now can exceed c. Because excess customers are rejected, the system can reach a steady state even when the capacity is inadequate to meet the total demand (i.e., $\lambda > c\mu$).

An interesting variation on this model is the no-queue situation, which occurs when no possibility exists for a customer to wait—because a waiting area is not provided. This situation can be modeled as a finite-queue system with

$N = c$. A parking lot is an illustration of this no-queue situation. If we consider each parking space as a server, then when the parking lot is completely full, an opportunity for further service no longer exists and future arrivals must be rejected. If c equals the number of parking spaces, then the parking lot system can be modeled as a no-queue variation of the finite-queue $M/M/c$ model.

General Self-Service M/G/∞ Model

If a multiple-server system has an infinite number of servers or arrivals serve themselves, then no arriving customer must wait for service. This, of course, describes exactly the concept that has made the modern supermarket so popular. At least during the shopping portion (excluding checkout), customers do not experience waiting. The number of customers in the process of shopping does vary because of random arrivals and differing service times, and the probability distribution of the number of customers in the system can be calculated by means of equation (IV.1), which is repeated here. Note that this distribution for P_n in fact is Poisson, with the mean, or L_s, being equal to ρ. Further, this model is not restricted to an exponential distribution of service times.

$$P_n = \frac{e^{-\rho}}{n!}\rho^n \qquad \text{where } L_s = \rho \tag{IV.1}$$

This model also is useful as an approximation to describe circumstances in which waiting only rarely may occur (e.g., emergency ambulance services). Using the Poisson distribution of the number of customers in the system, we can calculate the number of servers that are required to ensure that the probability of someone waiting is quite small.

Example 17.3: Supermarket

The typical supermarket can be viewed as two queuing systems in tandem. The arriving customer secures a shopping cart and proceeds to serve himself or herself by picking items from the shelves. On completing this task, the shopper joins a single queue (a new idea to reduce waiting caused by multiple queues) behind the checkout registers.

The checker tallies the bill, makes change, and sacks the groceries. The shopper then exits this system, perhaps with the assistance of a carryout person. T. L. Saaty's observation that departures from the standard $M/M/c$ queuing system also are Poisson-distributed suggests that the supermarket system can be analyzed as two independent systems in series.[2] The first is self-service shopping, or $M/M/\infty$, system, and the second (at the cash registers) is an $M/M/c$ system. Observation of customer behavior indicates that arrivals are Poisson-distributed, with a rate of 30 per hour, and that shopping is completed in 20 minutes on the average, with exponential distribution. Shoppers then join the single queue behind the three checkout registers and wait until a register becomes available. The checkout process requires 5 minutes on average, with exponential distribution.

For the shopping experience, the $M/M/\infty$ model applies, with $\rho = 30/3$, resulting in $L_s = 10$ customers on the average being engaged in the shopping

[2]T. L. Saaty, *Elements of Queuing Theory with Applications*, McGraw-Hill, New York, 1961.

activity. To study the checkout system we use Appendix B with $c = 3$ and $\rho = 30/12 = 2.5$, and find that $L_q = 3.5$. The average number of customers in the checkout area $L_s = L_q + \rho = 6$ customers. Together, we find on average a total of 16 shoppers in the store. The expected time that a customer spends in the supermarket is 20 minutes shopping plus 12 minutes (i.e., $L_s/\lambda = 6/30 = 0.2$ hour) checking out, for a total of 32 minutes.

GENERAL RELATIONSHIPS BETWEEN SYSTEM CHARACTERISTICS

In concluding the discussion of queuing models, it is necessary to point out some general relationships between the average system characteristics that exist across all models. The first two relationships are definitional in nature.

First, the expected number in the system should equal the expected number in queue plus the expected number in service, or

$$L_s = L_q + E\,(\text{number in service}) \tag{1}$$

Note that E (number in service) is not the number of servers. It equals ρ for all models except the finite-queue case.

Second, the expected time in the system should equal the expected time in queue plus the expected time in service, or

$$W_s = W_q + \frac{1}{\mu} \tag{2}$$

where $1/\mu$ is the reciprocal of the service rate.

The characteristics for a busy system are conditional values that are based on the probability that the system is busy, or $P(n \geq c)$. Thus, the expected number in queue for a busy system simply is the expected number under all system states divided by the probability of the system being busy, or

$$L_b = \frac{L_q}{P(n \geq c)} \tag{3}$$

Similarly, the expected waiting time in queue for a busy system is

$$W_b = \frac{W_q}{P(n \geq c)} \tag{4}$$

Further, the following relationship exists between the expected number in the system and the expected time in the system[3]:

$$W_s = \frac{1}{\lambda} L_s \tag{5}$$

[3]J. D. C. Little, "A Proof of the Queuing Formula: $L = \lambda W$," *Operations Research*, vol. 9, no. 3, May–June 1961, pp. 383–387; W. S. Jewell, "A Simple Proof of $L = \lambda W$," *Operations Research*, vol. 15, no. 6, November–December 1967, pp. 1109–1116; S. Stidham, Jr., "A Last Word on $L = \lambda W$," *Operations Research*, vol. 22, no. 2, March–April 1974, pp. 417–421.

The following relationship between the expected number in queue and the expected waiting time also exists:

$$W_q = \frac{1}{\lambda} L_q \tag{6}$$

When equations (5) and (6) are applied to systems with a finite queue, an effective arrival rate must be used for λ. For a system with a finite queue, the effective arrival rate is $\lambda(1 - P_N)$.

These relationships are very useful, because they permit all the average characteristics of a system to be derived from the knowledge of one characteristic obtained by analysis or the collection of data on actual system performance.

CAPACITY PLANNING CRITERIA

Queuing theory indicates that in the long run, capacity to serve must exceed the demand. If this criterion is not met, at least one of the following adjustments must occur:

1. Excessive waiting by customers will result in some reneging (i.e., a customer leaves the queue before being served) and, thus, in some reduction of demand.
2. Excessive waiting, if known or observed by potential customers, will cause them to reconsider their need for service and, thus, will reduce demand.
3. Under the pressure of long waiting lines, servers may speed up, spending less time with each customer, and, thus, increase service capacity. A gracious and leisurely manner, however, now becomes curt and impersonal.
4. Sustained pressure to hurry may result in eliminating time-consuming features and performing the bare minimum and, thus, service capacity is increased.

These uncontrolled situations result from inadequate service capacity, which can be avoided through rational capacity planning.

Several approaches to capacity planning are explored on the basis of different criteria for evaluating service system performance. Determining the desired level of service capacity implies a tradeoff between the cost of service and the cost of customer waiting, as suggested by Figure 17.1. Thus, capacity analysis will utilize the queuing models to predict customer waiting for various levels of service.

Average Customer Waiting Time

The criterion of average customer waiting time for capacity planning can be appropriate in several circumstances. For example, a restaurant owner may wish to promote liquor sales in the bar and, therefore, stipulates that customers be kept waiting 5 minutes on average for a table. It has been suggested that because the face of a watch typically is divided into 5-minute increments, people who are waiting in line may not realize how long they have been waiting until at least 5 minutes have passed. Therefore, in designing a drive-in bank facility, it may be advisable to have customers wait no more than 5 minutes on average for service. In a study of a health clinic, the appointment system was changed to meet increasing demand, but the same average waiting time for patients was maintained.[4] In these cases, use of the $M/M/c$ model would be appropriate to identify the service capacity in terms of the number of servers that would guarantee the desired expected customer waiting time.

Example 17.4: Drive-in Bank

Excessive congestion is a problem during the weekday noon hour at a downtown drive-in bank facility. Bank officials fear customers may take their accounts elsewhere unless service is improved. A study of customer arrivals during the noon hour indicates an average arrival rate of 30 per hour, with Poisson distribution. Banking transactions take 3 minutes on average, with exponential distribution. Because of the layout of the drive-in facility, arriving customers must select one of three lanes for service. Once a customer is in a lane, it is impossible for him or her to renege or jockey between lanes because of separating medians. Assuming that arriving customers select lanes at random, we can treat the system as parallel, independent, single-channel queuing systems with the arrival rate divided evenly among the tellers. If the bank officers agree to a criterion that customers should wait no more than 5 minutes on average, how many drive-in tellers are required? Because we are concerned only with customers who actually wait, equation (I.9), which is repeated here, is appropriate:

$$W_b = \frac{1}{\mu - \lambda} \tag{I.9}$$

For the current three-teller system, arrivals per teller $\lambda = 30/3 = 10$ per hour. Thus, $W_b = 1/(20 - 10) = 0.1$ hour, or 6 minutes. Table 17.3 indicates that one additional teller is required to meet the service criterion.

Probability of Excessive Waiting

For public services that have difficulty identifying the economic cost of waiting, a service level often is specified. This service level is stated in a manner such that P or more percent of all customers should experience a delay of less than T time units. For example, a federal guideline states that the response time for 95 per-

[4] E. J. Rising, R. Baron, and B. Averill, "A Systems Analysis of a University Health-Service Outpatient Clinic," *Operations Research*, vol. 21, no. 5, September 1973, pp. 1030–1047.

TABLE 17.3. Expected Time in Queue for Bank Teller Alternatives

Tellers (n)	λ per Teller	μ	W_b (min)
3	10	20	6
4	7.5	20	4.8

cent of all ambulance calls should be less than 10 minutes for urban and less than 30 minutes for rural systems. The Public Utilities Commission gives a similar performance criterion for telephone service, directing that telephone service must be provided at a resource level such that 89 percent of the time, an incoming call can be answered within 10 seconds. A probability distribution of delays is required to identify service levels that will meet these probabilities of not exceeding a certain excessive delay, and equations for these delay probabilities are available for the standard $M/M/c$ model.[5] For the case when no delay is desired ($T = 0$), equation (II.3) can be used to find a value for c such that the probability of immediate service is at least P percent.

Example 17.5: Self-Serve Gas Station

A retail gasoline distributor plans to construct a self-service filling station on vacant property leading into a new housing development. On the basis of the traffic in that area, the distributor forecasts a demand of 48 cars on average per hour. Furthermore, this demand will be divided equally between those seeking regular and those seeking unleaded fuels. Time studies that have been conducted at other sites reveal an average self-service time of 5 minutes for a driver to fill the tank, pay the cashier, and drive away. The service times are distributed exponentially, and past experience justifies assuming an arrival rate with a Poisson distribution. Because of the two types of fuel being offered, the queuing system can be modeled as two independent $M/M/c$ systems in parallel, each with a mean arrival rate of $\lambda = 24$ customers per hour. The distributor believes that the success of self-service stations results from competitive gasoline prices and the customers' desires for fast service. Therefore, the distributor would like to install enough regular and unleaded pumps to guarantee that arriving customers will find a free pump at least 95 percent of the time. We use equation (II.3) to calculate the probability that a customer waits for various values of c, and results for up to six-pumps are summarized in Table 17.4. When $c = 6$, the $P(n \geq c)$ reaches a value of 0.02 and, thus, meets the criterion that fewer than 5 percent of arriving customers having to wait. This result suggests that six pumps should be installed for regular gas and six for unleaded.

Minimizing the Sum of Customer Waiting Costs and Service Costs

If both customers and servers are members of the same organization, then the costs of providing service and employee waiting are equally important to the or-

[5]Saaty, op. cit.

TABLE 17.4. Probability of Finding All Gas Pumps in Use

c	P_0	$P(n \geq c)$
3	0.11	0.44
4	0.13	0.27
5	0.134	0.06
6	0.135	0.02

ganization's effectiveness. This situation arises, for example, when organizations rely on a captive service, such as a secretarial pool or a computer facility. In these cases, the cost of employees' waiting time is at least equal to their average salary, and in fact, this cost could be considerably more if all the implications of waiting, such as the frustration of not completing a task or the effect of delays on others in the organization, are assessed.

The economic tradeoff depicted in Figure 17.1 best describes this situation in which the capacity to serve may be increased by adding servers. As servers are added, the cost of service increases, but this cost is offset by a corresponding decrease in the cost of waiting. Adding both costs results in a convex total-cost curve for the organization that identifies a service capacity with minimum combined costs. The queuing models are used to predict the expected waiting time of employees for different levels of capacity, and the values are substituted in the total-cost function here.

Assuming linear cost functions for service and waiting and comparing alternatives based on steady-state performance, we calculate the total cost per unit of time (hour) as:

$$\begin{aligned} \text{Total cost per hour} &= \text{hourly cost of service} + \text{hourly waiting cost} \\ TC &= C_sC + C_w\lambda W_s \\ &= C_sC + C_wL_s \end{aligned} \qquad (7)$$

where

C = number of servers,
C_s = hourly cost per server, and
C_w = hourly cost of waiting customer.

Recall that equation (5) converts λW_s, the number of arriving customers per hour times the average waiting time per customer, to its equivalent, L_s. For equation (7), waiting is defined as time in system; however, if waiting in queue is more appropriate, then L_q is substituted for L_s. In situations in which service is self-service, such as using a copying or a fax machine, waiting in queue might be justified.

Example 17.6: Computer Terminal Selection

The director of a large engineering staff is considering the rental of several computer terminals that will permit the staff to interact directly with the computer. On the basis of a survey of the staff, the director finds that the department will generate, on average, eight requests per hour for service, and the engineers estimate that the average computer analysis will require 15 minutes. A computer terminal that is adequate for these needs rents for $10 per hour. When the average salary of the engineering staff is considered, the cost of keeping an engineer idle is $30 per hour. For a "quick and dirty" analysis, the director assumes that requests for service are Poisson distributed and that user times are exponentially distributed. Further, the engineering staff is large enough to assume an infinite calling population. Using the $M/M/c$ model with $\rho = 8/4 = 2$ and Appendix B to calculate L_q, the director obtains the results shown in Table 17.5.

Note that L_q is used instead of L_s in the calculations, because the computer terminals are self-serve devices. The results indicate that four termi-

TABLE 17.5. Total Cost of Computer Terminal Alternatives

C	L_q	C_sC (\$)	C_wL_q (\$)	TC (\$)
3	0.88	30	26.4	56.4
4	0.17	40	5.1	45.1
5	0.04	50	1.2	51.2
6	0.01	60	0.3	60.3

nals will minimize the combined costs of rent for the terminals and salary for the waiting engineers.

Our assumption of waiting costs being linear with time, as shown in equation (7), is suspect, because as the delay increases, a larger percentage of customers become dissatisfied and vocal, possibly creating a mass exodus. Taguchi's concept of a quadratic quality loss function as described in Chapter 10, "Service Quality" seems to be more appropriate, particularly when alternative service is available from a competitor. First, the longer the wait, the more irritated customers become and the greater the probability that they will take their future business elsewhere. In addition, they will tell friends and relatives of their bad experiences, which also will affect future sales. Finally, the loss of an immediate sale is small compared with the future stream of lost revenues when a customer is lost forever. In practice, however, the linear assumption usually is made because of the difficulty of determining a customer waiting cost function.

Probability of Sales Lost Because of Inadequate Waiting Area

This planning criterion concerns capacity of the waiting area rather than capacity to serve. An inadequate waiting area may cause potential customers to balk and seek service elsewhere. This problem is of particular concern where arriving customers can see the waiting area, such as the parking lot at a restaurant or the driveway at a drive-in bank. Analysis of these systems uses the finite-queue $M/M/c$ model to estimate the number of balking customers.

If N is the maximum number of customers allowed in the system, then P_N is the probability of a customer arriving and finding the system to be full. Thus, P_N represents the probability of sales lost because of an inadequate waiting area, and λP_N represents the expected number of sales lost per unit of time. The cost of sales lost because of an inadequate waiting area now can be compared with the possible investment in additional space.

Example 17.7: Downtown Parking Lot

A parking lot is a multiple-server queuing system without a queue; that is, the lot can be considered a service system in which each parking space is a server. After the lot is full, subsequent arrivals are rejected, because the system has no provision for a queue. Thus, a parking lot is a finite-queuing system with a queue capacity of zero, because $N = c$.

With this model in mind, an enterprising student notes the availability of a vacant lot in the central business district. The student learns from a real estate agent that the owner is willing to rent the property as a parking lot for \$50 a day until a buyer is found. After making some observations of traffic in the area, the student finds that approximately ten cars per hour have difficulty finding space in the parking garage of the department store across the street from the vacant lot. The garage attendant reports that customers spend approximately 1 hour shopping in the store. To calculate the feasibility of this venture, the student assumes that arrivals are Poisson distributed and that shopping times are exponentially distributed. The student is interested in what potential business is lost because the lot has room for only six cars.

This parking lot can be considered an $M/M/c$ finite-queuing system with no provision for a queue. Therefore, equations for the finite-queue $M/M/c$ model are calculated with $c = N$. Substituting for $c = N$ in equations (VI.1), (VI.2), (VI.4), and (VI.7) yields the following results for the no-queue case. No other equations are applicable.

$$P_0 = \frac{1}{\sum_{i=0}^{N} \frac{\rho^i}{i!}} \tag{8}$$

$$P_n = \frac{\rho^n}{n!} P_0 \tag{9}$$

$$L_s = \rho(1 - P_N) \tag{10}$$

$$W_s = \frac{1}{\mu} \left(\text{Note: } L_q = 0\right) \tag{11}$$

With $\lambda = 10$, $N = 6$, and $\mu = 1$ we calculate $P_0 = 0.000349$ using Equation (8) and calculate $P_6 = 0.48$ using Equation (9). Thus, of the ten arriving customers per hour, approximately one-half ($10 \times 0.48 = 4.8$) find the lot full. Therefore, this lot with a capacity of six cars serves approximately one-half the demand.

Requirement That Expected Profit on Last Unit of Capacity Should Just Exceed Expected Loss

This capacity planning criterion does not rely on use of queuing models; rather, it relies on an economic principle called *marginal analysis*, which was discussed in Chapter 12, "Managing Facilitating Goods." This approach is useful when a capacity decision must be made in which losses are associated both with inadequate and excess capacity. This capacity problem typically arises during the facility design phase, such as when decisions are made concerning the seating capacity of a restaurant or movie theater. In addition to an estimate of the unit profit per customer and possible loss, the analysis requires a probability distribution for the service demand.

The *critical fractile*, which was derived in Chapter 12, is shown here. It requires the expected revenue on the last sale to exceed the expected loss on the last sale.

$$P(d < x) \leq \frac{C_u}{C_u + C_o} \tag{12}$$

where

C_u = unit contribution from potential sale, cost of *under*estimating demand (inadequate capacity);
C_o = unit loss from idle capacity, cost of *over*estimating demand (excess capacity);
d = demand; and
x = capacity (e.g., airline seats, hotel rooms).

Example 17.8: Paradise Tours

For the past several years, Paradise Tours has offered a Hawaiian adventure package each summer that has attracted a good though variable-sized group of vacationers from the local university. A review of past records suggests that demand for this tour is distributed normally, with a mean of 50, standard deviation of 10, and no trend indicated. Paradise Tours reserves seats with a regularly scheduled airline at a special, reduced, affinity-group rate. This policy enables the airline to attract small groups that are not large enough to charter an entire plane. The airline also allows the travel agent to charge a $30 service fee in addition to the ticket price; however, a major concern of Paradise is the $10 charge by the airline for each unsold reserved seat. The airline is concerned about tying up seats during the peak season and also wants to prevent oversubscription by travel agents. Paradise has been reserving 50 seats and finds that it has no record of ever paying the $10 overbooking charge. Should it continue this reservation policy?

Using equation (12), we calculate the following critical fractile:

$$P(d < x) \leq \frac{30}{30 + 10} \leq 0.75$$

From Appendix A, "Areas of a Standard Normal Distribution," the z value for 0.75 is 0.68. Thus, the number of seats to reserve is determined as:

$$\begin{aligned} \text{Reserved seats} &= \mu + z\sigma \\ &= 50 + (0.68)(10) \\ &= 56 \text{ (rounded down because of inequality)} \end{aligned}$$

SUMMARY

When their assumptions are met, analytical queuing models can help service system managers to evaluate possible alternative courses of action by predicting waiting time statistics. The models also provide insights that help to explain such queuing phenomena as pooling, the effect of finite queues on realized demand, the nonproportional effects of adding servers on waiting time, and the importance of controlling demand as seen by reducing service time variance. The approach to capacity planning depends on the criterion of system performance being used. Further, queuing models are useful in the analysis because of their ability to predict system performance. If the queuing model assumptions are not met or the system is too complex, however, then computer-simulation modeling is required.

KEY TERMS AND DEFINITIONS

***A/B/C* classification of queuing models** where *A* stands for the arrival distribution, *B* for the service time distribution, and *C* for number of servers in a parallel-server queuing system.

Critical fractile a cumulative probability of customer demand that will be accommodated by an optimal level of capacity.

Finite queue a queue that is limited physically (e.g., a limited number of parking spaces).

Steady state the condition of a system when distribution of its characteristics, such as the number of customers in queue, becomes stationary regarding time (i.e., the system has moved out of an initial transient state and reached statistical equilibrium).

TOPICS FOR DISCUSSION

1. For a queuing system with a finite queue, the arrival rate can exceed the capacity to serve. Use an example to explain how this is feasible.
2. What are some disadvantages associated with the concept of pooling service resources?
3. Capacity planning using queuing models usually is applied to strategic decisions rather than to day-to-day operations. Explain.
4. Discuss how the $M/G/\infty$ model could be used to determine the number of emergency medical vehicles that are required to serve a community.
5. Discuss how one could determine the economic cost of keeping customers waiting.

Service Benchmark

Simulation Modeling for Process Reengineering in the Telecommunications Industry

Traditionally, firms have used simulation modeling to analyze manufacturing processes and to evaluate production management strategies. More recently, they have used it to analyze various service processes. U S WEST Communications has used a service process model to analyze the installation (provisioning) process of a high-capacity fiber-optic telecommunications service. This process is a sequence of tasks that includes interaction with the customer, verification of available facilities, changes to billing information, and testing equipment. Managers who need to design and improve the process frequently make decisions based on intuition, historical patterns, or descriptive statistics drawn from insurmountable amounts of raw data. We developed a process simulation model to support the managers in designing and reengineering the service process. The model enables managers to gain insight that will help them control the current complex service flow. This insight and an analysis of the process help them to identify areas that need reengineering and to predict the quantitative impact of reengineering efforts.

Business process reengineering, a term coined by Hammer and Champy,[6] is the managerial paradigm that many businesses need to radically change the organizational structure of a business process and the policies and methods by which the process operates in order to achieve significant improvements. It is an alternative to "continuous improvement," which aims to incrementally improve existing outdated structures within the process, leaving the fundamental framework of the process intact. Process reengineering, in contrast, emphasizes the overall improvement of a process with respect to its quality, cost, and efficiency. Process simulation modeling allows us to observe the work flows within a service process in their entirety. We can thus easily identify key service functions and subsequently improve, consolidate, or dissolve them through process reengineering.

The modeling group used simulation modeling to reflect the current status of a service process and to quantify the impact of changes imposed on the process by tracking performance measures. By reflecting the dynamics of a service process, our simulation model has helped managers determine why and where they should reengineer processes. It also helps them to establish tangible management goals. For example, it can help them determine when and how much to increase the work force to maintain or to improve current service cycle times. It can also help them determine how much to spend for improvements to information systems that automate or simplify tasks within the process. Simulation modeling provides us with quantitative service performance measures, such as queue length, total cycle time, and idle time at each service center, that help managers allocate their resources.

DS1 (digital signal level 1) networks are high-capacity, high-speed (1.5 Mb/sec) data transfer pathways used primarily by long distance carriers, large businesses, and government agencies. As shown in the figure, the DS1 service process originates with the arrival of a service request from a long distance carrier at the interexchange carrier service center (ICSC) or from a business or government customer at the market unit (MU) service center. ICSC (or MU) confirms the request and issues a service order to a high-capacity provisioning center (HCPC) that generates an engineering specification "work order record details" (WORD). However, if the customer or the service representative at the ICSC or the MU made errors in receiving or issuing the service order, the HCPC issues a "supplement order" and sends it back to the ICSC or the MU for correction. At the HCPC, we have three pathways for the WORD.

First, if the necessary facilities are already in place to handle the request (a preprovisioned request), we send the WORD directly to the digital services operations center (DSOC) for execution. Second, we may send the WORD to the interoffice facilities current planning center (IFCPC), which orders the materials necessary to fill the request. Third, we may send the WORD to the construction management center (CMC), which is responsible for building new conduits or for attaching new facilities to existing conduits. Once the IFCPC has or-

[6]Michael Hammer and James Champy, *Reengineering the Corporation*, Harper Business, New York, 1994.

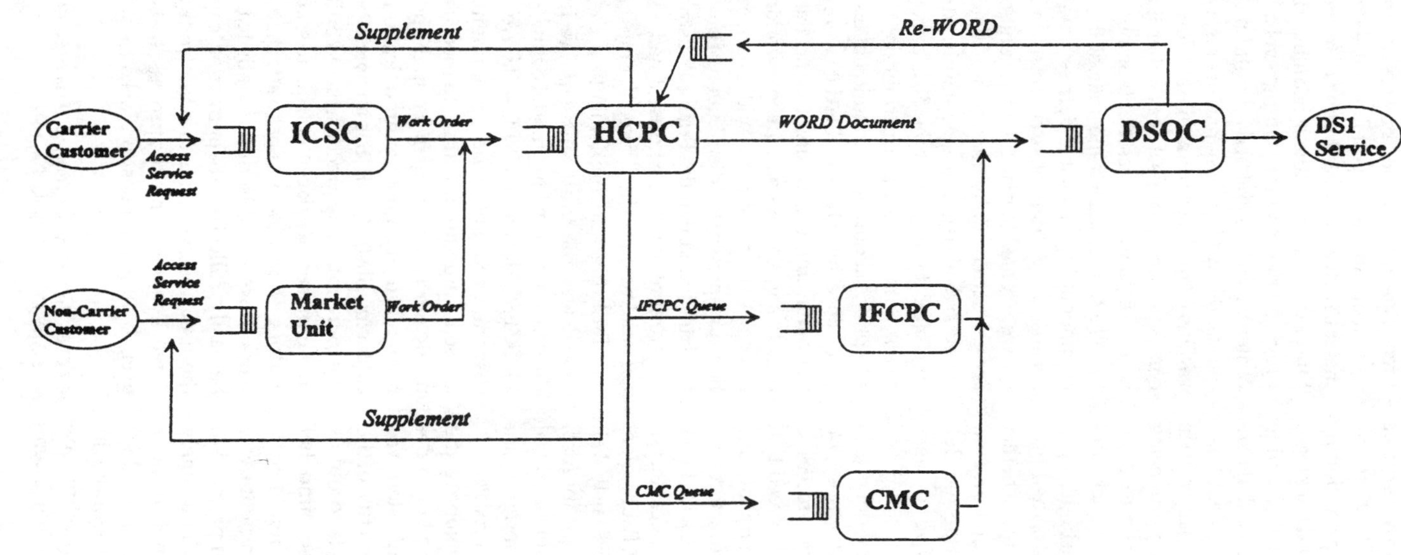

U S WEST high-capacity digital signal queuing network. (Youngho Lee and Amie Elcan, "Simulation Modeling for Process Reengineering in the Telecommunications Industry," *Interfaces*, vol. 26, no. 3, May–June 1996, p. 3.)

dered the materials or CMC has completed, we notify the DSOC to execute the work order to install the service. However, if the DSOC discovers errors made by the HCPC, it sends "re-WORD" to the HCPC for modification. Because this provisioning process includes both forward flows and backward flows, we conceptualized it as a stochastic queuing network model. In the model, we assumed that handling an error takes 50 percent of the time it takes to handle a normal order at each processing center. We also experimented with several sequencing rules, including the shortest-processing-time rule, to assign priorities to service requests at each processing center. That is, we assigned the highest priority to preprovisioned requests because their processing time is shortest. We did this to test whether we could reduce overall average cycle time and improve the percentage of customer-requested due date commitments. Below, we discuss five key steps of process simulation modeling in turn.

Our first step in constructing the model was to determine its primary objective and scope. We talked to the managers supervising the process to gather the modeling requirements and agreed that the primary focus of the model should be analyzing the impact of changes in demand, work force, or error rate on the cycle time of connecting a DS1 line, from the service request to the final physical installation. The scope is the Minneapolis/St. Paul region, because this region represents U S WEST fairly well in terms of demand pattern and service quality. Also, we decided to model only the centers most critical to the provisioning process, with small insignificant processes being aggregated as a single process.

Our second crucial step in developing the model was gathering the data we needed to develop a stochastic queuing model. This step was closely tied in with determining the objective of the model, because the lack of detailed data forced us to reevaluate the scope of the model. We found that the lack of relevant data prevented us from modeling the true service process. Collecting data was one of the most challenging steps in our project. We initially had difficulty obtaining data in a timely manner because many managers did not consider gathering data important until they were pressured by their supervisors. Also, getting those working in the service centers to agree on common definitions was challenging and time-consuming. For example, we spent a lot of time coming to an agreement on exactly what a "supplement order" is or on the precise meaning of the "processing time" of a task.

In our model, we established several key parameters, such as the distribution of service processing times, the error rate, the scheduling rules, the preprovision rate, and the staffing level at each process center as well as the arrival pattern of service requests. By varying these parameters, we performed various what-if scenario analyses. However, since the complete input data set was either inaccessible or would require an unreasonable amount of resources to collect, we adjusted the scale of the model to accommodate the available data sets. As an example, because arrival data were collected on a daily basis, we were forced to make the time unit of the request arrival pattern daily, though we would have preferred arrival data collected hourly. After collecting suitable data sets, we fit the distribution of daily arrivals with a Weibull distribution and made assumptions about the distribution of task-processing times since the only available data were estimates for the minimum, the maximum, and the mean times based on interviews with people working within the centers. We experimented with exponential distributions to represent the distribution of processing times but later found that the Erlang II distribution was a better representation because it had a smaller right tail and less mass distributed at times close to zero.

Building and implementing the simulation model was the third key step. We implemented the conceptual queuing model on the PC with SIMPROCESS, developed by CACI.[7] We selected this discrete event simulation programming tool because its animation feature helped us to communicate with the managers. From the beginning, we recognized that good communication was a critical factor. SIMPROCESS is an object-based modeling tool containing preconstructed building blocks that represent work centers, queues, and item generators. These blocks may be attached to represent work flows, and descriptive statistical results may be easily collected. Its animation capabilities let the user observe items moving from work center to work center within the process. It also allows the user to attach queues to blocks to capture work-

[7]CACI Products Company, *Reference Manual for SIMFACTORY II.5 and SIMPROCESS*, La Jolla, CA, 1992.

center delay times. The fourth key step in implementing our simulation model was to maintain close contact with the managers at the process centers to verify that the model's intermediate results were valid. This required several visits to interview people working in the centers. Their feedback during the preliminary stages of model development was crucial in verifying that the model accurately represented work flow through the centers.

The fifth and final step was to analyze the model results and present recommendations to managers. Once we had verified that the model output closely reflected previously known estimates of cycle times, we conducted what-if experiments by varying key process parameters. This analysis enabled us to predict the quantitative impact of the process parameters on the cycle time. To do the analysis, we had to develop an appropriate experimental design. We ran the model five to 10 times under each scenario and computed 95-percent confidence intervals for average cycle times, utilization rates, and work-center delay times under steady-state conditions.

We ran the models using a set of five what-if scenarios provided by U S WEST process managers. We carried out these five scenarios under three different error rates, 5, 20, and 50 percent. We ran the simulation model for a period of six months using daily time intervals, while we observed the total average cycle time as a key performance measure. A primary observation was that a decrease in error rate diminishes the impact of increases in demand and decreases in the work force. Also, we measured the performance of the process centers by tracking their queue lengths and utilization rates. These observations led us to believe that the error rate is a driving force in process improvement. Accordingly, we recommended that process reengineering teams should focus on decreasing error rates and on mechanizing certain manual processes to compensate for the increase in cycle times under various scenarios.

Source: Adapted from Youngho Lee and Amie Elcan, "Simulation Modeling for Process Reengineering in the Telecommunications Industry," *Interfaces*, Vol. 26, No. 3, May–June 1996, pp. 1–9.

EQUATIONS FOR SELECTED QUEUING MODELS

Definition of Symbols

n = number of customers in the system
λ = mean arrival rate (e.g., customer arrivals per hour)
μ = mean service rate per busy server (e.g., service capacity in customers per hour)
ρ = traffic intensity (λ/μ)
N = maximum number of customers allowed in the system
c = number of servers
P_n = probability of exactly n customers being in the system
L_s = mean number of customers in the system
L_q = mean number of customers in queue
L_b = mean number of customers in queue for a busy system
W_s = mean time customer spends in the system
W_q = mean time customer spends in the queue
W_b = mean time customer spends in the queue for a busy system

I. Standard M/M/1 Model[8]

$$P_0 = 1 - \rho \tag{I.1}$$

$$P(n \geq k) = \rho^k \tag{I.2}$$

[8]Note: $0 < \rho < 1.0$.

$$P_n = P_0 \rho^n \tag{I.3}$$

$$L_s = \frac{\lambda}{\mu - \lambda} \tag{I.4}$$

$$L_q = \frac{\rho\lambda}{\mu - \lambda} \tag{I.5}$$

$$L_b = \frac{\lambda}{\mu - \lambda} \tag{I.6}$$

$$W_s = \frac{1}{\mu - \lambda} \tag{I.7}$$

$$W_q = \frac{\rho}{\mu - \lambda} \tag{I.8}$$

$$W_b = \frac{1}{\mu - \lambda} \tag{I.9}$$

II. Standard M/M/c Model[9]

$$P_0 = \frac{1}{\left(\sum_{i=0}^{c-1} \frac{\rho^i}{i!}\right) + \frac{\rho^c}{c!\,(1 - \rho/c)}} \tag{II.1}$$

$$P_n = \begin{cases} \frac{\rho^n}{n!} P_0 & \text{for } 0 \le n \le c \\ \frac{\rho^n}{c!\,c^{n-c}} P_0 & \text{for } n \ge c \end{cases} \tag{II.2}$$

$$P(n \ge c) = \frac{\rho^c \mu c}{c!\,(\mu c - \lambda)} P_0 \tag{II.3}$$

$$L_s = \frac{\rho^{c+1}}{(c-1)!\,(c-\rho)^2} P_0 + \rho \tag{II.4}$$

$$L_q = L_s - \rho \tag{II.5}$$

$$L_b = \frac{L_q}{P(n \ge c)} \tag{II.6}$$

$$W_s = \frac{L_q}{\lambda} + \frac{1}{\mu} \tag{II.7}$$

[9]Note: $0 < \rho < c$.

$$W_q = \frac{L_q}{\lambda} \tag{II.8}$$

$$W_b = \frac{W_q}{P(n \geq c)} \tag{II.9}$$

III. *Standard* M/G/1 *Model*[10]

$$L_s = L_q + \rho \tag{III.1}$$

$$L_q = \frac{\rho^2 + \lambda^2 V(t)}{2(1-\rho)} \tag{III.2}$$

$$W_s = \frac{L_s}{\lambda} \tag{III.3}$$

$$W_b = \frac{L_q}{\lambda} \tag{III.4}$$

IV. *Self-Service* M/G/∞ *Model*[11]

$$P_n = \frac{e^{-\rho}}{n!}\rho^n \qquad \text{for } n \geq 0 \tag{IV.1}$$

$$L_s = \rho \tag{IV.2}$$

$$W_s = \frac{1}{\mu} \tag{IV.3}$$

V. *Finite-Queue* M/M/1 *Model*

$$P_0 = \begin{cases} \dfrac{1-\rho}{1-\rho^{N+1}} & \text{for } \lambda \neq \mu \\ \dfrac{1}{N+1} & \text{for } \lambda = \mu \end{cases} \tag{V.1}$$

$$P(n > 0) = 1 - P_0 \tag{V.2}$$

$$P_n = P_0\rho^n \qquad \text{for } n \leq N \tag{V.3}$$

$$L_s = \begin{cases} \dfrac{\rho}{1-\rho} - \dfrac{(N+1)\rho^{N+1}}{1-\rho^{N+1}} & \text{for } \lambda \neq \mu \\ \dfrac{N}{2} & \text{for } \lambda = \mu \end{cases} \tag{V.4}$$

$$L_q = L_s - (1 - P_0) \tag{V.5}$$

[10]Note: $V(t)$ = service time variance.
[11]$e = 2.718$, the base of natural logarithms.

$$L_b = \frac{L_q}{1 - P_0} \tag{V.6}$$

$$W_s = \frac{L_q}{\lambda(1 - P_N)} + \frac{1}{\mu} \tag{V.7}$$

$$W_q = W_s - \frac{1}{\mu} \tag{V.8}$$

$$W_b = \frac{W_q}{1 - P_0} \tag{V.9}$$

VI. Finite-Queue M/M/c *Model*

$$P_0 = \frac{1}{\left(\sum_{i=0}^{c} \frac{\rho^i}{i!}\right) + \left(\frac{1}{c!}\right)\left(\sum_{i=c+1}^{N} \frac{\rho^i}{c^{i-c}}\right)} \tag{VI.1}$$

$$P_n = \begin{cases} \frac{\rho^n}{n!} P_0 & \text{for } 0 \le n \le c \\ \frac{\rho^n}{c!\, c^{n-c}} P_0 & \text{for } c \le n \le N \end{cases} \tag{VI.2}$$

$$P(n \ge c) = 1 - P_0 \sum_{i=0}^{c-1} \frac{\rho^i}{i!} \tag{VI.3}$$

$$L_s = \frac{P_0 \rho^{c+1}}{(c-1)!\,(c-\rho)^2}\left[1 - \left(\frac{\rho}{c}\right)^{N-c} - (N-c)\left(\frac{\rho}{c}\right)^{N-c}\left(1 - \frac{\rho}{c}\right)\right] + \rho(1 - P_N) \tag{VI.4}$$

$$L_q = L_s - \rho(1 - P_N) \tag{VI.5}$$

$$L_b = \frac{L_q}{P(n \ge c)} \tag{VI.6}$$

$$W_s = \frac{L_q}{\lambda(1 - P_N)} + \frac{1}{\mu} \tag{VI.7}$$

$$W_q = W_s - \frac{1}{\mu} \tag{VI.8}$$

$$W_b = \frac{W_q}{P(n \ge c)} \tag{VI.9}$$

SOLVED PROBLEMS

1. Calculating System Characteristics

Problem Statement

Sunset Airlines is reviewing its check-in procedures in anticipation of its "two for the price of one" fare promotion. Presently, a single clerk spends an average of 3 minutes per passenger checking luggage and issuing boarding passes. Service times have a negative exponential distribution, and passenger arrivals are Poisson distributed, with an anticipated mean of 15 per hour during flight operations.

a. What is the probability that an arriving passenger will be served immediately without waiting?

Solution

Note that we have an $M/M/1$ system with $\lambda = 15$ per hour and $\mu = 60/3 = 20$ per hour. Using equation (I.1):

$$\begin{aligned} P(\text{system idle}) = P_0 &= 1 - \rho \\ &= 1 - (15/20) \\ &= 0.25. \end{aligned}$$

b. The area immediately in front of the Sunset counter can accommodate only three passengers, including the one being served. What percentage of time will this area be inadequate for waiting passengers?

Solution

Using equation (I.2):

$$\begin{aligned} P(\text{inadequate waiting space}) = P(n \geq 4) &= \rho^4 \\ &= (15/20)^4 \\ &= 0.316 \end{aligned}$$

Thus, the waiting area is inadequate 32 percent of the time.

c. Anticipating an increase in demand, Sunset has decided to add another clerk when passengers begin to experience an average wait time in queue of 17 minutes. Since arrival rates are monitored at the check-in counter, determine what arrival rate per hour would indicate the need for another clerk.

Solution

Set equation (I.8) equal to 17/60 hours, substitute $\mu = 20$, and solve for λ:

$$W_q = \frac{\rho}{\mu - \lambda}$$

$$= \frac{\lambda}{20}\left[\frac{1}{20 - \lambda}\right]$$

$$= \frac{\lambda}{400 - 20\lambda}$$

$$= \frac{17}{60}$$

Therefore,

$$\lambda = 17 \text{ per hour.}$$

2. Capacity Planning

Problem Statement

Average arrival rate of customers has reached 20 per hour, and Sunset Airlines must increase the capacity of its check-in system with the addition of one clerk. Based on a customer survey, $15 per hour is considered to be the opportunity cost of waiting in queue. Clerks are paid $10 per hour and still process a passenger in 3 minutes. Evaluate the following check-in system alternatives to find the least expensive arrangement using total hourly costs of clerks and customers waiting in queue.

a. Consider a multiple-queue configuration with separate waiting lines and no customer jockeying. Assuming demand is divided equally among the two clerks, what is the total hourly cost of this arrangement?

Solution

Treat each line as independent $M/M/1$ queues, with total system cost being twice the single-line cost. Calculate the value for L_q using equation (I.5), and substitute in equation (7) to determine the line cost:

$$L_q = \frac{\rho\lambda}{\mu - \lambda}$$

$$= \frac{10}{20}\left[\frac{10}{20 - 10}\right]$$

$$= 0.5$$

Therefore, total system cost = 2[10 + 15(.5)] = $35 per hour.

b. Consider adding one self-serve automatic ticketing machine (ATM) with a constant service time of 3 minutes to help the single clerk. Assume demand is divided equally between the single live clerk and the ATM. What is the total hourly cost of this arrangement if the ATM operating costs are negligible?

Solution

Treat each line as independent, with one being an $M/M/1$ as in part **a**, with $L_q = 0.5$ and the other being an $M/D/1$ (constant service of ATM). First, calculate the L_q for the ATM line using equation (III.2) with $V(t) = 0$:

$$L_q = \frac{\rho^2 + \lambda^2 V(t)}{2(1 - \rho)}$$
$$= \frac{0.5^2 + 10^2(0)}{2(1 - .5)}$$
$$= 0.25$$

Therefore, total system cost = single clerk + ATM = 10 + 15(0.5) + 0 + 15(0.25) = \$21.25 per hour.

c. Consider a single-queue arrangement with two live tellers. What is the total hourly cost of this arrangement?

Solution

From Appendix B, $c = 2$, and $\rho = 20/20 = 1$. Thus, we find $L_q = 0.333$, so the total system cost = 10(2) + 15(0.333) = \$25 per hour.

EXERCISES

17.1. A general-purpose auto-repair garage has one mechanic who specializes in muffler installations. Customers seeking service arrive at an average rate of two per hour, with a Poisson distribution. The average time to install a muffler is 20 minutes, with negative exponential distribution.

a. On arrival at the garage, how many customers should one expect to find in the system?

b. The management is interested in adding another mechanic when the customer's average time in the system exceeds 90 minutes. If business continues to increase, at what arrival rate per hour will an additional mechanic be needed?

17.2. A business school is considering replacing its old minicomputer with a faster model. Past records show that the average student arrival rate is 24 per hour, Poisson distributed, and that the service times are distributed exponentially. The computer selection committee has been instructed to consider only machines that will yield an average turnaround time (i.e., expected time in the system) of 5 minutes or less. What is the smallest computer-processing rate per hour that can be considered?

17.3. The Lower Colorado River Authority (LCRA) has been studying congestion at the boat-launching ramp near Mansfield Dam. On weekends, the arrival rate averages five boaters per hour, Poisson distributed. The average time to launch or retrieve a boat is 10 minutes, with negative exponential distribution. Assume that only one boat can be launched or retrieved at a time.

a. The LCRA plans to add another ramp when the average turnaround time (i.e., time in the system) exceeds 90 minutes. At what average arrival rate per hour should the LCRA begin to consider adding another ramp?

b. If there were room to park only two boats at the top of the ramp in preparation for launching, how often would an arrival find insufficient parking space?

17.4. On average, four customers per hour use the public telephone in the sheriff's detention area, and this use has a Poisson distribution. The length of a phone call varies according to a negative exponential distribution, with a mean of 5 minutes. The sheriff will install a second telephone booth when an arrival can expect to wait 3 minutes or longer for the phone.

a. By how much must the arrival rate per hour increase to justify a second telephone booth?

b. Suppose the criterion for justifying a second booth is changed to the following: install a second booth when the probability of having to wait at all exceeds 0.6. Under this criterion, by how much must the arrival rate per hour increase to justify a second booth?

17.5. A company has a central document-copying service. Arrivals are assumed to follow the Poisson probability distribution, with a mean rate of 15 per hour. Service times are assumed to follow the exponential distribution. With the present copying equipment, the average service time is 3 minutes. A new machine is available that will have a mean service time of 2 minutes. The average wage of the people who bring the documents to be copied is $3 an hour.

a. If the new machine can be rented for $4 per hour more than the old machine, should the company rent the new machine? Consider lost productive time of employees as time spent waiting in queue only because the copying machine is a self-serve device.

b. For the old copying machine, what is the probability when a person arrives that he or she will encounter people already waiting in line for service? (Be careful to identify properly the number of customers who might be present for this situation to arise.)

c. Suppose the new copying machine is rented. How many chairs should be provided for those waiting in line if we are satisfied when there will be enough chairs at least 90 percent of the time?

17.6. Sea Dock, a private firm, operates an unloading facility in the Gulf of Mexico for supertankers delivering crude oil for refineries in the Port Arthur area of Texas. Records show that on average, two tankers arrive per day, with a Poisson distribution. Supertankers are unloaded one at a time on a first-come, first-served (FCFS) basis. Unloading requires approximately 8 hours of a 24-hour working day, and unloading times have a negative exponential distribution.

a. Sea Dock has provided mooring space for three tankers. Is this sufficient to meet the U.S. Coast Guard requirement that at least 19 of 20 arrivals should find mooring space available?

b. Sea Dock can increase its unloading capacity to a rate of four ships per day through additional labor at a cost of $480 per day. Considering the $1000-per-day demurrage fee charged to Sea Dock for keeping a supertanker idle (this includes unloading time as well as time spent waiting in queue), should management consider this expansion opportunity?

17.7. Last National Bank is concerned about the level of service at its single drive-in window. A study of customer arrivals during the window's busy period revealed that on average, 20 customers per hour arrive, with a Poisson distribution, and they are given FCFS service, requiring an average of 2 minutes, with service times having a negative exponential distribution.

a. What is the expected number of customers waiting in queue?

b. If Last National were using an automated teller machine with a constant service time of 2 minutes, what would be the expected number of drive-in customers in the system?

c. There is space in the drive for three cars (including the one being served). What is the probability of traffic on the street being blocked by cars waiting to turn into the bank driveway?

d. Last National is considering adding tellers at the current drive-in facility. It has decided on $5 per hour as the imputed cost of customer waiting time in the system. The hourly cost of a teller is $10. The average arrival rate of customers has reached 30 per hour. On the basis of the total hourly cost of tellers and customer waiting, how many tellers do you recommend? Assume that with use of pneumatic tubes, tellers can serve customers as though there were a single queue.

17.8. Green Valley Airport has been in operation for several years and is beginning to experience flight congestion. A study of airport operations revealed that planes arrive at an average rate of 12 per hour, with a Poisson distribution. On the single runway, a plane can land and be cleared every 4 minutes on average, and service times have a negative exponential distribution. Planes are processed on an FCFS basis, with take-offs occurring between landings. Planes waiting to land are asked to circle the airport.

a. What is the expected number of airplanes circling the airport, waiting in queue for clearance to land?

b. A new ground-approach radar system approved by the Federal Aviation Administration is being considered as a means of reducing congestion. Under this system, planes can be processed at a constant rate of 15 per hour (i.e., the variance is zero). What would be the expected number of airplanes circling the airport, waiting in queue for clearance to land, if this system were to be used?

c. Assume that the cost of keeping an airplane in the air is approximately $70 per hour. If the cost of the proposed radar system were $100 per hour, would you recommend its adoption?

17.9. Lakeside Community College has been using a medium-sized computer, donated by a local firm, to support its computer science program. The director of the computer center notes that students submit batch jobs at an average rate of 20 per hour, with a Poisson distribution. Jobs are processed on an FCFS basis and take, on average, 2 minutes of processing time, with a negative exponential distribution. Students are requested to remain in the ready room as their jobs are processed.

a. What is the expected number of students waiting in queue to have their jobs processed?

b. If only three chairs are provided in the ready room for students, what is the probability that an arriving student will find no chair available? (Assume that all students will sit if given the opportunity.)

c. The college plans to consider replacing the computer when increases in demand result in an average waiting time in queue exceeding 6 minutes. If the computer center tracks the average arrival rate of students per hour, at what point should a new computer be considered?

d. Lakeside has an opportunity to get another computer, which is identical to the current one, for its computation center. Assume that the arrival rate still is 20 per hour, with a Poisson distribution. What is the average number of jobs in the system if the computers operate in parallel to select jobs from a single queue?

e. As an alternative, the college decides to dedicate one computer to research computation and the other to teaching. If the demand of 20 jobs per hour were divided equally between research and teaching, how many jobs on average would be in the total system?

f. What savings in student waiting time could be achieved by pooling the computers?

17.10. Community Bank is planning to expand its drive-in facility. Observations of the existing single-teller window reveal that customers arrive at an average rate of 10 per hour, with a Poisson distribution, and that they are given FCFS service, with an average transaction time of 5 minutes. Transaction times have a negative exponential distribution. Community Bank has decided to add another teller and to install four remote stations with pneumatic tubes running from the stations to the tellers, who are located in a glassed-in building. The cost of keeping a customer waiting in the system is represented as a $5-per-hour loss of goodwill. The hourly cost of a teller is $10.

a. Assume that each teller is assigned two stations exclusively, that demand is divided equally among the stations, and that no customer jockeying is permitted. What is the average number of customers waiting in the entire system?

b. If, instead, both tellers work all the stations and the customer waiting the longest is served by the next available teller, what is the average number of customers in the system?

c. What hourly savings are achieved by pooling the tellers?

17.11. Consider a one-pump gas station that satisfies the assumptions for the $M/M/1$ model. It is estimated that on average, customers arrive to buy gas when their tanks are one-eighth full. The mean time to service a customer is 4 minutes, and the arrival rate is six customers per hour.

a. Determine the expected length of the queue and the expected time in the system.

b. Suppose that customers perceive a gas shortage (when there is none) and respond by changing the fill-up criterion to more than one-eighth full on average. Assuming that changes in λ are inversely proportional to changes in the fill-up criterion, compare results when the fill-up criterion is one-quarter full with the results in part **a**.

c. Making the same assumption as in part **b**, compare the results obtained if the fill-up criterion is one-half full. Do we have the makings of a behaviorally induced gasoline panic?

d. It is reasonable to assume that the time to service a customer will decrease as the fill-up criterion increases. Under "normal" conditions, it takes, on average, 2 minutes to pump the gasoline and 2 minutes to clean the windshield, check the oil, and collect the money. Rework parts **b** and **c** if the time to pump the gasoline changes proportionally to changes in the fill-up criterion.

CASE: HOUSTON PORT AUTHORITY

The Houston Port Authority has engaged you as a consultant to advise it on possible changes in the handling of wheat exports. At present, a crew of dockworkers using conventional belt conveyors unloads hopper cars containing wheat into cargo ships bound overseas. The crew is known to take an average of 30 minutes to unload a car. The crew is paid a total wage of $10 per hour. Hopper car arrivals have averaged 12 per 8-hour shift. The railroad assesses a demurrage charge from time of arrival to release at a rate of $4 per hour on rolling stock not in service. Partially unloaded cars from one shift are first in line for the following shift.

A chi-square "goodness-of-fit" analysis of arrival rates for the past months indicates a Poisson distribution. Data on unloading times for this period may be assumed to follow a negative exponential distribution.

Because of excessive demurrage charges, adding another work crew has been proposed. A visit to the work area indicates that both crews will be unable to work together on the same car because of congestion; however, two cars may be unloaded simultaneously with one crew per car.

During your deliberations, the industrial engineering staff reports that a pneumatic handling system has become available. This system can transfer wheat from cars to cargo ships at a constant rate of three cars per hour, 24 hours per day, with the assistance of a skilled operator earning $8 per hour. Such a system would cost $400,000 installed. The Port Authority uses a 10-percent discount rate for capital improvement projects. The port is in operation 24 hours per day, 365 days per year. For this analysis, assume a 10-year planning horizon, and prepare a recommendation for the Port Authority.

CASE: FREEDOM EXPRESS

Freedom Express (FreeEx), affectionately known as the Filibuster Fly, is a small commuter airline based in Washington, D.C., that serves the U.S. east coast. It runs nonstop flights between several cities and Washington National Airport (DCA).

DCA frequently is congested, and at such times, planes are required to fly in a "stack" over the field. In other words, planes in the process of landing and those waiting for permission to land are deployed above the field.

FreeEx management is interested in determining how long its planes will have to wait so that an adequate amount of fuel can be loaded before departure from the outlying city to cover both the intercity flying time and the time in the stack. Excess fuel represents an unnecessary cost, however, because it reduces the payload capacity. Equally important is the present cost of aviation fuel, $1.80 per gallon, and an average consumption rate of 20 gallons per minute.

The rate of arrival for all planes at DCA varies by the hour. The arrival rate and time in the stack are greatest each weekday between 4 and 5 PM and so FreeEx selected this time period for an initial study.

The study indicated that the mean arrival rate is 20 planes per hour, or one every 3 minutes. The variance about this mean, resulting from flight cancellations as well as charter and private flights, is characterized by a Poisson distribution.

During clear weather, the DCA control tower can land one plane per minute, or 60 planes per hour. Landings cannot exceed this rate in the interest of air safety. When the weather is bad, the landing rate is 30 per hour. Both good- and bad-weather landing rates are mean rates with a Poisson distribution. FreeEx's flights are short enough that management usually can tell before takeoff in an outlying city whether or not the rate of landings in DCA will be reduced because of weather considerations.

When a plane runs short of fuel while in the stack, it is given priority to land out of order. DCA rules, however, make clear that the airport will not tolerate abuse of this consideration. Therefore, FreeEx ensures that its planes carry enough fuel so that it will take advantage of the policy no more than 1 time in 20.

Questions

1. During periods of bad weather, as compared with periods of clear weather, how many additional gallons of fuel on average should FreeEx expect its planes to consume because of airport congestion?

2. Given FreeEx's policy of ensuring that its planes

do not run out of fuel more than 1 in 20 times while waiting to land, how many reserve gallons (i.e., gallons over and above expected usage) should be provided for clear-weather flights? For bad-weather flights?

3. During bad weather, FreeEx has the option of instructing the Washington air controller to place its planes in a holding pattern from which planes are directed to land either at Washington National or at Dulles International, whichever becomes available first. Assume that the Dulles landing rate in bad weather also is 30 per hour, Poisson distributed, and that the combined arrival rate for both airports is 40 per hour. If FreeEx must pay $100 per flight to charter a bus to transport its passengers from Dulles to Washington National, should it exercise the option of permitting its aircraft to land at Dulles during bad weather? Assume that if the option is used, FreeEx's aircraft will be diverted to Dulles about one-half the time.

CASE: CEDAR VALLEY COMMUNITY COLLEGE

Founded only 2 years ago, Cedar Valley Community College has experienced enrollment beyond its expectations. The large number of students in the computer-science program has placed such demands on the college's small computer that complaints of excessive turnaround time have reached the president's office.[12]

As director of the computer center, you have been asked to identify the new computer models that are available and to recommend a replacement for the existing batch processor. After talking to several computer-hardware vendors, you have settled on a compatible system with six models available that differ only in their processing speed and, of course, their price.

On the basis of historical records, you estimate that an average program can be processed in 1, 2, 3, 4, 5, or 6 minutes depending on whether model A, B, C, D, E, or F, respectively, is chosen. The rental cost of a particular model depends on its speed. The rental rate per minute is 90 cents/S, where S is the service time for the average program (e.g., model A, which completes a program in 1 minute, rents for 90 cents per minute and model B for 45 cents per minute).

A statistical analysis of the distribution of historical processing times reveals that they follow a negative exponential distribution. During the past month, you installed a time clock to gather information on the time of arrival of computer-center users to plan the staffing of the ready desk. A study of the clock times indicates that on average, 12 users arrive per hour, with a Poisson distribution.

The president has suggested that a criterion of minimizing the average total cost per hour (i.e., rental plus waiting) be used in the analysis. For this analysis, the cost of keeping a user waiting for output is estimated to be 50 cents per minute. At your suggestion, the president also agrees to an acceptable service level that does not exceed an average turnaround time of 5 minutes.

Which computer model(s) and configuration would you recommend?

[12]Turnaround time for batch processing is the elapsed time from submitting a computer job to the time that output is available for pick-up.

CASE: PRONTO PIZZA

Pronto Pizza is a delivery-only pizza service promising delivery within 40 minutes of receiving a call for an order or the customer gets $2 off the price. Pronto employs a single pizzamaker, who is paid $10 per hour, and who can make, on average, one pizza every 3 minutes. This service time has a negative exponential distribution. Pizzas are placed in a large oven with a capacity for ten pizzas to bake for approximately 12 minutes. A team of six delivery persons serves the neighboring population within a maximum drive of 10 minutes from the store. The travel time to deliver a pizza in the market area and then return averages 10 minutes, with a negative exponential distribution. Calls for pizza average one every 5 minutes, with a negative exponential distribution. Pizzas are delivered one at a time to customers by drivers who use their own cars and are paid $8 per hour.

Assignments

1. Draw a process flow diagram, and identify the bottleneck operation.

2. Using the queuing equations, evaluate the delivery guarantee. What is the probability of paying off on the guarantee?

3. Determine the number of delivery persons required to ensure that the average waiting time for a completed pizza to be picked up for delivery is limited to 1 minute.

4. What do you think of this service guarantee policy?

5. What other design or operating suggestions could improve Pronto Pizza's performance and customer service?

SELECTED BIBLIOGRAPHY

BLEUEL, W. H.: "Management Science's Impact on Service Strategy," *Interfaces,* vol. 6, no. 1, November 1975, part 2, pp. 4–12.

CRABILL, T. B., D. GROSS, and M. J. MAGAZINE: "A Classified Bibliography of Research on Optimal Design and Control of Queues," *Operations Research,* vol. 25, no. 2, March–April 1977, pp. 219–232.

DRAKE, A. W., R. L. KEENEY, and P. N. MORSE, editors: *Analysis of Public Systems,* M.I.T. Press, Cambridge, Mass., 1972.

ERIKSON, WARREN J.: "Management Science and the Gas Shortage," *Interfaces,* vol. 4, no. 4, August 1974, pp. 47–51.

FOOTE, B. L.: "A Queuing Case Study of Drive-In Banking," *Interfaces,* vol. 6, no. 4, August 1976, pp. 31–37.

GRASSMAN, W. K.: "Finding the Right Number of Servers in Real-World Queuing Systems," *Interfaces,* vol. 18, no. 2, 1988, pp. 94–104.

MAGGARD, MICHAEL J.: "Determining Electronic Point-of-Sale Cash Register Requirements," *Journal of Retailing,* vol. 57, no. 2, Summer 1981, pp. 64–86.

PARIKH, S. C.: "On a Fleet Sizing and Allocation Problem," *Management Science,* vol. 23, no. 9, May 1977, pp. 972–977.

RISING, E. J., R. BARON, and B. AVERILL: "A Systems Analysis of a University Health-Service Outpatient Clinic," *Operations Research,* vol. 21, no. 5, September 1973, pp. 1030–1047.

ROTHKOPF, M. H., and P. RECH: "Perspectives on Queues: Combining Queues Is Not Always Beneficial," *Operations Research,* vol. 35, no. 6, November–December 1987, pp. 906–909.

CHAPTER 18

Linear Programming Models in Services

LEARNING OBJECTIVES

After completing this chapter, you should be able to:

1. Describe the features of constrained optimization models.
2. Formulate linear programming models for computer solution.
3. Use graphics to solve a two-variable linear programming model, and explain the nature of sensitivity analysis.
4. Use Excel Solver to solve a linear programming model, and interpret the results, including the sensitivity analysis.
5. Formulate a goal programming model and interpret the solution.

Linear programming (LP) is a general computer-based modeling tool for making resource allocation decisions that transcend all aspects of service operations management. Linear programming is not computer programming; it refers to planning that uses mathematical models consisting of linear expressions.

A model is a selective abstraction of reality. Modeling is an art, because judgments are made when selecting the important features of reality for the problem at hand. Modeling also is a science, however, because data are collected to measure the relationship between decision variables, objectives desired, and resources available. The process of identifying decision variables and clarifying objectives imposes a discipline that is useful in itself.

Use of models such as LP springs from a belief that the decision-making process can be enhanced by applying the scientific method. Scientists study nature and conduct controlled experiments to understand better the phenomena of interest. Decision models are the laboratory of managers who are interested in testing the outcomes of decisions before their actual implementation. In this way, potential disasters may be avoided, and the decision-making process may be improved through a better understanding of the environment.

CHAPTER PREVIEW

This chapter emphasizes the art of formulating LP models and interpreting computer output. The mathematical details involved in solving an LP model are not discussed. The availability of computer programs to solve such models is extensive, and users need not be concerned about the mechanics of how optimal solutions are found any more than one need know the theory of the internal combustion engine to drive an automobile. The chapter concludes with a discussion of an extension of LP called goal programming, which is useful when one is dealing with the multiple objectives that often are present in service decision making. We begin by discussing the concept of an optimum solution to a constrained model.

CONSTRAINED OPTIMIZATION MODELS

Each day, we are faced with making decisions in which our potential set of alternatives is restricted by money, time, physical limitations, or some other element. For example, suppose we wish to buy a car, we can qualify for a $10,000 loan, and we want a vehicle with an EPA rating of at least 30 miles per gallon. The set of possible cars is constrained by time, budget, and mileage performance. These constraints are restrictions that reduce the allowable set of solutions to our problem. Thus, constraints actually help us to make decisions by limiting our search for a solution to cars that meet the stipulated requirements.

If economy were our goal, we could measure this by calculating the cost per mile for each car that meets our constraints. The car with the lowest cost-per-mile value would be considered the optimum solution to our constrained decision problem.

Constrained optimization problems are common to service operations. For example, a potential location for a service facility is constrained by the available sites. Scheduling telephone operators is constrained by variations in demand for the service and by the personnel policies regarding split shifts.

Linear programming models are a special class of constrained optimization models. In LP, all relationships are expressed as linear functions, and all LP models have the following algebraic form:

$$\text{Maximize (or minimize)} \qquad c_1x_1 + c_2x_2 + \cdots + c_nx_n$$

$$\text{subject to} \qquad a_{11}x_1 + a_{12}x_2 + \cdots + a_{1n}x_n \begin{Bmatrix} \leq \\ = \\ \geq \end{Bmatrix} b_1$$

$$a_{21}x_1 + a_{22}x_2 + \cdots + a_{2n}x_n \begin{Bmatrix} \leq \\ = \\ \geq \end{Bmatrix} b_2$$

$$\vdots$$

$$a_{m1}x_1 + a_{m2}x_2 + \cdots + a_{mn}x_n \begin{Bmatrix} \leq \\ = \\ \geq \end{Bmatrix} b_m$$

and nonnegativity constraints

$$x_1, x_2, \ldots, x_n \geq 0$$

Note that each system constraint is limited to only one of the conditions ≤ or = or ≥ (strictly > or < is not permitted). This problem structure contains the following characteristics:

1. *Decision variables.* The variables $x_1, x_2, \ldots, x_n$ are called decision variables, which take on real values greater than or equal to zero. These variables represent actions the decision maker can take, such as assigning ten telephone operators to the Tuesday afternoon shift.
2. *Objective function.* The function $c_1x_1 + c_2x_2 + \ldots + c_nx_n$ is called the objective function, which is either maximized (e.g., profits) or minimized (e.g., costs) depending on the nature of the coefficients $c_1, c_2, \ldots, c_n$. The problem states that this function is made as large or as small as possible provided that a system of constraints is met.
3. *Constraint functions.* As numerical values are assigned to the decision variables $x_1, x_2, \ldots, x_n$ to influence the objective function, these values also are assigned to each constraint function. The model requires that numerical values be assigned such that no constraint is violated. The numbers $b_1, b_2, \ldots, b_m$ taken together are called the *right-hand sides* (RHS). These numbers indirectly limit the possible values of the decision variables. For example, these RHS values could be resource constraints, such as total worker hours available.
4. *Parameters.* The coefficients in the objective function and the RHS values are parameters. Parameters are entities whose values remain fixed during the problem solution but could be changed later. Examples are unit profit contributions for the objective-function coefficients and the availability of resources for the RHS values.

5. *Constants.* The coefficients $a_{11}, a_{12}, \ldots, a_{1n}$ represent the consumption of the first RHS resource per unit of each decision variable. These coefficients reflect a constant rate of resource use (e.g., the ounces of beef required to make a hamburger).

Example 18.1: Stereo Warehouse

The retail outlet of Stereo Warehouse, a discount audio-components store, is planning a special clearance sale. The showroom has 400 square feet of floor space available for displaying this week's specials, a model X receiver and series Y speakers. Each receiver has a wholesale cost of $100, requires 2 square feet of display space, and will sell for $150. The wholesale cost for a pair of speakers is $50; the pair requires 4 square feet of display space and will sell for $70. The budget for stocking the stereo items is $8000. The sales potential for the receiver is considered to be no more than 60 units; however, the budget-priced speakers appear to have an unlimited appeal. The store manager, desiring to maximize gross profit, must decide how many receivers and speakers to stock.

This problem can be formulated as an LP problem in the following manner:

Let x = number of receivers to stock
y = number of speakers to stock

Maximize	$50x + 20y$	gross profit
subject to	$2x + 4y \leq 400$	floor space
	$100x + 50y \leq 8000$	budget
	$x \leq 60$	sales limit
	$x, y \geq 0$	

The decision variables x and y appear in both the objective function and the constraint functions to ensure that the optimum solution does not violate resource limits. The objective is to maximize gross profit, which represents the difference between the selling price and the wholesale cost for each receiver and speaker sold. Thus, the objective becomes maximize $(150 - 100)x + (70 - 50)y$, or $50x + 20y$. The first two constraints account for resources that cannot be exceeded (i.e., available floor space and budget dollars). Thus, the 400 square feet of floor space represents a less-than-or-equal-to constraint, with each receiver occupying 2 square feet and each speaker occupying 4 square feet. Likewise, the $8000 budget is consumed by the expenditure of $100 for each receiver and $50 for each pair of speakers stocked. Finally, the sale of receivers is limited to 60 units.

The solution to this problem will increase the values of x and y until some, but not necessarily all, of the resources are depleted. The solution to the Stereo Warehouse example is deferred until a later section.

Before leaving the topic of constrained optimization models, a few caveats are in order. When a constrained optimization model is solved, the solution is called optimal, meaning that the best values for the decision variables have been found. This so-called optimal solution, however, is optimal relative to the model but may not be optimal in reality. Recall that the model is only an abstraction and cannot include all the elements of reality. There can be a vast difference between the optimal solution of the model and what finally is implemented by the decision maker for reasons ranging from political considerations to personal preference. An optimal site selection for company headquarters could be vetoed by the corporate president, who refuses to live in the selected city. When used with care, however, LP models provide an excellent vehicle to structure a problem in explicit detail for all to see and question. Constraints can be modified, added, or eliminated, and objective functions can be changed. Further, the cost of pursuing a nonoptimal solution can be determined.

Next, we discuss the art of formulating LP models and consider examples of classic LP model structures as applied to services.

FORMULATING LINEAR PROGRAMMING MODELS

The ability to recognize a potential LP problem and to structure it for computer solution is an art that is acquired from experience. Some exposure to examples of classical forms of LP models can help, however. For example, recognizing that a problem is like the classical "diet problem" suggests the likely mathematical structure that will evolve, and experience with formulating LP problems suggests that the following strategy can be helpful:

1. Draw a diagram or construct a table showing the relationships in the problem, including the parameters and constraints.
2. Identify and invent symbolic notation for the decision variables.
3. State the objective in words.
4. Express each constraint in words, identify the RHS values, and note the direction of the inequality.
5. Write the complete model in algebraic form. Begin with the objective function; then list the right-hand sides, followed by the inequality signs; and finish by filling in the left-hand algebraic expressions for each constraint.
6. Note the nonnegativity conditions for the decision variables.
7. Using possible solutions, test the problem for internal consistency and completeness.

These guidelines are followed in formulating the example problems.

Diet Problem

This class of problems is illustrated by the selection of various food items for a meal that meets certain nutritional requirements. Given that each item selected contributes to the nutritional requirements at different rates, the objective is to identify the food and amounts that minimize costs.

Example 18.2: Lakeview Hospital

The dietitian at Lakeview Hospital is preparing a special milkshake as a "treat" for pediatric care patients recovering from surgery. The dietitian wants to ensure that the level of cholesterol will not exceed 175 units and the level of saturated fat 150 units. The protein content should be at least 200 units, and the calorie content should exceed 100 units. The dietitian has selected three possible ingredients: an egg custard base, ice cream, and butterscotch-flavored syrup. One unit of the egg custard base costs 15 cents and contributes 50 units of cholesterol, no fat, 70 units of protein, and 30 calories. One unit of ice cream costs 25 cents and contributes 150 units of cholesterol, 100 units of fat, 10 units of protein, and 80 calories. One unit of butterscotch-flavored syrup costs 10 cents and contributes 90 units of cholesterol, 50 units of fat, no protein, and 200 calories. How many units of each ingredient should be included in the milkshake if costs are to be minimized?

The information from the problem statement is organized and displayed in Table 18.1.

The problem suggests the following decision variables:

Let E = units of egg custard base in the shake
C = units of ice cream in the shake
S = units of butterscotch syrup in the shake

The object is to minimize the total cost of the milkshake. Table 18.1 identifies the constraints as a cholesterol content less than or equal to 175 units, fat content less than or equal to 150 units, protein content equal to or more than 200 units, and calorie content equal to or more than 100 units. The algebraic expression of the model then becomes:

$$\begin{array}{llllllll} \text{Minimize} & 0.15E & + & 0.25C & + & 0.10S & & \\ \text{subject to} & 50E & + & 150C & + & 90S & \leq 175 & \text{cholesterol} \\ & & & 100C & + & 50S & \leq 150 & \text{fat} \\ & 70E & + & 10C & & & \geq 200 & \text{protein} \\ & 30E & + & 80C & + & 200S & \geq 100 & \text{calories} \\ & & & & & E, C, S & \geq 0 & \end{array}$$

Note that as formulated, the problem could yield a solution using egg custard base alone (i.e., $E = 3.5$, $C = 0$, and $S = 0$). Because such a solution would hardly be considered a milkshake, additional constraints should be added to the problem that preclude this from occurring.

TABLE 18.1. Lakeview Hospital Diet Problem
(Units of nutritional element per unit of ingredient)

Nutritional Element	Egg Custard	Ice Cream	Syrup	Nutritional Requirement
Cholesterol	50	150	90	≤ 175
Fat	0	100	50	≤ 150
Protein	70	10	0	≥ 200
Calories	30	80	200	≥ 100
Cost per unit (cents)	15	25	10	

Shift-Scheduling Problem

This problem arises when an operation must be staffed for a period of time during which the requirements for service vary. The objective is to schedule staff assignments to meet the requirements during that period using the minimum number of people.

Example 18.3: Gotham City Police Patrol

Unable to hire new police officers because of budget limitations, the Gotham City police commissioner is trying to utilize the force better. The minimum requirements for police patrols on weekdays are:

Period	Time	Patrol Officers (minimum)
1	Midnight–4 AM	6
2	4–8 AM	4
3	8–Noon	14
4	12–4 PM	8
5	4–8 PM	12
6	8–Midnight	16

Patrol officers are assigned in pairs to a patrol car, and they work an 8-hour shift. Currently, patrol officers report for duty at midnight, 8 AM, and 4 PM. The commissioner believes that better use of officers could be achieved if they also were permitted to report for duty at 4 AM, noon, and 8 PM. Of course, this might require some officers to switch partners after 4 hours of duty. How many officers should report for their 8-hour shifts at each of the six reporting times? The assignments must minimize the total number of officers yet still meet the minimum staffing requirements.

The shaded areas in Figure 18.1 show the periods of overstaffing that result from the current practice of officers reporting for 8-hour shifts at three reporting times (i.e., $x_1 = 6$, $x_3 = 14$, and $x_5 = 16$).

The decision variables for the staffing problem are defined as:

Let x_i = number of officers reporting at period i for $i = 1, 2, 3, 4, 5, 6$

The problem is directed at minimizing the total number of patrol officers, with constraints on the minimum number required for each 4-hour time interval during the day. The algebraic expression of the model also accounts for the implied constraint that once an officer reports for duty, he or she remains on duty for a complete 8-hour shift.

$$\text{Minimize} \quad x_1 + x_2 + x_3 + x_4 + x_5 + x_6$$

$$\begin{aligned}
\text{subject to} \quad & x_1 + x_6 \geq 6 && \text{period 1} \\
& x_1 + x_2 \geq 4 && \text{period 2} \\
& x_2 + x_3 \geq 14 && \text{period 3} \\
& x_3 + x_4 \geq 8 && \text{period 4} \\
& x_4 + x_5 \geq 12 && \text{period 5} \\
& x_5 + x_6 \geq 16 && \text{period 6}
\end{aligned}$$

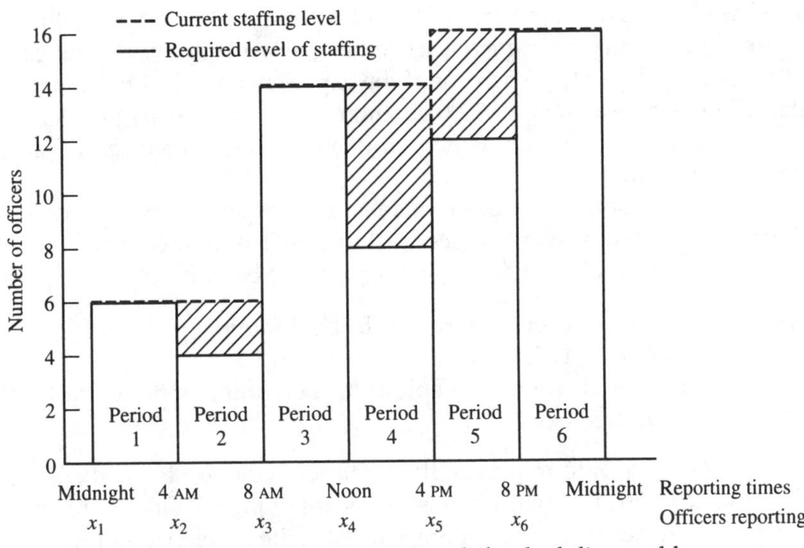

FIGURE 18.1. Gotham City Police shift-scheduling problem.

Note that each decision variable appears in exactly two constraints to account for the 8-hour shift. For example, officers reporting at 4 AM (i.e., x_2) contribute to the staffing requirements for both the second and third period, because each period is 4 hours in duration. Because we are dealing with numbers of patrol officers, the decision variables must be restricted to integer values. Fortunately, because of the problem structure, the LP solution will be integer. In general, however, such a solution yields nonnegative real (integer or fractional) numbers.

Workforce-Planning Problem

Employee turnover is common among service occupations; for example, bank tellers and airline attendants often leave their jobs. Further, new employees require a training period before they are ready to meet the public. The level of staff that is required also varies in response to changes in consumer demand, such as during summer or holiday vacation periods for airlines. Workforce planning involves identifying when and how many people to recruit to meet future staffing requirements and replace employees who leave. The objective is to meet staff requirements in a dynamic setting at a minimum personnel cost.

Example 18.4: Last National Drive-In Bank

Last National Bank must decide how many new tellers to hire and train over the next 6 months. The teller requirements, expressed as the number of teller-hours needed, are 1500 in January, 1800 in February, 1600 in March, 2000 in April, 1800 in May, and 2200 in June. One month of training is necessary before a teller can be assigned to duty; thus, tellers must be hired 1 month before they actually are needed. Also, each trainee requires 80 hours of simulated job experience, supervised by a regular teller, during the month of training. Hence, for each trainee, 80 fewer hours are available from a regular teller. Each experienced teller works 160 hours per month, whether he or she is needed or not. Last National has 12 experienced tellers available at the beginning of January. Past experience has shown that by the end of each month, approximately 10 percent of the experienced tellers have quit. Regular tellers receive a salary of \$600 per month, and trainees are paid \$300 during their month of training. How many tellers should be hired for each of the next 6 months?

Figure 18.2 captures the essential relationships for this time-phased planning model. The decision variables are the number of trainees to hire for each period and the number of tellers available at the beginning of each period.

Let T_t = number of trainees hired at the beginning of period t for $t = 1, 2, 3, 4, 5, 6$

A_t = number of tellers available at the beginning of period t for $t = 1, 2, 3, 4, 5, 6$

The objective is to minimize the total personnel costs for the 6-month planning horizon. Two sets of constraints are required. One represents the required teller-hours for each of the 6 months; the other, beginning with the second month, tracks the number of available tellers carried from one month to the next, which accounts for new hires and employee turnover. The following model uses some shorthand algebraic notations:

$$\text{Minimize} \sum_{t=1}^{6} (600A_t + 300T_t)$$

$$\begin{aligned}
\text{subject to}\quad & 160A_1 - 80T_1 \geq 1500 && \text{January}\\
& 160A_2 - 80T_2 \geq 1800 && \text{February}\\
& 160A_3 - 80T_3 \geq 1600 && \text{March}\\
& 160A_4 - 80T_4 \geq 2000 && \text{April}\\
& 160A_5 - 80T_5 \geq 1800 && \text{May}\\
& 160A_6 - 80T_6 \geq 2200 && \text{June}\\
& A_1 = 12 &&\\
& 0.9A_{t-1} + T_{t-1} - A_t = 0 && \text{for } t = 2, 3, 4, 5, 6\\
& A_t, T_t \geq 0 \text{ and integer for } t = 1, 2, 3, 4, 5, 6 &&
\end{aligned}$$

FIGURE 18.2. Monthly teller transition diagram.

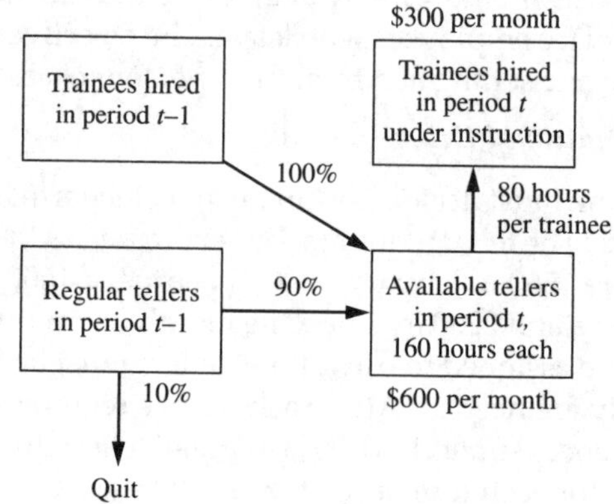

Note that when this model is used, only the value for January hiring is of immediate interest. The trainee hires for the other months can be treated as estimates for now. Before the start of February, the model is run again, with the requirements for January dropped and the July requirements added. In this manner, each hiring decision is based on a 6-month projected requirement plan, which permits a gradual adjustment in the size of the workforce. Also, as in the police patrol example, the decision variables must be restricted to integers. Unfortunately, this problem structure does not necessarily yield integer results. This problem illustrates a special class of LP models called *integer programming,* which requires a special computer code that guarantees integer results.

Transportation Problem

Transportation problems are a special class of LP models called networks. The problem structure also ensures an integer solution. The problem essentially is one of shipping goods from origins, or supply points, to destinations, or demand points. Each destination has a particular demand and each origin a particular supply. The number of origins need not equal the number of destinations. To facilitate a solution, a dummy origin or destination is added to balance the total demand and supply. Given a unit cost for shipping between each origin and destination pair, the objective is to minimize the total shipping cost. This problem structure also arises in nontransportation situations, such as when assigning personnel to jobs.

Example 18.5: Lease-a-Lemon Car Rental

Lease-a-Lemon Car Rental has discovered an imbalance in the distribution of rental cars within its northeast territory. The following surpluses exist: 26 cars in New York, 43 in Washington, and 31 in Cleveland. Shortages include 32 cars in Pittsburgh, 28 in Buffalo, and 26 in Philadelphia. The distance in miles to transfer a car between each city is:

	Pittsburgh	Buffalo	Philadelphia
New York	439	396	91
Washington	296	434	133
Cleveland	131	184	479

Develop a plan to redistribute the cars at a minimum cost on the basis of a transportation charge of $1 per mile.

Figure 18.3 is a network representation of the problem, with origin nodes showing a positive supply and destination nodes a negative demand. The supply and demand are balanced with the addition of a dummy destination node showing a –14 (i.e., 86 – 100) demand. The dummy represents cars not redistributed and, thus, has unit transportation costs of zero. Decision variables are the numbers of cars sent from the supply cities to the demand cities, including the dummy destination.

The objective is to minimize the total redistribution cost. Two sets of constraints are required: one limiting the supply from each origin, and the other

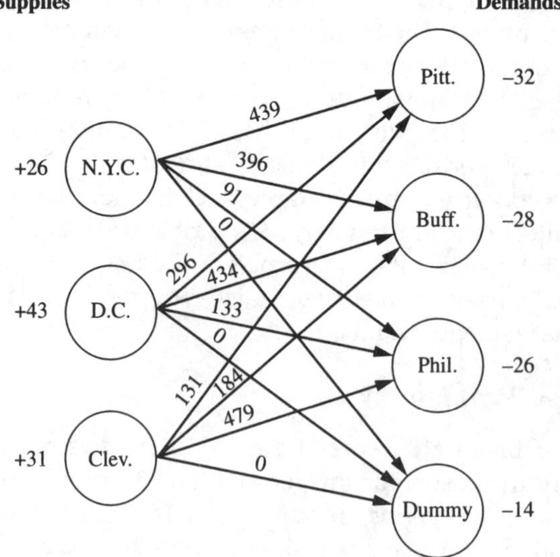

FIGURE 18.3. Lease-a-Lemon car redistribution network.

limiting the demand at each destination. All the constraints will be equalities, because supply and demand are balanced.

Let x_{ij} = number of cars sent from city i to city j for $i = 1, 2, 3$ and $j = 1, 2, 3, 4$

Minimize $439x_{11} + 396x_{12} + \ldots + 479x_{33} + 0x_{34}$
subject to

$$
\begin{array}{llllllllllllr}
x_{11} + & x_{12} + & x_{13} + & x_{14} & & & & & & & & & = 26 \\
 & & & & + x_{21} + & x_{22} + & x_{23} + & x_{24} & & & & & = 43 \\
 & & & & & & & & x_{31} + & x_{32} + & x_{33} + & x_{34} & = 31 \\
x_{11} & & & & + x_{21} & & & & + x_{31} & & & & = 32 \\
 & x_{12} & & & & + x_{22} & & & & + x_{32} & & & = 28 \\
 & & x_{13} & & & & + x_{23} & & & & + x_{33} & & = 26 \\
 & & & x_{14} & & & & + x_{24} & & & & + x_{34} & = 14
\end{array}
$$

$$x_{ij} \geq 0 \quad \text{for all } i, j$$

Note the characteristic structure of the constraints that is common to all transportation problems. This structure and appearance of only coefficients of 1 in the constraint equations assure an integer solution.

OPTIMAL SOLUTIONS AND COMPUTER ANALYSIS

The Stereo Warehouse problem (Example 18.1) is used to illustrate graphically the nature of LP models and their solutions. Because this problem has only the two decision variables x and y, we can draw a picture of the model and see how an optimal solution is achieved. This geometric representation of the model also is used to explain the computer-generated solution.

Graphical Solution of Linear Programming Models

Recall the formulation of the Stereo Warehouse model, in which x and y represent the number of receivers and speakers to be stocked. In this formulation, Z represents the value of the objective function.

Maximize	$Z = 50x + 20y$	gross profit
subject to	$2x + 4y \leq 400$	floor space
	$100x + 50y \leq 8000$	budget
	$x \leq 60$	sales limit
	$x, y \geq 0$	nonnegativity

The set of inequalities or constraints defines a region of permissible values for x and y. Note that letting $x = 0$ and $y = 0$ satisfies all the inequalities, as it should, because that is the "do-nothing" alternative. Our interest, however, is in finding the best, or optimal, values of x and y that maximize the objective function. For a two-variable problem, the permissible, or *feasible*, region can be identified if we plot each constraint inequality. The procedure for drawing the feasible region is:

1. Assign one variable to the x axis and the other to the y axis.
2. Note that the nonnegativity constraints on the variables limit the feasible region to the first quadrant (i.e., upper right-hand corner).
3. Temporarily change each inequality constraint to an equality.
4. Plot each constraint as an equation using the x and y intercepts (i.e., assume that $x = 0$ and solve for the y intercept, repeat for $y = 0$ to find the x intercept, then draw a straight line joining these two axis intercepts). If (0, 0) happens to be a solution of the equation (e.g., $2x - 3y = 0$), however, then another arbitrary point must be selected and the line drawn from that point through the origin.
5. Identify the feasible side of the inequality. This can be accomplished by substituting $x = 0$ and $y = 0$ into the inequality constraint, unless (0, 0) happens to be on the line, in which case some other arbitrary point must be selected. If the inequality is satisfied, then the side containing $x = 0$ and $y = 0$ should be shaded; otherwise, the opposite side of the line is shaded (i.e., it represents a feasible region).
6. Note that each constraint further reduces the feasible region into a geometric figure called a *convex polygon* (i.e., from inside the space looking outward, all the corners point outward).

This procedure is followed for Stereo Warehouse to create the feasible region, as shown in Figure 18.4. Note for the first constraint that the x intercept ($y = 0$) is $400/2 = 200$ and the y intercept ($x = 0$) is $400/4 = 100$. Also note that the test point $x = 0, y = 0$ satisfies all three constraints; thus, the shaded area is either below or to the left of each constraint. Further, note that any point (i.e., combination of x and y values) within the feasible region simultaneously satisfies all three constraints and the nonnegativity condition.

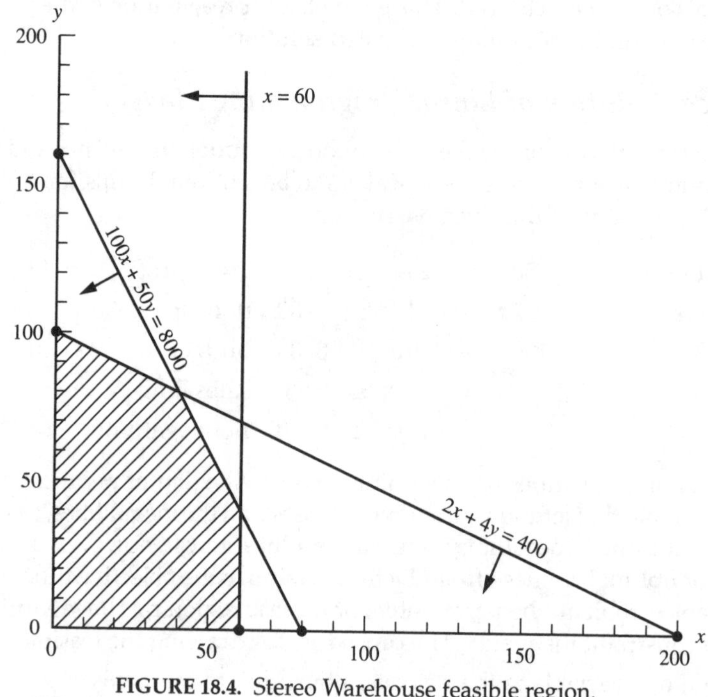

FIGURE 18.4. Stereo Warehouse feasible region.

The optimal solution to the problem now can be found graphically. Recall that the objective is to make Z as large as possible provided that the values of x and y are in the feasible region. If we let Z take on a trial value (e.g., 2000), then we can plot Z as a straight line using the intercept approach. For $Z = 2000$, the x intercept ($y = 0$) is $2000/50 = 40$ and the y intercept ($x = 0$) is $400/4 = 100$. Figure 18.5 shows the objective function $Z = 2000$ plotted on the graph of the feasible region. As the value of Z is increased to 3000, 3600, and, finally, 3800, the objective function moves out from the origin in parallel lines, or contours. The maximum value of $Z = 3800$ occurs at point C (i.e., $x = 60$, $y = 40$), a corner of the polygon. If Z moves out any further, no point on the contour line will be common to the feasible region, and we have just demonstrated an axiom of LP. An optimal solution to an LP model always will occur at a corner, or *extreme point*, of the feasible region. In the special case in which the slope of the objective function is identical to the slope of a constraint, the optimal solution also will include any point between the extreme points along the constraint line.

Linear Programming Model in Standard Form

Realizing that an optimal solution will be found at an extreme point reduces our search for a feasible region to a finite set of points. Further, each extreme point is defined as the simultaneous solution of a pair of constraints that are stated as equations.

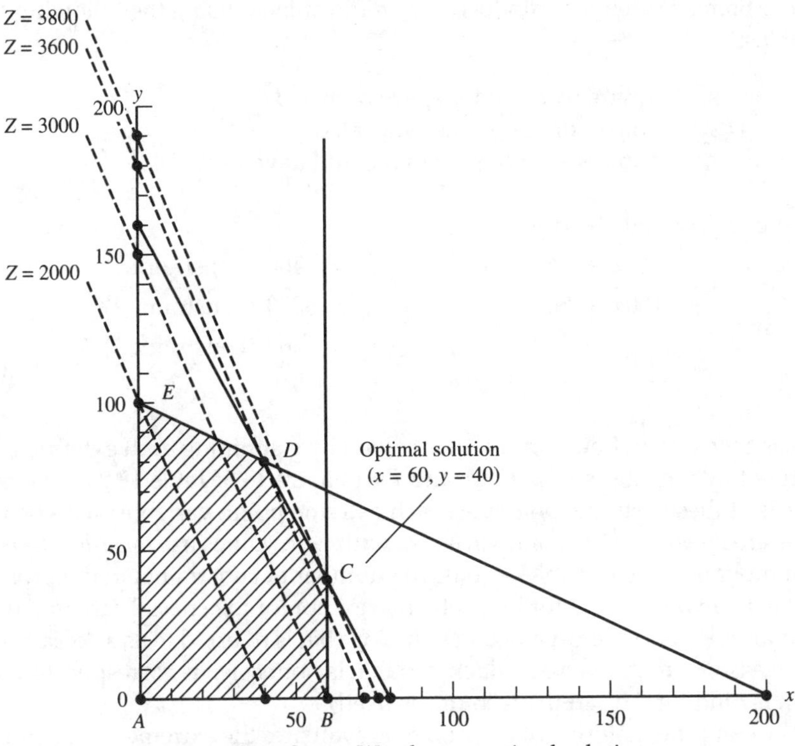

FIGURE 18.5. Stereo Warehouse optimal solution.

A formal way of restating an inequality constraint as an equation in LP models is accomplished with the use of a *slack,* or *surplus,* variable. For constraints of the ≤ variety, a nonnegative slack (i.e., resources not used) variable is added to the left-hand side. For example, the Stereo Warehouse floor-space constraint would be restated as:

$$2x + 4y + s_1 = 400$$

The slack variable s_1 would represent available floor space not used by the receivers and speakers stocked. For constraints of the ≥ variety, a nonnegative surplus (i.e., results produced in excess of requirements) variable is subtracted from the left-hand side. For example, in the Gotham City Police Patrol problem, the first-period patrol officer requirement would be restated as:

$$x_1 + x_6 - s_1 = 6$$

In this case, the surplus variable s_1 would represent the number of patrol officers assigned to the first period in excess of the requirement of six officers. Note that the subscript number for the slack or surplus variable corresponds to the constraint number.

The Stereo Warehouse model can be reformulated using the following slack variables:

Let s_1 = square feet of floor space not used
s_2 = dollars of budget not allocated
s_3 = number of receivers that could have been sold

$$
\begin{aligned}
\text{Maximize } Z &= 50x + 20y \\
\text{subject to } \quad & 2x + 4y + s_1 = 400 \text{ (constraint 1)} \\
& 100x + 50y + s_2 = 8000 \text{ (constraint 2)} \\
& x + s_3 = 60 \text{ (constraint 3)} \\
& x, y, s_1, s_2, s_3 \geq 0
\end{aligned}
$$

The Stereo Warehouse problem is solved by examining each extreme point, identified by the letters *A*, *B*, *C*, *D*, and *E* in Figure 18.5. Table 18.2 contains the analysis of these extreme points. At each extreme point, variables with positive values are labeled as *basic* and variables with zero values as *nonbasic*. Note that the number of basic variables equals the number of constraints in the problem. This result always is true for LP problems, except for the special case in which a basic variable also is zero-valued (a situation that is referred to as a *degenerate solution*). Also, note that when a slack variable is nonbasic, its corresponding constraint is binding (i.e., all the resource is used).

The computer solution of LP problems evaluates the extreme points in a systematic way. This procedure is called the *simplex algorithm*. In our Stereo Warehouse example, the simplex algorithm starts at point *A*, proceeds to extreme point *B* (because variable x contributes more than variable y does to the objective function), and stops at extreme point C (the optimum). The algorithm is able to identify optimality; thus, all the extreme points need not be examined. Details of the

TABLE 18.2. Stereo Warehouse Extreme-Point Solutions

Extreme Point	Nonbasic Variables	Basic Variables	Variable Value	Objective-Function Value(Z)
A	x, y	s_1	400	0
		s_2	8000	
		s_3	60	
B	s_3, y	s_1	280	3000
		s_2	2000	
		x	60	
C	s_3, s_2	s_1	120	3800
		y	40	
		x	60	
D	s_1, s_2	s_3	20	3600
		y	80	
		x	40	
E	s_1, x	s_3	60	2000
		y	100	
		s_2	3000	

simplex algorithm are not discussed here, but they can be found in any of the operations research texts listed in the Selected Bibliography.

Computer Analysis and Interpretation

The following illustrations of computer input and output reports result from using Excel Solver 7.0 for personal computers.

The computer input for the Stereo Warehouse example shown in Table 18.3 is an illustration of the Excel Add-ins Solver feature provided by Paul A. Jensen.[1]

The computer solution and sensitivity report for the Stereo Warehouse problem is shown in Table 18.4. Each decision variable x and y and the slack variable s_1 have a nonzero solution value. The zero values for s_2 and s_3 indicate that these are nonbasic variables; thus, the corresponding constraints are binding.

The *shadow price* shown in the sensitivity table has an important managerial interpretation. Recall that a nonbasic slack variable means that the corresponding constraint is binding at optimality. For the Stereo Warehouse problem, the budget constraint of \$8000 (corresponding slack variable s_2) and limit of 60 units for receiver sales (corresponding slack variable s_3) are restricting the profit to a maximum of \$3800. The floor-space constraint is no problem, because at optimality, 120 square feet (value of s_1) of the available 400 square feet is not being used. If profits are to be increased, more of the limiting resources must be obtained. The shadow price of \$10 associated with the slack variable s_3 represents the increase in the objective-function value if one more receiver could be sold.

[1]Paul A. Jensen, *Operations Research Add-ins for Microsoft Excel*, Operations Research/Industrial Engineering Program, Department of Mechanical Engineering, University of Texas at Austin, June 1996.

TABLE 18.3 Formulation of the Stereo Warehouse Problem in Excel 7.0 Using Linear Programming Add-in

Linear Model

Name:	Stereo
Type:	LP
No. Var.:	2
Int. Var.:	0
No. Con.:	3
Nonlinear:	0

Objective Value: 0

Model	Variables	Num.	1	2
		Name	X	Y
0		Values	0	0
2		Linear Obj. Coef.	50	20
TRUE		Lower Bounds	0	0
TRUE		Upper Bounds	99999	99999

Model	Constraints Num.	Name	Value	Constraint Bounds Lower	Upper	Constraint Coefficients X	Y
TRUE							
TRUE							
100	1	Floor	0	0	400	2	4
	2	Budget	0	0	8000	100	50
	3	Sales	0	0	60	1	0

TABLE 18.4 Microsoft Excel 7.0 Solution and Sensitivity Report for Stereo Warehouse

Target Cell (Max)

Cell	Name	Original Value	Final Value
H5	Stereo_Obj	0	3800

Changing Cells

Cell	Name	Final Value	Reduced Cost	Objective Coefficient	Allowable Increase	Allowable Decrease
G8	Values X	60	0	50	1E+30	10
H8	Values Y	40	0	20	5	20

Constraints

Cell	Name	Final Value	Shadow Price	Constraint R.H. Side	Allowable Increase	Allowable Decrease
D14	Floor Value	280	0	400	1E+30	120
D15	Budget Value	8000	0.4	8000	1500	2000
D16	Sales Value	60	10	60	20	20
D14	Floor Value	280	0	0	280	1E+30
D15	Budget Value	8000	0	0	8000	1E+30
D16	Sales Value	60	0	0	60	1E+30

Note that if the limit on receiver sales is increased by 1, the budget constraint and limit on x sales define the new extreme point:

$$100x + 50y = 8000$$

$$x = 61$$

The solution of these simultaneous equations yields $x = 61$ and $y = 38$. Substituting these values into the objective function provides a revised profit of $3810, which is an increase of $10. A similar analysis explains the $0.40 increase in the objective-function value if the RHS of the budget constraint is increased by $1 to $8001 and the limit on x remains at 60 (the solution becomes $x = 60$ and $y = 40.02$).

The shadow price represents the imputed price of a unit of the limited resource. Shadow prices can be used by managers to decide on the value of securing more resources. For example, if money can be borrowed for less than 40 cents on the dollar during the period of the sale, the difference will become additional profit.

Most computer programs use the convention that if a unit increase in the RHS value improves the objective function (i.e., increases it for maximization or decreases it for minimization), then the shadow price is positive and represents the amount of objective-function change. In some problems, however, increasing an RHS could result in impairing the objective function. For example, if the protein constraint in the Lakeview Hospital diet problem were increased, then contrary to the minimization desired, the objective function could increase. The shadow price would be negative for this constraint if it were binding at optimality.

Finally, note that the shadow price of a resource in excess (corresponding slack variable is basic) is considered to be zero. In the Stereo Warehouse problem, the value to the manager of securing additional floor space is zero, because not all the available floor space is being used.

SENSITIVITY ANALYSIS

What happens to the optimal solution of an LP problem if the values of the model parameters change? This question is of great interest to a decision maker in an uncertain environment. The sensitivity of a solution regarding the objective-function coefficients is discussed first, and then constraint RHS ranging is analyzed.

Objective-Function Coefficient Ranges

The permissible range of each objective-function coefficient is shown in the "changing cells" portion of Table 18.4. The y-variable coefficient may range from a low of 0 to a high of 25; the x-variable coefficient may range from 40 to infinity. Within these ranges, the optimal solution remains at extreme point C, as shown by Figure 18.6, in which the objective-function slope changes with different coefficient values and essentially pivots about extreme point C.

Note that with a y coefficient of 0, the objective function lies along the line segment BC of constraint 3. When the y coefficient is 25, the objective function lies along the line segment DC, which is parallel to constraint 2. Note also that if the coefficient of y exceeds 25, the optimal solution moves to the extreme point D. A similar analysis can be made for the x objective-function coefficient. The decision maker must be cautioned that the range for each coefficient is limited to changing one parameter at a time while holding all others fixed. Further, the value of the objective function changes as these coefficients are changed.

Right-Hand-Side Ranging

The allowable RHS range for each constraint is shown in the "constraints" portion of Table 18.4. The RHS for the budget constraint ranges from 6000 to 9500; the RHS for the sales constraint ranges from 40 to 80. Within these ranges, the optimal solution contains the same basic variables s_1, x, and y. The values of these variables as well as the objective-function value will change. It should be noted that the shadow price for each resource applies only within these ranges. For example, recall that the shadow price for constraint 3 is a \$10-per-unit increase in the RHS. Note that the objective-function value increases from \$3800 to \$4000 when the RHS increases from 60 to 80 [i.e., (80 – 60)(10) = 200]. Likewise, the objective-function value is reduced by \$200 when the RHS of constraint 3 decreases from 60 to 40.

Note in Figure 18.7 what happens graphically when the RHS of constraint 3 is changed. As the RHS increases, the extreme point C moves along the line seg-

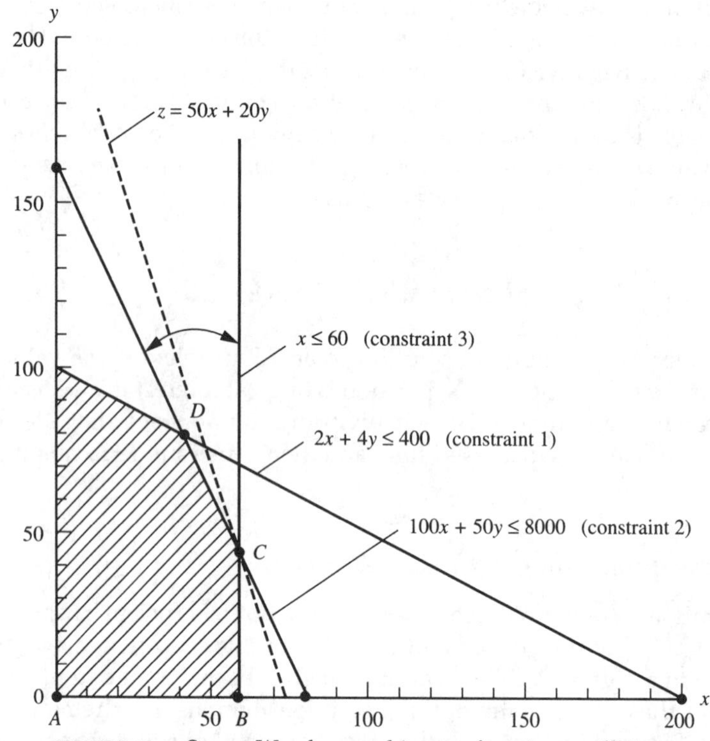

FIGURE 18.6. Stereo Warehouse objective-function coefficient ranging.

ment CI until it becomes coincident with I at RHS = 80. The values of the basic variables at extreme point I are $s_1 = 240$, $x = 80$, and $y = 0$. This is a degenerate solution, because variable $y = 0$ but it still remains in the basis.

If the RHS of constraint 3 is reduced, the extreme point C moves along the line segment CD until it becomes coincident with D at RHS = 40. The values of the basic variables at extreme point D are $s_1 = 0$, $x = 40$, and $y = 80$. This is a degenerate solution, because variable $s_1 = 0$ but it still remains in the basis. A similar analysis for binding constraint 2 can be made to show the movement of extreme point C along the line segment BII as the RHS is changed from 6000 to 9500.

The concept that the resource shadow price is limited to the RHS range is important in *postoptimality analysis.* For example, in the Stereo Warehouse problem, suppose that additional money can be obtained at a cost that is less than the shadow price of 40 cents per dollar. The question of how much to obtain at this price is answered by the RHS range on the budget constraint. Secure \$9500 – \$8000, or \$1500, in additional financing to maximize profits. The same caution raised earlier, however, about treating the sensitivity analysis as being limited to changing one parameter at a time while holding all others fixed, is true for RHS ranging.

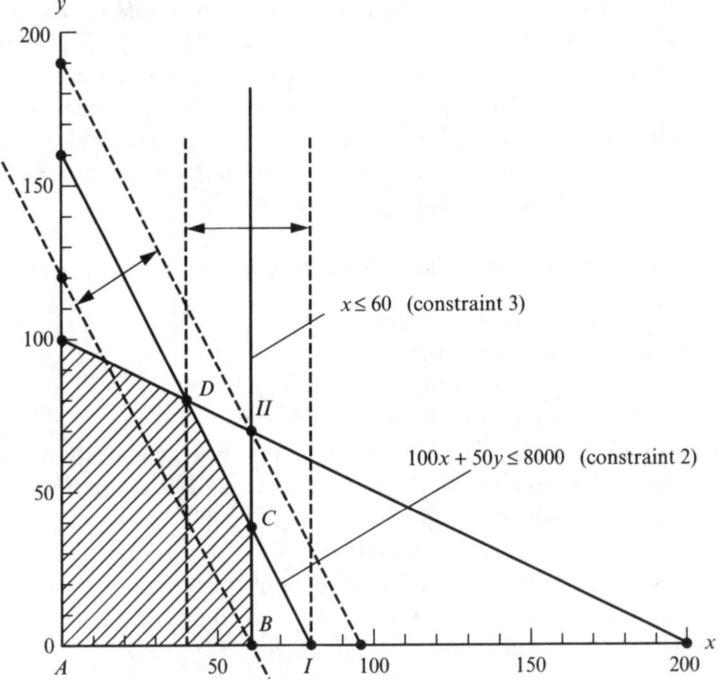

FIGURE 18.7. Stereo Warehouse right-hand-side ranging.

GOAL PROGRAMMING

Linear programming models allow for only one objective, and all constraints must be met absolutely. Many problems, however, particularly in the public sector, have multiple objectives in different units of measure. This makes construction of a consolidated single objective difficult, if not impossible. For example, an emergency ambulance system could have the following objectives:

1. Maintain an average response time of approximately 4 minutes.
2. Ensure that 90 percent of all calls receive aid in less than 10 minutes.
3. Try not to exceed a budget of $100,000 per year.
4. Allocate calls to ambulance crews in an equitable manner.

Goal programming is a variation of LP that permits multiple and conflicting goals with different dimensions. Multiple goals are rank-ordered and treated as *preemptive priorities.* In the solution procedure, higher-ranked goals are not sacrificed to achieve lower-ranked goals. The solution approach is equivalent to solving a series of nested LP problems in which higher-ranked goals become constraints on lower-ranked goals. While LP optimizes a single objective, goal programming minimizes deviations from goals. This solution approach is known as *satisficing,* because not all goals necessarily will be met. Instead, the goals will be achieved as closely as possible.

The objective function will contain only deviational variables (i.e., plus or minus deviations from goals), which also can be given *deviational weights* to distinguish relative importance within a priority level. The objective always is to minimize the sum of the deviations at each priority level, with consideration being given to the hierarchy of preemptive priorities. All constraints are stated as equalities and contain both plus and minus deviational variables in addition to decision variables. To illustrate a goal programming model, the Stereo Warehouse example is reformulated as a goal program.

Example 18.6: Stereo Warehouse as a Goal Program

Let x = number of receivers to stock
y = number of speakers to stock
d_1^- = amount by which profit falls short of \$99,999
d_1^+ = amount by which profit exceeds \$99,999
d_2^- = amount by which floor space used falls short of 400 square feet
d_2^+ = amount by which floor space used exceeds 400 square feet
d_3^- = amount by which budget falls short of \$8000
d_3^+ = amount by which budget exceeds \$8000
d_4^- = amount by which sales of receivers fall short of 60
d_4^+ = amount by which sales of receivers exceed 60
P_k = priority level with rank k

$$\text{Minimize } Z = P_1 d_4^+ + P_2\left(d_1^- + 2d_3^+\right) + P_3\left(d2_1^- + 2d_2^+\right)$$

subject to

$$\begin{aligned} 50x + 20y + d_1^- - d_1^+ &= 99{,}999 && \text{profit goal} \\ 2x + 4y + d_2^- - d_2^+ &= 400 && \text{floor-space goal} \\ 100x + 50y + d_3^- - d_3^+ &= 8000 && \text{budget goal} \\ x + d_4^- - d_4^+ &= 60 && \text{sales-limit goal} \\ x, y, d_1^-, d_1^+, d_2^-, d_2^+, d_3^-, d_3^+, d_4^-, d_4^+ &\geq 0 \end{aligned}$$

This formulation has translated the profit objective into a goal at the second priority level. Note that only d_1^- is included in the objective function to be minimized. Minimizing d_1^-, which is the underachievement of the goal, forces the profit to approach 99,999, a large number far in excess of expected profit. The floor space used for display now becomes a third priority, in which both deviational variables are minimized. In other words, we want to use approximately 400 square feet. The goal programming model permits a previous absolute constraint on available space to be treated as a more realistic approximate requirement. Exceeding the budget is to be avoided, so only d_3^+ is found in the objective function. The deviational weight of 2 indicates that meeting the budget is twice as important as maximizing profit. Finally, exceeding the sales limit of 60 receivers is found at the first priority. This illustrates how system or physical constraints are treated in goal programming. Thus, the typical LP absolute constraints, such as ≤ or ≥, have their appropriate deviational variable at the first priority level. The goal hierarchy ensures that no solution will violate these system constraints.

Table 18.5 shows the Excel formulation for the Stereo Warehouse goal pro-

TABLE 18.5 Excel 7.0 Goal Programming Formulation for Stereo Warehouse

Linear Model

Name:	Stereo
Type:	LP
No. Var.:	10
Int. Var.:	0
No. Con.:	4
Nonlinear:	0

Objective Value
0

Model	Variables	Num.	1	2	3	4	5	6	7	8	9	10
		Name	X	Y	DM1	DM2	DM3	DM4	DP1	DP2	DP3	DP4
0		Values	0	0	0	0	0	0	0	0	0	0
10		Linear Obj. Coef.	0	0	100	1	0	0	0	1	200	1000
TRUE		Lower Bounds	0	0	0	0	0	0	0	0	0	0
TRUE		Upper Bounds	99999	99999	99999	99999	99999	99999	99999	99999	99999	99999

Model	Constraints Num.	Name	Value	Constraint Bounds Lower	Upper	Constraint Coefficients									
TRUE															
FALSE															
100	1	Profit	0	99999	99999	50	20	1	0	0	0	-1	0	0	0
	2	Floor	0	400	400	2	4	0	1	0	0	0	-1	0	0
	3	Budget	0	8000	8000	100	50	0	0	1	0	0	0	-1	0
	4	Sales	0	60	60	1	0	0	0	0	1	0	0	0	-1

gramming model. To ensure that the goal hierarchy is not violated, priority ranks have been given increasingly large weights (i.e., $P_1 = 1000$, $P_2 = 100$, and $P_3 = 1$). The variables labeled DM represent underachievement deviations (d^-), and the variables labeled DP represent overachievement deviations (d^+).

The goal programming solution to the Stereo Warehouse example is found in Table 18.6. Note that the values for the decision variables x and y are identical to the values in the previous LP solution. When the value for DM1 is subtracted from its RHS of 99,999, the profit is found to be \$3800, as before. The deviational variable DM2 takes on a value of 120, indicating the underachievement of our goal to use approximately 400 square feet of floor space. Our budget of \$8000 is completely exhausted, because DP3 = 0. The deviational variable DM4 is zero, as is required to achieve the constraint on

TABLE 18.6 Excel 7.0 Goal Programming Solution and Sensitivity Report for Stereo Warehouse

Target Cell (Min)

Cell	Name	Original Value	Final Value
\$H\$5	Stereo_Goal_Obj	0	9620020

Changing Cells

Cell	Name	Final Value	Reduced Cost	Objective Coefficient	Allowable Increase	Allowable Decrease
\$G\$8	Values X	60	0	0	994	6
\$H\$8	Values Y	40	0	0	3	497
\$I\$8	Values DM1	96199	0	100	0.6	99.4
\$J\$8	Values DM2	120	0	1	165.6666667	1
\$K\$8	Values DM3	0	40.08	0	1E+30	40.08
\$L\$8	Values DM4	0	994	0	1E+30	994
\$M\$8	Values DP1	0	100	0	1E+30	100
\$N\$8	Values DP2	0	2	1	1E+30	2
\$O\$8	Values DP3	0	159.92	200	1E+30	159.92
\$P\$8	Values DP4	0	6	1000	1E+30	6

Constraints

Cell	Name	Final Value	Shadow Price	Constraint R.H. Side	Allowable Increase	Allowable Decrease
\$D\$14	Profit Value	99999	0	99999	1E+30	0
\$D\$15	Floor Value	400	0	400	1E+30	0
\$D\$16	Budget Value	8000	-40.08	8000	1500	0
\$D\$17	Sales Value	60	-994	60	20	0
\$D\$14	Profit Value	99999	100	99999	0	96199
\$D\$15	Floor Value	400	1	400	0	120
\$D\$16	Budget Value	8000	0	8000	0	1E+30
\$D\$17	Sales Value	60	0	60	0	1E+30

receiver sales. In summary, all goals are met, except for the desire to utilize 400 square feet of floor space. The objective-function value is of little consequence, because it simply is the sum of all the weighted deviations. Unfortunately, the shadow prices are of no interest in this case, because the objective function has no economic meaning.

SUMMARY

Linear programming is one of the most popular computer-based modeling techniques available to the modern service operations manager. The power of LP to find optimal solutions and conduct sensitivity analyses is invaluable to the decision maker. Further, the structure of the constrained optimization model fits well with the real world of the service operations manager.

The art of formulating LP models is developed through examples and practice using a systematic approach. Many examples of LP models illustrate the general problem-solving nature of LP. We find that the discipline of formulating LP models helps decision makers to clarify objectives and to identify resource constraints.

The procedure for solving LP models was demonstrated by use of graphics. Because no one solves real LP models by hand, interpretation of computer solutions was stressed. Again, using graphics, the concepts of shadow prices and sensitivity analysis were demonstrated. Because many service operations managers are faced with multiple objectives, the concept of goal programming was introduced. With goal programming, the manager attempts to satisfy goals rather than to optimize a single objective.

KEY TERMS AND DEFINITIONS

Basic variables variables that solve a set of constraint equations when a set of nonbasic variables are set to zero.

Convex polygon the geometric figure defined by the set of constraint functions stipulating the feasible region of possible solutions.

Degenerate solution an occasion when a basic variable also is zero-valued.

Deviational weights weights given to goals within a priority level to show their relative importance.

Extreme point any corner of a convex polygon in which at least one point will define the optimal solution that maximizes (or minimizes) the objective function.

Goal programming a variation of linear programming that is useful when dealing with multiple objectives.

Objective function an algebraic statement measuring the performance of a system when decision variables take on values.

Preemptive priorities a condition in goal programming where higher-ranked goals are not sacrificed to achieve lower-ranked goals.

Postoptimality analysis use of the shadow prices of limited resources and their right-hand-side ranging to evaluate the opportunities for investment in more resources.

Shadow price an opportunity cost (or imputed price) assigned to a limited resource.

Simplex algorithm a systematic procedure to evaluate the extreme points in search of an optimal solution.

TOPICS FOR DISCUSSION

1. Give some everyday examples of constrained optimization problems.
2. How can the validity of LP models be evaluated?
3. Interpret the meaning of the opportunity cost for a nonbasic decision variable that did not appear in the LP solution.
4. Explain graphically what has happened when a degenerate solution occurs in an LP problem.
5. Using Figure 18.6, analyze the x objective-function coefficient that ranges from a value of 40 to infinity.
6. Using Figure 18.7, explain what happens to the LP solution as the RHS of binding constraint 2 ranges from \$6000 to \$9500.
7. Linear programming is a special case of goal programming. Explain.
8. What are some limitations to the use of LP?

Service Benchmark

An Analysis of Alternative Locations and Service Areas of American Red Cross Blood Facilities

The blood service of the American Red Cross (ARC) is divided into a number of regions. Each region has responsibility for blood collection, testing, and distribution. The mid-Atlantic ARC region has responsibility for most of Virginia and northeastern North Carolina.

The ARC collects, tests, and sells blood throughout the mid-Atlantic region, except in the immediate vicinity of Richmond. It owns and operates facilities for collecting, testing, and distributing blood. The mid-Atlantic region of ARC has three facilities, each performing some of these functions. They are located in Norfolk and Charlottesville, Virginia, and in Greenville, North Carolina. Currently, the Norfolk and Greenville facilities both collect and distribute blood in their assigned areas, while Charlottesville only collects. The Norfolk facility does all the testing.

The ARC uses site-specific drives to collect the blood. The three fixed facilities send out vans (called "mobiles") to collect blood at various sites. These mobiles generally carry the necessary equipment and staff and stay at one site all day. All collections are arranged by entities called chapters. There are a number of chapters responsible for collection sites in each county within a facility's area. Each chapter has an established collection goal, which determines the number of collections and the assigned resources. Blood is also collected from walk-in donors at the fixed facilities.

Nightly "shuttles" from Greenville and Charlottesville transport the blood collected each day to be tested at Norfolk. ARC is not interested in duplicating or relocating the testing facility because it has invested heavily in specialized equipment.

After the blood is tested, the Norfolk and Greenville facilities distribute it to regional hospitals and medical centers, which are ARC's main customers. The number of distributions to customers remains fairly constant except in emergency situations. Typically, volunteer drivers make three deliveries a week to each customer.

To remain competitive and reduce costs, the mid-Atlantic ARC assessed its entire system to explore alternatives for its major activities. Its managers considered relocating the Charlottesville facility to the Richmond area with the goal of attracting new customers and collection sites. However, before making a final decision, they wanted to understand the financial implications.

DECISION ALTERNATIVES FOR COLLECTIONS

To evaluate the feasibility of opening a collection facility in the Richmond area, three location decision alternatives were generated:

(1) Retain the three existing collection facilities, Norfolk, Greenville, and Charlottesville, without expanding into Richmond.

(2) Close the Charlottesville collection facility, and open a new collection facility in Richmond. Re-

tain the existing collection facilities in Norfolk and Greenville.

(3) Retain the Charlottesville collection facility, and open a new collection facility in Richmond. Consider Norfolk, Greenville, Charlottesville, and Richmond facilities for collections.

For each of these location alternatives, three allocation scenarios were used to analyze the financial implications:

(A) Retain the current allocation of resources and allocation of collection sites to facilities. Using this scenario with alternative (1) creates a "do nothing" or baseline case.

(B) Within the existing resource constraints, optimize the allocation of collection sites to facilities.

(C) Remove the resource constraints, and optimize the allocation of collection sites among facilities. This scenario could cause some shifting of both collection sites and resources among facilities, resulting in the biggest change from the current structure.

DECISION ALTERNATIVES FOR DISTRIBUTION

Two location decision alternatives were developed to evaluate the feasibility of opening a distribution facility in the Richmond area:

(4) Retain the two existing distribution facilities in Norfolk and Greenville, without expansion into Richmond.

(5) Open a new facility in Richmond for distributions. Retain distribution facilities in Norfolk and Greenville.

Two allocation scenarios were proposed to analyze the financial implications:

(D) Retain the current allocation of customers to facilities. Using this scenario with alternative (1) creates a "do nothing" or baseline case.

(E) Optimize the allocation of customers to facilities.

INTEGER PROGRAMMING MODELS

Based on this framework, the integer programming models shown here were developed. In each case the objective was to minimize transportation costs for each combination of alternative and scenario for collection decisions and distribution decisions. The number of variables and constraints for each model varied depending upon the alternative and scenario being considered.

Collection Model

The model is formulated as follows:

$$\text{Min} \sum_{i=1}^{m} \sum_{j=1}^{n} x_{ij} D_{ij}$$

subject to

$$\sum_{i=1}^{m} \sum_{j=1}^{n} x_{ij} y_{ij} \le A_i$$

$$\sum_{i=1}^{m} \sum_{j=1}^{n} x_{ij} w_{ij} \le B_i$$

$$\sum_{i=1}^{m} \sum_{j=1}^{n} x_{ij} z_{ij} \le C_i$$

$$\sum_{i=1}^{m} \sum_{j=1}^{n} x_{ij} = 1$$

where m = number of facilities

n = number of chapters

$x_{ij} = \begin{cases} 1 \text{ if chapter } j \text{ is assigned facility } i \\ 0 \text{ if not} \end{cases}$

D_{ij} = distance between facility i and chapter j

y_j = number of operations required for chapter j

A_i = total number of operations facility i can conduct

w_j = the pints of blood chapter j needs to collect

B_i = total pints of blood facility i can collect

z_j = number of staff chapter j requires

C_i = total number of staff available at facility i

Distribution Model

The model is formulated as follows:

$$\text{Min} \sum_{i=1}^{m} \sum_{j=1}^{n} x'_{ij} D'_{ij}$$

subject to

$$\text{Min} \sum_{i=1}^{m} \sum_{j=1}^{n} x'_{ij} = 1$$

where m = number of facilities

n = number of customers

D'_{ij} = distance between facility i and chapter j

$$x_{ij} = \begin{cases} 1 \text{ if customer } j \text{ is assigned facility } i \\ 0 \text{ if not} \end{cases}$$

ANALYSIS OF RESULTS FOR COLLECTION MODELS

The results of the collection models were quite surprising. Comparison of retaining the current collection facilities, Norfolk, Greenville, and Charlottesville (alternative 1) and relocating Charlottesville to Richmond (alternative 2) provides an unexpected result: opening a collection facility in Richmond causes increased transportation costs under all three scenarios. The reason that the move to Richmond does not immediately generate savings is that a number of the existing collection sites are very close to Charlottesville. However, retaining Charlottesville and opening a new facility in Richmond for collections (alternative 3, scenario C) provides noticeable savings in transportation costs. This is because Charlottesville can still serve most of its collection sites while the Richmond facility can incorporate some of Norfolk's and Greenville's collection sites. From examining these three alternatives, ARC should keep Charlottesville as a collection facility and open a new collection facility in Richmond, as shown in the following table:

	Scenario A Retain Current Capacity and Allocations of Collection Sites	**Scenario B** Retain Current Capacity but Optimize Allocation of Collection Sites	**Scenario C** Remove Capacity Constraints and Optimize Allocation of Collection Sites
Alternative 1 Norfolk, Greenville, Charlottesville	$207,437	$197,984	$197,984
Alternative 2 Norfolk, Greenville, Richmond	$237,514	$215,187	$214,294
Alternative 3 Norfolk, Greenville, Charlottesville, Richmond	—	—	$173,254

ANALYSIS OF RESULTS FOR DISTRIBUTION MODELS

The ARC should consider opening a distribution facility in Richmond and realize transportation cost savings. Even without a facility in Richmond, it could still reduce distribution costs by reallocating its customers between the current Norfolk and Greenville facilities, as shown in the table below:

	Scenario D Retain Current Allocations of Customers to Facilities	Scenario E Optimize Allocation of Customers to Facilities
Alternative 4		
Norfolk	$128,016	$125,568
Greenville		
Alternative 5		
Norfolk	—	$95,904
Greenville		
Richmond		

Source: Adapted from D. A. Jacobs, M. N. Silan, and B. A. Clemson, "An Analysis of Alternative Locations and Service Areas of American Red Cross Blood Facilities," *Interfaces*, vol. 26, no. 3, May–June 1996, pp. 40–50.

SOLVED PROBLEMS

1. Formulating a Linear Programming Model

Problem Statement

Moonstruck Country Store packages and sells three blends of coffee labeled (A)maretto, (B)reakfast blend, and (C)hicory, at prices of $2.60, $2.50, and $2.30 per pound, respectively. The blends are made from two coffee beans, Colombian and Mexican. The percentage of Colombian beans in blends A, B, and C is 80 percent, 50 percent, and 30 percent, respectively, with the remaining percentage being Mexican beans. At present, Moonstruck has an inventory of 20 pounds of Colombian beans purchased at 90 cents per pound and 30 pounds of Mexican beans purchased at 50 cents per pound. The roasting and packaging cost for all three brands is $1.20 per pound. Formulate a linear programming model to determine the pounds of each brand to mix that will maximize profits.

Solution

First, formulate the objective function by determining the profit per pound for each blend using the following relationship:

Profit per pound = selling price − packaging cost −
Columbian bean cost as percentage − Mexican bean cost as percentage.

$$\begin{aligned}\text{Max } Z &= [2.60 - 1.20 - (.8)(.9) - (.2)(.5)]A + [2.50 - 1.20 - (.5)(.9) - \\ &\quad (.5)(.5)]\,B + [2.30 - 1.20 - (.3)(.9) - (.7)(.5)]C \\ &= .58A + .60B + .48C\end{aligned}$$

Second, formulate the constraints:

$$\begin{aligned} .8A + .5B + .3C &\le 20 \quad \text{Colombian-bean inventory} \\ .2A + .5B + .7C &\le 30 \quad \text{Mexican-bean inventory} \\ A, B, C &\ge 0 \end{aligned}$$

2. Computer Solution and Interpretation of Results

Problem Statement

Use Excel Solver to find the optimal product mix and to perform postoptimality analysis.

Solution

From Table 18.7, we find that the optimal solution yields a profit of $27 with a product mix of 25 pounds of (B)reakfast blend and 25 pounds of (C)hicory blend. Note that with two constraints, only two variables can be basic; thus, it is not optimal to produce all three blends.

Considering the objective function coefficient sensitivity, we see that the (A)maretto blend will be produced only if the unit profit contribution exceeds 78 cents (or a selling price of $2.80). The shadow prices indicate that we are overpaying for Mexican beans, because they are only worth 30 cents per pound in our solution but we paid 50 cents per pound.

EXERCISES

18.1. The Economy Cab Company wants to mix two fuels (A and B) for its taxicabs to minimize operating costs. The company needs at least 3000 gallons to operate its cabs next month. There are only 2000 gallons of fuel A available, but fuel B is unlimited in supply. The mixed fuel must have an octane rating of at least 80.

When fuels are mixed, the amount of the fuel that is obtained equals the sum of the amounts put in, assuming that no spillage or evaporation occurs. The resulting octane rating is the average of the individual octane ratings, weighted in proportion to the respective volumes. Fuel A costs 20 cents per gallon and has an octane rating of 90; fuel B costs 10 cents per gallon and has an octane rating of 75.

a. Formulate this blending problem (a variation on the diet problem) as an LP model to minimize the cost of the blended fuel.

b. Using the graphical method, determine the amount of each fuel that is required for an optimum blend.

18.2 Springdale has been ordered by a federal district court to desegregate its school system. The city is divided into seven school districts and is served by three elementary, one junior high, and one high school. The table here gives the distance from each district to each elementary school and the number of both minority and white children in each district. Ideally, minorities should represent 40 percent of enrollment

	Distance to School (miles)			*Numbers in District*	
District	A	B	C	Minorities	Whites
1	10	18	32	90	40
2	0	25	38	110	20
3	20	13	24	50	60
4	8	22	33	70	70
5	35	0	16	40	130
6	26	14	24	30	120
7	38	7	0	10	160
Total				400	600

TABLE 18.7 Moonstruck Formulation, Solution, and Sensitivity Report Using Excel 7.0

Linear Model

			Name:	Moonstruck					
			Type:	LP					
			No. Var.:	3					
			Int. Var.:	0				Objective Value	
			No. Con.:	2				0	
	Variables	Num.	Nonlinear:	0			1	2	3
Model		Name					A	B	C
0		Values					0	0	0
3	Linear Obj. Coef.						0.58	0.6	0.48
TRUE	Lower Bounds						0	0	0
TRUE	Upper Bounds						99999	99999	99999
TRUE	Constraints				Constraint Bounds				
TRUE	Num.	Name	Value		Lower	Upper	Constraint Coefficients		
100	1	Col	0		0	20	0.8	0.5	0.3
	2	Mex	0		0	30	0.2	0.5	0.7

Target Cell (Max)

Cell	Name	Original Value	Final Value
H5	Moonstruck_Obj	0	27

Changing Cells

Cell	Name	Final Value	Reduced Cost	Objective Coefficient	Allowable Increase	Allowable Decrease
G8	Values A	0	-0.2	0.58	0.2	1E+30
H8	Values B	25	0	0.6	0.2	0.08
I8	Values C	25	0	0.48	0.133333333	0.12

Constraints

Cell	Name	Final Value	Shadow Price	Constraint R.H. Side	Allowable Increase	Allowable Decrease
D14	Col Value	20	0.9	20	10	7.142857143
D15	Mex Value	30	0.3	30	16.66666667	10
D14	Col Value	20	0	0	20	1E+30
D15	Mex Value	30	0	0	30	1E+30

in each elementary school. Achieving perfect desegregation is not practical, however, so the school board is willing to settle for a percentage of minorities in each school that is not less than 30 percent or more than 50 percent. Each school has a capacity of 400 students. Formulate an LP model to minimize the total number of student miles traveled by bus. Do not solve.

18.3 The computer input for the Lakeview Hospital example is shown in Table 18.8, with *E*, *C*, and *S* defined as units of egg custard base, ice cream, and butterscotch syrup. The results of the computer solutions are given in Table 18.9.

a. What is the cost of the special milkshake?

b. How many units of each ingredient are required for this minimum-cost shake? If you feel that this mixture is unacceptable, suggest a constraint that would guarantee an acceptable milkshake.

c. What would be the cost of including one unit of ice cream in the mixture? Explain why this cost is less than 25 cents.

d. What is the cholesterol, fat, protein, and calorie content of this milkshake?

e. What are the ranges of acceptable unit costs for the egg custard base and butterscotch syrup for the computer solution to remain optimal?

f. What would the milkshake cost if the protein requirement were increased to its RHS limit?

g. Why are there no upper limits on the requirements for cholesterol and fat?

18.4. The computer input for the Gotham City Police Patrol example is shown in Table 18.10, with x_j defined as the number of patrol officers reporting for duty at the beginning of period *j*. The results of the computer solution are given in Table 18.11.

a. How many patrol officers are required to meet the staffing requirements? Is this solution an improvement over the current practice of officers reporting at only three times during the day?

b. In what period is there an excess of officers? As the police commissioner, how could you make full use of their time?

c. Using Figure 18.1, sketch the results of this optimum staffing schedule.

d. What does the reduced cost of zero for variable x_4 suggest?

e. A police officer, unhappy about reporting for duty at midnight, suggests the following schedule: $x_1 = 0$, $x_2 = 8$, $x_3 = 6$, $x_4 = 2$, $x_5 = 10$, and $x_6 = 6$. Show that this schedule is both feasible and optimal.

TABLE 18.8 Excel 7.0 Formulation for Lakeview Hospital

Linear Model

Name:	Lakeview
Type:	LP
No. Var.:	3
Int. Var.:	0
No. Con.:	4
Nonlinear:	0

Objective Value: 0

Model	Variables	Num.	1	2	3
		Name	E	C	S
0		Values	0	0	0
3		Linear Obj. Coef.	0.15	0.25	0.1
TRUE		Lower Bounds	0	0	0
TRUE		Upper Bounds	99999	99999	99999
TRUE	Constraints				
TRUE					
100					

Constraints Num.	Name	Value	Constraint Bounds Lower	Constraint Bounds Upper	Constraint Coefficients E	C	S
1	Chol	0	0	175	50	150	90
2	Fat	0	0	150	0	100	50
3	Protein	0	200	99999	70	10	0
4	Calories	0	100	99999	30	80	200

TABLE 18.9 Excel 7.0 Solution and Sensitivity Report for Lakeview Hospital

Target Cell (Min)

Cell	Name	Original Value	Final Value
H5	Lakeview_Obj	0	0.435714286

Changing Cells

Cell	Name	Final Value	Reduced Cost	Objective Coefficient	Allowable Increase	Allowable Decrease
G8	Values E	2.857142857	0	0.15	1.335	0.135
H8	Values C	0	0.190714286	0.25	1E+30	0.190714286
I8	Values S	0.071428571	0	0.1	0.503773585	0.1

Constraints

Cell	Name	Final Value	Shadow Price	Constraint R.H. Side	Allowable Increase	Allowable Decrease
D14	Chol Value	149.2857143	0	175	1E+30	25.71428571
D15	Fat Value	3.571428571	0	150	1E+30	146.4285714
D16	Protein Value	200	0	99999	1E+30	99799
D17	Calories Value	100	0	99999	1E+30	99899
D14	Chol Value	149.2857143	0	0	149.2857143	1E+30
D15	Fat Value	3.571428571	0	0	3.571428571	1E+30
D16	Protein Value	200	0.001928571	200	33.33333333	200
D17	Calories Value	100	0.0005	100	57.14285714	14.28571429

TABLE 18.10 Excel 7.0 Formulation for Gotham City

Linear Model

Name:	Gotham_City
Type:	LP
No. Var.:	6
Int. Var.:	0
No. Con.:	6
Nonlinear:	0

Objective Value

0

Model	Variables	Num.	1	2	3	4	5	6
		Name	X 1	X 2	X 3	X 4	X 5	X 6
0		Values	0	0	0	0	0	0
6		Linear Obj. Coef.	1	1	1	1	1	1
TRUE		Lower Bounds	0	0	0	0	0	0
TRUE		Upper Bounds	99999	99999	99999	99999	99999	99999
TRUE								
FALSE								
100								

Constraints

Num.	Name	Value	Constraint Bounds Lower	Upper	Constraint Coefficients					
1	Period 1	0	6	99999	1	0	0	0	0	1
2	Period 2	0	4	99999	1	1	0	0	0	0
3	Period 3	0	14	99999	0	1	1	0	0	0
4	Period 4	0	8	99999	0	0	1	1	0	0
5	Period 5	0	12	99999	0	0	0	1	1	0
6	Period 6	0	16	99999	0	0	0	0	1	1

TABLE 18.11 Excel 7.0 Solution and Sensitivity Report for Gotham City

Target Cell (Min)

Cell	Name	Original Value	Final Value
H5	Gotham_City_Obj	0	32

Changing Cells

Cell	Name	Final Value	Reduced Cost	Objective Coefficient	Allowable Increase	Allowable Decrease
G8	Values X 1	2	0	1	0	1
H8	Values X 2	6	0	1	0	0
I8	Values X 3	8	0	1	0	0
J8	Values X 4	0	0	1	1E+30	0
K8	Values X 5	12	0	1	0	1
L8	Values X 6	4	0	1	1	0

Constraints

Cell	Name	Final Value	Shadow Price	Constraint R.H. Side	Allowable Increase	Allowable Decrease
D14	Period 1 Value	6	0	99999	1E+30	99993
D15	Period 2 Value	8	0	99999	1E+30	99991
D16	Period 3 Value	14	0	99999	1E+30	99985
D17	Period 4 Value	8	0	99999	1E+30	99991
D18	Period 5 Value	12	0	99999	1E+30	99987
D19	Period 6 Value	16	0	99999	1E+30	99983
D14	Period 1 Value	6	1	6	99991	2
D15	Period 2 Value	8	0	4	4	1E+30
D16	Period 3 Value	14	1	14	99985	4
D17	Period 4 Value	8	0	8	4	8
D18	Period 5 Value	12	1	12	4	2
D19	Period 6 Value	16	0	16	2	4

18.5. The computer input for the Last National Drive-In Bank example is shown in Table 18.12, with A_j and T_j representing the number of tellers available and trainees hired at the beginning of period j. The results of the computer solution are given in Table 18.13.

a. The solution did not result in integer values as required. On the basis of the fractional solution, how many trainees would you recommend be hired in each of the coming six periods?

b. Is your recommendation in part **a** feasible?

c. Why are you not surprised to find that T_6 is nonbasic?

d. How much overstaffing results from your solution?

e. Explain why this LP formulation cannot be solved as an integer program.

TABLE 18.12 Excel 7.0 Formulation for Last National Bank

Linear Model

Model
0
12
TRUE
TRUE
TRUE
FALSE
100

Name: National_Bank
Type: LP
No. Var.: 12
Int. Var.: 0
No. Con.: 12
Nonlinear: 0

Objective Value
0

Variables	Num.	1	2	3	4	5	6	7	8	9	10	11	12
	Name	A1	A2	A3	A4	A5	A6	T1	T2	T3	T4	T5	T6
	Values	0	0	0	0	0	0	0	0	0	0	0	0
	Linear Obj. Coef.	600	600	600	600	600	600	300	300	300	300	300	300
	Lower Bounds	0	0	0	0	0	0	0	0	0	0	0	0
	Upper Bounds	99999	99999	99999	99999	99999	99999	99999	99999	99999	99999	99999	99999

Constraints Num.	Name	Value	Constraint Bounds Lower	Upper	Constraint Coefficients											
1	Jan	0	1500	99999	160	0	0	0	0	0	-80	0	0	0	0	0
2	Feb	0	1800	99999	0	160	0	0	0	0	0	-80	0	0	0	0
3	Mar	0	1600	99999	0	0	160	0	0	0	0	0	-80	0	0	0
4	Apr	0	2000	99999	0	0	0	160	0	0	0	0	0	-80	0	0
5	May	0	1800	99999	0	0	0	0	160	0	0	0	0	0	-80	0
6	June	0	2200	99999	0	0	0	0	0	160	0	0	0	0	0	-80
7	Initial A	0	12	12	1	0	0	0	0	0	0	0	0	0	0	0
8	Feb-A	0	0	0	0.9	-1	0	0	0	0	1	0	0	0	0	0
9	Mar-A	0	0	0	0	0.9	-1	0	0	0	0	1	0	0	0	0
10	Apr-A	0	0	0	0	0	0.9	-1	0	0	0	0	1	0	0	0
11	May-A	0	0	0	0	0	0	0.9	-1	0	0	0	0	1	0	0
12	June-A	0	0	0	0	0	0	0	0.9	-1	0	0	0	0	1	0

TABLE 18.13 Excel 7.0 Solution and Sensitivity Report for Last National Bank

Target Cell (Min)

Cell	Name	Original Value	Final Value
H5	National_Bank_Obj	0	46865.35692

Changing Cells

Cell	Name	Final Value	Reduced Cost	Objective Coefficient	Allowable Increase	Allowable Decrease
G8	Values A1	12	0	600	1E+30	330
H8	Values A2	11.67432039	0	600	1E+30	630
I8	Values A3	11.35552913	0	600	1E+30	847.2413793
J8	Values A4	12.93103448	0	600	1E+30	922.1521998
K8	Values A5	12.5	0	600	1E+30	947.9835172
L8	Values A6	13.75	0	600	1E+30	1226.890868
M8	Values T1	0.87432039	0	300	366.6666667	300
N8	Values T2	0.848640781	0	300	700	750
O8	Values T3	2.711058264	0	300	941.3793103	858.6206897
P8	Values T4	0.862068966	0	300	1024.613555	896.0760999
Q8	Values T5	2.5	0	300	1053.315019	908.9917586
R8	Values T6	0	913.445434	300	1E+30	913.445434

Constraints

Cell	Name	Final Value	Shadow Price	Constraint R.H. Side	Allowable Increase	Allowable Decrease
D14	Jan Value	1850.054369	0	99999	1E+30	98148.94563
D15	Feb Value	1800	0	99999	1E+30	98199
D16	Mar Value	1600	0	99999	1E+30	98399
D17	Apr Value	2000	0	99999	1E+30	97999
D18	May Value	1800	0	99999	1E+30	98199
D19	June Value	2200	0	99999	1E+30	97799
D20	Initial A Value	12	0	12	1E+30	0
D21	Feb-A Value	2.33147E-15	0	0	1E+30	0
D22	Mar-A Value	2.77556E-15	0	0	1E+30	0
D23	Apr-A Value	-3.10862E-15	0	0	1E+30	0
D24	May-A Value	3.44169E-15	0	0	1E+30	0
D25	June-A Value	0	0	0	1E+30	0
D14	Jan Value	1850.054369	0	1500	350.0543688	1E+30
D15	Feb Value	1800	2.715517241	1800	218.7607346	202.8423306
D16	Mar Value	1600	3.651902497	1600	698.8505747	285.4827586
D17	Apr Value	2000	3.974793964	2000	222.2222222	827.9
D18	May Value	1800	4.08613585	1800	644.4444444	290
D19	June Value	2200	7.668067925	2200	49517.3608	580
D20	Initial A Value	12	330	12	0	1.508855038
D21	Feb-A Value	2.33147E-15	300	0	0	0.87432039
D22	Mar-A Value	2.77556E-15	517.2413793	0	0	1.230529132
D23	Apr-A Value	-3.10862E-15	592.1521998	0	0	3.568534483
D24	May-A Value	3.44169E-15	617.9835172	0	0	1.25
D25	June-A Value	0	626.890868	0	0	3.625

18.6. The computer input for the Lease-a-Lemon Car Rental example is shown in Table 18.14, with x_{ij} representing the number of cars to send from city i to city j. The results of the computer solution are given in Table 18.15.

a. What is the recommended schedule of car movements?

b. Is this solution degenerate?

18.7. A certain company is planning to introduce a new product that will be promoted by specially trained agents. The new-product campaign will be guided by the following considerations: (1) the training session for special agents should be as close to 20 working days as possible, (2) sales during the first quarter, it is hoped, will be near 5 million units, and (3) under no circumstances can training costs exceed $600,000. Write the objective function and constraints if the sales target is considered to be twice as important as the training time target. The training cost is $20,000 per day, and each day of training will produce 150,000 units of sales during the first quarter. The decision to be made concerns the number of days that should be spent training sales agents. Let x = the number of days devoted to training. Define other variables as necessary, and formulate a goal programming model.

18.8. Tennis World carries three lines of its Toe-brand tennis racket: the Student, the Weekender, and the Professional. The more expensive the line, the greater the mark-up, but the more expensive lines also require more floor space for increasingly elaborate displays. Pertinent data can be summarized as:

Tennis Racket	Cost per Racket to Tennis World ($)	Tennis World Mark-up (%)	Display Space per Racket (ft²)
Student	10	10	1
Weekender	15	20	2
Professional	30	50	5

In deciding on the optimal merchandising plan, the manager states the following goals in order of preference: (1) avoid overrunning the purchasing budget of $2000, (2) achieve a gross margin (i.e., the sum of mark-ups for each racket) of at least $500, (3) avoid using more than 300 square feet of floor space for displays, and (4) ensure that the entire purchasing budget is spent. Formulate a goal programming model to determine the number of each type of tennis racket to stock. Recall the following retailing relationship: selling price = cost + (markup)(cost).

TABLE 18.14 Excel 7.0 Formulation for Lease-a-Lemon

Linear Model

Name: Lease_A_Lemon
Type: LP
No. Var.: 12
Int. Var.: 0
No. Con.: 7
Nonlinear: 0

Objective Value: 0

Model	Variables	Num.	1	2	3	4	5	6	7	8	9	10	11	12
0		Name	X 11	X12	X13	X 14	X21	X22	X 23	X24	X31	X 32	X 33	X 34
12		Values	0	0	0	0	0	0	0	0	0	0	0	0
TRUE		Linear Obj. Coef.	439	396	91	0	296	434	133	0	131	184	479	0
TRUE		Lower Bounds	0	0	0	0	0	0	0	0	0	0	0	0
TRUE		Upper Bounds	99999	99999	99999	99999	99999	99999	99999	99999	99999	99999	99999	99999
FALSE														
100														

Constraints

Num.	Name	Value	Constraint Bounds Lower	Constraint Bounds Upper	Constraint Coefficients											
1	NYC	0	26	26	1	1	1	1	0	0	0	0	0	0	0	0
2	DC	0	43	43	0	0	0	0	1	1	1	1	0	0	0	0
3	Clev	0	31	31	0	0	0	0	0	0	0	0	1	1	1	1
4	Pitt	0	32	32	1	0	0	0	1	0	0	0	1	0	0	0
5	Buff	0	28	28	0	1	0	0	0	1	0	0	0	1	0	0
6	Phil	0	26	26	0	0	1	0	0	0	1	0	0	0	1	0
7	Dummy	0	14	14	0	0	0	1	0	0	0	1	0	0	0	1

TABLE 18.15 Excel 7.0 Solution and Sensitivity Report for Lease-a-Lemon

Target Cell (Min)

Cell	Name	Original Value	Final Value
H5	Lease_A_Lemon_Obj	0	16495

Changing Cells

Cell	Name	Final Value	Reduced Cost	Objective Coefficient	Allowable Increase	Allowable Decrease
G8	Values X 11	0	143	439	1E+30	143
H8	Values X12	0	47	396	1E+30	47
I8	Values X13	26	0	91	42	1E+30
J8	Values X 14	0	0	0	47	42
K8	Values X21	29	0	296	47	74
L8	Values X22	0	85	434	1E+30	85
M8	Values X 23	0	42	133	1E+30	42
N8	Values X24	14	0	0	42	47
O8	Values X31	3	0	131	74	47
P8	Values X 32	28	0	184	47	184
Q8	Values X 33	0	553	479	1E+30	553
R8	Values X 34	0	165	0	1E+30	165

Constraints

Cell	Name	Final Value	Shadow Price	Constraint R.H. Side	Allowable Increase	Allowable Decrease
D14	NYC Value	26	0	26	1E+30	0
D15	DC Value	43	0	43	1E+30	0
D16	Clev Value	31	0	31	1E+30	0
D17	Pitt Value	32	0	32	1E+30	0
D18	Buff Value	28	0	28	1E+30	0
D19	Phil Value	26	-74	26	0	0
D20	Dummy Value	14	-165	14	0	0
D14	NYC Value	26	165	26	0	0
D15	DC Value	43	165	43	0	0
D16	Clev Value	31	0	31	0	1E+30
D17	Pitt Value	32	131	32	0	0
D18	Buff Value	28	184	28	0	0
D19	Phil Value	26	0	26	0	1E+30
D20	Dummy Value	14	0	14	0	1E+30

CASE: MUNICH DELICATESSEN

Among the most popular items served by the Munich Delicatessen is its bratwurst. This sausage is based on an original Old World recipe combining beef, chicken, lamb, and assorted spices in a pure animal casing. By U.S. Department of Agriculture regulations, the Munich Deli must display on the sausage label certain content information and adhere to those content specifications in the processing and packaging of the sausage. Because of the popularity of its bratwurst, Munich Deli can sell all the bratwurst it can make. Potential variability of the costs of the major ingredients, however, causes a continuing problem for the processing manager, who must determine the amount of each ingredient to mix into the sausage.

Bratwurst is prepared in 100-pound batches. According to the label, which cannot be altered except through a lengthy and costly procedure, each batch consists of at least 30-percent lamb by weight, with no specific requirement on beef or chicken. Moreover, the label indicates that each batch, by weight, is at most 24-percent fat, at least 12-percent protein, and at most 64-percent water and other ingredients. It can be reasonably assumed that the spices and casing add an insignificant amount to the total sausage weight and almost nothing in terms of the elements being controlled.

A recent Department of Agriculture study has shown that the major ingredients in bratwurst contain the label-controlled elements in the following proportions:

	Percentage of Weight		
Element	Beef	Chicken	Lamb
Fat	20	15	25
Protein	20	15	15
Water and others	60	70	60

Currently, the costs of the principal ingredients are \$1.00, \$0.50, and \$0.70 per pound for beef, chicken, and lamb, respectively. At these costs, there seem to be unlimited supplies. Thus, the processing manager at Munich Deli must decide how much of each principal ingredient to mix into each batch of bratwurst to meet the labeling requirements at the lowest cost.

A preliminary analysis suggests that this decision problem can be formulated as an LP model, with:

x_1 = number of pounds of beef per batch,
x_2 = number of pounds of chicken per batch, and
x_3 = number of pounds of lamb per batch.

Formulate this problem as an LP problem and solve.

Questions

1. Suppose that the early, unseasonably cold weather reduces the production of lamb and that the price for new supplies rises to 85 cents per pound. What effect will this situation have on the optimum contents of the sausage found originally? What effect will this situation have on Munich Deli's production costs for each batch of bratwurst?
2. The Department of Agriculture is considering the adoption of new regulations that would restrict the water content in all sausage. For what range of water-content values would Munich Deli continue to use the same ingredients in its sausage as in the original optimum (i.e., the same basic variables)?
3. Suppose that a meat supplier advises Munich Deli of the availability of veal tongues. The original recipe for bratwurst reveals that veal tongues could be used, and technically, this ingredient already is covered on the sausage label under the generic category "beef and beef by-products." Unlike the regular beef originally considered, these tongues are 30-percent fat, 15-percent protein, and 55-percent water, all by weight. The meat supplier is willing to sell Munich Deli these tongues for \$0.40 per pound. Should this new ingredient be included in the optimal sausage composition? Why?

CASE: SEQUOIA AIRLINES

Sequoia Airlines is a well-established regional airline serving California, Nevada, Arizona, and Utah. Sequoia competes against much larger carriers in this regional market, and its management feels that the price, frequency of flight service, ability to meet schedules, baggage handling, and image projected by its flight attendants are the most important marketing factors that airline passengers consider when deciding to use a particular carrier.

In each of these areas, Sequoia is attaining its desired objectives. Maintaining its flight-attendant staff at desired levels has been difficult in the past, however, and many times, it has had to ask flight attendants to work overtime because of worker shortages. This has resulted in excessive personnel costs and some morale problems among the attendants. One reason for these worker shortages is a higher-than-industry-average turnover rate resulting from experienced attendants being hired away by other airlines. This is not totally due to morale problems; that cause seems to become important only during seasonal peak-demand periods, when shortages are particularly bad. By interviewing the existing personnel, Sequoia has discovered that competing regional carriers (whose training programs are not as highly developed) have been hiring away from Sequoia a significant proportion of its staff by offering slightly higher direct salaries, attractive indirect benefit packages, and guarantees of a minimum number of flying hours in off-peak demand periods.

As a beginning, Sequoia's management has asked for a 6-month hiring and training analysis of the flight-attendant staff requirements beginning next month (July). An investigation of the operations schedule indicates that 14,000 attendant-hours are needed in July, 16,000 in August, 13,000 in September, 12,000 in October, 18,000 in November, and 20,000 in December. Sequoia's training program for new personnel requires an entire month of classroom preparation before they are assigned to regular flight service. As junior flight attendants, they remain on probationary status for 1 additional month. Periodically, there is some personnel movement from the working flight attendant staff to the staff that supervises the training of new employees. Figure 18.8 shows the relationships and percentages of interstaff movements.

When no personnel shortages occur, each junior flight attendant normally works an average of 140 hours per month and is paid a salary of $1050 during the probationary period. During the training period, each new employee is paid $750. Experienced flight attendants receive an average salary of $1400 per month and work an average of 125 hours per month. Each instructor receives a salary of $1500 per month.

The poorly kept secret of Sequoia's personalized training program is that the number of trainees is limited to no more than five per instructor. Instructors not needed in a particular month (i.e., surplus) may be used as flight attendants. To ensure a high level of quality in flight service, Sequoia requires that the proportion of junior flight attendant hours not exceed 25 percent of any month's total (i.e., junior plus experienced) attendant-hours.

FIGURE 18.8. Sequoia Airlines flight-attendant flows.

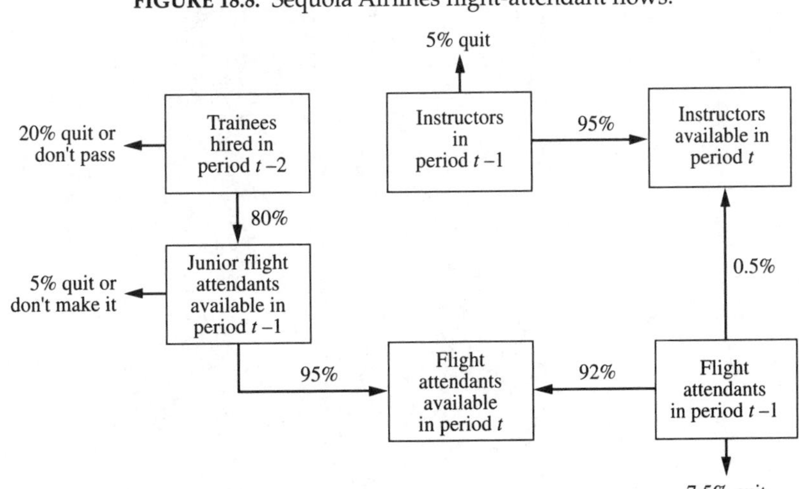

In May, Sequoia hired 10 new employees to enter the training program, and this month, it hired 10 more. At the beginning of June, there were 120 experienced flight attendants and six instructors on Sequoia's staff.

Let T_t = number of trainees hired at the beginning of period t, with $t = 1, 2, 3, 4, 5, 6$

J_t = number of junior flight attendants available at the beginning of period t, with $t = 1, 2, 3, 4, 5, 6$

F_t = number of experienced flight attendants available at the beginning of period t, with $t = 1, 2, 3, 4, 5, 6$

I_t = number of instructors available at the beginning of period t, with $t = 1, 2, 3, 4, 5, 6$

S_t = number of surplus instructors available as flight attendants at the beginning of period t, with $t = 1, 2, 3, 4, 5, 6$

Questions

1. For the forecast period (i.e., July–December), determine the number of new trainees who must be hired at the beginning of each month so that total personnel costs for the flight-attendant staff and training program are minimized. Formulate the problem as an LP model and solve.

2. How would you deal with the noninteger results?

3. Discuss how you would use the LP model to make your hiring decision for the next 6 months.

SELECTED BIBLIOGRAPHY

ANDERSON, D. R., D. J. SWEENEY, and T. A. WILLIAMS: *An Introduction to Management Science*, 7th ed., West Publishing Co., New York, 1994.

HILLIER, F. S., and G. J. LIEBERMAN: *Introduction to Operations Research*, 4th ed., Holden-Day, Inc., San Francisco, 1986.

JENSEN, PAUL A.: *Operations Research Add-ins for Microsoft Excel*, Operations Research/Industrial Engineering Program, Dept. of Mechanical Engineering, University of Texas at Austin, 1996.

Microsoft® Excel for Windows 95, Version 7.0, Microsoft Corporation, Redmond, WA, 1996.

Appendix A: Areas of a Standard Normal Distribution

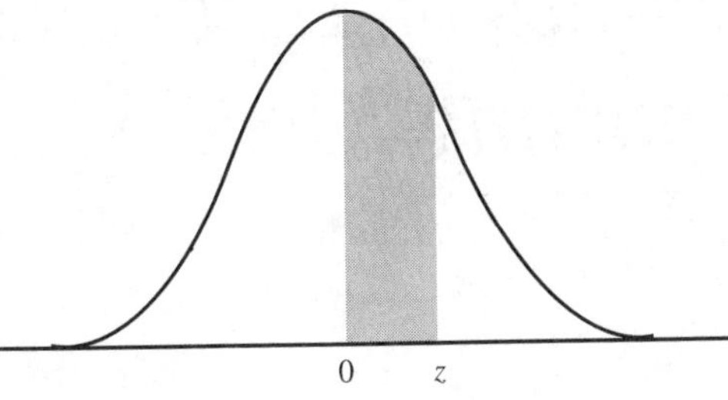

An entry in the table is the proportion under the entire curve which is between $z = 0$ and a positive value of z. Areas for negative values of z are obtained by symmetry.

z	0.00	0.01	0.02	0.03	0.04	0.05	0.06	0.07	0.08	0.09
0.0	0.0000	0.0040	0.0080	0.0120	0.0160	0.0199	0.0239	0.0279	0.0319	0.0359
0.1	0.0398	0.0438	0.0478	0.0517	0.0557	0.0596	0.0636	0.0675	0.0714	0.0753
0.2	0.0793	0.0832	0.0871	0.0910	0.0948	0.0987	0.1026	0.1064	0.1103	0.1141
0.3	0.1179	0.1217	0.1255	0.1293	0.1331	0.1368	0.1406	0.1443	0.1480	0.1517
0.4	0.1554	0.1591	0.1628	0.1664	0.1700	0.1736	0.1772	0.1808	0.1844	0.1879
0.5	0.1915	0.1950	0.1985	0.2019	0.2054	0.2088	0.2123	0.2157	0.2190	0.2224
0.6	0.2257	0.2291	0.2324	0.2357	0.2389	0.2422	0.2454	0.2486	0.2517	0.2549
0.7	0.2580	0.2611	0.2642	0.2673	0.2703	0.2734	0.2764	0.2794	0.2823	0.2852
0.8	0.2881	0.2910	0.2939	0.2967	0.2995	0.3023	0.3051	0.3078	0.3106	0.3133
0.9	0.3159	0.3186	0.3212	0.3238	0.3264	0.3289	0.3315	0.3340	0.3365	0.3389
1.0	0.3413	0.3438	0.3461	0.3485	0.3508	0.3531	0.3554	0.3577	0.3599	0.3621
1.1	0.3643	0.3665	0.3686	0.3708	0.3729	0.3749	0.3770	0.3790	0.3810	0.3830
1.2	0.3849	0.3869	0.3888	0.3907	0.3925	0.3944	0.3962	0.3980	0.3997	0.4015
1.3	0.4032	0.4049	0.4066	0.4082	0.4099	0.4115	0.4131	0.4147	0.4162	0.4177
1.4	0.4192	0.4207	0.4222	0.4236	0.4251	0.4265	0.4279	0.4292	0.4306	0.4319
1.5	0.4332	0.4345	0.4357	0.4370	0.4382	0.4394	0.4406	0.4418	0.4429	0.4441
1.6	0.4452	0.4463	0.4474	0.4484	0.4495	0.4505	0.4515	0.4525	0.4535	0.4545
1.7	0.4554	0.4564	0.4573	0.4582	0.4591	0.4599	0.4608	0.4616	0.4625	0.4633
1.8	0.4641	0.4649	0.4656	0.4664	0.4671	0.4678	0.4686	0.4693	0.4699	0.4706
1.9	0.4713	0.4719	0.4726	0.4732	0.4738	0.4744	0.4750	0.4756	0.4761	0.4767
2.0	0.4772	0.4778	0.4783	0.4788	0.4793	0.4798	0.4803	0.4808	0.4812	0.4817
2.1	0.4821	0.4826	0.4830	0.4834	0.4838	0.4842	0.4846	0.4850	0.4854	0.4857
2.2	0.4861	0.4864	0.4868	0.4871	0.4875	0.4878	0.4881	0.4884	0.4887	0.4890
2.3	0.4893	0.4896	0.4898	0.4901	0.4904	0.4906	0.4909	0.4911	0.4913	0.4916
2.4	0.4918	0.4920	0.4922	0.4925	0.4927	0.4929	0.4931	0.4932	0.4934	0.4936
2.5	0.4938	0.4940	0.4941	0.4943	0.4945	0.4946	0.4948	0.4949	0.4951	0.4952
2.6	0.4953	0.4955	0.4956	0.4957	0.4959	0.4960	0.4961	0.4962	0.4963	0.4964
2.7	0.4965	0.4966	0.4967	0.4968	0.4969	0.4970	0.4971	0.4972	0.4973	0.4974
2.8	0.4974	0.4975	0.4976	0.4977	0.4977	0.4978	0.4979	0.4979	0.4980	0.4981
2.9	0.4981	0.4982	0.4982	0.4983	0.4984	0.4984	0.4985	0.4985	0.4986	0.4986
3.0	0.4987	0.4987	0.4987	0.4988	0.4988	0.4989	0.4989	0.4989	0.4990	0.4990

Source: Donald H. Sanders, A. Franklin Murph, and Robert J. Eng: *Statistics—A Fresh Approach*, McGraw-Hill Book Company, New York, 1976.

Appendix B: Values of L_q for the M/M/c Queuing Model

ρ	$c = 1$	$c = 2$	$c = 3$	$c = 4$	$c = 5$	$c = 6$	$c = 7$	$c = 8$
0.15	0.026	0.001						
0.20	0.050	0.002						
0.25	0.083	0.004						
0.30	0.129	0.007						
0.35	0.188	0.011						
0.40	0.267	0.017						
0.45	0.368	0.024	0.002					
0.50	0.500	0.033	0.003					
0.55	0.672	0.045	0.004					
0.60	0.900	0.059	0.006					
0.65	1.207	0.077	0.008					
0.70	1.633	0.098	0.011					
0.75	2.250	0.123	0.015					
0.80	3.200	0.152	0.019					
0.85	4.817	0.187	0.024	0.003				
0.90	8.100	0.229	0.030	0.004				
0.95	18.050	0.277	0.037	0.005				
1.0		0.333	0.045	0.007				
1.1		0.477	0.066	0.011				
1.2		0.675	0.094	0.016	0.003			
1.3		0.951	0.130	0.023	0.004			
1.4		1.345	0.177	0.032	0.006			
1.5		1.929	0.237	0.045	0.009			
1.6		2.844	0.313	0.060	0.012			

ρ	c = 1	c = 2	c = 3	c = 4	c = 5	c = 6	c = 7	c = 8
1.7		4.426	0.409	0.080	0.017			
1.8		7.674	0.532	0.105	0.023			
1.9		17.587	0.688	0.136	0.030	0.007		
2.0			0.889	0.174	0.040	0.009		
2.1			1.149	0.220	0.052	0.012		
2.2			1.491	0.277	0.066	0.016		
2.3			1.951	0.346	0.084	0.021		
2.4			2.589	0.431	0.105	0.027	0.007	
2.5			3.511	0.533	0.130	0.034	0.009	
2.6			4.933	0.658	0.161	0.043	0.011	
2.7			7.354	0.811	0.198	0.053	0.014	
2.8			12.273	1.000	0.241	0.066	0.018	
2.9			27.193	1.234	0.293	0.081	0.023	
3.0				1.528	0.354	0.099	0.028	0.008
3.1				1.902	0.427	0.120	0.035	0.010
3.2				2.386	0.513	0.145	0.043	0.012
3.3				3.027	0.615	0.174	0.052	0.015
3.4				3.906	0.737	0.209	0.063	0.019
3.5				5.165	0.882	0.248	0.076	0.023
3.6				7.090	1.055	0.295	0.019	0.028
3.7				10.347	1.265	0.349	0.109	0.034
3.8				16.937	1.519	0.412	0.129	0.041
3.9				36.859	1.830	0.485	0.153	0.050
4.0					2.216	0.570	0.180	0.059
4.1					2.703	0.668	0.212	0.070
4.2					3.327	0.784	0.248	0.083
4.3					4.149	0.919	0.289	0.097
4.4					5.268	1.078	0.337	0.114
4.5					6.862	1.265	0.391	0.133
4.6					9.289	1.487	0.453	0.156
4.7					13.382	1.752	0.525	0.181
4.8					21.641	2.071	0.607	0.209
4.9					46.566	2.459	0.702	0.242
5.0						2.938	0.810	0.279
5.1						3.536	0.936	0.321
5.2						4.301	1.081	0.368
5.3						5.303	1.249	0.422
5.4						6.661	1.444	0.483
5.5						8.590	1.674	0.553

ρ	$c = 1$	$c = 2$	$c = 3$	$c = 4$	$c = 5$	$c = 6$	$c = 7$	$c = 8$
5.6						11.519	1.944	0.631
5.7						16.446	2.264	0.721
5.8						26.373	2.648	0.823
5.9						56.300	3.113	0.939
6.0							3.683	1.071
6.1							4.394	1.222
6.2							5.298	1.397
6.3							6.480	1.598
6.4							8.077	1.831
6.5							10.341	2.102
6.6							13.770	2.420
6.7							19.532	2.796
6.8							31.127	3.245
6.9							66.055	3.786
7.0								4.447
7.1								5.270
7.2								6.314
7.3								7.675
7.4								9.511
7.5								12.109
7.6								16.039
7.7								22.636
7.8								35.898
7.9								75.827

Indexes

Name Index

Subject Index